Oxford Medical Publications

Oxford Textbook of
Public Health

VOLUME 3

Oxford Textbook of
Public Health

FIFTH EDITION

The practice of
public health

Roger Detels

Distinguished Professor of Epidemiology and Infectious Diseases, Schools of
Public Health and Medicine, University of California, Los Angeles, Los Angeles,
California, USA

Robert Beaglehole

Professor Emeritus, University of Auckland, Auckland, New Zealand

Mary Ann Lansang

Professor of Medicine and Clinical Epidemiology, College of Medicine,
University of the Philippines, Manila, The Philippines

Martin Gulliford

Professor of Public Health, Department of Public Health Sciences,
King's College London, London, United Kingdom

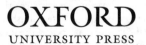

OXFORD
UNIVERSITY PRESS

OXFORD

UNIVERSITY PRESS

Great Clarendon Street, Oxford ox2 6DP

Oxford University Press is a department of the University of Oxford.
It furthers the University's objective of excellence in research, scholarship,
and education by publishing worldwide in

Oxford New York

Auckland Cape Town Dar es Salaam Hong Kong Karachi
Kuala Lumpur Madrid Melbourne Mexico City Nairobi
New Delhi Shanghai Taipei Toronto

With offices in

Argentina Austria Brazil Chile Czech Republic France Greece
Guatemala Hungary Italy Japan Poland Portugal Singapore
South Korea Switzerland Thailand Turkey Ukraine Vietnam

Oxford is a registered trademark of Oxford University Press
in the United Kingdom and in certain other countries.

Published in the United States
by Oxford University Press Inc., New York

© Oxford University Press 2009

The moral rights of the author have been asserted
Database right Oxford University Press (maker)

First edition 1984
Second edition 1991
Third edition 1997
Fourth edition 2002 (reprinted in paperback 2004, 2005 twice)
Fifth edition 2009

British Library Cataloguing in Publication Data

Data available

Library of Congress Cataloguing in Publication Data

Data available

Typeset by Cepha Imaging Pvt. Ltd., Bangalore, India
Printed by L.E.G.O.S.p.A.

ISBN 978–0–19–921870–7 (Set)
ISBN 978–0–19–957943–3 (Vol. 1)
ISBN 978–0–19–957944–0 (Vol. 2)
ISBN 978–0–19–957945–7 (Vol. 3)

1 3 5 7 9 10 8 6 4 2

Available as a set only

Preface to the fifth edition

Much has happened in the world and in the field of public health since the publication of the 4th edition of the *Oxford Textbook of Public Health*. Sudden acute respiratory syndrome (SARS) has come and gone, H5N1, H1N1 and the probability of new variant influenzas are the emerging infectious diseases of greatest concern, the health gap between rich and poor countries and within many countries has widened, HIV continues to be a major problem despite the development of effective treatments and strategies to prevent mother-to-child transmission, wars continue to be waged causing massive loss and disruption of human life and displacement of people, violence and terrorism have increased, and the epidemics of obesity and asthma have intensified. Our inability to effectively meet disasters has been demonstrated with the tsunami devastating northern Indonesia, Sri Lanka, and southern Thailand (2004), although the rapid, effective response by the Chinese to the Sichuan earthquake (2008) gives evidence that our ability to respond to natural disasters is improving.

On the positive side, the World Health Organization and member states are in the process of developing international reporting systems for emerging diseases, we have made strides in preventing chronic diseases such as cancer and heart disease (although these diseases are already a major cause of morbidity and mortality in low- and middle-income countries), polio has been eliminated in much of the world through effective new immunization strategies, and environmental pollution and global warming are now recognized as major problems and have attracted political concern—a major step in implementing effective solutions. Further, the burgeoning field of genomics holds promise of transforming both medicine and public health, but we must be concerned that it is applied to the improvement of the health of individuals and society and not used to discriminate against genetically vulnerable persons. Although private organizations have long contributed to public health, there has been a recent surge in private support of public health, particularly in the field of HIV/AIDS. While these contributions have had very positive effects on the health of people, particularly in low- and middle-income countries, they have also had unexpected impacts.

Public health continues to be a dynamic, exciting field which challenges creative thinking and demands implementation of innovative strategies. For the 5th edition of the Textbook, we have outlined these continuing and new public health problems and have recruited authors who are leaders in recognizing and addressing them. Although we have continued dividing the basic structure of the Textbook into three major topic areas, the scope of public health, the methods of public health, and the practice of public health, we have added chapters to reflect the growth and changes in the field since 2002 and the emergence of new public health strategies. Thus, we have added new chapters on management of public health disasters, collective violence including war, applications of genomics to the field of public health, gene–environment interactions, clinical epidemiology, private support of public health, and the global health agenda for the twenty-first century, among others. All other chapters have been updated, most of them by new leaders in their respective fields. Further, we have recruited public health professionals from all the major regions of the world, reflecting the global scope of public health and the textbook.

We hope that this 5th edition will contribute to the advancement of the field of public health through its presentation of the scope, concerns, strategies, and applications of the field. The Textbook is intended for public health researchers, practitioners, students of the field, and other health professionals who wish to understand the field and their opportunities for contributing to the health and well-being of the people of the world.

Roger Detels
Robert Beaglehole
Mary Ann Lansang
Martin Gulliford

Introduction to Volume 3: The practice of public health

Public health is what we, as a society, do collectively to assure the conditions for people to be healthy. This requires that continuing and emerging threats to the health of the public be successfully countered . . . through effective, organised, and sustained efforts led by the public sector. Institute of Medicine (1988)

Volume 3 of the Textbook provides a state-of-the-art account of the practice of public health through forty-seven chapters written by leading experts. The contents of this volume continue the shift in thinking, already introduced in Volumes 1 and 2, that considers public health not only as a matter of local and national concern and a key responsibility of governments and public agencies, but also as an international issue that must be addressed through optimal global governance. This change in thinking has led to the inclusion of new chapters that reassess priorities, recognize the evolving burden of disease, and recommend new strategies for intervention.

Volume 3 begins with a discussion of the major groups of non-communicable disorders (Section 9). This section includes, for the first time, separate chapters on obesity and diabetes, reflecting the growing concern for the increasing impact of these conditions on global health. Current estimates suggest that there are about 1.1 billion overweight and obese adults in the world, with an estimated 10% of all children now being overweight. More than half of those affected are in middle- or low-income countries.

The series of chapters on communicable diseases has been similarly expanded, with new chapters on tuberculosis, malaria, hepatitis, and emerging diseases. Together, these conditions represent major priorities: tuberculosis accounts for an estimated 1.6 million deaths worldwide each year, with 8.8 million new cases; malaria accounts for 46.5 million disability-adjusted life years lost annually; while one out of every 40 deaths is attributed to liver cirrhosis or primary liver cancer. In addition to outlining problems and their causes, each of these chapters discusses potential solutions, including national and international strategies for disease control and prevention.

The emphasis on intervention for prevention of disease and promotion of health is continued in the volume's second section on public health hazards, including tobacco, alcohol, drug abuse, injuries, and violence (Section 10). The proposed intervention strategies encompass both population-based approaches—including,

for example, regulation, the use of deterrents and incentives, and public education—and strategies targeted at individuals at high risk through health care services. It remains clear, however, that the greatest risks are generally found among those groups for whom interventions are least accessible.

In keeping with the equity orientation of public health, Section 11 considers the public health needs of different population groups, paying particular attention to groups that, for a range of reasons, are vulnerable to public health hazards and disease risks. Separate chapters outline the needs of families, women, children, adolescents, older people, ethnic minorities, people with disabilities, and forced migrants and displaced populations. Collectively, these chapters emphasize the importance of the public health role in analysing the health needs of these often marginalized populations and advocating for their rights to health.

Section 12 presents an analysis of the core public health skills required for improving population health and reducing inequalities in health. This section begins with a discussion of the concept of need, as a capacity to benefit from health intervention. This is accompanied by a practical guide to the assessment of need in public health practice. Needs must often be met through a combination of intervention strategies, and this is exemplified by chapters on current strategies for control of non-communicable and infectious diseases. A series of chapters then outlines opportunities for intervention through the health sector, including health care services, population screening, and environmental health practice. However, addressing the main determinants of health requires the development and implementation of public health interventions that extend well beyond the health sector. The difficulties of multi-sectoral intervention are illustrated by the complex problems of tackling health inequalities in either high-income or middle- and low-income countries. As Davidson Gwatkin observes, achieving change is critically dependent on political will.

In the final section of the book, Roger Detels and Sheena Sullivan question the assumption that intervention on public health problems must be led by the public sector. They describe a re-emerging role for powerful private sector advocates of public health intervention, while at the same time drawing attention to some of the difficulties of this approach and the importance of the stewardship role of governments. The final chapter by Margaret Chan and colleagues summarizes many of the key issues that have been raised in earlier chapters of the book. The authors conclude that technical skills will be insufficient to achieve the public health goals of improving population health and reducing inequalities. 'Efforts to provide good health for all' must be underscored by an ethical focus driven by recognition that 'the highest attainable standard of health is one of the fundamental rights of every human being'.

Institute of Medicine (1988). *The future of public health*. Washington DC. National Academies Press. Page 19.

Brief Contents

Contents

List of contributors

Quarraisha Abdool Karim Columbia University (Department of Epidemiology), University of KwaZulu Natal (School of Family Medicine and Public Health) and CAPRISA (Centre for the AIDS Programme of Research in South Africa), South Africa.
Chapter 9.13 Acquired immunodeficiency syndrome

Salim S. Abdool Karim, Pro Vice Chancellor (Research), University of KwaZulu-Natal; Director, Centre for the AIDS Programme of Research in South Africa (CAPRISA); Professor in Clinical Epidemiology, Columbia University Adjunct; Professor in Medicine, Cornell University, South Africa.
Chapter 9.13 Acquired immunodeficiency syndrome

Maia Ambegaokar London School of Hygiene and Tropical Medicine, London, UK.
Chapter 3.4 Leadership in public health

Ian Anderson Professor for Indigenous Health, Centre for Health and Society & Onemda VicHealth Koori Health Unit, School of Population Health, University of Melbourne, Melbourne, Australia.
Chapter 11.5 Ethnic minorities and indigenous peoples

Roy M. Anderson Rector, Imperial College London, London, UK.
Chapter 6.16 Mathematical models of transmission and control

Samira Asma Associate Director, Global Tobacco Control, Centers for Disease Control and Prevention, USA.
Chapter 10.1 Tobacco

Gunilla Backman Senior Researcher, Human Rights Centre, University of Essex, UK.
Chapter 4.1 The right to the highest attainable standard of health

Rajiv Bahl Medical Officer, Department of Child and Adolescent Health and Development, World Health Organization, Geneva, Switzerland.
Chapter 11.3 Child health

Dean Baker Professor and Director, Center for Occupational and Environmental Health, University of California, Irvine, CA, USA.
Chapter 8.5 Occupational health

Hilary J. Bambrick Senior Lecturer, School of Medicine, University of Western Sydney, Campbelltown NSW Australia; Visiting Fellow, National Centre for Epidemiology and Population Health, The Australian National University, Canberra ACT, Australia.
Chapter 2.8 The global environment

Catherine R. Bateman School of Public Health and Community Medicine, University of New South Wales, Sydney, Australia.
Chapter 11.8 Forced migrants and other displaced populations

Robert Beaglehole Professor Emeritus, University of Auckland, Auckland, New Zealand.
Chapter 12.5 Prevention and control of chronic, non-communicable diseases

Ruth L. Berkelman Department of Epidemiology, Rollins School of Public Health, Emory University, Atlanta, GA, USA.
Chapter 6.17 Public health surveillance

Douglas Bettcher Director, Tobacco Free Initiative, World Health Organization, Geneva, Switzerland.
Chapter 4.3 International public health instruments
Chapter 10.1 Tobacco

Zulfiqar Ahmed Bhutta Husein Lalji Dewraj Professor of Pediatrics, and Chairman, Department of Pediatrics & Child Health, The Aga Khan University, Karachi, Pakistan.
Chapter 2.7 Infectious diseases

Stella Bialous President, Tobacco Policy International, San Francisco, USA.
Chapter 10.1 Tobacco

Fred Binka Dean School of Public Health, College of Health Sciences, University of Ghana, Legon, Ghana.
Chapter 5.2 Information systems and community diagnosis in low- and middle-income countries

Jennifer Bishop Department of Food Safety, Zoonoses and Foodborne Diseases, World Health Organization, Geneva, Switzerland.
Chapter 4.3 International public health instruments

Marike Boezen Unit Chronic Airway Diseases (head), Department of Epidemiology, University Medical Center Groningen, University of Groningen, Groningen, The Netherlands.
Chapter 9.4 Chronic obstructive pulmonary disease and asthma

Paolo Boffetta International Agency for Research on Cancer, Lyon, France.
Chapter 9.3 Neoplasms

Diana Bonta Vice President, Public Affairs, Kaiser Foundation Health Plans and Hospitals, Southern California Region, USA.
Chapter 7.5 Governance and management of public health programmes

Cynthia Boschi-Pinto Medical Officer, Department of Child and Adolescent Health and Development, World Health Organization, Geneva, Switzerland.
Chapter 11.3 Child health

James Bowen Center at Evergreen, Kirkland, WA, USA.
Chapter 9.10 Neurologic diseases, epidemiology, and public health

James W. Buehler Department of Epidemiology, Rollins School of Public Health, Emory University, Atlanta, GA, USA.
Chapter 6.17 Public health surveillance

Wylie Burke Professor and Chair, Department of Medical History and Ethics, University of Washington, Seattle, WA, USA.
Chapter 2.4 Genomics and public health

Jason W. Busse Assistant Professor, Department of Clinical Epidemiology & Biostatistics, McMaster University, Hamilton, Ontario, Canada; Scientist, Institute for Work & Health, Toronto, Ontario, Canada.
Chapter 6.11 Clinical epidemiology

Julie E. Byles Director, Research Centre for Gender, Health and Ageing Faculty of Health, University of Newcastle, NSW, Australia.
Chapter 11.7 Health of older people

Meredith Cagle Cagle Consulting Services.
Chapter 7.5 Governance and management of public health programmes

Simon Carroll Associate Director, Centre for Community Health Promotion Research, University of Victoria, Canada.
Chapter 7.3 Health promotion, health education, and the public's health

Margaret Chan Director General, World Health Organization, Geneva, Switzerland.
Chapter 12.14 Global health agenda for the twenty-first century

Venkatraman Chandra-Mouli Head, Adolescent Health and Development, Department of Child and Adolescent Health and Development (CAH), World Health Organization, Geneva, Switzerland.
Chapter 11.4 Adolescent health

Leda Chatzi Department of Social Medicine, Medical School, University of Crete, Heraklion, Greece.
Chapter 6.3 Cross-sectional studies

Chien-Jen Chen Academician and Distinguished Research Fellow, Genomics Research Center, Academic Sinica, National Taiwan University School of Medicine, Taipei, Taiwan.
Chapter 8.1 Environmental health issues in public health

Virasakdi Chongsuvivatwong Professor of Community Medicine, Epidemiology Unit, Faculty of Medicine, Prince of Songkla University, Hatyai, Thailand.
Chapter 12.5 Prevention and control of chronic, non-communicable diseases

Aileen Clarke Associate Clinical Professor in Public Health & Health Services Research, Health Sciences Research Institute, Warwick Medical School, University of Warwick, Coventry, UK.
Chapter 12.2 Needs assessment: A practical approach

Thomas Clasen Department of Infectious and Tropical Diseases, London School of Hygiene and Tropical Medicine, London, UK.
Chapter 2.5 Water and sanitation

Myles Cockburn Associate Professor, Department of Preventive Medicine, Keck School of Medicine; Department of Geography, College of Letters, Arts and Sciences, University of Southern California, USA.
Chapter 8.2 Radiation and public health

Bernadette Daelmans Department of Child and Adolescent Health and Development, World Health Organization, Geneva, Switzerland.
Chapter 11.3 Child health

Peter Davis Department of Sociology, University of Auckland, New Zealand.
Chapter 7.6 Public health sciences and policy in high-income countries

Manuel M. Dayrit Director, Human Resources for Health, World Health Organization, Geneva, Switzerland.
Chapter 3.4 Leadership in public health

Judith Bueno de Mesquita Senior Researcher, Human Rights Centre, University of Essex, UK.
Chapter 4.1 The right to the highest attainable standard of health

Katherine DeLand Senior Technical Officer, Tobacco Free Initiative, World Health Organization, Geneva, Switzerland.
Chapter 4.3 International public health instruments
Chapter 10.1 Tobacco

Rodolfo Dennis Head, Departments of Medicine and Research, Fundacion Cardioinfantil; Professor of Medicine, Pontificia Universidad Javeriana, Bogota, Colombia.
Chapter 6.11 Clinical epidemiology

Roger Detels Distinguished Professor of Epidemiology and Infectious Diseases, Schools of Public Health and Medicine, University of California, Los Angeles, Los Angeles, CA, USA.
Chapter 1.1 The scope and concerns of public health
Chapter 6.1 Epidemiology: The foundation of public health
Chapter 9.13 Acquired immunodeficiency syndrome
Chapter 12.13 Private support of public health

Ana V. Diez-Roux Department of Epidemiology, University of Michigan School of Public Health, Ann Arbor, MI, USA.
Chapter 6.2 Ecologic variables, ecologic studies, and multilevel studies in public health research

Allan Donner Department of Epidemiology and Biostatistics, Schulich School of Medicine and Dentistry, University of Western Ontario London, Ontario, Canada.
Chapter 6.8 Methodological issues in the design and analysis of community intervention trials

Manjit Dosanjh Advisor to the Director General, Life Sciences and International Organisations, CERN, Geneva.
Chapter 8.2 Radiation and public health

John M. Douglas, Jr Director, DSTDP, NCHHSTP, CDC, Atlanta, GA, USA.
Chapter 9.12 Sexually transmitted infections

Jeroen Douwes Associate Director, Centre for Public Health Research, Massey University Wellington Campus, Wellington, New Zealand.
Chapter 9.4 Chronic obstructive pulmonary disease and asthma

Lesley Doyal Professor of Gender and Health, School for Policy Studies, University of Bristol, Bristol, UK; Visiting Professor, University of Cape Town, South Africa.
Chapter 11.2 Women, men, and health

Shah Ebrahim Professor of Public Health, Department of Epidemiology & Population Health, London School of Hygiene and Tropical Medicine, London, UK.
Chapter 11.7 Health of older people

Matthias Egger Professor of Epidemiology and Public Health, Institute of Social & Preventive Medicine (ISPM), University of Bern, Switzerland.
Chapter 6.14 Systematic reviews and meta-analysis

Marcos Espinal Executive Secretary, Stop TB Partnership, Geneva, Switzerland.
Chapter 9.14 Tuberculosis

Daniel Ferrante World Health Organization, Geneva, Switzerland.
Chapter 10.1 Tobacco

Josep Figueras Director, European Observatory on Health Systems and Policies, Head, WHO Centre for Health Policy, Brussels.
Chapter 12.10 Strategies for health services

J. Peter Figueroa Chief, Epidemiology & AIDS, Ministry of Health, Kingston, Jamaica.
Chapter 7.7 Public health sciences and policy in low- and middle-income countries

Louise Finer Senior Researcher, Human Rights Centre, University of Essex, UK.
Chapter 4.1 The right to the highest attainable standard of health

Baruch Fischhoff Howard Heinz University Professor, Department of Social and Decision Sciences, Department of Engineering and Public Policy; Department of Social and Decision Sciences, Carnegie Mellon University, Pittsburgh, PA, USA.
Chapter 8.8 Risk perception and communication

Olivier Fontaine Department of Child and Adolescent Health and Development, World Health Organization, Geneva, Switzerland.
Chapter 11.3 Child health

Sven Francque Division of Gastroenterology and Hepatology, University Hospital Antwerp, Belgium.
Chapter 9.16 Chronic hepatitis and other liver disease

Melvyn Freeman Extraordinary Professor, University of Stellenbosch, South Africa.
Chapter 9.7 Public mental health

Julio Frenk Dean, Harvard School of Public Health, Boston, USA.
Chapter 3.3 Health policy in developing countries

Lawrence M. Friedman Independent Consultant, Rockville, MD, USA.
Chapter 6.7 Methodology of intervention trials in individuals

Fu Paul Fu, Jr. Associate Professor of Pediatrics and Public Health, David Geffen School of Medicine at UCLA, and UCLA School of Public Health, CA, USA.
Chapter 5.1 Information systems in support of public health in high-income countries

Michelle Funk Michelle Funk, Coordinator, Mental Health Policy and Service Development (MHP), Department of Mental Health and Substance Abuse, World Health Organization, Geneva, Switzerland.
Chapter 9.7 Public mental health

Gary Giovino Senior Research Scientist and Director, Tobacco Control Program, Roswell Park Cancer Institute, Buffalo, USA.
Chapter 10.1 Tobacco

Lynn R. Goldman Professor, Environmental Health Sciences, Johns Hopkins University, Bloomberg School of Public Health, Baltimore, MD, USA.
Chapter 12.8 Environmental health practice

Bernard D. Goldstein Professor, Department of Environmental and Occupational Health, University of Pittsburgh Graduate School of Public Health, Pittsburgh, PA, USA.
Chapter 8.7 Toxicology and risk assessment in the analysis and management of environmental risk

Octavio Gómez-Dantés Researcher, National Institute of Public Health, Mexico.
Chapter 3.3 Health policy in developing countries

Miguel Angel González-Block Executive Director of the Center for Health Systems Research, INSP—National Public Health Institute, Mexico.
Chapter 3.3 Health policy in developing countries

Fernando González-Martín International Health Regulations Secretariat, World Health Organization, Geneva, Switzerland.
Chapter 4.3 International public health instruments

Sherwood L. Gorbach Professor of Public Health, Medicine, and Molecular Biology/Microbiology, Tufts University School of Medicine, Boston, MA, USA.
Chapter 2.7 Infectious diseases

Lawrence W. Green Adjunct Professor, Department of Epidemiology and Biostatistics, School of Medicine, University of California at San Francisco, CA, USA.
Chapter 2.3 Behavioural determinants of health and disease

Manfred S. Green Center for the Study of Bioterrorism, Tel Aviv University, Israel Center for Disease Control, Ministry of Health, Israel.
Chapter 10.8 Public health aspects of bioterrorism

Sander Greenland Professor, Department of Epidemiology and Department of Statistics University of California, Los Angeles, CA, USA.
Chapter 6.12 Validity and bias in epidemiological research
Chapter 6.13 Causation and causal inference

Emily Grundy Centre for Population Studies, London School of Hygiene and Tropical Medicine, London, UK.
Chapter 7.2 Demography and public health

Martin Gulliford Department of Public Health Sciences, King's College London, London, UK.
Chapter 2.9 Health services as determinants of population health
Chapter 11.5 Ethnic minorities and indigenous peoples

Davidson R. Gwatkin The World Bank, Washington, DC, USA.
Chapter 12.4 Reducing health inequalities in developing countries

Davidson H. Hamer Associate Professor of International Health and Medicine, Department of International Health, Boston University School of Public Health, Department of Medicine, Boston University School of Medicine; Adjunct Associate Professor of Nutrition, Tufts University Friedman School of Nutrition Science and Policy, Boston, MA, USA.
Chapter 2.7 Infectious diseases

Christopher Hamlin Professor, Department of History, and in the Program of History and Philosophy of Science, University of Notre Dame, Notre Dame, IN, USA; Honorary Professor, Department of Public Health and Policy, London School of Hygiene and Tropical Medicine, London, UK.
Chapter 1.2 The history and development of public health in developed countries

Summer Hammide Student researcher, UCLA School of Public Health.
Chapter 4.3 International public health instruments

Marian T. Hannan Associate Professor of Medicine, Harvard Medical School, Co-Director of Musculoskeletal Research, Institute for Aging Research, Hebrew SeniorLife, Boston, MA, USA.
Chapter 9.9 Musculoskeletal diseases

Piya Hanvoravongchai Lecturer in Health Policy, Department of Public Health and Policy, London School of Hygiene and Tropical Medicine, London, UK.
Chapter 12.11 Public health workers

David Heymann Assistant Director General, Health Security and Environment, and Polio Eradication, World Health Organization, Geneva, Switzerland.
Chapter 9.17 Emerging and re-emerging infections

Robert A. Hiatt Co-Chair, Department of Epidemiology and Biostatistics, School of Medicine, University of California at San Francisco, CA, USA.
Chapter 2.3 Behavioural determinants of health and disease

Marcia Hills Professor, School of Nursing, Director, Centre for Community Health Promotion Research President, Canadian Consortium for Health Promotion Research University of Victoria, Canada.
Chapter 7.3 Health promotion, health education, and the public's health

Katherine J. Hoggatt Assistant Professor, Department of Epidemiology, University of Michigan, Ann Arbor, MI, USA.
Chapter 6.13 Causation and causal inference

Walter W. Holland Emeritus Professor of Public Health Medicine, Visiting Professor, LSE Health and Social Care, London School of Economics and Political Science, London, UK.
Chapter 3.1 Overview of policies and strategies
Chapter 12.7 Population screening and public health

T. Déirdre Hollingsworth Department of Infectious Disease Epidemiology, Faculty of Medicine, Imperial College London, London, UK.
Chapter 6.16 Mathematical models of transmission and control

Robert L. Hubbard Director, National Development and Research Institutes, Raleigh, NC, USA.
Chapter 10.2 Drug abuse

Paul Hunt UN Special Rapporteur on the right to the highest attainable standard of health (2002–2008); Professor, Human Rights Centre, University of Essex (England); Adjunct Professor, University of Waikato, New Zealand.
Chapter 4.1 The right to the highest attainable standard of health

Adnan A. Hyder Johns Hopkins University, Bloomberg School of Public Health, Department of International Health; Center for Injury Research & Policy, Baltimore, MD, USA.
Chapter 10.4 Injury prevention and control: The public health approach

Sopon Iamsirithaworn International Field Epidemiology Training Program, Bureau of Epidemiology, Department of Disease Control, Ministry of Public Health, Thailand.
Chapter 6.4 Principles of outbreak investigation

Alec Irwin Associate Director, François-Xavier Bagnoud Center for Health and Human Rights, Harvard School of Public Health, Boston, USA.
Chapter 2.2 Overview and framework

Philip James London School of Hygiene and Tropical Medicine, London, UK; International Obesity TaskForce, IASO, London, UK.
Chapter 9.5 Obesity

Dean T. Jamison Professor, Department of Global Health, University of Washington, Seattle, WA, USA.
Chapter 7.4 Cost-effectiveness analysis: Concepts and applications

Stephen Jan Senior Health Economist, The George Institute for International Health; Associate Professor, Faculty of Medicine, University of Sydney, NSW, Australia.
Chapter 12.1 Need: What is it and how do we measure it?

Don C. Des Jarlais Director of Research, Baron Edmond de Rothschild Chemical Dependency Institute, Beth Israel Medical Center, New York, NY, USA; Professor of Epidemiology and Population Health, Albert Einstein College of Medicine, Bronx, NY, USA.
Chapter 10.2 Drug abuse

Mary L. Kamb International Coordinator, Division of STD Prevention, Centers for Disease Control & Prevention (CDC), USA.
Chapter 9.12 Sexually transmitted infections

Nancy Kass Phoebe R. Berman Professor of Bioethics and Public Health, Berman Institute of Bioethics, Johns Hopkins Bloomberg School of Public Health, Baltimore, USA.
Chapter 4.4 Ethical principles and ethical issues in public health

Jennifer L. Kelsey Professor Emeritus, Stanford University School of Medicine, Department of Health Research and Policy, Stanford, CA, USA; Professor (part-time), University of Massachusetts Medical School, Departments of Medicine and of Family Medicine and Community Health, Worcester, MA, USA.
Chapter 9.9 Musculoskeletal diseases

Leeka Kheifets Professor, UCLA School of Public Health, Department of Epidemiology, Los Angeles, CA, USA.
Chapter 8.2 Radiation and public health

Rajat Khosla Senior Researcher, Human Rights Centre, University of Essex, UK.
Chapter 4.1 The right to the highest attainable standard of health

Muin J. Khoury Director, National Office of Public Health Genomics, Centers for Disease Control and Prevention, Atlanta, GA, USA.
Chapter 2.4 Genomics and public health

Robert J. Kim-Farley Professor, Departments of Epidemiology and Community Health Sciences, UCLA School of Public Health, Los Angeles, USA.
Chapter 12.6 Principles of infectious disease control

Mary Kindhauser Office of the Director General, World Health Organization, Geneva, Switzerland.
Chapter 12.14 Global health agenda for the twenty-first century

Richard S.G. Knight Professor of Clinical Neurology, National CJD Surveillance Unit, University of Edinburgh, Western General Hospital, Edinburgh, UK.
Chapter 9.11 The transmissible spongiform encephalopathies

Manolis Kogevinas Professor and co-Director, Centre for Research in Environmental Epidemiology (CREAL) Municipal Institute of Medical Research (IMIM), Barcelona, Spain.
Chapter 6.3 Cross-sectional studies

David Koh Head, Department of Community, Occupational and Family Medicine; Yong Loo Lin School of Medicine, National University of Singapore, Singapore.
Chapter 8.5 Occupational health

Dragana Korljan Human Rights Officer, Office of the High Commissioner for Human Rights.
Chapter 4.1 The right to the highest attainable standard of health

Walter A. Kukull Professor, Epidemiology, Director, Nat'l Alzheimer's Coord Ctr (NACC), Department of Epidemiology, University of Washington, Seattle, WA, USA.
Chapter 9.10 Neurologic diseases, epidemiology, and public health

Vipat Kuruchittham Lecturer, College of Public Health Sciences, Chulalongkorn University, Bangkok, Thailand.
Chapter 5.2 Information systems and community diagnosis in low- and middle-income countries

Kamakshi Lakshminarayan Assistant Professor, Department of Neurology, School of Medicine, University of Minnesota, Minneapolis, USA.
Chapter 9.2 Cardiovascular and cerebrovascular diseases

Mary Ann Lansang Professor of Medicine and Clinical Epidemiology, College of Medicine, University of the Philippines, Manila.
Chapter 7.7 Public health sciences and policy in low- and middle-income countries
Chapter 12.2 Needs assessment: A practical approach

Kelley Lee Head, Public and Environmental Health Research Unit, London School of Hygiene and Tropical Medicine, London, UK.
Chapter 2.1 Globalization

June Leung Intern, Hospital Authority, Hong Kong Special Administrative Region, People's Republic of China.
Chapter 10.1 Tobacco

Barry S. Levy Adjunct Professor of Public Health, Tufts University School of Medicine, Sherborn, MA, USA.
Chapter 10.6 Collective violence: War

Khanchit Limpakarnjanarat Communicable Disease Surveillance and Response (CSR), Department of Communicable Diseases (CDS), WHO SEARO.
Chapter 12.12 Planning for and responding to public health needs in emergencies and disasters

Annette Lin A candidate for a JD (juris doctorate) and MPH (masters of public health) joint degree at the University of California in Los Angeles, CA, USA.
Chapter 4.3 International public health instruments

Paul J. Lioy Professor and Vice Chair, Department of Environmental and Occupational Medicine, RWJMS, Deputy Director of Government Relations and Director of the Exposure Science Division of the Environmental and Occupational Health Sciences Institute (EOHSI), Robert Wood Johnson Medical School (RWJMS), UMDNJ and Rutgers University, Piscataway, NJ, USA.
Chapter 8.4 The science of human exposures to contaminants in the environment

Alexander Lo Dak Wai Solicitor, Hong Kong; Solicitor, England and Wales (non-practising); Chinese Medical Practitioner, Hong Kong; Professional Consultant, School of Law, The Chinese University of Hong Kong.
Chapter 4.2 Comparative national public health legislation

Donald Lollar Senior Research Scientist, National Center on Birth Defects and Developmental Disabilities, Centers for Disease Control and Prevention, United States Department of Health and Human Services, Atlanta, GA, USA.
Chapter 11.6 People with disabilities

A.D. Lopez School of Population Health, University of Queensland, Brisbane, Australia.
Chapter 2.10 Assessing health needs: The global burden of disease approach

Adetokunbo Lucas Adjunct Professor, Harvard University, Cambridge, MA, USA.
Chapter 3.3 Health policy in developing countries

Jeff Luck Department of Health Services, UCLA School of Public Health, CA, USA.
Chapter 5.1 Information systems in support of public health in high-income countries

Russell V. Luepker Mayo Professor, Division of Epidemiology and Community Health School of Public Health University of Minnesota, Minneapolis, USA.
Chapter 9.2 Cardiovascular and cerebrovascular diseases

Johan P. Mackenbach Department of Public Health, Erasmus MC, University Medical Centre Rotterdam, Rotterdam, The Netherlands.
Chapter 12.3 Socioeconomic inequalities in health in high-income countries: The facts and the options

Dermot Maher Senior Clinical Epidemiologist, Medical Research Council/Uganda Virus Research Institute, Entebbe, Uganda.
Chapter 9.14 Tuberculosis

Lindiwe Makubalo Chief Director, Health Information, Epidemiology, Evaluation & Research, Department of Health, South Africa.
Chapter 7.7 Public health sciences and policy in low- and middle-income countries

Zoe Marshman Clinical Lecturer in Dental Public Health School of Clinical Dentistry, Claremont Crescent, Sheffield, UK.
Chapter 9.8 Dental public health

Robyn Martin Professor of Public Health Law, Centre for Research in Primary and Community Care, University of Hertfordshire, Hatfield, UK; Visiting Professor, The Chinese University of Hong Kong; Honorary Professor, London School of Hygiene and Tropical Medicine, London, UK; Director, European Public Health Law Network.
Chapter 4.2 Comparative national public health legislation

Jose Martines Department of Child and Adolescent Health and Development, World Health Organization, Geneva, Switzerland.
Chapter 11.3 Child health

Elizabeth Mason Director Department of Child and Adolescent Health and Development (CAH), World Health Organization, Geneva, Switzerland.
Chapter 11.3 Child health

Colin Douglas Mathers Coordinator, Mortality and Burden of Disease, Department of Health Statistics and Informatics, World Health Organization, Geneva, Switzerland.
Chapter 2.10 Assessing health needs: The global burden of disease approach

Di McIntyre Professor and South African Research Chair in 'Health and Wealth', Health Economics Unit, School of Public Health and Family Medicine, University of Cape Town.
Chapter 12.1 Need: What is it and how do we measure it?

Martin McKee European Centre on Health of Societies in Transition, London School of Hygiene and Tropical Medicine, London, UK.
Chapter 12.10 Strategies for health services

Anthony J. McMichael NHMRC Australia Fellow, National Centre for Epidemiology and Population Health, The Australian National University, Canberra ACT Australia.
Chapter 2.8 The global environment

Pierre-André Michaud, Médecin chef, Unité multidisciplinaire de santé des adolescents, Lausanne, Switzerland.
Chapter 11.4 Adolescent health

Peter Michielsen, Division of Gastroenterology and Hepatology, University Hospital Antwerp, Belgium.
Chapter 9.16 Chronic hepatitis and other liver disease

Edward Mills Canada Research Chair, Global Health, Faculty of Health Sciences, University of Ottawa, Ottawa, Ontario, Canada.
Chapter 6.11 Clinical epidemiology

Mark R. Montgomery Professor of Economics, Stony Brook University; and Senior Associate, Population Council, NY, USA.
Chapter 10.7 Urban health in low- and middle-income countries

Gavin Mooney Professor of Health Economics, Department of Public Health, University of Sydney, Australia and Health Economics Unit, University of Cape Town, South Africa.
Chapter 12.1 Need: What is it and how do we measure it?

Myfanwy Morgan Professor of Sociology and Health, Department of Public Health Sciences, King's College London, London, UK.
Chapter 7.1 Sociology and psychology in public health
Chapter 11.5 Ethnic minorities and indigenous peoples

Richard Morrow Professor of International Health, Johns Hopkins Bloomberg School of Public Health, Baltimore, MD, USA.
Chapter 9.15 Malaria

William Moss Associate Professor of Epidemiology, Johns Hopkins Bloomberg School of Public Health, Baltimore, MD, USA.
Chapter 9.15 Malaria

Alvaro Muñoz Professor of Epidemiology, Johns Hopkins Bloomberg School of Public Health, Baltimore, MD, USA.
Chapter 6.6 Cohort studies

C.J.L. Murray Institute for Health Metrics and Evaluation, University of Washington, Seattle, USA.
Chapter 2.10 Assessing health needs: The global burden of disease approach

F. Javier Nieto Professor and Chair, Department of Population Health Sciences, University of Wisconsin School of Medicine and Public Health, Madison, WI, USA.
Chapter 6.6 Cohort studies

D. James Nokes KEMRI-Wellcome Trust Programme, Kilifi, Kenya; Reader, Department of Biological Sciences, University of Warwick, Coventry, UK.
Chapter 6.16 Mathematical models of transmission and control

Ellen Nolte Senior Lecturer, European Centre on Health of Societies in Transition, London School of Hygiene and Tropical Medicine, London, UK.
Chapter 12.10 Strategies for health services

Don Nutbeam Provost and Deputy Vice Chancellor, University of Sydney, NSW, Australia.
Chapter 12.9 Structures and strategies for public health intervention

Roderico H. Ofrin Technical Officer, Emergency and Humanitarian Action, WHO SEARO.
Chapter 12.12 Planning for and responding to public health needs in emergencies and disasters

Jane Ogden Professor of Health Psychology, Department of Psychology, University of Surrey, Guildford, UK.
Chapter 7.1 Sociology and psychology in public health

Lisa Oldring Special Advisor to Mary Robinson, GAVI Fund Board of Directors.
Chapter 4.1 The right to the highest attainable standard of health

Jørn Olsen Professor and Chair, Department of Epidemiology, School of Public Health, UCLA, CA, USA.
Chapter 12.5 Prevention and control of chronic, non-communicable diseases

Adrian Ong Office of the Director General, World Health Organization, Geneva, Switzerland.
Chapter 12.14 Global health agenda for the twenty-first century

Krishna M. Palipudi Senior Survey Statistician, Office on Smoking and Health, Centers for Disease Control and Prevention (CDC), Atlanta, Georgia, USA.
Chapter 10.1 Tobacco

George C. Patton VicHealth Professor of Adolescent Health, Centre for Adolescent Health, Murdoch Children's Research Institute, Melbourne, Australia.
Chapter 11.4 Adolescent health

Sarah Payne Reader in Social Policy, School for Policy Studies, University of Bristol, Bristol, UK.
Chapter 11.2 Women, men, and health

Neil Pearce Director, Centre for Public Health Research, Massey University Wellington Campus, Wellington, New Zealand.
Chapter 9.4 Chronic obstructive pulmonary disease and asthma

Corinne Peek-Asa Professor, University of Iowa, Occupational and Environmental Health, Injury Prevention Research Center, Iowa City, IA, USA.
Chapter 10.4 Injury prevention and control: The public health approach

John Powell Associate Clinical Professor of Epidemiology and Public Health, Health Sciences Research Institute, Warwick Medical School, University of Warwick, Coventry, UK.
Chapter 12.2 Needs assessment: A practical approach

John Powles Senior Lecturer in Public Health Medicine, Department of Public Health and Primary Care, Institute of Public Health, Robinson Way, Cambridge, UK.
Chapter 3.2 Public health policy in developed countries

Deborah Prothrow-Stith Professor, Harvard University School of Public Health, Boston, Mass, USA.
Chapter 10.5 Interpersonal violence prevention: A recent public health mandate

Denis J. Protti Professor, Health Information Science, Human & Social Development Building, University of Victoria, Victoria, Canada; Visiting Professor, Health Informatics, City University, London, UK.
Chapter 5.1 Information systems in support of public health in high-income countries

Laura Punnett Professor, Department of Work Environment; Director, Center to Promote Health in the New England Workplace (CPH-NEW); Senior Associate, Center for Women and Work (CWW), University of Massachusetts Lowell, MA, USA.
Chapter 8.6 Ergonomics and public health

Pekka Puska Director General, National Public Health Institute (KTL), Helsinki, Finland.
Chapter 6.9 Community-based intervention studies in high-income countries

Mario Raviglione Director, Stop TB Department, World Health Organization, Geneva, Switzerland.
Chapter 9.14 Tuberculosis

K. Srinath Reddy President, Public Health Foundation of India, New Delhi, India.
Chapter 1.4 The development of the discipline of public health in countries in economic transition: India, Brazil, China

Margaret Reid Professor of Women's Health, Public Health and Health Policy, Community Based Sciences, University of Glasgow, Glasgow, UK.
Chapter 7.1 Sociology and psychology in public health

Peter G. Robinson School of Clinical Dentistry, University of Sheffield, UK.
Chapter 9.8 Dental public health

Robin Room Professor, School of Population Health, University of Melbourne; and Director, AER Centre for Alcohol Policy Research, Turning Point Alcohol & Drug Centre, Fitzroy, Victoria, Australia.
Chapter 10.3 Alcohol

Julia Royall Chief, Office of International Programs, US National Library of Medicine, USA.
Chapter 5.3 Web-based public health information dissemination and evaluation

Jonathan Samet Professor, University of Southern California, Los Angeles, California, USA.
Chapter 10.1 Tobacco

Rodolfo Saracci Director of Research in Epidemiology, IFC-National Research Council, Pisa Italy.
Chapter 9.1 Gene–environment interactions and public health

Benedetto Saraceno Director, Department of Mental Health and Substance Abuse, Acting Director, Department of Chronic Diseases and Health Promotion, World Health Organization, Geneva, Switzerland.
Chapter 9.7 Public mental health

Jorgen Schlundt Director, Department of Food Safety, Zoonoses and Foodborne Diseases, World Health Organization, Geneva, Switzerland.
Chapter 4.3 International public health instruments

Eleanor B. Schron Program Director, National Heart, Lung, and Blood Institute, National Institutes of Health ,Bethesda, MD, USA.
Chapter 6.7 Methodology of intervention trials in individuals

John C. Scott President, Center for Public Service Communications, Arlington, Virginia, USA.
Chapter 5.3 Web-based public health information dissemination and evaluation

Than Sein Director, Noncommunicable Diseases and Mental Health, World Health Organization, Regional Office for Southeast Asia, New Delhi, India.
Chapter 1.3 The history and development of public health in low- and middle-income countries

Shira Shafir Department of Epidemiology, School of Public Health, UCLA, CA, USA.
Chapter 8.3 Control of microbial threats: Population surveillance, vaccine studies, and the microbiological laboratory

Prakash S. Shetty Professor of Public Health Nutrition, Institute of Human Nutrition, School of Medicine, University of Southampton, Southampton, UK.
Chapter 2.6 Food and nutrition

Daniel Shouval Liver Unit, Hadassah-Hebrew University Hospital, Jerusalem, Israel.
Chapter 9.16 Chronic hepatitis and other liver disease

Victor W. Sidel Distinguished University Professor of Social Medicine, Montefiore Medical Center and the Albert Einstein College of Medicine, Bronx, NY, USA; Adjunct Professor of Public Health at Weill Medical College of Cornell University in New York City, NY, USA.
Chapter 10.6 Collective violence: War

Elliot R. Siegel Associate Director for Health Information Programs Development, US National Library of Medicine, US National Institutes of Health, US Department of Health and Human Services, Bethesda, MD, USA.
Chapter 5.3 Web-based public health information dissemination and evaluation

Chitr Sitthi-Amorn Professor and Senior Consultant, College of Public Health Sciences, Chulalongkorn University, Bangkok, Thailand.
Chapter 5.2 Information systems and community diagnosis in low- and middle-income countries

George Davey Smith Professor of Clinical Epidemiology, Department of Social Medicine, University of Bristol, UK.
Chapter 6.14 Systematic reviews and meta-analysis

Ian Smith Office of the Director General, World Health Organization, Geneva, Switzerland.
Chapter 12.14 Global health agenda for the twenty-first century

Orielle Solar Ministry of Health, Chile; and World Health Organization, Geneva, Switzerland.
Chapter 2.2 Overview and framework

Frank Sorvillo Department of Epidemiology, School of Public Health, UCLA, CA, USA.
Chapter 8.3 Control of microbial threats: Population surveillance, vaccine studies, and the microbiological laboratory

Jonathan Sterne Professor of Medical Statistics and Epidemiology, Department of Social Medicine, University of Bristol, UK.
Chapter 6.14 Systematic reviews and meta-analysis

Alison Stewart Principal Associate, Foundation for Genomics and Population Health, Cambridge, UK.
Chapter 2.4 Genomics and public health

Allison Streetly Programme Director, NHS Sickle Cell and Thalassaemia Screening Programme, Department of Public Health Sciences, King's College London, London, UK.
Chapter 12.7 Population screening and public health

Steven Sugden The Hygiene Centre, Department of Infectious and Tropical Diseases, London School of Hygiene and Tropical Medicine, London, UK.
Chapter 2.5 Water and sanitation

Patrick S. Sullivan Department of Epidemiology, Rollins School of Public Health, Emory University, Atlanta, GA, USA.
Chapter 6.17 Public health surveillance

Sheena G. Sullivan National Center for AIDS/STD Control and Prevention, Chinese Center for Disease Control and Prevention, Beijing China; Edith Cowan University, Perth, Australia.
Chapter 6.10 Community-based intervention trials in low- and middle-income countries
Chapter 12.13 Private support of public health

Julien O. Teitler Associate Professor of Social Work and Sociology, Columbia University, New York, NY, USA.
Chapter 11.1 The changing family

Tim Tenbensel School of Population Health, University of Auckland, New Zealand.
Chapter 7.6 Public health sciences and policy in high-income countries

Puja Thakker Research Associate, Public Health Foundation of India, New Delhi, India.
Chapter 1.4 The development of the discipline of public health in countries in economic transition: India, Brazil, China

Elma B. Torres Director, Health Safety and Environmental Management Consultancy Services, Inc., Philippines.
Chapter 12.8 Environmental health practice

Peter Tugwell Canada Research Chair in Health Equity; Director, Centre for Global health, Institute of Population Health, University of Ottawa, Canada.
Chapter 6.11 Clinical epidemiology

Kumnuan Ungchusak Director, Bureau of Epidemiology and International Health Regulation (IHR) Focal point Department of Diseases Control, Ministry of Public Health, Thailand.
Chapter 6.4 Principles of outbreak investigation

Nigel Unwin Professor of Epidemiology, Institute of Health and Society, Newcastle University, UK.
Chapter 9.6 The epidemiology and prevention of diabetes mellitus

Pierre van Damme Centre for the Evaluation of Vaccination, Vaccine & Infectious Disease Institute, University of Antwerp, Belgium.
Chapter 9.16 Chronic hepatitis and other liver disease

Koen Van Herck Centre for the Evaluation of Vaccination, Vaccine & Infectious Disease Institute, University of Antwerp, Belgium.
Chapter 9.16 Chronic hepatitis and other liver disease

Erkki Vartiainen Director, Department of Health Promotion and Chronic Disease Prevention, Helsinki, Finland.
Chapter 6.9 Community-based intervention studies in high-income countries

Carlo La Vecchia Head, Laboratory of General Epidemiology, Istituto di Ricerche Farmacologiche 'Mario Negri', Milano, Italy.
Chapter 9.3 Neoplasms

Jeanette Vega Vice Minister of Health, Chile.
Chapter 2.2 Overview and framework

Gemma Vestal World Health Organization, Geneva, Switzerland.
Chapter 10.1 Tobacco

Paolo Vineis Chair in Environmental Epidemiology, Imperial College London, UK.
Chapter 9.1 Gene–environment interactions and public health

Hester J.T. Ward Consultant in Epidemiology and Public Health, National CJD Surveillance Unit, University of Edinburgh, Western General Hospital, Edinburgh, UK.
Chapter 9.11 The transmissible spongiform encephalopathies

Noel S. Weiss School of Public Health and Community Medicine, University of Washington, WA, USA.
Chapter 6.5 Case–control studies

Vivian Welch Institute of Population Health, University of Ottawa, Ottawa, Canada.
Chapter 6.11 Clinical epidemiology

Suwit Wibulpolprasert Senior Advisor on Disease Control, Ministry of Public Health, Thailand.
Chapter 12.11 Public health workers

Gail Williams School of Population Health, Faculty of Health Sciences, University of Queensland, Australia.
Chapter 6.15 Statistical methods

Marilyn Wise School of Public Health, University of Sydney, NSW, Australia.
Chapter 12.9 Structures and strategies for public health intervention

Fred B. Wood Office of Health Information Programs Development, US National Library of Medicine, US National Institutes of Health, Bethesda, MD, USA.
Chapter 5.3 Web-based public health information dissemination and evaluation

Zunyou Wu Director, National Center for AIDS/STD Control and Prevention, Chinese Center for Disease Control and Prevention, Beijing, China.
Chapter 6.10 Community-based intervention trials in low- and middle-income countries

Derek Yach Vice-President, Global Health Policy, PepsiCo Foundation, USA.
Chapter 10.1 Tobacco

Gonghuan Yang Deputy Director, China Center for Disease Prevention and Control, Beijing, China.
Chapter 10.1 Tobacco

Ron Zimmern Executive Director, Foundation for Genomics and Population Health, Cambridge, UK.
Chapter 2.4 Genomics and public health

Paul Zimmet Director Emeritus and Director of International Research, Baker IDI Heart and Diabetes Institute, Melbourne Australia.
Chapter 9.6 The epidemiology and prevention of diabetes mellitus

Anthony B. Zwi School of Public Health and Community Medicine, University of New South Wales, Sydney, Australia.
Chapter 11.8 Forced migrants and other displaced populations

SECTION 9

Major health problems

Gene–environment interactions and public health

Paolo Vineis and Rodolfo Saracci

Searching for disease genes

Twentieth-century developments

The establishment of the role of genes in the hereditary causation of disease followed almost immediately the independent rediscovery in 1900, after 35 years of oblivion, of Mendel's laws by three botanists, de Vries, Correns, and Tschermak (1950). In 1902, Archibald Garrod published in *The Lancet* a paper titled 'The incidence of alkaptonuria, a study of chemical individuality', in which he noted both the all-or-none character of the disease and its familial and discontinuous inter-generational distribution. Each day, affected subjects excreted several grams of homogentisic acid, a metabolite of tyrosine which imparts a black colour to deposited urine, while normal subjects did not excrete any. Garrod consulted William Bateson, one of the first British geneticists who propounded the general relevance of Mendel's laws across the living world (he also coined the word 'genetics'). He pointed out that the observed data could be readily explained in terms of a Mendelian inheritance pattern. Alkaptonuria became the first recognized example of a recessive condition in humans (Harris 1959). Garrod subsequently produced a considerable body of research on inherited biochemical disorders, culminating in the publication of the book *Inborn Errors of Metabolism*, in which the concept of genetically determined biochemical variations in humans was developed. The nature of these variations brings into focus the complementary and necessary role of the environment in disease causation: Alkaptonuria requires the presence of tyrosine and phenylalanine in the diet and, at least in theory, could be relieved by a selectively restricted diet. Porphyrias, conditions also investigated by Garrod, are now known to depend on the deficiency of any of the seven enzymes in the biosynthetic pathway of the haeme, the oxygen-carrying moiety of haemoglobin: Crises are precipitated by external factors like the absorption of barbiturates or sulphonamides that accelerate the synthesis of the haeme above the catalytic capacity of the defective enzyme, resulting in the accumulation of noxious precursor metabolites.

Garrod had opened a new field of research which by the middle of the past century had thrown light on a substantial number of inherited diseases, identified phenotypically by characteristic biochemical disorders and genetically by Mendelian patterns of familial segregation and transmission. Among these of particular importance were early pharmacogenetic observations (Harris 1959). Abnormal sensitivity to the muscle relaxant succinylcholine, used in anaesthesia, resulted in prolonged apnoea due to inadequate inactivation of the drug by a defective cholinesterase enzyme: The defect appeared inherited as an autosomal recessive trait. Plasmatic level of the antituberculosis drug isoniazid showed a wide inter-individual variation for a fixed administered dose: Subjects could be divided into fast and slow acetylators (inactivators) of the drug, with slow acetylator behaving as an autosomal recessive trait. Primaquine, an antimalarial drug, caused haemolytic crises in subjects defective in glucose-6-phospahate dehydrogenase (G-6-PD), an enzyme central to the aerobic metabolism of red cells: In this case, the defective trait appeared X-linked with incomplete dominance.

In the first years of the twentieth century also, the blood groups of the ABO system were recognized as individually different and inheritable traits. By the mid-1920s, the pattern of inheritance had become clear, involving only one locus with three alleles (A, B, and O), the first demonstrable case of multiallelic inheritance in humans. These firmly identified heritable traits, either normal like the blood groups or pathological like a host of biochemical disorders, are almost always monogenic, with a direct and constant, or marginally variable, correspondence between phenotype and genotype (in a given environment). The same applies to the vast number of (uncommon) clinical syndromes, from Tay–Sachs disease to Marfan's syndrome to neurofibromatosis, inventoried in McKusick's reference book *Mendelian Inheritance in Man* (McKusick 1998). The persistence in a population of rare alleles with pathological effects could be understood in terms of history of mutation of normal alleles balanced by selective pressure keeping the abnormal alleles at low equilibrium level (say a frequency of <1 per cent). It was much less clear, however, whether selection could play any role in the persistence of frequent polymorphic alleles, like those of the ABO blood groups, with no obvious pathological effects. Association studies were carried out to search for subtler effects, in the form of increased risk of (or 'susceptibility to') common diseases.

These consistently showed, for instance, an association of blood groups O with gastric, duodenal, and stomal ulcer, findings that can today be related to differential affinity of *Helicobacter pylori* for the gastric mucosa mediated by blood group antigens (Borén *et al.* 1993). A paper by Lower *et al.* (reprinted in 2007) marked in 1979 a clear step forward in the investigation of susceptibility to a common disease, bladder cancer, when exposure to an environmental pathogen occurs. Lower *et al.* argued, on the basis of a detailed consideration of the activation and inactivation (detoxification) metabolism of aromatic amines, that slow N-acetylators of aromatic amines, a phenotype with a Mendelian segregation, should have—other things been equal—a higher risk of bladder cancer than fast acetylators when exposed to aromatic amines in the environment. They tested the hypothesis in a case–control study in urban Denmark and rural Sweden finding an odds ratio of 1.7 for the association of the slow acetylator phenotype with bladder cancer in urban Denmark and an odds ratio of 1.1 in rural Sweden. They attributed the difference to the different levels of exposure to aromatic amines from occupational and environmental sources in the two study locations. As noted in a commentary (Vineis 2007), this explanation is questionable since studies have generally failed to show an association between air pollution and bladder cancer and occupational exposure to aromatic amines is uncommon. However, the argument underlying the explanation is of interest as it stresses the role of environmental exposures to detect an increase susceptibility to disease development.

The contemporary scene

Advances in molecular genetic technologies in the last quarter of the twentieth century have remarkably improved the ability to locate genes in chromosomes and allowed for the first time to clone and sequence genes in DNA samples. This has led to the completed sequence of the human genome in 2003 and has opened new avenues for the study of common diseases, such as ischaemic heart disease, diabetes, and cancers, whose complex determination results from the interplay of heritable polygenic and environmental factors. Genetic epidemiology linkage studies of these diseases, in which the co-segregation within families of the disease with genetic markers of known segregation pattern and chromosomal location is analysed, are being largely superseded by association studies. These may investigate the association of disease with an allele presumed, from existing biological knowledge, to functionally affect the disease (candidate gene) or, often, with some allele in 'linkage disequilibrium' with it (i.e. tightly associated with it because it is located at a closely proximate site, no recombination occurring between the loci of the two alleles). With this approach and the availability of a dense chromosomal map of marker alleles, like the single-nucleotide polymorphisms (SNPs), the exploration of all regions of the genome has become feasible. The efficiency of the search is being further facilitated by the fact that SNPs in linkage disequilibrium with each other tend to be passed together in a block (haplotype) from parents to offspring. The International HapMap Project has completed a map of haplotypes making possible to choose for testing only selected single SNPs ('tagging' SNPs) within each haplotype, as these imply the presence of all other SNPs in the block as well of any functionally disease-related mutation. Concurrently the testing technology has undergone a vertiginous advancement: High-throughput platforms allowing the simultaneous determination of half a million SNPs are available

and this, combined with the tagging SNP approach, has paved the way to 'genome-wide association' (GWA) studies. In these the search of disease-related alleles is not any more focused on candidate genes but covers bit by bit the whole genome.

A successful story concerning the use of high-throughput genetic technologies to screen for new associations is represented by the region 8q24. Family-based linkage studies, association studies, and studies of tumours had already highlighted human chromosome 8q as a genomic region of interest for a prostate cancer susceptibility loci. Recently, a locus at 8q24, characterized by both a SNP and a microsatellite marker, has been shown to be associated with prostate cancer risk in Icelandic, Swedish, and US samples (Witte 2007). These data suggest that the locus on chromosome 8q24 harbours a genetic variant associated with prostate cancer and that the microsatellite marker is a stronger risk factor for aggressive prostate cancers defined by poorly differentiated tumour morphology. Evidence has now been provided that colon cancer might also be associated with the same region. Using a multistage genetic association approach comprising 7480 affected individuals and 7779 controls, researchers have identified markers in chromosomal region 8q24 associated with colorectal cancer (Zanke *et al.* 2007). This example is interesting for several reasons, including (a) 'reverse genetics', i.e. the possibility that aetiologic pathways for cancers that elude epidemiological research can be discovered starting from the observation of genetic susceptibility; and (b) 'pleiotropy', the ability of certain gene variants to increase or modulate the risk for different diseases.

Recently the results of a large genome-wide association study have been published (The Wellcome Trust Case Control Consortium 2007), involving 2000 cases of each of seven common diseases and 3000 shared controls. Case–control comparisons identified 24 independent association signals at a high level of statistical significance ($P < 5 \times 10^{-7}$): One in bipolar disorder, one in coronary heart disease, nine in Crohn's disease, three in rheumatoid arthritis, seven in type 1 diabetes, and three in type 2 diabetes. On the basis of prior findings and of the limited replication already performed the authors interpret almost all of the signals as reflecting genuine susceptibility effects. Also in this study some loci identified by the signals are implicated in more than one disease, i.e. show pleiotropy.

Given the strong momentum that this high-tech research has gained more GWA studies will come forward in the near future. In addition important new sources of variability have been discovered all along the human genome, notably the copy-number variants (CNV), involved in gene expression, ready to be explored in relation to disease. A recent comment stated: 'The avalanche of recent data provided by genome-wide association studies represents a quantum leap in information about the inherited component of certain diseases' (Hunter & Kraft 2007). No doubt the environmental components can be submerged and lost sight of within the avalanche.

Genes or environment?

Genes and heredity

Genes have to do with heredity, but what is the relationship between the two? A confusion, still largely present in the literature and regularly echoed in the lay press, concerning heredity vs. genetic causation is emblematically represented by the debate that took place around IQ after the publication of The Bell Curve by Herrnstein and Murray (1994). As it was pointed out by Block (1995), the basic confusion in this book and in many other similar papers was between heritability and genetic determination. Heritability has to do with similarity of observable traits between parents and the off-spring, while a characteristic is 'genetically determined' if it is coded in and caused by the genes within a 'normal' environment. Two extreme examples are the following: (a) the number of fingers in humans is totally genetically determined and the rare deviations from five fingers are caused by defects of development, e.g. from thalidomide; they are congenital but not heritable; (b) wearing skirts among European populations has a very strong heritability, as it occurs only in women (with the exception of the odd Scotsmen). Hence, it is related to having an XX rather than a XY chromosomal pair but it is not genetically determined (Block 1995). Such mis-conceptions are clearly relevant to the discussion about the herita-bility vs. genetic determination of diseases. For example, studies of twins which often do not rule out similar environmental exposures for the pair, cannot be used to automatically infer that cancer or schizophrenia are due to pathologic genetic variants in DNA. In fact the environment itself is inherited, for example in the case of the propensity to wear skirts. The same argument applies to claims that IQ has 60 per cent heritability, academic performance 50 per cent or occupational status 40 per cent: These figures do not mean that such characteristics are inherited through genes (DNA), i.e. there is genetic determination, but only that there is a substantial association between the characteristic in the index subject and the same characteristic in the parents.

Genes and disease

The role of genes in causing human disease is often misunderstood. In 1972, a key paper by Lewontin drew attention on the mistakes of partitioning nature and nurture (Lewontin 1972). Genetic determinism, namely the contention that the causal determination of a disease is due to a gene and nothing else, is a fundamental misconception.

There are several objections to it, in particular:

(1) The sequence of information in genes is 'per se' insufficient to dictate how gene products give origin to a new organism; much depends on a cascade of interacting events, pre-mRNA alternative splicing, a large number of different types of RNA, gene–gene interactions and the pre-natal environment, i.e. biological phenomena that encompass but expand much beyond the gene sequence.

(2) Genetic pathways completely specify an abnormal function of the organism only on rare occasions, namely for 'monogenic' diseases like sickle-cell anaemia or Huntington's chorea. In these cases the cell does not have compensatory mechanisms to overcome the metabolic alteration and influences from environmental variations within the range experienced by the human species are negligible. These are the only situations in which the simplified paradigm 'one gene-one disease' is valid. In all other cases diseases are due to the interplay of gene vari-ations with environmental variations, the latter being often dominant. The phenomenon of availability of multiple meta-bolic pathways, controlled by different genes, that allow the cell and the organism to adequately overcome damages caused by the environment, represents an early conquest of human evolution. As the geneticist Bailey stated, the implication of gene *robustness* is the inability of many genes (or signals, or

regulatory interactions) to have any significant effect over the phenotype unless a number of other genes are simultaneously altered (Fox Keller 2000). This is a complementary phenome-non to the already mentioned *pleiotropy* by which most genes have multiple functions.

A simple correspondence between genotype and phenotype subsumed when exploring the role of genes in disease may in fact almost completely break down. For example, some African populations—such as the Ethiopians, show multiple gene copies (multiduplication) of genes such as CYP2D6. This phenomenon has been attributed to diet-related selection during the evolution-ary history of these populations (famine and the need to adapt their detoxifying metabolic capacities to toxicants in the only food available). However, often they tend to have a slow rather than a rapid metabolizer phenotype, as would be expected. To reconcile the genotype–phenotype gap, and to determine if environmental factors are responsible for the observed differences, the genotype and phenotype of CYP2D6 among Ethiopians living in Sweden were assessed and compared to data from Ethiopians living in Ethiopia and Swedish Caucasians (Aklillu *et al.* 2002). A compari-son of the debrisoquine metabolizing ability among individuals of the same CYP2D6 genotype revealed that Swedes exhibited the highest rate of debrisoquine metabolism, followed by Ethiopians in Sweden and Ethiopians in Ethiopia. It has been speculated that inhibitory dietary factors may explain the differences seen between the different groups and that these components in the past might have contributed to dietary stress-mediated selection of duplicated and multiduplicated active CYP2D6 genes, as frequently seen in Ethiopians. These results indicate a significant influence of envi-ronmental factors in shaping the difference in the relation between CYP2D6 genotype and phenotype (metabolic capacity) between Caucasians and Black Africans.

Notwithstanding these considerations genetic determinism is still at least implicit in a large number of investigations, when certain traits or diseases are straightaway attributed to genes or even to a single gene.

A clear example is the so called 'fragile X syndrome', a condition in which 1 out of 1000 males develops a serious mental retardation (Abbeduto *et al.* 2007; Penagarikano *et al.* 2007). When their X chromosome is observed under the microscope, it appears as lacking a fragment, a characteristic named 'fragile site'. These obser-vations led to the conclusion that chromosome X carries a gene implicated in the development of the central nervous system. Several research groups started work to isolate the gene also in the hope that new prenatal screening strategies could be developed to avoid the birth of children with the syndrome. The gene was identi-fied in 1991 and it received the name of FMR-1 (fragile X mental retardation-1). In the meantime, the syndrome was assigned a spectrum that went much beyond reality to include anti-social and criminal behaviours: The denomination 'crime gene' ensued. However, after the isolation of the gene it became evident that things were much more complex. Expressivity of the gene turned out to be variable: Children with the same defect (repetition of three letters in the DNA sequence, CGG) may have very serious neurological defects, while others may be absolutely normal. These children are sometimes hyperkinetic, or have difficulties in concen-trating, but—contrary to some claims—there is no firm evidence of criminal behaviour. Currently the disorder is interpreted as mainly caused by the expansion of the trinucleotide sequence CGG located in the 5′ UTR of the FMR1 gene on the X chromosome. The abnormal expansion of this triplet leads to hypermethylation and consequent silencing of the FMR1 gene, and the absence of the encoded protein (FMRP) is the basis for the phenotype. FMRP appears to play an important role in synaptic plasticity by regulating the synthesis of proteins encoded by certain mRNAs localized in the dendrite. Around the one specific and clearly genetically based condition (lack of FMRP) there are a number of minor forms and other phenotypes that have little resemblance to the genetically based disorder.

Genes and environment

There is a large consensus among scientists that only a minor fraction of diseases, of the order of about 5 per cent is monogenic while the vast majority of cases are due to the interplay or 'interaction' of genetic and environmental factors, the latter being often dominant.

Models of gene–environment interactions

Some useful models describing gene–environment interactions as they manifest at the level of disease occurrence have been proposed by Ottman (Fig. 9.1.1) (Ottman 1996): These models portray five different and general biological situations, rather than entering in the details of disease-specific pathogenetic mechanisms. A similar approach has been used by Yang and Khoury (1997) who present a typology of six models describing in terms of relative measures of association in epidemiological studies (relative risks) different ways in which genes and the environment can interact.

In Ottman's Model A the effect of the genotype is to produce or increase expression of an environmental 'risk factor' that can also be produced non-genetically. For example, in phenylketonuria (PKU) subjects homozygous for the autosomal recessive allele are deficient in the enzyme necessary to convert dietary phenylalanine into tyrosine. If left untreated, i.e. without dietary restriction, these subjects develop high levels of blood phenylalanine (regarded as the internal environment 'risk factor') which causes mental retardation. High blood levels of phenylalanine and mental retardation may, however, even occur in subjects without the deficient genotype, e.g. children who had intrauterine exposure to high blood levels because the mother is affected by the enzyme deficiency. In the pathway from gene to disease the high blood level of phenylalanine is an intermediate variable which can however also be induced by *a separate and independent mechanism*. Model A therefore typifies an absence of interaction.

In Model B, the genotype exacerbates the effect of the environmental factor, but there is no effect of genotype in unexposed persons. For example, xeroderma pigmentosum (XP) is an autosomal recessive disorder in which exposure to UV light causes a large number of skin cancers because of a defect of DNA repair enzymes. However, the risk of skin cancer is increased with UV exposure also in people without XP.

In Model C, the environmental factor exacerbates the effect of genotype but there is no effect of the environmental factor in persons with the low-risk genotype. For example, an autosomal dominant disorder, porphyria variegata, is characterized by skin problems of variable severity. Exposure to barbiturates, which is innocuous in persons without the condition, precipitates an acute crisis that may involve even paralysis and death.

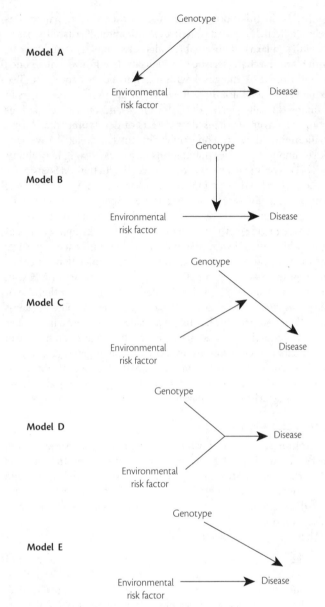

Fig. 9.1.1 Five general models of gene–environment interaction (from Ottman).

In Model D, both genotype and the environmental factor are required to increase risk. As already mentioned, G-6-PD deficiency is an X-linked recessive disorder with incomplete penetrance: Individuals are asymptomatic unless, for example, they eat fava beans, in which case they develop severe haemolytic anaemia. Fava beans, however, do not produce any symptoms without the deficiency.

Finally, in Model E, both the genotype and the environmental factor have a separate effect in disease risk, but when they occur together the risk is higher or lower than when they occur alone. For example, COPD risk is increased in smokers without alpha-1-antitrypsin deficiency and in non-smokers with the deficiency, but risk is increased to a greater extent in smokers with the deficiency. It is likely that many cases of gene–environment interactions relevant to common diseases belong to this category.

A population story: Native Americans and the metabolic syndrome

Investigating gene–environment interactions may play a role not only in elucidating disease development and individual susceptibility, but also in understanding why certain populations or subgroups show high risks of disease. A classical example, worth some detailed consideration, is represented by 'Native Americans' and other genetically well-defined population.

Native American (NA) populations have rates of chronic diseases such as those encompassed by the 'metabolic syndrome' that are higher than in other populations with similar lifestyles. It had been suggested that this is due to a genetic predisposition coupled with rapid environmental changes as their lifestyle became more Westernized (Wendorf 1989). More recently, it has been hypothesized that Native Americans have a relatively large number of gene variants that modify environmental factors to cause chronic disease (Nagi *et al.* 1998). Accordingly, the Native American population could be considered to be a 'natural laboratory' for the thesis that chronic diseases are caused by gene–environment interactions. The metabolic syndrome is a good example of a complex of chronic conditions. Its prevalence has been increasing and is higher in Native Americans than in other populations living a similar lifestyle (Ford *et al.* 2002; Resnick 2002).

In 1999, the World Health Organization defined metabolic syndrome as the presence of diabetes or impaired glucose tolerance or insulin resistance, plus two of the following: Obesity, dyslipidaemia, hypertension, or microalbuminuria (Isomaa 2003). Having one of these traits increases the risk of having another, and there is a consequential high risk of cardiovascular disease and increased incidence of type 2 diabetes mellitus (T2DM) (Greenlund *et al.* 1999).

The metabolic syndrome is a complex condition and many genes could contribute to its development (Reilly & Rader 2003). Genes that have been reported to be involved are those controlling both energy metabolism and storage and inflammatory pathways. Genes that improve the efficiency of energy storage, especially as fat, are often referred to as 'thrifty genes'. These would have been selected when our ancestors were hunter–gatherers and lived in times of alternating feast and famine (Zimmet & Thomas 2003). It has also been suggested that physical inactivity may alter gene expression in some way that leads to derangement of metabolism and metabolic syndrome (Booth *et al.* 2002). There are various genes that have shown differences in expression due to exercise, including genes that encode for intermediates in insulin signalling and energy metabolism and enzymes that are involved in lipid metabolism. These genes could also be candidate genes for causing metabolic syndrome (Bray 2000).

It has been hypothesized that when modern humans began to spread across the globe 100 000 years ago these genetic divergences occurred due to the selection pressures of the different geographical areas and social groups in which they were living. Genes/mutations that made it more likely for an individual in a group to reach reproductive age and be successful in finding a mate became more common in that group (Olson 2002). Concerning Native Americans, there is some debate surrounding the settlement of the Americas. It is likely that the initial settlers migrated from Asia probably through Siberia and then moved south. It is also possible that some settlers also came from Europe (Olson 2002). When the ancestors of the Native Americans migrated south, they did so in a particularly harsh environment, so it is possible that those genes giving an efficient energy metabolism would have been selected for in this population (Wendorf 1989).

Over the past 50 years, Native American populations have become increasingly Westernized. The main changes that have come with the Western lifestyle are those in physical activity and diet. For example, a community initiative in Mohawk Native Americans has shown that over the last 50 years they had become less physically active and that the availability of foods high in fat and calories has increased (Hood *et al.* 1997).

A study of diabetes prevalence and behavioural risk factors in Native Americans showed that their prevalence of diabetes was 2.5 times higher than in whites. The prevalence of obesity was also higher. However the prevalence of risk factors such as a sedentary lifestyle and smoking were similar in Native Americans and Caucasian populations (Muneta *et al.* 1993). This suggests that Native Americans might have a higher frequency of gene variants that interact with the environment causing them to have the high prevalence of metabolic syndrome. Or, alleles that are beneficial with a traditional lifestyle (and so would have been selected in these populations) may be disadvantageous in the context of a Western lifestyle.

In light of these hypotheses the exploration has developed of genetic causes of cardiovascular disease, obesity or type 2 diabetes in Native Americans populations. At the time of writing there are already more than 25 published papers investigating a spectrum of genes. Four papers (Aguilar *et al.* 1999; Kataoka *et al.* 1996; Thompson *et al.* 1997; Vozarova *et al.* 2003) found variation between Native Americans and Caucasians in the frequency of an allele associated with metabolic syndrome. In each case the frequency of the allele positively associated with metabolic syndrome was higher in the Native American population. Additionally, Knowler *et al.* (1988) found an allele with a negative association with type 2 diabetes that was associated with the presence of Caucasian admixture.

Methodological issues

The investigation of the effects, separate and joint, of genes and environment confronts a number of methodological issues (Thomas 2004).

Errors of measurement

First, measurement of genes (genotyping) and of environmental agents are usually prone to different degrees of error. Genotyping is in general more accurate than the majority of methods used to measure environmental exposures. This implies a lower degree of classification error that in turn means an easier identification of associations with disease. Table 9.1.1 (Armstrong *et al.* 1994) shows the attenuation that a true association, expressed as true odds ratio, undergoes as a consequence of errors of measurement, expressed as imperfect (i.e. less than 1 per cent or less than 100 per cent) sensitivity and specificity; the error is assumed to be non-differential, applying equally to cases and controls. The observable odds ratio for an environmental exposure is likely to be markedly attenuated, as in the first line of the table, as a sensitivity of 60 per cent and a specificity of 90 per cent are realistic, and perhaps even optimistic for measurements of environmental exposures. The attenuation for the genetic exposure, i.e. for genotyping, is more likely to be as in the last lines of the table (for example, the common genotyping method Taqman has 96 per cent sensitivity and 98 per cent specificity): The observable odds ratios are materially higher than those in the first line and much closer to the true ones, making a true association, namely the point estimate of the odds ratio, more likely to show-up for the genetic than for the environmental variable. Whether the estimate is statistically significant at a chosen probability level depends also on the prevalence of the exposure (whose effect on the attenuation of the true odds ratio is shown in Table 9.1.1): The power of the study to detect an odds ratio as significantly deviating from unity is higher for exposures with frequencies of 40–50 per cent (as for the slow acetylator phenotype of NAT2 or the GSTM1 null variant of GSTM) than for rare exposures, of the order of 1–10 per cent, as is often the case for environmental exposures in the general population. Again this favours the detectability of associations of disease with genetic traits more than with environmental exposures and has obvious consequences for the size of studies. When both genetic traits and environmental exposure are investigated within the same study, as typically occurs when one of the aims is to explore gene–environment interactions, the size of the study which has a good power for detecting gene–disease associations may be vastly underpowered for detecting associations of environmental exposures with disease, and the study may become 'de facto' worthless for this purpose and, related to this, for an adequate exploration of the interaction.

Testing of multiple hypotheses

While accurate genotyping measurements make easier the detection of gene–disease associations it also contributes to enhancing the chance of false positive results if, as is more and more the case, associations between each of the hundred or thousands of genetic variants and disease phenotype are tested. If a thousand association tests are performed and the conventional level of statistical significance of, say, $P = 0.01$, is used one expects merely by chance to find 10 associations with $P < 0.01$ when none is real. The problem becomes dramatic with the genome-wide association studies in which hundred of thousands or even millions of SNP-to-disease association tests are performed. As pointed out in recent papers (Wacholder *et al.* 2004; Thomas & Clayton 2004), the issue is not one of finding an appropriate level of statistical significance for the multiple testing of a single global null hypothesis (as in the classical theory of multiple testing) but for multiple hypotheses, one for each SNP-to-disease association. In the light of reasonable assumptions on the 'a priori' probability of an association being real and of the power of the study, values of P of the order of 10^{-7} have been worked out as significance threshold to separate real from false associations (however associations with less extreme P values may still be worth considering for replication studies, particularly when supported by information on biological mechanism).

Interactions

Further problems arise when the joint effects of genes and environment are considered, namely 'gene–environment interactions'. This label—GEI—has become current for any study involving genotyping as well as some measures of environmental factors. The term interaction lends itself to confusion as it has several meanings: Biological, statistical, and public health (Saracci 1980).

In a biological sense, it indicates how two or more agents—genetic and/or environmental—cooperate in a biological mechanism to produce an effect. Specific mechanistic models of interactions translating into observable patterns of disease occurrence have been developed for communicable diseases but much less commonly for non-communicable diseases: The multistage carcinogenesis model is one example.

In a statistical sense the presence of an interaction indicates that the observed data actually deviate in respect to a model of joint effect assumed to adequately summarize the data. The interaction is designated as 'qualitative' or 'non-removable' if the deviation consists of the reversal of the effect of an agent, for example, the hypotensive effect of a drug being changed into an hypertensive effect in the presence of a genetic variant controlling a metabolizing enzyme. If the deviation consists instead of an amplification or reduction of the effect expected under the model, the interaction is designated as 'quantitative' and can be removed by an appropriate change of the scale of measurement on which the effect is expressed, for instance changing the scale from arithmetic to logarithmic. The additive and the multiplicative models are the two summarizing models most employed in epidemiology. Unfortunately, it has been

Table 9.1.1 Effect of non-differential misclassification of a dichotomous exposure on the observable odds ratio (ORobs) (from Armstrong *et al.* 1994)

Exposure sensitivity	Exposure specificity	Prev.	OR true = 1.5 OR obs.	OR true = 2 OR obs.	OR true = 4 OR obs.
0.6	0.9	0.1	1.17	1.34	1.93
0.6	0.9	0.5	1.24	1.42	1.86
0.6	0.99	0.1	1.40	1.79	3.20
0.6	0.99	0.5	1.30	1.54	2.12
0.9	0.9	0.1	1.24	1.48	2.41
0.9	0.9	0.5	1.38	1.73	2.85
0.9	0.99	0.1	1.45	1.89	3.61
0.9	0.99	0.5	1.43	1.82	3.11

Note: 'Prev.' is the exposure prevalence among non-diseased subjects.

shown that each of them may arise from a variety of underlying mechanistic models so that, contrary to hopes, the observation of joint responses to several agents, e.g. a gene and an environmental exposure, throws scarce light on the biological pathways involved. Even the different models outlined by Ottman and by Khoury *et al.* previously mentioned, which are more specific than the additive and multiplicative models may prove difficult to distinguish by means of epidemiological data.

In the additive model, the incidence rate resulting from the joint exposure to several agents equals the sum of the basic population rate (no agent present) plus the excess rate associated with each of the agents: The incidence rate is the fundamental expression of the disease occurrence in a population, hence anything larger or smaller than this baseline sum can be regarded as an interaction, notably in a public health sense.

In the multiplicative model, the relative risk due to the two exposures is simply the product of the relative risk for the separate exposures. In a case–control study, the same relationship holds for the odds ratios. This multiplicative relation is the basis of the logistic regression, commonly used in the analysis of epidemiological data from studies with multiple exposure variables. In the context of a GEI study, it presents an additional interesting feature: If the distributions in the source population of the genotypes and of the environmental factors are independent, errors in environmental exposure measurement have as the only effect the driving of the data toward a multiplicative relation (probably this being the reason why in practice the data very often conform to a multiplicative model) (Clayton & McKeigue 2001). Under the same assumption of independent distributions of genotypes and environmental exposures in the source population it becomes possible to explore the GEI only among cases ('case-only' study design). If in this type of study no association is found (namely an odds ratio of 1) between genotype and environmental exposure among the cases of a disease, the inference can be made that the joint effect of the two agents is multiplicative: Hence, the 'case-only' design can be used to screen for genes and environmental factors acting (at least) multiplicatively, a point not always clearly understood. In fact both from a biological and a public health viewpoint this multiplicative, i.e. more than merely additive, joint effect may be in itself of interest.

Focusing on the joint effect of a gene and an environmental agent could also help in detecting weak overall effects. If the gene variant acts only in the presence of an environmental exposure, i.e. exhibits a supramultiplicative interaction, the possibility of detecting its effects depends on having correctly measured the environmental variable as well. Suppose the gene variant has an odds ratio of 4 for the association with a disease among subjects who also are exposed (in an independent way) to an environmental agent, and an odds ratio of 1 among those not so exposed. If there is no information on the environmental exposure, which is in fact present in 50 per cent of the subjects, the odds ratio for the main effect of the gene variant will show up as 2.5; if however the environmental exposure is present in only 10 per cent of the subjects (a more realistic situation for many environmental agents) the odds ratio for the main effect will be reduced to 1.3, a weak effect hardly detectable. Knowledge of environmental variables may thus enhance the power of detecting the effects of genetic variables (and vice versa). This advantage, however, needs to be looked at with caution: Unless existing biological knowledge allows one to pinpoint the subgroups where one should expect to observe the highest risks a mere blind search will contribute to inflate the problem of multiple hypotheses testing previously discussed (Clayton & McKeigue 2001).

The importance of measuring environmental exposures

Many investigations labelled as studies on 'gene–environment interactions' are under way in different parts of the world, and the subject also currently appears as one of the leading items in grant calls from NIH or EU. Most of these studies employ similar methods and technological supports for genotyping while the assessment of exposure to environmental agents is extremely variable, being for example state of the art for dietary intake in the EPIC investigation, but not in other studies, nor for other exposures. Unless the size of these studies is calculated to achieve an adequate power of detection for associations of disease with the variables most affected by classification errors, i.e. the environmental ones (diet, pollutants, etc.) it can be safely predicted that such studies will come up with a number of genetic associations but very few credible environmental associations with disease. In addition as the majority of genetic polymorphisms are believed to act through biological interaction with environmental agents, it may also become difficult to make sense of genetic observations if the environmental component is substantially misclassified.

Accurate and precise measurements of environmental exposures meet objective problems as they are targeted on free-living populations with great variability of exposures and changes in time. These measurements often involve recall of complex information—such as diet—or extrapolation from few points in space and time—such as for air pollution data. For rare exposures (that may be relevant for the involved subjects) these difficulties are even greater. The solution lies in empowering exposure assessment, by investing—much more than many investigators have done until now—in robust and validated exposure measurement procedures. This implies that epidemiologists collaborate not only with geneticists and molecular biologists, but also with environmental scientists. Large efforts have already been made in the field of nutrition, but not yet in other areas of environmental exposures. Novel research-based measurement methods should be developed, for example those derived from metabolomics or the identification of specific DNA adducts, to detect signatures left within body fluids by metabolic processes and/or external exposures e.g. air pollutants. Also in the actual measurement process repeated measurements of the same environmental variables, as well as combined measurements of different variables, will reduce misclassification.

Mendelian randomization

Not only exposures to environmental agents are imperfectly measured but the relation of environmental exposures to disease is prone to confounding. Mendelian randomization (MR) is a way to exploit genetic testing in epidemiology to overcome some of the limitations of observational epidemiology. MR has been suggested (Davey Smith & Ebrahim 2003) as a way to overcome confounding by exploiting the random allocation of alleles from parents to the offspring. Because of chromosome separation at meiosis and of recombination, at long-term equilibrium—i.e. after many generations—alleles at different loci on the same or on different chromosomes become (under some reasonable assumptions about the mating pattern in the population) all independently and randomly distributed in the population. Hence one should not expect that alleles, in general, are associated with any particular exposure and as a consequence an association between a gene variant and a disease should not be subject to the confounding by environmental, behavioural or socioeconomic factors that plague observational epidemiological studies. Also 'reverse causation' (the disease inducing the exposure rather than the exposure inducing the disease) would be excluded by MR.

An interesting example of MR concerns dairy products, lactase and prostate cancer. It has been suggested that the intake of milk could increase the risk of prostate cancer. In an international ecological study in 42 countries, Ganmaa *et al.* (2002) found a strong correlation between milk intake and the incidence of prostate cancer ($r = 0.71$). Analytical studies are overall positive, with odds ratios in the order of 1.6–5.1 in both case–control and cohort studies (Chan *et al.* 1998). The mechanism which is hypothesized is the inhibitory effect of calcium on the conversion of 25 (OH) vitamin D to 1,25 (OH)2 vitamin D. The latter has an antiproliferation effect in human prostate cells (Skowronski *et al.* 1993). Also, a protective effect of ultraviolet radiation on prostate cancer has been suggested and is consistent with this proposed mechanism (Hanchette & Schwartz 1992). However, milk intake is subject to considerable measurement error and the association with prostate cancer could be due to confounders such as dietary habits or exposures/behaviours associated with social class.

If it can be shown that a genetic variant (e.g. related to lactase persistence) that affects milk intake is associated with prostate cancer, this will be indirect but unconfounded evidence on the role of milk in prostate carcinogenesis. The autosomal lactase gene (LTC) presents a two allele T and C polymorphism and lends itself to this exercise as it controls the lactose metabolizing lactase enzyme and its persistence or non-persistence in adults. In a study on the geographic distribution of allele frequencies for the lactase gene (Sacerdote *et al.* 2007) it was hypothesized: (a) a north-to-south gradient for the T allele frequency for LTC in Italy, based on previous observations of such a gradient in Europe; (b) a lower intake of milk (but not yoghurt or cheese, in which lactose is hydrolysed) among carriers of the CC genotype for LTC. Overall, the LTC gene T allele frequency was around 21 per cent in Northern Italy and 9 per cent in Southern Italy, i.e. much lower than in Northern Europe (80 per cent in the UK). Food intake was associated with gene variants. A statistically significant association was evident for ice-cream and LTC variants ($P = 0.004$), less so for milk intake. The next step will be to examine the association between lactase and prostate cancer. If an association between the T allele and cancer will be found, then the 'MR triangle' will have been completed, i.e. it will be reasonable to infer that the involvement of milk in prostate cancer aetiology is real and not confounded, or biased because of inaccurate measurement. The concept of 'MR triangle' refers to the fact that the strategy implies looking at the association between: (a) exposure and disease (usually the first to be investigated and found), (b) exposure or its metabolites and gene variants and (c) gene variants and disease.

Like for any method there are, however, limitations with this approach, whose real relevance will become clearer as the method becomes applied in different circumstances. The Achilles heel of MR is probably the fact that many genes are pleiotropic, i.e. have multiple effects: Hence an association gene variant-disease may occur not via the path involving the exposure of interest but via one of the other gene-dependent paths. Confounding thrown out

by the door using MR would reenter by the window through pleiotropy. The opposite case of no association found between the gene variant and the disease would also be open to several possibilities: (a) the relationship between exposure and disease was in fact confounded or biased; (b) the phenotype is only partially related to the tested allele, and other haplotypes/gene variants are also involved; (c) penetrance/expression of the gene depends on circumstances, including for example diet (as the example of CYP2D6 in Ethiopians suggests); (d) the power of the study could be too limited to show an association.

Public health applications and perspectives

A number of potential public health applications flowing from the investigation of gene–environment interactions may be imagined, the common element of which is by definition the identification of subjects carrying different gene variants through genetic testing within families already known to be at high risk of disease or genetic screening in the general population The former is well established within clinical genetics (though the new developments may pose new specific problems) while the latter opens perspectives worth discussion.

Preventing disease in high-risk subjects: Rose's framework for prevention

A theoretical and practical discussion took place several years ago about the selection of high-risk subjects groups for the implementation of preventive measures. Particularly important in this discussion was Geoffrey Rose's setting out the main advantages and disadvantages of such a 'high-risk group' preventive strategy. The strategy presents two main advantages:

♦ It produces interventions that are appropriate to the particular individuals identified and consequently has the potential advantage of enhanced subject motivation in complying with the intervention requirements (e.g. changing diet, taking a drug, etc.)

♦ It offers in principle a more cost-effective use of limited resources and a more favourable ratio of benefits to risks.

However the 'high-risk' strategy has some serious disadvantages and limitations. First, as in all screening, it may meet problems with compliance, with a tendency for the response to be greatest amongst those who are often least at risk of the disease (this, however, is unlikely to apply for genetic screening). A second disadvantage is that this strategy is palliative and temporary. It does not seek 'to alter the underlying causes of the disease but rather to identify individuals who are particularly susceptible to those causes' (Rose 1985). There is another, third, related and more crucial reason why the predictive basis of the 'high-risk' strategy of prevention could be weak, as well illustrated, for example, by the case of breast cancer in relation to parity and other reproductive factors. Women at the highest risk for these factors generate a relatively small proportion of the cases, too few to justify pre-screening for the identification of high-risk women to whom to offer mammography. The lesson from this and numerous other examples is that *a large number of people at a small risk may give rise to more cases of disease than the small number who are at a high risk*. To the extent that this situation is common—as it appears to be—it limits the utility of the 'high-risk' approach to prevention, and is certainly relevant to the issue of screening for 'low-penetrant' gene variants. How far it is relevant needs some closer consideration, through specific examples, as Rose's concepts were formulated when the field of gene–environment interactions and susceptibility due to low-penetrance genes was in its infancy, at least for major chronic diseases.

Screening for genetic susceptibility: Number needed to screen and treat

To assess the role of a gene–environment interaction and screening in a population knowledge of the penetrance of the genetic trait (variant allele) and of its frequency is needed. Penetrance is expressed by the absolute risk of disease among individuals carrying the gene variant. So, high penetrance means high individual risk, which tends to be a feature of rarer gene variants or mutations. A useful measure for assessing the utility of an intervention is to estimate the number needed to treat (NNT) to prevent an event, which is equal to the inverse of the absolute risk reduction (Vineis *et al.* 2001). If screening is applied before intervening, NNT and frequency may be combined to compute the number needed to screen (NNS) to prevent one case of, say, cancer. The NNS in high-risk families for a high-penetrant gene (BRCA1) of breast cancer has been calculated (the expression 'genetic testing' rather than 'genetic screening' would be more appropriate in this situation). The cumulative (lifetime) risk of breast cancer was found as high as 80 per cent in some studies and in some populations among mutation carriers (in high-risk families) and the frequency of mutations in high-risk families is about 50 per cent. Based on results from randomized trials it can be assumed that tamoxifen or raloxifene halve this risk. In this situation it can be calculated that one needs to treat 2.5 (i.e. $1/[0.8 \times 0.5]$) mutation carriers and test 5 (i.e. $1/[0.8 \times 0.5 \times 0.5]$) family members to prevent one cancer. If instead the general population would be screened the NNS would change greatly. In the general population, however, the cumulative risk in carriers of mutations that do not all confer the same very high risk, turns out to be lower than 80 per cent and in the order of 40 per cent: This implies, with tamoxifene or raloxifene halving it, an absolute risk reduction of 20 per cent and a number needed to treat of five mutation carriers. However, since only 0.2 per cent of the general population are mutation carriers, the NNS is 2500 to prevent one cancer. One might discuss whether this substantial NNS (which even with a highly specific test may involve a number of false-positives) would make BRCA1 a realistic target for screening in the general population. However, with dwindling cost and ease of high throughput genotyping technology this calculus may change in future, at least among certain populations known to be at higher risk of carrying mutations.

Calculations along similar lines have been considered for low-penetrance genes (Vineis *et al.* 2001). For example, in the occupational context workers exposed to polycyclic aromatic hydrocarbons (PAHs) might hypothetically be screened for the null variant of the GSTM1 gene, which through a deficit of detoxification of the PAHs may entail an increased risk, of the order of 30 per cent, of lung cancer. Through screening subjects found to have the null genotype can be excluded from jobs that expose them to PAHs (maybe not hiring them at all). From a prevention viewpoint there is, however, a basic though subtle difference of this scenario in respect to the just mentioned case of BRCA1. In the latter the aim is to identify women who test positive and are at (much) higher risk of breast cancer than other women in order to offer them intensive treatment (e.g. continuous surveillance plus mastectomy when it

becomes necessary); no demonstrable benefit would follow instead by the same treatment (unless universal prophylactic mastectomy would be adopted) for women testing negative. In contrast, in the workplace scenario the treatment would be radical—no exposure at all to PAHs—for those testing positive, while workers testing negative, who could also obviously benefit from the same measure (or in any case from a reduction in exposure) would not receive the treatment and be left at risk. In this situation a comparison of different preventive strategies simply in terms of NNT and NNS is not adequate and needs to be expanded taking into account costs, direct and indirect, tangible and intangible.

For example in a simulation study, Bartell and colleagues showed that genetic screening for chronic beryllium disease with HLA-DPB1*0201 may give health benefits that outweighed financial costs only if avoidance of one case of the disease is valued at US$1 million or higher in a US context (Bartell *et al.* 2000). Yet, their estimate of the predictive value of the screening might have been unrealistically high and might not have correctly weighed the harmful effects of false-positive results.

Screening for genetic susceptibility to environmental exposure to arsenic

Arsenic is an exposure that is important both for industrial workers and for the general population in wide areas of the world. The identification of high-risk groups could in principle be extremely useful to overcome the practical difficulties and the costs of primary prevention in affected populations.

Chronic exposure to arsenic is known to cause non-melanocytic skin and internal tumours in humans. Exposure to arsenic commonly occurs in occupational and environmental settings. Although occupational exposure to arsenic occurs in a variety of industrial settings the predominant source of arsenic exposure for more than 100 million people worldwide, including nearly 70 million in Bangladesh and the adjoining part of India, has been from contaminated drinking water (Rahman *et al.* 2001). Given the magnitude of the problem, which the WHO labelled as the largest mass poisoning in human history, the issue of risk reduction of arsenic-induced health problems has become an important research and policy topic. Since millions of people already accrued chronic exposure, and their risk of cancer has increased several fold, measures of secondary and even tertiary prevention also become pertinent in addition to primary prevention. The ability to isolate 'high-risk' groups would contribute enormously to the development of an effective preventive strategy. For this reason the knowledge of mechanisms of arsenic carcinogenesis can help. Several studies have examined the role of oxidative stress and DNA repair genes on the susceptibility to arsenic carcinogenicity as expressed by premalignant skin lesions. In these studies, carriers of certain polymorphisms in oxidative stress genes of myeloperoxidase (MPO) and catalase (CAT) as well as in the DNA repair gene xeroderma pigmentosum complementation group D (XPD) have been shown to have a 3 to 11-fold higher risk of premalignant skin lesions than the non-carriers (Ahsan *et al.* 2003).

Arsenic has a dose-dependent effect on skin and internal tumours. The risk of cancer among arsenic exposed population is ~1 per cent but the risk for premalignant skin lesions is much higher, up to more than 10 per cent, depending on the dose and duration of exposure.

Let us make an extreme assumption, i.e. the relative risk for premalignant lesions is 11, the highest estimate in literature, and that the cumulative risk of such lesions is 10 per cent in subjects with wildtype (normal) polymorphisms. Also assume two kinds of interventions: (a) one that leads to a 50 per cent decrease in the risk of skin lesions, and (b) one leading to a 100 per cent decrease. (These assumptions, useful for the sake of the example, are probably too extreme and unrealistic, since a relative risk of 11 is more compatible with a high-penetrant gene than with a low-penetrant gene.) As the calculations in Table 9.1.2 show: (a) if an intervention is implemented (improving the quality of water) that reduces the risk of premalignant lesions by 50 per cent, 20 subjects with wildtype genotype need to be 'treated' (NNT) to prevent one lesion, given that the cumulative risk of lesions is 10 per cent for the wildtype; (b) if the intervention is 100 per cent effective, then the NNT is 10, i.e. for every 10 treated persons (wildtype) one case is prevented. If screening for a gene variant that multiplies the risk of skin lesions by 11 (entailing a cumulative risk close to 100 per cent) is applied and a preventive intervention 50 per cent effective, the NNT is 2 for subjects testing positive, i.e. for every two persons screened and found positive one is 'saved'. However, in order to identify the subjects with the variant gene one needs to actually screen the population: With a prevalence of 20 per cent of the variant, the NNS is 10 for an intervention with 50 per cent efficacy and 5 with an intervention of 100 per cent. In the absence of screening, the NNT in the total population is the weighted mean of the NNT among subjects testing negative and subjects testing positive: 16.4 for 50 per cent efficacy and 8.2 for 100 per cent efficacy of the preventive effort. Hence even with (unrealistically) extreme assumptions the screening strategy would entail, with a 50 per cent effective intervention, screening 10 people and treating 2 to prevent one premalignant lesion to be contrasted with treating 16.4 without the screening: These comparative figures (and the same applies for those for a 100 per cent effective intervention) offer no support for the screening strategy unless the costs of screening and targeted

intervention on the subjects testing positive would be orders of magnitude inferior to the intervention for everybody, i.e. general improvement of the water quality entailing a substantial reduction of exposure to arsenic.

In this particular example if a high-risk strategy would be considered as an option, rather than genetic screening (because of uncertainties in NNT and NNS), identification of the at-risk population through screening for arsenic exposure of the population by testing drinking water and biological samples (urine, hair or nail) for arsenic would be more practical. Since the distribution of arsenic exposure is somewhat less individual-specific (unlike genetic polymorphisms), instead of genetically tailored individual-level interventions household-level interventions (provision of safe wells) may turn out to be more promising. For many arsenic affected areas where 50–90 per cent of the population are exposed (e.g. in Bangladesh, West Bengal, India, inner Mongolia, and certain provinces of China) several community-level interventions (e.g. community wells, supply water, and, in addition, food fortification with antioxidants or other anti-arsenic nutrients) are warranted. Needless to say, provision of good-quality water, a primary good, entails also a number of other benefits for the population.

Screening for subjects claimed to be genetically susceptible: The NicoTest

A recent example illustrates how weakly supported findings might translate into shaky 'predictive medicine' under the pressure of commercial interests. In 2004, a private firm from Oxford (G-Nostics) put on the market a kit for the identification of the carriers of a genetic variant of the gene DRD2, involved in the syndrome of nicotine addiction. The carriers of the variant would be more susceptible to developing addiction, but also to responding to a treatment with nicotine patches, and then should be treated as really 'sick' people. There were some observations from studies of the DRD2 gene that genetic variants related to relatively decreased dopaminergic tone in the mesocorticolimbic system are associated with increased risk for relapse to smoking following a cessation attempt. The offer of the test was, however, mainly based on the results of a randomized experiment, the most persuasive type of clinical investigation. Overall 1532 heavy smokers had been randomly allocated to two arms, the first receiving the nicotine patch, and the second other types of anti-smoking treatments. Subsequently (after 8–10 years), 755 (49.3 per cent) of these subjects agreed to donate a blood sample for genetic determinations. At this point, the researchers noted that those who quit smoking with the use of a patch were predominantly subjects with the genetic variant of DRD2, who came to be regarded as the best target for this kind of dissuasion intervention. The difference between carriers of the variant and 'normal' subjects was strong (a proportion of quitting two–three times higher) and statistically significant. However, the effectiveness of the dissuasion intervention, i.e. quitting smoking, was evaluated at short time (between 1 and 12 weeks) (Johnstone et al. 2004), while it is well known that relapses occur in a substantial proportion within the first 6–12 months. Also, in two other randomized trials, carried out in two culturally very diverse populations (African Americans and Japanese) (McBride et al. 2002; Hamajima et al. 2004), knowledge of genotype did not influence the success rate of smoking cessation.

It is worth noting the potential problems and the slippery slope that could be created on the basis of premature introduction into

Table 9.1.2 Calculation of the number needed to screen for a hypothetical highly penetrant gene among subjects exposed to arsenic. Two assumptions are made, that the preventive intervention has 50% (a) or 100% (b) efficacy (from Vineis et al.).

	Gene			
	Wildtype		Variant	
	(a)	(b)	(a)	(b)
Relative risk for gene	1.0	1.0	11	11
Cumulative risk of premalignant lesions (%)	10	10	100	100
Risk reduction (%)	50	100	50	100
Cumulative risk after intervention (%)	5	0	50	0
Absolute risk reduction (%)	5	10	50	100
NNT	20	10	2	1
Carrier frequency (%)	80	80	20	20
NNS	25	12.5	10	5
NNT in the absence of screening	16.4	8.2		

practice, based on wholly inadequate evidence, of a test like the NicoTest (incidentally, the DRD2 genotype seems of relevance also to the propensity to develop obesity) (Morton *et al.* 2006). It is not far-fetched to imagine that there might be a category of people who, being told that they have a greater genetic resistance to the effectiveness of the nicotine patch and other anti-smoking devices, will end up with thinking they have no hope of quitting; other people might instead wrongly come to think that, based on their genetic make-up, they are generally protected from the effects of smoking and for the same reason may not give up. A worrying scenario would develop if this type of testing based on flimsy evidence would extend to other characteristics, for example the propensity to develop obesity or antisocial behaviours. An approach that is typical of clinical medicine (pharmacogenetics) would be automatically extended to behaviours like smoking, thus suggesting that these complex behaviours simply belong to the category of 'disease'. Addictions and behaviours that are hazardous to health, and even antisocial, arise from an interaction between the environment and individual susceptibility, including the genetic form. The two aspects cannot be simplistically disentangled, and to dissociate them may lead to a dangerous slippery slope including: A stigma towards minorities (for carriers of the susceptibility genes); increasing conflicts around the eligibility for insurance of carriers of such genes; a widespread climate of irresponsibility, since the fault for diseases and behaviours is attributed to genes; and the diffusion of a model of causality more and more influenced by hard natural sciences rather than social and political determinants of the most significant events in people's lives.

Ethical issues (Vineis *et al.* 2005)

Screening for low-penetrant genes also raises a number of important ethical and social issues which need to be considered in any decision about implementation. The following analysis of arguments for and against such screening is centred on workers but similar considerations apply to environmentally exposed populations.

Arguments in favour of the availability of genetics testing in the workplace

The use of genetic screening in employment is hardly objectionable when it aims at directly protecting a wider 'public interest', i.e. public safety. An example might be screening those who are to be responsible for flying planes or working in air traffic control for mutations conferring a low risk of fatal cardiac arrhythmia on the rationale that whilst unlikely, the occurrence of such failure would have serious implications for public safety.

Apart from such cases there are some ethical arguments which have been put forward in favour of the use, or at least the availability, of genetic screening of workers. Perhaps the strongest of these draws its strength from a long-standing belief that employers and indeed legislators, have a duty, where this is possible, to protect employees, particularly those who are vulnerable, from avoidable risks in the workplace. Duties of this kind have been stressed in employment legislation in the United Kingdom and many other countries for well over a century; e.g., in the Factory Act 1851 (outlawing child labour under the age of 8) and the Mines Act 1842 (outlawing women, girls, and boys under 10 working in mines).

If employers have a duty of care for their employees it follows that when a test or screen is known to be effective, employers have

an obligation to use it to improve the safety of workers and potential workers. This may also imply that where such tests or screens do exist, but are not used, the employers may be vulnerable to legal challenge. Indeed such a case has recently occurred in the United States where the Dow Chemical Company was sued by the widow of a deceased employee for failing to include the employee in a cytogenetic testing programme which might have detected his development of leukaemia from exposure in the workplace to benzene at an early stage (Brandt-Rauf & Brandt-Rauf 2004).

A second set of ethical arguments in favour of the availability of screening or testing arises from the broad duty of respect for freedom of choice, i.e. autonomy. It could be argued that making an informative test available, either commercially or in the workplace, would enable workers to make informed choices about the kinds of jobs they take—about whether or where to work. In at least one legal jurisdiction this right has been established legally. In the case of *International Union UAW v Johnson Controls Inc.*, it was decided that the choice of whether or not to work in a hazardous environment—while pregnant in this case—was reserved for workers to make themselves and was not for their potential employers to decide (Desmond & Gardner-Hopkins 2001). Freedom of choice arguments claim that to deny workers access to informative tests is unacceptably paternalistic. On the other side, the concern has been raised that creating a situation in which workers are free to use tests but employers are not would lead to 'adverse selection' (Human Genetics Commission 2002), i.e. employees who know about their risks (while employers, and insurers, do not) may use this asymmetry to their advantage. This may be particularly relevant in contexts, such as the United States, where healthcare insurance is related to employment. As a consequence, 'genetic transparency' has been advocated, where both parties should have access to such information (Diver & Cohen 2001).

A third argument for the use of genetic screening in the workplace might be that this has the potential to bring about important economic advantages through increased safety and reduced healthcare costs. Again, this might be of particular relevance to companies operating in a country such as the United States where health insurance is tied to employment. But, taking economic advantage in the broader sense, such an argument might also be made in the context of countries with publicly funded healthcare (Vineis *et al.* 2005, p. 139).

Arguments against the use of genetic testing in the workplace

Despite the arguments put forward for the availability and use of genetic screening in the workplace under certain conditions, there are a number of important arguments against it which provide grounds for concern and extreme caution should such screening be contemplated for implementation.

The first and strongest argument against the use of genetic testing in employment is that it carries the potential to lead to increased discrimination. There is indeed, good evidence that this is already happening. Recently, for example, the US Equal Employment Opportunity Commission filed suit against the Burlington Northern Santa Fe Railroad Co. for defying the 'Americans with Disability' Act (case settled in 2002 for US$2.2 million) on the grounds that the company required employees to submit blood samples to test them for genes predisposing to the carpal tunnel syndrome. It was also argued, successfully, that the company failed to obtain adequate informed consent and in some cases threatened employees with dismissal for failing to comply (Vineis *et al.* 2005, p. 139). This is one amongst many examples of such discrimination (p. 146).

Discrimination might also arise out of the *selective* use of genetic screening. For example, if there is a shortage of people willing to work in a particularly dangerous process, testing may be withheld for economic reasons in order to maintain a needed workforce.

In general, arguments about discrimination arise out of concern that genetic screening in employment may lead to a situation in which a person's genetic make-up determines work opportunities (Davis 2004): Individuals who test 'positive' may as a result become less employable, less insurable, and vulnerable in a number of different and important respects. Such concerns do not arise solely out of the nature of genetics or of genetic information but also out of the social and political realities of the world in which people live and work. Arguments about freedom of choice, for example, may sound attractive in the abstract, but policies based on freedom of choice divorced from an awareness of the broader social context have the potential to favour the wealthy, the highly educated, and the 'genetically normal'. Not everyone, for example, has the choice about where to work: Lack of skills, lack of mobility, living in an area of high unemployment, may make it impossible for those who are rejected from local employment to find a job elsewhere.

Second, in addition to its potential to lead to increased discrimination, the use of genetic screening in the workplace may lead to an increased likelihood of invasion of privacy and confidentiality of workers, for example in the writing of references or the provision of information for the purposes of insurance. Moreover, the standards of security and confidentiality in relation to the use of genetic information and samples may be less rigorously monitored in the context of employment than in, for example, medical research. Indeed, examples already exist of samples being tested for outcomes other than that for which they were taken. For example, in the case of *Norman-Bloodsaw v Lawrence Berkeley Laboratory employees* provided blood and urine samples for cholesterol testing but in fact some of these samples were subsequently tested for syphilis, pregnancy and sickle-cell trait (Michie *et al.* 2003).

A third set of arguments against the use of genetic screening for low-penetrant genes in the workplace arises out of concerns that the information provided by such tests is likely to be extremely difficult to interpret and/or to communicate. To begin with there is the question about the extent to which such testing is likely to produce information of any real value for use in the workplace. In addition the question arises of how risk information, particularly in the case of low-penetrant genes associated with a mild increase in disease risk, is to be communicated to employers and to employees in a way that is understandable or usable. Finally there is a good deal of evidence that even in the case of single gene disorders where the mode of inheritance and risk are, by comparison, clear, those tested have a tendency to misunderstand the implications of test results, especially when these are negative.

The fourth and final set of arguments against the use of genetic screening in the workplace is that it may easily become a diversion from the responsibility of employers and legislators to ensure that the working environment is safe for all of those who work there. Instead of using resources to identify workers who may be genetically at lesser risk, the focus should be on finding ways to make the workplace safe for all. Of course, quite similar arguments apply to environmentally exposed populations, with the added proviso that these include subjects often particularly vulnerable, like children, very old people, or pregnant women.

Conclusion

At present, knowledge of gene–environment interactions and of genetic susceptibility to disease in presence of environmental exposures does not support the view that screening for genetic variants—especially of low-penetrance genes—in order to identify subjects and subgroups at higher risk in the general population may be a practical and useful (or ethically recommendable) prevention strategy. Research in this area, however, is undergoing an extremely fast evolution and a reassessment of the evidence at short intervals is necessary.

Acknowledgements

This work was made possible by a grant to ECNIS (Environmental Cancer Risk, Nutrition and Individual Susceptibility), a network of excellence operating within the European Union 6th Framework Program, Priority 5: 'Food Quality and Safety' (Contract No 513943). We wish to acknowledge Sarah Teague, Michael Parker, and Habibul Ahsan for thoughtful contributions.

References

Abbeduto L., Brady N., Kover S.T. (2007) Language development and fragile X syndrome: profiles, syndrome-specificity, and within-syndrome differences. *Mental Retardation and Development Disabilities Research Review*, 13, 36–46.

Aguilar C.A., Talavera G., Ordovas J.M. *et al.* (1999). The apolipoprotien E4 allele in not associated with an abnormal lipid profile in a Native American population following its traditional lifestyle. *Atherosclerosis*, 142, 409–14.

Ahsan H., Chen Y., Wang C. *et al.* (2003) DNA repair gene XPD and susceptibility to arsenic-induced hyperkeratosis. *Toxicology Letters*, 143, 123–31.

Aklillu E., Herrlin K., Gustafsson L.L. *et al.* (2002) Evidence for environmental influence on CYP2D6-catalysed debrisoquine hydroxylation as demonstrated by phenotyping and genotyping of Ethiopians living in Ethiopia or in Sweden. *Pharmacogenetics*, 12, 375–83.

Armstrong B.K., White E., and Saracci R. (1994) *Principles of exposure measurement in epidemiology*. 2nd edition. Oxford University Press, Oxford.

Bartell S.M., Ponce R.A., Takaro T.K. *et al.* (2000) Risk estimation and value-of-information analysis for three proposed genetic screening programs for chronic beryllium disease prevention. *Risk Analysis*, 20, 87–99.

Block N. (1995) How heritability misleads about race. *Cognition*, 56, 99–128.

Booth F.W., Chakravarthy M.V., and Spanenberg E.E. (2002) Exercise and gene expression: physiological regulation of the human genome through physical activity. *Journal of Physiology*, 543, 399–411.

Borén T., Falk P., Roth K.A. *et al.* (1993). Attachment of *Helicobacter pylori* to human gastric epithelium mediated by blood group antigens. *Science*, 262, 1892–5.

Brandt-Rauf P.W. and Brandt-Rauf S.I. (2004) Genetic testing in the workplace: ethical, legal and social implications. *Annual Review of Public Health*, 25, 139–53.

Bray M.S. (2000) Genomics, genes, and environmental interaction: the role of exercise. *Journal of Applied Physiology*, 88, 788–92.

Chan J.M., Giovannucci E., Andersson S.O. *et al.* (1998) Dairy products, calcium, phosphorous, vitamin D, and risk of prostate cancer (Sweden). *Cancer Causes & Control*, 9, 559–66.

Clayton D. and McKeigue P.M. (2001) Epidemiological methods for studying genes and environmental factors in complex diseases. *Lancet*, **358**, 1356–60.

Davey Smith G. and Ebrahim S. (2003) 'Mendelian randomization': can genetic epidemiology contribute to understanding environmental determinants of disease? *International Journal of Epidemiology*, **32**, 1–22.

Davis D.S. (2004) Genetic research and communal narratives. *Hastings Center Report*, **34**, 40–9.

Desmond J. and Gardner-Hopkins J.D. (2001) Unemployable genes: genetic discrimination in the workplace. *Auckland University Law Review*, **9**, 435–68.

Diver C.S. and Cohen J.M. (2001) Genephobia: what is wrong with genetic discrimination? *University PA Law Review*, **149**, 1439–82.

Ford E.S., Giles W.H., and Dietz W.H. (2002) Prevalence of the metabolic syndrome among US adults: findings from the Third National Health and Nutrition Examination Survey. *JAMA*, **287**, 356–9.

Fox Keller E. (2000) *The century of the gene*. Harvard University Press, Cambridge, MA.

Ganmaa D., Li X.M., Wang J. *et al.* (2002) Incidence of testicular and prostate cancers in relation to world dietary practices. *International Journal of Cancer*, **98**, 262–7.

Greenlund K.J., Valdez R., Casper M.L. *et al.* (1999) Prevalence and correlates of the insulin resistance syndrome among Native Americans. The Inter-Tribal Heart Project. *Diabetes Care*, **22**, 441–7.

Hamajima N., Atsuta Y., Goto Y. *et al.* (2004) A pilot study on genotype announcement to induce smoking cessation by Japanese smokers. *Asian Pacific Journal for Cancer Prevention*, **5**, 409–13.

Hanchette C.L. and Schwartz G.G. (1992) Geographic patterns of prostate cancer mortality. Evidence for a protective effect of ultraviolet radiation. *Cancer*, **70**, 2861–9.

Harris H. (1959) *Human biochemical genetics*. Cambridge University Press, Cambridge.

Herrnstein R.J. and Murray C. (1994) *The Bell Curve: Reshaping of American Life by Differences in Intelligence*. Simon and Schuster, New York.

Hood V.L., Kelly B., Martinez C. *et al.* (1997) A Native American community initiative to prevent diabetes. *Ethnicity & Health*, **2**, 277–85.

Human Genetics Commission. (2002) Inside Information: balancing interests in the use of personal genetic data. (Accessed on 1 July 2008 on: www.hgc.gov.uk)

Hunter D.J. and Kraft P. (2007) Drinking from the fire hose – statistical issues in genomewide association studies. *New England Journal of Medicine*, **357**, 436–9.

Isomaa B. (2003) A major health hazard: the metabolic syndrome. *Life Sciences*, **73**, 2395–411.

Johnstone E.C., Yudkin P.L., Hey K. *et al.* (2004) Genetic variation in dopaminergic pathways and short-term effectiveness of the nicotine patch. *Pharmacogenetics*, **14**, 83–90.

Kataoka S., Robbins D.C., Cowan L.D. *et al.* (1996) Apolipoprotein E polymorphism in American Indians and its relation to plasma lipoproteins and diabetes. The Strong Heart Study. *Arteriosclerosis, Thrombosis & Vascular Biology*, **16**, 918–25.

Knowler W.C., Williams R.C., Pettitt D.J. *et al.* (1988) Gm3;5,13,14 and type 2 diabetes mellitus: an association in American Indians with genetic admixture. *American Journal of Human Genetics*, **43**, 520–6.

Lewontin R. (1972) The analysis of variance and the analysis of causes. *American Journal of Human Genetics*, **26**, 400–11.

Lower G.M., Jr, Nilsson T., Nelson C.E. *et al.* (2007). N-acetyltransferase phenotype and risk in urinary bladder cancer: approaches in molecular epidemiology. Preliminary results in Sweden and Denmark. *International Journal of Epidemiology*, **36**, 11–17.

McBride C.M., Bepler G., Lipkus I.M. *et al.* (2002) Incorporating genetic susceptibility feedback into a smoking cessation program for African-American smokers with low income. *Cancer Epidemiology Biomarkers & Prevention*, **11**, 521–8.

McKusick V.A. (1998) *Mendelian inheritance in man*, 12th edn. Johns Hopkins University Press, Baltimore.

Michie S., Smith J.A., Senior V. *et al.* (2003) Understanding why negative genetic test results sometimes fail to reassure. *American Journal of Medical Genetics*, **119**, 340–7.

Morton L.M., Wang S.S., Bergen A.W. *et al.* (2006) DRD2 genetic variation in relation to smoking and obesity in the Prostate, Lung, Colorectal, and Ovarian Cancer Screening Trial. *Pharmacogenetics and Genomics*, **16**, 901–10.

Muneta B., Newman J., Wetterall S. *et al.* (1993) Diabetes and associated risk factors among Native Americans. *Diabetes Care*, **16**, 1619–20.

Nagi D.K., Foy C.A., Mohamed-Ali V. *et al.* (1998) Angiotensin-1-converting enzyme (ACE) gene polymorphism, plasma ACE levels, and their association with the metabolic syndrome and electrocardiographic coronary artery disease in Pima Indians. *Metabolism*, **47**, 622–6.

Olson S. (2002) *Mapping human history: unravelling the mystery of Adam and Eve*. Bloomsbury Publishing, London.

Ottman R. (1996) Gene-environment interaction: definitions and study designs. *Preventive Medicine*, **25**, 764–70.

Penagarikano O., Mulle J.G., Warren S.T. (2007) The pathophysiology of fragile X syndrome. *Annual Review of Genomics and Human Genetics*. May 3, **8**, 109–29.

Rahman M.M., Chowdhury U.K., Mukherjee S.C. (2001) Chronic arsenic toxicity in Bangladesh and West Bengal, India--a review and commentary. *Journal of Toxicology and Clinical Toxicology*, **39**, 683–700.

Reilly M.P. and Rader D.J. (2003) The metabolic syndrome: more than the sum of its parts? *Circulation*, **108**, 1546–51.

Resnick H. (2002) Metabolic Syndrome in American Indians. *Diabetes Care*, **25**, 1246–7.

Rose G. (1985) Sick individuals and sick populations. *International Journal of Epidemiology*, **14**, 32–8.

Sacerdote C., Guarrera S., Smith G.D. *et al.* (2007) Lactase persistence and bitter taste response: instrumental variables and Mendelian randomization in epidemiologic studies of dietary factors and cancer risk. *American Journal of Epidemiology*, **166**, 576–81.

Saracci R. (1980) Interaction and synergism. *American Journal of Epidemiology*, **112**, 465–6.

Skowronski R.J., Peehl D.M., and Feldman D. (1993) Vitamin D and prostate cancer: 1,25 dihydroxyvitamin D3 receptors and actions in human prostate cancer cell lines. *Endocrinology*, **132**, 1952–60.

The Wellcome Trust Case Control Consortium. (2007). Genome-wide association study of 14,000 cases of seven common diseases and 3,000 shared controls. *Nature*, **447**, 661–84.

Thomas D.C. (2004) *Statistical Methods in Genetic Epidemiology*. Oxford University Press, New York.

Thomas D.C. and Clayton D. (2004) Betting odds and genetic associations. *JNCI*, **96**, 421–3.

Thompson D.B., Ravussin E., Bennet P.H. *et al.* (1997). Structure and sequence variation at the human leptin receptor gene in lean and obese Pima Indians. *Human Molecular Genetics*, **6**, 675–9.

Tschermak E. (1950). Concerning artificial crossing in 'Pisum Sativum'. *Genetics*, **35**, 42–7 (translation of the original 1900 publication in German).

Vineis P. (2007). Commentary: First steps in molecular epidemiology: Lower *et al.* 1979. *International Journal of Epidemiology*, **36**, 20–22.

Vineis P., Ahsan H., Parker M. (2005) Genetic screening and occupational and environmental exposures. *Occupational and Environmental Medicine*, **62**, 657–62.

Vineis P., Schulte P., and McMichael A.J. (2001) Misconceptions about the use of genetic tests in populations. *Lancet*, **357**, 709–12.

Vozarova B., Fernandez-Real J.M., Knowler W.C. *et al.* (2003). The interleukin-6 (-174) G/C promoter polymorphism is associated with type-2 diabetes mellitus in Native Americans and Caucasians. *Human Genetics*, **112**, 409–413.

Wacholder S., Chanock S., Garcia-Closas M. *et al.* (2004) Assessing the probability that a positive report is false: an approach for molecular epidemiology studies. *JNCI*, **96**, 434–42.

Wendorf M. (1989) Diabetes, the ice free corridor, and the Paleoindian settlement of North America. *American Journal of Physical Anthropology*, **79**, 503–20.

Witte J.S. (2007) Multiple prostate cancer risk variants on 8q24. *Nature Genetics*, **39**, 579–80.

Yang Q. and Khoury M.J. (1997) Evolving methods in genetic epidemiology. III. Gene-environment interaction in epidemiologic research. *Epidemiological Review*, **19**, 33–43.

Zanke B.W., Greenwood C.M., Rangrej J. *et al.* (2007). Genome-wide association scan identifies a colorectal cancer susceptibility locus on chromosome 8q24. *Nature Genetics*, **39**, 989–94.

Zimmet P. and Thomas C.R. (2003) Genotype, obesity and cardiovascular disease—has technical advancement outstripped evolution? *Journal of Internal Medicine*, **254**, 114–25.

Cardiovascular and cerebrovascular diseases

Russell V. Luepker and Kamakshi Lakshminarayan

Abstract

Cardiovascular diseases, conditions of the heart and blood vessels, are leading causes of morbidity and mortality throughout the world. Largely diseases of lifestyle and affluence, they account for a majority of deaths in some industrialized countries. They are a coming epidemic in the developing world as communities and individuals attain richer and less healthy lifestyles. The leading cardiovascular diseases are coronary heart disease, hypertension, stroke, and heart failure. They are frequently interconnected with the underlying pathology atherosclerosis, a condition damaging medium and large arteries. There are also other important diseases which, while less common, present considerable health burden including rheumatic heart disease, peripheral artery disease, cardiomyopathy, and congenital heart disease.

Unlike many lifestyle related conditions, the causes or risk factors for the leading cardiovascular diseases are well known. They are diet resulting in hyperlipidemia, elevated blood pressure leading to hypertension, diabetes mellitus, physical inactivity, and cigarette smoking. There are also other identified characteristics but this group of risk factors underlies the epidemic. As well studied conditions, much is known about the pathophysiology of risk factors and cardiovascular disease. In addition, knowledge from clinical trials dictates treatment of risk for primary and secondary prevention. Few chronic diseases had such an extensive scientific basis for the prevention and treatment. Prevention starts at the community level where unhealthy diets, smoking and physical inactivity can be confronted and reduced. Clinical presentations of individual risk factors such as hypertension, hyperlipidemia and diabetes mellitus can be treated with lifestyle modification and/or medication. The implementation of prevention programmes at the community and clinic level results in population-wide changes and disease reduction. The potential for continuing improvement in the industrialized world and blunting the epidemic in the developing world is substantial.

Introduction

Cardiovascular and cerebrovascular diseases are the leading causes of death and disability in most industrialized countries and they are increasingly prevalent in the developing world. The principal cardiovascular diseases are related to atherosclerosis: Coronary heart disease, athero-thrombotic stroke, and peripheral vascular disease. Hypertension, haemorrhagic stroke, heart failure, rheumatic heart disease, cardiomyopathy, and congenital heart disease are also common. The patterns on distributions of these diseases vary in different regions; however, coronary heart disease, stroke and heart failure are frequently pre-eminent, leading to widespread population morbidity and mortality.

The rise of the cardiovascular diseases is attributed to a number of factors. The gradual reduction and elimination of infectious disease leading to increased longevity. Cardiovascular diseases are usually chronic conditions mainly affecting older populations. Additionally, atherosclerotic-related diseases are associated with affluent lifestyles. The widespread availability of rich foods leads directly to elevated blood lipids. Surplus food and reduction in habitual physical activity results in obesity, also encouraging hyperlipidaemia, hypertension and diabetes. In countries where affluence is growing, these diseases are found first among the wealthy. However, cardiovascular disease gradually affects all segments of the population as affluent living conditions prevail.

These shifts have led to changing patterns of cardiovascular diseases worldwide. In many industrialized countries, the rates of cardiovascular disease are falling, in others still rising. In most developing countries, the rates are rising associated with greater affluence and reduced infectious diseases.

The rise in cardiovascular and cerebrovascular diseases was a phenomenon of the twentieth century in the industrialized world. It threatens to be the leading cause of death and disability worldwide in the twenty-first century. Public health can and does play a leading role in the prevention of these diseases. Since risk factors for these diseases are identifiable and readily modified in healthy individuals at the population level, the sources of this epidemic can be confronted. The elimination of these diseases is possible and is a major public health challenge for the coming period.

Burden of cardiovascular diseases mortality

Cardiovascular disease is the leading cause of death in many countries and rising in many others. Figure 9.2.1 depicts mortality for cardiovascular disease including stroke, cancer, and all causes in 2002 for men and women combined in selected countries. Cardiovascular diseases account for around 50 per cent of the deaths in many countries (WHO 2007). For example, in the United States,

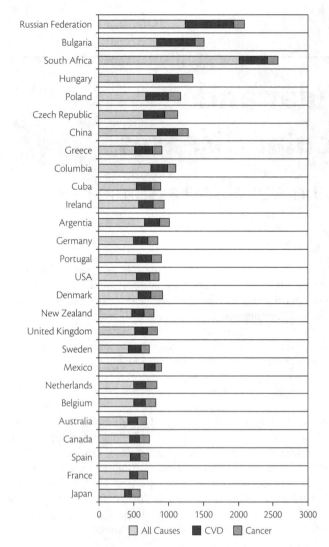

Fig. 9.2.1 Mortality for CVD, cancer, and all causes by selected country, age standardized to WHO population (age 35–74) (Year 2002).

Morbidity

While death is a common outcome of cardiovascular disease, non-fatal disease is also prevalent. As shown in Table 9.2.1, the total population with prevalent cardiovascular disease is estimated to be over 71 million in the United States in 2003 (NHLBI 2006). Hypertension is most common, but there are over 13 million people with coronary heart disease and 5 million with congestive heart failure. Stroke is estimated to include 5.5 million current victims in the population.

The magnitude of this problem is also shown in Fig. 9.2.2, which describes trends in non-fatal and fatal coronary heart disease hospital admissions over time in Southeastern New England in the United States. The rates reflect the age and sex differences in coronary heart disease (Derby *et al.* 2000). More people are surviving previously fatal attacks.

These common diseases now have many high-technology procedures designed to ameliorate the conditions and reduce symptoms. Many can prolong life. These medical procedures and treatments include cardiac surgery, angioplasty, angiography, pacemakers, implanted defibrillators, sophisticated diagnostic testing, and pharmaceuticals. Between the cost of this care and the lost productivity resulting from morbidity and mortality, cardiovascular disease represents an enormous economic burden, as shown in Fig. 9.2.3, for the United States in 2006 (AHA 2007). The total is over US$430 billion.

Disease trends

The epidemic of cardiovascular disease is largely a phenomenon of the twentieth century, and trends within this century are apparent. The Monitoring Trends and Determinants in Cardiovascular Disease (MONICA) study demonstrated that coronary heart disease rose or fell in different nations during the 1980s and 1990s (Tunstall-Pedoe *et al.* 1999). In selected countries, different patterns continue to be observed for coronary heart disease from 1970 to 2005 (Fig. 9.2.4) (NHLBI 2006). A downward trend was noted in the United States with coronary heart disease rates peaking in the mid-1960s and falling substantially since that time (Table 9.2.2) (NHLBI 2006). Stroke peaked earlier, declined slowly and then began a precipitous age-adjusted decline in the 1970s. Non-cardiovascular disease

as in many Western European countries, coronary heart disease accounts for approximately half of the cardiovascular deaths, while stroke and other causes provide the remainder. In Sweden, coronary heart disease and stroke are about equal. In Japan, stroke is more common. In Egypt, infectious cardiac diseases are important causes, however, atherosclerotic diseases are increasing (WHO 2007; AHA 2007). These differences in distributions of cardiovascular disease mortality are associated with different circumstances in those countries and differing methods of classifying death. They also reflect age and sex distributions of the populations, as most cardiovascular diseases are strongly associated with increasing age.

Although rarely appreciated by clinicians, the majority of cardiovascular disease mortality occurs outside of hospitals as 'sudden' death (McGovern *et al.* 1996; Tunstall-Pedoe *et al.* 1996). It may occur at home, in a public place, at work and during ambulance transport. Even those who reach the hospital alive have high rates of mortality which may approach 100 per cent in some categories (e.g. myocardial rupture).

Table 9.2.1 Prevalence of common cardiovascular and lung diseases, US, 2004

Disease	Number
Cardiovascular diseases[a]	79 400 000
Hypertension[b]	72 000 000
Coronary heart disease	15 800 000
Heart failure	5 200 000
Stroke	5 700 000
Congenital heart disease[c]	1 000 000

[a] Includes hypertension, CHD, heart failure, and stroke.

[b] Systolic blood pressure ≥140 mm Hg, diastolic blood pressure ≥90 mm Hg, on antihypertensive medication, or told twice of having hypertension.

[c] Range from 650 000 to 1 300 000 (Am Hrt J 2004;147:425–439).

Sources: National Health and Nutrition Examination Survey (NHANES) of NCHS and National Health Interview Survey of NCHS, except as noted.

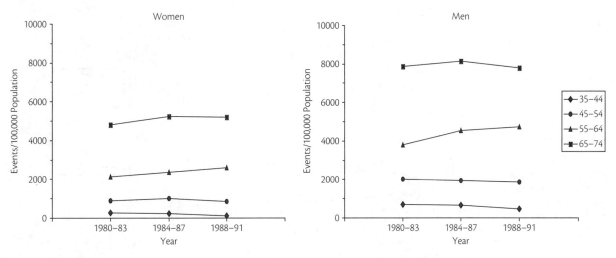

Fig. 9.2.2 Total discharges and deaths with ICD-9 code 410-414 in men and women, by age, Southeastern New England, 1980–91.

declined somewhat, but accounted for only a small fraction of the improvements in age-adjusted population mortality. With age-adjusted mortality falling, driven by a decline in cardiovascular disease, the result has been increased longevity in many populations. However, absolute mortality (not adjusted for age) has not fallen as much, as the disease is pushed into older age groups (Luepker 1994).

Disease definitions and classification

Cardiovascular disease

The leading cause of cardiovascular disease is atherosclerosis, a pathology affecting the walls of large and medium arteries. This disease process begins with injury and deposits of cholesterol in the arterial wall associated with inflammation and cellular infiltration. The arterial channel narrows with these deposits sometimes becoming 'hardened' with calcification. The result is an obstruction of blood flow and inadequate perfusion with diminished oxygen supply. Acute obstruction may occur with clots forming on the diseased vessel walls. In organs such as the heart or brain, which are dependent on a constant blood supply and oxygen, an acute obstruction can lead to irreversible damage to the tissue dependent

on that supply. Temporary interruption or diminished flow will result in other symptoms. In the heart, loss of blood supply leads to myocardial infarction with death of heart muscle. In blood vessels of the extremities, atherosclerotic disease can limit blood flow resulting in symptoms of pain on exertion. In extreme cases, loss of blood supply can lead to gangrene and loss of a limb.

Other cardiovascular diseases have their own pathology which is described in later sections.

Stroke

Stroke is a heterogeneous entity and can be broadly divided into ischaemic strokes caused by blockage or occlusion of blood vessels and haemorrhagic stroke caused by a rupture of blood vessels. Ischaemic strokes are further subdivided based on mechanism of causation into those due to (i) atherosclerotic stenosis or occlusion of large cervico-cerebral vessels, (ii) cardio-embolism, (iii) small vessel disease, i.e. lacunes caused by the lipohyalinosis of and micro-atheromata from small penetrating arteries and (iv) less common, miscellaneous group of mechanisms including non-atherosclerotic vasculopathies, central nervous system infections such as *Cryptococcus*, certain hypercoagulable states, and disorders

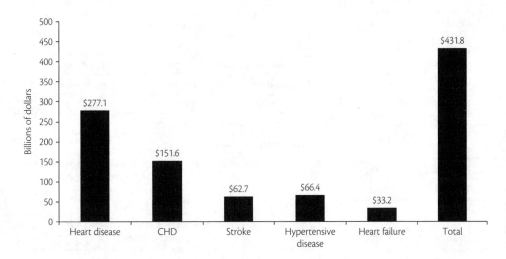

Fig. 9.2.3 Estimated direct and indirect costs of cardiovascular disease (CVD) and stroke in the United States, 1998.

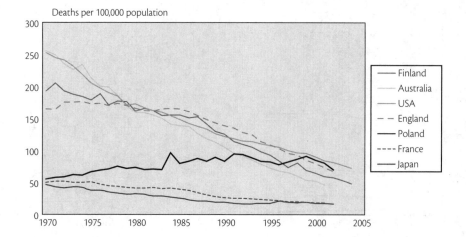

Deaths per 100,000 population

Fig. 9.2.4 Death rates* for coronary heart disease in women ages 35–74 years, selected countries, 1970–2004 *Age-adjusted to the European Standard Population.

of the cellular components of blood including sickle cell disease and polycythemia vera. Up to a third of all ischaemic strokes do not have an identified mechanism despite extensive evaluation. Haemorrhagic strokes can be subdivided based on location of haemorrhage into (i) subarachnoid haemorrhages commonly caused by the rupture of berry aneurysms into the subarachnoid space and (ii) intra-parenchymal haemorrhages caused by bleeding into the substance of the brain from a variety of reasons (Table 9.2.3).

Coronary heart disease

A vast body of research enhances the understanding of the aetiology, prevention, and treatment of coronary heart disease (AHA 2007). Important observations are summarized below:

1. Population-based studies show wide differences between countries and groups within those countries (Fig. 9.2.1).

2. Between and within populations, lipids, blood pressure, cigarette smoking, diabetes, and other characteristics are highly predictive of coronary heart disease events in individuals (Keys 1980). These risk factors are first evidenced in youth and track into adulthood. That is, high-risk youth are likely to become high-risk adults (Luepker *et al.* 1999).

3. Studies of large-scale migrations from one culture to another demonstrate that an increase in risk factors and coronary heart disease is observed when individuals migrate from a low- to high-risk culture and assume the lifestyle of that new culture (Kagan *et al.* 1974).

4. Population patterns in coronary heart disease are changing rapidly (Fig. 9.2.5).

5. Changes in coronary heart disease patterns are associated with a reduction in risk characteristics leading to decreased incidence

Table 9.2.2 Death rates[a] for cardiovascular and non-cardiovascular diseases, US, 1963, 1984, and 2004

Cause of death	1963	Rate[a] 1984	2004	Percent Change 1963–2004	Percent Change 1983–2004
All causes	1346	982	801	−40	−18
Cardiovascular diseases	805	488	289	−64	−41
Coronary heart disease	478	268	150	−69	−44
Stroke	174	83[b]	50	−71	−40
Other	153	137	88	−42	−36
Noncardiovascular diseases	541	495	512	−5	4
COPD and asthma	16	34[c]	42	153	24
Other	524	462	471	−10	2

[a] Age-adjusted; rate per 100 000 populations.
[b] Comparability ratio (1.0502) applied.
[c] Comparability ratio (1.0411) applied.
Source: Vital Statistics of the United States, NCHS.

Table 9.2.3 Stroke subtypes and pathophysiological causes

Ischemic strokes
Large vessel atherosclerosis or stenosis of cranio-cerebral vessels
Cardio-embolism
Small vessel disease (Lacunar strokes)
Miscellaneous
Non-atherosclerotic vasculopathies—e.g. vasculitis, dissection
Infectious—e.g. *Cryptococcus*
Hypercoagulable states—e.g. antiphospholipid syndrome
Blood dyscrasias causing increased viscosity—e.g. polycythemia vera
Drugs of abuse—e.g. cocaine
Cryptogenic—Up to 30% of ischaemic strokes
Haemorrhagic strokes
Intracerebral haemorrhage—hypertension leading to microaneurysms, amyloid angiopathy, arteriovenous malformations, trauma, blood dyscrasias (e.g. acute leukaemia)
Subarachnoid haemorrhage—aneurysms, arteriovenous malformations, sinus thrombosis

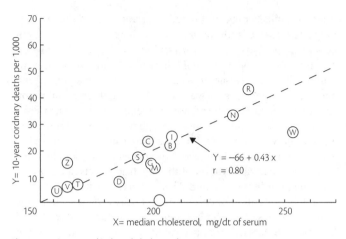

Fig. 9.2.5 Coronary death and cholesterol.
E=East Finland, R=American railroad, N=Zutphen, W=West Finland, I=Italian railroad, B=Belgrade, C=Crevalcore, S=Slavonia, G=Corfu, M=Montegiorgio, D=Dalmatia, K=Crete, Z=Zrenjanin, T=Tanushimaru, V=Velika Krsna, U=Ushibuka
Coronary heart disease age-standardized 10-year death rates of the cohorts versus the median serum cholesterol levels (mg per dl) of the cohorts. All men judged free of coronary heart disease at entry.
Source: Keys, A. Seven Countries 1980.

and to improved medical care, leading to increased survival after an initial clinical event.

6. Clinical trials demonstrate conclusively that a reduction in coronary heart disease mortality and morbidity results from the lowering of traditional risk factors (cholesterol, blood pressure, cigarette smoking) by either behavioural and/or pharmaco-logical methods. This occurs in both primary and secondary trials.

The rationale for disease prevention is found in many observations. Environmental factors encourage population-wide changes in behaviour resulting in mass elevations of risk. As populations live longer, this chronic disease is manifest following prolonged and sustained exposure to risk factors. Widespread genetic susceptibility also plays an important role in the setting of an unfavourable environment. Prevention of coronary heart disease is well founded based on these scientific observations. It begins with primary prevention or prevention of risk factor elevation in the first place (Luepker 1999). It includes identification and reduction of risk in high-risk individuals without manifest disease signs or symptoms. Finally, it rests on the identification of those who continue to be at high-risk after a coronary heart disease diagnosis. Well-established population and medical strategies are tested to implement prevention and the epidemic could be controlled with widespread and effective implementation of current knowledge.

Risk factors for atherosclerosis and coronary heart disease

There are numerous known risk factors playing a role in the development of atherosclerosis. Risk factors are characteristics discovered initially in prospective epidemiological studies. The aetiological role of risk factors is supported by laboratory experimental data and confirmed in clinical trials reducing risk in humans. Risk factors predict disease and frequently play a causal role in the

pathological process. These include diet, lipids, obesity, physical inactivity, diabetes, hypertension, tobacco smoking, and others.

Diet
There is substantial evidence to support a causal association of habitual dietary intake with coronary heart disease. Much of that evidence is found in studies comparing populations. However, there is also evidence within populations to suggest the role of individual dietary intake in coronary heart disease morbidity and mortality. Human feeding experiments add evidence as do animal studies. A number of components of habitual diet have been considered. These include fats, dietary cholesterol, carbohydrates, fibre, alcohol, protein, and caloric excess. Information regarding diet and coronary heart disease is summarized here:

1. Habitual food intake varies greatly between populations. These differences are related to population prevalence of coronary heart disease (Keys 1980).

2. While more difficult to study, individual eating patterns are also associated with coronary heart disease (Keys 1980).

3. When all components of diet are considered, the type and amount of fat intake is the most important component in preventing coronary heart disease.

4. The association of dietary fat with coronary heart disease is predominantly through the effects of saturated fats and cholesterol on blood lipids.

5. Eating patterns are changing in many cultures, leading to improving coronary heart disease rates in some and worsening in others.

6. Clinical trials of secondary prevention find diet change useful in lowering coronary heart disease.

7. Laboratory animal studies of non-human primates are congruent with human diet–disease relationships.

Fat
The evidence is strong for the effect of diet between populations. The best known is the Seven Countries Study. This research compared habitual food intake in samples from among seven national populations (Keys 1980). This study demonstrated great variability in habitual food intake and a clear association of fatty acids and dietary cholesterol with blood cholesterol levels. Those blood cholesterol levels were a strong predictor of coronary heart disease in initially healthy populations followed more than 25 years (Blackburn & Jacobs 1984).

So central is the association of diet with blood cholesterol level, that many investigators suggest a cholesterol-raising diet is essential for mass expression of coronary heart disease (Blackburn & Jacobs 1984). These conclusions rest on data showing a diet with increased animal fats, specifically saturated fat and cholesterol, is found in populations where disease rates are high. Conversely, populations where these dietary components are low show a decreased incidence of coronary heart disease. Changes in diet seem to precede rising or falling coronary heart disease rates. Such is the case in the United States where diet is changing associated with falling blood cholesterol and coronary heart disease (CDC 2006) (Table 9.2.4). Additional evidence comes from observations in other international studies, where countries such as Japan have elevated levels of blood pressure and cigarette smoking, important coronary heart disease risk factors,

Table 9.2.4 Nutrient intake in the United States (1971–2002)

	1971–1975	1976–1980	1988–1994	1999–2002
Saturated fat (g/day)	31	31	27	25
Total fat (g/day)	87	87	80	78

but fail to manifest high rates of coronary heart disease. The Japanese have lower population levels of blood cholesterol (Keys 1980).

Observations on migrating populations show the same conclusions. The Japanese living in Japan have low cholesterol levels and low rates of coronary heart disease. As they move to Hawaii and the United States, they progressively assume the lifestyle of those Westernized cultures and experience elevations in blood cholesterol, obesity and coronary heart disease rates similar to the local population (Kagan *et al.* 1974). Again, the assumption of a high-fat Western diet is associated with increased coronary heart disease.

While the associations between diet and coronary heart disease are very strong in between population comparisons, the data are more conflicting in studies within populations. Here, studies of food intake or eating patterns of individuals modestly predict subsequent disease, if at all. There are several well-recognized reasons for this apparent paradox.

Supportive evidence comes from metabolic ward feeding studies. Here, individuals fed controlled diets of known composition for prolonged periods, show a clear relationship between type and quantity of fat intake and blood cholesterol levels. This relationship is best described by the Keys' formula which relates the intake of saturated fats, polyunsaturated fats, and dietary cholesterol to blood cholesterol levels (Keys *et al.* 1974). The Keys formula is calculated using the formula: $1.35 (2S - P) + 1.5Z$ where S is the percentage of dietary calories from saturated fatty acids, P is the percentage of dietary calories from polyunsaturated fatty acids, and Z is the square root of dietary cholesterol in mg/1000 kcal.

More recent studies have provided increased detail including information on monounsaturated fats, and specific fatty acids including *trans*-fatty acids (Ascherio *et al.* 1994; Ginsberg *et al.* 1998). Trans-fatty acids, often the result of the chemical saturation process to harden fats, have a significant cholesterol raising effect.

Given clear and consistent associations in between population studies and feeding experiments involving fat, why has such an association not emerged in free-living populations? There are several reasons postulated. Among these is the difficulty of measurement of habitual food intake in individuals. While this measure is relatively simple in societies which have little variation in foods, it is particularly difficult in societies where unlimited foods are available and composition is highly variable on a daily basis. Individual data collection, such as 24-h recalls, fail to characterize usual intake adequately. Food frequency approaches which characterize longer periods of time are susceptible to recall bias and difficulty in determining 'average intake'.

There are also individual factors in the response to dietary intake. Even when food intake is carefully controlled, the digestion and absorption process may vary between individuals and genetic factors may play a role. Thus, two individuals eating the same diet may have a different cholesterol response.

It is generally acknowledged that a large-scale trial of reducing dietary fat intake for the primary prevention of coronary heart disease is unlikely to be performed (Gordon 1988). Although coronary heart disease is common in populations, the enormous numbers of individuals needed for randomization, the challenges to effective control of food intake in a free-living population, the number of years necessary to accumulate adequate endpoint events, and the cost, precludes such a study. However, there are numerous congruent sources of information that lend strength to the validity of dietary fat recommendations through reduced blood cholesterol and coronary heart disease. Prominent are clinical trials of secondary prevention using diet. Supportive evidence may also be found in the consistent observation of the beneficial effects of cholesterol lowering regardless of method. This is widely recognized in trials of secondary prevention of coronary heart disease through lipid lowering (Lipid Research Clinics Program 1984; Buchwald *et al.* 1990; Scandinavian Simvastatin Survival Study Group 1994; Sacks *et al.* 1996; LIPID Study Group 1998), but also studies of primary prevention with lipid-lowering medications (Shepherd *et al.* 1995; Downs *et al.* 1998).

The recognition that usual food intake is a behaviour strongly related to culture and food availability has resulted in community-based public health strategies to improve dietary intake. The North Karelia and Stanford Three Town Studies were among the first to use public and health professional education about dietary fat to reduce blood cholesterol (Farquhar *et al.* 1977; Puska *et al.* 1995). In both studies, an improved eating pattern with reduced animal fats (saturated fats and cholesterol) resulted in reduced average blood cholesterols in these small communities. Larger studies in medium-sized cities in Europe and the United States showed similar results. Strong favourable secular trends in control communities resulted in modest differences in blood cholesterol levels (GCP Research Group 1988; Farquhar *et al.* 1990; Luepker *et al.* 1994; Carleton *et al.* 1995).

Protein

Comparisons between populations in countries show an ecological correlation between dietary proteins, particularly animal protein and mortality from coronary heart disease. However, there is little evidence that this association is causal. Metabolic ward experiments of men under isocholoric condition, with fat intake held constant while protein intake varied between 5 and 20 per cent of daily calories, found no change in blood cholesterol levels (University of Minnesota, unpublished data).

These observations and others suggest that associations observed between populations are the result of animal fat associated with animal protein, rather than the effect of the protein itself. Specifically, consumption of fat from animals and high-fat milk products result in elevated blood cholesterol, rather than their high protein content. In coronary heart disease, it is generally agreed that dietary protein is not a factor in coronary heart disease.

Carbohydrates

A positive association is found between population intake of refined sugars and coronary heart disease. This relationship is confounded by many other dietary components and, importantly, the association of high levels of refined sugars with the usual diet of Westernized industrial countries. In the absence of a plausible biological connection between refined sugars and atherosclerosis, the association may actually be that of the high animal fat intake also found in those societies. However, refined sugars have other deleterious effects such as dental disease.

Complex carbohydrates are negatively associated with coronary heart disease. Higher intake is found with low coronary heart disease mortality. These are also confounded by fat intake and other dietary factors. There is a plausible biological mechanism by which complex carbohydrates may affect coronary heart disease. Foods having high levels of carbohydrates, such as fruits and vegetables, also contain fibre including pectins in fruit, bran fibre, and guar gum. These play a role in the absorption of fat and cholesterol in the intestines. Observational studies and clinical trials have demonstrated that increased fibre intake is associated with lower cholesterol levels (Jenkins *et al.* 1993). It is important to note that increased fibre intake is best attained by consumption of healthy fruits and vegetables, rather than dietary supplements.

Alcohol

There is a continuing debate regarding the effects of alcohol consumption on cardiovascular disease including coronary heart disease. Alcohol has several associations with coronary heart disease including: (1) the association of alcohol consumption with increased blood pressure and the risk of stroke (Criqui 1987); (2) the association of alcohol consumption with increased high-density lipoprotein cholesterol and levels of triglycerides (Gordon *et al.* 1981); (3) the effect of alcohol on haemostatic factors including fibrinogen, platelet aggregation and fibrinolysis (Meade *et al.* 1987); (4) Large doses of alcohol lead to addiction and other severe diseases. These include cardiovascular diseases such as congestive cardiomyopathy, cardiac arrhythmias, and sudden death (Regan 1990).

Given these findings, why is there controversy about alcohol intake? It principally stems from epidemiological research which shows moderate intake of alcohol is associated with lower risk of coronary heart disease when compared to non-drinkers. Numerous studies support this observation after adjusting for other risk factors and confounders, which stimulates this debate. One controversy focuses on the type of alcoholic beverage containing this benefit. Some have suggested wine is the essential form, while others find that other alcoholic beverages such as beer and spirits are equally implicated (Colditz 1990). It is still not certain whether it is the ethanol or some other component in the beverage. Studies of alcohol consumption are also fraught with difficulties. In many, report of consumption is inaccurate with long-term consumption as difficult to ascertain as for other foods. There is also a suggestion that people who are ill eliminate their alcohol consumption as the result of their illness, confusing cause and effect. Finally, there are social factors associated with the intake of certain beverages, particularly the use of wine among the more affluent.

In summary, while there are observational studies associating alcohol intake with lower coronary heart disease rates and plausible biological mechanisms are available, there are also concerns regarding the recommendation of alcoholic beverages as a preventive strategy for coronary heart disease. These rest in the potential for addiction, vehicular accidents, and negative effects on a number of organ systems, including the cardiovascular system.

Vitamins, minerals, and food supplements

Coronary heart disease has many advocates of oral supplements for treatment and prevention. Vitamins, minerals, and other food supplements are promoted as a simple easy way to avoid disease. There are numerous manufacturers who are willing to fulfil this 'need'. However, most of these substances are untested in a rigorous and controlled manner. Among those considered are vitamins C and E, β-carotene, copper, iron, selenium, fish oil, and fibre.

Observational studies show benefit and/or harm for some supplements (Ascherio & Hunter 1994; Kritchevsky *et al.* 1995; Stampfer & Rimm 1995; Ascherio *et al.* 1999). Very few have been submitted to clinical trials. When this has occurred, either in healthy subjects or those with coronary heart disease, the results have been mixed and usually negative (Omenn *et al.* 1996; Hennekens *et al.* 1996; Collins *et al.* 2002; Lee *et al.* 2005). The need for more trials is recognized.

Homocysteine has been evaluated as a risk factor for coronary heart disease. It is a product of methionine metabolism and observational studies consistently show elevated blood homocysteine in association with coronary heart disease (Boushey *et al.* 1995). The exact mechanism for this association is uncertain. Supplementation with vitamins B6, B12, and folate appears to lower homocysteine levels (Osganian *et al.* 1999). Recently in the United States and other nations, folate supplementation was added to many grain products to prevent birth defects. This should result in lower population levels of homocysteine (Boushey *et al.* 1995; Osganian *et al.* 1999). Unfortunately, several large clinical trials of vitamin supplementation in patients with known cardiovascular disease and stroke failed to show treatment advantages (Toole *et al.* 2004; Lonn *et al.* 2006; Bonaa, *et al.* 2006).

Blood lipids

The preponderance of population, clinical, and experimental data indicate that blood lipids play a causal role in atherosclerosis and resulting coronary heart disease. Mass elevations in blood lipids appear to be a necessary factor for mass coronary heart disease. The research underlying these statements is summarized below.

1. Mean levels and distributions of blood lipids which vary widely between populations (Keys 1980) demonstrate a strong graded relationship between levels of total serum or plasma cholesterol and coronary heart disease. The low-density lipoprotein fraction of cholesterol is most atherogenic.

2. High-density lipoprotein cholesterol is inversely related to coronary heart disease. Higher levels are associated with less disease. High-density lipoprotein cholesterol is strongest as a predictor of coronary heart disease in populations where total cholesterol and disease risk is high (NIH 2002).

3. Although the mechanisms are poorly understood, there is a growing consensus that serum triglycerides, as measured in the fasting state, are associated with coronary heart disease (NIH 2002).

4. Blood cholesterol levels among youth after puberty parallel those of the adult population (Luepker 1999).

5. Blood cholesterol levels continue to be predictive among adults over the age of 65 years, although the relative risk is reduced (Abbott *et al.* 1997).

6. Blood cholesterol can be lowered among adults with moderate changes in diet and loss of weight.

7. Clinical trials with lipid-lowering agents among those with moderate to severe blood cholesterol elevations demonstrate reduced coronary heart disease associated with lower cholesterol levels. This occurs both in individuals with coronary heart disease and those without evidence of clinical disease. It is particularly true

of the newer statin drugs, but also with other methods (Scandinavian Simvastatin Survival Study 1994; Shepherd *et al.* 1995; Multiple Risk Factor Intervention Trial Research Group 1996; Sacks *et al.* 1996; Downs *et al.* 1998; LIPID Study Group 1998).

8. A progressive fall in blood cholesterol in the United States is associated with changes in the habitual diet during the last 25 years (Carroll *et al.* 2005; Arnett *et al.* 2005).

Population studies of blood lipids consistently show a positive association of mean blood cholesterol with coronary heart disease. As shown in Fig. 9.2.5, comparisons between different national groups show a significant association between blood cholesterol levels in health and coronary heart disease events among middle-aged men (Keys 1980). Similarly, data from the Multiple Risk Factor Intervention Trial, where over 356 000 healthy middle-aged men were followed over time, blood cholesterol predicted coronary heart disease outcomes in a progressive and continuous way as shown in Fig. 9.2.6 (Neaton *et al.* 1992). This continued gradation of blood cholesterol levels and disease suggest that lower blood cholesterol is better but there is no discrete point at which relative risk is sharply higher.

Lipids are insoluble in a water medium, namely blood. They are carried as lipoprotein particles in combination with proteins. Total cholesterol is the most widely used blood measure. It represents that chemical entity regardless of the carrier protein. Total cholesterol is commonly divided into three major components based on the density of the particles: Low-density lipoprotein cholesterol, high-density lipoprotein cholesterol, and very low-density lipoprotein cholesterol. Each of these fractions is associated with specific protein carrier molecules. Low-density lipoprotein is the largest component of total cholesterol and is the atherogenic fraction. High-density lipoprotein comprises a smaller fraction and is inversely related to coronary heart disease, with higher levels of high-density lipoprotein associated with less disease. The very low-density lipoprotein contains modest amounts of cholesterol, but is the main carrier for triglycerides. Triglycerides are the major method by which fat is transported and stored in the body.

There is considerable research on subfractions of these lipoproteins and the protein carriers which transport them. While important in research, these subfractions—including lipoprotein A, apolipoprotein E, B-lipoprotein, high-density lipoprotein 2, and high-density lipoprotein 3—and many others are not established measures

for clinical use nor are they relevant for public health strategies at this time.

There are numerous trials designed to lower blood cholesterol or its subfractions. Dietary trials are noted above. The majority of trials have been in high-risk individuals by virtue of elevated blood cholesterol or known coronary heart disease. The trials take many years and are costly; however, the results are consistent and clear. The Coronary Drug Project enrolled men between 30 and 64 years old who had a previous myocardial infarction. The nicotinic acid treatment group showed significant lower mortality compared to those on placebo at 15 years after the study began (Canner *et al.* 1986). Many early trials occurred before the more powerful cholesterol lowering drugs—the statins. With the use of statins, much larger effects of cholesterol reduction are observed with accompanying greater reductions in coronary heart disease events. In primary prevention, the West of Scotland Coronary Prevention Study is of particular interest (Shepherd *et al.* 1995). Randomizing 6595 men with moderately elevated cholesterol to placebo or pravastin, investigators observed significant reductions in serum total cholesterol and low-density lipoprotein cholesterol concentrations. Significantly fewer major coronary events were observed with lower total mortality in the treatment group compared to the controls. Similarly, the Airforce/Texas Coronary Atherosclerosis Prevention Study studied healthy subjects with modest increases in blood cholesterol. With lovastatin, significant reductions in cholesterol, coronary events and all causes of mortality were observed (Downs *et al.* 1998).

A number of large secondary prevention trials using statin therapy to lower cholesterol have also been completed, including the Scandinavian Simvastatin Survival Study (Scandinavian Simvastatin Survival Study 1994). It demonstrated a significant reduction in all causes of mortality, coronary heart disease mortality, coronary events and revascularization procedures in patients with known coronary heart disease. The Cholesterol and Recurrent Events trial and the Long-Term Intervention with Fibrostatin in Ischaemic Disease trial also demonstrated lipid reductions associated with fewer major coronary events (Sacks *et al.* 1996; LIPID Study Group 1998). The MRC/BHF Heart Protection Study resulted in a 25 per cent reduction in cardiovascular events with simvastatin in 20 536 high-risk adults (Collins *et al.* 2002).

There have also been two important secondary prevention trials with gemfibrozil, a fibric acid derivative. A Finnish trial among men with known coronary heart disease resulted in a significant reduction of coronary events associated with increased high-density lipoprotein cholesterol and decreased triglycerides. Total cholesterol results were variable (Frick *et al.* 1987). A more recent treatment study of men with average total and low-density lipoprotein cholesterol but low high-density lipoprotein cholesterol with gemfibrozil also produced positive results. High-density lipoprotein cholesterol increased in the treatment group compared to placebo. Coronary events were reduced. Serum triglycerides also fell significantly, raising questions about the relative importance of the two lipid effects (Rubins *et al.* 1999).

There is consistent evidence from clinical trials of the benefits of lower total cholesterol and low-density lipoprotein cholesterol. There is also a suggestion that raising high-density lipoprotein cholesterol and lowering triglycerides add to these beneficial effects.

While recognizing that population-wide reductions in blood cholesterol would have the greatest benefits, there are also clinical indicators of elevated blood cholesterol requiring aggressive and

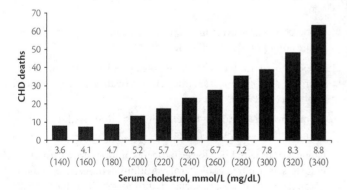

Fig. 9.2.6 CHD deaths and cholesterol.
Source: Neaton *et al.* (1992).

pharmacological management. This includes both high-risk individuals who are disease free and those who have known coronary heart disease. The Adult Treatment Panel (ATP III) of the United States National Cholesterol Education Program has suggested levels appropriate for further diagnosis and treatment (NIH 2002). These are seen in Table 9.2.5. This report also adds 'coronary heart disease risk equivalents'. In addition to prevalent coronary heart disease, peripheral artery disease, carotid artery disease, abdominal aortic aneurysm, and diabetes are considered as factors requiring more aggressive treatment. The report also includes other risk factors for coronary heart disease (e.g. smoking) in a combined risk score which directs prevention strategies. The European Society of Cardiology made similar recommendations for prevention (Wood *et al.* 1998).

Blood pressure

Considerable epidemiological, clinical, and experimental data find high blood pressure or hypertension to be a major risk factor for coronary heart disease. Hypertension is also strongly predictive of other diseases including stroke, renal failure, and congestive heart failure. It is also widely recognized that treatment of hypertension to lower blood pressure reduces cardiovascular disease. The problem is common, and large portions of the population have hypertension and/or are currently under treatment. The important observations about hypertension are as follows:

1. Population studies find a modest relationship between hypertension and coronary heart disease mortality between countries (Keys 1980) but within populations, coronary heart disease is strongly related to both systolic and diastolic blood pressures.

2. Levels of blood pressure among youth track into adulthood.

3. For those with fixed hypertension, clinical trials demonstrate that treatment to reduce blood pressure reduces stroke, coronary heart disease, congestive heart failure, cardiovascular disease, and total mortality.

4. Treatment for hypertension is widely available; however, many individuals are neither diagnosed nor effectively treated (Chobanian *et al.* 2003).

Elevated blood pressure plays an important role in a number of diseases. The effect of sustained mechanical forces associated with

Table 9.2.5 ATP III classification of total cholesterol, LDL cholesterol, and triglycerides

Total cholesterol (mg/dL)		LDL cholesterol (mg/dL)		Triglycerides (mg/dL)	
		<100	Optimal	<150	Normal
<200	Desirable	100–129	Near optimal/ above optimal	150–199	Borderline high
200–239	Borderline high	130–159	Borderline high	200–499	High
≥240	High	160–189	High	≥500	Very high
		≥190	Very high		

Source: National Cholesterol Education Program. Third Report of the National Cholesterol Education Program Expert Panel on: Detection, Evaluation, and Treatment of High Blood Cholesterol in Adults (Adult Treatment Panel III). NIH Pub. 02-5215. Bethesda, MD: National Heart, Lung, and Blood Institute, 2002.

elevations in blood pressure leads to target organ damage in the heart, brain, kidneys, and other organs. The origins of high blood pressure are not well understood, however, associations with obesity, physical inactivity, salt intake, and alcohol intake suggest behavioural factors play an important role. Genetic factors are also apparent, but the considerable prevalence of hypertension suggests that any hereditary characteristics are very common in most populations.

In international studies, systolic blood pressure predicts coronary heart disease outcomes between populations in a modest but linear fashion (Keys 1980). Many populations worldwide have highly prevalent hypertension including the Japanese, Chinese, Africans, and others (over 50 per cent in some adult groups).

Within populations, blood pressure is predictive of cardiovascular disease outcomes including coronary heart disease (Chobanian *et al.* 2003). Early studies focused on diastolic blood pressure, but more recently systolic blood pressure, which appears to be more reliably measured, has assumed increasing importance for diagnosis and treatment (Fig. 9.2.7).

While hypertension is common, its prevalence has not changed significantly in recent years. However, in the past 20 years, detection, treatment and control of high blood pressure has progressively improved. As shown in Table 9.2.6, awareness, treatment and control of blood pressure have substantially increased. In the 1990s, however, there was an apparent levelling of effect in the United States with many still unaware and ineffectively treated (Chobanian *et al.* 2003; Luepker 2006).

Lifestyle modifications including weight, exercise, and diet offer the potential for preventing hypertension. They have also been found to be effective at lowering moderate hypertension with little risk and minimal cost. Even though lifestyle factors alone may not control high blood pressure, they can reduce the amount of antihypertensive drugs deemed necessary (Neaton *et al.* 1993). Excess body weight is associated with elevation in blood pressure. Weight reduction can reduce blood pressure in obese individuals with hypertension (Neaton *et al.* 1993). Therefore, it is widely recommended that weight reduction is an important part of hypertension control. Physical inactivity also plays a role in hypertension with unfit individuals having up to 50 per cent increased risk of developing high blood pressure. Moderate physical activity aids in controlling weight and may actually lower blood pressure (NIH 1996). Dietary factors may also play a role in precipitating or reducing hypertension. Alcohol use raises blood pressure. The National High Blood Pressure Education Program recommends no more than 30 ml of ethanol as beer, wine, or whisky per day for men and 15 ml per day for women (Chobanian *et al.* 2003).

Salting of food as a method of preservation is well established over many centuries. However, modern food preservation methods do not require salt and it is mainly an acquired taste. Unfortunately, the human kidney was developed in the setting of low sodium and high potassium diets. Hence, the body is well designed to retain, but not excrete sodium, which it effectively does. The need for sodium is quite small and many times the amount required is consumed in processed food (Blackburn & Prineas 1983).

Salt intake is particularly relevant to hypertension. Population surveys demonstrate strong associations between population blood pressure and salt intake (INTERSALT Cooperative Research Group 1988). Migration studies where salt intake is greatly increased among people who migrate from low to high salt cultures is associated with increasing prevalence of hypertension (Joseph *et al.* 1983).

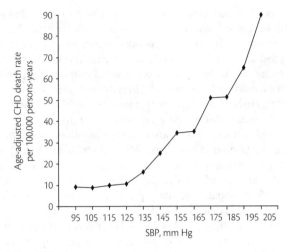 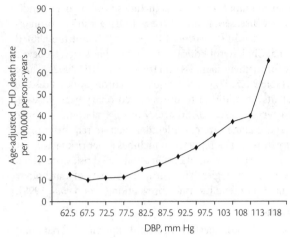

Fig. 9.2.7 CHD and blood pressure.
Source: Neaton *et al.* (1992).

Clinical studies have found that restriction in salt results in lower blood pressure. Marked sodium depletion, as practised in an earlier era, can even reduce blood pressure among severe hypertensives, and sodium restriction enables high blood pressure to be controlled with lower doses of antihypertensive drugs. In some patients, salt restriction may control mild-to-moderate hypertension without resorting to drugs.

Despite widespread information about the role of salt, considerable debate remains. The US National Dietary Goals recommend no more than 6 g of sodium chloride daily (Chobanian *et al.* 2003). This remains significantly more than humans need, but well below the average intake. As the use of processed foods increases, salt may play an undiminished or even increasing role in hypertension.

The decision to initiate pharmacological treatment of high blood pressure depends on a variety of factors, including the absolute level of blood pressure, the presence of cardiovascular disease, target organ damage and the presence of other coronary heart disease risk factors. The benefits of pharmacological treatment have been demonstrated for coronary heart disease, stroke, heart failure, renal disease, and all causes of mortality (Furberg 2002). There was debate over the generalizability of hypertension trials

to older adults and other groups; it is generally believed that all populations will benefit from blood pressure lowering. There are many medications currently available for hypertension treatment, however, diuretics are recommended for initiating treatment as they have the longest clinical trial experience and a proven record of reducing morbidity and mortality in clinical trials (Chobanian *et al.* 2003; Furberg 2002). Other agents may be added if blood pressure is not adequately controlled (Chobanian *et al.* 2003).

There is some debate regarding what constitutes a normal blood pressure and, hence, what requires pharmacological treatment. Most agree that 120/80 represents a normal blood pressure in an adult. The recommendations for blood pressure classification and treatment among adults over the age of 18 years of the United States National High Blood Pressure Education Program are shown in Table 9.2.7 (Chobanian *et al.* 2003). The European recommendations are somewhat different, but in a similar range (Wood *et al.* 1998).

Cigarette smoking

Tobacco use is a worldwide problem associated with many diseases. While best known for causing lung cancer, cigarette use has a larger

Table 9.2.6 Trends in awareness, treatment, and control of high blood pressure in adults with hypertension aged 18–74 years*

	National Health and Nutrition Examination Surveys, weighted %			
	1976–1980	1988–1991	1991–1994	1999–2000
Awareness	51	73	68	70
Treatment	31	55	54	59
Control†	10	29	27	34

* Data from the National Heart, Lung, and Blood Institute and data for National Health and Nutrition Examination Surveys.

† Systolic blood pressure of less than 140 mm Hg and diastolic blood pressure of less than 90 mm Hg.

Source: Chobanian *et al.* (2003).

Table 9.2.7 Classification and management of blood pressure for adults aged 18 years or older

BP classification	Systolic BP, mm Hg*		Diastolic BP, mm Hg*
Normal	<120	and	<80
Prehypertension	120–139	or	80–89
Stage 1 hypertension	140–159	or	90–99
Stage 2 hypertension	≥160	or	≥100

* Treatment determined by highest BP category.

Source: Chobanian *et al.* (2003).

effect on mortality and morbidity from coronary heart disease. Some of the salient observations on tobacco use are as follows:

1. Cigarette smoking addicts 20–80 per cent of adult men worldwide, with a somewhat lower proportion of adult women addicted.

2. Comparisons between populations often find no association between coronary heart disease and the prevalence of cigarette smoking. However, the individual association of cigarette smoking to coronary heart disease is strong.

3. Cigarette smoking is falling in some countries but rising in many, and is a growing epidemic in developing nations.

4. Cigarette smoking begins in youth and gradually increases until it becomes nicotine addiction.

5. The main mechanisms by which cigarette smoking affects coronary heart disease are as a chronic promoter of atherosclerotic lesions and as an acute risk factor increasing sympathetic stimulation and enhancing clotting.

6. While randomized population trials of cigarette use have not been performed, cigarette smoking cessation is associated with reduced coronary heart disease mortality.

7. There is growing evidence that environmental tobacco smoke or second-hand smoke has a deleterious effect on exposed non-smokers.

Tobacco use through cigarette smoking is one of the major causes of disease and disability in the world. In the United States, there are approximately 47 million adult smokers, and it is estimated that 430 000 deaths annually are associated with cigarette smoking (USDHHS 1998a). These victims are replaced by the teenagers who begin the smoking habit. In the United States, the direct medical costs of smoking are estimated to be over US$60 billion/year, with similar indirect costs.

Cigarette smoking is linked to the major cardiovascular diseases including myocardial infarction, sudden death, stroke and peripheral vascular disease (USDHHS 1997). These associations are found across age, gender and ethnic groups (USDHHS 1997; Neaton & Wentworth 1992). The relationship of coronary heart disease mortality to smoking status is shown in Fig. 9.2.8. One of the most important findings is the association of cigarette smoking with

sudden unexpected death among younger individuals. Similarly, acute myocardial infarction in younger individuals (less than 50 years of age) is very strongly associated with tobacco use. The interaction of cigarette smoking with other risk factors such as cholesterol, diet, obesity, hypertension, lipids, diabetes, and ECG abnormalities is also well demonstrated (Multiple Risk Factor Intervention Trial Research Group 1996). Among the strongest pieces of evidence is the observation that continued cigarette smoking after myocardial infarction is predictive of recurrent events and death (Hermanson et al. 1988), and those who quit smoking dramatically reduce their chance of a second event or death (Hermanson et al. 1988; USDHHS 1990).

The mechanisms by which tobacco and the constituents of tobacco smoke affect cardiovascular disease are still debated. Both acute and chronic mechanisms probably contribute. Firstly, there is evidence that smoking plays a direct role in the atherosclerotic process. This is shown by the Pathological Determinants of Atherosclerosis in Youth Study of 1443 autopsies of men and women aged 15–34 years who died of trauma (McGill et al. 1997). Fatty abdominal and aortic streaks and raised lesions were associated with cigarette use in this otherwise healthy population. This may be the result of injury to the arterial endothelium from smoking (McGill et al. 1997). More acutely, the immediate pharmacological effects of nicotine and carbon monoxide are well known. Platelet adhesion, acute coronary constriction and tachycardia are commonly cited (Meade et al. 1987). Finally, there is the rapid improvement in patients observed after smoking cessation.

In recent years, the focus has shifted to environmental tobacco smoke which affects non-smokers in public and private settings. A number of recent studies suggest consistent and increased relative risk of cardiovascular disease among those exposed to environmental tobacco smoke (Table 9.2.8). While it is difficult to measure exposure to environmental tobacco smoke, the consistency of these studies is suggestive and reinforces the effort to control cigarette smoking in public settings (Steenland et al. 1996).

Programmes to control tobacco use have focused on prevention and cessation. Smoking prevention programmes in the schools have received considerable attention and met some success (Perry

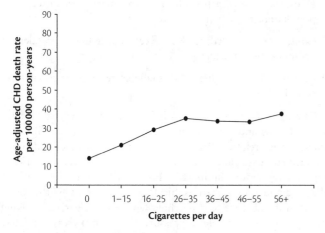

Fig. 9.2.8 Cigarette smoking and CHD
Source: Neaton et al. (1992).

Table 9.2.8 Cohort studies of environmental tobacco smoke and CHD

Source	Year	Location	Cases/ population	Adjusted RR (CI)
Garland	1985	United States	19/695	2.7 (0.7–10.5)
Svendsen	1987	United States	88/1245	2.2 (0.72–6.92)
Helsing	1988	United States	1358/19 035	M 1.31 (1.05–1.64)
				F 1.24 (1.10–1.40)
Hole	1989	United Kingdom	53/7987	2.01 (1.2–3.4)
Layard	1995	United States	1389/2916	M 0.97 (0.73–1.28)
				F 0.99 (0.84–1.16)
Tunstall–Pedoe	1995	United Kingdom	70/2,278	2.7 (1.3–5.6)
Steenland	1996	United States	3819/309 599	M 1.22 (1.07–1.40)
				F 1.10 (0.96–1.27)
Kawachi	1997	United States	152/32 046	F 1.91 (1.11–3.28)

et al. 1992). Cessation interventions among adults have emphasized behavioural and pharmacological strategies (Fiore *et al.* 1996). These have included nicotine replacement therapy, medications, social support, and skills training/problem solving. In addition, widespread restriction of smoking reduces the societal support for the behaviour.

In summary, cigarette smoking is an addictive behaviour leading to many health-impairing effects including coronary heart disease. Elimination of cigarette smoking would significantly improve the health of any population.

Overweight and obesity

Excess body weight as fat is increasingly recognized for its importance in the development of cardiovascular diseases. On a population level, overweight and obesity have become common among all adults in industrialized countries and the affluent in developing countries. Several important observations include the following:

1. Overweight and obesity are associated with increased mortality.

2. Obesity is associated with elevated blood pressure, hyperlipidaemia, diabetes mellitus, and insulin resistance. Reduction in body fat diminishes the level of each of these risk factors.

3. Increasing body weight is a worldwide problem and is the result of excess food in the setting of reduced physical activity.

Obesity is commonly described as excess body fat; however, the exact proportion of fat rendering one overweight or obese is debated. Body mass index, which is weight in kilograms divided by height in meters squared, is a commonly used standard. Expert panels suggest a body mass index above 25 is classified as overweight and above 30 as obese (Eckel & Krauss 1998; USDHHS 1998*b*). More recently, visceral adiposity has been proposed as a better marker for obesity as a predictor of cardiac risk (Freedman 1995). Visceral adiposity is simply measured by the waist to hip ratio, using the circumference of these two sites. Other more complex methods to determine body fat are available but require sophisticated instruments.

Overweight and obesity are an increasing problem in much of the world. In recent years, overweight and obesity measured in national surveys have substantially increased in the United States (Ogden *et al.* 2006). Men are more likely to be overweight (body mass index greater than 25 kg/m^2) but women are more likely to be obese (body mass index greater than 30 kg/m^2). Ethnic minorities, such as African Americans, and Mexican Americans living in the United States, have similar, if not greater, adiposity (Ogden *et al.* 2006).

The association of obesity with mortality is well established. For the severe or morbidly obese, lifespan is significantly reduced (Sjostrom 1992). For the less severely obese, the debate is that of obesity as an independent risk factor for cardiovascular disease or as one which operates through other known risk factors (Harris *et al.* 1997; Solomon & Manson 1997). The question is a scientific one rather than one of public health.

Obesity and overweight affects lipoprotein metabolism through higher low-density lipoprotein cholesterol, increased triglycerides and lower levels of high-density lipoprotein cholesterol. Weight reduction accomplished through diet is associated with significant improvement in lipids (Dattilo & Kris-Etherton 1992). The association of weight and blood pressure is also well established. In the

Nurses Health Study, one unit in body mass index was associated with a 12 per cent increase in the risk of hypertension (Huang *et al.* 1998). Other observational studies consistently show this relationship (Dyer & Elliott 1989). Weight loss is well demonstrated to reduce blood pressure. This includes even modest reductions in weight (Trials of Hypertension Prevention Collaborative Research Group 1997). In addition, recent research suggests that a diet lower in fat and higher in fruits and vegetables also results in lower blood pressure among the mildly hypertensive (Krauss *et al.* 1998). In each of these studies, weight reduction via diet allows the reduction of antihypertensive medications.

Insulin resistance is the underlying condition associated with adult-onset or type II diabetes. Obesity is a crucial factor in the development of insulin insensitivity and increased interabdominal fat is implicated (Krauss *et al.* 1998). The current epidemic of diabetes is associated with the increase in obesity. Weight loss can be critical to the control of adult-onset diabetes. Both insulin resistance and hyperglycaemia are significantly reduced when patients lose weight (Paisey *et al.* 1998). This may result in the ability to reduce diabetic therapy.

Clinicians are well aware of the difficulty of obtaining significant and sustained weight loss among patients, consequently obesity prevention is a better strategy. By reducing the increased adiposity that occurs with age, many of the sequelae and difficulty of losing weight as an adult would be avoided (National Task Force on Prevention and Treatment of Obesity 1994). For those who are obese, both control of calorie intake and increase in calorie expenditure through physical activity is essential.

Diabetes, hyperglycaemia, and hyperinsulinaemia

The insulin era, allowing patients to live longer, revealed a strong association between diabetes and cardiovascular diseases, particularly those caused by atherosclerosis. Large vessel disease associated with diabetes results in myocardial infarction, stroke, and peripheral vascular disease. Microvascular disease is associated with retinopathy, renal disease and cardiomyopathy. In addition to strong associations with known cardiovascular risk factors, diabetes is an independent predictor of disease (Stamler *et al.* 1993). Salient observations regarding diabetes are as follows:

1. Diabetes and hyperglycaemia are strongly related to atherosclerosis, obesity, and abnormal lipid patterns.

2. Diabetes is increasing along with obesity in susceptible populations.

3. Control of associated risk factors can reduce the atherosclerotic complications of diabetes.

4. Control of blood glucose in diabetes reduces microvascular complications.

The association of clinical diabetes mellitus with coronary heart disease and other atherosclerotic conditions is well documented with relative risks at two or three times that for diabetic subjects compared to non-diabetic individuals (Stamler *et al.* 1993). Figure 9.2.9, shows Multiple Risk Factor Intervention Trial data for diabetic and non-diabetic subjects. It is apparent that diabetes alone in the absence of hypercholesterolaemia, cigarette smoking and elevated systolic blood pressure results in increased relative risk of cardiovascular disease mortality. The effect of diabetes is magnified when associated with these other risk characteristics.

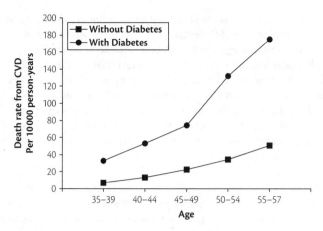

Fig. 9.2.9 CVD mortality and diabetes.
Source: Stamler *et al.* (1993).

It was believed that diabetes combined with the use of a high-fat, low-carbohydrate, and low-fibre diet increased vascular complications. It is now clear that the deleterious effects of the disease itself on the endothelium and coagulation abnormality play an important direct role (Sowers *et al.* 1994). It was also observed that diabetes is strongly associated with classical risk factors. People with diabetes have elevated levels of triglycerides and low-density lipoprotein cholesterol with decreased levels of high-density lipoprotein cholesterol. There is also a high prevalence of obesity and hypertension among people with diabetes (Lehto *et al.* 1997).

Cross-cultural comparisons present a more complicated picture. They indicate that factors other than the glucose insulin disorder itself result in atherosclerosis. Evidence is presented in the apparently low rates of atherosclerosis in diabetic Eastern Jews, Chinese, and south-west American Indians. The Pima Indians are a classical example of a population exposed to calorie abundance, excessive obesity, and diabetes, but little cardiovascular disease.

In healthy people, glucose intolerance alone is weak and inconsistently associated with cardiovascular disease risk. However, increased insulin levels were found to predict coronary heart disease in Australia, France, and Finland, and it is postulated to be the cause of excess coronary heart disease among South Asian immigrants to the United Kingdom (Hughes 1990).

The treatment of diabetes is based on control of blood glucose and treatment of associated risk factors. Lifestyle strategies, weight loss, and physical activity can be effective at reducing blood glucose and controlling the associated risk factors. This is particularly true in type II diabetes. For type I diabetes, insulin for glucose control and control of associated risk factors can reduce some diabetic complications.

Pharmacological control of type II diabetes has produced mixed results. The original University Group Diabetes Program reported an increased rate of myocardial infarction with the use of first-generation sulphonylureas in the setting of effective blood glucose control (UGDP 1975). Later trials with newer oral agents did not observe this complication (UKPDS 1995). The Diabetes Control and Complication Trial studied glucose control in insulin dependent diabetes. Microvascular complications were significantly reduced (DCCT Research Group 1993). Large vessel disease was also reduced, but the differences were not significant. More recently,

a meta-analysis of clinical trials of a popular oral hypoglycemic, rosiglitazone, revealed a significant increase in myocardial infarction and an increase in death from cardiovascular causes (Nissen & Wolski 2007).

The control of blood lipids in diabetes has been shown to be particularly effective in the setting of increased LDL cholesterol. This is true for primary prevention (Downs *et al.* 1998) and secondary prevention in type 2 diabetes (Pyorala *et al.* 1997; Goldberg *et al.* 1998).

The relationship between diabetes, atherosclerosis and coronary heart disease is well established in people with clinical diabetes living in affluent industrialized cultures. Data from other cultures suggest that other factors are at work. The use of lifestyle strategies, control of other risk factors and pharmacological measures in diabetes is the standard of care and may reduce cardiovascular complications of this disease.

Physical inactivity

Physical inactivity has assumed increasing importance as a risk factor for cardiovascular disease. As society has become more mechanized, sedentary lifestyle is the norm. Operating through other risk factors such as obesity, hypertension, hyperlipidaemia and diabetes, physical inactivity is associated with cardiovascular disease. However, it may be independently associated as well. Several important observations regarding physical inactivity include the following:

1. Physical inactivity is associated with acute myocardial infarction and sudden death both for the initial event and recurrent events. Regular activity is associated with reduced events.

2. Physical activity at work is declining.

3. Physical activity in leisure time, while increasing, is still not widespread.

4. Physical inactivity begins with declining exercise among youth as they reach teenage years.

5. Physical inactivity is associated with known risk factors including hyperlipidaemia, hypertension, diabetes mellitus, and obesity.

Two of the primary activities of human beings are obtaining and consuming food. Historically, this took considerable physical energy in hunting or farming activities, only a few very affluent were spared from activity. The past two centuries have witnessed a dramatic transition as farming has become more efficient. Mechanized transportation has eliminated the use of physical activity to move from place to place and in the workplace machines do most or all heavy labour. The result has been a rising tide of physical inactivity.

Much of the information on physical inactivity comes from observational studies. A meta-analysis of observational studies selected for quality, measurement and follow-up showed a significant and graded relationship between physical inactivity and the risk of first coronary heart disease event. They calculated a relative risk of 1.9 compared with sedentary individuals (Powell *et al.* 1987). The Multiple Risk Factor Intervention Trial of over 12 000 men demonstrated similar relationships with those with regular leisure time physical activity having lower risk of coronary heart disease and death (Leon *et al.* 1987) (Table 9.2.9). While there are many observational studies, there is general agreement that a primary prevention trial of physical activity is unlikely to be feasible and public health recommendations must come from available data.

Table 9.2.9 Mortality and leisure-time physical activity—men

End points	Tertile of LTPAs		
	1 (lowest)	2	3 (highest)
	Age-adjusted risk ratios		
CHD death	1.00	0.63‡(0.43–0.86)	0.64‡(0.47–0.88)
Sudden death	1.00	0.63‡(0.42–0.93)	0.65‡(0.44–0.96)
All-cause deaths	1.00	0.71‡(0.57–0.88)	0.83‡(0.67–1.01)

Source: Leon et al. (1987).

There are more data for secondary prevention. Observational studies find that individuals who continue with regular physical activity after myocardial infarction have lower relative risk than those who are sedentary (NIH 1996). These studies are confounded by disease severity associated both with physical inactivity and mortality. Those who are most ill are less likely to exercise and more likely to have increased recurrent events and mortality. For this reason, a number of randomized clinical trials of cardiac rehabilitation after myocardial infarction have been performed. These demonstrate lower mortality associated with exercise, but most studies have been small and underpowered. A meta-analysis by Oldridge et al. of 10 randomized trials found significant improvement associated with cardiac rehabilitation programmes lasting at least 6 weeks (Oldridge et al. 1988).

Physical activity is believed to function through a number of biological and physiological mechanisms. It operates through other cardiovascular risk factors including lipoproteins, carbohydrate metabolism, clotting factors, and obesity. It may result in lower blood pressure and aid in smoking cessation. In addition to its effects on other risk characteristics, physical activity is thought to increase epicardial artery diameter, increase coronary blood flow, and decrease myocardial work and oxygen demand. The heart may work more efficiently and be better able to function under stressful circumstances.

There is considerable debate over public health recommendations for physical activity. Some of the issues include the amount, type, and duration of physical activity needed to obtain beneficial cardiovascular effects. There is also the independent issue of fitness. Finally, the association of vigorous physical activity with sudden death has increased concerns regarding advice. Considering these factors, several recommendations have emerged in recent years (NIH 1996). These suggest that moderate physical activity such as brisk walking for 30 min on most days of the week is adequate to produce significant benefit in a sedentary society. More vigorous physical activity can be recommended; however, only moderate cardiovascular gains accrue from this addition (NIH 1996). The activity should be of sufficient vigour to increase the heart rate and breathing rate. Regular physical activity will lead to increased fitness; however, much of the association with fitness may be genetically determined rather than the result only of training (Blair et al. 1989). Nonetheless, observational studies do show that physical fitness is associated with lower rates of cardiovascular disease (Blair et al. 1989).

Finally, safety considerations are crucial in advising physical activity for individuals or public health recommendations. Research has shown an excess risk of sudden death during and shortly after strenuous exercise (Mittleman et al. 1993). However, the overall benefit of regular exercise far outweighs the acute excess risk.

Physical inactivity is epidemic in most industrialized societies and becoming more so in the developing world. It is associated with cardiovascular disease through myocardial infarction and sudden death. Regular physical activity involving daily exertion is an important public health recommendation. The type of physical activity recommended is that which involves large muscle groups for sustained periods of at least 30 min.

Psychosocial factors

Psychosocial factors including personality characteristics and the social environment are popularly believed to play an important role in cardiovascular disease. There are also many professionals who believe that these factors influence the major diseases of modern life. Despite this widespread belief, it has been difficult to demonstrate causal connections to coronary heart disease or other diseases. This may be due to difficulties in measurement, confounders, or less than convincing biological mechanisms. Nonetheless, emotional states of anger, aggression, fear, anxiety, and depression are associated with physiological changes which may affect cardiovascular disease. Certain personality types may precipitate or aggravate these factors. There are three major areas that have received attention and will be briefly discussed here. They are type A behaviour, hostility and social support.

Type A behaviour

Type A behaviour is characterized by aggressiveness, competitive drive, preoccupation with deadlines, and time urgency. Historically, it is measured by a structured interview (Friedman & Rosenman 1959). There are also other methods including self-reported inventories and questionnaires. Data in the 1980s found type A behaviour to be associated with coronary heart disease in the Western Collaborative Group Study and the Framingham Study (Rosenman et al. 1975; Haynes et al. 1980). In the Western Collaborative Group Study, a prospective cohort of 3000 men was assessed by the structured interview. The relative risk of fatal and non-fatal coronary heart disease was approximately 2 for type A men. The Framingham Study used a self-administered questionnaire to evaluate type A behaviour. Relative risk for coronary heart disease was similar to that found in the Western Collaborative Group Study (Haynes et al. 1980).

Following these initial observations, a number of other studies attempted to replicate these results. A summary of 14 angiography studies found an equal balance of positive and null associations (Dimsdale et al. 1981). Several larger prospective studies done in the 1980s failed to confirm earlier findings using either self-administered instruments or the structured interview (Case et al. 1985; Shekelle et al. 1985a,b). A reanalysis of the original Western Collaborative Group data also questioned the original results (Ragland & Brand 1988). In an intervention study to look at behaviour patterns and recurrent coronary heart disease, performed by the originators of the type A behaviour interview, coronary heart disease outcomes were reduced, but this study has not been replicated (Friedman et al. 1984).

Current evidence for type A behaviour is mixed and while there continues to be widespread belief about its importance, there is inadequate evidence to make public health or clinical recommendations regarding its detection and treatment.

Hostility

Initial enthusiasm about type A behaviour findings led to an attempt to find critical elements accounting for the observed coronary heart disease differences. Studies in selected groups found an association between hostility and coronary heart disease (Barefoot *et al.* 1983). Many studies used parts of the type A behaviour construct. Others used the Minnesota Multi-Phasic Personality Index and its 'Cook Medley Hostility Subscore'. Six prospective studies using the Cook Medley instrument have been published with three positive and three negative findings (Shekelle *et al.* 1983; McCranie *et al.* 1986; Hecker *et al.* 1988; Hearn *et al.* 1988; Leon *et al.* 1988; Barefoot *et al.* 1989).

Recent research suggests that anger or hostility is an acute rather than a chronic risk factor and associated with plaque rupture (Muller *et al.* 1997). This research may provide further insights into this characteristic.

Social support

A number of observational studies find social support or a supportive environment associated with lower coronary heart disease risk. Scandinavian studies found a strong relationship between social support and mortality in men (Orth-Gomer & Johnson 1987). Disentangling the role of social support from prevalent illness, economic factors and personality types is difficult but it is apparent from observational studies that those who report substantial support network, including a supportive spouse, have better coronary heart disease outcomes.

An intervention study of 2481 post MI patients (ENRICHD) evaluated cognitive behaviour therapy to improve social support (Berkman *et al.* 2003). Measures of psychosocial outcomes were significantly improved but there were no differences in recurrent myocardial infarction or mortality.

Acute coronary heart disease risk factors

Most of the risk factors discussed are associated with the underlying disease process, atherosclerosis. If atherosclerosis is prevented, then coronary heart disease, as a clinical event, is rare. However, since many individuals have atherosclerosis by middle-age or older years, there has been an increasing search for factors which lead to the transition from chronic atherosclerotic disease to acute ischaemia, myocardial infarction, and sudden death. These are indicators of sub-clinical arterial disease burden and acute risk factors or triggers.

There were two initial observations leading to these insights. The first related to the pathophysiology of the atherosclerotic plaque. While large and obstructing plaques are clearly related to disease, it was also found that small non-obstructive lesions can rupture, form a nidus for clot, and ultimately obstruct the coronary artery. This phenomenon was more likely to result in death than traditional obstructive lesions causing chronic ischaemia and angina pectoris (Fuster *et al.* 1992). The second observation was that of a morning peak in acute myocardial infarction, sudden death, and stroke. This suggested there were identifiable circumstances associated with disease manifestation (Muller *et al.* 1987). Further work in this field suggested that sympathetic stimulation with activation of clotting as a potential underlying mechanism. A number of factors were implicated. They included heavy exertion, sexual activity, anger, and other factors (Mittleman *et al.* 1993). Some of the characteristics are modified with aspirin use or β-blockers (Willich *et al.* 1993).

In summary, it is likely that more will be learned about these risk factors and treatment found to prevent events in individuals with established atherosclerotic disease. This should not be confused with true primary prevention where the atherosclerotic process is prevented.

Stroke risk factors

Risk factors for stroke can be broadly classified into non-modifiable risk factors such as age, gender, race and ethnicity, and genetic factors, and, modifiable risk factors such as hypertension, hyperlipidemia, smoking, diabetes, and others discussed below. There are several salient observations about stroke including:

1. Stroke rates vary between ethnic groups and countries as do stroke subtypes.

2. Hypertension is the strongest modifiable risk factor for stroke.

3. Drug treatment of hypertension can significantly reduce stroke incidence and recurrence.

Age

Stroke is a disease of older adults and advanced age is associated with increased stroke incidence, prevalence, and mortality. The United States Framingham study (Wolf *et al.* 1991) showed that the risk of stroke increased with age and that this increased risk persisted after adjustment for risk factors associated with increased age including blood pressure, diabetes, smoking, heart disease and atrial fibrillation. The adjusted relative risk for every decade increase in age after 55 years was 1.66 in men and 1.93 in women. This association with increased age has been shown in other geographic/ethnic cohorts. A population-based study from Taiwan estimated an annual incidence of 2.6/100 000 in those in the 36–44 years age group and 1417/100 000 in those aged 75 and older (Hu *et al.* 1992). Data from a stroke registry in Malmö, Sweden similarly showed incident stroke rates of 10/100 000 in those younger than 45 years of age to rates greater than 1700/100 000 in the very elderly (85 years and older) (Jerntrop *et al.* 1992). The association of increased stroke incidence with age is most marked for ischaemic stroke and intra-parenchymal haemorrhages and less so for strokes due to sub-arachnoid haemorrhages (Jerntrop *et al.* 1992). The rise in stroke incidence with age contributes to increased age-associated stroke prevalence and stroke mortality. For example, the stroke prevalence in the NHANES study increased from 0.5 per cent to those in the 20–39-year age category to 12-15 per cent among those in the 80+ age groups. Similarly, stroke mortality increased from 0.5 per 100 000 in those 15–24 years of age to 360/100 000 in those 65 years and older according to United States census data. This association of stroke risk with age has public health implications as the population ages.

Sex

Stroke incidence is higher in men with an overall male/female ratio ranging from 1.15 to 1.3 depending on the population studied (Sacco *et al.* 2001) There appears to be an age effect with the male/female difference shrinking or even reversing in older age groups (Brown *et al.* 1996). Stroke prevalence and mortality are also modestly higher in men than in women though stroke survival per se appears to be higher in men (Brown *et al.* 1996).

Geography and ethnicity

Stroke mortality shows a wide geographic variation with the highest rates reported in Eastern European countries (Fig. 9.2.10)

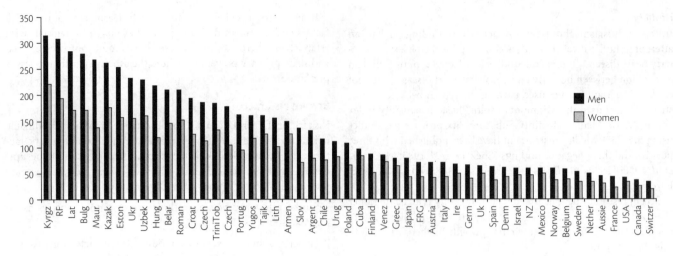

Fig. 9.2.10 Age-standardized stroke mortality per 100 000 men and women in the 1990s.
Source: Sarti *et al.* (2000).

(Sarti *et al.* 2000). The high mortality is a reflection of both higher incidences as well as higher case fatality rates (WHO 2003). There are ethnic differences in stroke mortality even within the same geographical area. For example, there is an excess of stroke mortality among African-Americans compared to Whites in the United States, even after adjustment for county of residence (Howard *et al.* 2001). Stroke mortality has continued to decline in many western countries over the last few decades though a few eastern European countries have shown a rising mortality trend (WHO 2003).

The distribution of stroke subtypes shows geographic and ethnic differences as well. For example, in the United States, pooled data from various population-based studies estimate that ischaemic strokes comprise 87 per cent of all strokes and haemorrhagic strokes comprise the remaining 13 per cent (AHA 2007). Studies from Japan (Sankai *et al.* 1991) and China (Zhang *et al.* 2003) have shown an estimated higher proportion of haemorrhagic strokes in those populations, in the range of 30–48 per cent. An epidemiological study from Malmö, Sweden examined the relative proportion of different subtypes in sub-populations defined by country of birth. This study found that while 12 per cent of all strokes were haemorrhages in those born in Sweden, up to 34 per cent were haemorrhages in immigrants to Malmö who were born in China (Khan *et al.* 2004). These variations in geographic and ethnic groups may be due to different risk profiles including genetic, dietary, or other environmental factors.

Genetic factors

Various genetic epidemiological studies have shown familial aggregation of stroke, though, many traditional stroke risk factors such as diabetes, hypertension, hyperlipidemia and cardiac disease also aggregate in families. Brass *et al.* (1992) analysed male twin pairs and found a fivefold increase in stroke prevalence in monozygotic twins compared to dizygotic twins. The Danish Twin study on the other hand reported a more modest effect in the range of 2.1 for relative risk of stroke death in mono vs. dizygotic twins (Bak *et al.* 2002). A recent systematic review focusing on ischaemic stroke also suggests a modest effect with monozygotic twins being 1.6 times more likely to be concordant for stroke than dizygotic twins (Flossmann *et al.* 2004). Many of the twin studies did not subtype stroke and this may have diluted the effect. There are

well-documented monogenic disorders associated with stroke such as the Notch-3 mutation on chromosome 19 leading to cerebral autosomal dominant arteriopathy with subcortical infarcts and leukoencephalopathy, the Icelandic form of amyloid angiopathy due to a Cystatin C point mutation on chromosome 20 associated with hereditary intra-cerebral haemorrhage. However, the overall contribution of monogenic disorders to the burden of stroke appears to be small (Sacco *et al.* 2001). The exact contribution of genetic factors to stroke risk as well as the interaction of genetic and environmental factors is still under investigation.

Hypertension

Hypertension is the most important modifiable stroke risk factor. The age-adjusted relative risk for stroke was increased at least 3-fold in hypertension with a blood pressure ≥ 160/95 and 1.5-fold with blood pressure between 140/90 and 160/95 (Wolf *et al.* 1998). The stroke risk is proportional to the level of hypertension. The Framingham study estimated the relative risk of stroke associated with every 10 mmHg increase in systolic blood pressure was 1.9 for men and 1.7 for women, even after adjustment for other risk factors (Wolf *et al.* 1991). Hypertension increases the risk in both ischaemic and haemorrhagic strokes. Both systolic and diastolic blood pressure levels are related to increased stroke risk. In people with diastolic hypertension (diastolic BP ≥ 95 mmHg) increase in levels of systolic blood pressure is associated with increased stroke risk. However, the converse is not true. In patients with systolic hypertension (systolic BP ≥ 160 mmHg) stroke risk does not increase with increasing levels of diastolic blood pressure (Wolf *et al.* 1998). Control of hypertension has been shown to reduce the risk of stroke in multiple clinical trials using a wide variety of anti-hypertensive agents. A review of eighteen long-term clinical trials examining beta-blockers and diuretics found that low-dose diuretics, high-dose diuretics and beta-blockers were all effective in reducing stroke risk when compared to placebo. The relative risk of stroke for various anti-hypertensive agents versus placebo ranged from 0.49 to 0.71 (Psaty *et al.* 1997). Other studies have shown angiotensin converting enzyme inhibitors, angiotensin receptor blockers and calcium channel blockers to be effective in reducing stroke risk in people with hypertension. The treatment of isolated systolic hypertension in the elderly has been shown to reduce overall stroke risk as well as the risk of ischaemic and haemorrhagic strokes separately (Perry *et al.* 2000; Staessen *et al.* 1997). The INDANA meta-analysis showed that blood pressure lowering drug interventions reduced the risk of stroke recurrence in stroke survivors consistently across multiple studies, (relative risk of stroke in those treated with anti-hypertensive therapy versus placebo controls = 0.72).

Diabetes

Diabetes mellitus is an independent risk factor for ischaemic stroke. The Honolulu Heart Program found a twofold increase in the relative risk of thrombo-embolic stroke in those with diabetes mellitus compared to those without even after adjustment for other risk factors (Abbott *et al.* 1987). There was no association between diabetes and haemorrhagic stroke. Similarly, the Framingham study showed diabetes to be an independent risk factor for stroke with a relative risk ranging from 1.4 to 1.7 (Wolf *et al.* 1991). Tight glycemic control in both type 1 and type 2 diabetes has been shown to delay the onset of microvascular complications such as diabetic retinopathy, nephropathy and neuropathy (UKPDS 1998; DCCT 1993). The effect of such glycemic control on stroke prevention has not been reported though recent results from the Diabetes Control and Complications Trial indicate significant reduction in a combined end-point of non-fatal myocardial infarction, stroke, or cardiovascular death with intensive diabetes therapy in patients with Type I diabetes (risk reduction 57 per cent; Nathan *et al.* 2005). The United Kingdom Prospective Diabetes Study showed that tight blood pressure control reduced stroke risk by 44 per cent in patients with type 2 diabetes (UKPDS 1998). Other studies have shown the beneficial effect of angiotensin converting enzyme inhibitors and angiotensin receptor blockers in reducing cardiovascular mortality and stroke rates in patients with diabetes (HOPE 2000; Dahlof *et al.* 2002).

Blood lipids

The relationship between lipid levels and stroke risk is complex and the nature of the relationship varies by stroke subtype. There is epidemiological evidence for increased haemorrhagic stroke risk with very low cholesterol levels. The Honolulu Heart Study showed that there was an inverse relationship between serum cholesterol levels and the risk of intra-cranial haemorrhage after adjustment for other risk factors (Kagan *et al.* 1980). Similar results were reported in a 10-year study of a rural population from Japan (Tanaka *et al.* 1982) and in the Multiple Risk Factor Intervention Trial (Iso *et al.* 1989). The MRFIT trial showed an interaction between high diastolic blood pressure and low serum cholesterol. The relation between total cholesterol and ischaemic stroke has been equivocal. There was a modest association between elevated serum cholesterol and thrombo-embolic stroke in the Honolulu Heart Program with a relative risk of 1.4 between the highest and lowest cholesterol quartiles (Benfante *et al.* 1994). The Framingham study did not find a significant relationship between ischaemic stroke and total cholesterol or its sub-fractions (Wolf *et al.* 1991). Other studies have shown associations between cholesterol sub-fractions and ischaemic stroke. The Northern Manhattan Stroke Study and the Oxfordshire Community Study both found a protective effect of high HDL-cholesterol levels on ischaemic stroke risk (Sacco *et al.* 2001; Qizilbash *et al.* 1991). Extra-cranial carotid atherosclerosis, an important risk factor for ischaemic stroke has been shown to be associated with elevated LDL-cholesterol levels and inversely related to HDL-cholesterol levels (Salonen *et al.* 1988). The recently published Stroke Prevention by Aggressive Reduction in Cholesterol Levels trial showed that treatment with a 3-hydroxy-3-methylglutaryl coenzyme A reductase inhibitor (atorvastatin) reduced the risk of recurrent strokes despite a small increase in the incidence of haemorrhagic stroke (Amarenco *et al.* 2006).

Cardiovascular disease

Cardiovascular disease is an independent risk factor for stroke with a relative risk estimated at 1.7 after adjustment for other risk factors (Wolf *et al.* 1991). Cardiovascular disease is primarily associated with ischaemic stroke. Specific entities associated with stroke include atrial fibrillation, coronary artery disease, acute myocardial infarction, congestive heart failure, dilated cardiomyopathy, significant right-to-left intra-cardiac shunts, left ventricular hypertrophy, and valvular heart disease. Atrial fibrillation, an independent risk factor for stroke, is estimated to increase the ischaemic stroke risk 5-fold. Rheumatic heart disease with mitral and tricuspid valvular involvement is the most common pre-disposing factor for atrial fibrillation in developing countries where rheumatic fever is common (Vora 2006). In contrast, atrial fibrillation is a disease related to atherosclerosis in western countries. For example, in the United States where rheumatic heart disease is uncommon, the incidence of atrial fibrillation in the United States ranges from less than 1 per 1000 patient years in those under 40–19.2 per 1000 patient years in those over 65. The aging of the population and the improved survival after myocardial infarction has led to projections of an increased atrial fibrillation burden in developed countries over the next few decades (Go *et al.* 2001). The risk of thromboembolism in atrial fibrillation patients with rheumatic valvular heart disease is in the order of 17–18 per cent per year (Vora 2006). In non-rheumatic atrial fibrillation, stroke risk varies from <2 per cent per year in otherwise healthy individuals in the 50–59 age range to over 10 per cent in the elderly in the presence of other co-morbidities such as hypertension and diabetes mellitus. Warfarin anti-coagulation has been shown to reduce stroke risk by 60–65 per cent in unselected patients with non-valvular atrial fibrillation and such anti-coagulation is recommended in eligible patients with risk factors for thromboembolism (Hart *et al.* 2003). This therapy, however, remains under-utilized (Lakshminarayan *et al.* 2006).

Cigarette smoking

Tobacco smoking is a worldwide problem, and cigarettes are associated with a substantial increase in stroke risk. The effect of tobacco smoking on stroke risk varies by stroke sub-type. Comparing current smokers to never smokers in the Nurses Health Study, Kawachi *et al.* estimate an adjusted relative risk of 4.85 for sub-arachnoid haemorrhage, 2.53 for ischaemic stroke and 1.24 for cerebral haemorrhage (Kawachi *et al.* 1993). A meta-analysis examining cigarette smoking and stroke risk also estimates a higher relative risk for sub-arachnoid haemorrhage compared (2.9), compared to ischaemic stroke (1.9) and intra-cerebral haemorrhage (0.7). The stroke risk due to tobacco smoking declines after smoking cessation and approaches that of non-smokers 2–4 years post-cessation.

Alcohol

Like tobacco smoking, the association between alcohol consumption and stroke risk appears to vary by stroke subtype. The Honolulu Heart Program study showed that both light and heavy alcohol use were associated with a significant increase in haemorrhagic stroke risk after adjustment for other risk factors (relative risk 2–3 compared to non-drinkers). The association was stronger for sub-arachnoid haemorrhages. In contrast, moderate alcohol consumption (up to two drinks per day) was associated with a decreased ischaemic stroke risk (odds ratio 0.51) in the NOMASS study (Sacco *et al.* 1999). The NOMASS study also found an increased risk of ischaemic stroke associated with heavy alcohol use (odds ratio 2.96) and the data suggested a J-shaped relation between alcohol consumption and ischaemic stroke risk.

Physical activity

Physical activity has been shown to reduce stroke risk in both men and women. The Framingham study showed that medium and high levels of physical activity were protective against stroke when compared to low levels of activity, but did not show a similar protective effect in women (Kiely *et al.* 1994). The Nurses Health Study however showed that physical activity was associated with a significant reduction in the risk of total stroke as well as ischaemic stroke and that the reduction was dose-related, i.e. the effect was more substantial at higher levels of activity (Hu *et al.* 2000).

Heart failure

Heart failure is a clinical constellation of signs and symptoms resulting from circulatory and neural responses to cardiac dysfunction. It is increasing in prevalence in many areas of the world. Manifest by inadequate pumping ability by the heart, heart failure can have multiple underlying aetiologies including ischaemic heart disease, hypertension, non-ischaemic cardiomyopathy, infection, diabetes mellitus, and others (Cowie *et al.* 1999). Several observations about the population patterns of include:

1. Population prevalence of heart failure is directly related to the prevalence and types of underlying cardiovascular conditions. Coronary heart disease is a leading cause in developed countries.

2. Population rates of heart failure vary widely because of the differing definitions and classification systems used to describe cases.

3. Population levels of heart failure are rising as more individuals survive acute myocardial infarction and chronic hypertension.

4. Heart failure is predominantly a disease of older adults and the mortality is similar to serious cancers.

5. Treatment of heart failure has improved as randomized clinical trials have demonstrated the utility of new drugs.

Research into heart failure is hampered by variability in case definition. Symptoms, signs, radiological studies, tests of ventricular performance, and tests of exercise capacity have all been utilized. All methods have limitations and are particularly poor in the classification of mild heart failure. The diagnosis may be commonly confused with obesity-related dyspnoea, poor physical condition, myocardial ischaemia, pulmonary disease, or other conditions.

There are several studies of heart failure incidence. The Framingham Study and the Gothenberg Study are examples of the cohort approach (Eriksson *et al.* 1989; Ho *et al.* 1993a). These were able to identify incident cases prospectively and characterize them at the time of diagnosis. Studies in Finland, Holland, and Rochester, Minnesota, are examples of a population approach (Mosterd *et al.* 1999; Remes *et al.* 1992; Senni *et al.* 1998). These studies find

significant differences in incidence, which ranges from 100 to 500 per 100 000 population per year, and that incidence increases sharply with age.

There are more data available on heart failure prevalence. Rates also vary widely due to differences in methodology and case definition. Observed prevalence in industrialized societies ranges from 300 to 2000 individuals per 100 000 population (unadjusted for age) and 3000 to 13 000 per 100 000 population for those over the age of 65 years (Cowie *et al.* 1997). Of particular interest are the data from the American National Health Interview Survey which show a self-report prevalence ranging from 0.1 per cent for adults aged 18–39 to 5.5 per cent for those 75 years and above (Ni 2003). Self-report may underestimate true prevalence. Heart failure prevalence appears to be rising, largely attributed to increased survival from acute myocardial infarction (Graves & Gillum 1996).

Mortality from heart failure is substantial with the Framingham Study reporting 5-year survival of 25 per cent for men and 38 per cent for women in an early analysis (Ho *et al.* 1993b). Among individuals with heart failure (age greater than 55 years), 61 per cent of women and 28 per cent of men were still alive 15 years later. However, the validity of heart failure diagnosis on death certificates has been questioned (Cowie *et al.* 1997). Because heart failure is a constellation of signs, symptoms and physiological changes, it is often not considered among the underlying causes of death. For example, in the United Kingdom, heart failure is never used as an underlying cause of death (Cowie *et al.* 1997). In the United States, heart failure is categorized as a cause of death and rose from 10 000 in 1968 to 58 000 deaths in 2004 (NHLBI 2006).

Previously, hypertension was the most common underlying cause of heart failure, but there has been a shift to coronary heart disease as a more common aetiology. Hypertensive cardiovascular disease with left ventricular hypertrophy results in a 15-fold greater risk of developing heart failure (Kannel *et al.* 1994). Coronary heart disease, particularly when manifested as myocardial infarction, also leads to increased heart failure with damaged and dysfunctional myocardial muscle. In the Framingham Study, approximately 20 per cent of those who survived myocardial infarction developed heart failure within 5–6 years (Kannel 1987). Diabetes mellitus with heart failure also increased in prevalence (Ho *et al.* 1993a; Levy *et al.* 1996; Davis *et al.* 1997). While these are the major causes of heart failure in industrialized societies, in many nations other diseases play an important role including rheumatic heart disease, cardiomyopathy and pulmonary heart disease.

As most heart failure is a late consequence of an underlying cardiovascular disease, primary treatment should consist of prevention of that underlying disease whether it is hypertension, coronary heart disease, rheumatic heart disease, or other conditions. If these conditions are adequately controlled, heart failure is uncommon. However, there are currently many individuals with these diseases who have heart failure as the primary cause of their limitation and disability. Treatment with diuretics and digitalis are widely used, however, these are aided by modern drugs (Cohn 1996). In recent clinical trials, heart failure treated with vasodilators, beta blockers and angiotensin-converting enzyme inhibitors has reduced mortality and increased function, leading to optimism for long-term therapy for heart failure (Johnson *et al.* 1993; Cohn 1996).

Rheumatic fever and heart disease

For centuries, rheumatic fever with resulting rheumatic heart disease was the leading cause of cardiovascular morbidity and mortality worldwide. It continues as an important problem in areas where poverty, overcrowding, malnutrition, and lack of medical care are found (Hanna *et al.* 2005; Kurahara *et al.* 2006; WHO 2004). Although much less common than previously, it is still a problem even in industrialized countries where outbreaks can occur.

During the 1960s, the incidence of acute rheumatic fever ranged from 23 to 55 per 100 000 urban children aged 2–14 years in the United States. Currently, it is less than 2 per 100 000 with a prevalence of rheumatic heart disease of less than 1 per 1000 school-aged children (Dajani 1991). In other parts of the industrialized world, such as Scandinavia, similar low rates are found (WHO 1988). However, in some areas of South America, the prevalence of acute rheumatic fever is significantly higher, ranging from 1 to 10 per cent of school-aged children (PAHO 1970). Similar high rates are seen in areas of Asia and Africa (WHO 2004). Reported prevalence of rheumatic heart disease in school children in these areas ranges from 1 to 78/1000 (WHO 2004). The mechanisms by which this infection produces the clinical syndrome of acute rheumatic fever and subsequent rheumatic heart disease is well studied (WHO 2004). A group A streptococcal infection of the throat (tonsillopharyngitis) can be followed, in approximately 3 weeks, by an episode of acute rheumatic fever. In outbreak situations, rheumatic fever occurs in up to 3 per cent of those with a throat infection; however, it is usually much lower (Siegel *et al.* 1961). The rheumatic fever attack results in an inflammatory reaction which involves the heart, joints and/or the central nervous system. Of those with acute rheumatic fever, at least 50 per cent develop some manifestation of carditis, and this proportion rises when more sophisticated diagnostic methods are used (Dajani 1991). The diagnosis of acute rheumatic fever is made principally from the clinical findings using the revised Jones Criteria. These include combinations of the major manifestations of carditis, polyarthritis, chorea, erythema marginatum, and/or subcutaneous nodules. Other manifestations include arthralgias and fever. Laboratory findings of acute phase reactants including elevated erythrocyte sedimentation rate and C-reactive proteins are common. A positive throat culture for streptococcal antigen and/or increased streptococcal antibody titre aid in making the diagnosis. These criteria may not be sufficiently sensitive in industrialized countries where clinical patterns have changed significantly so that arthritis may be the only presentation. In addition, a significant portion of individuals do not have a symptomatic preceding infection (Wannamaker 1973).

Rapid antigen tests for the diagnosis of group A streptococcal throat infections are highly specific, but less sensitive. While a positive test suggests the need for treatment, a negative test indicates the need for a throat culture (Dajani *et al.* 1995). Antibody tests can confirm a recent group A streptococcal infection.

Primary prevention of acute rheumatic fever is the recommended approach. Throat cultures should be performed on all patients with tonsillopharyngitis and those with a positive culture for group A streptococcal infections treated (Dajani *et al.* 1995). Antibiotic treatment can effectively prevent acute rheumatic fever even when given up to 9 days from the onset of the infection (Denny *et al.* 1950). The recommended treatment schedule by the American Heart Association is found at http://www.americanheart.org. Antibiotic treatment can be either oral or by injection.

In individuals with a history of acute rheumatic fever, the likelihood of secondary attacks with additional damage is common, estimated to be approximately 50 per cent of those with streptococcal infections. For this reason, prophylaxis with an antibiotic is recommended (Dajani *et al.* 1995).

If group A streptococcal infections are appropriately detected and treated, rheumatic heart disease can be effectively prevented. In those where it is not prevented, lifelong valvular heart disease results in diminishing function and premature mortality.

Congenital heart disease

Malformations of the heart and cardiovascular system present at birth are among the more common of congenital defects. They are the result of genetic and/or environmental factors. These malformations frequently have significant haemodynamic consequences and may result in severe illness and/or death (Friedman 1997).

Congenital heart disease includes a wide variety of malformations of the cardiovascular system including the septal, heart valve, and great vessels defects. The true incidence of moderate-to-severe congenital heart disease is difficult to determine but approximates 6 per 1000 live births in the United States (Friedman 1997; Hoffman & Kaplan 2002). This is probably an underestimate, as much congenital heart disease is not discovered until adulthood, is mild, or is fatal prior to birth (Hoffman & Kaplan 2002). In addition, the 0.6 per cent incidence does not include mitral valve prolapse or non-obstructive bicuspid aortic valves, both of which are common. Males are more likely to have congenital heart disease than females, but the pattern differs by defect type (Samanck 1994).

Genetic transmission plays an important role in congenital heart disease. Family studies find that the offspring of parents with congenital heart disease have an increased malformation incidence ranging from 1.4 to 16.1 per cent (Ferencz 1986). Identical twins are both affected 25–30 per cent of the time. However, despite the known genetic clustering and the identification of disorders associated with single genes, it is estimated that only 10 per cent of congenital heart disease has an identifiable genetic origin (Noonan 1978).

Maternal infections are an important etiology of congenital heart disease. Rubella is commonly implicated when it occurs in the first 2 months of pregnancy with congenital malformations in about 80 per cent of live births. Subclinical maternal Coxsackie and other virus infections are also implicated in congenital heart disease.

There are many exposures associated with increased incidence of congenital heart disease. Acute hypoxia, residence at high altitudes, high carboxyhaemoglobin levels and cigarette smoking are among potential causes. X-ray exposure is associated with Down syndrome and other congenital defects. Metabolic defects including diabetes and phenylketonuria are associated with increases in congenital defects.

Diet- and drug-associated exposures are also implicated. They include the well-known examples of thalidomide and folic acid antagonists. Dextroamphetamines, anticonvulsants, lithium chloride, alcohol and progesterone/oestrogen are suspected as teratogens acting in the first trimester of pregnancy. Certain pesticides and herbicides are implicated (Zierler 1985).

The overall incidence of congenital heart disease appears to have remained stable although the distribution of defect types may be changing. There are unexplained increases in ventricular septal defect and patent ductus arteriosis. Rubella-related disease is declining, perhaps the result of widespread vaccination for that disease.

The most effective strategy for congenital heart disease is prevention including genetic counselling for families with congenital heart disease, rubella immunization, and avoidance of exposure to known teratogens. Of particular importance are avoidance of alcohol abuse and cigarette smoking.

For many that were born with congenital heart disease, modern medical and surgical techniques can provide palliation, if not a cure. For the most severe cases, heart and heart–lung transplants are assuming increasing importance.

Cardiomyopathy and myocarditis

Cardiomyopathy and myocarditis are a diverse set of diseases that have, as a central feature, pathological involvement of the heart muscle. Heart failure is the frequent outcome of this condition. Cardiomyopathies account for a substantial portion of cardiovascular disease related deaths in developing countries. However, they are becoming more common in industrialized nations with increasing rates of ischaemic cardiomyopathy associated with coronary heart disease.

There are numerous known causes of myopathy as detailed in a recent report by the WHO (Richardson *et al.* 1996). The WHO advocates that the term 'cardiomyopathy' be reserved for myocardial dysfunction of unknown aetiology; however, it is commonly applied even when the aetiology is known (Richardson *et al.* 1996).

The natural history of cardiomyopathy varies according to the type. Many cases begin with an acute phase where inflammation of the myocardium is common (myocarditis). The widespread use of endomyocardial biopsy has been of some assistance in identifying and classifying myocarditis (Fowles 1985). In many cases, the initial myocarditis is probably undetected because it is mild. There are clinical courses ranging from minimal heart failure to a brief rapid course leading to death. Investigators at the Mayo Clinic in Olmsted County, Minnesota, found an incidence of idiopathic dilated cardiomyopathy of 6 per 100 000 person years (Shabeter 1983). Overall prevalence in the United States was 35.3 per 100 000 population (Gillum 1986).

The prevalence of cardiomyopathy appears to be increasing in the United States. However, it is uncertain whether this is an actual increase or improved diagnostic methods and greater clinical sensitivity. For many cases, a specific cause is not known.

Cardiomyopathy is grouped into three major types: (a) dilated, characterized by dilatation of the ventricles and contractual dysfunction with heart failure; (b) hypertrophic, with left ventricular hypertrophy and well-preserved cardiac function; (c) restrictive, with impaired diastolic filling frequently due to scarring of the myocardium of the ventricle. The dilated cardiomyopathy pattern is most commonly observed, although there is considerable overlap between types (Keren & Popp 1992).

Alcohol abuse is an important environmental cause of cardiomyopathy in the United States accounting for approximately 8 per cent of all cases (Okada & Wakafuji 1985). This may operate through a direct toxic effect, thiamine deficiency, or additives such as cobalt in alcoholic beverages. Abstinence may halt or reverse this disease (Okada & Wakafuji 1985). Viral infections are a very commonly observed cause of cardiomyopathy. Coxsackie virus, echo virus,

influenza, and polio are frequently implicated (Levine 1979). These diseases begin as acute myocarditis and then progress to a chronic condition which results in dilated cardiomyopathy.

Hypertrophic cardiomyopathy is detected by the use of echocardiographic techniques. This condition uncommonly causes difficulty for patients and is usually well managed with medication (Wigle 1988). Chagas' disease is caused by the protozoan *Trypanosoma cruzi*. Beginning as a myocarditis, its clinical manifestations are manifest many years later. The disease is most prevalent in Central and South America with over 20 million thought to be infected with the parasite (Morris *et al.* 1990; Hagar & Rahimtoola 1995). This disease may also be found in non-endemic areas through migration, contaminated blood products and tourism (Hagar & Rahimtoola 1995). Treatment is available for the acute parasitic infections; however, the cardiomyopathy cannot be directly treated.

Schistosomiasis is a parasitic infection epidemic in the Nile and Yangtze basins. It may involve a majority of the population in certain endemic areas. Chronic pulmonary embolization of the parasite leads to pulmonary hypertension, right ventricular hypertrophy and right ventricular heart failure. Direct involvement of the myocardium is rare. New medications can be of assistance in controlling the infection and prevention is the principal strategy employed.

Prevention programmes for cardiovascular disease and stroke

Research in the prevention of cardiovascular diseases and stroke at the individual level resulted in more advanced programmes at the individual and community level than any other chronic disease. Core to this understanding is the risk factor model and the identification of disease predictors using epidemiological techniques. The finding of modifiable risk factors such as hypertension and demonstration of modification by interventions forms the basis for causality, treatment, and public policy recommendations. The demonstration of environmental and behavioural factors in the genesis of increased disease risk also points to specific strategies. For the high-risk individual patient, smoking cessation, blood pressure control, and cholesterol reduction form the basis of medical therapy to prevent disease events. For the high-risk community, facilitation of smoke-free buildings, healthy diets, regular physical activity are among the prevention strategies (Farquhar *et al.* 1990; Luepker *et al.* 1994; Carleton *et al.* 1995; Puska *et al.* 1995). The dramatic reduction in cardiovascular disease and stroke observed in some industrialized countries is directly linked to community wide and individual patient changes.

Summary

Cardiovascular disease and stroke is a leading cause of morbidity and mortality worldwide. While rates are declining in some industrialized nations, they are rising in the developing world resulting in a continued epidemic. Much is known about the prevention of cardiovascular disease and stroke. The major risk factors are known and effective interventions at the community and individual levels available. If these preventive strategies were widely applied, the epidemic could be controlled. There is an important role for public health in the prevention of cardiovascular disease and stroke.

References

Abbott R.D., Donahue R.P., MacMahon S.W. *et al.* (1987). Diabetes and the risk of stroke. The Honolulu Heart Program. *Journal of the American Medical Association*, **257**, 949.

Abbott R.D., Sharp D.S., Burchfiel C.M. *et al.* (1997). Cross-sectional and longitudinal changes in total and high-density-lipoprotein cholesterol levels over a 20-year period in elderly men: the Honolulu Heart Program. *Annals of Epidemiology*, **7**, 417–24.

Amarenco P., Bogousslavsky J., Callahan A. *et al.* (2006). High-dose Atorvastatin after stroke or transient ischemic attack. *New England Journal of Medicine*, **355**, 549.

American Heart Association (2007). *Heart Disease and Stroke Statistics - 2007 Update*. Dallas, Texas.

Arnett D.K., Jacobs Jr., D.R., Luepker R.V. *et al.* (2005). Twenty-year trends in serum cholesterol, hypercholesterolemia, and cholesterol medication use: the Minnesota Heart Survey, 1980-1982 to 2000-2002. *Circulation*, **112**, 3884–91.

Ascherio A. and Hunter D.J. (1994). Iron and myocardial infarction. *Epidemiology*, **5**, 135–7.

Ascherio A., Hennekens C.H., Buring J.E. *et al.* (1994). Trans-fatty acids intake and risk of myocardial infarction. *Circulation*, **89**, 94–101.

Ascherio A., Rimm E.B., Hernan M.A. *et al.* (1999). Relation of consumption of vitamin E, vitamin C, and carotenoids to risk for stroke among men in the United States. *Annals of Internal Medicine*, **130**, 963–70.

Bak S., Gaist D., Sindrup S.H. *et al.* (2002). Genetic liability in stroke: a long-term follow-up study of Danish twins. *Stroke*, **33**, 769.

Barefoot J.C., Dahlstrom W.G., and Williams R.B. (1983). Hostility, coronary heart disease incidence and total mortality: a 25-year follow-up study of 255 physicians. *Psychosomatic Medicine*, **45**, 59–63.

Barefoot J.C., Dodge K.A., Peterson B.L. *et al.* (1989). The Cook-Medley hostility scale: item content and ability to predict survival. *Psychosomatic Medicine*, **51**, 46–57.

Benfante R., Yano K., Hwang L.J. *et al.* (1994). Elevated serum cholesterol is a risk factor for both coronary heart disease and thromboembolic stroke in Hawaiian Japanese men. Implications of shared risk. *Stroke*, **25**, 814.

Berkman L.F., Blumenthal J., Burg M. *et al.* (2003) Effects of treating depression and low perceived social support on clinical events after myocardial infarction: the Enhancing Recovery in Coronary Heart Disease Patients (ENRICHD) Randomized Trial. *Journal of the American Medical Association*, **289**, 3106–16.

Blackburn H. and Jacobs D. (1984). Sources of the diet–heart controversy: confusion over population versus individual correlations. *Circulation*, **70**, 775–80.

Blackburn H. and Prineas R.J. (1983). Diet and hypertension: anthropology, epidemiology, and public health implications. *Progress in Biochemical Pharmacology*, **19**, 31–79.

Blair S.N., Kohl H.W., Paffenbarger Jr R.S. *et al.* (1989). Physical fitness and all-cause mortality: a prospective study of healthy men and women. *Journal of the American Medical Association*, **262**, 2395–401.

Bonaa K.H., Njolstad I., Ueland P.M. *et al.* (2006). Homocysteine lowering and cardiovascular events after acute myocardial infarction. *New England Journal of Medicine*, **354**, 1578–88.

Boushey C.J., Beresford S.A., Omenn G.S. *et al.* (1995). A quantitative assessment of plasma homocysteine as a risk factor for vascular disease. Probable benefits of increasing folic acid intakes. *Journal of the American Medical Association*, **274**, 1049–57.

Brass L.M., Isaacsohn J.L., Merikangas K.R. *et al.* (1992). A study of twins and stroke. *Stroke*, **23**, 221.

Brown R.D., Whisnant J.P., Sicks J.D. *et al.* (1996). Stroke incidence, prevalence, and survival: secular trends in Rochester, Minnesota, through 1989. *Stroke*, **27**, 373.

Buchwald H., Matts J.P., Fitch L.L. *et al.* for the Program on the Surgical Control of the Hyperlipidemias (POSCH) Group (1992). Changes in sequential coronary arteriograms and subsequent coronary events. *Journal of the American Medical Association*, **268**, 1429–33.

Buchwald H., Varco R.L., Matts J.P. *et al.* (1990). Effective lipid modification by partial ileal bypass reduced long-term coronary heart disease mortality and morbidity: five year post-trial follow-up report from POSCH. *New England Journal of Medicine*, **323**, 946–55.

Canner P.L., Berge K.G., Wenger N.K. *et al.* (1986). Fifteen year mortality in Coronary Drug Project patients: long-term benefit with niacin. *Journal of the American College of Cardiology*, **8**, 1245–55.

Carleton R.A., Lasater T.M., Assaf A.R. *et al.* and the Pawtucket Heart Health Program Writing Group (1995). The Pawtucket Heart Health Program: community changes in cardiovascular risk factors and projected disease risk. *American Journal of Public Health*, **85**, 777–85.

Carroll M.D., Lacher D.A., Sorlie P.D. *et al.* (2005). Trends in serum lipids and lipoproteins of adults, 1960–2002. *Journal of the American Medical Association*, **294**, 1773–81.

Case R.B., Heller S.S., Case N.B. *et al.* (1985). Type A behavior and survival after acute myocardial infarction. *New England Journal of Medicine*, **312**, 737–41.

Centers for Disease Control and Prevention, National Center for Health Statistics. National Health and Nutrition Examination Survey (NHANES): NHANES I, II, III, 1999–2000 and 2001–2002.

Chobanian A.V., Bakris G.L., Black H.R. *et al.* (2003). Seventh report of the Joint National Committee on Prevention, Detection, Evaluation, and Treatment of High Blood Pressure. *Journal of the American Medical Association*, **289**, 2560–2571.

Cohn J.N. (1996). The management of chronic heart failure. *New England Journal of Medicine*, **335**, 490–8.

Colditz G.A. (1990). A prospective assessment of moderate alcohol intake and major chronic diseases. *Annals of Epidemiology*, **1**, 167–77.

Cowie M.R., Mosterd A., Wood D.A. *et al.* (1997). The epidemiology of heart failure. *European Heart Journal*, **18**, 208–25.

Cowie M.R., Wood D.A., Coats A.J. *et al.* (1999). Incidence and aetiology of heart failure; a population-based study. *European Heart Journal*, **20**, 421–8.

Criqui M.H. (1987). The roles of alcohol in the epidemiology of cardiovascular diseases. *Acta Medica Scandinavica*, **717** (Suppl), 73–85.

Dahlof B., Devereux R.B., Kjeldsen S.E. *et al.* (2002). Cardiovascular morbidity and mortality in the Losartan Intervention For Endpoint reduction in hypertension study (LIFE): a randomised trial against atenolol.see comment. *Lancet*, **359**, 995.

Dajani A., Taubert K., Ferrieri P. *et al.* (1995). Treatment of acute streptococcal pharyngitis and prevention of rheumatic fever: a statement for health professionals. Committee on Rheumatic Fever, Endocarditis, and Kawasaki Disease of the Council on Cardiovascular Disease in the Young, The American Heart Association. *Pediatrics*, **96**, 758–64.

Dajani A.S. (1991). Current status of nonsupportive complications of group A streptococci. *Pediatric Infectious Disease Journal*, **105**, S25–7.

Dattilo A.M. and Kris-Etherton P.M. (1992). Effects of weight reduction on blood lipids and lipoproteins: a meta-analysis. *American Journal of Clinical Nutrition*, **56**, 320–8.

Davis R.C., Hobbs F.D.R., McLeod S. *et al.* (1997). Heart failure prevalence in patients in 'high-risk' groups. *European Heart Journal*, **18**, 597.

DCCT (Diabetes Control and Complications Trial) Research Group (1993). The effect of intensive treatment of diabetes on the development and progression of long-term complications in insulin-dependent diabetes mellitus. *New England Journal of Medicine*, **329**, 977–86.

Denny F.W., Wannamaker L.W., Brink W.R. *et al.* (1950). Prevention of rheumatic fever: treatment of the preceding streptococcic infection. *Journal of the American Medical Association*, **143**, 151–3.

Derby C.A., Lapane K.L., Feldman H.A. *et al.* (2000). Sex-specific trends in validated coronary heart disease rates in Southeastern New England, 1980–1991. *American Journal of Epidemiology*, **151**, 417–29.

Dimsdale J.E., Gilbert J., Hutter A.M. *et al.* (1981). Predicting cardiac morbidity based on risk factors and coronary angiographic findings. *American Journal of Cardiology*, **47**, 73–6.

Downs J.R., Clearfield M., Weis S. *et al.* (1998). Primary prevention of acute coronary events with lovastatin in men and women with average cholesterol levels: results of AFCAPS/TexCAPS. Air Force/Texas Coronary Atherosclerosis Prevention Study. *Journal of the American Medical Association*, **279**, 1615–22.

Dyer A.R. and Elliott P. (1989). THE INTERSALT Study: relations of body mass index to blood pressure. *Journal of Human Hypertension*, **3**, 299–308.

Eckel R.H. and Krauss R.M. (1998). American Heart Association call to action: obesity as a major risk factor for coronary heart disease. *Circulation*, **97**, 2099–100.

Eriksson H., Svardsudd K., Larsson B. *et al.* (1989). Risk factors for heart failure in the general population: the study of men born in 1913. *European Heart Journal*, **10**, 647–56.

Farquhar J.W., Fortmann S.P., Flora J.A. *et al.* (1990). Effects of community-wide education on cardiovascular disease risk factors: the Stanford Five-City Project. *Journal of the American Medical Association*, **264**, 359–65.

Farquhar J.W. Maccoby N. Wood P.D. *et al.* (1977). Community education for cardiovascular health. *Lancet*, **1**, 1192–5.

Ferencz C. (1986). Offspring of fathers with cardiovascular malformations. *American Heart Journal*, **111**, 1212–13.

Fiore M.C., Bailey W.C., Cohen S.J. *et al.* (1996). *Smoking cessation*. Clinical practice guideline No. 18. United States Department of Health and Human Services, Public Health Service, Agency for Health Care Policy and Research. AHCPR Publication No. 96–0692.

Flegal K.M. (1996). Trends in body weight and overweight in the US population. *Nutrition Reviews*, **54**, S97–S100

Flossmann E., Schulz U.G., and Rothwell P.M. (2004). Systematic review of methods and results of studies of the genetic epidemiology of ischemic stroke. *Stroke*, **35**, 212.

Fowles R.E. (1985). Progress of research in cardiomyopathy and myocarditis in the USA. International Symposium on Cardiomyopathy and Myocarditis. *Heart Vessels*, **1**, 5–7.

Freedman D.S. (1995). Relation of body fat distribution to ischemic heart disease. The National Health and Nutrition Examination Survey I (NHANES I) Epidemiologic Follow-up Study. *American Journal of Epidemiology*, **142**, 53–63.

Frick M.H., Elo O., Haapa K. *et al.* (1987). Helsinki Heart Study: primary-prevention trial with gemfibrozil in middle-aged men with dyslipidemia. *New England Journal of Medicine*, **317**, 1237–45.

Friedman M. and Rosenman R.H. (1959). Association of specific overt behavior pattern with blood and cardiovascular findings: blood cholesterol level, blood clotting time, incidence of arcus senilis, and clinical coronary artery disease. *Journal of the American Medical Association*, **169**, 1286–96.

Friedman M., Thorensen C.E., Gill J.J. *et al.* (1984). Alteration of type A behavior and reduction in cardiac recurrences in post-myocardial infarction patients. *American Heart Journal*, **108**, 237–48.

Friedman W.F. (1997). Congenital heart disease in infancy and childhood. In *Heart disease: a textbook of cardiovascular medicine* (ed. E. Braunwald), (5th ed), pp. 877–962. Saunders, Philadelphia.

Furberg C.D., Wright J.T., Davis B.R. *et al.* (2002). Major outcomes in high-risk hypertensive patients randomized to angiotensin-converting enzyme inhibitor or calcium channel blocker vs diuretic - The Antihypertensive and Lipid-Lowering Treatment to Prevent Heart Attack Trial (ALLHAT). *Journal of the American Medical Association*, **288**, 2981–2997

Fuster V., Badimon L., Badimon J. *et al.* (1992). Mechanisms of disease: the pathogenesis of coronary artery disease and the acute coronary syndromes. *New England Journal of Medicine*, **326**, 310–18.

GCP Research Group (1988). GCP German Cardiovascular Prevention study. *Design, methods, results*. Program Report. Scientific Institute of the German Medical Association (WIAD), Bonn, Germany.

Gillum R.F. (1986). Idiopathic cardiomyopathy in the United States, 1970–1982. *American Heart Journal*, **111**, 752–5.

Ginsberg H.N., Kris-Etherton P., Dennis B. *et al.* (1998). Effects of reducing dietary saturated fatty acids on plasma lipids and lipoproteins in healthy subjects: the DELTA Study, protocol 1. *Arteriosclerosis, Thrombosis and Vascular Biology*, **18**, 441–9.

Go A.S., Hylek E.M., Phillips K.A. *et al.* (2001). Prevalence of diagnosed atrial fibrillation in adults: national implications for rhythm management and stroke prevention: the Anticoagulation and Risk Factors in Atrial Fibrillation (ATRIA) Study. *Journal of the American Medical Association*, **285**, 2370.

Goldberg R.B., Mellies M.J., Sacks F.M. *et al.* (1998) Cardiovascular events and their reduction with pravastatin in diabetic and glucose-intolerant myocardial infarction survivors with average cholesterol levels: subgroup analyses in the cholesterol and recurrent events (CARE) trial. The Care Investigators. *Circulation*, **98**, 2513–9.

Gordon T. (1988). The diet–heart idea. *American Journal of Epidemiology*, **127**, 220–5.

Gordon T., Ernst N., Fisher M. *et al.* (1981). Alcohol and high-density lipoprotein cholesterol. *Circulation*, **64**, (Supplement III), 63–7.

Graves E.J. and Gillum B.S. (1996). 1994 Summary: National hospital discharge survey: advance data. *National Center for Health Statistics*, **278**, 1–12.

Hagar J.M. and Rahimtoola S.H. (1995). Chagas' heart disease. *Current Problems in Cardiology*, **20**, 825–924.

Hanna J.N., Heazlewood R.J. (2005). The epidemiology of acute rheumatic fever in Indigenous people in north Queensland. *Australia and New Zealand Journal of Public Health*, **29**, 313–7.

Harris T.B., Launer L.J., Madans J. *et al.* (1997). Cohort study of effect of being overweight and change in weight on risk of coronary heart disease in old age. *British Medical Journal*, **314**, 1791–4.

Hart R.G., Halperin J.L., Pearce L.A. *et al.* (2003). Lessons from the Stroke Prevention in Atrial Fibrillation trials. *Annals of Internal Medicine*, **138**, 831–8.

Haynes S.G., Feinleib M., and Kannel W.B. (1980). The relationship of psychosocial factors to coronary heart disease in the Framingham Study. III. Eight-year incidence of coronary heart disease. *American Journal of Epidemiology*, **111**, 37–58.

Hearn M.D., Murray D.M., and Luepker R.V. (1988). Hostility, coronary heart disease, and total mortality. A 33-year follow-up study of university students. *Journal of Behavioral Medicine*, **12**, 105–21.

Heart Outcomes Prevention Evaluation Study Investigators (2000). Effects of ramipril on cardiovascular and microvascular outcomes in people with diabetes mellitus: results of the HOPE study and MICRO-HOPE substudy. *Lancet*, **355**, 253–9.

Hecker M.H.L., Chesney M.A., Black G.W. *et al.* (1988). Coronary prone behaviors in the Western Collaborative Group Study. *Psychosomatic Medicine*, **50**, 153–64.

Hennekens C.H., Buring J.E., Manson J.E. *et al.* (1996). Lack of effect on long-term supplementation with beta carotene on the incidence of malignant neoplasms and cardiovascular disease. *New England Journal of Medicine*, **334**, 1145–9.

Hermanson B., Omenn G.S., Kronmal R.A. *et al.* (1988). Beneficial six-year outcome of smoking cessation in older men and women with coronary artery disease: results from the CASS registry. *New England Journal of Medicine*, **319**, 1365–9.

Ho K.K., Pinsky J.L., Kannel W.B. *et al.* (1993a). The epidemiology of heart failure: the Framingham Study. *Journal of the American College of Cardiology*, **22**, 6A–13A.

Ho K.K., Anderson K.M., Kannel W.B. *et al.* (1993b). Survival after the onset of congestivec heart failure in Framingham Heart Study subjects. *Circulation*, **88**, 107–15.

Hoffman J.I. and Kaplan S. (2002). The incidence of congenital heart disease. *Journal of the American College of Cardiology*, **39**, 1890–900.

Howard G., Howard V.J. for the Reasons for Geographic And Racial Differences in Stroke Investigators (2001). Ethnic disparities in stroke: the scope of the problem. *Ethnicity & Disease*, **11**, 761.

Hu F.B., Stampfer M.J., Colditz G.A. *et al.* (2000). Physical activity and risk of stroke in women. *Journal of the American Medical Association*, **283**, 2961.

Hu H.H., Sheng W.Y., Chu F.L. *et al.* (1992). Incidence of stroke in Taiwan. *Stroke*, **23**, 1237.

Huang Z., Willett W.C., Manson J.E. *et al.* (1998). Body weight, weight change, and risk for hypertension in women. *Annals of Internal Medicine*, **128**, 81–8. 1150.

Hughes L.O. (1990). Insulin, Indian origin and ischemic heart disease (editorial). *International Journal of Cardiology*, **26**, 1–4.

INTERSALT Cooperative Research Group (1988). INTERSALT: an international study of electrolyte excretion and blood pressure: results for 24 h urinary sodium and potassium excretion. *British Medical Journal*, **297**, 319–28.

Iso H., Jacobs D.R., Jr., Wentworth D. *et al.* (1989). Serum cholesterol levels and six-year mortality from stroke in 350,977 men screened for the multiple risk factor intervention trial. *New England Journal of Medicine*, **320**, 904.

Jenkins D.J.A., Wolever T.M.S., Rao A.V. *et al.* (1993). Effect on blood lipids of very high intakes of fiber in diets low in saturated fat and cholesterol. *New England Journal of Medicine*, **329**, 21–6.

Johnson G., Carson P., Francis G.S. *et al.* (1993). Influence of prerandomization (baseline) variables on mortality and on the reduction of mortality by enalapril: Veterans Affairs Cooperative Study on Vasodilator Therapy of Heart Failure (V-HeFT II). *Circulation*, **87**, VI32–VI39.

Joseph J.G., Prior I.A.M., Salmond C.E. *et al.* (1983). Elevation of systolic and diastolic blood pressure associated with migration: the Tokelau Island Migrant Study. *Journal of Chronic Disorders*, **36**, 507–16.

Kagan A., Popper J.S., and Rhoads G.G. (1980). Factors related to stroke incidence in Hawaii Japanese men. The Honolulu Heart Study. *Stroke*, **11**, 14.

Kagan A., Harris B.R., Winkelstein W. *et al.* (1974). Epidemiologic studies of coronary heart disease and stroke in Japanese men living in Japan, Hawaii and California: demographic, physical, dietary and biochemical characteristics. *Journal of Chronic Disorders*, **27**, 345–64.

Kannel W.B. (1987). Epidemiology and prevention of cardiac failure: Framingham Study insights. *European Heart Journal*, **8**, 23–6.

Kannel W.B., Ho K., and Thom T. (1994). Changing epidemiological features of cardiac failure. *British Heart Journal*, **72**, S3–9.

Kawachi I., Colditz G.A., Stampfer M.J. *et al.* (1993). Smoking cessation and decreased risk of stroke in women. *Journal of the American Medical Association*, **269**, 232.

Keren A. and Popp R.L. (1992). Assignment of patients into the classification of cardiomyopathies. *Circulation*, **86**, 1622–33.

Keys A. (ed.) (1980). *Seven countries: a multivariate analysis of death and coronary heart disease.* Harvard University Press, Cambridge, MA.

Keys A., Grande F., and Anderson J.T. (1974). Bias and misrepresentation revisited—'perspective' on saturated fat. *American Journal of Clinical Nutrition*, **27**, 188–212.

Khan F.A., Zia E., Janzon L. *et al.* (2004). Incidence of stroke and stroke subtypes in Malmo, Sweden, 1990–2000: marked differences between groups defined by birth country. *Stroke*, **35**, 2054.

Kiely D.K., Wolf P.A., Cupples L.A. *et al.* (1994). Physical activity and stroke risk: the Framingham Study. *American Journal of Epidemiology*, **140**, 608.

Krauss R.M., Wonston M., Fletcher R.N. *et al.* (1998). Obesity: impact of cardiovascular disease. *Circulation*, **98**, 1472–6.

Kritchevsky S.B., Shimakawa T., Tell G.S. *et al.* (1995). Dietary antioxidants and carotid artery wall thickness: the ARIC Study. *Circulation*, **92**, 2142–50.

Kurahara D.K., Grandinetti A., Galario J. *et al.* (2006). Ethnic Differences for Developing Rheumatic Fever in a Low-Income Group Living in Hawaii. *Ethnicity and Disease*, **16**, 357–361.

Lakshminarayan K., Solid C.A., Collins A.J. *et al.* (2006). Atrial fibrillation and stroke in the general medicare population: a 10-year perspective (1992 to 2002). *Stroke*, **37**, 1969.

Lee I.M., Cook N.R., Gaziano J.M. *et al.* (2005). Vitamin E in the primary prevention of cardiovascular disease and cancer: the Women's Health Study: a randomized controlled trial. *Journal of the American Medical Association*, **294**, 56–65.

Lehto S., Ronnemaa T., Haffner S.M. *et al.* (1997). Dyslipidemia and hyperglycemia predict coronary heart disease events in middle-aged patients with NIDDM. *Diabetes*, **48**, 1354–9.

Leon A.S., Connett J., Jacobs Jr. D.R. *et al.* (1987). Leisure time physical activity levels and risk of coronary heart disease and death: the Multiple Risk Factor Intervention Trial. *Journal of the American Medical Association*, **258**, 2388–95.

Leon G.R., Finn S.E., Murray D. *et al.* (1988). Inability to predict cardiovascular disease from hostility scores of MMPI items related to type A behavior. *Journal of Consulting and Clinical Psychology*, **56**, 597–600.

Levine H.D. (1979). Virus myocarditis: a critique of the literature from clinical, electrocardiographic and pathologic standpoints. *American Journal of Medical Sciences*, **277**, 132–43.

Levy D., Larson M.G., Vasan R.S. *et al.* (1996). The progression from hypertension to congestive heart failure. *Journal of the American Medical Association*, **275**, 1557–62.

Long-term Intervention with Pravastatin in Ischaemic Disease (LIPID) Study Group (1998). Prevention of cardiovascular events and death with pravastatin in patients with coronary heart disease and a broad range of initial cholesterol levels. *New England Journal of Medicine*, **339**, 1349–57.

Lonn E., Yusuf S., Arnold M.J. *et al.* (2006). Homocysteine lowering with folic acid and B vitamins in vascular disease. *New England Journal of Medicine*, **354**, 1567–77.

Luepker R.V. (1994). Epidemiology of atherosclerotic diseases in population groups. In *Primer in preventive cardiology* (ed. T.A. Pearson, M.H. Criqui, R.V. Luepker, A. Oberman, and M. Winston), pp. 1–10. American Heart Association, Dallas, TX.

Luepker R.V. (ed.) (1999). Proceedings from primordial prevention of cardiovascular disease risk factors: an international symposium honoring the career and research of Henry Blackburn, MD. *Preventive Medicine*, **29**.

Luepker R.V., Arnett D.K., Jacobs Jr, D.R. *et al.* (2006). Trends in blood pressure, hypertension control, and stroke mortality: The Minnesota Heart Survey. *American Journal of Medicine*, **119**, 42–49.

Luepker R.V., Jacobs D.R., Prineas R.J. *et al.* (1999). Secular trends of blood pressure and body size in a multi-ethnic adolescent population: 1986 to 1996. *Journal of Pediatrics*, **134**, 668–74.

Luepker R.V., Murray D.M., Jacobs Jr. D.R. *et al.* (1994). Community education for cardiovascular disease prevention: risk factor changes in the Minnesota Heart Health Program. *American Journal of Public Health*, **84**, 1383–93.

McCranie E.W., Watkins L.O., Brandsma J.M. *et al.* (1986). Hostility, coronary heart disease incidence, and total mortality: lack of an association in a 25-year follow-up study of 478 physicians. *Journal of Behavioral Medicine*, **9**, 119–25.

McGill H.C., McMahan C.A., Malcom G.T. *et al.* for the PDAY Research Group (1997). Effects of serum lipoproteins and smoking on atherosclerosis in young men and women. *Arteriosclerosis and Thrombosis Vascular Biology*, **17**, 95–106.

McGovern P.G., Pankow J.S., Shahar E. *et al.* for the Minnesota Heart Survey Investigators (1996). Recent trends in acute coronary heart disease mortality, morbidity, medical care and risk factors. *New England Journal of Medicine*, **334**, 884–90.

Meade T.W., Imeson J., and Stirling Y. (1987). Effects of changes in smoking and other characteristics on clotting factors and the risk of ischaemic heart disease. *Lancet*, **2**, 986–8.

Mittleman M.A., Maclure M., Tofler G.H. *et al.* for the Determinants of Myocardial Infarction Onset Study Investigators (1993). Triggering of acute myocardial infarction by heavy physical exertion: protection against triggering of regular exertion. *New England Journal of Medicine*, **329**, 1677–83.

Morris S.A., Tanowitz H.B., Wittner M. *et al.* (1990). Pathophysiological insights into the cardiomyopathy of Chagas' disease. *Circulation*, **82**, 1900–9.

Mosterd A., Hoes A.W., de Bruyne M.C. *et al.* (1999). Prevalence of heart failure and left ventricular dysfunction in the general population; The Rotterdam Study. *Eur Heart J*, **20**, 447–55.

Muller J.E., Kaufmann P.G., Luepker R.V. *et al.* (1997). Mechanisms precipitating acute cardiac events: Review and recommendations of an NHLBI workshop. *Circulation*, **96**, 3233–9.

Muller J.E., Ludmer P.L., Willich S.N. *et al.* (1987). Circadian variation in the frequency of sudden cardiac death. *Circulation*, **75**, 131–8.

Multiple Risk Factor Intervention Trial Research Group (1996). Mortality after 16 years for participants randomized to the Multiple Risk Factor Intervention Trial. *Circulation*, **94**, 946–51.

Nathan D.M., Cleary P.A., Backlund J.Y. *et al.* for the Diabetes Control and Complications Trial/Epidemiology of Diabetes Interventions and Complications (DCCT/EDIC) Study Research Group (2005). Intensive diabetes treatment and cardiovascular disease in patients with type 1 diabetes. *New England Journal of Medicine*, **353**, 2643–53.

National Task Force on Prevention and Treatment of Obesity (1994). Towards prevention of obesity: research directions. *Obesity Research*, **2**, 571–84.

Neaton J.D. and Wentworth D. for the Multiple Risk Factor Intervention Trial Research Group (1992). Serum cholesterol, blood pressure, cigarette smoking, and death from coronary heart disease: Overall findings and differences by age for 316 099 white men. *Archives of Internal Medicine*, **152**, 56–64.

Neaton J.D., Grimm Jr R.H., Prineas R.J. *et al.* (1993). Treatment of mild hypertension study: final results. *Journal of the American Medical Association*, **270**, 713–24.

NHLBI (National Heart, Lung, and Blood Institute) (2006). Morbidity and Mortality: 2006 Chart book on cardiovascular, lung, and blood diseases. Bethesda, MD: National Institutes of Health.

NIH (2003). Prevalence of self-reported heart failure among US adults: results from the 1999 National Health Interview Survey. *American Heart Journal*, **146**, 121–8.

NIH (2002). *Third Report of the* National Cholesterol Education Program *Expert Panel on Detection, Evaluation, and Treatment of High Blood Cholesterol in Adults (Adult Treatment Panel III)*. US Department of Health and Human Services.
NIH Publication No. 02–5215. National Institutes of Health, Washington, DC.

NIH Consensus Conference (1996). Physical activity and cardiovascular health. *Journal of the American Medical Association*, **276**, 241–6.

Nissen S.E. and Wolski K. (2007). Effect of rosiglitazone on the risk of myocardial infarction and death from cardiovascular causes. *New England Journal of Medicine*, **356**, 2457–71.

Noonan J. (1978). Twins, conjoined twins and cardiac defects. *American Journal of Diseased Children*, **132**, 17–18.

Ogden C.L., Carroll M.D., Curtin L.R. *et al.* (2006). Prevalence of overweight and obesity in the United States, 1999-2004. *Journal of the American Medical Association*, **295**, 1549–55.

Okada R. and Wakafuji S. (1985). Myocarditis in autopsy. International Symposium on Cardiomyopathy and Myocarditis. *Heart Vessels*, **1**, 23–9.

Oldridge N.B., Guyatt G.H., Fischer M.E. *et al.* (1988). Cardiac rehabilitation after myocardial infarction. Combined experience of randomized clinical trials. *Journal of the American Medical Association*, **260**, 945–50.

Omenn G.S., Goodman G.E., Thornquist M.D. *et al.* (1996). Effects of a combination of beta carotene and vitamin A on lung cancer and cardiovascular disease. *New England Journal of Medicine*, **334**, 1150–5.

Orth-Gomer K. and Johnson J.V. (1987). Social network interaction and mortality: a six year follow-up study of a random sample of the Swedish population. *Journal of Chronic Disorders*, **40**, 949–57.

Osganian S.K., Stampfer M.J., Spiegelman D. *et al.* (1999). Distribution of and factors associated with serum homocysteine levels in children: Child and Adolescent Trial for Cardiovascular Health. *Journal of the American Medical Association*, **281**, 1189–96.

PAHO (Pan American Health Organization) (1970). *Fourth Meeting of the Working Group on Prevention of Rheumatic Fever*, Quito, Ecuador.

Paisey R.B., Harvey P., Rice S. *et al.* (1998). An intensive weight loss programme in established type 2 diabetes and controls: effects on weight and atherosclerosis risk factors at 1 year. *Diabetic Medicine*, **15**, 73–9.

Perry H.M., Jr., Davis B.R., Price T.R. *et al.* (2000). Effect of treating isolated systolic hypertension on the risk of developing various types and subtypes of stroke: the Systolic Hypertension in the Elderly Program (SHEP). *Journal of the American Medical Association*, **284**, 465.

Perry C.L., Kelder S.H., Murray D.M. *et al.* (1992). Community-wide smoking prevention: long-term outcomes of the Minnesota Heart Health Program and the Class of 1989 Study. *American Journal of Public Health*, **82**, 1210–16.

Powell K.E., Thompson P.D., Caspersen C.J. *et al.* (1987). Physical activity and the incidence of coronary heart disease. *Annual Review of Public Health*, **8**, 253–87.

Psaty B.M., Smith N.L., Siscovick D.S. *et al.* (1997). Health outcomes associated with antihypertensive therapies used as first-line agents. A systematic review and meta-analysis. *Journal of the American Medical Association*, **277**, 739–45.

Puska P., Tuomilehto J., Nissinen A. *et al.* (ed.) (1995). *The North Karelia Project: 20 year results and experiences.* Helsinki University Printing House.

Pyorala K., Pedersen T.R., Kjekshus J. *et al.* (1997). Cholesterol lowering with simvastatin improves prognosis of diabetic patients with coronary heart disease. A subgroup analysis of the Scandinavian Simvastatin Survival Study (4S). *Diabetes Care*, **20**, 614–20.

Qizilbash N., Jones L., Warlow C. *et al.* (1991). Fibrinogen and lipid concentrations as risk factors for transient ischaemic attacks and minor ischaemic strokes. *British Medical Journal*, **303**, 605.

Ragland D.R. and Brand R.J. (1988). Coronary heart disease mortality in the Western Collaborative Group Study. Follow-up experience of 22 years. *American Journal of Epidemiology*, **127**, 462–75.

Regan T.J. (1990). Alcohol and the cardiovascular system. *Journal of the American Medical Association*, **264**, 377–81.

Remes J., Reunanen A., Aromaa A., and Pyorala K. (1992). Incidence of heart failure in Eastern Finland: a population-based surveillance study. *European Heart Journal*, **13**, 588–93.

Richardson P., McKenna W., Bristow M. *et al.* (1996). Report of the 1995 World Health Organization/International Society and Federation of Cardiology Task Force on the Definition and Classification of cardiomyopathies. *Circulation*, **93**, 841–2.

Rosenman R.H., Brand R.J., Jenkins C.D. *et al.* (1975). Coronary heart disease in the Western Collaborative Group Study: final follow-up experience of 8.5 years. *Journal of the American Medical Association*, **233**, 872–7.

Rubins H.B., Robins S.J., Collins D. *et al.* (1999). Gemfibrozil for the secondary prevention of coronary heart disease in men with low levels of high-density lipoprotein cholesterol. Veterans Affairs High-Density Lipoprotein Cholesterol Intervention Trial Study Group. *New England Journal of Medicine*, **341**, 410–18.

Sacco R.L., Benson R.T., Kargman D.E. *et al.* (2001). High-density lipoprotein cholesterol and ischemic stroke in the elderly: the Northern Manhattan Stroke Study. *Journal of the American Medical Association*, **285**, 2729.

Sacco R.L. and Boden-Albala B. (2001). Stroke Risk Factors. In M. Fisher (ed). *Stroke Therapy*. Boston Butterworth-Heinemann, 1–23.

Sacco R.L., Elkind M., Boden-Albala B. *et al.* (1999). The protective effect of moderate alcohol consumption on ischemic stroke. *Journal of the American Medical Association*, **281**, 53.

Sacks F.M., Pfeffer M.A., Moye L.A. *et al.* (1996). The effect of pravastatin on coronary events after myocardial infarction in patients with average cholesterol levels. Cholesterol and Recurrent Events Trial Investigators. *New England Journal of Medicine*, **335**, 1001–9.

Salonen R., Seppanen K., Rauramaa R. *et al.* (1988). Prevalence of carotid atherosclerosis and serum cholesterol levels in eastern Finland. *Arteriosclerosis* **8**, 788–92.

Samanck M. (1994). Boy:girl ratio in children born with different forms of cardiac malformation: a population-based study. *Pediatric Cardiology*, **15**, 53–7.

Sankai T., Miyagaki T., Iso H. *et al.* (1991). A population-based study of the proportion by type of stroke determined by computed tomography scan. *Nippon Koshu Eisei Zasshi - Japanese Journal of Public Health*, **38**, 901.

Sarti C., Rastenyte D., Cepaitis Z. *et al.* (2000). International trends in mortality from stroke, 1968 to 1994. *Stroke*, **31**, 1588–1601.

Scandinavian Simvastatin Survival Study (1994). Randomized trial of cholesterol lowering in 4444 patients with coronary heart disease: the Scandinavian Simvastatin Survival Study (4S). *Lancet*, **344**, 1383–9.

Senni M., Tribouilloy C.M., Rodeheffer R.J. *et al.* (1998). Congestive heart failure in the community: a study of all incident cases in Olmsted County, Minnesota, in 1991. *Circulation*, **98**, 2282–9.

Shabeter R. (1983). Cardiomyopathy: How far have we come in 25 years? How far yet to go? *Journal of the American College of Cardiology*, **1**, 252–63.

Shekelle R.B., Hulley S.B., Neaton J.D. *et al.* (1985a). The MRFIT behavior pattern study. I. Type A behavior and incidence of coronary heart disease. *American Journal of Epidemiology*, **122**, 559–70.

Shekelle R.B., Gale M., and Norusis M. (1985b). Type A score (Jenkins Activity Survey) and risk of recurrent coronary heart disease in the Aspirin Myocardial Infarction Study. *American Journal of Cardiology*, **56**, 221–5.

Shekelle R.B., Gale M., Ostfeld A.M. *et al.* (1983). Hostility, risk of coronary heart disease, and mortality. *Psychosomatic Medicine*, **45**, 109–14.

Shepherd J., Cobbe S.M., Ford I. *et al.* for the West of Scotland Coronary Prevention Study Group (1995). Prevention of coronary heart disease with pravastatin in me with hypercholesterolemia. *New England Journal of Medicine*, **333**, 1301–7.

Siegel A.C., Johnson E.E., and Stollerman G.H. (1961). Controlled studies of streptococcal pharyngitis in a pediatric population: 1. factors related to the attack rate of rheumatic fever. *New England Journal of Medicine*, **265**, 559–66.

Sjostrom L.V. (1992). Mortality of severely obese subjects. *American Journal of Clinical Nutrition*, **55**, 516S–23S.

Solomon C.G. and Manson J.E. (1997). Obesity and mortality: a review of the epidemiologic data. *American Journal of Clinical Nutrition*, **66**, 1044S–50S.

Sowers J.R., Sowers P.S. and Peuler J.D. (1994). Role of insulin resistance and hyperinsulinemia in development of hypertension and atherosclerosis. *Journal of Laboratory and Clinical Medicine*, **123**, 647–52.

Staessen J.A., Birkenhager W.H. and Fagard R. (1997). Implications of the Systolic Hypertension in Europe (Syst-Eur) Trial for clinical practice. *Nephrology Dialysis Transplantation*, **12**, 2220.

Stamler J., Vaccaro O., Neaton J.D. *et al.* (1993). Diabetes, other risk factors, and 12-year cardiovascular mortality for men screened in the Multiple Risk Factor Intervention Trial. *Diabetes Care*, **16**, 434–44.

Stampfer M.J. and Rimm E.B. (1995). Epidemiologic evidence for vitamin E in prevention of cardiovascular disease. *American Journal of Clinical Nutrition*, **62**, 1365S–9S.

Steenland K., Thun M., Lally C. *et al.* (1996). Environmental tobacco smoke and coronary heart disease in the American Cancer Society CPS-II cohort. *Circulation*, **94**, 622–8.

Tanaka H., Ueda Y., and Hayashi M. (1982). Risk factors for cerebral hemorrhage and cerebral infarction in a Japanese rural community. *Stroke*, **13**, 62.

Toole J.F., Malinow M.R., Chambless L.E. *et al.* (2004). Lowering homocysteine in patients with ischemic stroke to prevent recurrent stroke, myocardial infarction, and death: the Vitamin Intervention for

Stroke Prevention (VISP) randomized controlled trial. *Journal of the American Medical Association*, **291**, 565–75.

Trials of Hypertension Prevention Collaborative Research Group (1997). Effects of weight loss and sodium reduction intervention on blood pressure and hypertension incidence in overweight people with high normal blood pressure: the Trials of Hypertension Prevention, phase II. *Archives of Internal Medicine*, **157**, 657–67.

Tunstall-Pedoe H., Kuulasmaa K., Mahonen M. *et al.* (1999). Contribution of trends in survival and coronary-event rates to changes in coronary heart disease mortality: 10-year results from 37 WHO MONICA project populations: monitoring trends and determinants in cardiovascular disease. *Lancet*, **353**, 1547–57.

Tunstall-Pedoe H., Morrison C., Woodward M. *et al.* (1996). Sex differences in myocardial infarction and coronary deaths in the Scottish MONICA population of Glasgow 1985 to 1991: presentation, diagnosis, treatment, and 28-day case fatality of 3991 events in men and 1551 events in women. *Circulation*, **93**, 1981–92.

UGDP (University Group Diabetes Program) (1975). A study of the effects of hypoglycemic agents on vascular complications in patients with adult onset diabetes. V. Evaluation of phenoformin therapy. *Diabetes*, **24**, 65–184.

UKPDS (United Kingdom Prospective Diabetes Study) Group (1995). UKPDS 13: relative efficacy of randomly allocated diet, sulphonylurea, insulin, or metformin in patients with newly diagnosed non-insulin dependent diabetes followed for three years. *British Medical Journal*, **310**, 83–8.

UK Prospective Diabetes Study Group (1998). Tight blood pressure control and risk of macrovascular and microvascular complications in type 2 diabetes: UKPDS 38. *British Medical Journal*, **317**, 703.

USDHHS (United States Department of Health and Human Services) (1990). *The health benefits of smoking cessation: a report of the Surgeon General*. DHHS Publication No. CDC-90–8416. USDHHS, Centers for Disease Control, Center for Chronic Disease Prevention and Health Promotion, Office on Smoking and Health, Washington, DC.

USDHHS (United States Department of Health and Human Services) (1997). *Changes in cigarette-related disease risks and their implication for prevention and control*. NIH Publication No. 97–4213. Monograph 8. USDHHS, Public Health Services, National Institutes of Health, National Cancer Institute, Washington, DC.

USDHHS (United States Department of Health and Human Services) (1998a). *Targeting tobacco use: the nation's leading cause of death: at-a-glance*. Centers for Disease Control and Prevention, Washington, DC.

USDHHS (United States Department of Health and Human Services) (1998b). *Clinical guidelines on the identification, evaluation, and treatment of overweight and obesity in adults: the evidence report*. USDHHS, Public Health Service, National Institutes of Health, National Heart, Lung, and Blood Institute, Washington, DC.

USDHHS (United States Department of Health and Human Services). National Heart, Lung, and Blood Institute. National High Blood Pressure Education Program (2003). Available at: http://www.nhlbi.nih.gov/about/nhbpep/index.htm. Accessed March 5, 2003.

Vora A. (2006). Management of atrial fibrillation in rheumatic valvular heart disease. *Current Opinion in Cardiology*, **21**, 47.

Wannamaker L.W. (1973). The chain that links the heart to the throat. *Circulation*, **48**, 9–18.

WHO (World Health Organization) (1988). *Cardiomyopathies*. Technical Report Series No. 764. Report of a WHO Expert Committee. WHO, Geneva.

WHO (World Health Organization) (2004). *Rheumatic fever and rheumatic heart disease*. Technical Report Series No. 923. WHO, Geneva.

WHO (World Health Organization) (2003). *MONICA Monograph Multimedia Sourcebook*. Tunstall-Pedoe H (ed). Geneva, Switzerland.

WHO/Europe, European mortality database (MDB), June 2007.

Wigle E.D. (1988). Hypertrophic cardiomyopathy 1988. *Modern Concepts in Cardiovascular Disease*, **57**, 1–6.

Willich S.N., Maclure M., Mittleman M. *et al.* (1993). Sudden cardiac death. Support for a role of triggering in causation. *Circulation*, **87**, 1442–50.

Wolf P.A. and D'Agostino R.B. (1998). Epidemiology of stroke. In Barnett H.J.M., Mohr J.P., Stein B.M., Yatso F.M. (eds). *Stroke - pathophysiology, diagnosis and management*. New York: Churchill-Livingstone, 3–28.

Wolf P.A., D'Agostino R.B., Belanger A.J. *et al.* (1991). Probability of stroke: a risk profile from the Framingham Study. *Stroke*, **22**, 312.

Wood D., De Backer G., Faergeman O. *et al.* (1998). Prevention of coronary heart disease in clinical practice. *European Heart Journal*, **19**, 1434–1503.

Zhang L.F., Yang J., Hong Z. *et al.* for the Collaborative Group of China Multicenter Study of Cardiovascular E (2003). Proportion of different subtypes of stroke in China. *Stroke*, **34**, 2091.

Zierler S. (1985). Maternal drugs and congenital heart disease. *Obstetrics and Gynecology*, **65**, 155–65.

9.3

Neoplasms

Paolo Boffetta and Carlo La Vecchia

Abstract

Neoplasms are a group of diverse diseases with complex distributions in human populations and with different aetiological factors. Current knowledge of the causes of human neoplasms and the development of control strategies have led to the elaboration of lists of recommendations for their prevention. A comprehensive strategy for cancer control might lead to the avoidance of a sizeable proportion of human cancers, and the greatest benefit can be achieved via tobacco control.

Nevertheless, neoplasms will continue to be a major source of human disease and death. Considerable efforts are made in the public and private domains to develop effective therapeutic approaches. Even if major discoveries in the clinical management of cancer patients will be accomplished in the near future, the changes will mainly affect the affluent part of the world population. Prevention of the known causes of cancer remains the most promising approach in reducing the consequences of cancer, in particular in countries with limited resources. Control of tobacco smoking and of smokeless tobacco products, reduced overweight and obesity, moderation in alcohol intake, increased physical activity, avoidance of exposure to solar radiation and control of known occupational carcinogens are the main approaches we currently have to reduce the burden of human neoplasms.

Introduction

Neoplasms include a family of diseases, several hundreds of which can be distinguished in humans by localization, morphology, clinical behaviour, and response to therapy. Whether considered from a biological, clinical or public health viewpoint, it is the invasive nature of many of these diseases which is of dominant importance.

Benign neoplasms represent localized growths of tissue with predominantly normal characteristics: In many cases they cause minor symptoms and are amenable to surgical therapy. Benign tumours, however, can become clinically very important when they occur in organs in which compression is possible and surgery cannot be easily performed (e.g. the brain), and when they produce hormones or other substances with a systemic effect (e.g. epinephrine produced by benign pheochromocytoma). Relatively little is known about the distribution and causes of most benign neoplasms and, with the exception of benign brain neoplasms, they will not be further discussed in this chapter.

Malignant neoplasms are characterized by progressive growth of tissue with structural and functional alterations with respect to the normal tissue. In some cases, the alterations can be so important that it becomes difficult to identify the tissue of origin. A peculiarity of most malignant tumours is the ability to migrate and colonize other organs (metastatization) via blood and lymph vessel penetration. The presence and extension of metastases are often the critical factors to determine the success of therapy and the survival of cancer patients.

The pace of growth of malignant neoplasms varies widely, and asymptomatic neoplasms are often found at autopsy of individuals deceased from other causes. The long process of carcinogenesis justifies the efforts to develop and apply screening approaches for early detection of selected subclinical neoplasms in healthy individuals.

At the molecular level, the process of malignant transformation is characterized by alterations in several genes that are responsible for the control of the replication cycle of the cell and other regulatory functions. Many cancer-related genes have been identified, and the distribution of their alterations varies among different neoplasms. However, neoplasms which are morphologically and clinically identical often include different genetic alterations, showing that the malignant transformation may result from the accumulation of genetic damage through different pathways.

Most malignant neoplasms in adults arise from epithelial tissues and are defined as carcinomas. In practice, however, the terms 'malignant neoplasm', 'malignant tumour' and 'cancer' are used interchangeably. Neoplasms are classified according to the International Classification of Diseases—Oncology (WHO 1990) into topographical categories (according to the organ where the neoplasm arises) and morphological categories (according to the characteristics of the cells). More and more often, neoplasms are characterized at the clinical level according to phenotypic aspects (e.g. presence of receptors, expression of genes) and genetic alterations (e.g. mutation in a given gene).

The identification of the determinants of cancer relies on two complementary approaches, the epidemiological and the experimental. The epidemiological approach has produced both general and specific evidence for the role of different types of agents in

Table 9.3.1 Ratio of the 20th and 80th percentile in the ranking of country-specific estimated age-standardized incidence rates of selected cancers (Globocan 2002)

Cancer	Men	Women
Oral cavity	3.5	2.7
Nasopharynx	5.5	5.1
Oesophagus	4.4	7.3
Stomach	3.9	3.1
Colon-rectum	6.1	6.0
Liver	5.1	4.2
Pancreas	5.5	4.2
Lung	9.3	6.4
Melanoma	8.5	9.0
Breast	–	2.8
Cervix	–	3.5
Corpus uteri	–	4.8
Ovary	–	2.3
Prostate	5.8	–
Bladder	4.2	3.4
Kidney	6.6	4.8
Nervous system	6.0	4.4
Non-Hodgkin's lymphoma	2.1	1.8
Leukaemia	2.8	2.4

cancer causation. The evidence of a more general nature derives from the observations of considerable variation of the incidence rates of most cancers in different populations, defined according to geographical area. Table 9.3.1 reports the ratio of the 80th to the 20th percentile of the ranking of country-specific incidence rates of selected cancers, as estimated in the Globocan 2002 project (Ferlay *et al.* 2004). For all gender-specific rates but one, the ratio is above 2, and for several neoplasms it is close to 10. This comparison is based on stable figures, but masks ever larger variations among very-high-risk and very-low-risk areas, which for many neoplasms may reach 100- or even 1000-fold differences. Variations are also shown within countries or according to other characteristics such as ethnic group, religion, social class. For instance, when contrasted with other religious groups, the Mormons of Utah and the Seventh-Day Adventists of California exhibit low rates for cancers of the respiratory, gastrointestinal, and genital systems. This marked variation in rates according to different axes of exploration is unlikely to be explained chiefly by concomitant genetic variations, and points to the role of lifestyle determinants.

Finally, changes in incidence rates in time, particularly when they take place over a few decades, are incompatible with a genetic explanation, as changes in the genes of a population pool require longer intervals. Recorded incidence rates are affected by diagnostic changes and mortality rates are, in addition, affected by changes in treatment effectiveness; however, marked trends like the one for lung cancer (Fig. 9.3.1) are most likely to reflect real changes in cancer rates, pointing to the importance of non-genetic factors.

Genetic determinants of cancer have also been demonstrated. Several inherited conditions carry a very high risk of one or several cancers. High-penetrance genes are identified through family-based and other linkage studies. These conditions, however, are rare and explain only a small proportion of human cancers. Genetic factors, however, are likely to play an important role in interacting with non-genetic factors to determine individual cancer risk.

The understanding of the molecular and cellular mechanisms of carcinogenesis has greatly advanced in recent years. According to a widely accepted model, cells have to acquire six characteristics to become fully malignant (Hanahan *et al.* 2000). These include the ability to produce growth signals (several known oncogenes mimic growth signalling), the lack of sensitivity to antigrowth signals [the Retinoblastoma (RB) protein and its homologues play a key role in the ability of the cell to decide whether to proliferate, to be quiescent, or to enter into a postmitotic state, based on external signalling], resistance towards programmed cell death or apoptosis (in many cases via inactivation of the p53 protein), immortalization (normal cells have a limited replication potential, that is related to the length of the telomeres: In malignant cells overexpression of telomerases circumvents it), stimulation of blood vessel production (by changing the balance of angiogenesis inducers and countervailing inhibitors) and ability to invade and metastasize. The acquisition of these neoplastic characteristics typically occurs by alterations of relevant genes, but an inability to maintain genomic integrity (so-called genomic instability, which includes reduced ability to repair DNA damage) is an additional feature of malignant cells, as accumulation of random mutations in genes involved in all the functions mentioned above would be a too rare event for the development of cancer during the normal lifespan. A final point to consider is the heterogeneity of neoplastic genetic alterations: The acquisition of the different biological capabilities of the neoplastic cell can appear at different times, and the particular sequence in which capabilities are acquired can vary widely, even among the same type of tumours.

The identification of carcinogens via the laboratory relies on three types of tests: (i) long-term (often lifetime) carcinogenicity tests in experimental animals, most commonly rodents (mice, rats, hamsters), (ii) short-term tests assessing the effect of chemical agents on a variety of endpoints belonging to three general classes: DNA damage, mutagenicity and chromosome damage, and (iii) mechanistic test, aimed at identifying the intermediate steps in the compound-specific carcinogenic process.

These tests are valuable to the extent that such effects may reflect underlying events in the carcinogenic process. Indeed, consistent positivity in tests measuring DNA damage, mutagenicity and chromosomal damage is usually regarded as indicating potential carcinogenicity of the tested agent. Results of laboratory tests constitute useful supporting evidence when adequate epidemiological data for the carcinogenicity of an environmental agent exist (for example, vinyl chloride), but they become all the more essential when the epidemiological evidence is non-existent or inadequate in quality or in quantity. In the latter case, although no universally accepted criteria exist to automatically translate data from long-term animal tests or short-term tests in terms of cancer risk in humans, an evaluation of the risk can be made on a judgmental basis using all available scientific evidence. This policy has been applied by the International Agency for Research on Cancer (IARC) in a systematic programme of evaluation of the carcinogenic risk of chemicals to man. Within this programme of IARC Monographs, agents are classified in group 1

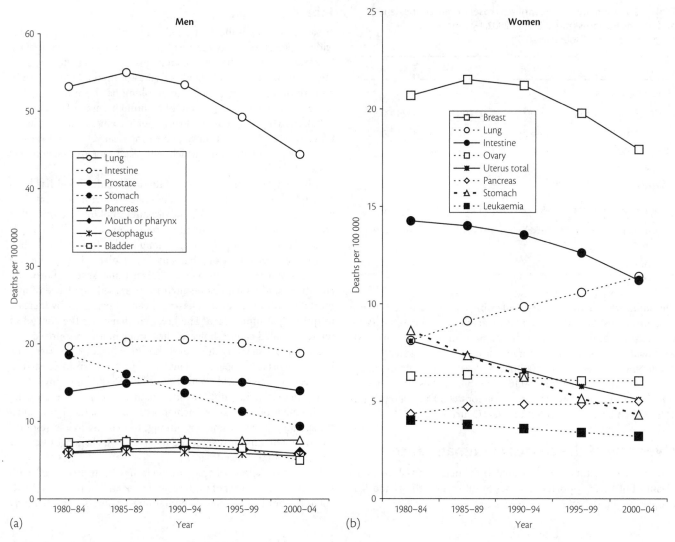

Fig. 9.3.1 Trends in mortality from major cancers in the European Union, 1980–2002.
Source: Levi *et al.* (2004a).

(established human carcinogen), 2A (probable human carcinogens), 2B (possible human carcinogens) and 3 (not classifiable as to carcinogenicity to humans) (http://monographs.iarc.fr/index.php). Agents are commonly classified in group 1 when the evidence of their carcinogenicity in humans, derived from epidemiological studies, is considered sufficient, and are classified in group 2A when the evidence in humans is limited and the agent is an experimental carcinogen. Agents in group 2B include mainly experimental carcinogens for which the human evidence is inadequate or non-existent. Between 1972 and 2006, 96 volumes presenting evaluations (and re-evaluations) for 932 chemical, physical and biological agents and groups of agents, as well as exposure circumstances such as occupations, have been published. A total of 101 agents have been classified in group 1, 69 in group 2A, and 245 in group 2B. The complete list of agents, with their evaluations can be found on the Monographs web site.

The global burden of neoplasms

The number of new cases of cancer which occurred worldwide in 2002 has been estimated at about 10 860 000 (Table 9.3.2) (Ferlay *et al.* 2004).

Of these, 5 800 000 occurred in men and 5 060 000 in women. About 5 020 000 cases occurred in high-resource countries (North America, Japan, Europe including Russia, Australia, and New Zealand) and 5 830 000 in low- and medium-resource countries. Among men, lung, stomach, colorectal, prostate, and liver cancers are the most common malignant neoplasms (Fig. 9.3.2), while breast, colorectal, cervical, lung, and ovarian cancers are the most common neoplasms among women (Fig. 9.3.3).

The number of deaths from cancer was estimated at about 6 720 000 in 2002 (Table 9.3.2) (Ferlay *et al.* 2004). No global estimates of survival from cancer are available: Data from selected cancer registries suggest wide disparities between high- and low-resource countries for neoplasms with effective but expensive treatment, such as leukaemia, while the gap is narrow for neoplasms without an effective therapy, such as lung cancer (Berrino *et al.* 1999; Kosary *et al.* 1995; Sankaranarayanan *et al.* 1998) (Fig. 9.3.4). The overall 5-year survival of cases diagnosed during 1985–1989 in European Union countries was 41 per cent (Berrino *et al.* 1999).

One complementary approach in assessing the global burden of neoplasms is to estimate the loss in disability-adjusted life-years.

Table 9.3.2 Estimated number of new cases of cancer (incidence) and of cancer deaths (mortality) in 2002, by gender and geographical area (Globocan 2002)

	Men	Women	Total
Incidence			
High-income countries	2 700 000	2 320 000	5 020 000
Low- and middle-income countries	3 090 000	2 740 000	5 830 000
Total	5 800 000	5 060 000	10 860 000
Mortality			
High-income countries	1 500 000	1 190 000	2 690 000
Low- and middle-income countries	2 280 000	1 740 000	4 020 000
Total	3 790 000	2 930 000	6 720 000

This indicator weighs the years of life with disability and adds them to the years lost because of premature death. An estimate for 1990 resulted in about 70 000 000 disability-adjusted life-years lost worldwide because of malignant neoplasms, of which 48 000 000 in developing countries and 22 000 000 in developed countries. Lung cancer was responsible for 8 900 000 disability-adjusted life-years, stomach cancer for 7 700 000, liver cancer for 6 600 000, leukaemia for 4 600 000, and breast cancer for 4 200 000 (Murray *et al.* 1996).

Overview of the causes of human cancer

A number of factors are associated with increased risk of neoplasms, but their importance varies in different settings and for neoplasms at different sites (Table 9.3.3).

Tobacco smoking

Tobacco smoking is the main single cause of human cancer worldwide (IARC 2004a). It is a cause of cancers of the lung, nasal cavity, larynx, oral cavity, pharynx, oesophagus, stomach, pancreas, uterine cervix, kidney and bladder, as well as of myeloid leukaemia. In high-resource countries, tobacco smoking has been estimated to cause approximately 30 per cent of all human cancers (Doll & Peto 2005). In many medium- and low-resource countries, the burden of tobacco-related cancer is lower, given the relatively recent start of the epidemics of smoking, which will result in a greater numbers of cancer in the future.

A benefit of quitting tobacco smoking in adulthood has been shown for all major cancers causally associated with the habit. This result emphasizes the need to devise anti-smoking strategies that address avoidance of the habit among the young as well as reduction of smoking and quitting among adults. In fact, the decline in tobacco consumption that has taken place during the last 20 years among men in North America and several European countries, and which has resulted in decreased incidence of and mortality from lung cancer, has been caused primarily by increase in quitting at middle age. The great challenge for the control of tobacco-related cancer, however, lies today in low-resource countries, in particular in China and the other Asian countries: The largest increase in tobacco-related cancers has been forecasted in this region of the world (Peto *et al.* 1999). Despite growing efforts from medical and public health institutions and the growing involvement of non-governmental organizations, the fight against the spread of tobacco smoking among women and in low-resource countries remains the biggest and most difficult challenge of cancer prevention in the next decades.

Use of smokeless tobacco products has been associated with increased risk of cancer of the head and neck and the pancreas (IARC 2004c). Chewing of tobacco-containing products is particularly

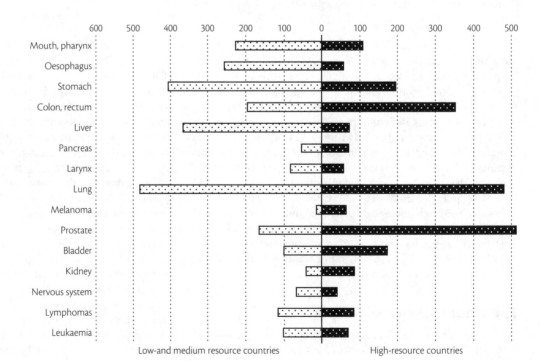

Fig. 9.3.2 Estimated number of new cancer cases (x1000), 2002. Men.

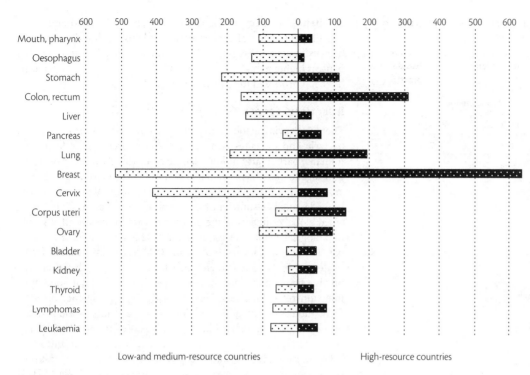

Fig. 9.3.3 Estimated number of new cancer cases (x1000), 2002. Women.

prevalent in Southern Asia, where it represents a major cause of oral and pharyngeal cancer.

Dietary factors

Despite considerable research efforts in recent years, the exact role of dietary factors in causing human cancer remains largely obscure. For no dietary factor other than alcohol and aflatoxin (a carcinogen produced by some fungi in certain tropical areas) there is sufficient evidence of an increased or decreased risk of cancer. In particular, a role of intake of fat or other nutrients in determining breast and

colorectal cancer risk has not been confirmed by recent studies (Marques-Vidal *et al.* 2006; Michels *et al.* 2007). There is limited evidence for a protective role of vegetable and fruit intake for cancers of the mouth and pharynx, oesophagus, stomach, colorectum, larynx, lung, ovary (vegetables only), bladder (fruit only), and bladder (IARC 2003), and there is evidence suggestive lack of cancer-preventive activity for preformed vitamin A (IARC 1998b) and for β-carotene when used at high doses (IARC 1998a). Systematic reviews have concluded that nutritional factors may be responsible for about one fourth of human cancers in high-resource countries, although,

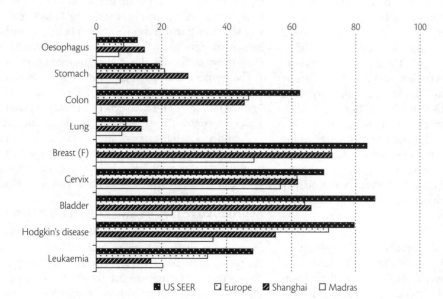

Fig. 9.3.4 Five-year relative survival from cancer in selected populations.

Table 9.3.3 Estimate of the proportion of cancers attributable to major risk factors in the United Kingdom

Risk factor	Attributable proportion (%)		Avoidable in practice (%)
	Best estimate	Range of acceptable estimates	
Tobacco smoking	30	27–33	30
Alcohol drinking	6	4–8	6*
Ionizing radiation	5	4–6	<1
Ultraviolet light	1	1	<1
Infections	5	4–15	1
Medical drugs	<1	0–1	<1
Occupation	2	1–5	<1
Pollution	2	1–5	<1
Diet and obesity	25	15–35	2
Reproduction and other hormonal factors	15	10–20	<1
Physical inactivity	<1	0–1	<1

* Total avoidance of alcohol would increase overall mortality as the increase in cardiovascular mortality would exceed the reduction in cancer mortality.
Source: Doll & Peto (2005).

because of the limitations of the current understanding of the precise role of diet in human cancer, the proportion of cancers known to be avoidable in practicable ways is much smaller (Doll & Peto 2005). The only justified dietary recommendation for cancer prevention is to reduce total caloric intake, which would contribute to a decrease in obesity, an established risk factor for human cancer.

Obesity and physical exercise

There is sufficient evidence for a cancer preventive effect of avoidance of weight gain, based on a decreased risk of cancers of the colon, gall-bladder, post-menopausal breast, endometrium, kidney, and oesophagus (adenocarcinoma) (IARC 2002b). It is likely that obesity exerts a carcinogenic effect in conjunction with other factors such as insulin resistance, low physical activity and menopausal status. The magnitude of the excess risk is not very high (for most cancers the RR ranges between 1.5 and 2 for body weight higher than 35 per cent above the ideal weight). Estimates of the proportion of cancers attributable to overweight and obesity in Europe range from 2 per cent (Doll & Peto 2005) to 5 per cent (Bergstrom *et al.* 2001). However, this figure is likely to larger in North American, where the prevalence of overweight and obesity is higher.

Increased workplace or recreational physical activity decreased the risk of colon and breast cancers and that of endometrial and prostate cancers (IARC 2002b). The RR of colon and breast cancers for regular versus no activity is in the order of 1.5–2. Increasing physical activity should be part of any comprehensive cancer prevention strategy.

Alcohol drinking

Alcohol drinking increases the risk of cancers of the oral cavity, pharynx, larynx, oesophagus and liver, colorectum, and female breast (Baan *et al.* 2007). For all cancer sites, risk is a function of the amount of alcohol consumed. Alcohol drinking and tobacco smoking show

an interactive effect on the risk of cancers of the head and neck. The global burden of cancer attributable to alcohol drinking has been estimated at 3.6 per cent (Boffetta *et al.* 2006b), although this figure is higher in high-resource countries; e.g. the figure of 6 per cent has been proposed for United Kingdom (Doll & Peto 2005).

Infectious agents

There is growing evidence that chronic infection with some viruses, bacteria and parasites represents a major carcinogenic factor for humans, particularly in low-income countries. A number of infectious agents have been evaluated within the IARC Monograph programme (Table 9.3.4), and the evidence of a causal association has been classified as sufficient for several of them. Parkin (2006) provided global estimates of the number of cases of cancer attributable to biological agents. His estimate for 2002 is 1 900 000 cases, or 17.8 per cent of total cancers. HBV- and HCV-related liver cancer, HPV-related cervical cancer and Helicobacter-related stomach cancer each provide between 20 per cent and 30 per cent of the total number of infection-related cancers. Because of the high prevalence of HBV, HCV and HPV in medium- and low-resource countries, the estimate of the attributable risk is higher in this part of the world (26.3 per cent of total cancer versus 7.7 per cent in high-resource countries).

Use of safe, effective, and cheap vaccines represents the best preventive strategy for cancers caused by viruses, and HBV and HPV infection can be effectively prevented today. Chronic infection with *Helicobacter pylori* can be prevented by eradication treatment and sanitation measures, and changes in dietary practices (e.g. avoidance of raw fish) can prevent infection by carcinogenic parasites.

Occupation and pollution

Approximately 40 occupational agents, groups of agents and mixtures have been classified as carcinogenic by IARC (Table 9.3.5). While some (e.g. *bis*-chloro methylethers) represent today a historic curiosity, exposure is still widespread for carcinogens such as asbestos, arsenic, and silica. Estimates of the global burden of cancer attributable to occupation in high-resource countries result in figures in the order of 2–3 per cent (Doll & Peto 2005; Steenland *et al.* 2003). However, these cancers concentrate in some sectors of the population (mainly male blue-collar workers), among whom they may represent a sizable proportion of total cancers. Furthermore, unlike lifestyle factors, exposure is involuntary. In fact, reduction of exposure to occupational and environmental carcinogens has taken place in high-resource countries during recent decades. Efforts should be made to avoid exposure also in low- and medium-resource countries.

The available evidence suggests, in most populations, a small role of air, water and soil pollutants. Global estimates are in the order of 1 per cent or less of total cancers (Boffetta 2006; Doll & Peto 2005). This is in contrast with public perception, which often identifies pollution as a major cause of human cancer. However, in selected areas (e.g. residence near asbestos processing plants or in areas with drinking water contaminated by arsenic), environmental exposure to carcinogens may represent an important cancer hazard.

Reproductive factors and exogenous hormones

There is a strong association between reproductive history and risk of cancer of the breast, ovary, and endometrium, which reflects changes in hormonal secretion. However, the role played by specific hormones and the mechanisms by which they act are still unclear. The reproductive factors with the strongest effect on breast cancer

Table 9.3.4 Assessment of associations between infections and human cancer, from IARC 1994a (Monographs Vol. 59), 1994b (Vol. 61), 1996 (Vol. 67), 1997b (Vol. 70), and in press (Vol. 90)

	Evidence[a]	Target organs[b]	IARC Monographs Vol.
Viruses			
Hepatitis B virus	S	Liver	59
Hepatitis C virus	S	Liver	59
Hepatitis D virus	I	Liver	59
Human papilloma virus type 16	S	Cervix, vulva, vagina, penis, anus, oral cavity, oropharynx	90
Human papillomavirus types 18, 31, 33, 35, 39, 45, 51, 52, 56, 58, 59, 66	S	Cervix	90
Human papilloma virus types 6, 11	L	(Larynx, vulva, penis, anus)	90
Human papilloma virus, genus-beta types	L	(Skin)	90
Human immunodeficiency virus 1	S	Kaposi's sarcoma, non-Hodgkin's lymphoma	67
Human immunodeficiency virus 2	I		67
Human T-cell lymphotrophic virus I	S	Adult T-cell leukaemia/ lymphoma	67
Human T-cell lymphotrophic virus II	I		67
Epstein–Barr virus	S	Burkitt's lymphoma, Hodgkin's disease, nasopharynx	70
Human herpes virus 8	L	(Kaposi's sarcoma)	70
Bacterium			
Helicobacter pylori	S	Stomach	61
Parasites			
Schistosoma haematobium	S	Bladder	61
Schistosoma japonicum	L	(Liver, stomach)	61
Schistosoma mansoni	I		61
Opistorchis viverrini	S	Liver	61
Opistorchis felineus	I		61
Clonorchis sinensis	L	Liver	61

[a] I, inadequate; L, limited; S, sufficient.
[b] Established target organs without brackets; suspected target organs in brackets.

risk are parity and age at first full-term pregnancy. Nulliparity or low parity is also related to increased risk of endometrial and ovarian cancer. In contrast, high parity is associated to an increased risk of cervical cancer. Oestrogenic stimulation is probably a major cause of breast cancer, as shown by the strong reduction in breast cancer risk among women enrolled in randomized trials of tamoxifen, and antioestrogenic drug. Exogenous oestrogens and progestins given in combination as hormone replacement therapy (HRT) in menopause and in steroid contraceptives increase the risk of breast and ovarian cancer (IARC 2005b). The risk is present, but considerably smaller, for use of oestrogen-only HRT. In contrast, unopposed oestrogens are strongly related to endometrial cancer. OC exert a consistent and long-term protection against ovarian and endometrial cancer, but current used of OC is associated to an increased risk of cervical and liver cancer (IARC 2005b). No detailed estimates are available of the contribution of reproductive factors to the global burden of cancer, and given the uncertainties in the definition of the relevant circumstances of exposure, proposed figures for high-resource countries range from 3 per cent (Harvard Center for Cancer Prevention 1996) to 15 per cent (Doll *et al.* 2005). An effect of sex hormones on testicular

and prostate cancer is plausible, but the epidemiological evidence is currently inadequate to draw any conclusion.

Perinatal and growth factors

Excess energy intake early in life is probably associated with an increased risk breast and colon cancer. The role of attained height, growth factors and other factors such as insulin resistance in this association is unclear. In addition, high birth weight has been associated with an increased risk of breast and prostate cancer. The implications of these findings for preventive strategies will be clarified by a more complete understanding of the underlying carcinogenic mechanisms.

Ionizing and non-ionizing radiation

Ionizing radiation causes several neoplasms, including in particular acute lymphocytic leukaemia, acute and chronic myeloid leukaemia and cancers of the breast, lung, bone, brain and thyroid (IARC 2000). Theoretical considerations and extrapolations from high doses lead to the conclusion that is a threshold below which no excess cancer risk is present is unlikely, although the quantification

Table 9.3.5 Occupational agents, classified by the IARC Monographs programme as carcinogenic to humans (www.monographs.iarc.fr)

Agents, mixture, circumstance	Main industry, use
Agents, groups of agents	
4-Aminobiphenyl	Pigment
Arsenic and arsenic compounds	Glass, metal, pesticide
Asbestos	Insulation, filter, textile
Benzene	Chemical, solvent
Benzidine	Pigment
Benzo[a]pyrene	Combustion processes
Beryllium and beryllium compounds	Aerospace
Bis(chloromethyl)ether and chloromethyl methyl ether	Chemical intermediate
1,3 Butadiene	Chemical
Cadmium and cadmium compounds	Dye/pigment
Chromium[VI] compounds	Metal plating, dye/pigment
Ethylene oxide	Sterilant
Formaldehyde	Chemical
Gallium arsenide	Microelectronics
2-Naphthylamine	Pigment
Nickel compounds	Metallurgy, alloy, catalyst
Radon-222 and its decay products	Mining
Silica, crystalline	Stone cutting, mining, glass, paper
Talc containing asbestiform fibres	Paper, paints
2,3,7,8 Tetrachlorodibenzo-para-dioxin	Chemical
Vinyl chloride	Plastics
X- and γ-radiation	Medical
Mixtures	
Coal-tar pitches	Construction, electrode
Coal-tars	Fuel
Mineral oils, untreated and mildly treated	Metal
Shale oils	Shale oil production
Soot	Pigment
Wood dust	Wood
Exposure circumstances	
Aluminium production	
Auramine, manufacture of	
Boot and shoe manufacture and repair	
Chimney sweeping	
Coal gasification	
Coal-tar distillation	
Coke production	
Furniture and cabinet making	
Haematite mining (underground) with exposure to radon	
Iron and steel founding	
Isopropyl alcohol manufacture (strong-acid process)	
Magenta, manufacture of	
Painter (occupational exposure as a)	
Paving and roofing with coal-tar pitch	
Rubber industry	
Strong-inorganic-acid mists containing sulphuric acid (occupational exposure to)	

of the excess risk at low doses, at which most people are commonly exposed, is difficult. For most individuals, the main exposure is natural radiation, including indoor radon, although artificial sources (e.g. radiotherapy) might be important in particular cases. The estimates of the contribution of ionizing radiation to human cancer in high-resource countries are in the order of 3 per cent (Harvard Center for Cancer Prevention 1996) to 5 per cent (Doll & Peto 2005).

Solar (ultraviolet, UV) radiation is carcinogenic to the skin. Over 90 per cent of skin neoplasms are attributable to sunlight; because of the low fatality of non-melanocytic skin cancer, solar radiation is responsible for only about 1 per cent of total cancer deaths (Doll & Peto 2005). Avoidance of sun exposure, in particular during childhood, is an important cancer preventive behaviour. The evidence of a carcinogenic effect of other types of non-ionizing radiation, in particular electric and magnetic fields, is inconclusive.

However, high rates of cancer motility have been observed in regions with low UV radiation, and among African-Americans. This has been related to anti-cancers effects of vitamin D, which is produced by the skin through solar UV-B radiation exposure. Vitamin D, and in particularly its most active forms 1,25 $(OH)_2D$, has been inversely related to the risk of colorectal, breast and prostate cancers (Giovannucci 2005b; Tuohimaa *et al.* 2007). There are also suggestion that sunlight exposure, and hence vitamin D, may favourably influence cancer prognosis and survival (Lim *et al.* 2006).

Medical procedures and drugs

The drugs that may cause or prevent cancer fall into several groups. Many cancer chemotherapy drugs are active on the DNA, which might also result in damage to normal cells. The main neoplasm associated with chemotherapy treatment is leukaemia, although the risk of solid tumours might also be increased. A second group of carcinogenic drugs includes immunosuppressive agents, notably used in transplanted patients. NHL is the main neoplasm caused by these drugs. The carcinogenic effects of HRT and OC are discussed above. Phenacetin-containing analgesics increase the risk of cancer of the renal pelvis.

No precise estimates are available for the global contribution of drug use to human cancer. It is unlikely, however, that they represent more than 1 per cent in high-resource countries (Doll & Peto 2005). Furthermore, the benefits of therapies are usually much greater than the potential cancer risk.

Use of ionizing radiation for diagnostic purposes is likely to carry a small risk of cancer, which has been demonstrated only for childhood leukaemia following intrauterine exposure. Radiotherapy increases the risk of cancer in the irradiated organs. There is no evidence of an increased cancer risk following other medical procedures, including mammography and surgical implants.

Genetic factors

A number of inherited mutations of a high-penetrance cancer gene increase dramatically the risk of some neoplasms (see sections on specific neoplasms). However, these are rare conditions in most populations and the number of cases attributable to them is rather small.

Familial aggregation has been shown for most types of cancers, in non-carriers of known high-penetrance genes. This is notably the case for cancers of the breast, colon, prostate and lung. The RR is in the order of 2–4, and is higher for cases diagnosed at young age. Although some of the aggregation can be explained by shared risk factors among family members, it is plausible that a true genetic component exists for most human cancers. This takes the forms of an increased susceptibility to endogenous and exogenous carcinogens. The knowledge of low-penetrance genes responsible for such susceptibility is still very limited, although research has currently focused on genes encoding for metabolic enzymes, DNA repair, cell cycle control and hormone receptors. Current estimates of the global contribution of genetic factors to human cancer are in the range of 5–10 per cent, of which less than 1 per cent is attributable to high-penetrance genes.

Principles of cancer prevention

Primary prevention

Many determinants of malignant neoplasms, including UV radiation, ionizing radiation, tobacco smoking, alcohol drinking, a number of viruses and parasites, and a number of chemicals, industrial processes and occupational exposures, are sufficiently well established to constitute logical priorities for preventive action. Two more reasons add weight to this priority: Some of the agents are responsible for sizeable proportions of the cancers occurring today, and for many agents it is in principle feasible to reduce or even to completely eliminate exposure. If this is taken as the objective of preventive action, some practical points are helpful in guiding such action.

First, although epidemiological data in most cases do not allow a direct estimate of the risk of cancer at low doses, it is reasonable (at least from a preventive point of view) to assume that the dose (exposure)–risk relationships for agents acting through damage to DNA is linear with no threshold (Peto et al. 1991). Second, the carcinogenic effect is not equally dependent on the dose rate (dose per unit of time) and on duration of exposure. For example, in regular smokers, the incidence rate of lung cancer depends more strongly on duration of exposure, increasing with the fourth power of it, than on dose rate, increasing only with the first or second power of it (Peto 1977).

Furthermore, as illustrated above, the carcinogenic process may be represented as a succession of stages, taking place in the time span from first exposure to a carcinogenic agent to the appearance of clinical cancer. In its simplest form, as first brought out in mouse skin carcinogenesis experiments, the multistage process reduces to two stages: An irreversible 'initiation' stage inducing malignant cells, and a 'promotion' stage which propagates these cells into a malignant growth. A third stage of 'progression', characterized by an increased rate of growth and metastases, as well as an increase in chromosomal changes in the cell, has also been observed. Formal statistical multistage models of carcinogenesis have provided a useful framework to interpret on a common basis of (postulated) mechanism both experimental and epidemiological observations. As the stages are assumed to occur in a specific sequence, some may be described as 'early' and some as 'late'. Epidemiological observations indicate that, for example, smoking has both an early stage effect, as indicated by the existence of a minimum interval of several years before an increase in risk of lung cancer becomes manifest, and a late stage effect, as indicated by the decrease in risk (with respect to continuous smokers) soon after stopping smoking.

The attribution of causality to specific agents (as done when, for instance, smoking is said to be the cause of some 30 per cent of all cancers) is complicated by their interactive effects. This is particularly relevant when considering the relative effectiveness of removing (or reducing) exposure to one of two (or more) jointly-acting agents. Whenever a positive interaction (synergism) occurs between two (or more) hazardous exposures, there is an enlarged possibility of preventive action; the effect of the joint exposure can be attacked in two (or more) ways, each requiring the removal or reduction of one of the exposures; moreover, the larger the size of the interaction relative to the total effect, the more these ways of attack tend to become equal in effectiveness.

Finally, reducing exposure to carcinogens can be implemented in two major ways: By elimination of the carcinogen or its substitution with a non-carcinogen, or by impeding by various means the contact between the carcinogen and people. Reduction of exposure depends in each case on technical and economical considerations.

Cancer prevention strategies have evolved from a predominant environmental and lifestyle approach to a model that matches individual-oriented actions with public health interventions. Advances in identifying, developing and testing agents with the potential either to prevent cancer initiation, or to inhibit or reverse the progression of initiated lesions support this approach. Encouraging laboratory and epidemiologic studies, along with studies of secondary endpoints in prevention trials, have provided a scientific rationale for the hypothesis. Promising results have been reported for various types of cancer, in particular among high-risk individuals (Greenwald 2005).

Secondary prevention

Given the limitations still constraining the primary prevention of many cancers, early detection needs to be considered as a secondary and alternative option, based on the reasonable expectation that the earlier the diagnosis and the stage at which a malignancy is discovered, the better the prognosis. This implies that an effective treatment for the disease exists and that the less advanced the cancer at the pre-clinical stage, the better the scope for treatment, and the better the prognosis. This latter aspect cannot be taken for granted.

Before a screening programme can be adopted on a large scale, a number of other requirements need to be fulfilled. First of all, a screening test (that is, a relatively simple and rapid test aimed at the presumptive identification of pre-clinical disease) must be available that is capable of correctly identifying cases and non-cases. In other words, both sensitivity and specificity should be high, approaching 100 per cent. While high sensitivity is obviously important, given that the very purpose of screening is to pick up, if possible, all cases of a cancer in its detectable pre-clinical phase, it is specificity that plays a dominant role in the practical utilization of the test within a defined population. As the prevalence of a pre-clinical cancer to be screened in well-defined populations is often in the range of 1 to 10 per 1000, if a test is used with a specificity of 95 per cent, then 5 per cent of results will be false-positives. In other words, for every case which will turn out at the diagnostic work-up to be a true cancer (assuming 100 per cent sensitivity), there will be 5–50 cases falsely identified as such and ultimately found not to be cancers. This situation is likely to prove unacceptable due to too high psychological and economical costs. One solution is an increase in specificity, for example by developing better tests or combinations of tests, or by changing the criterion of positivity of a given test to make it more stringent (this necessarily decreases sensitivity). In addition, one might select populations with relatively high prevalence of the cancer ('high-risk' groups), so as to increase the number of the true positives. Whatever the group on which the programme operates, additional requirements are that the test is safe, easily and rapidly applicable, and acceptable in a broad sense to the population to be examined. It has also to be cheap, but what is or is not cheap is better evaluated within a cost-effectiveness analysis of different ways of preventing a cancer case or death, an issue not further discussed here.

If these requirements are met, still nothing is known about the possible net benefit in outcome deriving from the screening programme (in fact, screening test plus diagnostic work-up plus treatment, as applied in a given population). To evaluate benefit, several measures of outcome can be assessed. An early one, useful but not sufficient, is the distribution by stage of the detected cancer cases which, if the programme is ultimately to be beneficial, should be shifted to earlier, less invasive stages of the disease in comparison with the distribution of the cases discovered through ordinary medical care. A second measure of outcome is the survival of cases detected at screening compared with the survival of cases detected through ordinary medical care. This is a superficially attractive but usually equivocal criterion, to the extent that a screening may only advance the time of diagnosis (and therefore the apparent survival time), without postponing the time of death ('lead-time bias'). A final outcome (and the main test of the programme) is the site-specific cancer mortality in the screened population compared with the mortality in the unscreened population.

Correct, unbiased comparison of this outcome, and thus unbiased measure of the effect of the screening programme, should in principle be made within the framework of a randomized controlled trial, in which two groups of subjects are randomly allocated to the screening programme and to no screening (that is, receiving only the existing medical care system) or to two alternative screening programmes, for instance, entailing different tests or different intervals between periodical examinations. Unfortunately, largely due to pressures to adopt a large scale screening programmes hoped to be effective, a situation has often arisen where withholding screening to a group has been regarded as unethical or socially unacceptable, thus preventing the conduct of a proper experiment. Very few randomized trials evaluating the effectiveness of screening programmes are available. Comparisons made through non-randomized experiments or through observational studies.

In addition to lead-time bias, three types of bias are peculiar to the assessment of screening programmes. Because of self-selection, persons who elect to receive early detection may be different from those who do not: For instance, they may belong to better educated classes, be generally healthier and health conscious, and this could produce a longer survival independent of any effect of early detection. In addition, cancers with longer pre-clinical phases, which

may mean less biological aggressiveness and better prognosis, are, in any case, more likely to be intercepted by a programme of periodical screening than cancers with a short pre-clinical phase, and a rapid, aggressive clinical course (length bias). Finally, because of criteria of positivity adopted to maximize yield of early cases, a number of lesions which in fact would never become malignant growths are included as 'cases', thus falsely improve the survival statistics (over-diagnosis bias).

Distribution, causes, and prevention of selected neoplasms

This section includes a review of the descriptive epidemiology of the most important malignant neoplasms. It also includes an overview of the current state of knowledge about the risk factors and the strategies for primary and secondary prevention. We chose a global approach, which excludes important local aspects of the descriptive epidemiology, the aetiology and the prevention of neoplasms. All incidence and mortality rates are standardized to the world population. We report estimates for 2002 since more recent data are available only for selected regions and countries.

Cancer of the stomach

Stomach cancer was the fourth most frequent cancer worldwide in 2002, accounting for approximately 930 000 new cases or 8.5 per cent of the global cancer burden (Ferlay et al. 2004). High incidence areas, with rates above 25/100 000 in men and 15/100 000 in women, are found in Central and Eastern Europe, Portugal, Eastern Asia and parts of South America. The highest observed rates are found in Japan, with an incidence rate in 1990 of 78/100 000 in men and 33/100 000 in women. Low-incidence areas include Eastern and Northern Africa, North America and South and Southeast Asia (IARC 2002a). The rates are approximately twice as high among men as among women and are also 2–3 times higher among groups of low socioeconomic status.

Migrants tend to maintain the high risk of their home country; their offspring tend to acquire a risk closer to their host country. The most striking feature of the epidemiology of stomach cancer is the dramatic decline in its incidence and mortality which has been observed in most countries over the past century. The decline is apparent for both sexes, and has occurred earlier in countries which currently have a low risk. This continuous dramatic decline, as well as the results from migrant studies, suggests a strong environmental influence on the disease.

The reasons for the generalized decline in gastric cancer rates are complex and not completely understood. Almost certainly, these include a more varied and affluent diet and better food conservation, including refrigeration, as well as the control of *Helicobacter pylori* infection. Whether improved diagnosis and treatment has also played some role on the favourable trends in gastric cancer, particularly over most recent calendar periods, however, remains open to question.

Several intervention trials have also been conducted involving nutrient supplements and stomach cancer. In one of these trials, which was conducted in a Chinese population known to be micronutrient deficient, a combination supplement of β-carotene, vitamin E and selenium did result in a small reduction in the risk of stomach cancer (Blot 1997), but recent findings on the issue on other, better nourished populations, are largely negative (Plummer et al. 2007).

Regarding beverages, no evidence has been found that black tea, coffee or alcohol influence the risk of stomach cancer. Throughout the world there is a strong and consistent correlation between consumption of salt and salted foods and stomach cancer incidence. A large number of studies that have examined this relationship have generally found an increased risk of approximately twofold for frequent consumption of salt and salted foods. The relationship is biologically plausible given that salt may lead to damage of the protective mucosal layer of the stomach.

An increased risk of gastric cancer is associated with *H. pylori*. The biological plausibility of a causal association is also supported by a strong association between *H. pylori* and precancerous lesions, including chronic and atrophic gastritis and dysplasia. Given that the prevalence of infection is very high, especially in developing counties and among older cohorts, *H. pylori* can explain over 50 per cent of all new cases of gastric cancer that occur, or over 5 per cent of all cancer cases globally (Parkin 2006). There are, however, still some uncertainties regarding this association. The extent to which different strains of *H. pylori*, for example those containing the *cagA* gene, have different carcinogenic potential is unclear (Kato *et al.* 2007).

Another important cause of stomach cancer is tobacco smoking. Smokers have a 50–60 per cent increased risk of stomach cancer, as compared to non-smokers. This relationship would indicate that smoking is responsible for approximately 10 per cent of all cases (IARC 2004a).

Primary prevention of stomach cancer by dietary means is feasible by encouraging high-risk populations to decrease consumption of cured meats and salt preserved foods. Prevention may also be feasible through eradication of *H. pylori* infection, particularly in childhood and adolescence, by avoiding mother to child transmission. Screening and early detection of stomach cancer have been developed in Japan with use of X-ray photofluorography to identify possible early lesions, followed by gastroscopy.

Colon cancer

Cancer of the intestine is the most frequent human neoplasm in non-smokers of both sexes combined and its rates are high in particular in developed countries. Most cancers of the intestine occur in the large intestines, while cancer of the small intestine is rare. Of colorectal cancers, approximately two-thirds originate from the colon and one third from the rectum and the rectosigmoid junction. Most cancers of the intestine are of adenocarcinoma type, that is, originate from the glandular cells. Other histological types include carcinoids, sarcomas and lymphomas.

When taken together, cancers of the colon and rectum accounted in 2002 for an estimated 1 020 000 new cases and 530 000 deaths worldwide (Ferlay *et al.* 2004). They represent the fourth most frequent malignant disease in terms of incidence and the third for mortality.

The highest rates of colon cancer (around or above 30/100 000 in men and 25/100 000 in women) are recorded in Oceania, the United States (in particular among Blacks) and Western Europe. Rates in developing countries are lower (5–15/100 000) (IARC 2002a). In most populations, rates are higher in men than in women, with a ratio in the order of 1.5; however, given the predominance of women at older ages, the number of cases is similar in the two genders. A small increase in the incidence of colon cancer has been observed during the last decades in most populations, but mortality has been declining in North America and Western Europe over the last two decades (Fernandez *et al.* 2005).

The predominant histological type of malignant neoplasms of the colon is adenocarcinoma. This neoplasm is usually preceded by a polyp, or adenoma, less frequently by a small area of flat mucosa exhibiting various grades of dysplasia. The malignant potential of an adenoma is increased by a surface diameter greater than 1 cm, by villous (rather than tubular) organization and by severe cellular dysplasia. Carriers of one adenoma larger than 1 cm have a 2–4 times increased risk of developing colon cancer; this risk is further doubled in carriers of multiple adenomas. On a geographical basis, the prevalence of adenomas detected during colonoscopy closely parallels the incidence of colon cancer.

Migrant studies suggest that dietary factors are responsible for a substantial proportion of colorectal cancer; however, recent evidence from perspective studies provides only limited evidence in favour of a role of specific foods and nutrients (Marques-Vidal *et al.* 2006). The strongest evidence concerns an increased risk for high intake of meat and of smoked, salted or processed foods. A protective role of high intake of fruits and vegetables has been reported, but is still open to discussion Vitamin D, and in particular its most active form, 25(OH) D has been inversed related to colorectal cancer risk (Giovannucci 2005).

Several studies have associated tobacco smoking with an increased risk of colonic adenoma. For colon cancer, a modest increased risk following prolonged heavy smoking has been shown in some of the largest prospective studies (IARC 2004a).

Increased use of aspirin and other anti-inflammatory drugs is likely to have reduced the incidence of colorectal cancer (Bosetti *et al.* 2006). Hormone therapy in menopause and other female hormones, including OC, have been inversely related to colon cancer risks, and hence may also play some protective role. In addition life-style factors, such as physical activity, and avoidance of overweight and obesity reduce the risk of the disease.

Patients with ulcerative colitis and Crohn's disease are at increased risk of colon cancer. The overall RR has been estimated in the range of 5–20, and it is higher for young age at diagnosis, severity of the disease, and presence of dysplasia. The contribution of shared genetic and environmental factors in the genesis of the two inflammatory conditions and of colon cancer is not known. Diabetes and cholecystectomy have been associated with a moderate (1.5–2-fold) increased risk of (right-sided) colon cancer, possibly due to continuous secretion of bile. Patients with one cancer of the colon have a double risk to develop a second primary tumour in the colon or rectum, and the relative (though not the absolute) risk is greater for early age at first diagnosis. In women, an association has been shown also with cancers of the endometrium, ovary and breast, possibly due to shared hormonal or dietary factors.

There are several rare hereditary conditions that are characterized by a very high incidence of colon cancer. Familial adenomatous polyposis, due to inherited or de-novo mutation in the adenomatous polyposis colon gene on chromosome 5, is characterized by a very high number of colonic adenomas and a cumulative incidence of colon or rectal cancer close to 100 per cent by age 55. Other, rarer, diseases characterized by colonic polyposis, among other features, are Gardner's syndrome, Turcot syndrome and juvenile polyposis. All these hereditary conditions, although very serious for the affected patients, account for no more than 1 per cent of colon cancers in the general population.

Two syndromes characterized by hereditary non-polyposis colon cancer, that is, with increased familial risk of colon cancer in the absence of adenomas, have been described. Lynch syndrome I is characterized by increased risk of cancer of the proximal (right) colon, and is due to inherited mutation in one of two genes involved in DNA repair. Patients of Lynch syndrome II have also an increased risk of extra-colonic neoplasms, mainly of the endometrium and the breast. As a whole, hereditary non-polyposis colon cancer may account for a sizeable proportion of cases of colon cancer in Western populations. In addition to these hereditary conditions, first-degree relatives of colon cancer patients have a 2–3-fold increased risk of developing a cancer of the colon or the rectum.

Cancer of the rectum

The distribution of cancer of the rectum, including the recto-sigmoid junction and the anus, parallels the distribution of colon cancer: The highest rates are recorded in Oceania, North America and central Europe and are in the order of 20/100000 in men and 10/100000 in women (IARC 2002a). In most populations, incidence rates have been stable in recent decades. The male-to-female ratio is close to 2.

Most biological and epidemiological features of rectal cancer resemble those described for colon cancer, including the pre-neoplastic role of adenomas and non-polypoid dysplastic mucosa, the presence of familial syndromes, the increased risk among patients with chronic inflammatory bowel diseases, and the likely protective role of dietary factors and physical activity. In addition, several studies have provided evidence, although not fully consistent, of an association between elevated intake of alcohol, and increased risk of colorectal adenoma and adenocarcinoma (Baan et al. 2007).

Surveillance via flexible colonoscopy, involving removal of adenomas, is a secondary preventive measure for colorectal cancer. An additional approach consists in the detection of faecal occult blood. The method suffers from low specificity and, to a lesser extent, low sensitivity, in particular in the ability to detect adenomas. However, trials have shown a reduced mortality from colorectal cancer after annual test, although this is achieved at a high cost due to an elevated number of false positive cases. Current recommendations for individuals aged 50 and over include either annual faecal occult blood testing or once colonoscopy (Boyle et al. 2003).

Cancer of the liver and biliary tract

The epidemiology of liver cancer is made complex by the large number of secondary tumours, which are difficult to separate from primary liver cancers without histological verification. The most common histological type of liver malignant neoplasm is hepatocellular carcinoma (HCC). Other forms include: (i) childhood hepatoblastoma, and (ii) adult cholangiocarcinoma (originating from the intrahepatic biliary ducts) and (iii) angiosarcoma (from the intrahepatic blood vessels). Cancers of the extrahepatic biliary ducts are of the adenocarcinoma type. Most HCC originate from cirrhotic tissue.

The incidence of liver cancer is high in all low-resource regions of the world, with the exception of Northern Africa and Western Asia. The highest rates (above 40/100000 in men and above 10/100000 in women) are recorded in Thailand, Japan and certain parts of China. In most high-resource countries, age-standardized rates are below 5/100000 in men and 2.5/100000 in women. Intermediate rates (5–10/100000 in men) are observed in areas of Southern and Central Europe (IARC 2002a). Rates are 2–3-folds higher in men than women, and the difference is stronger in high-incidence than

in low-incidence areas. The estimated worldwide number of new cases of liver cancer in 2002 is 630000, of which more than 80 per cent are from developing countries (55 per cent from China alone) (Ferlay et al. 2004). Given the poor survival from this disease, the estimated number of deaths is similar to that of new cases (600000): Liver cancer is the second most frequent cause of neoplastic death in low-resource countries.

Incidence and mortality from primary liver cancer have been rising among middle age men in the United States (El Serag 2004), but not consistently in Europe (Bosetti et al. 2008), over the last few decades.

Incidence rates of biliary tract cancer are high (above 3/100000 in men and above 5/100000 in women) in Central Europe, South America, Japan, and Western Asia. In the United States, rates are higher among people of American-Indian, Hispanic, and Japanese origin than in other groups. Most of the geographical variation is accounted for by cancer of the gall-bladder, which represents the majority of biliary tract cancers. Rates of gall-bladder cancer in women are generally higher than in men, while other biliary tract cancers are slightly more frequent in men.

Hepatocellular carcinoma

Chronic infections with hepatitis B virus (HBV) and hepatitis C virus (HCV) are the main causes of HCC (Fig. 9.3.5). The risk increases with early age at infection (in high-risk countries, most HBV infections occur perinatally or in early childhood), and the presence of cirrhosis is a pathogenic step. HBV is the main agent in China, Southeast Asia and Africa, while HCV is the predominant virus in Japan and Southern Europe. The most frequent routes of HCV transmission are parenteral HCC and sexual, while perinatal infection is rare. The estimated risk of developing HCC among infected subjects, relative to uninfected, ranged between 10 and 50 in different studies. On a global scale, the fraction of liver cancer cases attributable to HBV is 54 per cent, the one attributable to HCV is 31 per cent (Parkin 2006).

Ecological studies have shown that the incidence of HCC correlates not only with HBV and HCV infection, but also with contamination of foodstuff with aflatoxins, a group of mycotoxins produced by the fungi Aspergillus flavus and Aspergillus parasiticus, which cause liver cancer in many species of experimental animals. Contamination originates mainly from improper storage of cereals, peanuts and other vegetables and is prevalent in particular in Africa, Southeast Asia and China (London et al. 2006).

Alcohol intake increases the risk of HCC. The most likely mechanism is through development of cirrhosis, although alternative mechanisms such as alteration in activation and detoxification of carcinogens may also play a role. Alcoholic cirrhosis is probably the most important risk factors for HCC in populations with low prevalence of HBV and HCV infection and low exposure to aflatoxins, such as North America and Northern Europe (La Vecchia 2007). The association between tobacco smoking and HCC is now established, with a RR of the order of 1.5 to 2 for tobacco smoking on liver carcinogenesis (IARC 2004a).

Use of oral contraceptives (OC) greatly increases the risk of liver adenomas, and is associated with the risk of HCC, although the absolute risk is likely to be small (IARC 2005b). Case reports have associated use of anabolic steroids with development of liver cancer, but the evidence is not conclusive at present. An increase in iron storage in the body is a likely cause of HCC: The evidence comes from studies of patients with hemochromatosis or other disorders of iron metabolism. The effect of iron overload seems to be

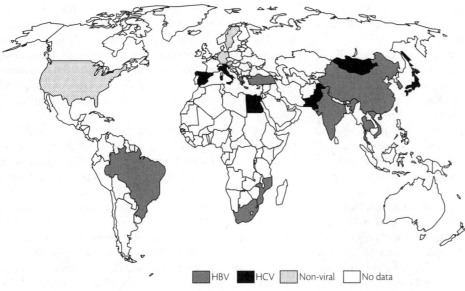

Fig. 9.3.5 Predominant causes of hepatocellular carcinoma (hepatitis B virus, hepatitis C virus, and seronegative for both) by country.*

HBV ■ HCV ▨ Non-viral □ No data

*Countries with more than 150 HCC cases using 2nd/3rd generation anti-HCV tests.

independent from development of cirrhosis and may interact with HBV infection.

Diabetes is also related to an excess risk of HCC and the increased prevalence of overweight and obesity, and consequently of diabetes, is several populations may have had some role in recent unfavourable trends in North America and other areas of the world.

Other types of primary liver cancer

Infestation with the liver flukes, *Opistorchis viverrini* and *Clonorchis sinensis*, is the main known cause of cholangiocarcinoma, that is rare in most populations but relatively frequent in infested areas in Southeast Asia. Infection occurs via consumption of improperly cooked fish. Exposure to thorotrast, a contrast medium containing radioactive thorium used for angiography in Europe and Japan during 1930–1955, resulted in an increase of cholangiocarcinoma and of liver angiosarcoma. Workers exposed to vinyl chloride, a monomer used in the chemical industry for production of the plastic polymer, polyvinyl chloride, experience an increased risk of angiosarcoma. The identification of clusters of cases of liver angiosarcoma in these workers has led to a drastic reduction in occupational exposure to vinyl chloride.

Cancer of extrahepatic biliary ducts

The main known risk factor for cancer of the gall-bladder is the presence of gallstones. The RR is in the order of 3, and it is higher in patients with large (>3 cm in diameter) rather than small (<1 cm) stones. In Western populations, most gallstones are formed by cholesterol, and their formation is associated with hypersecretion and saturation of cholesterol in the bile. The possible causes of cholesterol saturation (obesity, multiple pregnancies and other hormonal factors) are also associated with increased risk of gall-bladder cancer. An additional role of gall-bladder hypomotility in stone formation is likely. In Asia, the main types of gallstone are formed by bilirubin salts and have as risk factor bacterial infection of the biliary system: Their association with gall-bladder cancer, however, is not clear (Hsing *et al.* 2006).

Fewer data are available on risk factors for cancer of extrahepatic biliary ducts. Infestation with the liver flukes causing intrahepatic

cholangiocarcinoma, and history of ulcerative colitis are established risk factors but explain only a small proportion of these cancers. Tobacco smoking and diabetes have been suggested as additional causes. The incidence of gall-bladder cancer has increase in Europe during the last two decades (Jepsen *et al.* 2007).

Prevention

The strong role in liver carcinogenesis of infection with HBV, a virus for which effective and cheap vaccines are available, indicates that a large proportion of liver cancers are preventable. In high-prevalence areas, HBV vaccination has to be introduced in the perinatal period. In the last decades, many countries from Asia, Southern Europe and, to a lesser extent, Africa have expanded the national childhood vaccination programme to include HBV. A similar primary preventive approach is not available for HCV. Control of transmissions is however feasible and medical treatment of carriers with interferon might represent an alternative approach (which is also available for HBV carriers).

Control of aflatoxin contamination of foodstuffs represents another important preventive measure. While this is easily achieved in high-income countries, its implementation is limited by economic and logistic factors in many high-prevalence regions. Control of alcohol drinking and tobacco smoking represents additional primary preventive measures.

Cholecystectomy is an obvious mean to prevent gall-bladder cancer. The removal of the gall-bladder in asymptomatic patients, however, is not justified, with the possible exception of high-risk circumstances such as large stones and calcified gall-bladder. The increased rate of cholecystectomy in many high-resource countries is probably responsible for the temporal decreasing trend of gall-bladder cancer (Randi *et al.* 2006).

Lung cancer

Lung cancer was a rare disease until the beginning of the twentieth century. Since then, its occurrence has increased rapidly and this neoplasm has become the most frequent malignant neoplasm among men in most countries, and represents the most important cause of cancer death worldwide. It accounts for an estimated 960 000 new cases and 850 000 deaths each year among men and 390 000 cases and 330 000 deaths among women (Ferlay *et al.* 2004). Survival from lung cancer is poor (5–10 per cent at 5 years).

The geographical and temporal patterns of lung cancer incidence are to a large extent determined by consumption of tobacco. An increase in tobacco consumption is paralleled some decades later by an increase in the incidence of lung cancer; similarly, a decrease in consumption is followed by a decrease in incidence.

The highest incidence rates in men (>80/100 000) are recorded among Blacks from the United States and in some Central and Eastern European countries (IARC 2003). Rates are declining among men in and Europe. The lowest incidence rates are reported from Africa and Southern Asia.

Rates in women are high in the United States, Canada, Denmark, and the United Kingdom, and low in countries such as Japan, in which the prevalence of smoking in women increased only recently. The lowest rates (<3 cases per 100 000 people) are recorded in Africa and India. China is a notable exception, with relatively high rates recorded among women (e.g. 37/100 000 in Tianjin during 1993–1997; (IARC 2003), despite a low prevalence of smoking.

The main histological types of lung cancer are squamous cell carcinoma, small cell carcinoma, adenocarcinoma and large cell carcinoma. Over the last decades, the proportion of squamous cell carcinomas, which used to be the predominant type, has decreased and an increase of adenocarcinomas has taken place in both genders.

A carcinogenic effect of tobacco smoke on the lung has been demonstrated in the 1950s and has been recognized by public health and regulatory authorities since the mid 1960s (IARC 2004a). The risk of lung cancer among smokers relative to the risk among never-smokers is in the order of 30-fold or more. This overall risk reflects the contribution of the different aspects of tobacco smoking: Average consumption, duration of smoking, time since quitting, age at start, type of tobacco product and inhalation pattern, with duration being the dominant factor. As compared to continuous smokers, the excess risk decreases in ex-smokers after quitting, but a small excess risk is likely to persist in long-term quitters throughout life. In the United Kingdom, the cumulative risk of lung cancer of a continuous smoker is 16 per cent and it is reduced to 10, 6, 3, and 2 per cent among those who stopped at age 60, 50, 40, and 30, respectively (Peto *et al.* 2000). Smokers of black (air-cured) tobacco cigarettes are at higher risk of lung cancer than smokers of blond (flue-cured) tobacco cigarettes. A causal association with lung cancer has been shown also for consumption of cigars, cigarillos, pipe, bidis, water pipe, and other smoking tobacco products.

An association has been shown in many studies between exposure to involuntary smoking and lung cancer risk in non-smokers. The magnitude of the excess risk among non-smokers exposed to involuntary smoking is in the order 20 per cent (IARC 2004a).

There is limited evidence that a diet rich in vegetables and fruits exerts a protective effect against lung cancer (IARC 2003). In particular, a protective effect has been suggested for intake of cruciferous vegetables, possibly because of their high content in isothiocyanates (IARC 2004b). Despite the many studies of intake of other foods, such as cereals, pulses, meat, eggs, milk, and dairy products, the evidence is inadequate to allow a judgement regarding the evidence of a carcinogenic or a protective effect.

A positive familial history of lung cancer has been found to be a risk factor in several studies. Segregation analyses suggest that inheritance of a major gene, in conjunction with tobacco smoking, might account for more than 50 per cent of cases diagnosed below age 60 (Gauderman *et al.* 1997). A pooled analysis of high-risk pedigrees identified a major susceptibility locus to chromosome 6q23–25 (Bailey-Wilson *et al.* 2004). In addition, low-penetrance genes involved in the metabolism of tobacco carcinogens, DNA repair and cell cycle control might influence individual susceptibility to lung cancer (Spitz *et al.* 2006).

There is conclusive evidence that exposure to ionizing radiation increases the risk of lung cancer (IARC 2000). Atomic bomb survivors and patients treated with radiotherapy for ankylosing spondylitis or breast cancer are at moderately increased risk of lung cancer, while studies of nuclear industry workers exposed to relatively low levels, however, provided no evidence of an increased risk of lung cancer. Underground miners exposed to radioactive radon and its decay products, which emit α-particles, have been consistently found to be at increased risk of lung cancer (IARC 2001a). The risk increased with estimated cumulative exposure and decreased with attained age and time since cessation of exposure (Lubin *et al.* 1994).

The risk of lung cancer is increased among workers employed in several industries and occupations. For several of these high-risk workplaces, the agent (or agents) responsible for the increased risk have been identified. Of these, asbestos and combustion fumes are the most important. Occupational agents are responsible for an estimated 5–10 per cent of lung cancers in industrialized countries.

Patients with pulmonary tuberculosis are at increased risk of lung cancer; it is not clear whether the excess risk is due to the chronic inflammatory status of the lung parenchyma or to the specific action of the Mycobacterium. Chronic exposure to high levels of fibres and dusts might result in lung fibrosis (e.g. silicosis and asbestosis), a condition which entails an increase in the risk of lung cancer. Chronic bronchitis and emphysema have also been associated with lung cancer risk.

There is abundant evidence that lung cancer rates are higher in cities than in rural settings (Speizer *et al.* 1994). Although this pattern might result from confounding by other factors, notably tobacco smoking and occupational exposures, the combined evidence from analytical studies suggests that urban air pollution might be a risk factor for lung cancer, although the excess relative risk is unlikely to be larger than 20 per cent in most urban areas.

Indoor air pollution is thought to be responsible for the elevated risk of lung cancer experienced by non-smoking women living in several regions of China and other Asian countries. The evidence is strongest for coal burning in poorly ventilated houses, but also burning of wood and other solid fuels, as well as fumes from high-temperature cooking using unrefined vegetable oils such as rapeseed oil (IARC 2006). In other parts of the world, indoor exposure to radon decay particles may entail a sizeable increase of risk.

Control of tobacco smoking remains the key strategy for the prevention of lung cancer. Reduction in exposure to occupational and environmental carcinogens (in particular indoor pollution and radon), as well as increase in consumption of fruits and vegetables are additional preventive opportunities. No screening approaches are effective to reduce lung cancer mortality (Bach *et al.* 2007).

Cancer of the skin

There are four main types of skin cancer: SqCC, arising from the epidermal cells, basal cell carcinoma, from basal cells forming sebaceous glands, melanoma, arising from melanocytes, and Kaposi's sarcoma, arising from endothelial cells. SqCC and basal cell carcinoma share pathological, clinical and aetiological features, and are often combined under the definition of non-melanocytic skin cancer.

Non-melanocytic skin cancer

Given the simplified diagnostic and therapeutic procedures (often treated in outpatient clinics and physicians' offices) of most non-melanocytic skin cancers, reporting of cases to registries is frequently incomplete, and many cancer registries do not attempt to provide incidence figures. The very good prognosis (a more than 95 per cent survival rate in most populations) makes mortality figures useless to estimate incidence. Population-based data incidence derive therefore from ad-hoc surveys. A survey conducted in the United States in the late 1970s estimated an age-adjusted incidence rate of SqCC of 68/100 000 in White men and 24/100 000 in white women; corresponding figures for basal cell carcinoma were 258 and 155/100 000. Rates in Blacks were about 100 times lower than in Whites, and SqCC predominates. The comparison with a similar survey conducted in the early 1970s revealed a 4–5 per cent increase in incidence of basal cell carcinoma per year, which can be attributed, at least in part, to improved diagnostic and surveillance procedures. SqCC rates increased little during the same period. Rates in Whites approximate those of all other malignant neoplasms combined. Even higher rates have been recorded in Ireland and among Whites living in countries with high solar exposure, such as Australia and South Africa, while black populations have consistently low rates.

Between 75 per cent and 90 per cent of both SqCC and basal cell carcinomas in Whites are localized on the face, head and neck. In Blacks, the lower extremities are the most frequent location of SqCC.

Solar radiation is the main known risk factor for non-melanocytic skin cancer. For squamous cell carcinoma, the cumulative dose of ultraviolet radiation, disregarding dose rate, appears to be the predominant risk factor, while for basal cell carcinoma sun exposure and sunburning during childhood are the main determinants of subsequent risk. The effect of solar radiation has been shown following occupational, recreational and involuntary exposure. A strong excess of skin cancer has also been shown in psoriasis patients treated with psoralen in combination with ultraviolet radiation A. Solar keratosis is a precursor lesion of SqCC of the skin (not of basal cell carcinoma): It occurs in those areas of the skin exposed to solar radiation. The cumulative progression rate of keratosis to carcinoma (usually through a phase of carcinoma in situ, or Bowen's disease) is in the order of 5 per cent. Skin pigmentation is a modifying factor of the carcinogenic effect of ultraviolet radiation, with people with light pigmentation having the greatest risk (Karagas et al. 2006).

An excess risk of basal carcinoma, but not SqCC, has been shown following exposure to ionizing radiation (studies of medical personnel, uranium miners, radiotherapy patients and atomic bomb survivors): The shape of the dose–response appears to be linear without threshold (Levi et al. 2006). Exposure to arsenic and its inorganic compounds has been linked to an excess of skin cancer in people exposed occupationally, from drinking water or from drugs used in the past. Mixtures of polycyclic aromatic hydrocarbons (coal tar, tar pitch, soot, creosote, lubricating and cutting oils) are also carcinogenic to the skin: An excess of non-melanocytic cancer has been shown in classical occupational epidemiological studies among workers such as chimney sweeps, machine operators and roofers.

Skin cancer occurs in Asian countries as a consequence of burn scars produced by traditional heating devices kept in close contact to the skin: Kangri in Kashmir, India, kairo in some areas of Japan and kang in northern China. It is possible that polycyclic aromatic hydrocarbons released by the burning material interact with heat in causing the cancer.

Immunodeficiency increases the risk of SqCC of the skin, as it has been shown in patients treated with immunosuppressive drugs following renal transplant or other conditions. Xeroderma pigmentosum and the nevoid basal cell carcinoma syndrome are rare hereditary conditions characterized by a very high incidence of skin cancer. In the former syndrome, the mechanism is a reduced capacity to repair damage to DNA. The action of immunodeficiency and genetic predisposition may be via an enhancement of the carcinogenic effect of ultraviolet and ionizing radiation, since the neoplasms occur on parts of the body exposed to the sun.

Avoidance of sun exposure, in particular during the middle of the day, is the primary preventive measure to reduce the incidence of skin cancer. There is no adequate evidence of a protective effect of sunscreens, possibly because use of sunscreens is associated with increased exposure to the sun. The possible benefit in reducing skin cancer risk, however, should be balanced against possible favourable effects of ultraviolet radiation in promoting vitamin D metabolism. Control of occupational skin carcinogens has taken place in many industries, although high exposure circumstances may still take place in developing countries. Avoidance of drinking water with a high arsenic level should be a priority in contaminated areas. Secondary prevention can be achieved by regular skin examination, in particular for high-risk individuals: However, there is a lack of controlled trials on skin cancer screening.

Malignant melanoma

Malignant melanomas occur most frequently on the trunk in men and on the lower limbs in women. While pathologists distinguish several histological types of melanoma, these are likely to represent different stages of the same condition. A special type of melanoma, however, is the rare lentigo malignant melanoma, which occurs on the head and neck, in areas with sun damage.

An estimated 160 000 new cases of malignant melanoma occurred worldwide in 2002 (Ferlay et al. 2004). The incidence is highest (in the order of 25/100 000) in Australia, it ranges between 5 and 10/100 000 in other parts of Oceania, in North America and in Northern and Western Europe, and is below 5/1 000 000 in the other regions of the world. In general, the incidence is low in dark-skinned populations (IARC 2002a). In many White populations, there has been an increase in incidence until the 1990s, with a recent levelling off: This pattern was not observed in non-White populations.

There is strong evidence of a carcinogenic role of ultraviolet radiation in determining malignant melanoma. Intermittent exposure to the sun seems to play a more important role than total cumulative exposure.

Exposure to fluorescent lamp is not associated to the risk of melanoma, but artificial sources of Ultraviolet Radiation (UBV) have been related to excess risk.

Light colour of hair and eyes and skin complexion are risk factors for melanoma. Colour of hair seems to be the main predictor of risk, with RR in the range of 1.5–2 for blond hair and 2–4 for red hair as compared to dark or brown hair. Freckling is likely to be an additional risk factor. Skin response to sun exposure and propensity to burn (or poor ability to tan) have also been associated to melanoma risk, with a RR in the range 1.5–4. However, pale complexion and propensity to burn are strongly correlated, and the available data are inadequate to completely separate these two factors.

Presence of a high number of nevi is the strongest risk factor for melanoma. Assessment of the number and type of nevi is not straightforward, and misclassification is likely to affect studies on nevi and melanoma. The RR is in the order of 10 for the category at highest number of nevi. Their number depends on sun exposure, in particular intermittent exposure and sunburns: Exposure in childhood is more important than exposure in adulthood. In subjects with familial melanoma, large atypical nevi, referred to as dysplastic nevi, might be found. Individuals with dysplastic nevi and familial melanoma have a very high risk of melanoma. In subjects without familial melanoma, presence of dyspastic nevi seems to be a risk factor independent from number of total nevi (Gruber *et al.* 2006).

The number of atypical nevi and the risk of melanoma are increased among immunosuppressed patients. There is no clear evidence of a role of any other risk factor, including dietary factors and exogenous hormones, in the aetiology of melanoma. There is a 2 to 5 increased risk of melanoma in subjects with an affected relative, which is independent from exposure to solar radiation. Several putative high-risk genes have been proposed to explain the increased familial risk.

Reducing of solar and other sources of UBV exposure, especially in childhood, is the major primary preventive measure that can be recommended. Early diagnosis, in particular of thin lesions, is associated with better survival: Screening via medical examination is justified in high-risk individuals, defined according to familial history, type of skin and reaction to solar radiation.

Cancer of the breast

Over 80 per cent of the neoplasms of the breast originate from the ductal epithelium, while a minority originates from the lobular epithelium. However, the proportion of ductal carcinomas has been increasing over recent calendar periods. Five-year survival from breast cancer has slowly increased in high-resource countries, where it now achieves 85 per cent, following improvements in screening practices and treatments. Survival in low-resource countries remains poor, in the order of 50–60 per cent.

Breast cancer is the most common cancer among women worldwide: The estimated number of new cases in 2002 was 640 000 in developed countries and 510 000 in developing countries (Ferlay *et al.* 2004). It is also the most important cause of cancer deaths among women, causing an estimated 410 000 deaths worldwide. The incidence of breast cancer is low (less than 20/100 000) in most countries from sub-Saharan Africa, in China and in other countries of East Asia, except Japan. The highest rates (70–90/100 000) are recorded in North America, Australia, and Northern and Western Europe, in Brazil and Argentina (IARC 2002a). The incidence of breast cancer has grown rapidly during the last decades in many low-resource countries and slowly in medicinal high-resource countries. Mortality rates have remained fairly stable between 1960 and 1990 in most of Europe and the Americas, with however appreciable declines since the early 1990s. The incidence increases linearly with age up to menopause, after which a further increase is less marked (high-resource countries) or almost absent (low-resource countries) (Fig. 9.3.6). Women from high social class have consistently

higher rates than women from low social class, the difference being in the order of 30–50 per cent.

The cumulative number of ovarian cycles is a determinant of breast cancer risk, and there is an increased risk for early age at menarche and late age at menopause. Artificial menopause exerts a similar or somewhat stronger protective effect than natural menopause (Colditz *et al.* 2006).

Pregnancy increases in the short term the risk of breast cancer, probably because of increase in the level of free oestrogens during the first trimester. Overall, there is a protective role of early age at first pregnancy and a small residual protective effect of other pregnancies. An additional protective effect of lactation has been shown in several populations. In a collaborative reanalysis of 47 studies, breast cancer risk decreased by 4.3 per cent for each year of lactation (Collaborative Group on Hormonal Factors in Breast Cancer 2002). Epidemiological studies indicate a lack of association between spontaneous or induced abortions and breast cancer.

Current and recent users of OC have a modest increase (i.e. about 25 per cent) in risk of breast cancer as compared to never users. Furthermore, 10 or more years after stopping use of OC the risk levels off to approach that of never users (IARC 2008). This is of particular importance, since most women who use OC are young and have low baseline incidence of breast cancer. Therefore, their increased risk during and shortly after OC use is little relevant (La Vecchia *et al.* 2001). With further reference to exogenous hormones, the evidence derived both from observational epidemiological studies (cohort and case–control) and randomized clinical trials indicates that the risk of breast cancer (mainly ductal cancer) is elevated among women using (combined) Hormonal Replacement Therapy (HRT) (IARC 2005c). Several epidemiological investigations consistently reported higher risks among current users of HRT, increasing from 1.1 to 1.6 according to their duration of use. The risk of breast cancer is reduced after cessation of use, and levels off after 5 or more years since quitting HRT. The Women's Health Initiative, a randomized controlled trial conducted on postmenopausal women, provided comprehensive information on the risk of breast cancer in users of conjugated oestrogen alone or in combination with progestin. In the oestrogen-alone trial, after about 7 years of follow-up, there was no significant difference in

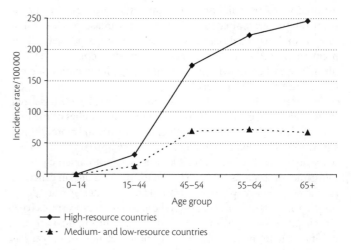

Fig. 9.3.6 Age-specific incidence rates of breast cancer by region of the world, 2002.

breast cancer incidence comparing conjugated oestrogen users to the placebo group (Stefanick *et al.* 2006). On the other hand, a higher incidence of invasive breast cancer was observed in the oestrogen plus progestin group as compared to women receiving placebo (Chlebowski *et al.* 2003).

The combined evidence from reproductive factors points towards an important role of endogenous hormones in breast carcinogenesis. A direct assessment of the role of oestrogen and testosterone is also available from recent prospective studies collecting data of biological samples. Oestradiol concentrations in the blood have been directly associated with breast cancer risk in post-menopausal women, whereas data are fewer and results are less consistent in pre-menopausal women. The association might be stronger with oestrogen and progesterone receptor positive tumours. Comparable findings have been reported for measures of testosterone and other androgens, but the data are inconsistent for all endogenous hormones across major cohort studies.

Women suffering from the two most common benign breast diseases, fibrocystic disease and fibroadenoma carry a 2–3-fold increased risk of breast cancer.

A history of breast cancer in first degree relatives is associated with a 2–3-fold increased risk of the disease. Most of the role of familial history is likely to result from low-penetrance genes associated with hormonal metabolism and regulation, DNA damage and repair. There is some evidence of an increased risk of breast cancer associated with polymorphisms of genes involved in the biosynthesis of oestradiol, particularly the CYP19 gene. Several other low-penetrance genes have been analysed, but studies have generally reported null or inconsistent findings. In addition, breast cancer risk is greatly increased in carriers of mutations of several high-penetrance genes, in particular BRCA1, BRCA2, ATM, CHECK2 and p53. Although the cumulative lifetime risk in carriers of these genes is over 50 per cent, they are rare in most populations and explain only a small fraction (2–5%) of total cases. There are exceptions, however, such as Ashkenazi Jews, among whom high-risk BRCA1 or BRCA2 mutations are responsible for an estimated 12 per cent of breast cancers.

Although a role of nutrition in breast cancer risk has been suggested by international comparisons, the combined evidence from epidemiological studies is inconclusive for most aspects of diet, including intake of fruit and vegetables, total fat, saturated fat and fibres (Michels *et al.* 2007). Similarly, results on micronutrients have been elusive, although there is some evidence of a protective role played by folate and phytooestrogens, particularly isoflavones and dietary lignans. Furthermore, vitamin D, and in particular serum 25(OH) D levels, have been inversely related to breast cancer risk (Giovannucci 2005). Hormonal levels and nutritional factors during the intrauterine period and childhood are also likely to be important in breast carcinogenesis (Lagiou *et al.* 2006). In fact, energy intake during childhood is one of the determinant of adult height, which in turn has been directly associated with breast cancer risk in most epidemiological studies.

Besides height, other anthropometric factors are involved in the aetiology of breast cancer (Lagiou *et al.* 2006). An increased risk with increasing weight during adult life has been consistently reported among women older than 60, but not among younger women. Body mass index is associated to breast cancer, the relation being inverse in pre-menopausal and direct in post-menopausal women (IARC 2002b). Several studies reported a modifying effect of HRT use on the relation between body weight and weight gain and breast cancer

in post-menopausal women. The increase in risk of breast cancer observed for a high body weight and/or weight gain was stronger or limited to non-users of HRT.

Many lifestyle factors have been investigated as possible causes of breast cancer. Alcohol drinking is an established aetiological factor. Consumption of three or more alcoholic drinks per day carries an increased risk in the order of 30–50 per cent, with each daily drink accounting for an about 10 per cent higher risk. It is likely that both overweight and heavy alcohol drinking act on breast cancer through mechanisms involving hormonal level or metabolism. Tobacco smoking does not carry an increased risk of breast cancer. A high level of physical activity, on the other hand, is likely to moderately decrease the risk. Studies of occupational factors and of exposure to organochlorine pesticides have failed to provide evidence of an aetiological role.

Less than 1 per cent of all cases of breast cancer occur in men. The incidence provides limited evidence of geographical and interracial variations, with no clear correlation with incidence in women. Conditions involving high oestrogen level, such as gonadal dysfunction, alcohol abuse and obesity, are risk factors for breast cancer in men. BRCA2 mutations are more frequent than BRCA1 in male familial breast cancers.

Control of weight gain and of overweight and obesity or postmenopausal women would have favourable implications in breast cancer risk.

Tamoxifen, an anti-oestrogen drug used in chemotherapy, has shown a chemopreventive action against breast cancer, although its use is recommended in women with a previous breast cancer only. Aspirin and other nonsteroidal anti-inflammatory drugs might also have a chemopreventive effect on breast cancer risk, although results from epidemiological studies are heterogeneous (Bosetti *et al.* 2006).

The most suitable approach for breast cancer control is secondary prevention through mammography. The effectiveness of screening by mammography in women older than 50 years has been demonstrated, and programmes have been established in various countries (Boyle *et al.* 2003). The effectiveness in women younger than 50 is not yet demonstrated, though there is some evidence for a reduction in risk of dying from breast cancer in women aged 40–49 years that undergo annual mammography. Other screening techniques, including breast self examination, have not been proven to reduce breast cancer mortality.

Cancer of the female genital organs

The female genital organs comprise the ovaries and their annexes, the uterus, the vagina and the external genitals. The uterus is composed of two parts, the cervix and the corpus, which have very distinct physiological and pathological features. Cancers of the cervix and corpus of the uterus are different histologically, clinically, and aetiologically. However, the distinction between cervix and corpus is often neglected in records used for epidemiological purposes, such as death certificates. Today in Europe and North America, most cancers of the uterus without further specification are likely to be cancer of the corpus. This, however, may not have been the case in the past and in other countries, and this fact complicates temporal and geographical comparisons.

Cancer of the uterine cervix

Cervical cancer is a major public health problem in many low- and medium-resource countries. Incidence rates are high

(20–40/100 000) in sub-Saharan African and Latin American countries, as well as in India and Southern Asia. In China, the Middle East, northern Africa and high-resource countries, rates are in the order of 5–15/100 000 (IARC 2002a). This results in a number of cases each year in excess of 370 000, 78 per cent of which occur in developing countries, where cervical cancer represents the second most common female neoplasm after breast cancer. The number of estimated cancer deaths in low- and medium-resource countries (230 000 in 2002) exceeds that from breast cancer (Ferlay *et al.* 2004). Incidence and mortality rates have decreased steadily in high-resource countries, but an upturn in incidence has been observed among young women. Few data on temporal trends are available from low-resource countries, but incidence has likely decreased during recent decades. In high-risk countries, rates increase up to age 60, while in low-resource countries there is little increase above age 50. In most countries, cervical cancer hits preferentially women of lower education and social class.

Most cervical cancers originate from the area of squamous metaplasia called transformation zone, which is adjacent to the junction between the columnar epithelium of endometrial origin and the cheratinizing epithelium of vaginal origin. Most invasive cancers are SqCC or mixed adeno-squamous tumours. Invasive carcinoma is preceded by inflammatory and condylomatous atypia, mild dysplasia (also called cervical intraepithelial neoplasia of grade 1, or CIN 1), moderate dysplasia (CIN 2), severe dysplasia, and carcinoma *in situ* (CIN 3) (Schiffman *et al.* 2006).

Chronic infection with HPV is a necessary cause of cervical cancer. Using sensitive molecular techniques, virtually all tumours are positive for the virus, while the prevalence in non-diseased women represents 5–40 per cent in the different populations (Clifford *et al.* 2005). Different types of HPV exist, and those associated with cervical cancer are mainly types 16, 18, 31, and 45. In particular, HPV 16 is a main carcinogen in many populations, while the distribution of other types varies by geographical region (Fig. 9.3.7). Differences in prevalence of HPV infection explain much of the descriptive epidemiology of cervical cancer (geographical patterns,

high risk in low social class, etc.). The host response to HPV infection is important in determining its possible carcinogenic effect; immunosuppression, as present in transplanted patients and Human Immunodeficiency Virus (HIV) infected individuals, increases the risk of dysplasia, carcinoma *in situ* and invasive neoplasms.

Sexual characteristics of women (early age at first intercourse and high number of sexual partners) and of their male partners (high number of sexual partners, presence of genital diseases and contact with prostitutes) are risk factors for cervical cancer in many populations. They reflect an increased likelihood of HPV infection, in particular at young age.

Studies of infection with other agents, in particular Chlamydia and Herpes Simplex 2, have failed to provide consistent evidence of an effect independent from HPV. An increased risk, of the order of twofold, has been detected among long-term current or recent users of OC, which is not completely explained by sexual behaviour or HPV infection. However, there is no residual association 5–10 years after stopping OC use. Consequently, the public health implications of OC use on cervical cancer risk are limited in time. Condom and diaphragm, on the other hand, exert a protective effect, possibly via prevention of HPV infection.

Tobacco smoking has also an independent effect, with a RR of 1.5–1.6 for current smokers, also once HPV infection was taken into account (IARC 2004a). A possible protective effect of a diet rich in fruits and vegetables has been suggested in a few studies, but the role of diet on cervical cancer risk is probably modest and largely undefined.

Cytological examination of exfoliated cervical cells (the Papanicolaou smear test) is effective in identifying precursor lesions, resulting in a decrease in incidence of and mortality from invasive cancer. Cytological smears are not applicable, however, in countries with limited availability of cytologists and pathologists, including in many countries with high prevalence of HPV infection and high incidence of invasive cancer. Alternative approaches for secondary prevention have therefore been proposed, including visual inspection of the cervix with possible enhancement of precursor lesions

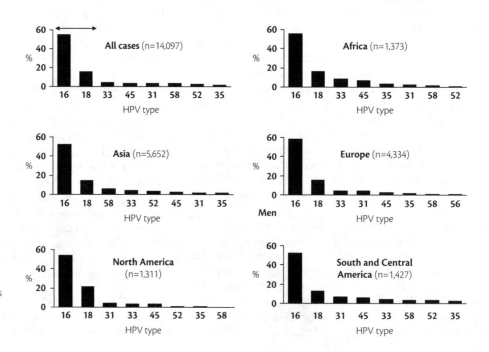

Fig. 9.3.7 Most common HPV types in 14 097 cases of invasive cervical cancer by region. *Source:* Clifford *et al.* 2005.

by acetic acid, but their efficacy on cervical cancer prevention remains unproven. Use of HPV testing as a screening method, either as a first choice for general application or as the triage method of inconclusive cytological diagnoses, is also under investigation. The primary method for prevention of cervical cancer for future generations, however, is likely to become HPV vaccination. One vaccine against HPV 16, 18, 6, and 11 is now available, and another against HPV 16 and 18 is in the late stage of testing (The Future II Study Group 2007). The final impact of the effect of such vaccination is complicated by the geographical variations in the distribution of HPV types (Clifford *et al.* 2005).

Cancer of the uterine corpus

Cancer of the endometrium is the most frequent malignant neoplasm of the uterine corpus, while sarcomas, originating from the muscular tissue, are relatively rare. The descriptive epidemiology of cancer of the uterine corpus is complicated by the large proportion of hysterectomized women in high-resource countries. The number of new cases occurring in 2002 worldwide was estimated in the order of 200 000, of which two thirds occurred in high-resource countries (Ferlay *et al.* 2004). The number of deaths is in the order of 50 000. Incidence rates are relatively high (10–15/100 000) in Europe and North America, while they are below 5/100 000 in most African countries, in the Caribbean, and in China. It is a cancer of postmenopausal women. In the United States, the incidence is higher in Whites as compared to Blacks, while the opposite applies to mortality (IARC 2002a).

Nulliparity, infertility and late age at menopause are associated with a 2–3-fold increased risk of endometrial cancer. The evidence regarding other reproductive factors, including age at menarche, is less consistent. Medical conditions resulting in high endogenous oestrogen levels (including oestrogen-secreting tumours and polycystic ovarian syndrome) have been consistently associated to an increased endometrial cancer risk. Studies of blood oestrogen levels, however, are too sparse to be conclusive (Cook *et al.* 2006).

An increased risk of endometrial cancer was reported in the 1970s, followed by a decline up to the 1990s. This trend in incidence parallels the patterns of postmenopausal unopposed oestrogen use. Combined contraceptives, on the other hands, reduce the risk of endometrial cancer by about 50 per cent (La Vecchia *et al.* 2001). Use of oestrogen replacement therapy is associated with a 2-fold increase in risk of endometrial cancer. The strength of the association depends on the dose and the duration of use. Addition of progestin to oestrogen replacement therapy may protect from the increased risk of endometrial cancer, but it may also reduce the beneficial effects of oestrogens on cardiovascular disease and osteoporosis (IARC 2005c). An increased risk of endometrial cancer has also been shown among breast cancer patients treated with tamoxifen at a relatively high dosage (30 to 40 mg) or for a long period of time (5 or more years), though results are not consistent for low dosages and short period of tamoxifen use.

An increased risk of endometrial cancer has been consistently reported among obese as compared to lean women (IARC 2002b) depending on the measure used to evaluate overweight, endometrial cancer risk increases 2–10-fold. An increased risk in the order of 50 per cent to 100 per cent has also been reported among women with diabetes and hypertension, which does not seem to be fully explained by increased weight in these patients. A decreased risk of endometrial cancer has been reported among smokers in many populations, particularly among post-menopausal women: This result has been attributed to an anti-oestrogenic activity of smoking. The results of studies of diet and endometrial cancer have been inconsistent. Several other potential risk factors have been addressed, including alcohol and coffee drinking, and history of gall-bladder disease, without conclusive evidence of an association.

Current knowledge suggests that an impact on primary prevention of endometrial cancer can be made by avoidance of overweight minimizing the use of unopposed oestrogens.

Ovarian cancer

Most malignant neoplasms of the ovary originate from the coelomic epithelium; less frequent tumours originate from the germ cells (dysgerminomas and teratomas) and the follicular cells (granulosa cell tumours). The estimated number of new cases worldwide in 2002 was in the order of 200 000, that of deaths 125 000 (Ferlay *et al.* 2004). High incidence rates (in the order of 10–12/100 000) are found in Western and Northern Europe and in North America; the lowest rates (below 3/100 000) are from China and Central Africa (IARC 2002a). In high-risk countries the rates have remained stable in recent decades.

Late age at menarche is a risk factor, but its effect on ovarian cancer risk is modest. Lifelong number of menstrual cycles has also been associated with ovarian cancer risk, suggesting that ovulation may be implicated in the process of ovarian carcinogenesis. Several studies showed a direct relation between risk of ovarian cancer and early menarche and late age at menopause (Hankinson *et al.* 2006).

Nulliparity and low parity are related to ovarian cancer. Most studies showed a decline in risk associated with number of full-term pregnancies beyond the first one, thus suggesting that additional risk reduction is conferred by events accompanying each pregnancy.

The protection afforded by combined OC is also established, and is most important from a public health perspective, feature of epithelial ovarian cancer. The overall estimated protection is approximately 40 per cent in ever OC users and increases with duration of use. The favourable effect of OC against ovarian cancer risk persists for at least 15–20 years after OC use has ceased, and it is not confined to any particular type of OC formulation (La Vecchia *et al.* 2001). The issue of fertility drugs and ovarian cancer has also attracted lively interest, but the findings of various studies remain inconsistent. Hormone therapy in menopause has also been related to increased ovarian cancer risk (Anderson *et al.* 2003).

Potential links between ovarian cancer and diet were originally suggested on the basis of international differences or correlation studies. The role of diet on ovarian cancer incidence and mortality rates and trends remains, however, unquantified.

There have long been clinical observations suggesting familial aggregations of ovarian cancer. Besides the clustering of ovarian cancer, an excess of breast cancer and a more general excess of several cancers (including colon and endometrium) have been described. These patterns are consistent with an autosomal dominant gene with variable penetration. The estimated RR from case–control studies that included data on family history range between 3 and 5. Two tumour-suppressor genes have been identified, BRCA1 on chromosome 17q and BRCA2 on chromosome 13q, whose autosomal dominant transmitted mutations confer a high risk of breast and ovarian cancer. BRCA1 may account for 5 per cent of ovarian cancers below age 50, and 2 per cent between age 50 and 70. The prevention of ovarian cancer is currently hampered by the limited knowledge of its causes and the lack of availability of early diagnostic techniques.

Cancer of the male genital organs

Prostate cancer

Cancer of the prostate is the most common malignant neoplasm in men from North America, where the incidence is as high as 100/100000. In other high-resource countries, the incidence is in the order of 20–40/100000, and in most low- and medium-resource countries it is below 30/100000, and it can be as low as 5/100000 in Southern and Eastern Asia (IARC 2002a). The estimated number of new cases occurring worldwide in 2002 is estimated to be about 680000 (Ferlay et al. 2004). Mortality rates show less variability among regions, suggesting that the number of non-fatal cases diagnosed in different countries varies depending on screening and other diagnostic procedures. The estimated number of deaths is 220000, 60 per cent of which occur in high-resource countries. The incidence of prostate cancer increased slowly during the last decades in most populations; in the United States and Canada, and subsequently in Europe and other high-resource regions of the world a very rapid increase has been observed since the mid-1980s. The disease is more common in African Americans than in European Americans. In most countries, it is more common among affluent groups of the population.

The descriptive epidemiology of prostate cancer is highly dependent on the adoption of Prostate Specific Antigen (PSA) testing. Prostate cancer incidence has shown substantial changes following the introduction of PSA testing, with major increases due to the detection of large number of prevalent cases, followed by substantial declines. The changes in trends have been much smaller for mortality, but both in the United States and in Western Europe, peak rates were observed in the early 1990s, with a levelling off thereafter (Levi et al. 2004b).

The recent trends in prostate cancer mortality in Europe are consistent with a favourable impact of improved diagnosis, and well as of advancements in therapy, on prostate cancer mortality in Western Europe and North America.

Carriers of BRCA1 and BRCA2 mutations have a 4–5-fold increased risk of prostate cancer. More in general, history of prostate cancer in first-degree relatives carries a 2–3-fold increased risk of developing the same neoplasm. Similar associations, of smaller magnitude, are also suggested for family history of breast and colon cancers (Negri et al. 2005). Recently, genetic variants entailing an increased risk of prostate cancer have been identified within the 8q24 region (Amundadottir et al. 2006; Gudmundsson et al. 2007a; Haiman et al. 2007; Yeager et al. 2007) and possibly the 17q12 region (Gudmundsson et al. 2007b).

It has been shown in several populations that the risk of the disease increases with number of sexual partners and number of encounters with prostitutes, and with previous history of syphilis and gonorrhoea. Serological studies of HPV 16 and HPV 18 have shown an increased risk among positive subjects. It is not clear at present, however, whether syphilis and HPV are causal factors or markers of infection with other sexually transmitted agents.

A possible protective role of high intake of vegetables has been suggested in several studies; high intake of meat, diary products, total fat, and saturated fat might represent a risk factor. The evidence concerning other dietary factors, including fruit intake and intake of specific micronutrients, is inconclusive at present, including that of lycopene, a retinoid present in particular in tomatoes which has been found to be associated with a reduced risk in a few (but not other) studies, and calcium which has been associated with elevated risk, possibly on account of its influence on vitamin D balance (Giovannucci 2005). An increased risk of the disease has been repeatedly reported among subjects with a high weight or body mass (Platz et al. 2006).

The wide geographical variability of prostate cancer strongly suggests that environmental factors likely related to diet and other lifestyle factors, such as physical activity, are important determinants of the disease. Primary prevention, however, is hampered by the fragmentary knowledge of its precise causes. Secondary prevention has been proposed, based on digital rectal examination and measurement of PSA. There is no evidence from controlled trials that either procedure decreases the mortality from prostate cancer (Boyle et al. 2003). Despite this lack of evidence, these procedures, in particular the PSA testing, have gained popularity in many countries, and are the cause of the steep increase in number of diagnosed cased since the mid-1980s in North America and other high-resource countries. It is unclear whether the decrease in mortality reported since the mid-1990s in the United States and in Western Europe can be partly attributed to a beneficial effect of unplanned use of PSA testing, but it is likely due mainly to improved treatment of the disease.

Testicular cancer

Some 95 per cent of malignant neoplasms of the testis arise from the germinal tissue. About half of the germinal neoplasms are seminomas, while the remaining comprise teratomas and a variety of rare lesions. Testicular cancer is common in young age, and its incidence decreases after age 30 (Fig. 9.3.8). Teratomas and other non-seminomatous neoplasms predominate before age 15, after which most tumours are seminomas. Incidence rates are high (3/100000 or more) in Latin America and Western Europe and are low (1/100000 or less) in most of Africa and in Eastern and Southern Asia (IARC 2002a). In the United States, rates are higher in European Americans than in African Americans. The global number of new cases in 2002 has been estimated at 50000, that of deaths at 9000 (Ferlay et al. 2004). The incidence has increased in most countries during the last decades, with evidence of a birth cohort effect. In many countries, the risk if higher in the more affluent groups of the population.

Cryptorchism is the best known cause of testicular cancer (Sarma et al. 2006). The RR is in the order of 2 to 5; this risk factor might

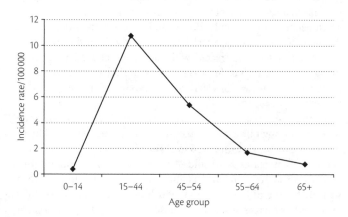

Fig. 9.3.8 Age-specific incidence rates of testicular cancer, United States 2002.

be responsible for up to 10 per cent of all cases of testicular cancer. The risk is lower when orchiopexy is performed before age 10 than at older ages (Pettersson *et al.* 2007). This suggests that micro-environmental factors might be responsible for the development of cancer in the undescended testis. Several rare diseases in gonadal differentiation, including Klinefelter's syndrome, increase the risk of non-germinal tumours of the testis. Exposure to elevated oestrogen levels during pregnancy, from either endogenous or exogenous origin, might be a risk factor for testicular cancer, although the evidence of an association is not fully consistent among studies. Familial aggregation has also been shown for different types of testicular cancer.

The limited knowledge about the causes of testicular cancer makes it difficult to devise effective preventive strategies, with the exception of early surgical treatment of cryptorchism.

Testicular cancer, particularly seminomas and teratomas in young men, is one of the most curable neoplasms if adequate treatment is adopted. Substantial differences in mortality from this neoplasm were found between Western and Eastern European countries, probably due to different availability of the expensive drugs required to treat testicular cancer (Levi *et al.* 2003). Likewise mortality from testicular cancer substantially declined in North America, but less so in Central and South America (Bertuccio *et al.* 2007). Widespread adoption of efficacious therapy worldwide is therefore a priority to avoid unnecessary deaths from testicular cancer in young men.

Childhood cancer

Acute lymphoblasts leukaemia and acute myeloid leukaemia account for the large majority of childhood leukaemias, and hence for over 50 per cent of all childhood cancers in most population.

Several chromosomal rearrangements are present in childhood leukaemia, and Down syndrome and ataxia-telangeciasia appreciably increase the risk of both types of leukaemia. In utero diagnostic radiation was associated to the risk of both types of childhood leukaemia, but the doses have substantially decreased over the last few decades, and consequently the public health implications are now minor. Childhood leukaemia is directly related to higher socioeconomic status, and both types of leukaemias have been related to a rare and late response to infection, though the pathogenic agent has and not been established. The role of other risk factors, including non-ionizing radiation, maternal smoking, paternal occupation, exposure to benzene or pesticides remains unclear (Ross *et al.* 2006).

Central nervous system cancers of various histologic types account for about one in six childhood cancers. They have been associated to nitrosamines, polyoma viruses, and pesticides, but the evidence is not conclusive and there is no established cause. Except for astrocitoma survival is relatively lower than for most other childhood cancers.

Hodgkin lymphoma (HL) in children has also been related to higher socioeconomics status, and shows a genetic predisposition. Its prognosis has substantially improved over the last few decades, and now survival is over 90 per cent in high-resource countries.

Most non-Hodgkin lymphoma (NHL) in children are high-grade tumours, including lymphoblastic lymphoma, Burkitt lymphoma and anaplastic lymphoma. Burkitt lymphoma accounts from most cases diagnosed in Africa, and is related to EBV infection. Apart from genetic factors (ataxia-telangectasia, Wiscott Aldrich syndrome), no other risk factor is known.

Table 9.3.6 European code against cancer

Many aspects of general health can be improved, and many cancer deaths prevented, if we adopt healthier lifestyles:

1. Do not smoke; if you smoke, stop doing so. If you fail to stop, do not smoke in the presence of non-smokers.

2. Avoid obesity.

3. Undertake some brisk, physical activity every day.

4. Increase your daily intake and variety of vegetables and fruits: eat at least five servings daily. Limit your intake of foods containing fats from animal sources.

5. If you drink alcohol, whether beer, wine, or spirits, moderate your consumption to two drinks per day if you are a man or one drink per day if you are a woman.

6. Care must be taken to avoid excessive sun exposure. It is specifically important to protect children and adolescents. For individuals who have a tendency to burn in the sun active protective+ measures must be taken throughout life.

7. Apply strictly regulations aimed at preventing any exposure to known cancer-causing substances. Follow all health and safety instructions on substances which may cause cancer. Follow advice of National Radiation Protection Offices.

There are public health programmes that could prevent cancers developing or increase the probability that a cancer may be cured:

8. Women from 25 years of age should participate in cervical screening. This should be within programmes with quality control procedures in compliance with *European Guidelines for Quality Assurance in Cervical Screening*.

9. Women from 50 years of age should participate in breast screening. This should be within programmes with quality control procedures in compliance with *European Guidelines for Quality Assurance in Mammography Screening*.

10. Men and women from 50 years of age should participate in colorectal screening. This should be within programmes with built-in quality assurance procedures.

11. Participate in vaccination programmes against hepatitis B virus infection.

Other types of childhood cancer include soft tissue sarcoma, neuroblastoma, renal cell cancers (Wilms tumour), bone tumours (osteosarcoma, Ewing sarcoma) germ cell cancers, hepatoblastoma and RB. The latter is related to the RB gene.

The advancements in treatment of childhood cancer were later and inadequate in Eastern Europe in South America, and in most all middle and low resource countries. At ages 15–19 years, a different proportional composition of various neoplasms is observed, with a rise of testicular cancer in boys, germ cell ovarian neoplasms in girls and, mostly, bone cancer in both genders combined. Nonetheless, mortality from all neoplasms, as well as from leukaemias, declined by over 50 per cent since the late 1960s in North America at in Western Europe, while in Eastern Europe and in other low and middle resource areas of the world some decline in cancer mortality was observed only during the last two decades, again reflecting the delayed and inadequate adoption of efficacious treatment for various cancers. This is reflected also within each neoplasm, including the ones most amenable to treatment, such as HL or leukaemia, and calls for urgent widespread adoption of modern and integrated treatment for childhood and adolescent cancers worldwide.

Conclusion

Neoplasms are a group of diverse diseases with complex distributions in human populations and with different aetiological factors. Current knowledge of the causes of human neoplasms and the development of control strategies have led to the elaboration of lists of recommendations for their prevention (Table 9.3.6). A comprehensive strategy for cancer control might lead to the avoidance of a sizeable proportion of human cancers, and the greatest benefit can be achieved via tobacco control. However, such a strategy would imply major cultural, societal, and economic changes. More modest objectives for cancer prevention should focus on the neoplasms and the exposures that are prevalent in any given population. For example, vaccination of children against HBV is likely to be the most cost-effective cancer prevention action in many countries of Africa and Asia.

Neoplasms will continue to be a major source of human disease and death. Considerable efforts are made in the public and private domains to develop effective therapeutic approaches. Even if major discoveries in the clinical management of cancer patients will be accomplished in the near future, the changes will mainly affect the affluent part of the world population. Prevention of the known causes of cancer remains the most promising approach in reducing the consequences of cancer, in particular in countries with limited resources. Control of tobacco smoking and of smokeless tobacco products, reduced overweight and obesity, moderation in alcohol intake, increased physical activity, avoidance of exposure to solar radiation, and control of known occupational carcinogens are the main approaches we currently have to reduce the burden of human neoplasms.

References

Amundadottir L.T., Sulem P., Gudmundsson J. et al. (2006). A common variant associated with prostate cancer in European and African populations. *Nat Genet*, **38**, 652–658.

Anderson G.L., Judd H.L., Kaunitz A.M. et al. (2003). Effects of estrogen plus progestin on gynecologic cancers and associated diagnostic procedures: the Women's Health Initiative randomized trial. *JAMA*, **290**, 1739–1748.

Baan R., Straif K., Grosse Y. et al. (2007). Carcinogenicity of alcoholic beverages. *Lancet Oncol*, **8**, 292–293.

Bach P.B., Jett J.R., Pastorino U., Tockman M.S., Swensen S.J., Begg C.B. (2007). Computed tomography screening and lung cancer outcomes. *JAMA*, **297**, 953–961.

Bailey-Wilson J.E., Amos C.I., Pinney S.M. et al. (2004). A major lung cancer susceptibility locus maps to chromosome 6q23-25. *Am J Hum Genet*, **75**, 460–474.

Bergstrom A., Pisani P., Tenet V., Wolk A., Adami H.O. (2001). Overweight as an avoidable cause of cancer in Europe. *Int J Cancer*, **91**, 421–430.

Berrino F., Capocaccia R., Esteve J. et al. (1999). Survival of Cancer Patients in Europe: the EUROCARE-2 Study. *IARC Sci. Publ.* No. 151. IARC, Lyon.11

Bertuccio P., Malvezzi M., Chatenoud L. et al. (2007). Testicular cancer mortality in the Americas, 1980-2003. *Cancer*, **109**, 776–779.

Blot W.J. (1997). Vitamin/mineral supplementation and cancer risk: international chemoprevention trials. *Proc Soc Exp Biol Med*, **216**, 291–296.

Boffetta P. (2006). Human cancer from environmental pollutants: the epidemiological evidence. *Mutat Res*, **608**, 157–162.

Boffetta P., Hashibe M. (2006a). Alcohol and cancer. *Lancet Oncol*, **7**, 149–156.

Boffetta P., Stayner L. (2006b). Pleural and Peritoneal Neoplasms. In Schottenfeld D., Fraumeni J.F., eds. Cancer Epidemiology and Prevention. Oxford University Press, New York. pp.659–673.

Bosetti C., Gallus S., La Vecchia C. (2006). Aspirin and cancer risk: an updated quantitative review to 2005. *Cancer Causes Control*, **17**, 871–888.

Bosetti C., Levi F., Boffetta P., Lucchini F., Negri E., La Vecchia C. (2008). Trend in mortality from hepatocellular carcinoma in Europe, 1980-2004. *Hepatol*, **48**, 137–145.

Boyle P., Autier P., Bartelink H. et al. (2003). European Code Against Cancer and scientific justification: third version (2003). *Ann Oncol*, **14**, 973–1005.

Chlebowski R.T., Hendrix S.L., Langer R.D. et al. (2003). Influence of estrogen plus progestin on breast cancer and mammography in healthy postmenopausal women: the Women's Health Initiative Randomized Trial. *JAMA*, **289**, 3243–3253.

Clifford G.M., Gallus S., Herrero R. et al. (2005). Worldwide distribution of human papillomavirus types in cytologically normal women in the International Agency for Research on Cancer HPV prevalence surveys: a pooled analysis. *Lancet*, **366**, 991–998.

Colditz G.A., Baer H.J., Tamimi R.M. (2006). Breast Cancer. In Schottenfeld D, Fraumeni JF, eds. Cancer Epidemiology and Prevention. Oxford University Press, New York. pp.995–1012.

Collaborative Group on Hormonal Factors in Breast Cancer (2002). Breast cancer and breastfeeding: collaborative reanalysis of individual data from 47 epidemiological studies in 30 countries, including 50302 women with breast cancer and 96973 women without the disease. *Lancet*, **360**, 187–195.

Cook L.S., Weis N.S., Doherty J.A., Chen C. (2006). Endometrial Cancer. In Schottenfeld D, Fraumeni JF, eds. Cancer Epidemiology and Prevention. Oxford University Press, New York. pp.1027–1043.

Doll R., Peto R. (2005). Epidemiology of cancer. In Warell D.A., Cox T.M., Firth J.D., eds. Oxford Textbook of Medicine. Volume 3. 4th Edition. Oxford University Press, New York. pp.193–218.

El Serag H.B. (2004). Hepatocellular carcinoma: recent trends in the United States. *Gastroenterology*, **127**, S27–S34.

Ferlay J., Bray F., Pisani P., Parkin M. (2004). Cancer Incidence, Mortality and Prevalence Worldwide. Globocan 2002. IARC CancerBase N°5, version 2.0. IARC Press, Lyon.

Fernandez E., La Vecchia C., Gonzalez J.R., Lucchini F., Negri E., Levi F. (2005). Converging patterns of colorectal cancer mortality in Europe. *Eur J Cancer*, **41**, 430–437.

Gauderman W.J., Morrison J.L., Carpenter C.L., Thomas D.C. (1997). Analysis of gene-smoking interaction in lung cancer. *Genet Epidemiol*, **14**, 199–214.

Giovannucci E. (2005). The epidemiology of vitamin D and cancer incidence and mortality: a review (United States). *Cancer Causes Control*, **16**, 83–95.

Greenwald P. (2005). Lifestyle and medical approaches to cancer prevention. *Recent Results Cancer Res*, **166**, 1–15.

Gruber S.B., Armstrong B.K. (2006). Cutaneous and ocular melanoma. In Schottenfeld D, Fraumeni JF, eds. Cancer Epidemiology and Prevention. Oxford University Press, New York. pp.1196–1229.

Gudmundsson J., Sulem P., Manolescu A. et al. (2007a). Genome-wide association study identifies a second prostate cancer susceptibility variant at 8q24. *Nat Genet*, **39**, 631–637.

Gudmundsson J., Sulem P., Steinthorsdottir V. et al. (2007b). Two variants on chromosome 17 confer prostate cancer risk, and the one in TCF2 protects against type 2 diabetes. *Nat Genet*, **39**, 977–983.

Haiman C.A., Patterson N., Freedman M.L. et al. (2007). Multiple regions within 8q24 independently affect risk for prostate cancer. *Nat Genet*, **39**, 638–644.

Hanahan D., Weinberg R.A. (2000). The hallmarks of cancer. *Cell*, **100**, 57–70.

Hankinson S.E., Danforth K.N. (2006). Ovarian. In Schottenfeld D., Fraumeni J.F., eds. Cancer Epidemiology and Prevention. Oxford University Press, New York. pp.1013–1026.

Harvard Center for Cancer Prevention (1996). Harvard report on cancer prevention, Volume 1: Causes of human cancer. *Cancer Causes Control*, 7, S3–S58.

Hsing A.W., Rashid A., Devesa S.S., Fraumeni J.F. (2006). Biliary tract cancer. In Schottenfeld D., Fraumeni J.F., eds. Cancer Epidemiology and Prevention. Oxford University Press, New York. pp.787–800.

IARC (1998a). IARC Handbooks of Cancer Prevention. Volume 3. Vitamin A. IARC Press, Lyon. pp.1–261.

IARC (1998b). IARC Handbooks of Cancer Prevention. Volume 2. Carotenoids. IARC Press, Lyon. pp.1–326.

IARC (2000). X-radiation and y-radiation. In IARC Monographs on the Evaluation of Carcinogenic Risks to Humans. Volume 75. Ionizing radiation, Part 1: X- and Gamma (y)-Radiation, and Neutrons. IARC, Lyon. pp.121–362.

IARC (2001a). IARC Monographs on the Evaluation of Carcinogenic Risks to Humans. Volume 78. Ionizing radiation, Part 2: Some internally deposited radionuclides. IARC Press, Lyon. pp.1–563.

IARC (2002a). Parkin DM, Whelan SL, Ferlay J, Teppo L, Thomas DB, eds. Scientific Publication No. 155. Volume 8. Cancer Incidence in Five Continents. IARC, Lyon. pp.1–781.

IARC (2002b). IARC Handbooks of Cancer Prevention. Volume 6. Weight Control and Physical Activity. IARC Press, Lyon. pp.1–315.

IARC (2003). IARC Handbooks of Cancer Prevention. Volume 8. Fruit and Vegetables. IARC Press, Lyon. pp.1–376.

IARC (2004a). Tobacco smoke. In IARC Monographs on the Evaluation of the Carcinogenic Risks to Humans. Volume 83. Tobacco Smoke and Involuntary Smoking. IARC, Lyon. pp.51–1187.

IARC (2004b). IARC Handbooks of Cancer Prevention. Volume 9. Cruciferous Vegetables, Isothiocyanates and Indoles. IARC Press, Lyon. pp.1–262.

IARC (2004c). IARC Monographs on the Evaluation of Carcinogenic Risks to Humans. Volume 89. Smokeless Tobacco Products. IARC, Lyon. pp.708–708.

IARC (2005b). Combined Estrogen-Progestogen Contraceptives. In IARC Monographs on the Evaluation of Carcinogenic Risks to Humans. Volume 91. Combined Estrogen-progestogen Contraceptives and Combined Estrogen-progestogen Menopausal Therapy. IARC, Lyon. pp.1–22. In press.

IARC (2005c). Combined Estrogen-Progestogen Menopausal Therapy. In IARC Monographs on the Evaluation of Carcinogenic Risks to Humans. Volume 91. Combined Estrogen-progestogen Contraceptives and Combined Estrogen-progestogen Menopausal Therapy. IARC, Lyon. pp.1–11. In press.

IARC (2006). IARC Monographs on the Evaluation of Carcinogenic Risks to Humans. Volume 95. Household Combustion of Solid Fuels and High-temperature Frying. IARC, Lyon. pp.977–978.

Jepsen P., Vilstrup H., Tarone R.E., Friis S., Sorensen H.T. (2007). Incidence rates of intra- and extrahepatic cholangiocarcinomas in Denmark from 1978 through 2002. *J Natl Cancer Inst*, 99, 895–897.

Karagas M.R., Weinstock M.A., Nelson H.H. (2006). Keratinocyte carcinomas (basal and squamous cell carcinomas of the skin). In Schottenfeld D, Fraumeni JF, eds. Cancer Epidemiology and Prevention. Oxford University Press, New York. pp.1230–1250.

Kato I., Canzian F., Plummer M. *et al.* (2007). Polymorphisms in genes related to bacterial lipopolysaccharide/peptidoglycan signaling and gastric precancerous lesions in a population at high risk for gastric cancer. *Dig Dis Sci*, 52, 254–261.

Kosary C.L., Ries L.A.G., Miller B.A., Hankey B.F., Harras A., Edwards B.K. (1995). SEER Cancer Statistics Review, 1973-1992: Tables and Graphs. NIH Publication No. 96-2789. National Cancer Institute, Bethesda.

La Vecchia C. (2007). Alcohol and liver cancer. *Eur J Cancer Prev*, 16, 495–497

La Vecchia C., Altieri A., Franceschi S., Tavani A. (2001). Oral contraceptives and cancer: an update. *Drug Saf*, 24, 741–754.

Lagiou P., Adami H.O., Trichopoulos D. (2006). Early life diet and the risk for adult breast cancer. *Nutr Cancer*, 56, 158–161.

Levi F., Lucchini F., Boyle P., Negri E., and La Vecchia C. (2003). Testicular cancer mortality in Eastern Europe. *Int J Cancer*, 105, 574–574.

Levi F., Lucchini F., Negri E., La Vecchia C. (2004a) Trends in mortality from major cancers in the European Union, including acceding countries. *Cancer*, 101, 2843–2850.

Levi F., Lucchini F., Negri E., Boyle P., La Vecchia C. (2004b). Leveling of prostate cancer mortality in Western Europe. *Prostate*, 60, 46–52.

Levi F., Randimbison L., Maspoli M., Te V.C., La Vecchia C. (2006). High incidence of second basal cell skin cancers. *Int J Cancer*, 119, 1505–1507.

Lim H.S., Roychoudhuri R., Peto J., Schwartz G., Baade P., Moller H. (2006). Cancer survival is dependent on season of diagnosis and sunlight exposure. *Int J Cancer*, 119, 1530–1536.

London W.T., McGlynn K.A. (2006). Liver Cancer. In Schottenfeld D., Fraumeni J.F., eds. Cancer Epidemiology and Prevention. Oxford University Press, New York. pp.763–786.

Lubin J.H., Liang Z., Hrubec Z. *et al.* (1994). Radon exposure in residences and lung cancer among women: combined analysis of three studies. *Cancer Causes Control*, 5, 114–128.

Marques-Vidal P., Ravasco P., Ermelinda C.M. (2006). Foodstuffs and colorectal cancer risk: a review. *Clin Nutr*, 25, 14–36.

Michels K.B., Mohllajee A.P., Roset-Bahmanyar E., Beehler G.P., Moysich K.B. (2007). Diet and breast cancer: a review of the prospective observational studies. *Cancer*, 109, 2712–2749.

Murray C.J., Lopez A.D. (1996). Evidence-based health policy--lessons from the Global Burden of Disease Study. *Science*, 274, 740–743.

Negri E., Pelucchi C., Talamini R. *et al.* (2005). Family history of cancer and the risk of prostate cancer and benign prostatic hyperplasia. *Int J Cancer*, 114, 648–652.

Parkin D.M. (2006). The global health burden of infection-associated cancers in the year 2002. *Int J Cancer*, 118, 3030–3044.

Pettersson A., Richiardi L., Nordenskjold A., Kaijser M., and Akre O. (2007). Age at surgery for undescended testis and risk of testicular cancer. *N Engl J Med*, 356, 1835–1841.

Peto R. (1977). Epidemiology, multistage models and short-term mutagenicity tests. In Origins of human cancer. In Hiatt H.H., Watson J.D., Winsten J.A., eds. Cold Spring Harbor Laboratory, *Cold Spring Harbor*, pp.1403–1428.

Peto J., Decarli A., La Vecchia C., Levi F., Negri E. (1999). The European mesothelioma epidemic. *Br J Cancer*, 79, 666–672.

Peto R., Darby S., Deo H., Silcocks P., Whitley E., Doll R. (2000). Smoking, smoking cessation, and lung cancer in the UK since 1950: combination of national statistics with two case-control studies. *BMJ*, 321, 323–329.

Peto R., Gray R., Brantom P., and Grasso P. (1991). Effects on 4080 rats of chronic ingestion of N-nitrosodiethylamine or N-nitrosodimethylamine: a detailed dose-response study. *Cancer Res*, 51, 6415–6451.

Platz E.A., Giovannucci E. (2006). Prostate Cancer. In Schottenfeld D., Fraumeni J.F., eds. Cancer Epidemiology and Prevention. Oxford University Press, New York. pp.1128–1150.

Plummer M., Vivas J., Lopez G. *et al.* (2007). Chemoprevention of precancerous gastric lesions with antioxidant vitamin supplementation: a randomized trial in a high-risk population. *J Natl Cancer Inst*, 99, 137–146.

Randi G., Franceschi S., La Vecchia C. (2006). Gallbladder cancer worldwide: geographical distribution and risk factors. *Int J Cancer*, 118, 1591–1602.

Ross J.A., Spector L.G. (2006). Cancers in Children. In Schottenfeld D., Fraumeni J.F., eds. Cancer Epidemiology and Prevention. Oxford University Press, New York. pp.1251–1268.

Sankaranarayanan R., Black R.J., Swaminathan R., Parkin D.M. (1998). An overview of cancer survival in developing countries. In: Sankaranarayanan R., Black R.J., and Parkin D.M., eds. Cancer Survival in Developing Countries. IARC Sci Publ No. 145, Lyon. pp.135–173.

Sarma A.V., McLaughlin J.C., Schottenfeld D. (2006). Testicular Cancer. In Schottenfeld D., Fraumeni J.F., eds. Cancer Epidemiology and Prevention. Oxford University Press, New York. pp.1151–1165.

Schiffman M.H., Hildesheim A. (2006). Cervical Cancer. In Schottenfeld D., Fraumeni J.F., eds. Cancer Epidemiology and Prevention. Oxford University Press, New York. pp.1044–1067.

Speizer F.E., Samet J.M. (1994). Air pollution and lung cancer. In Epidemiology of lung cancer. Volume 74. Lung Biology in Health Disease. Marcel Dekker, New York. pp.131–150.

Spitz M.R., Wu X., Wilkinson A., Wei Q. (2006). Cancer of the Lung. In Schottenfeld D, Fraumeni JF, eds. Cancer Epidemiology and Prevention. Oxford University Press, New York. pp.638–658.

Steenland K., Burnett C., Lalich N., Ward E., Hurrell J. (2003). Dying for work: The magnitude of US mortality from selected causes of death associated with occupation. *Am J Ind Med*, **43**, 461–482.

Stefanick M.L., Anderson G.L., Margolis K.L. *et al.* (2006). Effects of conjugated equine estrogens on breast cancer and mammography screening in postmenopausal women with hysterectomy. *JAMA*, **295**, 1647–1657.

The Future II Study Group (2007). Quadrivalent vaccine against human papillomavirus to prevent high-grade cervical lesions. *N Engl J Med*, **356**, 1915–1927.

Tuohimaa P., Pukkala E., Scelo G. *et al.* (2007). Does solar exposure, as indicated by the non-melanoma skin cancers, protect from solid cancers: Vitamin D as a possible explanation. *Eur J Cancer*, **11**, 1701–1712.

WHO (1990). International Classification of Diseases for Oncology (ICD-O). World Health Organization, Edition 2, Geneva.

Yeager M., Orr N., Hayes R.B. *et al.* (2007). Genome-wide association study of prostate cancer identifies a second risk locus at 8q24. *Nat Genet*, **39**, 645–649.

Chronic obstructive pulmonary disease and asthma

Jeroen Douwes, Marike Boezen, and Neil Pearce

Abstract

In this chapter, we will describe definitions of chronic obstructive pulmonary disease (COPD) and asthma, possible mechanisms, time trends, and population patterns of prevalence, and evidence regarding the causes of both diseases. COPD and asthma are highly prevalent non-malignant respiratory conditions that have increased dramatically in the past few decades, both in Western and non-Western societies. They have a profound impact on the quality of life for patients and their families, and COPD is also a major cause of death.

The major causal risk factor for COPD is tobacco smoke, although a substantial proportion of COPD is also caused by occupational exposures and indoor environmental exposures, particularly in middle- and low-income countries. Although cigarette smoking is the major risk factor for COPD, usually only a relatively small proportion of smokers develop COPD, a pattern which may be explained by genetic susceptibility factors. Similar to asthma, COPD prevalence differs greatly between countries and these differences are not explained by cigarette smoking alone. Nonetheless, smoking cessation is the most effective way to halt global increases in the prevalence of COPD. Improved indoor ventilation measures to reduce indoor pollutants in houses of most middle- and low-income countries are also effective ways to reduce morbidity and mortality, particularly in the developing world.

A large number of potential risk factors for asthma have been identified including genetic factors, allergen exposure, demographic parameters, diet, obesity, indoor and outdoor pollution, passive and active tobacco smoking, occupational exposures, viral infections, and the use of paracetamol (acetaminophen). However, none of these risk factors on their own appear to explain the substantial global increases in asthma prevalence observed over the last few decades. They also cannot explain the significant differences in asthma prevalence between countries. Interestingly, recent studies have shown that the increase in asthma prevalence appears to have levelled off in many high-income countries, with some even showing a decrease. The reasons for this are unclear. Understanding why these changes in prevalence are occurring, and ascertaining which elements of the 'package' of twentieth-century economic development and lifestyle changes are responsible, is essential in order to develop effective intervention programmes to halt the current global asthma epidemic.

Introduction

The most common non-malignant respiratory conditions characterized by airway dysfunction are often collectively referred to as obstructive airway diseases and comprise several clinical disease entities including chronic obstructive pulmonary disease (COPD) and asthma. Both conditions are highly prevalent and have increased dramatically in the past few decades, both in Western and non-Western societies (Douwes & Pearce 2002; Mannino & Buist 2007). They have a profound impact on the quality of life for patients and their families. In addition, COPD accounts for several million premature deaths per year worldwide (Lopez *et al.* 2006a).

COPD is usually defined as airflow obstruction due to inflammation of the peripheral airways and lung parenchyma, in which the airflow limitation is not fully reversible and progresses over time. Asthma is a heterogeneous chronic inflammatory disorder of the airways involving airflow limitation, which is variable and reversible. Thus, the critical difference between the definitions of the two conditions is whether airflow obstruction is reversible. However, it is now well recognized that airway obstruction in some asthmatics is only partially reversible. Also, acute and chronic reversibility of airway obstruction has been described in COPD patients. COPD and asthma are therefore partially overlapping conditions that share some clinical features. They also share some common risk factors including various environmental and occupational exposures. Based on these similarities, it has been suggested that COPD and asthma should not be considered as separate diseases rather as different expressions of the same disease entity. This theory, proposed in 1961 and known as the *Dutch hypothesis*, has since been heavily debated with compelling arguments both in favour (Kraft 2006) and against (Barnes 2006).

In this chapter, we will describe both conditions in parallel. We first consider definitions, possible mechanisms, time trends, and population patterns of prevalence. Then, we consider the evidence regarding risk factors for exacerbations as well as the initial development of both diseases.

Definitions

COPD

Traditionally, COPD has been defined as 'irreversible airflow obstruction due to chronic bronchitis and emphysema, which progresses over time' (Petty 2006). Emphysema was already described in the seventeenth and eighteenth century (Petty 2006), and one of the first reports of chronic bronchitis as a serious and disabling disorder appeared in 1814 (Badham 1814). It was only a few years later that Laënnec (1821) made the observation that chronic bronchitis and emphysema often occurred in the same subject at the same time (Petty 2002, 2006). However, it was not until about 150 years later that Burrows *et al.* (1966) suggested labelling the spectrum of chronic bronchitis and emphysema as 'chronic obstructive lung disease', or COPD as it is currently most often referred to. A few years before that, the CIBA Guest Symposium (1959) and the American Thoracic Society symposium (Committee on Diagnostic Standards for Nontuberculous Respiratory Diseases 1962) proposed the first definitions of chronic bronchitis and emphysema, respectively. Our current definitions are still largely based on these initial definitions; that is chronic bronchitis is defined clinically as 'the presence of chronic productive cough for at least three consecutive months in two consecutive years'; emphysema, on the other hand, is defined in pathological terms as 'an increase in the size of the distal airspaces and destruction of their walls without obvious fibrosis' (American Thoracic Society Committee on Diagnostic Standards 1962).

The most recent definitions of COPD as reported in the American Thoracic Society (ATS), European Respiratory Society (ERS), and the Global Initiative for Chronic Obstructive Lung Disease (GOLD) guidelines emphasize the inflammatory response to noxious particles and gases as the predominant pathological feature of the disease, and have parted from the definition of COPD as being a syndrome of chronic bronchitis and emphysema. The widely accepted GOLD definition states that COPD is:

A preventable and treatable disease with some significant extra pulmonary effects that may contribute to the severity in individual patients. Its pulmonary component is characterized by airflow limitation that is not fully reversible. The airflow limitation is usually progressive and associated with an abnormal inflammatory response of the lung to noxious particles or gases (Rabe *et al.* 2007)

Although no longer specifically included in the definition, it is still recognized that chronic bronchitis and emphysema are important causes of the chronic airflow limitation characteristic of COPD. The three main components (inflammation, airflow limitation that is not fully reversible, and a gradual loss of lung function over time) represent the major pathophysiological events leading to the symptoms typically expressed by those with COPD: Chronic and progressive cough, sputum production, and dyspnoea (difficult or laboured breathing). Cough and sputum production may precede the development of airflow limitation by many years, but fixed airflow obstruction may also develop without these symptoms (Petty 2006).

Clinical COPD

Spirometry is an essential tool in the clinical diagnosis of COPD and there are well-accepted standardized guidelines (Miller *et al.* 2005). In COPD, the maximum volume of air that can be forcibly expired (forced vital capacity [FVC]) is generally not affected, or only marginally affected; the volume of air exhaled in the first second of expiration (forced expiratory volume in one second [FEV_1]), on the other hand, is significantly reduced and is a clear marker of

airway obstruction. COPD is therefore defined based on the post-bronchodilator FEV_1/FVC ratio. A cut-off point of 0.7 (i.e. 70 per cent) is widely used (Rabe *et al.* 2007), but this has not been clinically validated. Also, it is well recognized that using a fixed FEV_1/FVC ratio to define COPD independent of age has the potential for significant misclassification, with underdiagnosis in younger adults and overdiagnosis in the elderly (Medbo & Melbye 2007). Bronchodilator treatment prior to spirometry is important because it establishes whether obstruction is irreversible and distinguishes it from asthma in which obstruction is mostly reversible.

The degree of severity of COPD (defined as a FEV_1/FVC < 70 per cent) is usually based on the patient's FEV_1. The 2006 GOLD criteria classify COPD severity into four stages (Rabe *et al.* 2007):

Stage I, mild: $FEV_1 \geq 80$ per cent predicted.

Stage II, moderate: 50 per cent $\leq FEV_1 \geq 80$ per cent predicted.

Stage III, severe: 30 per cent $\leq FEV_1 \geq 50$ per cent predicted.

Stage IV, very severe: $FEV_1 < 30$ per cent predicted *or* $FEV_1 < 50$ per cent predicted *plus* chronic respiratory failure (i.e. arterial pressure of oxygen [PaO_2] less than 8 kPa [60 mm Hg] with or without arterial pressure of CO_2 [$PaCO_2$] greater than 6.7 kPa [50 mm Hg] while breathing air at sea level).

Previous GOLD guidelines also listed a 'Stage 0, at risk' level, which included those with respiratory symptoms such as chronic cough and sputum production but normal lung function. This is no longer included in the 2006 guidelines as there is insufficient evidence that the individuals who meet these criteria necessarily progress on to Stage I.

Despite the well-accepted guidelines for diagnosis, and the availability of inexpensive and convenient hand-held spirometers, COPD remains a significantly underdiagnosed disease particularly in younger people and women (Halbert *et al.* 2006). This is largely because those with mild COPD often have no symptoms, or they have symptoms that are not perceived by patients and healthcare providers as abnormal, therefore not warranting a spirometric assessment. Similarly, subjects may be less likely to be diagnosed with COPD if there is no history of smoking, one of the best-known risk factors for COPD.

Defining COPD in epidemiological surveys

In population-based surveys, COPD is often defined on the basis of (1) self-report of a doctor diagnosis of COPD, bronchitis, or emphysema; (2) self-report of respiratory symptoms; and (3) spirometry with or without prior bronchodilator treatment. It has repeatedly been shown that self-reports of a clinical diagnosis significantly underestimate the true disease prevalence (Chapman *et al.* 2006). In a recent meta-analysis using population-based prevalence estimates during the period 1990–2004, it was shown that spirometric criteria resulted in an almost twofold higher prevalence estimate compared with patient-reported COPD; i.e., 9.2 per cent versus 4.9 per cent, respectively (Halbert *et al.* 2006). This is probably largely due to the general underdiagnosis of COPD by most general practitioners.

Spirometric assessment to define COPD is therefore superior to a clinical assessment without spirometry, or a self-report of doctor-diagnosed COPD. However, the use of bronchodilators significantly complicates large population-based spirometry surveys and many studies therefore do not collect post-bronchodilator measurements. The implications of failing to check for reversibility of airflow obstruction (using pre- and post-bronchodilator spirometry) may, however, result in an overestimation of the prevalence. For example, in a study in a random population sample of 2235 Norwegian adults aged 26–82 years, the prevalence of COPD based on post-bronchodilator measurements was 7 per cent compared to 9.6 per cent for pre-bronchodilator measurements (Johannessen *et al.* 2005). Thus, post-bronchodilator spirometry to determine the diagnosis of COPD in population-based studies is strongly recommended.

Asthma

The word 'asthma' comes from a Greek word meaning 'panting' (Keeney 1964), but reference to asthma can also be found in ancient Egyptian, Hebrew, and Indian medical writings (Unger & Harris 1974; Ellul-Micallef 1976). Asthma has puzzled and confused physicians and patients from the time of Hippocrates to the present day. There were clear observations of patients experiencing attacks of asthma in the second century and evidence of disordered anatomy in the lung as far back as the seventeenth century (Willis 1678).

The definition of asthma initially proposed at the Ciba Foundation conference in 1959 (CIBA Foundation Guest Symposium 1959) and endorsed by the American Thoracic Society in 1962 (American Thoracic Society Committee on Diagnostic Standards 1962) is that 'asthma is a disease characterized by wide variation over short periods of time in resistance to flow in the airways of the lung'. Although these features receive lesser prominence in some current definitions, as the importance of airways inflammation is appropriately recognized, they still form the basis of the recent Global Initiative for Asthma (GINA) description of asthma, as follows:

> *A chronic inflammatory disorder of the airways in which many cells and cellular elements play a role. The chronic inflammation is associated with airway hyperresponsiveness that leads to recurrent episodes of wheezing, breathlessness, chest tightness, and coughing, particularly at night or in the early morning. These episodes are usually associated with widespread, but variable, airflow obstruction within the lung that is often reversible either spontaneously or with treatment.* (Global Initiative for Asthma 2006)

These three components—chronic airways inflammation, reversible airflow obstruction, and enhanced bronchial reactivity—form the basis of current definitions of asthma. They also represent the major pathophysiological events leading to the symptoms of wheezing, breathlessness, chest tightness, cough, and sputum by which physicians clinically diagnose this disorder.

Clinical asthma

There is no single test or pathognomic feature that defines the presence or absence of asthma. Furthermore, the variability of the condition means that evidence of it may or may not be present on the day, or at the time, that someone is assessed. Thus, a diagnosis of asthma is made on the basis of the clinical history, combined with physical examination and respiratory function tests over a period of time. Several studies have found the prevalence of physician-diagnosed asthma to be substantially lower than the prevalence of asthma symptoms in the community (e.g. Asher *et al.* 1998). This is not surprising because a clinical diagnosis of asthma can only be made if a person presents him or herself to a doctor. This requires an initial self assessment of the symptoms (in terms of severity and frequency), as well as access to a doctor once a self-assessment has

been made. Several medical consultations may then be required. Thus, diagnosed asthma is dependent not only on morbidity but also on patient perception of their symptoms, physician practice, and the availability of healthcare.

There are a number of tests that may facilitate the diagnosis and monitoring of asthma. Measurements of lung function are the most frequently used and provide important information on airflow limitation including variability, reversibility, and severity. Airflow limitation is most often measured using spirometry or a peak flow (PEF) meter. Spirometry is the preferred method. Pre- and post-bronchodilator treatment is important because it will establish whether obstruction is irreversible and will distinguish it from COPD in which obstruction is mostly reversible. Reversibility of $FEV_1 \geq 12$ per cent and ≥ 200 mL from the pre-bronchodilator value is generally accepted as a valid indication of asthma (Global Initiative for Asthma 2006). However, due to the highly variable nature of the condition, repeated lung function tests are required. PEF meters are inexpensive and easy to use, but they are less precise and may underestimate the degree of airflow limitation (Aggarwal *et al.* 2006).

In subjects with asthma symptoms but normal lung function, bronchial hyperresponsiveness (BHR) testing is often used as a diagnostic aid. BHR constitutes airway narrowing to non-specific stimuli, such as exercise, cold air, and chemical irritants, and can be measured as airway responsiveness to histamine, methacholine, adenosine-5'-monophosphate (AMP), hypertonic saline or exercise challenge (de Meer *et al.* 2004a). However, although BHR is related to asthma, it may occur independently of asthma, and vice versa (Pearce *et al.* 2000a), which makes this test of limited use for individual asthma diagnostics.

More recently, an increasing number of tests are available to measure non-invasive markers of airway inflammation including sputum induction tests (Simpson *et al.* 2006), exhaled NO tests (Taylor *et al.* 2006), and measurements of inflammatory markers in exhaled breath condensate (Kharitonov & Barnes 2006). Although these may be useful in establishing asthma phenotypes (Simpson *et al.* 2006; Douwes *et al.* 2002a) and determining optimal treatment (Smith *et al.* 2005), they have as yet to be demonstrated to aid in asthma diagnosis. Also, with the exception of the exhaled NO test, all other tests require rigorous validation before they can be applied in clinical practice.

The degree of severity is commonly classified using GINA criteria (Global Initiative for Asthma 2006), which subdivide asthma into four categories:

Intermittent: Symptoms less than once a week, brief exacerbations, nocturnal symptoms not more than twice a month, FEV_1 or PEF ≥ 80 per cent predicted, FEV_1 or PEF variability < 20 per cent.

Mild persistent: Symptoms more than once a week but less than once a day, exacerbations may affect activity and sleep, nocturnal symptoms more than twice a month, FEV_1 or PEF ≥ 80 per cent predicted, FEV_1 or PEF variability < 20–30 per cent.

Moderate persistent: Symptoms daily, exacerbations may affect activity and sleep, nocturnal symptoms more than once a week, daily use of inhaled short-acting β2-agonist, FEV_1 or PEF = 60–80 per cent predicted, FEV_1 or PEF variability > 30 per cent.

Severe persistent: Symptoms daily, frequent exacerbations, frequent nocturnal asthma symptoms, limitation of physical activities, FEV_1 or PEF ≤ 60 per cent predicted, FEV_1 or PEF variability > 30 per cent.

Defining asthma in epidemiological surveys

Defining and diagnosing asthma in population-based epidemiological surveys of asthma prevalence or incidence poses even greater difficulties than defining asthma in individual patients. Thus, comparisons of diagnosed asthma between populations are fraught with difficulty as the differences in diagnostic practice may be as great in magnitude as the real differences in asthma morbidity.

Thus, asthma prevalence surveys usually focus on self-reported (or parental reported) 'asthma symptoms' rather than diagnosed asthma. Standardized questionnaires on asthma symptoms have therefore become the cornerstone of large studies of the incidence or prevalence of asthma (Burney *et al.* 1994; Asher *et al.* 1995). This approach allows a large number of participants to be surveyed without great cost, in a short time period. Wheezing, chest tightness, breathlessness, and coughing are all symptoms clinically associated with asthma, but epidemiological studies have shown that wheezing is the most important symptom for the identification of asthma, and the majority of questionnaires used to assess asthma prevalence are based on this symptom (Pearce *et al.* 1998).

An alternative approach to symptom questionnaires has been to use more 'objective' measures such as bronchial responsiveness testing, either alone or in combination with questionnaires. In particular, it has been suggested that asthma should be defined in epidemiological studies as symptomatic BHR (Toelle *et al.* 1992). However, some have criticized the use of BHR as a more valid assessment of asthma (Pearce *et al.* 2000a).

Mechanisms, prevalence, and risk factors of COPD

Mechanisms of COPD

Patients with COPD have an impaired ability to exhale air from their lungs. COPD includes emphysema, chronic bronchitis, or a combination of both conditions. Emphysema is characterized by loss of elasticity of the lung tissue and destruction of structures supporting the alveoli. As a result, the small airways collapse during exhaling, which leads to obstruction and trapping of air in the lungs. Chronic bronchitis involves an inflammation of the airways in the lungs resulting in thick mucus, which plugs up the airways and makes it difficult to efficiently inhale air into the lungs.

COPD is a major cause of death throughout the world and is accompanied by a large personal, societal, and economic burden. Patients experience poor physical functioning and live with distressing symptoms that require frequent hospital admission as the disease progresses. They are frequently unable to work and may become socially isolated and depressed. In the Confronting COPD survey, 80 per cent of the patients had two or more symptoms on most or all days, such as breathlessness (45 per cent), cough (46 per cent), and sputum production (40 per cent) (Rennard *et al.* 2002). Just over two thirds of the patients were breathless when walking up a flight of stairs, and one third were breathless getting washed or dressed. In addition, 39 per cent of the patients woke due to their symptoms at least a few nights each week.

As well as living with the daily symptoms of stable disease, patients live with the fear of exacerbations, which are common for all levels of lung disease. Exacerbations are associated with significant mortality, lead to frequent hospitalization, and are a major determinant of COPD costs.

Smoking is the major risk factor for its development, and therefore COPD is largely (but not exclusively) attributable to this environmental factor, with the exception of the genetic predominance of the alpa-1-antitrypsine (AAT) deficiency gene, in which carriers need no further environmental smoke exposure to develop a phenotypic expression of COPD. AAT deficiency accounts for only a minimal number of COPD cases worldwide (<1 per cent); thus, the majority of the COPD cases are due to smoking. However, genetics may also play a role in the development of COPD. In particular, although cigarette smoking is clearly the major risk factor for development of COPD, only a small proportion of smokers develop COPD. These 'susceptible smokers' show premature onset of lung function decline and, to a lesser extent, more rapid rates of decline later in life (Tager *et al.* 1988) In non-smokers, FEV_1 declines at a mean rate of approximately 30 mL/year during adult life, whereas in smokers this is increased to 30–45 mL/year. Within a subset of susceptible cigarette smokers, the rate of decline is 80–100 mL/year, and only 10–20 per cent of Caucasian chronic heavy cigarette smokers develop symptomatic COPD.

The deleterious effect of smoking is due to the fact that cigarette smoke contains a large amount of free radicals, which disturbs the reduction–oxidation balance in the lungs, leading to elevated oxidative stress (Kirkham & Rahman 2006). Such an oxidant overdose can injure lung tissue directly by oxidation of cellular components, or indirectly by promoting neutrophilic inflammation and tissue degradation, subsequently affecting lung function (Kirkham & Rahman 2006; MacNee 2005).

Prevalence of COPD

Up to 2001, only about 30 prevalence surveys of COPD had been reported. This is in sharp contrast with asthma, which has been much more extensively studied with hundreds of reported prevalence studies (Chapman *et al.* 2006). The establishment of the Burden of Obstructive Lung Disease (BOLD) initiative (described later in this subsection), and other recent international initiatives to assess the global burden of COPD, will allow more valid comparisons of the prevalence of COPD over time and across nations in the near future. In the following, we summarize the most important studies currently available.

European epidemiological studies of COPD show prevalence estimates of 4–11 per cent (Vestbo 2004). These differences in prevalence estimates are presumed to be attributable to differences in risk exposures or population characteristics, but methods and definitions used to measure COPD may also play a role. Definitions of COPD used in these studies vary from doctor's diagnosis of COPD to more rigid definitions based on pathology and/or pulmonary lung function testing. Definitions based on spirometry are the least influenced by local diagnostic practice, but are nevertheless subject to variation based on the lung function parameters selected (Vestbo 2004).

Halbert *et al.* (2006) assessed the reasons for conflicting prevalence estimates described in the literature. They selected studies that had (1) estimated population-based COPD prevalences and (2) clearly described the methods used to obtain these estimates. In total, 32 studies presenting prevalence data for COPD were identified and reviewed, representing 17 countries and 8 World Health Organization (WHO) regions. Prevalence estimates were based on spirometry (11 studies), respiratory symptoms (14 studies), patient-reported disease (10 studies), or expert opinion.

The reported prevalence of COPD ranged from 0.23 to 18.3 per cent, with the lowest prevalences (0.2–2.5 per cent) being those based on expert opinion. Sixteen studies had measured rates that could confidently be extrapolated to an entire region or country; all of these 16 studies were conducted in Europe or North America, and in most the prevalence was between 4 and 10 per cent. A recent analysis of the data of the Vlagtwedde and Vlaardingen population-based cohort of Dutch Caucasians (van Diemen *et al.* 2005) reported that based on spirometry 13.4 per cent of all subjects had COPD as defined by GOLD stage II or higher, corresponding to $FEV_1/FVC < 70$ per cent and $FEV_1 < 80$ per cent predicted (see the section title 'Definitions').

Although the most accurate prevalence data are from Western countries, estimates suggest that about half of the approximately 2.7 million deaths in 2000 were in the Western Pacific Region, with the majority occurring in China. About 400 000 deaths occur each year from COPD in industrialized countries (Lopez *et al.* 2006b). Lopez *et al.* recently noted that the increase in global COPD deaths between 1990 and 2000 (0.5 million) is partially real, and may partially be due to better diagnostic methods and more extensive data availability in 2000. The regional COPD prevalence in adults in 2000 was estimated to vary from 0.5 per cent in parts of Africa to 3–4 per cent in North America (Soriano *et al.* 2000).

Halbert *et al.* (2006) recently quantified the global prevalence of COPD by performing a systematic review and random effects meta-analysis. They searched for studies published during 1990–2004, and identified 101 prevalence estimates from 28 countries. The pooled prevalence of COPD was 7.6 per cent, the prevalence of chronic bronchitis alone was 6.4 per cent, and the prevalence of emphysema alone was 1.8 per cent. The pooled prevalence of COPD based on spirometry was 8.9 per cent, with the most commonly used spirometric definitions being those of the Global Initiative for Chronic Obstructive Lung Disease.

The BOLD initiative developed standardized methods for estimating COPD prevalence and is currently one of only a few studies with truly comparable international prevalence estimates (Buist *et al.* 2007). The study included 9425 participants from 12 centres in 12 countries including China, Turkey, Austria, South Africa, Iceland, Germany, Poland, Norway, Canada, the United States, the Philippines, and Australia. Using identical methods, the study showed considerable variation in COPD prevalences, with GOLD stage II or higher COPD (post-bronchodilator $FEV_1/FVC < 70$ per cent) in women ranging from 5.1 per cent in Guangzhou, China, to 16.7 per cent in Cape Town, South Africa. In men, it ranged from 8.5 per cent in Reykjavik, Iceland, to 22.2 per cent in Cape Town, South Africa. Using a similar study design, the Latin American Project for the Investigation of Obstructive Lung Diseases (PLATINO) studied the prevalence of COPD among 5315 study participants in five Latin American centres (Mexico, Venezuela, Brazil, Chile, and Uruguay) (Menezes *et al.* 2005). Crude prevalence rates of COPD ranged from 7.8 per cent in Mexico City, Mexico, to 19.7 per cent in Montevideo, Uruguay. Interestingly, age and smoking did not fully explain the international variation in disease prevalence, suggesting an important role of additional risk factors.

Although COPD is considered to be mainly present in the elderly, it is not a disease of the elderly alone. In the Confronting COPD study, the presence of COPD based on doctor's diagnosis and presence of symptoms in younger age groups has also been described (Rennard *et al.* 2002); a phenomenon that was confirmed in the European Community Respiratory Health Survey (ECRHS) which verified COPD diagnosis with spirometric testing in random population samples of younger age (<45 years) (Vestbo 2004).

Future prevalence and burden of COPD

Although it is recognized that the burden of COPD is high, an accurate estimate of COPD prevalence data is hampered by both underdiagnosis and misdiagnosis. Mortality data are also likely to underestimate the impact of COPD because many COPD patients do not have this recorded on their death certificate due to inconsistent use of International Classification of Disease (ICD) codes (Vestbo 2004). However, despite this under-reporting, it is clear that COPD is one of the most common causes of death.

Assessing the future prevalence and burden of COPD requires taking changing population distributions and smoking habits into account. For example, Feenstra *et al.* (2001) used a dynamic multi-stage life table model to compute projections for the Netherlands. Changes in the size and composition of the population were predicted to increase COPD prevalence from 21/1000 in 1994 to 33/1000 in 2015 for men, and from 10/1000 to 23/1000 for women. Changes in smoking behaviour would reduce the projected prevalence to 29/1000 for men, but would increase it to 25/1000 for women. The model estimated the unavoidable increase in the burden of COPD, an increase that is greater for women than for men (142 per cent and 43 per cent increase in prevalence, respectively) (Watson *et al.* 2003). This greater increase in prevalence of COPD in women compared to men might also be associated with more severe COPD in women.

Vestbo *et al.* examined survival after admission due to COPD in 267 men and 220 women who had participated in the Copenhagen City Health Study and who were hospitalized with a discharge diagnosis of COPD. The crude five-year survival rate after a COPD admission was higher in women (52 per cent) than in men (37 per cent). However, estimations of the overall mortality due to COPD in the next decade showed that COPD mortality of women was expected to exceed that of men. A similar trend was observed in the United States. Thus, with the expected global increase in female mortality from COPD, it is predicted that COPD mortality rates for females will soon equal or exceed those for males (Watson *et al.* 2003; Crockett *et al.* 1994; Mannino *et al.* 1997; Vestbo *et al.* 1998; Vestbo 2002).

Irrespective of the expected greater increase in prevalence of COPD in women compared to in men, women are less likely to receive a COPD diagnosis than men when presenting to a physician (Watson *et al.* 2003). This gender bias results in a further underdiagnoses of COPD in women, as shown by Chapman *et al.* (2001). They found that spirometry not only reduced the risk of underdiagnosis but also limited the effects of gender bias.

Risk factors for COPD

In the past few decades, the environmental risk factors for COPD—that is, smoking, air pollution, occupational exposure, childhood respiratory illness, diet, and exposure to respiratory allergens—have been studied in detail. Also, the presence of respiratory symptoms, increased numbers of eosinophils, and increased airway responsiveness were all found to be significant predictors of reduced level of FEV_1 (Wang *et al.* 2004).

Cigarette smoking

The WHO has estimated that 73 per cent of all COPD mortality in high-income countries is caused by smoking; the estimate for low- and middle-income countries was 40 per cent (Lopez et al. 2006a). Tobacco smoke, therefore, is the most important cause of COPD. In fact, there is a well-established association between current and cumulative smoking and COPD, and several cohort studies have shown that adult smokers experience a faster FEV_1 decline than non-smokers. This excess decline in lung function may return to normal levels of ageing-related decline after smoking cessation (Camilli et al. 1987).

Women and children are considered to be particularly sensitive to the effects of inhaled tobacco smoke (Xu et al. 1994). A recent study also demonstrated a significant (10.7 per cent) reduction in FEV_1 due to environmental tobacco smoke among children with smoking parents compared to children of non-smoking parents. This latter finding emphasizes the importance of environmental tobacco smoke in childhood (Tager et al. 1983).

What has been the most striking about the epidemiology of COPD is the change in prevalence in women over the past decade (Lopez & Murray 1998). As a result of changes in smoking habits in recent decades, the prevalence of COPD in women in the United Kingdom reached the same level as that of men in the previous decade (Lopez et al. 2006b). A similar pattern is seen in the United States with respect to female mortality and this is expected to be reflected in other European countries in the near future (Halbert et al. 2003). Nonetheless, as noted in the preceding subsection, women with COPD are less likely to be diagnosed and treated (Miravitlles et al. 2005). General practitioners, in particular, consider the diagnosis of COPD less frequently in women than in men although presenting with the same risk factors and clinical symptoms (Miravitlles et al. 2006).

The pattern, until recently, of greater COPD prevalence among males than females is likely to be explained by the traditionally higher rates of smoking among men (Watson et al. 2003). This is supported by an increase in the prevalence of COPD in the past ten years among females, which is attributed to the fact that the rates of smoking among women have significantly increased in more recent times (Kemm 2001). Moreover, females now take up smoking at younger ages, thereby increasing their risk of developing smoking-related disease.

Few data are available on the incidence of COPD according to smoking habits. Analysis of the Copenhagen City Heart Study confirmed a higher incidence of COPD among smokers than non-smokers with 27 per cent of the participants who continued to smoke over a 25-year period developing COPD as defined by GOLD stage II–IV COPD, compared with 5.7 per cent of the non-smokers (Lokke et al. 2006). The longitudinal Vlagtwedde and Vlaardingen cohort study with a follow-up of 25 years also showed that persistent cigarette smokers (OR = 1.99; 95% CI = 1.68,2.35), recidivist smokers (OR = 1.96; 95% CI = 1.34,2.86), variable pipe or cigar smokers (OR = 2.11; 95% CI = 1.52,2.91), and subjects who stopped smoking (OR = 1.39; 95% CI = 1.08,1.80) had an increased risk of developing COPD compared to never-smokers. The risks of developing COPD in sustained ex-smokers (OR = 0.98; 95% CI = 0.79,1.22), starters (OR = 1.62; 95% CI = 0.87,2.99), brief smokers (OR = 1.22; 95% CI = 0.76,1.94), and persistent pipe or cigar smokers (OR = 1.41; 95% CI = 0.98,2.04) were not significantly different from the risk in the never-smokers. Therefore, it was concluded that, taking longitudinal smoking habits into account, subjects who had quit smoking between two successive surveys still had an increased risk of developing COPD compared

with never-smokers, whereas sustained ex-smokers were no longer at risk of developing COPD.

Other environmental risk factors

In addition to smoking, the rate of decline in lung function is also determined by several other environmental factors. For example, occupational exposure to dusts, gases, and fumes has been shown to be associated with the rate of decline in FEV_1 and the development of COPD. In fact, a 2003 report by an ad hoc committee of the American Thoracic Society reviewing occupational studies on COPD estimated that 15–20 per cent of the COPD cases were caused by occupational factors (Balmes 2005). More recent studies suggest that these estimates could even be higher. For example, analyses of data collected in the Third National Health and Nutrition Examination Survey (NHANES III) suggest that approximately 20 per cent of the COPD cases in the United States are attributable to work-related exposures (Hnizdo et al. 2002). The proportion was even higher (approximately 30 per cent) among never-smokers. Combined exposures to smoking and occupational factors have been shown to have greater than additive effects (Trupin et al. 2003). Some examples of occupational risk factors for COPD are coal dust, silica dust, oil mists, welding fumes, and organic dusts including cotton, grain, and wood (Balmes 2005).

Indoor air pollutants are another important risk factor for COPD, particularly in low-income countries where biomass fuels (wood and crop residues) and coal fuels are often used for heating and cooking without appropriate ventilation (Liu et al. 2007). WHO estimates suggest that indoor smoke from biomass fuels may cause 35 per cent of all COPD cases in low- and middle-income countries (Lopez et al. 2006a). COPD is also related to outdoor pollution levels, but the attributable risk is expected to be relatively small (Tashkin et al. 1994).

Genetic risk factors

Genetic risk factors have been studied in detail only recently. COPD is a disease that is predominantly expressed at later ages and genetic factors are also more difficult to study, because the parents of individuals with COPD have often already died and the children of subjects with COPD are likely to be too young to have significant fixed airway obstruction (van Diemen & Boezen 2007). In the past decade, genetic studies on COPD have therefore usually included small numbers of subjects and applied various definitions of disease, hampering a valid comparison between studies. Also, small sample sizes increase the likelihood of spurious results, because genotyping in small sample sizes can lead to positive results in a predefined number of studies (e.g. 5 per cent, if = 0.05 is accepted). Thus, it is not surprising that many positive results from genetic studies of COPD have not been replicated (Boezen & Postma 2007). In addition, there may be a bias towards lack of publication of negative findings.

Lack of replication might also be due to the apparent difficulties of extrapolating results from one population to another. For example, associations found in Asians may be missed in Caucasian populations as a result of lower prevalences of the polymorphisms under study in Caucasians (Boezen & Postma 2007).

More recently, several large population-based cohort studies have been conducted in which excess decline in lung function leading to development of COPD was studied prospectively. These studies have the advantage of being able to assess different mechanisms that can lead to poor lung function. For example, subjects may have experienced an unusually high rate of decline in lung function, or alternatively they may not have attained the normal maximal level of lung function, or the age of onset of decline may have been unusually early. Genetic factors may affect any one, or a combination, of these different patterns of lung function loss. Therefore, it is of crucial importance to study the genetic contribution to lung function loss in a longitudinal population-based study design, covering the time span during which these different patterns and their underlying causes evolve (van Diemen & Boezen 2007).

To date, most studies on the genetics of COPD have focused on genes that are involved in the processing of various tobacco smoke products, affect the degree of oxidative stress, or are involved in the protease–anti-protease balance. In particular, variations in the enzymes that detoxify cigarette smoke products, and are thus protective against oxidative stress, might explain why only a small proportion of smokers develop COPD. For example, a polymorphism in exon 5 of the glutathione S1-transferase (GST) P1 that affects its catalytic activity was significantly more common in men with irreversible airway obstruction than in those without (Hayes et al. 2005). More recently, an association between COPD and a short tandem repeat polymorphism in the haeme oxygenase-1 gene promoter has been described, which results in an up-regulation of haeme oxygenase-1 upon exposure to reactive oxygen species in cigarette smoke (Takahashi et al. 2004). As haeme oxygenase is more expressed in lung tissue of individuals with COPD, a genetic variation in this gene may also contribute to its development. Moreover, mutations in enzymes that generate protective antioxidants have also been associated with the development of COPD.

Detoxifying enzymes such as microsomal epoxide hydrolase (mEH) and cytochrome P 4501A1 (CYP1A1) are important protective factors against oxidative stress and may also play a role in COPD. There are about 50 known CYP genes, and the CYP3 and CYP1 genes are expressed in lung tissue and have an important role in the detoxification of inhaled substances such as cigarette smoke. CYP3A5 and CYP3A4 may be of particular interest; CYP3A5 is the predominant CYP3A form in human airways and CYP3A4 is expressed in about 20 per cent of the individuals, with considerable variation of pulmonary expression occurring in both CYPs between individuals (Anttila et al. 1997; Yamada et al. 2000). Slow detoxification of epoxide derivatives of cigarette smoke components may contribute as well. In addition, enzymes affecting the degree of oxidative stress due to exogenous (cigarettes) or endogenous reactive oxygen species, as well as mutations in enzymes that generate protective antioxidants, may be associated with the development of COPD (Barnes 1999; Sandford et al. 2002; Boezen & Postma 2004). Finally, genes involved in the protease–anti-protease balance are likely to play a role in COPD development.

Mechanisms, prevalence, and risk factors of asthma

Allergy, atopy, and asthma

Asthma is almost universally regarded as an atopic disease involving allergen exposure, IgE-mediated sensitization with a Th_2 lymphocyte response, and subsequent IL 5-mediated eosinophilic airways inflammation, resulting in enhanced bronchial reactivity and reversible airflow obstruction (asthma) (Douwes et al. 2002a). As a consequence, asthma is often described as an allergic disease and grouped together with other 'allergic diseases' such as rhinitis

and eczema. This assumption is increasingly being challenged (Pearce et al. 1999; Ronchetti et al. 2007; Weinmayr et al. 2007), and there is growing interest in other (non-allergic and non-eosinophilic) inflammatory mechanisms that may be involved in producing the final common pathway of enhanced bronchial reactivity and reversible airflow obstruction that characterizes asthma (Simpson et al. 2006, 2007; Douwes et al. 2002a; Berry et al. 2007).

Respiratory allergy

Allergy can be defined as 'adverse acute or chronic hypersensitivity reactions resulting from immunologic sensitization with production of immunoglobulin (Ig) E against a specific agent or allergen'. Thus, the term allergy refers to symptomatic conditions (allergic asthma, rhinitis, etc.) whereas the term sensitization refers to an individual's immune status assessed by in vivo or in vitro diagnostic tests. Symptoms can be induced by inhalation of allergens, even at very low concentrations. Individuals who are not sensitized to these allergens will usually not show symptoms even with very high exposure. Symptoms in sensitized subjects are caused by inflammatory reactions initiated by allergen-specific IgE antibodies present in the airways. Only a proportion of sensitized subjects show symptoms and are thus also allergic. It can take weeks to years between first encounter with an allergen and the development of an allergy.

Allergic asthma is caused by IgE-mediated inflammatory mechanisms in which a large number of cells play a role including mast cells, eosinophils, T lymphocytes, dendritic cells, and macrophages. Briefly, the sensitization process involves the adaptive (or acquired) immune system wherein allergens interact with dendritic cells in the airway mucosa, which migrate to the regional lymph nodes where the allergens are presented to B and T cells. This results (through T helper-2 [Th_2] responses) in the production of allergen-specific IgE. Once allergic, a subject can develop symptoms minutes after being exposed. This is known as the early-phase allergic reaction and symptoms develop as a result of mast cell degranulation and release of inflammatory mediators through allergen IgE–antibody complexes on the surface of mast cells, causing contraction of bronchial smooth muscle and oedema in the airways. Clinically, this results in a decreased lung function and symptoms of wheeze, shortness of breath, chest tightness, and coughing.

During the late phase of the allergic reaction (4–8 h after exposure), eosinophil-related inflammatory reactions are particularly important. A critical step in this late-phase reaction is the activation of Th_2 cells, which release several pro-inflammatory cytokines including IL-5 resulting in the influx and activation of eosinophils. This reaction is characterized by the development of a non-specific bronchial hyperresponsiveness (BHR) that can continue for several days. Repeated exposures can result in more permanent BHR.

Atopy

'Atopy' (allergic sensitization) is a common term for IgE-mediated sensitization and/or allergic reaction. In population studies, this term is used to indicate the predisposition of individuals to produce increased levels of specific or total IgE after exposure to common allergens such as house-dust mite, pet and various food allergens. It is usually assessed by using skin prick tests or specific serum IgE against common allergens, and it can therefore be defined either in terms of skin prick text positivity or elevated serum IgE levels (Pearce et al. 1999). Depending on the definition, about 20–40 per cent of the people in affluent countries are atopic.

In population studies, atopy is often associated with an increased risk of asthma (Pearce *et al.* 1999), but the association is stronger in Westernized countries than in developing countries (Weinmayr *et al.* 2007).

Aeroallergens

Many macromolecules (particularly proteins) of non-human origin, including those of animals (e.g. arthropod proteins, animal dander, proteins in excreta), plants (e.g. pollens, latex dust), and microorganisms (e.g. spores of fungi such as *Alternaria*, *Aspergillus*, and *Penicillium*), can act as allergens by inducing a specific IgE response and provoke allergic reactions in sensitized subjects.

Dust mites produce the predominant inhalant allergens in many parts of the world. The most common mite species that produce allergens are *Dermatophagoides pteronyssisus* and *D. farinae*. The major allergens produced by *D. pteronyssisus* (called Der p 1 and Der p 2) are proteases present in high amounts in faecal pellets. *D. farinae* produces as its major allergen Der f 1. Elevated levels of these allergens have been detected in house dust, mattress dust, and bedding in damp homes (Van Strien *et al.* 1994).

Other important inhalant allergens include proteins associated with cats and dogs, cockroaches, grass and tree pollens, and fungi such as *Alternaria*. Allergens in the occupational environment can range from cow urinary proteins in farming situations to fungal enzymes in the biotechnology and bakery industry. Low molecular weight chemicals such as diisocyanates (e.g. tolueen diisocyanate, TDI) can also cause occupational allergic asthma, but the specific immunological mechanisms have not yet been resolved.

Is asthma an allergic disease?

Ten years ago, it was widely believed that asthma was an atopic disease caused by allergen exposure. The fundamental aetiological mechanism was that allergen exposure, particularly in infancy, produced atopic sensitization and continued exposure resulted in asthma through the development of eosinophilic airways inflammation, bronchial hyperresponsiveness, and reversible airflow obstruction. In recent years, it has become increasingly evident that this picture is, at best, too simplistic (Ronchetti *et al.* 2007; Weinmayr *et al.* 2007). A systematic review of population-based studies (Pearce *et al.* 1999) has shown that the proportion of asthma cases that are attributable to atopy (defined as skin prick test positivity) is usually less than one half (Table 9.4.1). Standardized comparisons across populations or time periods also show only weak and inconsistent associations between the prevalence of asthma and the prevalence of atopy. For instance, a comparison of asthma and atopy among 9–11-year-olds in Albania and the United Kingdom (Priftanji *et al.* 2001) showed large differences

in the prevalence of current wheeze (4.4 per cent and 9.7 per cent, respectively) and exercise-induced bronchial reactivity (0.8 per cent and 5.4 per cent) but not in skin prick test positivity (15 per cent and 17.8 per cent), suggesting that large variations in asthma prevalence can occur without differences in the frequency of atopy. This was confirmed by the International Study on Allergies and Asthma in Children (ISAAC; see subsection on the same), which showed that the association between atopy and asthma symptoms differed strongly among populations, but increased with economic development (Weinmayr *et al.* 2007). In this study, the fraction of current wheeze attributable to atopy ranged from 0 per cent in Ankara (Turkey) to 93.8 per cent in Guangzhou (China) (Figs. 9.4.1a and 9.4.1b); the overall proportion of asthma cases that were attributable to atopy was only 40.7 per cent in affluent countries and 20.3 per cent in non-affluent countries. Moreover, the ECRHS (see subsection on the same) showed that asthma attributable to atopy in adults ranged from 4 to 61 per cent between individual study centres with an overall estimate of only 30 per cent for all centres combined (Sunyer *et al.* 2004).

Also, Martinez (1998) questions whether the association of atopy with asthma is causal, on the basis that the development of sensitization after 8 years is not associated with an increased asthma risk, whereas if the association of sensitization and asthma was causal, one would not expect the age at which sensitization occurs to be of major importance.

Recent studies using sputum induction and/or bronchoalveolar lavage (BAL) techniques to measure and characterize airways inflammation in asthmatics have also demonstrated that less than 50 per cent of the asthma cases are attributable to eosinophilic airways inflammation, the hallmark of allergic asthma (Simpson *et al.* 2006; Douwes *et al.* 2002a). Thus, evidence from studies of eosinophilia and asthma is consistent with that from studies of atopy and asthma: In both instances, at most about one half of the asthma cases appear to be due to 'allergic' mechanisms. This further adds to the evidence that allergic mechanisms may not be the only, or the most important, underlying mechanism for asthma.

Non-allergic mechanisms

As noted earlier, a substantial proportion of all asthma cases have an underlying pathology that is clearly different from that observed in 'classic' allergic asthma (Simpson *et al.* 2006; Douwes *et al.* 2002a). Patients may have severe and persistent asthma in the absence of eosinophilic inflammation, and may experience an exacerbation of asthma without an increase in eosinophilic inflammation (Turner *et al.* 1995). Repeated assessments of airways inflammation over time have shown that the non-eosinophilic asthma phenotype is reproducible both in the short (4 weeks) and

Table 9.4.1 Summary of nine population-based studies in children and seven population-based studies in adults: proportions of asthmatics and non-asthmatics who are atopic, and per cent of asthma cases attributable to atopy

Age-group	Non-asthmatics atopic (per cent)	Asthmatics atopic (per cent)	Pooled relative risk	Cases attributable to atopy (per cent)
Children	29	58	3.4	38
Adults	24	54	3.7	37

Source: Adapted from Pearce *et al.* How much asthma is really attributable to atopy? *Thorax* 1999;**54**:268–72.

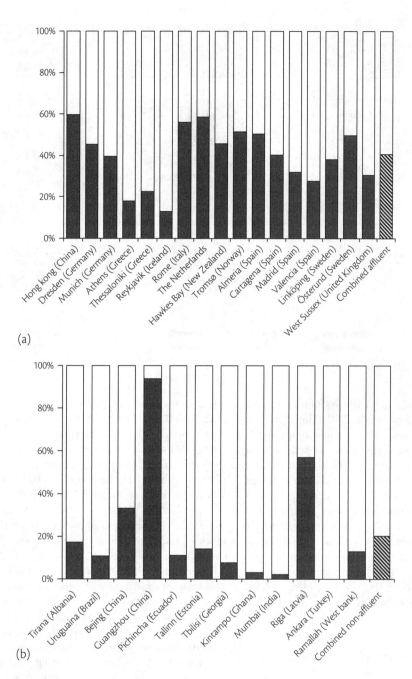

Fig. 9.4.1 The ISAAC Phase II-estimated fractions (per cent) of current wheeze attributable to atopy for all affluent countries (A) and non-affluent countries (B). (Adapted from Weinmayr *et al.* Atopic sensitization and the international variation of asthma symptom prevalence in children. *American Journal of Respiratory and Critical Care Medicine* 2007;**176**:565–74.).

long-term (1–5 years) (Simpson *et al.* 2006). However, the underlying mechanisms of non-eosinophilic and non-allergic asthma are not fully elucidated. One recent study in 93 non-smoking adult asthmatics found sputum airway eosinophilia in 41 per cent of all asthma cases, 20 per cent had elevated levels of neutrophils, 8 per cent had a mixed inflammatory profile with both cell types being elevated, and the remainder (31 per cent) had no signs of airway inflammation with both eosinophil and neutrophil levels within the normal range (Simpson *et al.* 2006). This suggests that asthma can be categorized into four inflammatory subtypes based on sputum eosinophil and neutrophil proportions: Eosinophilic asthma, neutrophilic asthma, mixed granulocytic asthma, and paucigranulocytic asthma (Simpson *et al.* 2006).

The common pathophysiological features of neutrophilic asthma involve an IL 8-mediated neutrophil influx and the subsequent

neutrophil activation is a potent stimulus to increased airway hyperresponsiveness (Simpson *et al.* 2007). Although the stimuli that trigger this response are diverse (endotoxin, ozone, particulates, virus infection), the common features are consistent with activation of innate immune mechanisms (involving Toll-like receptors and CD14) rather than IgE-mediated activation of acquired immunity (Fig. 9.4.2).

There is also the potential for combined activation of both innate and allergen-specific inflammatory mechanisms in asthma. This may be the case in mixed granulocytic asthma (Fig. 9.4.2), and may explain the ability of ozone and NO_2 to potentiate allergen-induced asthmatic responses (Jenkins *et al.* 1999). The pathophysiological mechanisms involved in paucigranulocytic asthma are not clear.

Clinically, the eosinophilic and non-eosinophilic phenotypes are very similar with only marginal differences in lung function, airway

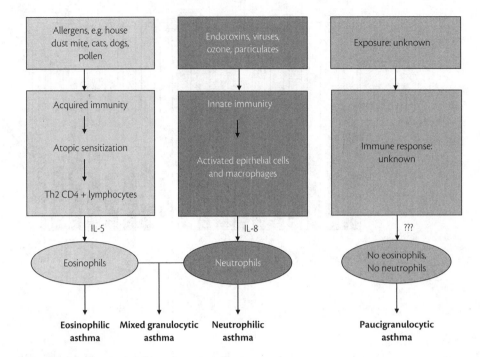

Fig. 9.4.2 The inflammatory pathways of various asthma phenotypes.

hyperreactivity, corticosteroid use, and β2 agonist-induced reversibility in FEV$_1$ (Simpson *et al.* 2006; Berry *et al.* 2007). However, there are also distinct differences: Non-eosinophilic asthmatics appear less atopic, have normal subepithelial-layer thickness, and perhaps most importantly, they have a poor short-term response to treatment with inhaled corticosteroids (Berry *et al.* 2007). Thus, despite clinical similarities, they represent distinct pathological phenotypes.

Non-allergic occupational asthma is also very common. For instance, in many occupational environments where workers are exposed to organic dust (e.g. farmers, grain workers), the majority of asthma cases are non-IgE-mediated, and are related to chronic exposure to environmental irritants. The underlying inflammatory mechanisms involve innate immune responses, which are often directed against constituents of bacteria and fungi (Douwes *et al.* 2002a,b).

Asthma time trends

It has long been suspected that the prevalence of asthma is increasing not only in industrialized countries but also in developing countries (Pearce *et al.* 2000c). However, this has been a particularly difficult issue to resolve because of the lack of systematic standardized studies measuring changes in asthma prevalence over time, and some reviewers have argued that the increases in reported prevalence are largely due to increased awareness, labelling, and diagnosis of asthma symptoms (Magnus & Jaakkola 1997). Nevertheless, most studies, which have determined the prevalence of asthma symptoms using the same methodology in the same community at different times, have reported that asthma prevalence has increased in the recent decades and that the magnitude of the increase has in some cases been substantial (Table 9.4.2). Although methodological differences in these studies make it difficult to compare the magnitude of the differences in asthma prevalence between countries, the trend of increasing prevalence among populations in countries of widely differing lifestyles and ethnic groups is generally consistent.

One of the most informative studies to date is that of Haahtela *et al.* (1990), who analysed the medical examination reports of approximately 900 000 conscripts to the Finnish defence forces during 1966–89, and a proportion of those examined in 1926–61. During 1926–61, the prevalence of asthma recorded at call-up examinations was in the range of 0.02–0.08 per cent. However, asthma prevalence increased from 0.29 per cent in 1966 to 1.79 per cent in 1989. The authors concluded that the increase was unlikely to be due to improved diagnostic methods, and that much of the increase was likely to be real. This conclusion was strengthened by a concomitant rise (from 0.12 per cent in 1966 to 0.75 per cent in 1989) in exemptions and discharges due to asthma. This study is consistent with other evidence that the increases in asthma prevalence in industrialized countries appear to have commenced after World War II, particularly in the 1960s and 1970s.

Thus, until recently, most studies reported that asthma prevalence has increased in the recent decades and that the magnitude of the increase had in some cases been substantial (Table 9.4.2).

However, several recent studies have reported either no increase or even a decrease in asthma prevalence over the last ten years. For instance, Bollag *et al.* (2005) examined time trends in consultations for asthma in primary care in Switzerland and found that overall consultation rates for asthma increased from 1989 to 1994, then stabilized, and have declined since 2000. The observation that asthma incidence might be falling is in agreement with several other studies that showed similar time trends for asthma and hay fever (Pearce & Douwes 2005). The best indication of what is currently happening globally is provided by the Phase III of the ISAAC study, the results of which are discussed in the following subsection.

International prevalence comparisons

The causes of the international time trends in the prevalence of asthma are unclear, and are currently a major focus for asthma epidemiology worldwide. An important component of this research process involves standardized international prevalence comparisons

Table 9.4.2 Changes in asthma prevalence in children and young adults

Country	Period	Asthma prevalence		Reference
		1st study	2nd study	
Australia	1964–1990	19.1%	46.0%	Robertson *et al.*
	1982–1992	10.4%	28.6%	Robertson *et al.*
	1992–2002	28.6%	23.7%	
	1987–1992	5.6%	9.3%	Campbell *et al.*
	1992–1995	9.3%	11.4%	Adams *et al.*
Canada	1980–1983	3.8%	6.5%	Infante-Rivard *et al.*
	1980–1990[c]	140/10 000	256/10 000[a]	Manfreda *et al.*
		125/10 000	254/10 000[b]	
England	1956–1975	1.8%	6.3%	Morrison Smith
	1966–1990	18.3%	21.8%	Whincup *et al.*
	1973–1986	2.4%	3.6%	Burney *et al.*
	1978–1991	11.1%	12.8%	Anderson *et al.*
England and Wales	1970–1981	11.6%	20.5%[a]	Fleming and Crombie
		8.8%	15.9%[b]	
Finland	1961–1986	0.1%	1.8%	Haahtela *et al.*
France	1968–1982	3.3%	5.4%	Perdrizet *et al.*
Germany	1991–1996	3.7%	4.1%	von Mutius *et al.*
Israel	1986–1990	7.9%	9.6%	Auerbach *et al.*
Italy	1983–1993/5	2.9%	4.4%	Ciprandi *et al.*
Japan	1982–1992	3.3%	4.6%	Nishima
Netherlands	1989–1993	13.4%	13.3%	Mommers *et al.*
	1993–1997	13.3%	11.9%	
	1997–2001	11.9%	9.1%	
New Zealand	1969–1982	7.1%	13.5%	Mitchell
	1975–1989	26.2%	34.0%	Shaw *et al.*
Papua New Guinea	1973–1984	0.0%	0.6%	Dowse *et al.*
Scotland	1964–1989	10.4%	19.8%	Ninan and Russell
	1989–1994	19.8%	25.4%	Omran and Russell
Spain	1994–2003	9.3%	9.3%	Garcia-Marcos *et al.*
Sweden	1971–1981	1.9%	2.8%	Aberg
	1979–1991	2.5%	5.7%	Aberg *et al.*
Tahiti	1979–1984	11.5%	14.3%	Liard *et al.*
Taiwan	1974–1985	1.3%	5.1%	Hsieh and Shen
United Kingdom	1991–1998	33.9%	27.5%	Anderson *et al.*
United States	1964–1983[d]	183/100 000	284/100 000	Yunginger *et al.*
	1971–1976	4.8%	7.6%	Gergen *et al.*
	1981–1988	3.1%	4.3%	Weitzman *et al.*
	1983–1992	9.2%	15.9%	Farber *et al.*
Wales	1973–1988	4.0%	9.0%	Burr *et al.*

[a]Men, [b]women, [c]prevalence rates per 10 000 subjects, [d]incidence rates per 100 000 subjects.

(Pearce *et al.* 1998). The key problem is to gain information on large numbers of people in random samples collected in a comparable manner across social groups, regions, and countries. Thus, comparisons of asthma prevalence are increasingly being based on a simple comparison of symptom prevalence in a questionnaire survey of a large number of people, followed by more intensive testing of factors related to asthma (e.g. BHR) and risk factors for asthma (skin prick test positivity, serum IgE, and environmental exposures) in a subsample, and a repeat of the prevalence survey over time. This approach has been used in the international survey of asthma prevalence in adults (Burney *et al.* 1994) and in the ISAAC study (Asher *et al.* 1995; Pearce *et al.* 1993; Ellwood *et al.* 2005).

The European Community Respiratory Health Survey (ECRHS)

In each centre of the ECRHS, a representative sample of 3000 adults, aged 20–44 years, completed a Phase-I screening questionnaire seeking information on asthma symptoms and medication use (Burney *et al.* 1994). Individuals answering 'yes' to waking with an attack of shortness of breath, an attack of asthma, or current asthma medications were defined as 'asthmatic'. A random subsample of 600 subjects and an additional sample of up to 150 'asthmatic' individuals were then studied in more detail in Phase II, with measurements of skin prick tests to common allergens, serum total and specific IgE, bronchial responsiveness to inhaled methacholine, as well as an additional questionnaire on asthma symptoms and medical history, occupation and social status, smoking, the home environment, and the use of medications and medical services. The Phase-I results (Burney *et al.* 1996) included data from 48 centres, predominantly in Western Europe, with only 9 centres from 6 countries (Algeria, Iceland, India, New Zealand, Australia, and the United States) being from outside Europe. Phase II was conducted in 37 centres in 16 countries (Burney *et al.* 1996).

The International Study of Asthma and Allergies in Childhood (ISAAC)

The ISAAC study (Asher *et al.* 1995; Ellwood *et al.* 2005) had a similar study design to that of the ECRHS study, with a simple Phase-I survey and a more in-depth Phase-II survey. However, in order to obtain the maximum possible participation across the world, Phase I (which was conducted in 155 centres in 56 countries) was separated from Phase II (which was conducted in a smaller number of centres), and the Phase-I questionnaire modules were designed to be simple and inexpensive to administer. In addition, a video presentation of clinical signs and symptoms of asthma was developed (Shaw *et al.* 1995) in order to minimize translation problems. The populations of interest were schoolchildren aged 6–7 years and 13–14 years within specified geographical areas. The Phase-I findings, involving more than 700 000 children, showed striking international differences in asthma symptom prevalence (Asher *et al.* 1998; Beasley *et al.* 1998). Figure 9.4.3 shows the international patterns of 12-month period prevalence of wheezing in 13–14 year olds (based on the question 'Have you had wheezing or whistling in the chest in the last 12 months?')

ISAAC Phase II was conducted in 30 centres in 22 countries and involved parental questionnaires ($n = 54\,439$), skin prick tests ($n = 31\,759$), and serum IgE measurements ($n = 8951$). House dust samples to measure indoor allergens were also collected (Weinmayr *et al.* 2007).

Phase III involved a repeat of the Phase-I survey after an interval of 5–10 years in 106 centres in 56 countries among children aged 13–14 years ($n = 304\,679$) and in 66 centres in 37 countries among children aged 6–7 years ($n = 193\,404$) (Asher *et al.* 2006; Pearce *et al.* 2007). It was found that international differences in asthma symptom prevalence have reduced, particularly among 13–14-year-olds, with decreases in prevalence in English-speaking countries and Western Europe and increases in prevalence in regions where prevalence was previously low (Fig. 9.4.4). Although there was little change in the overall prevalence of current wheeze, the percentage of children reported to have had asthma increased significantly, possibly reflecting greater awareness of this condition and/or changes in diagnostic practice. The asthma symptom prevalence increases in Africa, Latin America, and parts of Asia indicate that the global burden of asthma is continuing to rise, but the global prevalence differences are lessening.

What do the ECRHS and ISAAC studies show?

The ISAAC and ECRHS studies provide, for the first time, a picture of global patterns of asthma prevalence, and identify the key phenomena which future research must address and attempt to explain:

1. Both studies show a particularly high prevalence of reported asthma symptoms in English-speaking countries (Fig. 9.4.3); that is, the British Isles, New Zealand, Australia, the United States, and Canada (Asher *et al.* 1998; Burney *et al.* 1996). This is unlikely to be entirely due to translation problems, because the same pattern was observed in the ISAAC video questionnaire (Asher *et al.* 1998).

2. The ISAAC study showed that centres in Latin America also had particularly high symptom prevalence (Fig. 9.4.3). This finding is of particular interest in that the Spanish-speaking centres of Latin America showed higher prevalences than Spain itself, in contrast with the general tendency for more affluent countries to have higher prevalence rates.

3. Among the non-English-speaking European countries, both studies show high asthma prevalence in Western Europe, with lower prevalences in Eastern and Southern Europe. For example, in the ISAAC study, there is a clear northwest–southeast gradient within Europe, with the highest prevalence in the world being in the United Kingdom, and some of the lowest prevalences in Albania and Greece (Asher *et al.* 1998). The West–East gradient was particularly strong; in particular, there was a significantly lower prevalence in the former East Germany than in the former West Germany.

4. Africa and Asia generally showed relatively low asthma prevalence (Fig. 9.4.3). In particular, prevalence was low in developing countries such as China and Indonesia, whereas more affluent Asian countries such as Singapore and Japan showed relatively high asthma prevalence rates. Perhaps the most striking contrast is between Hong Kong and Guangzhou, which are close geographically and involve the same language and predominant ethnic group: Hong Kong (the more affluent city) had a 12-month period prevalence of wheeze of 10.1 per cent compared with 2 per cent in Guangzhou (the less affluent city).

5. In contrast to the asthma findings, the highest prevalences of rhinitis were reported from centres scattered throughout most regions of the world, including Western Europe, Africa, North America, and Southeast Asia; the highest prevalences of eczema were generally in centres of high latitude, including

Scandinavia and New Zealand, although there were some notable exceptions including some centres in South America and Africa (Ethiopia). Thus, although the prevalences of these conditions were correlated, the association was not particularly strong and there were numerous centres that had high prevalence for asthma but not for rhinitis and/or eczema, and vice versa, suggesting that the major risk factors are different for these related disorders, or that they involve different latency periods and time trends.

6. The ISAAC Phase II showed that the link between atopic sensitization and asthma symptoms differed strongly between populations

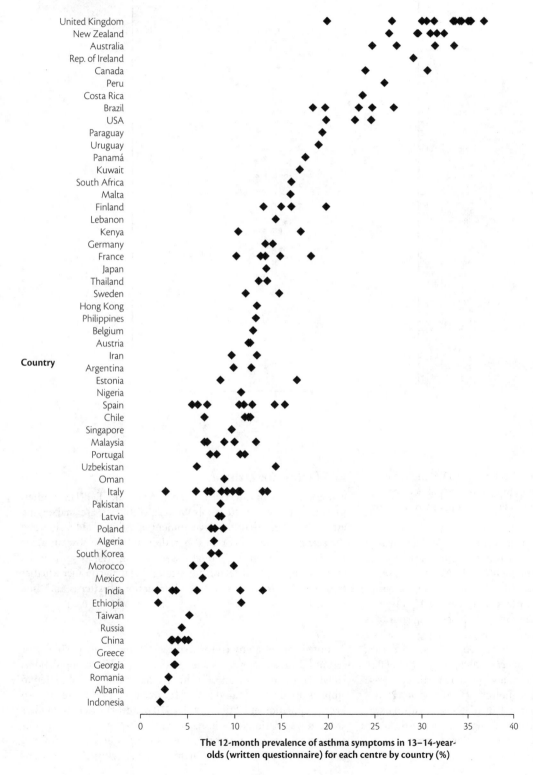

Fig. 9.4.3 Wheeze in the previous 12 months among 13–14-year-olds for each centre by country (per cent), ordered according to the mean prevalence for all centres in the country (from ISAAC 1998a).

The 12-month prevalence of asthma symptoms in 13–14-year-olds (written questionnaire) for each centre by country (%)

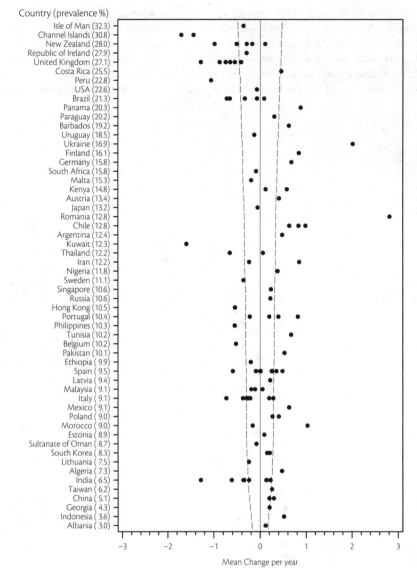

Fig. 9.4.4 Ranking plot showing the change per year in the 12-month prevalence (per cent) of current wheeze among 13–14-year-olds for each centre by country, with countries ordered by their average prevalence (for all centres combined) across Phase I and Phase III. The plot also shows the confidence interval about zero change (dashed lines) for a given level of prevalence (i.e. the average prevalence across Phase I and Phase III) given a sample size of 3000 and no cluster sampling effect. (From Pearce *et al.* Worldwide trends in the prevalence of asthma symptoms: Phase III of the International Study of Asthma and Allergies in Childhood (ISAAC). *Thorax* 2007;**62**:758-66.)

and increased with economic development (Weinmayr *et al.* 2007); the association between atopy and flexural eczema was also weak and positively linked to gross national income (Flohr *et al.* 2007).

7. The asthma prevalences in many affluent countries have peaked or even begun to decline, whereas asthma symptom prevalence continues to rise in less affluent countries. In particular, ISAAC Phase III showed that international differences in asthma symptom prevalence have reduced, particularly among 13–14-year-olds, with decreases in prevalence in English-speaking countries and Western Europe and increases in prevalence in regions where prevalence was previously low including Africa, Latin America, and parts of Asia (Fig. 9.4.4) (Asher *et al.* 2006; Pearce *et al.* 2007). Similarly, Phase II of the ECRHS study found no further increase in current or severe asthma symptoms (Chinn *et al.* 2004). Nonetheless, a significant increase in diagnosed asthma was observed, which most likely reflects changes in diagnostic labelling and/or medical treatment for mild and/or moderate asthma (Weiland & Pearce 2004).

Risk factors for asthma

These striking findings from the ISAAC and ECRHS studies, together with recent studies in Western countries, are challenging established theories of the development of asthma, and facilitating the search for new theoretical paradigms. In this subsection, we review evidence on traditional risk factors as well as some more recently suggested risk factors for asthma. We then consider whether these risk factors can explain the international patterns and time trends.

Atopy

As noted earlier, atopy (measured by skin prick test positivity or serum IgE) is strongly associated with asthma within populations. However, the proportion of asthma cases that are attributable to atopy is usually less than one half (Pearce *et al.* 1999), and an even lower population attributable risk (~20 per cent) was found in less affluent populations (Weinmayr *et al.* 2007). Also, comparisons across populations suggest that the association between atopy and asthma is relatively weak and highly variable between populations

(Weinmayr *et al.* 2007; Sunyer *et al.* 2004). Furthermore, although atopy may be a risk factor for asthma, it is not a classic environmental 'exposure' (e.g. indoor allergen exposure, smoking, air pollution), which could by itself explain increases in asthma prevalence; rather, it represents a biological response to various exposures (e.g. allergen exposure), which is modified by susceptibility factors (genetic and/or environmental).

Genetic factors

Asthma is multifactorial in origin and influenced by multiple genes and environmental factors. Thus, it is not inherited in the simple Mendelian fashion that is characteristic of single-gene disorders. A particular genetic factor may affect one or more aspects of the complex aetiological processes potentially involved in asthma including atopic sensitization, bronchial hyperresponsiveness (BHR), airway inflammation, innate immunity, and so on. Whether this genetic potential is expressed will depend upon various factors, including whether sufficient exposure to environmental factors occurs. Investigating possible genes for the individual aetiological factors is also fraught with difficulties, because control of these factors (e.g. IgE production and BHR) are also multifactorial (Zamel *et al.* 1996). Also, as noted earlier, asthma is an extremely heterogeneous disease including a variety of phenotypical and clinical manifestations, which are likely to be associated with different (combinations of) genes. Another potential source of phenotypic variability is that asthma development, exacerbations, and progression may involve different environmental triggers and genetic factors.

Currently, a number of genome-wide linkage studies have identified several chromosomal regions associated with asthma susceptibility; the regions with the strongest evidence include chromosome 2q, 5q, 6q, 11q, 12q, and 13q (Bierbaum & Heinzmann 2007). A large number of candidate genes have been described, with only some confirmed in subsequent independent studies; these include IL4, IL13, CD14, and ADRB2 on chromosome 5; HLA-DRB1, HLA-DBQ1, and TNF on chromosome 6; FCER1B on chromosome 11; IL4RA on chromosome 16; and ADAM33 on chromosome 20 (Bierbaum & Heinzmann 2007). However, some of these potentially interesting findings need further replication in other populations.

Demographic factors

There are a variety of demographic factors that are associated with asthma including age (Anderson *et al.* 1992), gender (Anderson *et al.* 1992), and ethnicity (Pattemore *et al.* 2004). Age is the demographic factor that is most strongly related to asthma symptom prevalence, with symptoms usually declining at or before the onset of puberty (Kimbell-Dunn *et al.* 1999).

Asthma incidence and prevalence are consistently lower among females than males before age 12 years, whereas during adolescence and adulthood there is evidence of higher incidence and prevalence among females (Kimbell-Dunn *et al.* 1999). One possible explanation is that the average age of onset in childhood and adolescence may be later for females. Levels of cord blood IgE are lower at birth in girls than in boys (Weeke 1992), indicating a lower risk of the subsequent development of asthma. Some authors have noted that boys have smaller airways relative to lung size than girls, and that this may explain the greater frequency and severity of lower respiratory tract illness in boys, even though infection rates are similar for both sexes (Martinez *et al.* 1988). Alternatively, it is possible that boys have more exposure to factors that increase asthma incidence or duration. On the other hand, the relatively higher prevalence (or smaller reduction in prevalence) among females than males after puberty could be due to hormonal influences on allergic predisposition, airway size, inflammation, and smooth muscle vascular functions (Redline & Gold 1994). Premenstrual asthma may be especially relevant to the hormonal involvement of asthma as it may not only cause asthma exacerbations but may thereby also affect the frequency and duration of asthma symptoms, resulting in an increase in the prevalence of 'current asthma'.

Studies in the 1960s and 1970s suggested that asthma is more common in children in the higher social classes. There has been less evidence of social class differences as the diagnosis of asthma has become more widespread (Littlejohns & Macdonald 1993), even though diagnostic labelling of wheezing in adults differs by social class (Littlejohns *et al.* 1989). However, severe asthma appears to be more common in children in the lower social classes (Stewart *et al.* 2001) and in some disadvantaged ethnic groups (Pattemore *et al.* 2004), and low socioeconomic status is associated with hospital admissions for asthma (Watson *et al.* 1996) and with reduced lung function in adults. This could represent either a greater prevalence of asthma in disadvantaged groups, increased severity due to environmental factors (e.g. environmental tobacco smoke, nutrition, occupational exposures) (Eagan *et al.* 2002; Ellison-Loschmann *et al.* 2007), or inadequate disease management and poor access to healthcare (Ellison-Loschmann & Pearce 2006).

Obesity

The specific mechanisms linking body weight and asthma are unclear, but several have been proposed including (1) common aetiologies, (2) co-morbidities, (3) mechanical factors, and (4) adipokines (i.e. cytokines secreted by adipose tissue) (Shore 2007). Similar to asthma, the prevalence of overweight and obesity have increased dramatically in the past few decades in many regions of the world (Burney 2002). Studies have shown associations between body weight and asthma in both adults (Braback *et al.* 2005) and children (von Mutius *et al.* 2001). Prospective studies of children suggest that obesity precedes asthma, signalling a causal link (Gilliland *et al.* 2003; Gold *et al.* 2003), as do studies showing associations between asthma and both weight gain and weight loss in adults (Hakala *et al.* 2000). Nonetheless, some studies have failed to show an association (Brenner *et al.* 2001) whereas others showed an association only in one gender (Mannino *et al.* 2006). Several reported an association only with respiratory symptoms (e.g. wheeze), but not BHR (Bustos *et al.* 2005), although this may merely indicate that obesity increases asthma risk through mechanisms other than BHR. Obesity may also increase severity in subjects with pre-existing asthma (Akerman *et al.* 2004).

Diet

Many studies have investigated the effects of breastfeeding on allergies and asthma with some studies showing protective effects, some showing no effect, and others suggesting that breastfeeding is a risk factor (Friedman & Zeiger 2005). A recent long-term longitudinal study found that exclusive breastfeeding was associated with a slightly reduced risk of asthma and atopy at age 7 years, but an increased risk at age 14 and 44 (Matheson *et al.* 2007). An infant cohort study in New Zealand showed that breastfeeding did not protect against atopy and asthma and may even increase the risk at age 9–26 years (Sears *et al.* 2002). A recent cluster randomized trial reported similar findings for allergies and asthma at age 6.5 years (Kramer *et al.* 2007).

Other nutritional factors may also play a role in the aetiology of asthma. In particular, it has been speculated that the increase in asthma prevalence may be due to a change in dietary patterns in the past few decades; that is, as cultures become more 'Westernized', they have shifted from a tradition of growing and consuming local foods to consuming more processed foods with an overall increase in the intake of refined sugars, fats, and additives, and a reduction in the intake of fresh fruits, vegetables, and fish. Several observational studies have shown protective effects of fruit and vegetables, whole grain products, and fish (Devereux 2007), and these findings are consistent with an ecologic analysis of the ISAAC Phase-I survey (Ellwood *et al.* 2001). Fruit, vegetables, and whole-grain products are rich in antioxidants and may reduce airway inflammation by protecting the airways against both endogenous and exogenous oxidants (Devereux 2007). Fish oils are rich in n-3 polyunsaturated fatty acids, which may also protect against airway inflammation and subsequent symptoms of asthma (Devereux 2007). However, recent dietary supplement studies focusing on antioxidants and n-3 fatty acids have not showed convincing evidence of a protective effect on allergies and asthma (Reisman *et al.* 2006; Almqvist *et al.* 2007).

Outdoor air pollution

The role of outdoor air pollutants (particulate matter, ozone, nitrogen dioxide, and sulphur dioxide) in asthma and other diseases has been extensively studied and debated. An association between measures of distance to major roads or traffic density and asthma symptoms has been demonstrated in a number of European countries (World Health Organization 2005). Also, a large number of studies have reported associations between direct measurements of air pollution levels and exacerbation of preexisting asthma, both in children and adults (World Health Organization 2005; Boezen *et al.* 1999). Some studies, including a recent birth cohort study (Brauer *et al.* 2007), have also suggested that air pollution may cause *new onset* of asthma and allergic disease. In particular, several large prospective studies have suggested a role of ozone (McDonnell *et al.* 1999, 2002), although significant associations with some asthma outcomes were also shown for PM2.5, soot, and NO_2 (Brauer *et al.* 2007). Nonetheless, although it is clear that air pollution can provoke exacerbations in preexisting asthma and a negative association between outdoor air pollution and asthma prevalence at the population level has been shown (Asher *et al.* 1998), the weight of evidence does not currently support a *major* role of outdoor air pollution as a cause of the initial development of asthma.

Tobacco

Similarly, the evidence for a role of tobacco smoke in asthma is strongest for increases in severity in children who already have asthma, whereas the evidence for the initial occurrence of asthma (incidence) is less conclusive. In particular, several recent reviews and meta-analyses differ in their conclusions about the role of second-hand tobacco smoke (SHS). The US Environmental Protection Agency (EPA) and the Californian EPA concluded that SHS was causally associated with the development of asthma in children (US Environmental Protection Agency 1992; Office of Environmental Health Hazard Assessment 1997). The 2006

Surgeon General's report on 'health effects from involuntary exposure to tobacco smoke' (US Department of Human Health and Human Services 2006) concluded that the evidence was suggestive but not sufficient to infer a causal relationship. This analysis was based on a previous meta-analysis conducted by Strachan and Cook (Strachan & Cook 1998) and did not include the most recent epidemiological studies. However, the most recent meta-analysis including studies published between 1970 and 2005 concluded that household SHS exposure was positively and consistently associated with the incidence of new-onset asthma (Vork *et al.* 2007) not only in younger but also older children.

The evidence on active smoking as a risk factor is also conflicting, with some studies reporting only exacerbations (Siroux *et al.* 2000) whereas others have also documented a dose-related risk of newonset asthma in adolescents and adults (Eagan *et al.* 2002).

Overall, it therefore appears that environmental tobacco smoke is a cause of asthma exacerbations, and that it may also be involved in the development of asthma itself.

Indoor air pollution

Little is currently known about the contribution of indoor air pollutants (other than environmental tobacco smoke) to the incidence and prevalence of asthma. The range of potential pollutants is large, the determinants of ambient levels involve a complex interaction of lifestyle and building factors, and precise measurement of airborne concentrations is difficult. Nitrogen dioxide from burning fossil fuels has by far received the most attention, and sulphur dioxide from burning sulphur-containing coal or gas, mosquito coil smoke, and formaldehyde from wood preparation have also been considered. Particulates from open or closed wood and coal-burning fires have received less attention in developed countries, but have been studied in developing countries, where very high indoor levels have been encountered.

Damp indoor environments and indoor fungal exposure may also play a role, as demonstrated in a large number of studies conducted across many geographical regions (Douwes & Pearce 2003). However, although it has been concluded that the evidence for a causal association between dampness and respiratory morbidity is strong, it is not clear whether indoor dampness *causes* or 'only' *exacerbates* pre-existing respiratory conditions such as asthma (Douwes & Pearce 2003).

Occupational exposures

Occupational asthma (OA) is the most common occupational respiratory disease in developed countries. For example, asthma accounted for 28 per cent of the cases reported to the United Kingdom Surveillance of Work-Related and Occupational Respiratory Diseases (SWORD) project (Meredith *et al.* 1991). Estimates of the total proportion of adult asthma thought to be occupational in origin range from 2 to 15 per cent in the United States, 15 per cent in Japan (Chan-Yeung & Malo 1994), 5 per cent in Spain (Kogevinas *et al.* 1996), 2 to 3 per cent in New Zealand (Fishwick *et al.* 1997), and 2 to 6 per cent in the United Kingdom (Meredith & Nordman 1966). More than 250 agents have been identified as causes of OA (see http://www.remcomp.com/asmanet/asmapro/asmawork.htm and http://www.state.nj.us/health/eoh/survweb/wra/agents.shtml). Some of the most common occupational asthmagens include flour and grain dusts, wood dusts, latex allergens, and isocyanates.

Respiratory viral infections

Viral infections are common causes of exacerbations of asthma (Johnston *et al.* 1995). In fact, respiratory viral infections are detected in the majority of asthma exacerbations (80–85 per cent in children and 75–80 per cent in adults); of these, about 60 per cent are rhinoviruses (Johnston 2007). There is also a strong association between viral infections and hospital admission for asthma among both children and adults.

Viral infections may also be involved in the development of asthma, but the evidence is less clear. Several long-term longitudinal studies have shown that respiratory syncytial virus (RSV) infections increase the risk of subsequent recurrent wheezing and asthma in early childhood (Stein *et al.* 1999; Sigurs *et al.* 2005). However, this risk may progressively decrease with increasing age (Stein *et al.* 1999). Other viruses have also been associated with asthma development including human rhinovirus (HRV), which may in fact be a more important risk factor than RSV (Lemanske *et al.* 2005). The mechanisms of viral-induced asthma are poorly understood, but it has been speculated that impaired innate immune responses may play a crucial role (Johnston 2007).

Paracetamol

It has been reported that prenatal paracetamol (or acetaminophen) use during pregnancy is a risk factor for asthma, wheezing, and total IgE in the offspring at 6–7 years of age (Shaheen *et al.* 2002, 2005). Similarly, several cross-sectional and longitudinal studies have reported that paracetamol use is associated in a dose-dependent manner with an increase in asthma in children and also new-onset asthma in adults (Shaheen *et al.* 2000; Barr *et al.* 2004). Furthermore, national per-capita consumption of acetaminophen was ecologically associated with the prevalence of wheeze, diagnosed asthma, and bronchial hyperresponsiveness in Western Europe (Newson *et al.* 2000). Some of these associations may have been due to confounding (e.g. confounding by indication), but this is unlikely to fully explain the positive associations in birth cohort studies (Shaheen *et al.* 2002; Shaheen *et al.* 2005), and longitudinal studies among adults that focused on new-onset asthma (Barr *et al.* 2004). The underlying mechanisms are unclear, but it has been suggested that paracetamol decreases glutathione levels in the lungs, which may predispose to oxidative injury, bronchospasm, and an increased Th_2 response (Shaheen *et al.* 2002). Interestingly, the use of paracetamol has increased considerably (replacing aspirin) since the 1970s and 1980s (Varner *et al.* 1998), suggesting that the increased used of paracetamol may account for some of the increasing prevalence of childhood asthma.

Allergens

Indoor allergens, particularly house-dust mite allergens, are perhaps the group of possible asthma risk factors that have received the greatest attention. It is well established that, in sensitized asthmatics, allergen exposure can trigger asthma attacks and that prolonged exposure can lead to the prolongation and exacerbation of symptoms. However, most studies among children show only weak associations between allergen exposure and current asthma, even when the analyses are restricted to atopic patients and allergen avoidance has been accounted for (Pearce *et al.* 2000b). Also, secondary intervention trials have had mixed results (Gotzsche *et al.* 1998).

In fact, although there is good evidence for asthma exacerbations, the evidence for new-onset asthma is much weaker (Pearce *et al.* 2000b). The key study linking allergen exposure in infancy to the subsequent development of asthma is that of Sporik *et al.* (1990), who followed 67 children with a family history of atopy. They found an association between dust mite allergen levels and mite sensitization, and an association between exposure to more than $10\ \mu g/g$ in the first year of life and a history of wheezing, although this association was not statistically significant (OR = 2.3, p = 0.17). There were marginally non-significant associations with 'active wheezing and BHR' (p = 0.08) and with 'receiving medication' (p = 0.10).

More recent longitudinal birth cohort studies found little or no association between early dust mite allergen exposure and asthma later in childhood (Burr *et al.* 1993; Corver *et al.* 2006; Tepas *et al.* 2006). For example, Burr *et al.* (1993) conducted a longitudinal study among 453 infants in South Wales with a family history of allergic diseases. Doctor-diagnosed asthma and wheezing at age 7 was neither associated with mite allergen exposure as determined in the first 12 months nor with dust mite levels measured at 7 years of age (odds ratios were not given). Similarly, in the German Multicentre Allergy Study, levels of mite and cat allergens in early life remained strongly related to specific sensitization at age 3–7 years, but no dose–response relationship between allergen exposure and any measure of asthma or wheeze at 7 years of age was found (Lau *et al.* 2000, 2002) Dust mite allergens are therefore unlikely to play a major role in the initial development of asthma.

There are several other indoor and outdoor allergens that have been suggested to be associated with the development of asthma, including cat, dog, cockroach, and *Alternaria* allergens. However, the evidence for a causal relationship is even weaker than for house-dust mite allergens (Pearce *et al.* 2000b). In fact, several studies even reported a protective effect on the development of asthma of pet keeping early in life.

Can the traditional risk factors explain the international patterns and time trends?

There is little evidence that the traditional risk factors can account for the global prevalence increases or the international prevalence patterns that have been observed. The increases in asthma prevalence cannot be due to genetic factors because they are occurring too rapidly, and the rapidity of the increases indicates that genetic factors alone are unlikely to account for a substantial proportion of asthma cases (Douwes & Pearce 2002), although genetic susceptibility to changing environmental exposures may play an important role.

The global patterns of asthma prevalence are also inconsistent with the hypothesis that air pollution is a major risk factor for the development of asthma (Asher *et al.* 1998, 2006; Beasley *et al.* 1998). Regions such as China and Eastern Europe, which have some of the highest levels of traditional air pollution such as particulate matter and SO_2, generally have lower asthma prevalence than the countries of Western Europe and North America, Australia, and New Zealand, which have lower levels of pollution. It also appears very unlikely that the international prevalence patterns can be explained by differences in smoking (Mitchell *et al.* 2001), or in occupational exposures.

Allergen exposure is the risk factor that has perhaps received the most attention as a possible cause of the global increases in prevalence of asthma and allergies. In particular, it has been suggested

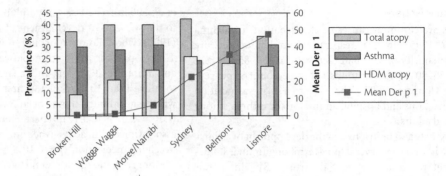

Fig. 9.4.5 Mean Der p 1 levels and prevalence (per cent) of house-dust mite (HDM) atopy, total atopy, and asthma in six areas of Australia.

that increases in indoor allergen exposures, through changes in lifestyle such as wall-to-wall carpeting, cold water washing, greater time spent indoors watching television, and so on, could account for the global increases in asthma prevalence (Sporik *et al.* 1990). However, the only study of English homes at two time points (1979 and 1989) did not demonstrate any change in house-dust mite allergen levels (Butland *et al.* 1997), but marked increases have been observed in Australian studies (Peat *et al.* 1996).

The ISAAC (Asher *et al.* 1998) and ECRHS (Burney *et al.* 1996) studies have consistently found uniformly high levels of asthma prevalence in centres in English-speaking countries, even though there is a wide variation in house-dust mite levels across these countries (Martinez 1997). In geographical areas in which dust mite exposure is very low or absent, including desert regions and mountainous regions, the prevalence of asthma is as high or even higher than that in other areas where house dust mite exposure is high (Martinez 1997).

Other available evidence on the association between allergen exposure and the subsequent risk of asthma at the population level is also less than persuasive. For example, Leung *et al.* (1997) reported that asthma prevalence was high in Hong Kong (6.6 per cent for asthma ever) and low in San Bu, China (1.6 per cent), but exposures to house-dust mite allergen were similar in Hong Kong and San Bu. Similarly, Fig. 9.4.5 shows data from six Australian surveys in centres with widely differing levels of mite allergen exposure; the overall prevalences of sensitization and asthma were both unrelated to the levels of house-dust mite allergen (Der p 1) exposure in the six centres. The dominant allergen varied between regions, but there was little overall difference in the prevalence of sensitization or of asthma despite the major differences in mite allergen levels. Similarly, Von Mutius *et al.* (1994) found that asthma was significantly higher in Munich, West Germany (5.9 per cent) than in Leipzig, East Germany (3.9 per cent), and this paralleled the pattern of skin prick test positivity (19.2 and 7.3 per cent); however, house-dust mite allergen levels were similar in the East and the West (Hirsch *et al.* 1998).

The other asthma risk factors (e.g. diet, obesity, and/or paracetamol) may significantly contribute to the observed time trends and international patterns of asthma prevalence, but the current evidence for this is scant.

Towards a new paradigm

Thus, for many of the traditional risk factors, there is evidence that they may exacerbate pre-existing asthma, but the evidence that they may be involved in the initial development of asthma is limited.

Also, there is little evidence that these factors account for the global prevalence increases.

Recent research has, therefore, shifted attention from allergens that may cause sensitization and/or provoke asthma attacks to factors that may 'programme' the initial susceptibility to asthma, through allergic or non-allergic mechanisms. This also, in part, involves a shift of attention from risk factors for asthma to protective factors, and the possible role of the loss of protective factors in the global increases in asthma prevalence (Pearce *et al.* 2000c).

The 'hygiene hypothesis' has been prompted by evidence that overcrowding and unhygienic conditions were associated with a lower prevalence of atopy, eczema, hay fever, and asthma (Strachan 1989). Having a large number of siblings (especially older siblings) and attendance at day-care centres were determined to be particularly protective (Ball *et al.* 2000). An increase in infections has been proposed as an explanation for these findings (Martinez 1994), and several studies have in fact shown a direct association between infections (e.g. hepatitis A, measles) or immunization with BCG and a lower prevalence of atopy and allergies (Shaheen *et al.* 1996; Matricardi *et al.* 1997). However, the results for airborne viruses (measles, mumps, rubella, and chickenpox) and BCG vaccination are inconsistent (Alm *et al.* 1998; Matricardi *et al.* 2000).

Exposure to specific microbial agents with strong pro-inflammatory properties such as bacterial endotoxin have also been suggested to be protective (Douwes *et al.* 2004). A study of 61 infants showed that allergen-sensitized infants had significantly lower house dust endotoxin levels than non-sensitized infants and levels correlated with IFN-γ producing T helper 1 cells (Th_1) but not with IL-4, IL-5, or IL-13 producing cell proportions (Th_2) (Gereda *et al.* 2000). Studies in both rural and non-rural environments reported a significant inverse association between indoor endotoxin levels and atopic sensitization (Gehring *et al.* 2001), hay fever, and atopic asthma (Braun-Fahrlander *et al.* 2002). In contrast, a birth cohort study conducted by the same researchers found that early endotoxin exposure was associated with an *increased* risk of atopy at the age of 2 years (Bolte *et al.* 2003) However, two similar birth cohort studies found a protective effect on atopy in 2-year-olds (Bottcher *et al.* 2003) and asthma symptoms in 4-year-olds (Douwes *et al.* 2006). Thus, despite some inconsistencies in the available evidence, which may be related to the hypothesized bimodal effect of endotoxin on the Th_1/Th_2 balance (Eisenbarth *et al.* 2002), it appears that endotoxin exposures may protect against atopy and allergic asthma.

Although most of the evidence points towards LPS, other pathogen-associated molecular patterns (PAMPs) may be equally (or more) important. There is evidence that exposure to peptidoglycans, CpG containing DNA, and certain viruses may also reduce the risk of atopic disease (Douwes *et al.* 2005). The evidence for these PAMPs is, however, scarce.

In addition to specific agents with potential protective effects, subpopulations have been identified with low atopy and asthma rates compared to the general populations. For instance, it has been documented that children with an anthroposophic lifestyle in Sweden (Alm *et al.* 1999) and children raised on farms with livestock in Europe, Canada, and Australia have less atopy and asthma (Braun-Fahrlander *et al.* 2002). Similar effects have also been shown in adult farmers (Douwes *et al.* 2007). Contact with animals was shown to be particularly protective. It is currently not clear which specific factors associated with animal contact confer protection, but specific microbial exposures have been hypothesized to be involved either through ingestion (lactobacilli) or inhalation (endotoxin). Ingestion of lactobacilli through consumption of unpasteurized milk may be important because they have the ability to colonise the human gut (Johansson *et al.* 1993), and may subsequently modify the immune development in a non-atopic Th$_1$ direction (Björkstén *et al.* 1999). However, various other microbes of the gut flora may play a role as well (Bottcher *et al.* 2000; Björkstén *et al.* 2001).

Furthermore, several studies in Europe have shown that the presence of pets in the home early in life was inversely associated with atopy (Hesselmar *et al.* 1999). Another study showed that having had a cat before the age of 18 protected against atopy to outdoor allergens, airway hyperreactivity, current wheeze, and current asthma (de Meer *et al.* 2004b). These results should, however, be interpreted with caution, because avoidance behaviour (removal of pets in the families with sensitized and/or symptomatic children) may have contributed to this inverse association. However, in a recent longitudinal study in which subjects with childhood asthma at enrolment were excluded from the analyses, the protective effects actually increased (de Meer *et al.* 2004b), whereas a decrease would be expected if selective avoidance was a major issue. At present, it is not clear which specific exposures and immunological mechanisms underlie the observed protective effects of pet ownership, but increased microbial exposure may play a role.

In other parts of the world (Guinea-Bissau and Nepal), it has been shown that pigs and cattle in the home are associated with less atopy (Shirakawa *et al.* 1997; Melsom *et al.* 2001). This is in line with observations that animal contact among farmers' children may confer protection, and as hypothesized for the farmers' children, increased endotoxin exposures may play a role (Douwes *et al.* 2002b).

Although the specific immune mechanisms are not clear, it is believed that microbial exposure may affect T lymphocytes, which have an important function in controlling immune responses including help for B-cell production of antibodies (IgE, IgG, IgA, IgM). T helper 2 (Th$_2$) cells stimulate B cells to produce IgE upon allergen stimulation whereas T helper 1 cells (Th$_1$) inhibit this process. The initial interpretation was that growing up in a more hygienic environment with less microbial exposure may enhance atopic (Th$_2$) immune responses, whereas microbial pressure would drive the response of the immune system—which is known to be skewed in an atopic Th$_2$ direction during foetal and perinatal life—into a Th$_1$ direction and away from its tendency to develop atopic immune responses (Martinez & Holt 1999). More recently, an alternative interpretation has been offered, which involves a reduction in activity of T regulatory cells resulting in a reduced immune suppression and subsequently an up-regulation of both Th$_1$ and Th$_2$ immunity. However, at this stage, the immunological mechanisms underlying the observed epidemiological associations (see the following subsection) remain largely unclear (Romagnani 2004).

Can the 'hygiene hypothesis' explain the international patterns and time trends?

With the large proportion of asthma that is not attributable to atopy or allergy, it is questionable whether the 'hygiene hypothesis' on its own can explain the large increases observed over the last decades or the global prevalence patterns, particularly because there is some evidence that non-atopic asthma may have increased more than atopic asthma (Thomsen *et al.* 2004). Also, although housing conditions are unlikely to have become more hygienic in US inner-city populations, asthma prevalence has increased significantly in those populations, particularly among African Americans living in poverty (Crater *et al.* 2001). Finally, the hygiene hypothesis is unlikely to explain why asthma prevalence is now apparently falling, as exposures to factors that have previously been identified as being 'protective' (family size, endotoxin exposure, infectious diseases, pets, etc.) are likely to have decreased in more recent times rather than increased. Also, there is no indication that exposures to suspected risk factors such as environmental tobacco smoke, house-dust mites, and air pollution have significantly decreased. These findings, thus, further emphasize the potential limitations of the current hygiene hypothesis. Nevertheless, whatever mechanism is involved, it is becoming increasingly clear that the 'package' of changes associated with Westernization may be contributing to the global increases in asthma susceptibility and prevalence.

Conclusion

What do these epidemiological findings tell us about the major causes of asthma and COPD?

The prevalence of COPD is still increasing particularly among women, and future projections indicate that the global burden of COPD will increase even further. The major causal risk factor is tobacco smoke, but a substantial proportion of COPD is also caused by occupational and indoor exposures, particularly in middle- and low-income countries. Only a minority of the persistent smokers develop COPD; that is, those who are likely to be genetically susceptible for cigarette smoking. Similar to asthma, large international differences are observed in COPD prevalence even when identical assessment methods are used, and these are not explained by age or cigarette smoking alone. Further understanding is required why some smokers develop COPD, and others do not, and what causes the striking differences in the global prevalence of COPD. However, we do know how to prevent COPD in the majority of cases; that is, smoking cessation is the most effective way to prevent the development of COPD and reduce disease progression.

In contrast, there are major gaps in our current understanding of asthma aetiology. Although atopic sensitization is strongly associated with asthma, it appears to account for less than one half of all cases, and there is little evidence that the traditional environmental asthma risk factors account for international prevalence increases. Recent decades have seen decreasing family size, increased hygiene, shift in dietary patterns, as well as increasing use of medical interventions such as immunization, antibiotics, and use of paracetamol. It seems that as a result of this 'package' of changes in the intrauterine and infant environment, we are seeing an increased susceptibility to the development of asthma and/or allergy. However, more recently, the increase in asthma prevalence appears to have levelled off in many high-income countries, with some even showing a decrease. The reasons for this are unclear. Understanding why these changes are occurring, and ascertaining which elements of the 'package' of twentieth-century economic development and lifestyle changes are responsible, is essential in order to develop effective intervention programmes to halt the current global asthma epidemic.

Key points

◆ COPD and asthma have increased dramatically in the past few decades, both in Western and non-Western societies.

◆ Smoking cessation and improved indoor ventilation measures to reduce indoor pollutants in houses of most middle- and low-income countries are the most effective ways to halt global increases in the prevalence of COPD.

◆ Asthma is a very heterogeneous disease with less than half of the asthma cases attributable to allergic mechanisms.

◆ Asthma prevalence differs greatly between countries with the highest prevalences in English-speaking countries and considerably lower prevalences in most low-income countries.

◆ The increases in asthma prevalence observed in the past few decades appear to have levelled off in many high-income countries in the last decade, with some even showing a decrease.

◆ Although risk factors for asthma exacerbations have been well identified, the main factors causing new-onset asthma are still only poorly understood, thus hampering the development of an effective prevention programme.

Acknowledgements

The Centre for Public Health Research is supported by a Programme Grant from the Health Research Council of New Zealand, and Jeroen Douwes is supported by a Sir Charles Hercus Research Fellowship from the Health Research Council (HRC) of New Zealand.

Author contributions

Jeroen Douwes has contributed to all sections of this chapter. Marike Boezen has primarily contributed to the COPD subsection, and Neil Pearce primarily to the asthma subsection.

References

Aberg N., Hesselmar B., Alberg B. *et al*. Increase in asthma, allergic rhinitis and eczema in Swedish schoolchildren between 1979 and 1991. *Clinical and Experimental Allergy* 1995;**25**:815–9.

Aberg N. Asthma and allergic rhinitis in Swedish conscripts. *Clinical and Experimental Allergy* 1989;**19**:59–63.

Adams R., Ruffin R., Wakefield M. *et al*. Asthma prevalence, morbidity and management practices in South Australia, 1992–1995. *Australian and New Zealand Journal of Medicine* 1997;**27**:672–9.

Aggarwal A.N., Gupta D., Jindal S.K. The relationship between FEV_1 and peak expiratory flow in patients with airways obstruction is poor. *Chest* 2006;**130**:1454–61.

Akerman M.J., Calacanis C.M., Madsen M.K. Relationship between asthma severity and obesity. *Journal of Asthma* 2004;**41**:521–6.

Alm J.S., Lilja G., Pershagen G. *et al*. BCG vaccination does not seem to prevent atopy in children with atopic heredity. *Allergy* 1998;**53**:537.

Alm J.S., Swartz J., Lilja G. *et al*. Atopy in children of families with an anthroposophic lifestyle. *Lancet* 1999;**353**:1485–8.

Almqvist C., Garden F., Xuan W. *et al*. Omega-3 and omega-6 fatty acid exposure from early life does not affect atopy and asthma at age 5 years. *Journal of Allergy and Clinical Immunology* 2007;**119**:1438–44.

American Thoracic Society Committee on Diagnostic Standards. Definitions and classification of chronic bronchitis, asthma and pulmonary emphysema. *American Review of Respiratory Disease* 1962;**85**:762–8.

Anderson H.R., Butland B.K., Strachan D.P. Trends in prevalence and severity of childhood asthma. *British Medical Journal* 1994;**308**:1600–4.

Anderson H.R., Pottier A.C., Strachan D.P. Asthma from birth to age 23—incidence and relation to prior and concurrent atopic disease. *Thorax* 1992;**47**:537–42.

Anderson H.R., Ruggles R., Strachan D.P. *et al*. Trends in prevalence of symptoms of asthma, hay fever, and eczema in 12–14 year olds in the British Isles, 1995–2002: questionnaire survey. *British Medical Journal* 2004;**328**:1052–3.

Anttila S., Hukkanen J., Hakkola J. *et al*. Expression and localization of CYP3A4 and CYP3A5 in human lung. *American Journal of Respiratory Cell and Molecular Biology* 1997;**16**:242–9.

Asher M.I., Anderson H.R., Stewart A. *et al*. Worldwide variations in the prevalence of asthma symptoms: International Study of Asthma and Allergies in Childhood (ISAAC). *European Respiratory Journal* 1998;**12**:315–35.

Asher M.I., Keil U., Anderson H.R. *et al*. International Study of Asthma and Allergies in Childhood (ISAAC): rationale and methods. *European Respiratory Journal* 1995;**8**:483–91.

Asher M.I., Montefort S., Bjorksten B. *et al*. Worldwide time trends in the prevalence of symptoms of asthma, allergic rhinoconjunctivitis, and eczema in childhood: ISAAC phases one and three repeat multicountry cross-sectional surveys. *Lancet* 2006;**368**:733–43.

Auerbach I., Springer C., Godfrey S. Total population survey of the frequency and severity of asthma in 17 year old boys in an urban area in Israel. *Thorax* 1993;**48**:139–41.

Badham C. An essay on bronchitis: with a supplement containing remarks on simple pulmonary abscess. 2nd ed. London: J Callow; 1814.

Ball T.N., Castro-Rodriguez J.A., Griffith K.A. Siblings, day care attendance and the risk of asthma and wheezing during childhood. *New England Journal of Medicine* 2000;**343**:538–43.

Balmes J.R. Occupational contribution to the burden of chronic obstructive pulmonary disease. *Journal of Occupational and Environmental Medicine* 2005;**47**:154–60.

Barnes P.J. Against the Dutch hypothesis: asthma and chronic obstructive pulmonary disease are distinct diseases. *American Journal of Respiratory and Critical Care Medicine* 2006;**174**:240–3.; discussion 243–4.

Barnes P.J. Genetics and pulmonary medicine. 9: Molecular genetics of chronic obstructive pulmonary disease. *Thorax* 1999;**54**:245–52.

Barr R.G., Wentowski C.C., Curhan G.C. *et al*. Prospective study of acetaminophen use and newly diagnosed asthma among women. *American Journal of Respiratory and Critical Care Medicine* 2004;**169**:836–41.

Beasley R., Keil U., Von Mutius E. *et al*. Worldwide variation in prevalence of symptoms of asthma, allergic rhinoconjunctivitis and atopic eczema: ISAAC. *Lancet* 1998;**351**:1225–32.

Berry M., Morgan A., Shaw D.E. *et al*. Pathological features and inhaled corticosteroid response of eosinophilic and non-eosinophilic asthma. *Thorax* 2007;**62**:1043–9.

Bierbaum S., Heinzmann A. The genetics of bronchial asthma in children. *Respiratory Medicine* 2007;**101**:1369–75.

Björkstén B., Naaber P., Sepp E. *et al.* The intestinal microflora in allergic Estonian and Swedish 2-year-old children. *Clinical and Experimental Allergy* 1999;**29**:342–6.

Björkstén B., Sepp E., Julge K. *et al.* Allergy development and the intestinal micro flora during the first year of life. *Journal of Allergy and Clinical Immunology* 2001;**108**:516–20.

Boezen H.M., Postma D.S. Genetics of COPD. In: Dekhuijzen PNR, editor. *Chronic obstructive pulmonary disease.* Alphen aan de Rhijn, the Netherlands: Van Zuijden Communications; 2004.

Boezen H.M., Postma D.S. Tumour necrosis factor and lymphotoxin A polymorphisms: a relationship with COPD and its progression? *European Respiratory Journal* 2007;**29**:8–10.

Boezen H.M., van der Zee S.C., Postma D.S. *et al.* Effects of ambient air pollution on upper and lower respiratory symptoms and peak expiratory flow in children. *Lancet* 1999;**353**:874–8.

Bollag U., Capkun G., Caesar J. *et al.* Trends in primary care consultations for asthma in Switzerland, 1989–2002. *International Journal of Epidemiology* 2005;**34**:1012–8.

Bolte G., Bischof W., Borte M. *et al.* Early endotoxin exposure and atopy development in infants: results of a birth cohort study. *Clinical and Experimental Allergy* 2003;**33**:770–6.

Bottcher M.F., Bjorksten B., Gustafson S. *et al.* Endotoxin levels in Estonian and Swedish house dust and atopy in infancy. *Clinical and Experimental Allergy* 2003;**33**:295–300.

Bottcher M.F., Nordin E.K., Sandin A. *et al.* Microflora-associated characteristics in faeces from allergic and non-allergic infants. *Clinical and Experimental Allergy* 2000;**30**:1590–6.

Braback L., Hjern A., Rasmussen F. Body mass index, asthma and allergic rhinoconjunctivitis in Swedish conscripts-a national cohort study over three decades. *Respiratory Medicine* 2005;**99**:1010–4.

Brauer M., Hoek G., Smit H.A. *et al.* Air pollution and development of asthma, allergy and infections in a birth cohort. *European Respiratory Journal* 2007;**29**:879–88.

Braun-Fahrlander C., Riedler J., Herz U. *et al.* Environmental exposure to endotoxin and its relation to asthma in school-age children. *New England Journal of Medicine* 2002;**347**:869–77.

Brenner J.S., Kelly C.S., Wenger A.D. *et al.* Asthma and obesity in adolescents: is there an association? *Journal of Asthma* 2001;**38**:509–15.

Buist A.S., McBurnie M.A., Vollmer W.M. *et al.* International variation in the prevalence of COPD (the BOLD Study): a population-based prevalence study. *Lancet* 2007;**370**:741–50.

Burney P., Chinn S., Luczynska C. *et al.* Variations in the prevalence of respiratory symptoms, self-reported asthma attacks, and use of asthma medication in the European Community Respiratory Health Survey (ECRHS). *European Respiratory Journal* 1996;**9**:687–95.

Burney P., Chinn S., Rona R.J. Has the prevalence of asthma increased in children? Evidence from a national study of health and growth, 1973–86. *British Medical Journal* 1990;**300**:1306–10.

Burney P. The changing prevalence of asthma? *Thorax* 2002;**57** Suppl 2: II36–II39.

Burney P.G.J., Luczynska C., Chinn S. *et al.* The European Community Respiratory Health Survey. *European Respiratory Journal* 1994; **7**:954–60.

Burr M.L., Butland B.K., King S. *et al.* Changes in asthma prevalence: two surveys 15 years apart. *Archives of Disease in Childhood* 1989;**64**: 1452–6.

Burr M.L., Limb E.S., Maguire M.J. *et al.* Infant-feeding, wheezing, and allergy—a prospective-study. *Archives of Disease in Childhood* 1993;**68**:724–8.

Burrows B., Fletcher C.M., Heard B.E. *et al.* The emphysematous and bronchial types of chronic airways obstruction. *A clinicopathological study of patients in London and Chicago. Lancet* 1966;**1**:830–5.

Bustos P., Amigo H., Oyarzun M. *et al.* Is there a causal relation between obesity and asthma? Evidence from Chile. *International Journal of Obesity (London)* 2005;**29**:804–9.

Butland B.K., Strachan D.P., Anderson H.R. The home environment and asthma symptoms in childhood: two population based case-control studies 13 years apart. *Thorax* 1997;**52**:618–24.

Camilli A.E., Burrows B., Knudson R.J. *et al.* Longitudinal changes in forced expiratory volume in one second in adults. Effects of smoking and smoking cessation. *American Review of Respiratory Disease* 1987;**135**:794–9.

Campbell D., Ruffin R., Mcevoy R. *et al.* South Australian asthma prevalence survey [abstract]. *Australian and New Zealand Journal of Medicine* 1992;**22**:A658.

Chan-Yeung M., Malo J.L. Epidemiology of occupational asthma. In: Busse W, Holgate ST, editors. *Asthma and rhinitis.* Oxford: Blackwell Scientific; 1994. p. 44–57.

Chapman K.R., Mannino D.M., Soriano J.B. *et al.* Epidemiology and costs of chronic obstructive pulmonary disease. *European Respiratory Journal* 2006;**27**:188–207.

Chapman K.R., Tashkin D.P., Pye D.J. Gender bias in the diagnosis of COPD. *Chest* 2001;**119**:1691–5.

Chinn S., Jarvis D., Burney P. *et al.* Increase in diagnosed asthma but not in symptoms in the European Community Respiratory Health Survey. *Thorax* 2004;**59**:646–51.

CIBA Foundation Guest Symposium. Terminology definitions, classification of chronic pulmonary emphysema and related conditions. *Thorax* 1959;**14**:286–99.

Ciprandi G., Vizzaccaro A., Cirillo I. *et al.* Increase of asthma and allergic rhinitis prevalence in young Italian men. *International Archives of Allergy and Immunology* 1996;**111**:278–83.

Committee on Diagnostic Standards for Nontuberculous Respiratory Diseases. Definitions and classification of chronic bronchitis, asthma and pulmonary emphysema. *American Review of Respiratory Disease* 1962;**85**:762–9.

Corver K., Kerkhof M., Brussee J.E. *et al.* House dust mite allergen reduction and allergy at 4 yr: follow up of the PIAMA-study. *Pediatric Allergy and Immunology* 2006;**17**:329–36.

Crater D.D., Heise S., Perzanowski M. Asthma hospitalization trends in Charleston, South Carolina, 1956 to 1997: twenty-fold increase among black children during a 30-year period. *Paediatrics* 2001;**108**:E97.

Crockett A.J., Cranston J.M., Moss J.R. *et al.* Trends in chronic obstructive pulmonary disease mortality in Australia. *Medical Journal of Australia* 1994;**161**:600–3.

de Meer G., Marks G.B., Postma D.S. Direct or indirect stimuli for bronchial challenge testing: what is the relevance for asthma epidemiology? *Clinial and Experimental Allergy* 2004a;**34**:9–16.

de Meer G., Toelle B.G., Ng K. *et al.* Presence and timing of cat ownership by age 18 and the effect on atopy and asthma at age 28. *Journal of Allergy and Clinical Immunology* 2004b;**113**:433–8.

Devereux G. Early life events in asthma—diet. *Pediatric Pulmonology* 2007;**42**:663–73.

Douwes J., Gibson P., Pekkanen J. *et al.* Non-eosinophilic asthma: importance and possible mechanisms. *Thorax* 2002a;**57**:643–8.

Douwes J., Le Gros G., Gibson P. *et al.* Can bacterial endotoxin exposure reverse atopy and atopic disease? *Journal of Allergy and Clinical Immunology* 2004;**114**:1051–4.

Douwes J., LeGros G., Gibson P. *et al.* On the hygiene hypothesis: regulation down, up, or sideways? [reply] *Journal of Allergy and Clinical Immunology* 2005;**115**:1326–1326.

Douwes J., Pearce N., Heederik D. Does environmental endotoxin exposure prevent asthma? [comment] *Thorax* 2002b;**57**:86–90.

Douwes J., Pearce N. Asthma and the Westernization 'package'. *International Journal of Epidemiology* 2002;**31**:1098–102.

Douwes J., Pearce N. Is indoor mold exposure a risk factor for asthma? [comment] *American Journal of Epidemiology* 2003;**158**:203–6.

Douwes J., Travier N., Huang K. *et al*. Lifelong farm exposure may strongly reduce the risk of asthma in adults. *Allergy* 2007;**62**:1158–65.

Douwes J., van Strien R., Doekes G. *et al*. Does early indoor microbial exposure reduce the risk of asthma? The Prevention and Incidence of Asthma and Mite Allergy birth cohort study. *Journal of Allergy and Clinical Immunology* 2006;**117**:1067–73.

Dowse G.K., Turner K.J., Stewart G.A. *et al*. The association between Dermatophagoides mites and the increasing prevalence of asthma in village communities within the Papua New Guinea highlands. *Journal of Allergy and Clinical Immunology* 1985;**75**:75–83.

Eagan T.M., Bakke P.S., Eide G.E. *et al*. Incidence of asthma and respiratory symptoms by sex, age and smoking in a community study. *European Respiratory Journal* 2002;**19**:599–605.

Eisenbarth S.C., Piggott D.A., Huleatt J.W. *et al*. Lipopolysaccharide-enhanced, toll-like receptor 4-dependent T helper cell type 2 responses to inhaled antigen. *Journal of Experimental Medicine* 2002;**196**:1645–51.

Ellison-Loschmann L., Pearce N. Improving access to health care among New Zealand's Maori population. *American Journal of Public Health* 2006;**96**:612–7.

Ellison-Loschmann L., Sunyer J., Plana E. *et al*. Socioeconomic status, asthma and chronic bronchitis in a large community-based study. *European Respiratory Journal* 2007;**29**:897–905.

Ellul-Micallef R. Asthma: a look at the past. *British Journal of Diseases of the Chest* 1976;**70**:112–6.

Ellwood P., Asher M.I., Beasley R. *et al*. The International Study of Asthma and Allergies in Childhood (ISAAC): phase three rationale and methods. *International Journal of Tuberculosis and Lung Disease* 2005;**9**:10–6.

Ellwood P., Asher M.I., Bjorksten B. *et al*. Diet and asthma, allergic rhinoconjunctivitis and atopic eczema symptom prevalence: an ecological analysis of the International Study of Asthma and Allergies in Childhood (ISAAC) data. ISAAC phase one study group. *European Respiratory Journal* 2001;**17**:436–43.

Farber H.J., Wattigney W., Berenson G. Trends in asthma prevalence: the Bogalusa Heart Study. *Annals of Allergy, Asthma and Immunology* 1997;**78**:265–9.

Feenstra T.L., van Genugten M.L., Hoogenveen R.T. *et al*. The impact of aging and smoking on the future burden of chronic obstructive pulmonary disease: a model analysis in the Netherlands. *American Journal of Respiratory and Critical Care Medicine* 2001;**164**:590–6.

Fishwick D., Pearce N., D'Souza W. *et al*. Occupational asthma in New Zealanders: a population based study [comment]. *Occupational and Environmental Medicine* 1997;**54**:301–6.

Fleming D.M., Crombie D.L. Prevalence of asthma and hay fever in England and Wales. *British Medical Journal (Clinical Research Edition)* 1987;**294**:279–83.

Flohr C., Weiland S.K., Weinmayr G. *et al*. The role of atopic sensitization in flexural eczema: findings from the International Study of Asthma and Allergies in Childhood phase two. *Journal of Allergy and Clinical Immunology* 2008;**121**:141–7.

Friedman N.J., Zeiger R.S. The role of breast-feeding in the development of allergies and asthma. *Journal of Allergy and Clinical Immunology* 2005;**115**:238–48.

Garcia-Marcos L., Quiros A.B., Hernandez G.G. *et al*. Stabilization of asthma prevalence among adolescents and increase among schoolchildren (ISAAC Phases I and III) in Spain. *Allergy* 2004;**59**:1301–7.

Gehring U., Bolte G., Borte M. *et al*. Exposure to endotoxin decreases the risk of atopic eczema in infancy: a cohort study. *Journal of Allergy and Clinical Immunology* 2001;**108**:847–54.

Gereda J.E., Leung D.Y., Thatayakitom A. Relation between house-dust endotoxin exposure, type 1 T-cell development, and allergen sensitisation in infants at high risk of asthma. *Lancet* 2000;**355**:1680–3.

Gergen P.J., Mullally D.I., Evans R., III. National survey of prevalence of asthma among children in the United States, 1976 to 1980. *Pediatrics* 1988;**81**:1–7.

Gilliland F.D., Berhane K., Islam T. *et al*. Obesity and the risk of newly diagnosed asthma in school-age children. *American Journal of Epidemiology* 2003;**158**:406–15.

Global Initiative for Asthma. Global strategy for asthma management and prevention. [Online]. 2006. Available from: *http://www.ginasthma.org*

Gold D.R., Damokosh A.I., Dockery D.W. *et al*. Body-mass index as a predictor of incident asthma in a prospective cohort of children. *Pediatric Pulmonology* 2003;**36**:514–21.

Gotzsche P.C., Hammarquist C., Burr M. House dust mite control measures in the management of asthma: meta-analysis. *British Medical Journal* 1998;**317**:1105–10.

Haahtela T., Lindholm H., Bjorksten F. *et al*. Prevalence of asthma in Finnish young men. *British Medical Journal* 1990;**301**:266–8.

Hakala K., Stenius-Aarniala B., Sovijarvi A. Effects of weight loss on peak flow variability, airways obstruction, and lung volumes in obese patients with asthma. *Chest* 2000;**118**:1315–21.

Halbert R.J., Isonaka S., George D. *et al*. Interpreting COPD prevalence estimates: what is the true burden of disease? *Chest* 2003;**123**:1684–92.

Halbert R.J., Natoli J.L., Gano A. *et al*. Global burden of COPD: systematic review and meta-analysis. *European Respiratory Journal* 2006;**28**:523–32.

Hayes J.D., Flanagan J.U., Jowsey I.R. Glutathione transferases. *Annual Review of Pharmacology and Toxicology* 2005;**45**:51–88.

Hesselmar N., Aberg N., Aberg B. *et al*. Does early exposure to cat or dog protect against allergy development? Clinical and Experimental Allergy 1999;**29**:611–7.

Hirsch T., Range U., Walther K.U. *et al*. Prevalence and determinants of house dust mite allergen in East German homes. *Clinical and Experimental Allergy* 1998;**28**:956–64.

Hnizdo E., Sullivan P.A., Bang K.M. *et al*. Association between chronic obstructive pulmonary disease and employment by industry and occupation in the US population: a study of data from the Third National Health and Nutrition Examination Survey. *American Journal of Epidemiology* 2002;**156**:738–46.

Hsieh K.H., Shen J.J. Prevalence of childhood asthma in Taipei, Taiwan and other Asian Pacific countries. *Journal of Asthma* 1991;**25**:73–82.

Infante-Rivard C., Esnaola Sukia S., Roberge D. *et al*. The changing frequency of childhood asthma. *Journal of Asthma* 1987;**24**:283–8.

Jenkins H.S., Devalia J.L., Mister R.L. *et al*. The effect of exposure to ozone and nitrogen dioxide on the airway response of atopic asthmatics to inhaled allergen: dose- and time-dependent effects. *American Journal of Respiratory and Critical Care Medicine* 1999;**160**:33–9.

Johannessen A., Omenaas E.R., Bakke P.S. *et al*. Implications of reversibility testing on prevalence and risk factors for chronic obstructive pulmonary disease: a community study. *Thorax* 2005;**60**:842–7.

Johansson M.L., Molin G., Jeppsson B. Administration of different Lactobacillus strains in fermented oatmeal soup: in vivo colonization of human intestinal mucosa and effect on the indigenous flora. *Applied Environmental Microbiology* 1993;**59**:15–20.

Johnston S.L., Pattemore P.K., Sanderson G. *et al*. Community study of role of viral-infections in exacerbations of asthma in 9–11 year-old children. *British Medical Journal* 1995;**310**:1225–9.

Johnston S.L. Innate immunity in the pathogenesis of virus-induced asthma exacerbations. *Proceedings of the American Thoracic Society* 2007;**4**:267–70.

Keeney E.L. The history of asthma from Hippocrates to Meltzer. *Journal of Allergy and Clinical Immunology* 1964;**35**:215–26.

Kemm J.R. A birth cohort analysis of smoking by adults in Great Britain 1974–1998. *Journal of Public Health Medicine* 2001;**23**:306–11.

Kharitonov S.A., Barnes P.J. Exhaled biomarkers. *Chest* 2006;**130**:1541–6.

Kimbell-Dunn M., Pearce N., Beasley R. Asthma. In: Hatch M, editor. *Women and health*. San Diego(CA): Academic Press; 1999. p. 724–39.

Kirkham P., Rahman I. Oxidative stress in asthma and COPD: antioxidants as a therapeutic strategy. *Pharmacology and Therapeutics* 2006;**111**:476–94.

Kogevinas M., Anto J.M., Soriano J.B. *et al.* The risk of asthma attributable to occupational exposures—a population-based study in Spain. *American Journal of Respiratory and Critical Care Medicine* 1996;**154**:137–43.

Kraft M. Asthma and chronic obstructive pulmonary disease exhibit common origins in any country! *American Journal of Respiratory and Critical Care Medicine* 2006;**174**:238–40.; discussion 243–4.

Kramer M.S., Matush L., Vanilovich I. *et al.* Effect of prolonged and exclusive breast feeding on risk of allergy and asthma: cluster randomised trial. *British Medical Journal* 2007;**335**:815.

Laënnec R. *A treatise on the disease of the chest* [translated from the French by J Forbes]. London: T and G Underwood; 1821.

Lau S., Illi S., Sommerfeld C. *et al.* Early exposure to house-dust mite and cat allergens and development of childhood asthma: a cohort study. Multicentre Allergy Study Group. *Lancet* 2000; **356**:1392–7.

Lau S., Nickel R., Niggemann B. *et al.* The development of childhood asthma: lessons from the German Multicentre Allergy Study (MAS). *Paediatric Respiratory Reviews* 2002;**3**:265–72.

Lemanske R.F., Jr., Jackson D.J., Gangnon R.E. *et al.* Rhinovirus illnesses during infancy predict subsequent childhood wheezing. *Journal of Allergy and Clinical Immunology* 2005;**116**:571–7.

Leung R., Ho P., Lam C.W.K. *et al.* Sensitization to inhaled allergens as a risk factor for asthma and allergic diseases in Chinese population. *Journal of Allergy and Clinical Immunology* 1997;**99**:594–9.

Liard R., Chansin R., Neukirch F. *et al.* Prevalence of asthma among teenagers attending school in Tahiti. *Journal of Epidemiology and Community Health* 1988;**42**:149–51.

Littlejohns P., Ebrahim S., Anderson R. Prevalence and diagnosis of chronic respiratory symptoms in adults. *British Medical Journal* 1989; **298**:1556–60.

Littlejohns P., Macdonald L.D. The relationship between severe asthma and social-class. *Respiratory Medicine* 1993;**87**:139–43.

Liu S., Zhou Y., Wang X. *et al.* Biomass fuels are the probable risk factor for chronic obstructive pulmonary disease in rural South China. *Thorax* 2007;**62**:889–97.

Lokke A., Lange P., Scharling H. *et al.* Developing COPD: a 25 year follow up study of the general population. *Thorax* 2006;**61**:935–9.

Lopez A., Mathers C., Ezzati M. *et al. Global burden of disease and risk factors.* Washington (DC): The World Bank; 2006a.

Lopez A.D., Murray C.C. The global burden of disease, 1990–2020. *Nature Medicine* 1998;**4**:1241–3.

Lopez A.D., Shibuya K., Rao C. *et al.* Chronic obstructive pulmonary disease: current burden and future projections. *European Respiratory Journal* 2006b;**27**:397–412.

MacNee W. Pulmonary and systemic oxidant/antioxidant imbalance in chronic obstructive pulmonary disease. *Proceedings of the American Thoracic Society* 2005;**2**:50–60.

Magnus P., Jaakkola J.J.K. Secular trend in the occurrence of asthma among children and young adults: critical appraisal of repeated cross sectional surveys. *British Medical Journal* 1997;**314**:1795–99.

Manfreda J., Becker A.B., Wang P.Z. *et al.* Trends in physician-diagnosed asthma prevalence in Manitoba between 1980 and 1990. *Chest* 1993;**103**:151–7.

Mannino D.M., Brown C., Giovino G.A. Obstructive lung disease deaths in the United States from 1979 through 1993. An analysis using multiple-cause mortality data. *American Journal of Respiratory and Critical Care Medicine* 1997;**156**:814–8.

Mannino D.M., Buist A.S. Global burden of COPD: risk factors, prevalence, and future trends. *Lancet* 2007;**370**:765–73.

Mannino D.M., Mott J., Ferdinands J.M. *et al.* Boys with high body masses have an increased risk of developing asthma: findings from the National Longitudinal Survey of Youth (NLSY). *International Journal of Obesity (London)* 2006;**30**:6–13.

Martinez F.D., Holt P.G. Role of microbial burden in aetiology of allergy and asthma. *Lancet* 1999;**354**:12–5.

Martinez F.D., Morgan W.J., Wright A.L. *et al.* Diminished lung-function as a predisposing factor for wheezing respiratory illness in infants. *New England Journal of Medicine* 1988;**319**:1112–7.

Martinez F.D. Complexities of the genetics of asthma. *American Journal of Respiratory and Critical Care Medicine* 1997;**156**:S117–22.

Martinez F.D. Gene by environment interactions in the development of asthma. *Clinical and Experimental Allergy* 1998;**28**:21–5.

Martinez F.D. Role of viral infections in the inception of asthma and allergies during childhood: could they be protective? *Thorax* 1994;**49**:1189–91.

Matheson M.C., Erbas B., Balasuriya A. *et al.* Breast-feeding and atopic disease: a cohort study from childhood to middle age. *Journal of Allergy and Clinical Immunology* 2007;**120**:1051–7.

Matricardi P.M., Rosmini F., Ferrigno L. Cross-sectional retrospective study of prevalence of atopy among Italian military students with antiboides against hepatitis A virus. *British Medical Journal* 1997;**314**:999–1003.

Matricardi P.M., Rosmini F., Riondino S. *et al.* Exposure to food borne and orofecal microbes versus airborne viruses in relation to atopy and allergic asthma. *British Medical Journal* 2000;**320**:412–7.

McConnell R., Berhane K., Gilliland F. *et al.* Asthma in exercising children exposed to ozone: a cohort study. *Lancet* 2002;**359**:386–91.

McDonnell W.F., Abbey D.E., Nishino N. *et al.* Long-term ambient ozone concentration and the incidence of asthma in non smoking adults: the AHSMOG Study. *Environmental Research* 1999;**80**:110–21.

Medbo A., Melbye H. Lung function testing in the elderly—can we still use $FEV_1/FVC < 70\%$ as a criterion of COPD? *Respiratory Medicine* 2007;**101**:1097–105.

Melsom T., Brinch L., Hessen J.O. Asthma and indoor environment in Nepal. *Thorax* 2001;**56**:477–81.

Menezes A.M., Perez-Padilla R., Jardim J.R. *et al.* Chronic obstructive pulmonary disease in five Latin American cities (the PLATINO study): a prevalence study. *Lancet* 2005;**366**:1875–81.

Meredith S., Nordman H. Occupational asthma: measures of frequency from four countries. *Thorax* 1966;**51**:435–40.

Meredith S.K., Taylor V.M., McDonald J.C. Occupational respiratory disease in the United Kingdom 1989—a Report to the British Thoracic Society and the Society of Occupational Medicine by the Sword Project Group. *British Journal of Industrial Medicine* 1991;**48**:292–8.

Miller M.R., Hankinson J., Brusasco V. *et al.* Standardisation of spirometry. *European Respiratory Journal* 2005;**26**:319–38.

Miravitlles M., de la Roza C., Naberan K. *et al.* Attitudes toward the diagnosis of chronic obstructive pulmonary disease in primary care. *Archives of Bronconeumology* 2006;**42**:3–8.

Miravitlles M., Ferrer M., Pont A. *et al.* Characteristics of a population of COPD patients identified from a population-based study. *Focus on previous diagnosis and never smokers. Respiratory Medicine* 2005;**99**:985–95.

Mitchell E.A., Stewart A.W., ISAAC Phase One Study Group. The ecological relationship of tobacco smoking to the prevalence of symptoms of asthma and other atopic diseases in children: The International Study of Asthma and Allergies in Childhood (ISAAC). *European Journal of Epidemiology* 2001;**17**:667–73.

Mitchell E.A. Increasing prevalence of asthma in children. *New Zealand Medical Journal* 1983;**96**:463–4.

Mommers M., Guekjens-Sijstermans C., Swaen G.M.H. *et al.* Trends in the prevalence of respiratory symptoms and treatment in Dutch children over a 12 year period: results of the fourth consecutive survey. *Thorax* 2005;**60**:97–9.

Morrison Smith J. The prevalence of asthma and wheezing in children. *British Journal of Diseases of the Chest* 1976;**70**:73–7.

Newson R.B., Shaheen S.O., Chinn S. *et al.* Paracetamol sales and atopic disease in children and adults: an ecological analysis. *European Respiratory Journal* 2000;**16**:817–23.

Ninan T.K., Russell G. Respiratory symptoms and atopy in Aberdeen school children: evidence from two surveys 25 years apart. *British Medical Journal* 1992;**304**:873–5.

Nishima S. A study on the prevalence of bronchial asthma in school children in western districts of Japan—comparison between the studies in 1982 and in 1992 with the same methods and same districts, the Study Group of the Prevalence of Bronchial Asthma and the West Japan Study Group of Bronchial Asthma. *Arerugi* 1993; **42**:192–204.

Office of Environmental Health Hazard Assessment. *Health effects of exposure to environmental tobacco smoke.* California Environmental Protection Agency; 1997.

Omran M., Russell G. Continuing increase in respiratory symptoms and atopy in Aberdeen schoolchildren. *British Medical Journal* 1996; **312**:34.

Pattemore P.K., Ellison-Loschmann L., Asher M.I. *et al.* Asthma prevalence in European, Maori, and Pacific children in New Zealand: ISAAC study. *Pediatric Pulmonology* 2004;**37**:433–42.

Pearce N., Ait-Khaled N., Beasley R. *et al.* Worldwide trends in the prevalence of asthma symptoms: phase III of the International Study of Asthma and Allergies in Childhood (ISAAC). *Thorax* 2007;**62**:758–66.

Pearce N., Beasley R., Burgess C. *et al. Asthma epidemiology: principles and methods.* New York (NY): Oxford University Press; 1998.

Pearce N., Beasley R., Pekkanen J. Role of bronchial responsiveness testing in asthma prevalence surveys. *Thorax* 2000a;**55**:352–4.

Pearce N., Douwes J., Beasley R. Is allergen exposure the major primary cause of asthma? *Thorax* 2000b;**55**:424–31.

Pearce N., Douwes J., Beasley R. The rise and rise of asthma: a new paradigm for the new millennium? *Journal of Epidemiology and Biostatistics* 2000c;**5**:5–16.

Pearce N., Douwes J. Asthma time trends—mission accomplished? International Journal of Epidemiology 2005:34:1018–9.

Pearce N., Pekkanen J., Beasley R. How much asthma is really attributable to atopy? *Thorax* 1999;**54**:268–72.

Pearce N., Weiland S., Keil U. *et al.* Self-reported prevalence of asthma symptoms in children in Australia, England, Germany and New Zealand: an international comparison using the ISAAC protocol. *European Respiratory Journal* 1993;**6**:1455–61.

Peat J.K., Tovey E., Toelle B.G. *et al.* House dust mite allergens—a major risk factor for childhood asthma in Australia. *American Journal of Respiratory and Critical Care Medicine* 1996;**153**:141–6.

Perdrizet S., Neukirch F., Cooreman J. *et al.* Prevalence of asthma in adolescents in various parts of France and its relationship to respiratory allergic manifestations. *Chest* 1987;**91**:104S-6S.

Petty T. The history of COPD. *International Journal of COPD* 2006;**1**:3–14.

Petty T.L. COPD in perspective. *Chest* 2002;**121**:116S-20S.

Priftanji A., Strachan D., Burr M. *et al.* Asthma and allergy in Albania and the UK. *Lancet* 2001;**358**:1426–7.

Rabe K.F., Hurd S., Anzueto A. *et al.* Global strategy for the diagnosis, management, and prevention of chronic obstructive pulmonary disease: GOLD executive summary. *American Journal of Respiratory and Critical Care Medicine* 2007;**176**:532–55.

Redline S., Gold D. Challenges in interpreting gender differences in asthma. *American Journal of Respiratory and Critical Care Medicine* 1994;**150**:1219–21.

Reisman J., Schachter H.M., Dales R.E. *et al.* Treating asthma with omega-3 fatty acids: where is the evidence? A systematic review. *BMC Complementary and Alternative Medicine* 2006;**6**:26.

Rennard S., Decramer M., Calverley P.M. *et al.* Impact of COPD in North America and Europe in 2000: subjects' perspective of Confronting COPD International Survey. *European Respiratory Journal* 2002; **20**:799–805.

Robertson C.F., Heycock E., Bishop J. *et al.* Prevalence of asthma in Melbourne schoolchildren: changes over 26 years. *British Medical Journal* 1991;**302**:1116–8.

Robertson C.F., Roberts M.F., Kappers J.H. Asthma prevalence in Melbourne schoolchildren: have we reached the peak? *Medical Journal of Australia* 2004;**180**:273–6.

Romagnani S. The increased prevalence of allergy and the hygiene hypothesis: missing immune deviation, reduced immune suppression, or both? *Immunology* 2004;**112**:352–63.

Ronchetti R., Rennerova Z., Barreto M. *et al.* The prevalence of atopy in asthmatic children correlates strictly with the prevalence of atopy among non-asthmatic children. *International Archives of Allergy and Immunology* 2007;**142**:79–85.

Sandford A.J., Joos L., Pare P.D. Genetic risk factors for chronic obstructive pulmonary disease. *Current Opinion in Pulmonary Medicine* 2002; **8**:87–94.

Sears M.R., Greene J.M., Willan A.R. *et al.* Long-term relation between breastfeeding and development of atopy and asthma in children and young adults: a longitudinal study. *Lancet* 2002;**360**:901–7.

Shaheen S.O., Aaby P., Hall A.J. Cell-mediated immunity after measles in Guinea-Bissau: historical cohort srudy. *British Medical Journal* 1996;**313**:969–74.

Shaheen S.O., Newson R.B., Henderson A.J. *et al.* Prenatal paracetamol exposure and risk of asthma and elevated immunoglobulin E in childhood. *Clinical and Experimental Allergy* 2005;**35**:18–25.

Shaheen S.O., Newson R.B., Sherriff A. *et al.* Paracetamol use in pregnancy and wheezing in early childhood. *Thorax* 2002;**57**:958–63.

Shaheen S.O., Sterne J.A., Songhurst C.E. *et al.* Frequent paracetamol use and asthma in adults. *Thorax* 2000;**55**:266–70.

Shaw R., Woodman K., Ayson M. *et al.* Measuring the prevalence of bronchial hyper-responsiveness in children. *International Journal of Epidemiology* 1995;**24**:597–602.

Shaw R.A., Crane J., O'Donnell T.V. *et al.* Increasing asthma prevalence in a rural New Zealand adolescent population: 1975–89. *Archives of Disease in Childhood* 1990;**65**:1319–23.

Shirakawa T., Enomoto T., Shimazu S. *et al.* The inverse association between tuberculin responses and atopic disorder. *Science* 1997;**275**:77–9.

Shore S.A. Obesity and asthma: lessons from animal models. *Journal of Applied Physiology* 2007;**102**:516–28.

Sigurs N., Gustafsson P.M., Bjarnason R. *et al.* Severe respiratory syncytial virus bronchiolitis in infancy and asthma and allergy at age 13. *American Journal of Respiratory and Critical Care Medicine* 2005;**171**:137–41.

Simpson J.L., Grissell T.V., Douwes J. *et al.* Innate immune activation in neutrophilic asthma and bronchiectasis. *Thorax* 2007;**62**:211–8.

Simpson J.L., Scott R., Boyle M.J. *et al.* Inflammatory subtypes in asthma: assessment and identification using induced sputum. *Respirology* 2006;**11**:54–61.

Siroux V., Pin I., Oryszczyn M.P. *et al.* Relationships of active smoking to asthma and asthma severity in the EGEA study. *Epidemiological study on the genetics and environment of asthma. European Respiratory Journal* 2000;**15**:470–7.

Smith A.D., Cowan J.O., Brassett K.P. *et al.* Use of exhaled nitric oxide measurements to guide treatment in chronic asthma. *New England Journal of Medicine* 2005;**352**:2163–73.

Soriano J.B., Maier W.C., Egger P. *et al.* Recent trends in physician diagnosed COPD in women and men in the UK. *Thorax* 2000;**55**:789–94.

Sporik R., Holgate S.T., Plattsmills T.A.E. *et al.* Exposure to house-dust mite allergen (Der-P-I) and the development of asthma in childhood—a prospective-study. *New England Journal of Medicine* 1990;**323**:502–7.

Stein R.T., Sherrill D., Morgan W.J. *et al.* Respiratory syncytial virus in early life and risk of wheeze and allergy by age 13 years. *Lancet* 1999;**354**:541–5.

Stewart A.W., Mitchell E.A., Pearce N. *et al.* The relationship of per capita gross national product to the prevalence of symptoms of asthma and other atopic diseases in children (ISAAC) [comment]. *International Journal of Epidemiology* 2001;**30**:173–9.

Strachan D.P., Cook D.G. Parental smoking and childhood asthma: longitudinal and case-control studies. *Thorax* 1998;**53**:204–12.

Strachan D.P. Hay fever, hygiene, and household size. *British Medical Journal* 1989;**299**:1259–60.

Sunyer J., Jarvis D., Pekkanen J. *et al.* Geographic variations in the effect of atopy on asthma in the European Community Respiratory Health Study. *Journal of Allergy and Clinical Immunology* 2004;**114**:1033–9.

Tager I.B., Segal M.R., Speizer F.E. *et al.* The natural history of forced expiratory volumes. Effect of cigarette smoking and respiratory symptoms. *American Review of Respiratory Disease* 1988;**138**:837–49.

Tager I.B., Weiss S.T., Munoz A. *et al.* Longitudinal study of the effects of maternal smoking on pulmonary function in children. *New England Journal of Medicine* 1983;**309**:699–703.

Takahashi T., Morita K., Akagi R. *et al.* Heme oxygenase-1: a novel therapeutic target in oxidative tissue injuries. *Current Medicinal Chemistry* 2004;**11**:1545–61.

Tashkin D.P., Detels R., Simmons M. *et al.* The UCLA population studies of chronic obstructive respiratory disease: XI. *Impact of air pollution and smoking on annual change in forced expiratory volume in one second. American Journal of Respiratory and Critical Care Medicine* 1994;**149**:1209–17.

Taylor D.R., Pijnenburg M.W., Smith A.D. *et al.* Exhaled nitric oxide measurements: clinical application and interpretation. *Thorax* 2006;**61**:817–27.

Tepas E.C., Litonjua A.A., Celedon J.C. *et al.* Sensitization to aeroallergens and airway hyperresponsiveness at 7 years of age. *Chest* 2006;**129**:1500–8.

Thomsen S.F., Ulrik C.S., Larsen K. *et al.* Change in prevalence of asthma in Danish children and adolescents. *Annals of Allergy, Asthma and Immunology* 2004;**92**:506–11.

Toelle B.G., Peat J.K., Salome C.M. *et al.* Toward a definition of asthma for epidemiology. *American Review of Respiratory Disease* 1992;**146**:633–7.

Trupin L., Earnest G., San Pedro M. *et al.* The occupational burden of chronic obstructive pulmonary disease. *European Respiratory Journal* 2003;**22**:462–9.

Turner M.O., Hussack P., Sears M.R. *et al.* Exacerbations of asthma without sputum eosinophilia. *Thorax* 1995;**50**:1057–61.

Unger L., Harris M.C. Stepping stones in allergy. *Annals of Allergy* 1974;**32**:214–30.

US Department of Human Health and Human Services. The health consequences of involuntary exposure to tobacco smoke: a report of the Surgeon General. Atlanta (GA): US Department of Human Health and Human Services, Centers for Disease Control and Prevention, Coordinating Centre for Health Promotion, Office on Smoking and Health; 2006.

US Environmental Protection Agency. *Respiratory health effects of passive smoking: lung cancer and other disorders.* Washington (DC): Office of Research and Development, US Environmental Protection Agency; 1992.

van Diemen C.C., Boezen H.M. Genetic epidemiology of reduced lung function. In: Postma D.S., Weiss S.T., editors. *Genetics of asthma and chronic obstructive pulmonary disease.* New York (NY): Informa Healthcare USA; 2007. p. 218.

van Diemen C.C., Postma D.S., Vonk J.M. *et al.* A disintegrin and metalloprotease 33 polymorphisms and lung function decline in the general population. *American Journal of Respiratory and Critical Care Medicine* 2005;**172**:329–33.

Van Strien R.T., Verhoeff A.P., Brunekreef B. *et al.* Mite antigen in house dust: relationship with different housing characteristics in The Netherlands. *Clinical and Experimental Allergy* 1994;**24**:843–53.

Varner A.E., Busse W.W., Lemanske R.F. Jr. Hypothesis: decreased use of pediatric aspirin has contributed to the increasing prevalence of childhood asthma. *Annals of Allergy, Asthma and Immunology* 1998;**81**:347–51.

Vestbo J., Prescott E., Lange P. *et al.* Vital prognosis after hospitalization for COPD: a study of a random population sample. *Respiratory Medicine* 1998;**92**:772–6.

Vestbo J. COPD in the ECRHS. *Thorax* 2004;**59**:89–90.

Vestbo J. Epidemiology. In: Voelkel NF, MacNee W, editors. *Chronic obstructive lung disease.* Hamilton, Canada: BC Decker Inc; 2002. p. 41–55.

Von Mutius E., Martinez F.D., Fritzsch C. Skin test reactivity and number of siblings. *British Medical Journal* 1994;**308**:692–5.

von Mutius E., Schwartz J., Neas L.M. *et al.* Relation of body mass index to asthma and atopy in children: the National Health and Nutrition Examination Study III. *Thorax* 2001;**56**:835–8.

von Mutius E., Weiland S.K., Fritzsch C. *et al.* Increasing prevalence of hay fever and atopy among children in Leipzig, East Germany. *Lancet* 1998;**351**:862–6.

Vork K.L., Broadwin R.L., Blaisdell R.J. Developing asthma in childhood from exposure to secondhand tobacco smoke: insights from a meta-regression. *Environmental Health Perspectives* 2007;**115**:1394–400.

Wang X., Mensinga T.T., Schouten J.P. *et al.* Determinants of maximally attained level of pulmonary function. *American Journal of Respiratory and Critical Care Medicine* 2004;**169**:941–9.

Watson J.P., Cowen P., Lewis R.A. The relationship between asthma admission rates, routes of admission, and socioeconomic deprivation. *European Respiratory Journal* 1996;**9**:2087–93.

Watson L., Boezen H.M., Postma D.S. Differences between males and females in the natural history of asthma and COPD. *European Respiratory Monthly* 2003;**25**:50–73.

Weeke E. Epidemiology of allergic diseases in children. *Rhinology* 1992;**30** Suppl **13**:5–12.

Weiland S.K., Pearce N. Asthma prevalence in adults: good news? *Thorax* 2004;**59**:637–8.

Weinmayr G., Weiland S.K., Bjorksten B. *et al.* Atopic sensitization and the international variation of asthma symptom prevalence in children. *American Journal of Respiratory and Critical Care Medicine* 2007;**176**:565–74.

Weitzman M., Gortmaker S.L., Sobol A.M. *et al.* Recent trends in the prevalence and severity of childhood asthma. *Journal of the American Medical Association* 1992;**268**:2673–7.

Whincup P.H., Cook D.G., Strachan D.P. *et al.* Time trends in respiratory symptoms in childhood over a 24 year period. *Archives of Disease in Childhood* 1993;**68**:729–34.

Willis T. Pharmaceutice rationalis [the operations of medicine in humane bodies]. London: Dring, Harper, and Leigh; 1678.

World Health Organization. *Air quality guidelines, global update 2005.* Particulate matter, ozone, nitrogen dioxide and sulphur dioxide. Copenhagen: WHO Regional office for Europe; 2005.

Xu X., Weiss S.T., Rijcken B. *et al.* Smoking, changes in smoking habits, and rate of decline in FEV_1: new insight into gender differences. *European Respiratory Journal* 1994;**7**:1056–61.

Yamada N., Yamaya M., Okinaga S. *et al.* Microsatellite polymorphism in the heme oxygenase-1 gene promoter is associated with susceptibility to emphysema. *American Journal of Human Genetics* 2000;**66**:187–95.

Yunginger J.W., Reed C.E., O'Connell E.J. *et al.* A community-based study of the epidemiology of asthma. *Incidence rates, 1964–1983. American Review of Respiratory Disease* 1992;**146**:888–94.

Zamel N., McClean P.A., Sandell P.R. *et al.* Asthma on Tristan de Cunha: looking for the genetic link. *American Journal of Respiratory and Critical Care Medicine* 1996;**153**:1902–6.

9.5

Obesity

Philip James

Abstract

Obesity is of increasing public health importance. Recent increases in life expectancy in high-income countries may be threatened by the rapid rise in the prevalence of obesity and associated health problems, including diabetes mellitus. Obesity has also emerged as an increasing concern in many middle-income countries. This chapter begins by analysing definitions of obesity, including older standard values of weight-for-height, more recent classifications based on body mass index (BMI) for adults and children, as well as classifications of abdominal obesity based on waist circumference. The association of anthropometric indices with ethnic origins is discussed and the rationale for population-specific criteria for abdominal obesity is outlined. Application of these criteria in population surveys from 191 countries around the year 2000 suggest that there were about 1.1 billion overweight and obese adults in the world of whom 320 million were obese with BMI of 30 kg/m^2 or more. More than half of overweight people are in middle- or low-income countries. About 10 per cent of boys and 9 per cent of girls aged 5–17 years are overweight, based on recently developed international standard criteria. Obesity is associated with a range of morbidity including well-known associations with diabetes and coronary heart disease and less appreciated impacts on respiratory function, sleep, and back and joint pains that contribute to diminished physical activity. Obesity is estimated to be one of the three risk factors that contribute most to the global burden of disability-adjusted life years lost (DALYs). Preventive interventions must target adults as well as children because it is in adult life that the greatest increases in obesity and its complications occur. Overweight and obesity result from small errors in energy balance, which lead to weight increments and the persistence of weight gain. In high-income countries, physical activity and energy expenditure have declined due to decrease in physical activity in work, commuting, and domestic activities while leisure-time physical activities have remained stable. Overall energy intakes have been declining. Interventions to reduce overweight and obesity must be made at individual, community, and societal levels. These may include changes in the physical environment that promote safe physical activity; economic measures using incentives or taxes to promote change; policy interventions to encourage, for example, breast feeding within healthcare settings; and sociocultural interventions including strategies for health promotion.

Introduction

The prevalence of obesity and overweight has been increasing rapidly in high-income countries, especially over the last decade. This increase is of great public health concern because projections suggest that as substantial further increases in obesity occur, the morbidity associated with obesity and its complications will threaten gains in life expectancy made as a result of the earlier decline in cardiovascular diseases. Overweight and obesity are also increasing rapidly in middle-income countries and in some low-income country populations. There is therefore a need to intervene on the growing epidemic of obesity with some urgency.

This chapter analyses the problem of obesity from the public health perspective. The chapter begins by considering definitions of overweight and obesity for adults and children. Definitions of abdominal obesity that are relevant in different populations are also described. The second section of the chapter presents estimates and projections for the prevalence of overweight and obesity, as well as estimates for the burden of disease and healthcare costs associated with obesity. The final section of the chapter outlines principles of energy balance in the context of trends in physical activity and energy intakes. This information may be used to inform potential interventions at the individual, community, and societal levels.

Definitions of obesity

The classification of obesity was originally based on analyses of death rates for those taking out life insurance policies with the US Metropolitan Life Insurance Company before the World War II. At that time, weights and heights were taken in light indoor clothing and wearing shoes with an additional subjective assessment by the doctor of whether the man or woman had a small, medium, or large frame size. It was then considered that somebody had a substantial increased risk if they were 20 per cent overweight but it was often unclear whether the normal weight should be the mid or upper level of the weight range for the man or woman of a particular frame size. These data were then recalculated by the UK Department of Health/MRC group in the early 1970s to provide BMI data after adjustments were made for the clothes and shoes (James 1976). To these data were later added those collected for the Build Study and the Royal College of Physicians (London) in their

1983 report highlighted for the first time the substantial public health significance of the prevailing rates of overweight and obesity based on taking a BMI of 30 as indicative of obesity. The value of 30 was 20 per cent above the now accepted upper normal BMI limit of 25, no specification now being made for using frame size in subcategorizing the risk. The upper normal limit of BMI 25 was taken from analyses of US (Royal College of Physicians 1983; Garrow 1981) mortality statistics but the separate analysis of male and female smokers then proved important in displaying the same U-shaped curves as those observed in non-smokers but with rates at a consistently higher level. Thus, the mortality risk of a smoker with a BMI of 22 was roughly equivalent to that of a non-smoker who had a BMI of 30. Then the World Health Organization (WHO) in 1995 accepted the BMI as the appropriate method for crudely assessing degrees of underweight and overweight but took a lower limit of 18.5 for distinguishing normal from underweight. This followed a series of earlier international analyses of adults' capacity to engage in heavy agricultural work which set the limit at 18.5, whereas the propensity to infections only became apparent in the available South American, African, and Asian studies when the BMI was below 17. This BMI value therefore became the next cut-off point signifying undernutrition (James et al. 1988) (Table 9.5.1) (National Institutes of Health 1998).

It was not until the WHO Expert Consultation on obesity in 1997 that the implications of overweight and obesity were accepted by WHO as a global problem (World Health Organization 2000). At that time, there was considerable discussion about the appropriateness of the choice of BMI cut-offs because in the United States it was accepted by physicians that there were so many heavy adults that perhaps one should only consider an individual overweight in national terms if their BMI was 28 or more. The Japanese, however, were pressing for a lower BMI cut-off and by the year 2000 the

WPRO branch of WHO had accepted an upper cut-off of 23 for Asians (WHO/IASO/IOTF 2000); above this value, the risks of diabetes and hypertension in particular were unacceptably high. This was generally accepted following the WHO Singapore meeting in 2002 (WHO Expert Consultation 2004) but has not been applied on a regional basis, although numerous national bodies in Asia take the lower BMI criteria for granted and use Table 9.5.1 as the approach to clinical and public health decision making.

More recently, mortality data from the United States involving nationally representative data from the NHANES series of surveys have produced controversial findings using new modelling techniques to assess whether modest degrees of overweight are inducing increased mortality rates (Flegal et al. 2007). The BMIs associated with the lowest death rates were about 25–28, and the risk of death associated with high BMIs seemed to be falling on a secular basis. These findings are intriguing but need to be taken with some caution because it was shown many years ago that identifying the mortality effects of overweight (BMIs 25–29.9) required many years of follow-up with very substantial numbers of subjects (James 1976) and in practice the apparent secular decline in death rates also involved progressively shorter periods of follow-up in Flegal's study (Flegal et al. 2007). The recent analyses take account of the first of two forms of statistical bias: (a) the reverse causation phenomenon whereby some of those with lower weights are already ill, and (b) the subjects' progressive increase in weight during the period of observation (Greenberg 2006). Once these corrections are made in other surveys, then more modest degrees of overweight are on a cohort basis associated with a clear increase in mortality. Thus, the British Whitehall study with over 18 000 men, but followed for up to 35 years, showed that all-cause and ischaemic heart disease mortality rates (but not stroke death rates) were increased in the overweight

Table 9.5.1 The NIH and Asian adaptations of the WHO criteria for classification of overweight and obesity with their associated risks

Classification	BMI kg/m²	Disease risk* Europids (NIH) Waist circumference ≤102 cm (M) ≤88 cm (W)	≥102 cm (M) >88 cm (W)	Asians Waist circumference <90 cm (M) <80 cm (W)	≥90 cm (M) ≥80 cm (W)
Underweight	<18.5		—	Low (but increased risk of other clinical problems)	Average
Asian normal	18.5–22.9		—	Average	Increased
Asian overweight	23–24.9			Increased	Moderate
Asian obesity grade I	25–29.9			Moderate	Severe
Asian grade II	≥30			Severe	Very severe
Europid normal	18.5–24.9				
Europid overweight	25–29.9	Increased	High		
Europid obese class 1	≥30	High	Very high		
Europid obese class 2	30–34.9	Very high	Very high		
Europid obese class 3	≥35	Extremely high	Extremely high		

* Disease risk specified by NIH as relating to type 2 diabetes, hypertension, and cardiovascular disease. M = Men W = Women.

group (Batty *et al.* 2006). Another recent integrated analysis of 33 cohorts involving nearly a third of a million adults, followed for an average of 7 years from the Asia-Pacific region and including Australasia and Pacific Islanders, showed that the risk of fatal and non-fatal cardiovascular disease, particularly ischaemic stroke and ischaemic heart disease increased progressively from a BMI of 20, whereas the impact on haemorrhagic stroke was not evident until BMIs were in the region of 30 (Asia Pacific Cohort Studies Collaboration 2004). As in many of these studies, the first 3 years of follow-up in all the cohorts had to be discarded because those who were already ill had lower BMIs and early deaths so without this adjustment the curves were J-shaped. Similarly when over half a million US subjects who had never smoked were followed for up to 10 years by the American Cancer Society there was a remarkably rapid increase in death rates related to earlier BMIs (albeit self reported) of ≥25 (Adams *et al.* 2006). This relationship was more evident when the follow-up periods were long; the avoidance of the marked confounding effects of smoking again proved important.

Given that the focus on specifying the disadvantages of excess weight gain was originally dependent on information from those who took out life insurance policies, it is not surprising that the mortality criteria dominated earlier thinking on classifying appropriate weights for height. Later, it will be shown that a somewhat different perspective emerges when account is taken of the physical impact of weight gain or that of diseases that either only develop or are amplified in their effects when weight gain occurs.

From a public health perspective the development of the original criteria for assessing the risk from excess weight neglected the fact that the classification of excess weight used a classic clinical categorical approach when in practice there are progressive increases in the risk as the BMI increases. Thus, the precise choice of cut-off point is arbitrary: The health hazards are progressive and not substantially changed at any particular cut-off point. Furthermore, there are age-dependent changes in the relationship of BMI to total mortality (see below) and the classic co-morbidities intrinsically linked to an excess BMI, e.g. diabetes, hypertension, gall stones, and coronary heart disease are linearly related to BMI from a BMI nadir of about 19 or 20 in prospective studies of professional groups of men and women. Thus, the choice of an upper normal value of 24.9 for individuals is very generous and this value is quite different from the optimum population mean BMI which, as in the latest WHO report, should be between 21 and 23. Non-smoking individuals are likely to have an optimum life expectancy and disability-free life if their BMIs remain at about 20 throughout life.

Other criteria for classifying excess weight gain: Abdominal obesity

It has been recognized for many decades that the distribution of body fat was a useful clinical guide to the likelihood of risk and the waist–hip ratio was frequently advocated as a valuable tool. More recently the INTERHEART international case–control study of coronary heart disease has shown that the waist–hip ratio (W/HR) was a far more sensitive measure of risk with several analyses then being cited to indicate that fat deposition on the hips was protective so that the risk associated with a high waist circumference was reduced by the extent to which fat was also laid down peripherally (Yusuf *et al.* 2005). The superiority of the WHR compared with other indices of risk in part relates to the fact that different

populations have very different skeletal and muscle masses so the ratio not only allows for the differential effect of central and peripheral fat distribution but also standardizes the risk for populations of very different sizes. From a simple clinical point of view and a practical public health approach, waist circumference alone is simpler to measure, does not require complex calculations, and overcomes the need to measure the hip circumference which in some societies is a culturally problematic measure to make except with female physicians taking considerable care.

The original choice of waist circumference (WC) was made so that the different values for men and women's waist cut-off points corresponded with the BMI cut-offs for overweight and obesity i.e. 25 and 30. These are the values which WHO then adopted (Table 9.5.1) for classifying—at least in Caucasians—excess abdominal fat. With the Asian focus on specifying lower normal BMI ranges, however, new WC values were proposed for Asians based on statistical calculations of the sensitivity and specificity of detecting hypertension or diabetes at different WC levels. More recently, the International Diabetes Federation in proposing new criteria for specifying the metabolic syndrome—which signifies a collection of risk factors including dyslipidaemia, hypertension, diabetes, and abdominal obesity—adapted the different values proposed for different ethnic groups despite their being derived very differently (Table 9.5.2). Thus, the women's WC limit for normality in Japan is based on the WC needed to find >100 cm² area of intra-abdominal fat on CT scanning, this value being taken as the marker of the absolute risk of men and women having a high risk

Table 9.5.2 Different waist circumference cut-off points selected by the International Diabetes Federation as part of their assessment of the metabolic syndrome

Country/ethnic group	Waist circumference (cm)	
Europids*		
In the United States, the ATP III values (102 cm male; 88 cm female) are likely to continue to be used for clinical purposes.	Male	≥94
	Female	≥80
South Asians		
Based on a Chinese, Malay, and Asian-Indian population	Male	≥90
	Female	≥80
Chinese	Male	≥90
	Female	≥80
Japanese**	Male	≥85
	Female	≥90
Ethnic South and Central Americans	Use South Asian recommendations until more specific data are available.	
Sub-Saharan Africans	Use European data until more specific data are available.	
Eastern Mediterranean and Middle East (Arab) populations	Use European data until more specific data are available.	

ATP—Adult Treatment Panel

* In future epidemiological studies of populations of Europid origin, prevalence should be given using both European and North American cut-points to allow better comparisons.

** Originally different values were proposed for Japanese people but new data support the use of the values shown above.

Source: International Diabetes Federation. A new worldwide definition of the Metabolic syndrome, 2005, 11. Available from: http://www.idf.org.

of a coronary artery diseases (James 2005). This contrasts with the general approach where the relative risk of a complication of a high WC determines the values chosen.

The criteria for specifying the metabolic syndrome differs markedly between different national and global groups but it is now generally accepted that different WC values are needed for different ethnic groups because of their increased absolute risk of diabetes and hypertension at the same WC. There is now increasing evidence that not only is there a strong genetic influence on fat distribution but in addition environmental factors including smoking and alcohol consumption amplify the propensity to abdominal obesity with early nutritional and other handicaps, demonstrated for example by low birth weights, being a marked promoter of subsequent abdominal obesity when even modest weight is gained in adult life. Thus, Indian, Chinese, and Hispanic populations with a marked history of early childhood malnutrition are particularly liable to display abdominal obesity even when their BMIs are within the normal WHO BMI range of <25. Thus, the unusual susceptibility of the major populations of the world to greater disability on adult weight gain than Caucasians living in Northern Europe or North America may require a much broader public health perspective involving the whole life cycle (see later).

Children's criteria for overweight and obesity

There were no acceptable criteria for overweight and obesity in children except those generated by WHO for the first time in 1995 when the same statistical criteria as those developed for underweight or childhood malnutrition were invoked. This essentially depended on arbitrarily classifying a child as underweight for their age, underheight for age, or underweight for height by defining any individual falling within the mean ±2 SDs as 'normal' and those outside these limits as 'abnormal'. Thus, the >2 SD for weight for height was taken as indicative of overweight and the reference data were based on a composite US data set which had become the WHO reference growth curves. They reflected the findings from a series of meticulous surveys of US children deemed to be healthy and growing adequately after World War II. No specific health criteria were therefore used in specifying the normal range. Furthermore, at that time WHO was wholly occupied with establishing national surveillance systems for monitoring only the under-5-year-olds so that they could assess progress in tackling the national and global prevalence of protein–energy malnutrition (PEM). PEM was originally specified as those having a low weight for age, but then more sophisticated approaches emerged in the 1970s to assess the prevalence of wasting i.e. low weight for heights and stunting—low heights for age. Thus, at that time, there were no coherent analyses of overweight in the under-5-year-olds and almost no data on older children. This reflected the paediatric view at that time that overweight and obesity in children was not a public health issue and any obese child needed clinical evaluation to see if they had an associated genetic disease.

Developing an international classification of overweight and obesity in children

The International Obesity Task Force (IOTF) group which had collected data on adult prevalences of overweight and obesity from

the developing as well as the developed world for the WHO consultation on obesity then recognized the need to develop a new classification system for overweight and obesity in children (Cole et al. 2000) because it had become clear that the obesity issue in children had been neglected. After a detailed analysis of the options (Dietz & Bellizzi 1999), the BMI index was again chosen as useful because it had already been applied to children (Must et al. 1991), and Cole's method (Cole & Green 1992) for developing smooth percentile BMI curves on a sex-specific basis throughout childhood made simpler analyses possible. Many countries, e.g. Japan, and some in Europe, North America, and the Middle East, were also beginning to use either a 90th, 95th, or 97th BMI percentile as the basis for distinguishing obese children from normal; only Australia used the 85th percentile as a cut-off point (Guillaume 1999). The IOTF concluded that one could develop an approach which linked the childhood and adult definitions by taking, at age 18 years, those percentiles which corresponded to BMIs of 25 and 30 and using these same percentiles throughout the childhood age range for specifying overweight and obesity in childhood in girls and boys separately. Table 9.5.3 sets out the cut-off points to be used for this classification. This assumes that individual boys and girls will tend to retain the same percentile as they grow (see below).

The IOTF chose data from six countries, i.e. the original NHANES I data from the United States, UK data, and surveys from the Netherlands, Hong Kong, Singapore, and Brazil. This choice could have been improved by the inclusion of data on well-fed children of Indian and African origin, but suitable data were not available. The composite percentile cut-off points chosen from the six data sets are now being used routinely in many parts of the world. These IOTF overweight cut-off points correspond approximately to the 90th and 95th centiles for British and Dutch males, respectively, but the obesity cut-off points are above the 97th centile for almost all the assessed national surveys. It is not surprising, therefore, that by selecting the much higher percentile value for obesity there is likely to be much greater variability at these extreme values.

There have been concerns about the use of BMI in a standardized form as an index of body fatness in children from different societies because of the different ages for the onset of puberty (Dietz & Bellizzi 1999). Reilly et al. (2000), however, using UK data and body impedance measures of total fat, assessed the sensitivity and specificity of the IOTF BMI cut-off points for overweight and obesity. They showed that there was excellent specificity and sensitivity for the overweight cut-off points, but lower sensitivity for the higher obesity cut-off point (Table 9.5.4).

Tracking of body fat and BMI into adult life

The usefulness of the age- and sex-specific BMI cut-off points in the IOTF reference values and the adult BMI 25 and 30 cut-off points would be amplified if children in practice do grow along the same percentiles for both body fat and BMI through childhood into adult life. This issue was not straight forward because Rolland-Cachera et al. (1987) produced a detailed study of 164 subjects monitored from the age of one month to adult life. Only 41–42 per cent of pre-school children remained into adult life in their original category of being lean, medium, or fat if these categories were defined based on the 25th and 75th centiles of BMI. Rolland-Cachera et al. therefore focused on the issue of 'fat-rebound' in

Table 9.5.3 The IOTF cut-off points by age and sex for children from 2 to 18 years designed to pass through BMIs of 25 and 30 when aged 18 years

Age years	Child's BMI percentile corresponding to BMI 25 when adult		Child's BMI percentile corresponding to BMI 30 when adult	
	Boys	Girls	Boys	Girls
2	18.41	18.02	20.09	19.81
2.5	18.13	17.66	19.60	19.55
3	17.89	17.56	19.57	19.36
3.5	17.69	17.40	19.39	19.23
4	17.55	17.28	19.29	19.15
4.5	17.47	17.19	19.26	19.12
5	17.42	17.15	19.30	19.17
5.5	17.45	17.20	19.47	19.34
6	17.55	17.34	19.78	19.65
6.5	17.71	17.53	20.23	20.08
7	17.92	17.75	20.63	20.51
7.5	18.16	18.03	21.09	21.01
8	18.44	18.39	21.60	21.57
8.5	18.76	18.69	22.17	22.18
9	19.10	19.07	22.77	22.81
9.5	19.46	19.45	23.19	23.36
10	19.84	19.86	24	24.11
10.5	20.20	20.29	24.57	24.77
11	20.55	20.74	25.10	25.42
11.5	20.89	21.20	25.58	26.05
12	21.22	21.68	26.02	26.67
12.5	21.56	22.14	26.43	27.24
13	21.91	22.58	26.84	27.76
13.5	22.27	22.98	27.25	28.20
14	22.62	23.34	27.63	28.87
14.5	22.96	23.66	27.98	28.87
15	23.29	23.94	28.10	29.11
15.5	23.60	24.17	28.60	29.29
16	23.90	24.34	28.68	29.43
16.5	24.19	24.54	29.14	29.56
17	24.46	24.70	29.41	29.69
17.5	24.73	24.85	29.70	29.84
18	25	25	30	30

Source: Cole et al. (2000).

pre-pubertal school children. Guo and Chumlea (1999), however, had shown from US longitudinal studies that the probability of children with high BMIs still being overweight and obese at the age of 35 rose markedly throughout childhood. Thus, the probability of being overweight when aged 35 was 0.3 in 5-year-old children

Table 9.5.4 Sensitivity and specificity of overweight and obesity based on the IOTF BMI cut-off points for boys and girls and based on impedance estimates of body fat

	Sensitivity (%, n)	Specificity (%, n)
Boys		
Overweight	90 (90/100)*	92 (1756/1910)
Obesity	46 (46/100)**	99 (1901/1910)
Girls		
Overweight	97 (94/97)	84 (1543/1841)
Obesity	72 (72/97)	99 (1813/1841)

Significant differences in sensitivity between the sexes *P < 0.05 **P < 0.01
Source: Reilly et al. (2000).

with a BMI on the 95th percentile, about 0.35 at 10 years, 0.5 at 15 years, and about 0.7 at the age of 18. Systematic reviews of the evidence, e.g. by Power et al. (1997) and Parsons et al. (1999), have not found much evidence for the value of selective monitoring in the pre-pubertal phase for predicting the emergence of obesity if this is based on detailed analyses of weight rebound. Power's analyses showed that the older the children studied, the greater was the risk of their continuing to be obese in adult life. Once children were over 5 years of age, being obese incurred a great risk of this persisting, with the majority remaining obese into adult life (Table 9.5.5). Barlow and Dietz (1998) have also emphasized the value of concentrating on children over at least the age of 3. IOTF therefore chose to concentrate on children aged 5 and over and a consensus seems to have emerged that, for the present, one should focus on children of school age for predicting the risk of obesity persisting into adult life.

New definitions of 'normal' weight gain in children

WHO has recently undertaken a new approach to defining the normal growth of children (WHO Child Growth Standards 2007) which traditionally has been seen by many paediatricians to be very different in different countries and ethnic groups. The original WHO criteria, based on US data, were used as a reference because it had become evident that when the environmental conditions improved in many societies, the growth of children increasingly conforms with that set out in the WHO reference tables. WHO then established a major multinational study involving children in California, Norway, India, Oman, Ghana, and Brazil. Normal babies delivered at full term by healthy, non-smoking mothers who agreed to breastfeed their babies exclusively for at least 4 months were monitored carefully, with specific advice being given relating to immunization and other rearing practices. Further cohorts of pre-school children from similar environments were also chosen so that, over a period of 6.5 years, it was possible to obtain data on 8400 children's growth patterns. It was surprising to find that whatever the ethnic background, the children's growth was almost identical and the variability in growth was far less than in the data bases normally used for producing growth charts. This implies that if one takes the latest WHO ±2 SD values, then the new estimates of underweight and overweight prevalences will be greater. This particularly applies to the prevalence of overweight children because

Table 9.5.5 The likelihood of children continuing to be overweight as adults ranked by age of first measurement

Study number	Age of monitoring		% still obese as adults	
	As children	As 'adults'	Males	Females
3	<1	20–30	36	-
5	1–5	19–26	27	-
7	7	14	90	87
7	7	16	63	62
11	7	33	43	63
6	7	35	40	20
9	1–14	10–23	42	66
8	2–14	10–24	43	-
4	9–10	31–35	57	64
11	11	33	54	64
2	9–13	42–53	63	-
1	10–13	29–34	74	72
6	13	35	40	30
4	13–14	31–35	77	70
10	13–17	27–31	58	-
11	16	33	64	78

Source: Data rearranged from Power *et al.* (1997) with study numbers as in their analysis. The proportion of obese adults who had been originally overweight as a child was usually 3–10 fold lower than the corresponding probability of overweight children maintaining their excess weight into adulthood.

in both children and adults there is an increasingly skewed distribution of weights as the average weight for age rises.

This new set of growth curves from WHO establishes for the first time a standard rather than a reference set of growth curves since it is being taken to imply that all children from any ethnic group, provided they have the advantages of exclusive breastfeeding and appropriate environmental conditions with suitable immunization and dietary patterns, will grow at almost identical rates. This is a proposition which is not accepted by many paediatricians or policy-makers in lower-income countries.

Later in 2007, WHO issued a further proposal on the appropriate growth of children from 5 to 20 years of age. This new set of criteria is surprisingly still based on US data, despite detailed examination of other growth curves from many international sources. However, the care with which the early US growth rates were monitored and the fact that the growth charts chosen link well with the charts for breastfed children <5 years is WHO's justification for now providing, for the first time, standard or reference growth charts for children throughout the world. As yet, only a few countries have begun to adapt their policies to incorporate the new concepts for the under-5-year-olds. What is already clear, however, is that with such small SDs for the variability in the growth of well-nourished non-infected children, the new WHO practice of taking the 85th and 95th percentiles corresponding very approximately to 1 SD and 2 SDs as cut-offs for 'at risk' and 'overweight' children will mean that far more children will be now designated as overweight. In fact, the cut-off points chosen are very close to those percentiles

chosen for the IOTF analyses at the age of 18–20 years, but there are differences in the actual BMI values between the different estimates at younger ages. The WHO charts are presented in Fig. 9.5.1.

The prevalence of adult overweight and obesity

The original assessment of the global prevalence of overweight and obesity for WHO in 1996 was based on crude analyses which showed that obesity had become a global problem. The Millennium analyses by IOTF and WHO, based on a sifting of data and some interpolation of data from 191 countries revealed that there were about 1.1 billion overweight and obese adults in the world, of whom about 320 million were obese with a BMI of 30 or more (James *et al.* 2004). Different regions varied markedly in their prevalence. Surprisingly the developing world is making an even greater contribution than the developed world: If the whole of the developing world comprises all countries other than Japan, and those in Europe, North America, and Australasia, then 54 per cent of the world's 1105 million overweight (i.e. BMI 25–29.9) and 46 per cent of the world's 312 million obese are in the lower-income countries. The problem in these countries is therefore beginning to match the problem of cardiovascular diseases where the developing countries have a far greater burden than that of the affluent world.

The nutrition transition

There is now a recognized major increase in obesity rates associated with the economic development of a country and particularly the urbanization of populations in the developing world (Popkin 2006). The development of overweight and obesity varies markedly. Early Brazilian studies showed that, in poorer communities, middle-aged women are the first to become overweight and then as the economy develops women become progressively heavier with men then also beginning to catch up. In poor societies, the more affluent have a higher prevalence of obesity with the average BMI of the population increasing progressively as national incomes rise to about a GDP of US$5000 then peaks in women at US$15 000 and in men at US$17 000 (Ezzati *et al.* 2005). Figure 9.5.3 shows that the average BMI rises with progressive urbanization and this also leads to a fall in the proportion of household income spent on food. Then, as societies develop, there is a progressive reversal of the socioeconomic gradient so that the more affluent women become slimmer and then both men and women in wealthy environments have lower obesity rates than the poor. Ethnic differences within countries are well documented but this often links to their socioeconomic status rather than to any relationship with ethnicity.

As the increase in the average weight of the population rises, the proportion of obese individuals goes up markedly because of the marked skewing of the BMI distributions as illustrated originally by Rose using data from the INTERSALT studies (Rose 1991). Figure 9.5.4 shows these data and also highlights the fact that the most genetically sensitive members of the community are those found in the upper distributions for their society.

Table 9.5.6 provides an illustration of the age-related adult changes in the prevalences in some of the regions of the world. It is noteworthy that the main increase occurs in the 20–40-year-old group.

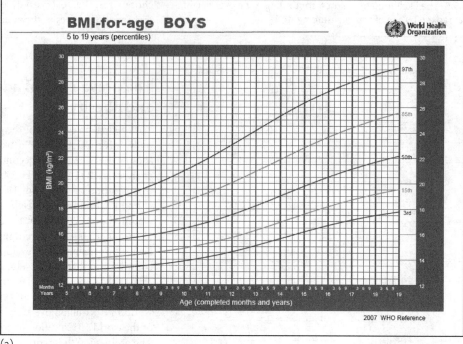

(a)

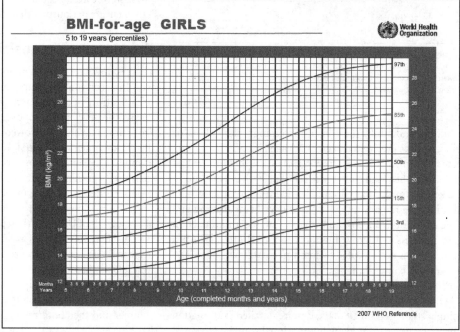

Fig. 9.5.1 New WHO children's growth charts.

(b)

Childhood prevalences on obesity

The preliminary analyses show that about 10 per cent of boys and 9 per cent of girls aged 5–17 years in the world are overweight, i.e. a total of 118 million overweight and obese children based on the IOTF criteria. The latest available regional prevalences for overweight and obesity using the IOTF international set of definitions (Wang & Lobstein 2006) are given in Table 9.5.7.

The health hazards associated with excess weight

Data relating to all the major risk factors were collected by different groups for WHO, the data then being collated according to standard protocols to take account of the different population age structures. These data were collated on a subregional basis by extrapolating to obtain estimates based on analogous countries and measured age

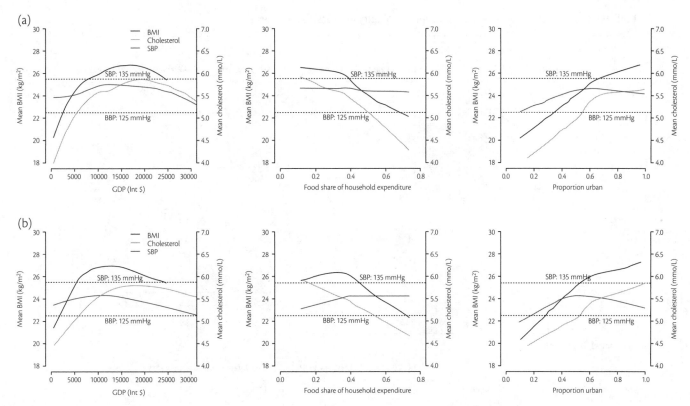

Fig. 9.5.2 (a) Males; (b) Females.
The relationship of mean population BMI, systolic blood pressure (SBP), and total cholesterol with average national income, food share of household expenditure, and proportion of population in urban areas. National income was measured as gross domestic product (GDP). Taken from Ezzati *et al.* (2005).

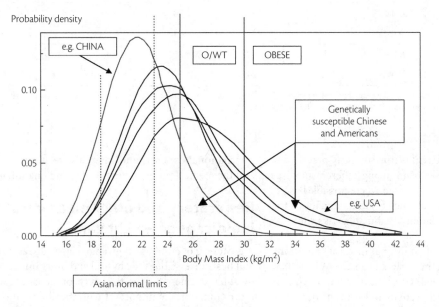

Fig. 9.5.3 The skewed distribution of BMI with increases in the average population BMI. Cross-sectional data taken from the INTERSALT study (Rose 1991) to illustrate the progressive marked increase in obesity rates for modest increases in mean BMI. Those in the upper BMI range for each population distribution represent the genetically susceptible individuals to weight gain. The usual Caucasian cut-offs for overweight and obesity are shown together with the Asian upper limit of 'normal' BMI.

Table 9.5.6 Regional prevalences of overweight and obesity in males and females

% Obese

		18–29 years	30–44 years	45–59 years	60–69 years	70+ years
Africa	Male	4.4	5.4	6.6	7.7	2.7
	Female	6.3	13.8	16.4	16	10.1
Northern America	Male	26.6	29.1	34.3	30.4	29.9
	Female	27.7	31.1	37.9	30.7	30.5
Latin America	Male	7.9	13.6	16.3	14.9	8.3
	Female	8.9	17.4	23.2	23.7	15.9
Europe	Male	4.9	12.5	20	16.6	7.8
	Female	6.8	16.3	27	26.7	14.1
Asia	Male	1.6	4.8	6	6.4	3.1
	Female	2.2	6	8.3	9.5	6.7
Oceania	Male	15	16.2	20.7	20.8	16.3
	Female	11.3	16.2	26.9	28.9	22.5

% Overweight (pre-obese)

		18–29 years	30–44 years	45–59 years	60–69 years	70+
Africa	Male	9.3	14.1	16.9	16.8	12.3
	Female	16.1	21.1	23.3	17.9	12.2
Northern America	Male	26.6	29.1	34.3	30.4	29.9
	Female	27.7	31.1	37.9	30.7	30.5
Latin America	Male	24.4	34.9	34.1	36.4	30.7
	Female	21.4	30.4	35.1	29	32.4
Europe	Male	27.2	42.4	47.7	47	45.8
	Female	17.2	28.7	36.4	38.8	38.1
Asia	Male	14.2	23.1	26	25.6	20.3
	Female	9.7	18.8	21.9	22.4	27
Oceania	Male	42.2	45.3	50.5	51.7	52.2
	Female	22.3	24.5	33.1	36.8	36.9

Unpublished updates of IOTF estimates using data from national or regional representative surveys with age standardization and allowances for national population differences as in the original WHO Millennium analyses (James *et al.* 2004).

and sex differences so that a coherent picture of likely prevalences could be obtained. Then the risks of inducing different medical problems with excess weight were estimated where possible by systematic analyses of epidemiological studies so that equations for deriving the proportion of population-attributable risks could be obtained.

Table 9.5.8 compares the list of additional medical conditions associated with excess weight gain as set out in the WHO 2000 (National Institutes of Health 1998) obesity consultation with an indication of those diseases which were included in the quantitative analyses for the WHO Millennium assessment of the risk factors contributing to the global burden of disease. The differences relate to the fact that quantitative estimates of the risks at different BMI levels could only be applied to conditions where there were

international data sets and where the relationships between BMI and the medical problem were robust and quantifiable.

Respiratory and other mechanical handicaps of weight gain

A great deal of emphasis is given to classic diseases such as diabetes and heart disease but the physical and other impacts of weight gain must be considered. Thus, the effects of increasing weight on respiratory function are important with the ability of overweight children and adults to engage in strenuous physical activity becoming more limited the greater their weight increase. Thus, very obese adults, when asked to walk slowly, are already using up to 60 per cent of their maximum exercise capacity, and this can only be sustained

Table 9.5.7 Prevalence of overweight and obesity in school-age children based on latest available data, and estimated for 2006 and 2010 based on population-weighted annualized increases in prevalence and the use of IOTF criteria for overweight and obesity

WHO region (dates of most recent surveys)	Most recent surveys		Projected 2006		Projected 2010	
	Overweight (inc obesity) %	Obesity %	Overweight (inc obesity) %	Obesity %	Overweight (inc obesity) %	Obesity %
Africa (1987–2003)	1.6	0.2	4.1	1.3	7.9	2.2
Americas (1988–2000)	29.7	11	44.4	15.4	50.8	17.4
Eastern Mediterranean (1992–2001)	22.1	4.2	37.9	8.9	44.3	10.9
Europe (1992–2003)	19.6	4.6	29.5	7.6	35.9	9.6
Southeast Asia (1997–2002)	10.9	1.9	18.1	4	24.4	6
West Pacific (1993–2000)	16.4	3.7	27.4	7.1	33.9	9.1

Source: Wang & Lobstein (2006).

for a while. It is therefore not surprising that obese adults are often found to be doing less than normal-weight individuals because their physical exertions are very energy consuming. For those with any degree of respiratory impairment, weight gain is also a marked handicap. Thus, asthmatic patients and those with chronic obstructive respiratory disease can show a marked improvement in exercise tolerance and comfort if they lose weight. One further feature of weight gain is the far greater tendency to develop sleep apnoea, which is associated with a large neck and a tendency to obstruct breathing. This leads to their stopping breathing for increasing

lengths of time, particularly at night. This seemingly innocuous problem is actually a major medical handicap associated with drug-resistant hypertension because of the persistent induction of the sympathetic nervous system by the repeated anoxia. When severe, it is not only associated with a higher mortality but can be the cause of traffic accidents as abdominally obese adults with thick necks fall asleep as they drive their vehicles.

Back and joint pains are another major problem leading to greater time off work for overweight and obese patients. The mechanical force on joints and the strain on the muscular skeletal system is marked leading to time off work and reactive depression among many overweight and obese subjects.

Table 9.5.8 The relative risk* of health problems associated with obesity

Greatly increased (relative risk much greater than 3)	Moderately increased (relative risk 2–3)	Slightly increased (relative risk 1–2)
NIDDM[†]	CHD[†]	Cancers: Breast[†] in postmenopausal women; endometrial[†]; colon[†]
Gallbladder disease	Hypertension[†]	Reproductive hormone abnormalities
Dyslipidaemia	Osteoarthritis (knees)[†]	Polycystic ovary syndrome
Insulin resistance	Hyperuricaemia and gout	Impaired fertility
Breathlessness		Low back pain due to obesity
Sleep apnoea		Increased risk of anaesthesia complications
		Fetal defects associated with maternal obesity

* All relative risk values are approximate;

[†] quantitative data in relation to different degrees of excess weight were available for these conditions which allowed them to be used in the assessment of the Millennium analyses of the global burden of disease. WHO Technical Report Series 894 (2000).

The medical and other costs of excess weight

There have been many estimates of the economic costs of obesity conducted by academic and government groups based on the direct costs of medical treatment of obesity and on the proportion of the other diseases, e.g. diabetes and hypertension which can theoretically be attributed to excess weight. A simpler scheme is shown in Fig. 9.5.5 where the observed medical costs of individuals was monitored on an annual basis as part of an assessment of the different annual medical costs at different extreme levels of obesity in the United States (Arterburn *et al.* 2005). It is clear that the least medical costs are incurred by individuals with BMIs within the normal range and that there is then a modest but steady increase in the costs at greater BMIs. If, however, the prevalences of these different groups is considered then the greatest absolute costs are incurred in the modest overweight group because this represents such a large proportion of the population.

The principal risk factors which affect both premature mortality and disability considered together as DALYs can then be assessed from data on mortality and national statistics for the prevalence of different medical conditions. Figure 9.5.6 provides the latest update on the dominance of different risk factors produced by the conjoint World Bank/WHO/CDC group in 2006 for the more affluent countries of the world (Lopez *et al.* 2006). By 2006, excess weight (calculated from the optimum of BMI 21) had climbed to the third most important factor and even if one includes all the poor countries

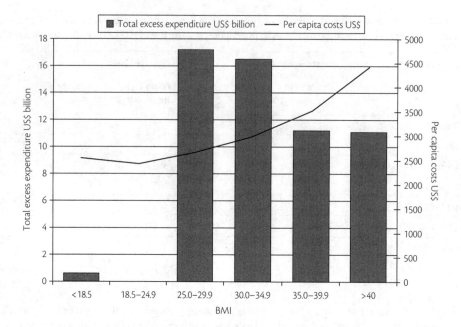

Fig. 9.5.4 The relationship between the annual costs per head of medical care in US adults and the estimated extra costs for the whole of each population group outside the normal weight range.

The curvilinear line reflects the increase in medical costs from about US$2500 per head per annum when at normal weight up to US$4500 for those with morbid obesity. The histograms then represent the impact of the different prevalences of the population within each BMI category on the total national cost in billions of US dollars for the BMI category within the population. Recalculated from data in Arterburn *et al.* (2005).

in analyses excess weight gain still comes out within the top 10 global risk factors. Further reappraisals are now being considered for the year 2010.

The estimations of the DALYs attributable to excess weight gain as conducted by WHO are sometimes considered unusual in that, as with blood pressure, total blood cholesterol, or any other risk factor, the challenge was to identify the optimum value to which the average population should ideally strive. For systolic blood pressure, the optimum value was estimated to be 115 mmHg, and for total blood cholesterol, 3.8 mmol/l. These values are very different from what one finds in clinical management guidelines, but illustrate the difference between pragmatic clinical judgements about what is possible on the basis of current management systems and what can be considered ideal from a public health perspective. So, the choice of BMI 21 as the optimum median population BMI was made in an analogous way.

Ethnic differences in susceptibility to chronic diseases on weight gain

Recently, Asian investigators have returned to this issue and considered with very large data sets whether the Asian community is really more susceptible to disease at different rates than Europids. This stems from the concern about the high prevalence of diabetes and hypertension at very modest increases in BMI. Figures 9.5.7a and b show that both type 2 diabetes and hypertension are markedly amplified by weight gain (Huxley *et al.* 2007). Similar relationships have been found in analyses of the Mexican national surveys which also showed that Mexicans as well as Asians are far more susceptible to increases in abdominal obesity at even normal BMIs than US non-Hispanic whites (Sanchez-Castillo *et al.* 2005).

While this ethnic difference is seen by most investigators as indicative of genetic factors, Barker and his colleagues suggested a

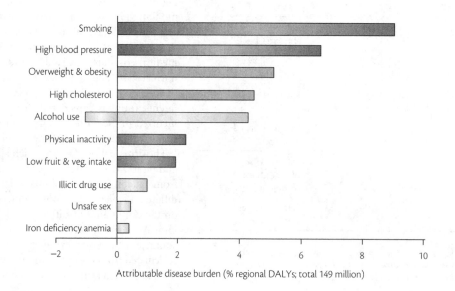

Fig. 9.5.5 The 2006 estimates of the relative importance of different risk factors contributing to the burden of diseases in high-income countries *Source:* Lopez *et al.* (2006).

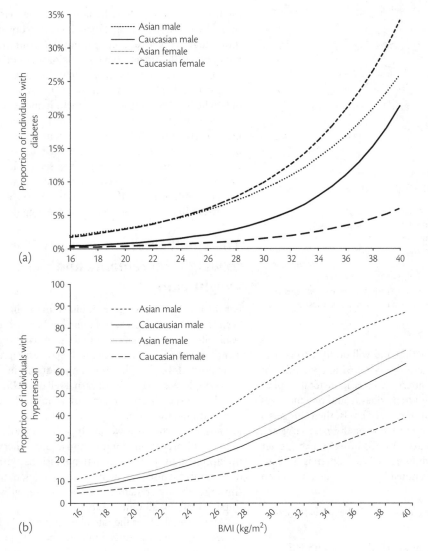

Fig. 9.5.6 The increased risk of (a) diabetes and (b) hypertension in Asian compared with Caucasian men and women in relation to their BMI. 7a) Diabetes 7b) Hypertension
Source: Huxley *et al.* (2007).

foetal nutrition hypothesis where environmental factors both in utero and early foetal life are of exceptional importance in amplifying the risk of abdominal obesity and the development of diabetes and hypertension and cardiovascular disease (Barker 2004). Thus, systematic analyses of the relationship between birth weight and the prevalence of adult hypertension have shown a clear inverse relationship between the two in the majority of more than 80 studies from all over the world, and this is very evident in children from both developed and developing countries (Law *et al.* 2001). New evidence suggests that even mental illness in adult life is perhaps amplified by events early in the life cycle through modulation of the stress and other responses to the programming of hypothalamic and other responses (Eero Kajantie *et al.* 2007). Although both diabetes and hypertension are amplified in adult life by increases in BMI the gradient of effect rather than the absolute differences may not be very different in differing societies. Therefore the amplification in the absolute but not relative risk in adult life of particular levels of BMI may well prove to be based on differences in foetal programming which in turn may be markedly affected by the mother's nutrition before and during pregnancy and subsequent changes in infantile and later childhood growth.

Projections of the obesity epidemic and its consequent morbidity and costs

Recently, the UK government in an unusual programme 'Foresight' has considered not only the basis of the epidemic but its likely evolution. They calculated costs on the basis of current trends, using national BMI data sets of high quality based on weights and heights measured by trained observers yearly over a 10-year period with 10 000–20 000 children and adults each year in England. These data provide the opportunity to project by non-linear regression analysis the changes in the distribution of BMI by age and sex in the years to come (Fig. 9.5.8) (McPherson *et al.* 2007). As in most countries, the progressive shift in the distribution of BMI seems to be unremitting; so, given the wealth of data and the proposed continued effects of the factors stimulating obesity, the future magnitude of the epidemic and its consequences and costs can be predicted with some confidence. The analyses also allow modelling to assess the potential value of different interventions, e.g. a selective approach to preventing obesity in different age groups.

Although the prevention of obesity on children is publicly and therefore politically appealing, it is not likely to bring rapid changes

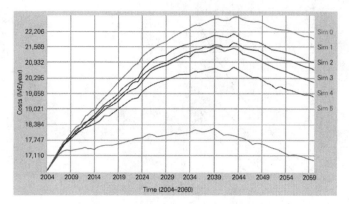

Fig. 9.5.7 The UK Foresight's modelling of the relative benefits in terms of the different effects of age related interventions for minimizing the impact of obesity related disease on the National Health costs in England.
Simulation 0 (top line): No interventions; and then simulations 1, 2, 3, and 4 reflect interventions where there were 1, 2, 4, and 8 BMI unit average reductions, respectively, achieved in the population aged 15–50 years only. Scenario 5 shows the comparison with scenario 4 but with all adults involved from ages 15 to 100 years. This highlights the importance of interventions in those >50 years.
Source: McPherson *et al.* (2007).

in the public health of the population and will do little to reduce the escalating health costs of the obesity-inducing epidemics of diabetes and hypertension now underway. Thus, if the total emphasis is put on the prevention of children's obesity and one manages to stop any further deterioration in obesity levels, then this has a negligible impact on the disease burden over the next 40 years, whereas intervention from 18 years onwards brings much greater benefits, Therefore, a focus on adults as well as children is particularly useful for several reasons, as noted by Seidel *et al.* (2005) and Gill (2002):

(a) The sharpest increase in the incidence of obesity is in (early) adulthood.

(b) Adults usually continue to gain weight during adulthood.

(c) Adult weight gain is almost always fat gain, except in athletes in training.

(d) The relative risks for many diseases associated with obesity decrease with age, but the absolute and population-attributable risks for disease increase with age.

(e) Interventions in children and adolescents need to be maintained for many more years or decades in order to have a considerable effect on the number of new cases of type 2 diabetes mellitus, heart disease, or cancer, compared with interventions in older individuals.

(f) Adults who are parents act as role models and have other responsibilities for the diet and physical activity behaviours of children.

These concepts have been reinforced by the UK's Foresight modelling (McPherson *et al.* 2007). Figure 9.5.8 shows that inducing such effective changes at the community level, so that the average BMI of the population is reduced by a whole 4 BMI units, produces a major and dramatic effect, but this has never been seen except perhaps in Cuba during their financial crisis when food deprivation was widespread throughout the country. Nevertheless, the remarkable differences in the medical burden and therefore

medical costs if substantial changes can be made in the population's BMI demonstrate that there is clearly considerable benefit for individuals as well as their employers, insurance companies, or national health budgets to have a major focus on adults.

Figure 9.5.8 also demonstrates that the focus should be on those most vulnerable to disease, which means, in practice, the >50 years olds. The logic would also be to include those below 50 years who can be considered most vulnerable to developing the disease, i.e. those with pre-diabetics or incipient hypertension. The development of diabetes is far more sensitive to weight change as one would expect than coronary heart disease. Given these different perspectives, one then needs to consider how to counteract the current epidemic and, if possible, to reverse it. This requires an understanding of the basis for the current epidemic.

The small errors in energy balance leading to weight increments and the persistence of weight gain

For the last 30 years or more, adults in many affluent societies have been trying to slim down, and there has been a huge increase in the availability of magazines, voluntary groups, and commercial slimming organizations, all aiming to help overweight adults return to their normal weight. The slimming industry in the United States, for example, is enormous and earns well over US$100 billion yearly. This huge expenditure is mainly by women who consider not only the health hazards of their excess weight, but the fact that they feel less attractive when overweight. It is likely that the marked increase in eating disorders with bulimia and anorexia nervosa has also been precipitated by these national obsessions with slimming. Yet, despite this intense and, in affluent societies, nation-wide effort to slim, the obesity epidemic becomes worse, with little sign of the impact of all this slimming effort.

When one calculates the rate of weight gain—which may amount to 0.5–1 kg per year in early adult life, this amounts to a yearly accumulation of about 3500–7000 kcal. This in turn means that, on average, the discrepancy between energy intake and energy expenditure is only in the range of 10–20 kcal/day—this now being called the 'energy gap'. The energy gap amounts to a discrepancy in energy balance of only about 0.4–0.8 per cent of normal food intake per day. This concept of only small changes in energy storage being responsible often leads to the idea that simple small measures—cutting down food a bit and going for a short walk daily—will stop this weight gain.

These small discrepancies actually show how remarkable the normal regulation of energy balance is. Thus, our expenditure in all activity may vary daily by 200–300 kcal, depending on how much walking or leisure time activity we undertake but the variation in food intake is much more marked and can vary easily by 1000 kcal/day. Hence, the discrepancies in energy balance with fat accumulation represent the residual effect of extremely complex neuro-hormonal regulatory mechanisms operating on a short-, medium-, and long-term basis to preserve energy balance. However, the mechanisms which avoid weight loss are multiple and much more robust than those that limit weight gain.

Physical inactivity

The obvious thermodynamic principles of energy balance require that one recognizes the influence of both dietary change and the reduction in physical activity. The collapse in the demand for physical exertion came with cheaper cars for personal transport and multiple mechanical and electrical aids to remove the physical demands in the home and at work. Then with the advent of computers and television it is now clear that in many affluent societies one can earn an excellent wage and have enjoyable leisure without any physical exertion at all.

The evidence for current trends in physical activity varies, but most affluent countries have noted relatively stable rates or slight declines in leisure time physical activity over recent decades (Brownson et al. 2005) and in general the rates of sedentariness, defined as an absence of leisure time physical activity (LTPA), have remained rather stable. Of more importance to total energy expenditure has been the decline in the other domains of physical activity. Thus, the number of people involved in heavy occupational physical activity has declined dramatically, with more than a 50 per cent reduction in 'heavy work' in Norwegian adults since the mid-1980s, this change being associated with increases in sedentary work (Anderssen et al. 2007). Other countries have noted marked increases in car usage and other motorized transport, at the expense of more active commuting through walking or cycling trips (Fox & Hillsdon 2007). One study even reported a 6 per cent increase in the risk of obesity for every hour spent commuting by car each day (Frank et al. 2004). Limited data are available on domestic settings, but with increases in technologically sophisticated labour-saving devices, and reduced time spent in preparing meals and carrying out household tasks (predominantly through increases in dual adult working households), it seems that energy expenditure on domestic tasks and yard/garden work is likely to have reduced as well (Brownson et al. 2005).

For some European countries, the increase in obesity was delayed by up to a decade, notably in the Netherlands and Scandinavian countries (IOTF slides 2007). This might have been due to high rates of active commuting, especially cycling, as nutritional differences are not apparent compared with several other Western European countries (UK Parliament Select Committee on Health Third Report 2007). A few countries have demonstrated increasing trends in LTPA. For example, Finland and Canada have shown increasing LTPA trends over 25 years, and Singapore over about 10 years (Barengo et al. 2006; Craig et al. 2004). These comparisons are reliable within-country, even if they are not comparable between countries, due to the different physical activity measures used (Craig et al. 2003). Yet, despite these increases in LTPA, all of these countries have observed increases in obesity rates that were similar to demographically matched countries which did not have increases in LTPA (Cutler et al. 2003; Borodulin et al. 2007; Belanger-Ducharme & Tremblay 2005). Thus, in Finnish adults, the rates of increase in obesity were marginally but not substantially faster among the inactive and in Norway (leisure time defined) active and inactive adults gained weight at roughly similar rates from 1990. Therefore, in spite of LTPA increases, the increasing obesity rates develop either because of the impact of increases in energy intake, or because of substantial reductions in energy expenditure for tasks during the normal non-leisure times of day.

Evidence for the transformation of our diets is easier to document but the mistake made by doctors, scientists, and policy makers is to assume that we can measure the diet with sufficient accuracy to discern an energy imbalance of 10–20 kcal/day, i.e. <1 per cent of normal daily intake and expenditure. Whatever the interplay of changes in intake and energy expenditure under the usual environmental conditions before 1980, children and adults on average were able to maintain their energy balance unless they became ill and anorexic. At that time, it also seems clear that there was sufficient demand for physical work both in the home and in the usual range of occupations for people's appetite regulatory centres to be repeatedly operating to ensure that sufficient food was eaten to satisfy energy needs.

It now seems clear that, with the removal of the need for physical activity to earn one's living, the prevailing pressure on most people's brain regulatory systems has been to attempt to limit intake. It seems reasonable to accept that we have already moved away from the fabled large meals of our ancestors. Indeed, within our lifetime in relatively sophisticated environments, the meals and portions served in restaurants—at least in Europe—have become smaller, because that is what consumers seem to want. Thus, data from national food surveys in the United Kingdom showed a progressive fall in consumption even when allowances were made for the greater amount of food now eaten outside the home. Similarly, there are many people now who do not bother with breakfast, and this may well be a behavioural adaptation to a brain system which is trying to stop us eating so much. However, there have been remarkable changes in the normal food systems with an ever-increasing tendency to eat outside the home and to buy rather than make at home the range of meals which busy women and men still wish to consume. This means that populations have become far more dependent on manufactured processed foods and on decisions based on information about the nature of the purchased food.

The biological as well as societal maintenance of obesity

Unfortunately, in addition to these social issues there is now very good evidence that, as weight gain occurs, particularly in older adults, there is a 'resetting' of the regulatory system, so that weight loss is resisted. As weight gain occurs, this extra weight includes 25 per cent lean tissues which once laid down require additional daily energy for their maintenance. Thus, people's weight should plateau as soon as their increased weight compensates for the small discrepancy in intake. Unfortunately, this is not as effective as we would wish because weight gain usually continues and slowly the neuroregulatory systems progressively adjust as though they prefer to maintain the excess weight. The adaptation is progressive so that in due course the additional 10 kg extra weight then demands a permanent extra daily intake of 200–300 kcal/day. This adaptive mechanisms does not occur after the acutely overfeeding of young adults because they spontaneously return after the overfeeding stops to their previous body weights but this is not seen when older adults are acutely overfed (Roberts et al. 1994; Roberts & Rosenberg 2006).

Putting overweight and obese individuals on a slimming diet then immediately leads to the switching on of acute hormonal, hypothalamic regulated responses involving both the thyroidal axis and the autonomic nervous system which simulate the response to semi-starvation within 2–4 days even though the obese may have 0.25–1 million extra kcal stored. The brain mechanism which increases the drive to eat is also activated immediately.

A reflection of this persistent adaptive change in the brain of obese people is that most slimming overweight individuals readily regain the weight which they have taken so much trouble to lose. Those who are successful in maintaining their weight loss find that

Table 9.5.9 The contributors to the development of obesity as set out by WHO and categorized by the level of evidence for each contributor

Evidence	Decreases risk	No relationship	Increases risk
Convincing	Regular physical activity High-dietary NSP (fibre) intake		High intake of energy-dense nutrient-poor foods Sedentary lifestyles
Probable	Home and school environments that support healthy food choices for children** Promoting linear growth Breastfeeding		Heavy marketing of energy-dense foods** and fast-food outlets Adverse social and economic conditions (in developed countries, especially for women) Sugar-sweetened soft drinks and fruit juices
Possible	Low-glycaemic index foods	Protein content of the diet	Large portion sizes High proportion of food prepared outside the home (Western countries) 'Rigid restraint/periodic disinhibition' eating patterns
Insufficient	Increasing eating frequency		Alcohol

** Associated evidence and expert opinion
Source: Table taken from Diet, Nutrition and the Prevention of Chronic Diseases, WHO 2003, TRS 916.

they have to obsessively monitor their food intake and purchasing habits and deliberately engage in 2000–3000 kcal per week exercise to avoid gaining weight (Wing 2004)! The individuals describe a continuous battle to maintain their normal weight, so on this basis it is far more likely that the biological adaptation observed experimentally contributes to and amplifies the continuing environmental pressures which in susceptible individuals promote weight regain. These adaptive problems therefore seem to explain why the obesity epidemic continues to increase despite the desire of so many adults to lose their excess weight. This indicates a need for prevention to become a very high priority.

An evaluation of all the principal factors contributing to the obesity epidemic was set out by WHO in an Expert Technical report (World Health Organization 2003) (Table 9.5.9), which became a politically sensitive document because it highlighted again the inappropriateness of the prevailing high sugar intakes which in the earlier WHO 797 report in 1990 had led to a sustained campaign by sugar organizations to pressure governments—particularly the United States—to negate its implications. Now, sugar intakes are being linked by WHO not only to the prevalence of dental caries but also to the development of obesity.

Preventive strategies: The options

The analyses already presented on the impact of changes in population BMIs at different ages have emphasized the importance of tackling not just obesity but also overweight. The strategies may initially be considered on the basis of rectifying the major societal forces which currently promote the epidemic. The multiplicity of factors promoting the epidemic is dramatically revealed in the UK Foresight exercise. The specific factors with seemingly the greatest impact were highlighted, and it then became clear that in terms of both physical activity and the intake of energy there are very powerful forces that the individual does not control. This analysis led to the United Kingdom's designation of obesity as a 'passive' normal response of humans to the prevailing inappropriate environment.

This then means that those who successfully remain lean throughout life are either genetically fortunate or they have the advantage in educative, social or financial terms to withstand the environmental forces and often create for themselves what is in effect a healthy 'microenvironment'.

The UK Foresight assessment of the key processes which contribute to the development of the epidemic cannot be used to simply specify that abolishing or reversing these forces will lead to useful prevention strategies. Thus, the introduction of the car, mechanical aids, the computerization of so many processes, and the advent of Internet-related communications have all contributed substantially to reducing the need of each of us to engage in physical activity by perhaps 750–1000 kcal or more on a daily basis. Nevertheless, nobody would consider reversing these developments as a coherent public health strategy for combating obesity. Hence, the issue is how best to combine current understanding of: (a) the most effective initiatives on the basis of either coherent trials or on the basis of a suitable model backed by an understanding of the underlying processes; (b) the most cost-efficient initiatives; (c) the most feasible initiatives on the basis of the features of the country's societal organization, cultural perceptions, and political system; and (d) whether there are other policy initiatives in the areas affecting food and physical activity which need to be integrated or, if conflicting, resolved.

Age-related issues: Childhood prevention

It was evident from Fig. 9.5.8 that successful measures in middle aged and older adults are likely to have an impact on public health rapidly: Selectively focusing primarily on the prevention of childhood overweight and obesity had very little impact on the burden of ill health nationally for decades. The current focus on childhood overweight/obesity has been justified, however, on several grounds:

(a) Public health measures are seen to be immediately relevant, given the fact that neither the public nor most policy makers blame the individual child for their predicament, and only a few try to assign blame to their parents. Therefore, this childhood focus has a politically useful place in persuading the public and politicians to do something other than advocating treatment.

(b) It is readily recognized that in older children excess weight gain confers on the affected group a far higher medical burden in their life time and a much greater probability of an early death than if one simply is concerned about the middle aged and older person. So a successful strategy can have a substantial impact for the individual concerned.

(c) The focus on children also chimes with the routine mantra that the key to the problem of obesity is 'education' so clearly there is merit in educating the child so that they 'do not behave' like their parents.

(d) If one is to focus on a group in society then school aged children are a useful choice because one is guaranteed to be able to reach them in most societies through a school mediated initiative.

Childhood prevention initiatives

These have been reviewed by Lobstein (2008) and by Brown *et al.* (2007). Table 9.5.10 summarizes the different types of programme which have shown some success as judged by short-term studies. This approach has been helped by the fact that the impact on weight gain of changes in children's environment can be documented relatively easily given their normal rates of growth. Studies lasting only a year or two are therefore valuable but whether the benefits can then be considered to last remains uncertain.

Table 9.5.10 Interventions for the prevention of overweight and obesity in school children*

Weight outcomes

1. The evidence of effectiveness of multi-component school-based interventions is equivocal.

2. School-based physical activity interventions (physical activity promotion and reduced television viewing) may help children maintain a healthy weight.

3. There is limited evidence from one UK-based study to suggest interventions to reduce consumption of carbonated drinks containing sugar.

Diet and physical activity outcomes

4. There is a body of evidence to suggest that school-based multi-component interventions addressing various aspects of diet and/or activity in the school, including the school environment (a 'whole-school approach'), are effective in improving physical activity and dietary behaviour, at least while the intervention is in place.

5. There is a body of evidence to suggest that short-term and long-term school-based interventions to improve children's dietary intake may be effective, at least while the intervention is in place. This includes interventions aiming to increase fruit and vegetable intake, improve school lunches, and/or promote water consumption.

6. UK-based evidence suggests that school children with the lowest fruit and vegetable intake at baseline may benefit the most from school-based dietary interventions.

7. There is a body of evidence from multi-component interventions to suggest that short-term and long-term school-based, physical activity-focused interventions may be effective, at least while the intervention is in place.

* Source: Brown et al. (2007).

Approaches to prevention: Is there a logic to the chosen initiatives?

A simpler overview than the United Kingdom's Foresight collation of different options is presented in Fig. 9.5.9, where the IOTF prevention group (Kumanyika *et al.* 2002) highlighted the different environmental systems which affect the environmental impact on both the diet and physical activity. Then, Swinburn (Egger & Swinburn 1997) developed the ANGELO framework for working out how to consider the different aspects of implementation at the different levels of influence on physical activity and diet. This depended on defining the options both at the micro and macro levels in terms of four overall areas of action:

(a) *Physical* changes, e.g. in the design of the environment for physical activity involving play areas, safe pedestrian and cycling friendly streets, or in terms of diet which is affected by food availability in shops within easy reach of poor families

(b) *Economic*, which might involve incentives or taxes or other economic measures at either a local or national level

(c) *Political*, e.g. specifying the requirement for baby-friendly hospitals to promote breastfeeding

(d) *Sociocultural*, e.g. involving changes to the health promotion and other national or local programmes and the involvement of major cultural figures to change perceptions of what is reasonable

This ANGELO approach was then taken further by WHO Euro (Robertson *et al.* 2004) to ensure that this approach to nutritional issues was integrated with other policy areas. On the energy expenditure side of energy balance there is a clear concordance of the need to promote physical activity with the new demand for societal mechanisms to limit climate change where national transport systems, e.g. trains and the use of buses is given much higher priority than car use. This then automatically requires more routine walking by the general public. In terms of food, Table 9.5.11 illustrates how the different levels of action can be classified and then how to consider the role of a ministry of government in taking responsibility for these actions.

This approach now allows a logical analysis of the options but still does not necessarily provide a clear approach to the choice of preventive measures. Some appear on the basis of collated evidence from previous initiatives to be good options whereas others are much more of an unknown entity. Given this uncertainty one can then develop a scheme of integrated public health actions judged on the basis of the likely impact and then the risk involved in implementing the various initiatives (Hawe & Shiell 1996). This approach, as illustrated in Table 9.5.12, was then used by Gill *et al.* (2006) to establish a set of obesity prevention priorities for New South Wales, Australia.

Identifying the evidence for effective prevention strategies by systematic review, if based on the demand to demonstrate conclusively the coherence of evidence from community or group interventions over a 12-month period at least, is sparse as set out in a recent review (Hawkes *et al.* in press) for the World Cancer Research Fund. Table 9.5.13 shows the current perceptions based on physiological studies, observational studies and mechanistic evidence, and Table 9.5.10 provided the outcome of one (in school children) of the five reviews of interventions. This illustrates how limited the data are when the criteria are based on having several properly controlled and preferably randomized groups in the community. It is also important to recognize that randomized controlled trials assess

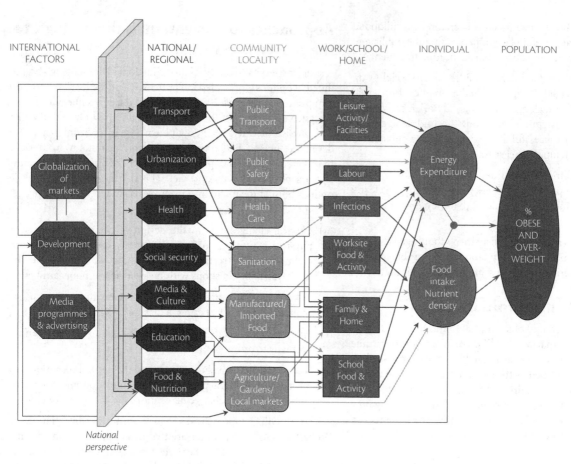

Fig. 9.5.8 Societal policies and processes influencing the population prevalence of obesity. *Source:* Modified from Kumanyika *et al.* (2002).

the efficacy of interventions but do not necessarily inform policy makers about their effectiveness when implemented on a wider public health basis. Even when this is undertaken, however, one still has to work out the cost effectiveness because initiatives, particularly at the grass roots level, can be very costly once one has taken into account all the checks and arrangements and training that are involved.

The State of Victoria, Australia, building on the NSW initiatives, undertook meticulous analyses of the costs having established a set of principles for determining effectiveness (Haby *et al.* 2006). Figure 9.5.10 shows the relative potential effectiveness of ten possible initiatives affecting school children in relation to the degree of uncertainty, and then Table 9.5.14 sets out the relative cost-effectiveness of these community-related initiatives in ranked order of cost-effectiveness (ACE Obesity 2006). The reason why TV advertising tops the list is because the options are calculated on the basis of the cost to the consumer or government and not to industry. Thus, restricting TV advertising has the benefit of modifying the input to practically all children because almost all watch TV—often for several hours a day. So, changes in the regulation, when implemented, will have an immediate potential impact on practically every child in most countries. Restricting access to the TV has also been shown to limit the development of obesity because it limits very sedentary behaviour during viewing time and the loss of the usual intense marketing of inappropriate foods may also play a role. This marketing has been shown to induce confusion about nutrition, alter attitudes favouring the advertised goods, change

purchasing practices in favour of the foods marketed and distort the children's diets (Hastings *et al.* 2003); the additional bonus of a government-directed ban on marketing is that the initiation of these measures simply requires a government regulation which then has to be followed. There is then no cost in terms of educating schools, parents, and children. This illustrates the fact that government intervention using conventional mechanisms for adjusting societal rules or habits usually automatically involve few direct costs. Thus, the more that can be undertaken by governmental processes which require industry or businesses or governmental workers to change their practices affecting food and activity, the lower the potential cost compared with individually related initiatives, e.g. involving health education or personal trainers or other focused and individually based advice to individual consumers.

Upstream measures for obesity prevention: The price, availability, and marketing of foods

In developing a food business, it is well recognized that, apart from producing a product that is attractive, there are three key features which determine their increasing turnover:

(a) The price of their product

(b) Its pervasive availability for consumers

(c) Intense marketing

Table 9.5.11 An illustration of the STEFANI (STrategies for Effective Food And Nutrition Initiatives) model developed by WHO (Euro) for action by (a) the Ministry of Health and (b) other ministries on diet

	Dietary quality; physical activity	Food safety	Environment
(A) Ministry of Health—direct responsibilities			
Physical	Appropriately accessible health centres Promoting access to appropriate self-monitoring, e.g. weight, BP	Catering in hospitals; monitoring facilities	Fluoridation systems for water Facilities for iodizing salt
Economic	Primary health payments for specific targets in management	Penalties for providing unsafe food	Subsidize iodine for iodination purposes
Policy	Baby-friendly hospitals Dietary guidelines establishing fortification policies Establish policies on health claims, e.g. functional foods	Health impact of multi-sectoral food safety policies	Establish specific guidelines for toxicants and contaminants in soil, water, and primary food products HIA of agrochemical use
Sociocultural	Health education	Promote concept of limited clinical antibiotic use	Promote new concept of health impact of new traffic policy
(B) Other ministries—specified on a national basis			
Physical	Ensuring playgrounds in schools, suitable cycling and road systems; urban planning; sports facilities. Designated urban areas for local food production	Provision of appropriate local abattoirs. Proper public toilet and sanitary facilities. Proper catering facilities based on stringent hygiene requirements	Urban planning: Green spaces, cycle paths, parks, playgrounds, lead free Establish facilities for farmers' markets
Economic	Re-evaluate taxation and subsidy policies	Establish appropriate penalties for inappropriate hygiene	Reform CAP. Finance new public transport systems. Promote urban agriculture, new outlets for high-quality, affordable foods in deprived areas
Policy	HIA of CAP Food labelling with appropriate, understandable health-related information	Establish criteria for ensuring pathogen- and contaminant-free access to the food chain. Establish systematic HACCP for food chain, systematic surveillance, and mechanisms for emergency response	Reform CAP Develop soil improvement, clean water, agricultural recycling, planting, fertilizer, pesticide, water use policies
Sociocultural	Promote physical activity in the workplace. Create breastfeeding time and space in the workplace with NGO help	Establish new criteria for excluding antibiotics as growth promoters and specifying veterinary use Educational initiatives for safety of fast-food outlets, and modifying nutrient composition, and limiting and ensuring appropriate food waste disposal	Change attitudes to cycle path use, pedestrian areas. Educational initiatives for caterers, communal use of school recreational facilities

Source: Taken from the WHO Euro report Robertson *et al.* (2004) and inspired by the ANGELO model Egger and Swinburn (1997).

Table 9.5.12. A planning approach to developing a portfolio of public health options: weighing up potential gains and risks

Increasing returns/health gains		
Very high gain—low uncertainty *Not found*	High gain—moderate uncertainty *1. Very promising*	High gain—high uncertainty *3. Promising*
Moderate gains—low uncertainty *Not found*	Moderate gain—moderate uncertainty *2. Promising*	Moderate gains—high uncertainty *4. Some promise*
Low gain—low uncertainty *Treatment options*	Low gain—moderate uncertainty *Inappropriate*	Low gain—high uncertainty *Inappropriate*
	Increasing uncertainty or risk	

Source: Hawe & Sheill (1996) by Gill *et al.* (2007).

Table 9.5.13 Components of diet and physical activity deemed to be important determinants of overweight and obesity based only on observational and mechanistic evidence

Evidence	Decreases risk of overweight and obesity	Increases risk of overweight and obesity
Convincing	Increased* total physical activity	
Probable	Breastfeeding (in terms of preventing obesity in child from 5 years of age); diets rich in low energy-dense foods (wholegrain cereals and cereal products; foods rich in non-starch polysaccharides and dietary fibre)	Frequent large portions of energy-dense foods; sugary drinks

*Increased over time, rather than simply 'high'.
Source: Brown *et al.* (2007).

These three factors—price, availability, and marketing—have also been repeatedly shown to be important in the public health initiatives for the effective limiting of smoking and alcohol consumption. The same clearly now applies to the issue of obesity because even children respond to cheaper options by purchasing more; e.g. of fruit in a school setting (French *et al.* 2001). It is also clear that the cost of foods in a Western environment is inversely related to the nutritional quality of the product; the greater the energy density of the food, i.e. in terms of kcal/g, the cheaper it is (Drewnowski & Specter 2004; Maillot *et al.* 2007).

The cost of foods in Western environments has been changing steadily over the last four to five decades as a result of government policies which were set out after World War II. The aim was to promote the production and consumption of ever cheaper meat, milk, butter, fats, and oils, as there was widespread disruption of food supplies during World War II, which rapidly became national

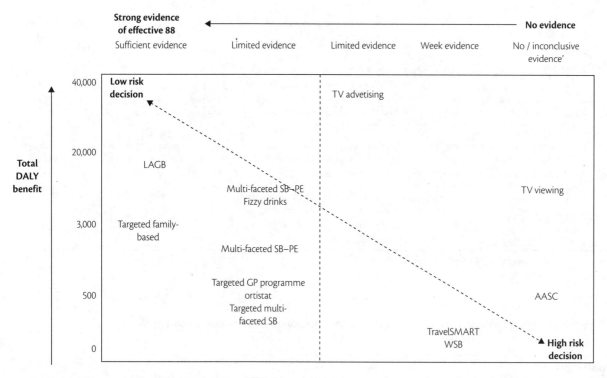

Fig. 9.5.9 The evaluation of different initiatives to prevent childhood obesity
The area to the left of the vertical dotted line signifies stronger evidence i.e. sufficient evidence or limited evidence that is unlikely to be due to chance. To the right of the line there is limited evidence of effectiveness but theoretical reasons why the intervention should work (Haby *et al.* 2006).
AASC—Active After School Communities programme
GP—General practitioner
LAGB—Laparoscopic adjustable gastric banding
PE—Active physical education
SB—School-based
WSB—Walking school bus

Table 9.5.14 Differences in estimated cost-effectiveness from different initiatives in the prevention of obesity in children in the state of Victoria, Australia

Intervention	Cost in AU$ for each DALY saved
Restrict TV advertising	4
Soft drink education intervention at school	3000
School education to reduce TV viewing	3000
School programme targeting overweight and obese children	3000
Family-based programme for the obese child	4000
Add physical education	7000
Gastric banding for severely obese adolescents	10 000
School multiple interventions, but no physical education	14 000
Medical treatment with drugs, e.g. orlistat	14 000
Doctors targeting the overweight children	32 000
After-school community programmes	90 000
Cycling (Travel SMART Schools)	260 000
Walking buses to school	770 000

Victoria State analyses announced by the Minister of Health, Australia, September 2006. *Source*: ACE Obesity (2006).

security issues. This led to a pervasive system of agriculture support involving direct grants, subsidies, free research and advisory services, guaranteed prices for food purchased by marketing boards for several decades, and continuing EU and US export subsidies (Elinder 2005; Shoonover & Muller 2006). It is not surprising therefore that there has been a remarkable transformation of food costs which have made fruits and vegetables more expensive in relative terms and fats, meat, sugars, and oils much cheaper. The poorer sections of the community in responding to their biological desire to satisfy their intrinsic energy needs purchase the cheapest products which are therefore richer in fat and sugars. This practice then tends to lead to 'passive over-consumption' because of the relatively poor satiety effects of fats and sugars—the latter particularly when provided in soft drinks between meals. The purchasing patterns of the poorer sections of society are much more price-sensitive; they are spending a much higher proportion of household income on food and normally attempt to minimize these costs to allow more flexibility for purchasing other household needs.

These economic constraints require an integrated approach before satisfactory dietary changes can be supported. Putting a higher price on fat- and sugar-rich foods will be a regressive measure, i.e. poorer households will pay more as with taxes on tobacco and alcohol. An integrated economic package needs to be developed, so that the poorer section of society obtains more financial support by other means. Then the alteration of relative food prices still induces changes, particularly in the poorer sections of the community. If the appropriate foods are then also made more readily available, the poorer sections of the community will respond.

Thus, in Finland, the vegetables provided with main meals at canteens and restaurants are included in the general price of the main meal. Thus, the poorer sectors of the community particularly benefited, and the combined public health measures in Finland led to a trebling in the average vegetable intake of the population over a 15-year period. In parallel with these changes, there was a marked reduction in the prevalence of hypertension and a progressive fall in cardiovascular diseases. Such practical measures at a community level will probably need reinforcing by changes in policies affecting the whole food chain from food labelling with appropriate instantly understandable symbols such as the traffic light labelling scheme proposed by the UK Food Standards Agency through to more complex arrangements affecting agricultural policies. These more upstream measures are only now being considered, but post-World War II policies relating to agriculture and other food policies, e.g. for school food, appear to have had marked and deleterious effects on public health over the last half century.

References

ACE Obesity (2006) Assessing the cost effectiveness of obesity interventions in children and adolescents. Summary of results. Published by the Victorian Government Department of Human Services Melbourne, Victoria 2006. www.health.vic.gov.au

Adams, K.F., Schatzkin, A., Harris, T.B., et al. (2006) Overweight, obesity, and mortality in a large prospective cohort of persons 50 to 71 years old. *New England Journal of Medicine*, **355**, 763–78.

Anderssen, S.A., Engeland, A., Sogaard, A.J., et al. (2007) Changes in physical activity behaviour and the development of body mass index during the last 30 years in Norway. *Scandinavian Journal of Public Health*, 1–9.

Arterburn, D.E., Maciejewski, M.L., Tsevat, J. (2005) Impact of morbid obesity on medical expenditures in adults. *International Journal of Obesity*, **29**, 334–9.

Asia Pacific Cohort Studies Collaboration (2004) Body mass index and cardiovascular disease in the Asia-Pacific Region: an overview of 33 cohorts involving 310 000 participants. *International Journal of Epidemiology*, **33**, 751–8.

Barengo, N.C., Nissinen, A., Pekkarinen, H., et al. (2006) Twenty-five-year trends in lifestyle and socioeconomic characteristics in Eastern Finland. *Scandinavian Journal of Public Health*, **34**, 437–44.

Barker, D.J. (2004) The developmental origins of well-being. *Phil Trans R Soc Lond B*, **359**, 1359–66.

Barlow, S.E., Dietz, W.H. (1998) Obesity evaluation and treatment: Expert committee recommendations. *Pediatrics*, **102**, 1–11.

Batty, G.D., Shipley, M.J., Jarrett, R.J., et al. (2006) Obesity and overweight in relation to disease-specific mortality in men with and without existing coronary heart disease in London: the original Whitehall study. *Heart*, **92**, 886–92.

Belanger-Ducharme, F., Tremblay, A. (2005) Prevalence of obesity in Canada. *Obesity Reviews*, **6**, 183–6.

Borodulin, K., Makinen, T., Fogelholm, M., et al. (2007) Trends and socioeconomic differences in overweight among physically active and inactive Finns in 1978–2002. Preventive Medicine, **45**, 157–62.

Brown, T., Kelly, S., Summerbell, C. (2007) Prevention of obesity: a review of interventions. *Obesity Reviews*, **8** (supp1), 127–30.

Brownson, R.C., Boehmer, T.K., Luke, D.A. (2005) Declining rates of physical activity in the United States: what are the contributors? *Annual Review of Public Health*, **26**, 421–43.

Cole, T.J., Green, P.J. (1992) Smoothing reference centile curves: the LMS method and penalized likelihood. *Statistics in Medicine*, **11**, 1305–19.

Cole, T.J., Bellizzi, M.C., Flegal, K.M., *et al.* (2000) Establishing a standard definition for child overweight and obesity worldwide: international survey. *British Medical Journal*, **320**, 1240–3.

Craig, C.L, Marshall, A.L., Sjostrom, M., *et al.* (2003) International Physical Activity Questionnaire: 12-country reliability and validity. *Medicine & Science in Sports & Exercise*, **35**, 1381–95.

Craig, C.L., Russell, S.J., Cameron, C., *et al.* (2004) Twenty–Year Trends in Physical Activity among Canadian Adults. *Canadian Journal of Public Health*, **95**, 59–63.

Cutler, D., Glaeser, E., Shapiro, J. (2003) Why have Americans become more obese?, *Journal of Economic Perspectives*, **17**, 93–118.

Dietz, W.H., Bellizzi, M.C. (1999) Assessment of childhood and adolescent obesity. *American Journal Clinical Nutrition*, **70**(suppl), 117–175S.

Drewnowski, A., Specter, S.E. (2004) Poverty and obesity: the role of energy density and energy costs. *American Journal of Clinical Nutrition*, **79**, 6–16.

Eero Kajantie, F., Feldt, K., Räikkönen, K., *et al.* (2007) Body size at birth predicts hypothalamic-pituitary-adrenal axis response to psychosocial stress at age 60 to 70 years. *Journal of Clinical Endocrinology and Metabolism.*, **92**, 4094–100. Epub 2007 Sep 11.

Egger, G., Swinburn, B. (1997) An "ecological" approach to the obesity pandemic. *British Medical Journal*, **315**, 477–80.

Elinder, L.S. (2005) Obesity, hunger and agriculture: the damaging role of subsidies. *British Medical Journal*, **331**, 1333–6.

Ezzati M., Hoorn S.V., Lawes C.M.M., *et al.* (2005) Rethinking the "diseases of affluence" paradigm: Economic development and global patterns of nutritional risks obesity and other cardiovascular risk factors 2005 in relation to economic development. *PLoS Medicine*, **2**, 0404–0412.

Flegal, K.M., Graubard, B.I., Williamson, D.F., *et al.* (2007) Cause-specific excess deaths associated with underweight, overweight, and obesity. *JAMA*, **298**, 2028–37.

Fox, K.R., Hillsdon, M. (2007) Physical activity and obesity. *Obesity Review*, **8**(S1), 115–21.

Frank, L.D., Andresen, M.A., Schmid, T.L. (2004) Obesity relationships with community design, physical activity, and time spent in cars. *American Journal of Preventive Medicine*, **27**, 87–96.

French, S.A., Story, M., Jeffery, R.W. (2001) Environmental influences on eating and physical activity. *Annual Review of Public Health*, **22**, 309–35.

Garrow, J.S. (1981) *Treat Obesity Seriously. A Clinical Manual.* Churchill Livingstone, New York.

Gill, T. (2002) The importance of preventing weight gain in adulthood. *Asia Pacific*, **11**(suppl), S632–6.

Gill, T., King, L., Webb, K. (2006) Best options for promoting healthy weight and preventing weight gain in NSW. NSW Dept of Health at www.health.nsw.gov.au

Greenberg, J.A. (2006) Correcting biases in estimates of mortality attributable to obesity 1. *Obesity*, **14**, 2071–9.

Guillaume, M. (1999) Defining obesity in childhood: current practice. *American Journal of Clinical Nutrition*, **70**(suppl), 126–30S.

Guo, S.S., Chumlea, W.C. (1999) Tracking of body mass index in children in relation to overweight in adulthood. *American Journal of Clinical Nutrition*, **70**, 145–148S.

Haby, M.M., Vos, T., Carter, R., *et al.* (2006) A new approach to assessing the health benefit from obesity interventions in children and adolescents: the assessing cost-effectiveness in obesity project. *International Journal of Obesity*, **30**, 1463–75.

Hastings, G., Stead, M., McDermott, L., *et al.* Review of research on the effects of food promotion to children. Final report prepared for the Food Standards Agency, 2003. http://www.food.gov.uk/multimedia/pdfs/foodpromotiontochildren1.pd

Hawe, P., Shiell, A. (1996) Preserving innovation under increasing accountability pressures. The health promotion investment portfolio approach. *Health Promotion Journal of Australia*, 5, 4–9.

Hawkes, C., Asfaw, A., Bauman, A., *et al.* Evidence on the determinants of dietary patterns, nutrition and physical activity, and the interventions to maintain or to modify them: A systematic review. WCRF (in press).

Huxley, R., James, W.P.T., Barzi, F., *et al.* on behalf of the Obesity in Asia Collaboration Ethnic comparisons of the cross-sectional relationships between measures of body size with diabetes and hypertension (2007) In James W.P.T. and Chen C.M. Obesity in China. *Obesity Reviews* (in press).

IOTF slides: Trends in obesity (Europe) http://www.iotf.org/database/TrendsinObesityPrevalence.htm [accessed July 2007].

James, W.P.T, Ferro-Luzzi, A., Waterlow, J.C. (1988) Definition of chronic energy deficiency in adults. Report of a Working Party of the International Dietary Energy Consultative Group. *European Journal of Clinical Nutrition*, **42**, 969–81.

James, W.P.T. (1976) (Compiler) *Research on Obesity.* A Report of the DHSS/MRC Group. H.M.S.O, London.

James, W.P.T. (1976) *Research on Obesity.* A Report of the DHSS/MRC Group. Compiled by James WPT, HMSO, London.

James, W.P.T. (2005) Assessing obesity: are ethnic differences in body mass index and waist classification criteria justified? *Obesity Reviews.*, **6**, 179–81.

James, W.P.T., Jackson-Leach, R., Ni Mhurchu, C., *et al.* (2004) Overweight and obesity (high body mass index). In: Ezzati M., Lopez A.D., Rodgers A., Murray C.J.L. (eds.) *Comparative Quantification of Health Risks. Global and Regional Burden of Disease Attributable to Selected Major Risk Factors*, Chapter 8, Volume 1. World Health Organization, Geneva.

Kumanyika, S., Jeffery, R.W., Morabia, A., *et al.* (2002) Public Health Approaches to the Prevention of Obesity (PHAPO) Working Group of the International Obesity Task Force (IOTF). Obesity prevention: the case for action. *International Journal of Obesity*, 26, 425–36.

Law, C.M., Egger, P., Dada, O., *et al.* (2001) Body size at birth and blood pressure among children in developing countries. *International Journal of Epidemiology.*, **30**, 52–7.

Lobstein T. (2008) The prevention of obesity in childhood and adolescence. In: Bray G.A., Bouchard C. (eds.) *Handbook of Obesity: Clinical Applications.* 3rd Edition. Informa Healthcare, New York, p. 131–156.

Lopez, A.D., Mathers, C.D., Ezzati, M., *et al.* (eds.) (2006) *Global Burden of Disease and Risk Factors.* New York: Oxford University Press.

Maillot, M., Darmon, N., Vieux, F., *et al.* (2007) Low energy density and high nutritional quality are each associated with higher diet costs in French adults. *American Journal of Clinical Nutrition*, 2007, **86**, 690–6.

McPherson, K., Marsh, T., Brown, M. (2007) Foresight. Tackling Obesities: Future choices – modelling future trends in obesity and the impact on health. www.foresight.gov.uk

Must, A., Dallal, G.E., Dietz, W.H. (1991) Reference data for obesity: 85th and 95th percentiles of body mass index (wt/ht2) and triceps skinfold thickness. *American Journal of Clinical Nutrition*, **53**, 839–46.

National Institutes of Health 1998: Clinical Guidelines on the Identification, Evaluation and Treatment of Overweight and Obesity in Adults: the Evidence Report. US Department of Health & Human Services, National Institutes of Health, National Heart, Lung and Blood Institute, USA.

Parsons, T.J., Power, C., Logan, S., *et al.* (1999) Childhood predictors of adult obesity: a systematic review. *International Journal of Obesity*, **23** (Suppl), S1–107.

Popkin, B.M. (2006) Global nutrition dynamics: the world is shifting rapidly toward a diet linked with noncommunicable diseases. *American Journal of Clinical Nutrition*, **84**, 289–98.

Power, C., Lake, J.K., Cole, T.J. (1997) Measurement and long-term health risks of child and adolescent fatness. *International Journal of Obesity*, **21**, 507–26.

Reilly, J.J., Dorosty, A.R., Emmett, P.M. and the ALSPAC Study Team (2000) Identification of the obese child: adequacy of the body mass index for clinical practice and epidemiology. *International Journal of Obesity*, **24**, 1623–7.

Roberts, S.B., Rosenberg, I. (2006) Nutrition and aging: changes in the regulation of energy metabolism with aging. *Physiological Review*, **86**, 651–67.

Roberts, S.B., Fuss, P., Heyman, M.B., *et al.* (1994) Control of food intake in older men. *JAMA*, **272**, 1601–6. Erratum in: *JAMA*, **273**, 702.

Robertson, A., Tirado, C., Lobstein, T., *et al.* Food and Health in Europe: a new basis of action. WHO 2004, European Series No 96.

Rolland-Cachera, M.F., Deheeger, M., Guilloud-Bataille, M., *et al.* (1987) Tracking the development of adiposity from one month of age to adulthood. *Annals of Human Biology*, **14**, 219–29.

Rose, G. (1991) Population distributions of risk and disease. *Nutrition Metabolism and Cardiovascular Diseases*, **1**, 37–40.

Royal College of Physicians (1983) Obesity – A Report of the Royal college of Physicians. *Journal of the Royal College of Physicians of London*, **17**.

Sanchez-Castillo, C.P., Velasquez-Monroy O., Lara-Esqueda A., *et al.* (2005) Diabetes and hypertension increases in a society with abdominal obesity: results of the Mexican National Health Survey 2000. *Public Health Nutrition.*, **8**, 53–60.

Seidell, J.C., Nooyens, A.J., Visscher, T.L.S. (2005) Cost-effective measures to prevent obesity: epidemiological basis and appropriate target groups. *Proceedings of the Nutrition Society*, **64**, 1–5.

Shoonover, H., Muller, M. (2006) Food without thought. How US food policy contributes to obesity. Institute for Agriculture and Trade Policy. Minneapolis, USA

UK Food Standards Agency. Signposting labelling scheme. http://www.food.gov.uk/foodlabelling/signposting

UK Parliament Select Committee on Health Third Report 2006–2007. http://www.publications.parliament.uk/pa/cm200304/cmselect/cmhealth/23/2306.htm. Accessed June 2007:. n 307, Sections 305–309

Wang, Y., Lobstein, T. (2006) Worldwide trends in childhood overweight and obesity. *International Journal of Pediatric Obesity*, **1**, 11–25.

WHO Child Growth Standards. WHO, Geneva, 2007.

WHO Expert Consultation (2004) Appropriate body-mass index for Asian populations and its implications for policy and intervention strategies. *Lancet*, **363**, 157–63.

WHO/IASO/IOTF (2000) The Asia-Pacific perspective: redefining obesity and its treatment. February 2000. Health Communications, Australia PTY Ltd. Full document available from: http://www.idi.org.au/obesity_report.htm

Wing, R.R. (2004) Behavioural approaches to the treatment of obesity. In *Handbook of Obesity. Clinical Applications.* (ed Bray, G.A. and Bouchard, C. 2nd Edition), Marcel Dekker, New York. pp. 147–67.

World Health Organization (WHO) (1995) *Physical Status: The Use and Interpretation of Anthropometry.* Tech. Rep. Series 854.

World Health Organization. (2000) *Obesity: Preventing and Managing the Global Epidemic.* WHO Technical Report Series No. 894. WHO, Geneva.

World Health Organization. *Diet, Nutrition and the Prevention of Chronic Diseases.* Report of a Joint WHO/FAO Expert Consultation. WHO Technical Report Series No. 916. World Health Organization, Geneva, 2003.

Yusuf, S., Hawken, S., Ôunpuu, S., *et al.* on behalf of the INTERHEART Study Investigators (2005) Obesity and the risk of myocardial infarction in 27 000 participants from 52 countries: a case-control study. *Lancet*, **366**, 1640–49.

The epidemiology and prevention of diabetes mellitus

Nigel Unwin and Paul Zimmet

Abstract

Diabetes mellitus is a heterogeneous disease characterized by raised blood glucose. The current classification recognizes two main types: Type 1, due to destruction of the insulin-producing cells of the pancreas and typically requiring exogenous insulin for survival; and type 2, representing 85–95 per cent of all diabetes, and due to a combination of resistance to the action of insulin and diminished insulin production. Currently, around 250 million people worldwide have diabetes, 6 per cent of the adult population, and this figure will increase markedly over the coming years as populations age and become increasingly overweight and sedentary, the major risk factors for type 2 diabetes. Contrary to popular perception over 70 per cent of people with diabetes live in low- or middle-income countries, and most new cases of diabetes over the coming decades will be in such countries. Diabetes reduces life expectancy by around 15 years in type 1 diabetes and 10 years in type 2 and in many populations is the major cause of lower limb amputation, visual loss and renal failure. It is a major source of expenditure in health systems the world over and also impacts upon economic productivity. It was recently estimated that in 2007 diabetes cost India 2.1 per cent of its gross domestic product. Prevention, or at least delayed onset, of type 2 diabetes through behavioural or pharmacological measures has been convincingly demonstrated in several trials. At best these trials were able to achieve a 60 per cent reduction in incidence. The prevention of type 1 diabetes remains the subject of research. Nonetheless, a substantial reduction in the incidence of complications in people with diabetes is possible, including reductions in cardiovascular disease events, visual loss, lower limb amputation and renal failure. However, achieving these reductions requires well organized and resourced health care, and good education and support to people with diabetes in managing their condition. Diabetes is one of the major public health challenges of the twenty-first century, a fact recognized in 2006 by a United Nations resolution.

Definition, classification, and diagnosis

Diabetes is a metabolic disease characterized by hyperglycaemia (raised blood glucose) resulting from defects in insulin secretion, insulin action, or both (American Diabetes Association 2004). Insulin, produced by the beta cells of the pancreatic islets of Langerhans, is the main hormone regulating blood glucose levels, and is released in response to rising blood glucose following eating or drinking. Insulin has wide-ranging metabolic effects, which include the stimulation of glucose uptake into skeletal muscle and liver, and key roles in lipid and protein metabolism.

Prior to the late 1970s, there was little consistency in the classification of, or diagnostic criteria for, diabetes. In the mid-1930s, Himsworth (1936) had proposed that there were at least two clinical types of diabetes, insulin-sensitive and insulin-insensitive, the former being due to insulin deficiency. Confirmation of his clinical observations came with Bornstein's development of a bioassay for insulin (Bornstein & Lawrence 1951). The Nobel Prize-winning discovery of a radioimmunoassay for insulin a decade later saw the confirmation of Bornstein's observations (Berson & Yalow 1963). The widespread acceptance of the terms *juvenile-onset* and *maturity-onset* diabetes at this time was affirmation of the concept that there were at least two major forms of the disease.

However, since 1979 and 1980, the American Diabetes Association (ADA) and the World Health Organization (WHO), respectively, have produced a series of recommendations on both classification and diagnosis. These recommendations have changed over time to reflect the latest scientific evidence. There are small but important differences between the WHO and ADA recommendations. Most parts of the world tend to follow the recommendations of WHO, but those of the ADA are also followed in many places outside the United States. In the description that follows, we therefore focus on the recommendations of WHO (World Health Organization 1999, 2006) but in appropriate places describe how those of the ADA differ.

The classification of diabetes is based on current understandings of its underlying aetiology. There are two main types of diabetes. Type 1 diabetes results from destruction of the insulin-producing cells (beta cells) in the pancreas. This is usually, but not always, associated with detectable auto-antibodies to components of the beta cell. Type 2 diabetes, which accounts for 85–95 per cent of all diabetes, results from a combination of resistance to the action of insulin, particularly at skeletal muscle, liver, and fat tissue, and insufficient insulin production by the pancreas. There are several other rarer types of diabetes with specific aetiologies, such as maturity onset diabetes of the young, associated with specific single gene defects, and diabetes associated with toxicity to certain drugs. Gestational diabetes refers to diabetes that is diagnosed for the first time during pregnancy.

A classification of diabetes is shown in Fig. 9.6.1 (World Health Organization 2006). It is worth remembering that, as is the case for many conditions, our current understandings of the aetiologies of diabetes remain incomplete, and the classification described here may well change in the future. For example, distinction between type 1 and type 2 diabetes is not always clear cut. The term 'double diabetes' has recently been used to describe the situation in some children and adolescents in which insulin resistance, associated with obesity, is accompanied by auto-antibodies to the beta-cell (Pozzilli & Buzzetti 2007), although rather than 'double diabetes', it is also hypothesized type 1 and type 2 diabetes are the same disorder of insulin resistance, set against different genetic backgrounds (Wilkin 2001), with one background leading to autoimmune destruction of the beta cells of the pancreas and what is currently called type 1 diabetes.

In adults, diabetes which clinically appears to be type 2 diabetes may be accompanied by auto-antibodies to the beta cells and follow a relatively rapid course to insulin dependency. This type of diabetes has received various names, including latent autoimmune diabetes of adults (LADA) (Tuomi et al. 1993) and type 1.5 (Palmer & Hirsch 2003). If all this seems a bit confusing, it makes the point that a classification of diabetes based on aetiology is work in progress, while at the present time the categories of type 1 and type 2 remain useful and widely used.

For clinical practice, it is often useful to stage people with diabetes according to their requirements for insulin as follows:

- Insulin required for survival (virtually all of these will have type 1 diabetes)

- Insulin required for adequate metabolic control but not survival (most of these will have type 2 diabetes, but some will have type 1 diabetes in which there remain some functioning beta cells)

- Insulin not required, and treatment adequate without drugs or drugs other than insulin (the vast majority will have type 2 diabetes, but some may have type 1 diabetes before the beta cell destruction has advanced very far)

The relationships between the current aetiological classification and clinical stages of diabetes are shown in Fig. 9.6.1. The clinical staging includes a category called 'intermediate hyperglycaemia', in which blood glucose is considered above normal but below the diagnostic thresholds for diabetes. This category should not be considered as a clinical entity but rather as a risk category, identifying as it does, people at high risk of developing type 2 diabetes and cardiovascular disease, and providing a potential target for preventive interventions.

Diagnosis

The diagnosis of diabetes is based on blood glucose levels. Diagnostic thresholds, following current WHO recommendations (World Health Organization, 1996, 2006 are shown in Table 9.6.1. The 'gold standard' diagnostic test or reference method is the oral glucose tolerance test (OGTT). In brief, an OGTT involves the measurement of fasting glucose, followed by a drink containing a fixed quantity of glucose, and the measurement of blood glucose 2 hours after that drink. Undertaking an OGTT is time consuming and relatively expensive (compared to fasting glucose alone). Largely for these pragmatic reasons, the ADA recommends using fasting glucose alone as the main diagnostic test. Unfortunately, however, around one-third of individuals who have diabetes will have an abnormal result after an OGTT but fasting glucose below the diabetes threshold (Decode Study Group 1999). In other words, using fasting glucose alone misses about one-third of individuals with diabetes. Similarly, with fasting glucose, it is impossible to identify those who fall into the category of intermediate hyperglycaemia based on the post glucose challenge result (impaired glucose tolerance (IGT)), and as is discussed later much of the evidence on preventing type 2 diabetes is in individuals with IGT.

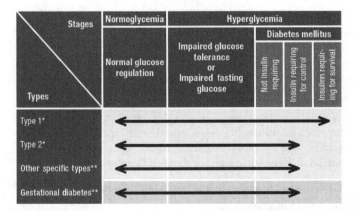

Fig. 9.6.1 The relationship between aetiological types of diabetes and clinical stages of hyperglycaemia.

* Even after presenting in an acute crisis, such as ketoacidosis, these patients can briefly return to normoglycaemia without requiring specific therapy

** In rare instances, patients in these categories (e.g. Vacor toxicity, type 1 diabetes presenting in pregnancy) may require insulin for survival.

Source: World Health Organization (2006).

Table 9.6.1 WHO criteria for the diagnosis of diabetes and intermediate hyperglycaemia

Diabetes	
Fasting plasma glucose	≥7 mmol/l (126 mg/dl) or
2-hour plasma glucose*	≥11.1 mmol/l (200 mg/dl)
Impaired glucose tolerance (IGT)	
Fasting plasma glucose	<7 mmol/l (126 mg/dl)
2-hour plasma glucose*	and
	≥7.8 and <11.1 mmol/l (140 mg/dl and 200 mg/dl)
Impaired fasting glucose (IFG)	
Fasting plasma glucose	6.1–6.9 mmol/l (110–125 mg/dl)
2-hour plasma glucose*	and (if measured) <7.8 mmol/l (140 mg/dl)

* Venous plasma glucose 2 hours after ingestion of 75 g oral glucose load (OGTT). If 2-hour plasma glucose is not measured, status is uncertain as diabetes or IGT cannot be excluded.

NB: The WHO criteria for gestational diabetes are diabetes (as defined above) or IGT.

Source: World Health Organization (2006).

There is also good evidence that the risk of cardiovascular disease associated with raised blood glucose is more strongly related to blood glucose after a glucose load than to fasting glucose (Decode Study Group 2001). It is for all these reasons that WHO continues to recommend using an OGTT as the main diagnostic test.

The thresholds for diabetes (Table 9.6.1) are based largely on epidemiological evidence that demonstrates an association between the diagnostic blood glucose levels and the presence of the typical small blood vessel complications of diabetes (e.g. diabetic retinopathy) (World Health Organization 2006). Because there is error in the measurement of blood glucose, and natural biological variation in its levels, the diagnosis of diabetes in someone without symptoms (such as polyuria and polydipsia) should only be made on the basis of two tests on separate occasions. In the presence of symptoms, the diagnosis of diabetes may be based on a casual (non-fasting, non OGTT) blood glucose level. It is worth noting that while the diagnostic cut points for diabetes are of necessity precisely defined (i.e. to the nearest tenth of a mmol per litre of glucose) different studies suggest somewhat different cut points often differing by at least one mmol per litre (Tapp et al. 2006).

The rationale for the cut points defining intermediate hyperglycaemia is less clear than that for those defining diabetes. Both fasting and 2 hours post challenge glucose are continuously related to the future risk of diabetes and cardiovascular disease—there is no evidence for thresholds and there is a strong argument for using the actual glucose value as part of a risk score for future diabetes or cardiovascular disease (Unwin et al. 2002; World Health Organization 2006). However, at present, this is not the case. The cut point for IGT is based on analyses published in the early 1980s on data from the Pima Indians on the risk of incident diabetes (Bennett et al. 1982). Impaired fasting glucose (IFG) was introduced in 1997 by the ADA (The Expert Committee on the Diagnosis and Classification of Diabetes Mellitus 1997), followed by WHO in 1999 (World Health Organization 1999). The cut point for IFG proposed in 1997, and still used by WHO, was based on physiological data of the level above which first phase insulin secretion is lost in response to intravenous glucose (The Expert Committee on the Diagnosis and Classification of Diabetes Mellitus 1997). However, in 2003, ADA recommended a lowering of the cut point for IFG, based partly on wishing to make the prevalence of IFG more similar to IGT and partly to improve the sensitivity of IFG as a predictor of future diabetes (American Diabetes Association 2004). WHO reviewed the classification of intermediate hyperglycaemia in 2006 and decided that the evidence was not strong enough to follow the ADA and lower the IFG cut point (World Health Organization 2006).

Incidence, prevalence, and trends

Both the WHO and the International Diabetes Federation (IDF) produce global estimates of the number of people with diabetes and how their numbers are expected to increase in the future (Wild et al. 2004; International Diabetes Federation 2006). These estimates are based on extrapolation from studies in which blood glucose was tested and thus include people with diagnosed and undiagnosed diabetes. This is important because in many populations more than half the people with diabetes (Harris 1993), sometimes as many as 80 or 90 per cent (Aspray et al. 2000), have not been diagnosed. The age specific prevalences of diabetes from these epidemiological studies are applied to United Nations population figures and

projections in order to give national, regional, and global estimates. The methodologies used by WHO and IDF are essentially the same, although relatively minor differences do exist in the criteria used to select the prevalence studies that are the basis of the estimates, and this leads to small differences in the estimated number of people with diabetes.

The most recent estimates are those of IDF, who estimate that in 2007 there were 246 million people globally with diabetes, 3.7 per cent of total global population, and that 5.9 per cent of the global adult population (age range 20–79 years) has diabetes. Figure 9.6.2 shows the prevalence of diabetes in adults across the world. The prevalence of diabetes rises steeply with age (see Fig. 9.6.3). Most people with diabetes, between 85 and 95 per cent depending on the population, have type 2 diabetes. Some studies have described differences in prevalence between men and women. For example, a pooled analysis of 13 European cohorts reported a higher prevalence in men than women in the age range 40–59, but higher in women above the age of 70 (The Decode Study Group 2003). However, such sex differences are not consistent across populations. For example, in Fig. 9.6.3, based on over 40 studies worldwide (Wild et al. 2004), the prevalence is similar in men and women across the age groups up to the age of 70. Above 70 the prevalence is marginally (1–2 per cent) higher in women.

IDF estimates that by 2025 the number of people with diabetes will have increased to 380 million. This estimate is based on demographic trends (increasing population size, and an increasing elderly population), and increasing urbanization. The projected increase does not specifically include trends in risk factor levels, such as obesity for type 2 diabetes, nor does it include the fact that people with diabetes may survive longer, at least in developed parts of the world, than in the past. Trends in risk factors will be partly accounted for by including trends in urbanization, but it is clear that obesity is increasing within urban centres the world over (Popkin 2002; Popkin & Gordon-Larsen 2004). Thus, the current global projections for the number of people with diabetes are likely to be conservative. Globally, most of the increase in the number of people with diabetes will occur in middle-aged adults in developing countries, illustrated in Fig. 9.6.4 using data available from the WHO.

At the present time, it is estimated that between 70 and 80 per cent of people with diabetes live in low- and middle-income (developing) countries. This proportion will increase as a result of population growth in developing countries, ageing of their populations, and increasing exposure to risk factors for type 2 diabetes associated with mechanization and urbanization (Unwin 2007). Diabetes, particularly type 2 diabetes, is often thought of as being a disease of affluence, and thus more prevalent in richer countries. This, however, is a misleading characterization, as Fig. 9.6.2 shows. Many middle- and even low-income countries have a prevalence that is similar or higher than some of the world's richest nations.

Differences in prevalence between different population groups

There are large differences in the prevalence of type 2 diabetes between different population groups. For example, in developing countries, the prevalence tends to be several fold higher in urban compared to rural areas (Wild et al. 2004). In most developed countries the prevalence is inversely related to socioeconomic position, with the highest prevalence in those of lowest socioeconomic

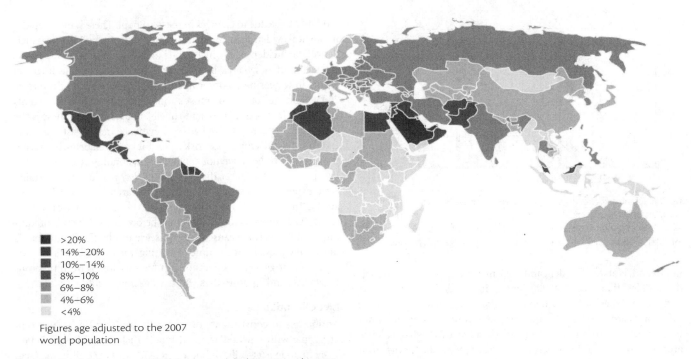

Fig. 9.6.2 The global prevalence (%) of diabetes in adults (20 in 79 years) in 2007. *Source: Diabetes Atlas,* third edition © International Diabetes Federation (2007).

position (Larranaga *et al.* 2005; Whitford *et al.* 2003; Evans *et al.* 2000; Connolly *et al.* 2000; Kumari *et al.* 2004). In some developing countries, there is evidence that diabetes prevalence is positively related to socioeconomic status, with the more affluent sections of society having the higher prevalence (Xu *et al.* 2006; Abu Sayeed *et al.* 1997; Herman *et al.* 1995). It is expected that with further economic development the socioeconomic patterning of type 2 diabetes will be similar in all countries, with the poorest groups having the highest prevalence. There is evidence from several middle-income countries that obesity, the strongest risk factor for type 2 diabetes, is now becoming more common in the less well off (Popkin 2004).

Finally, there are marked differences in diabetes prevalence between some ethnic groups living within the same regions and countries.

For example, in England, most studies have found that the prevalence in people of South Asian and African Caribbean origin is 2–4-fold higher than in people of European origin living in the same area (Oldroyd *et al.* 2005) (see Fig. 9.6.5). In North America, African and Hispanic Americans (Kenny *et al.* 1995) have higher levels of type 2 diabetes than white Americans, with some of the highest rates of all in the indigenous peoples of North America (Gohdes 1995).

Incidence of type 1 diabetes

Unlike type 2 diabetes, in which the incidence is highest in adults and rises with age, the incidence of type 1 diabetes is highest in children, and in most populations peaks between the ages of 5–14 years (International Diabetes Federation 2006; Karvonen *et al.* 2000). Internationally there are huge differences, up to 300-fold, in the incidence of type 1 diabetes. For example, an incidence of greater than 20 per 100 000 per year (in those aged 14 years or less) is found

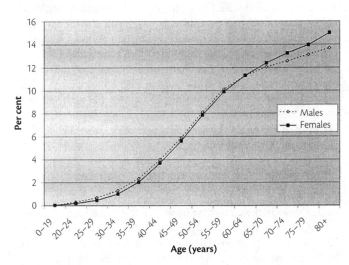

Fig. 9.6.3 The global prevalence of diabetes by age and sex in the year 2000. *Source:* Wild *et al.* (2004).

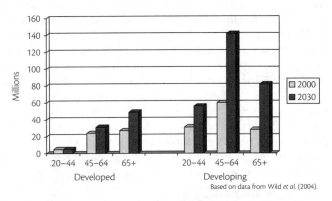

Fig. 9.6.4 Estimated number of adults by broad age group with diabetes in developed and developing countries.

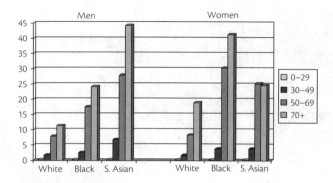

Fig. 9.6.5 Estimated prevalence (%) of diabetes by age, sex and ethnic group in England in 2007. Based on data from Yorkshire and Humber Public Health Observatory Diabetes Prevalence Model (http://www.yhpho.org.uk/PBS_diabetes.aspx), with special thanks to David Merrick for providing age-specific data.

in Finland, Norway, Sweden, and the United Kingdom, and an incidence of less than 1 per 100,000 per year in populations from China and South America (Karvonen *et al.* 2000). The reasons for these differences are incompletely understood, but the finding that rates tend to increase in migrants from low-incidence to high-incidence areas (Knip *et al.* 2005) suggests that environmental factors account for at least some of the difference. There is also evidence from several parts of the world, including the United Kingdom, that the incidence of type 1 diabetes is increasing (Onkamo *et al.* 1999), particularly in younger children, again suggesting the influence of environmental factors.

Risk factors

There are strong genetic and environmental (in its broadest sense) influences on the risk of both type 1 and type 2 diabetes, and it is the interaction between the two that results in the onset of the disease. The specific environmental influences on the risk of type 2 diabetes are relatively well understood (essentially certain behaviours and their physiological consequences), whereas those for type 1 diabetes remain frustratingly elusive.

Risk factors for type 1 diabetes

Familial and genetic

The lifetime risk of type 1 diabetes is roughly 6 per cent if a first degree relative has the condition, such as a sibling, compared to roughly 0.4 per cent (depending on the population) if a first degree relative is not affected. If a monozygotic twin has type 1 diabetes, the lifetime risk in the other twin is around 50 per cent (Hirschhorn 2003). There are well-established associations between combinations of human leukocyte antigen (HLA) genes and type 1 diabetes. Other genes involved in cell-mediated immunity, and therefore autoimmune disease, have also been associated with type 1 diabetes (Gillespie 2006; Hirschhorn 2003). More than 90 per cent of people with type 1 diabetes carry known genetic markers for the disease (Gillespie 2006). It is important to note, however, that while the presence of known genetic markers greatly increases the risk of the disease, the vast majority people with the genetic markers do not develop type 1 diabetes (Knip *et al.* 2005).

Environmental factors

The importance of environmental factors is indicated by the changing incidence of type 1 diabetes (described above) at a rate that is far

too rapid to be due to changes in the gene pool. There is much epidemiological evidence, including the seasonality of type 1 diabetes incidence, the incidence of which tends to be higher in winter, and the clustering of new cases in space and time, to implicate infective agents in triggering its onset in susceptible individuals (Knip *et al.* 2005; Gillespie 2006). The most strongly implicated infective agents are enteroviruses, rotavirus, and rubella, but for none of these is the evidence conclusive. There has been evidence in the past that early exposure to cow's milk was a risk factor for type 1 diabetes, but recent prospective studies have not supported this finding (Couper 2001). It is plausible that other dietary factors may play a role, including early exposure to cereals, but further research is needed (Couper 2001). In summary, identification of the likely environmental agent(s) has proved elusive. This may be because it (they) is ubiquitous and the hardest cause of any disease to identify is one that is universally present. At the time of writing, the frontrunners as environmental triggers are aspects of diet (cereals, toxins from tuberous vegetables) and enteroviruses (Rewers & Zimmet 2004).

Islet cell antibodies

Antibodies to constituents of islet cells are found in 90 per cent of people with newly diagnosed type 1 diabetes (Gillespie 2006). They include islet-cell antibodies (ICA), anti-GAD (glutamic acid decarboxylase), anti-insulin, and so called IA2 (anti-tyrosine-phosphatase-like protein **IA2**). In those without diabetes, the presence of two or more antibodies carries a high risk of progression to overt diabetes, whereas the presence of a single antibody appears to carry little additional risk (Kukko *et al.* 2005).

Identifying individuals at high risk of type 1 diabetes

A combination of family history, genotyping, and measurement of islet cell antibodies can identify a group of individuals in whom around half will develop type 1 diabetes over five years (Diabetes Prevention Trial—Type 1 Diabetes Study Group 2002). This, however, is a costly and labour intensive exercise and currently only worthwhile as a means of identifying high risk individuals for trials of preventive measures, and none of the measures for prevention so far tested have been found to work.

Risk factors for type 2 diabetes

It is useful to divide risk factors for type 2 diabetes into unmodifiable and modifiable. Unmodifiable risk factors include age, sex, family history, genetic markers, history of previous gestational diabetes, and ethnicity. The most important modifiable risk factors are obesity and physical inactivity; others include certain dietary constituents, smoking, and low birth weight. Biological risk factors are also important as they can be used to identify high-risk individuals. Biological risk factors include raised blood glucose and the presence of several cardiovascular risk factors (known collectively as 'the metabolic syndrome').

Unmodifiable risk factors for type 2 diabetes

Age and sex

As described in the section on incidence and prevalence, the risk of type 2 diabetes increases steeply with age. Most United Kingdom-based studies of previously diagnosed diabetes have found a slightly higher prevalence in men, whereas studies in which glucose is measured either find no sex difference or a slightly higher prevalence in women.

Familial and genetic

The strong familial clustering of type 2 diabetes, suggestive of important genetic influences, has been known for many years (Zimmet 1992). For example, the presence of type 2 diabetes in a parent or sibling tends to double the risk type 2 diabetes. Until recently, however, identifying genetic markers for type 2 diabetes has proved difficult, and the markers identified could account for only a few percent of the genetic risk (Permutt et al. 2005; Almind et al. 2001). The use of genome-wide approaches is likely to change this picture rapidly. Recently, for example, a genome-wide approach identified four genetic loci that accounted for 70 per cent of the genetic risk of type 2 diabetes in the populations studied (Sladek et al. 2007).

Previous gestational diabetes

Women with gestational diabetes tend to be older, more overweight, have a family history of diabetes, and be from an ethnic group with high prevalence of diabetes (Buchanan & Xiang 2005). Following delivery, glucose levels return to normal in around 90 per cent of women, but over the next 10 years, as many as 70 per cent go on to develop diabetes (Buchanan & Xiang 2005; Kim et al. 2002).

Ethnicity

As described previously, there are marked differences in the prevalence of type 2 diabetes by ethnic group. It is far from clear what underlies these differences, how much is related to differences in environment (including behaviours), and how much to differences in genetic susceptibility (Oldroyd et al. 2005).

Modifiable risk factors for type 2 diabetes

Obesity, physical inactivity, and aspects of diet

The relationship between overweight and obesity and the risk of type 2 diabetes is continuous, very strong, and is apparent below conventional cut points for overweight (Vazquez et al. 2007; Hartemink et al. 2006). There is a large body of evidence suggesting that it is the distribution of body fat that is particularly important in determining the risk of type 2 diabetes (and indeed cardiovascular disease), with the greatest risk associated with abdominal obesity (Despres 2001).

There is good evidence that physical activity lowers the risk of type 2 diabetes independently of obesity level. Regular moderate or vigorous activity has been associated with a 30–50 per cent reduction in the risk (Jeon et al. 2007) of developing type 2 diabetes. Physical activity is hard to measure accurately, particularly if assessed by questionnaire, as it is in most studies, and it is possible that its protective effect is even greater.

There is also evidence that the composition of the diet, over and above its calorific value, influences the risk of type 2 diabetes. Increased risk has been associated with diets low in fibre and high in saturated fat (Parillo & Riccardi 2004), and conversely intervention studies support the hypothesis that high-fibre–low-saturated-fat diets can help to prevent diabetes (Lindstrom et al. 2006b). High-glycaemic index foods have also been associated with an increased risk of type 2 diabetes (Hodge et al. 2004). There is evidence that moderate alcohol intake (Wannamethee et al. 2003; Parillo & Riccardi 2004) and coffee consumption (Salazar-Martinez et al. 2004; Smith et al. 2006) both reduce the risk of type 2 diabetes.

Smoking

Several studies have found that smoking increases the risk of type 2 diabetes by 50 per cent or more (Rimm et al. 1995; Sargeant et al. 2001; Carlsson et al. 2004; Foy et al. 2005).

Birth weight and intrauterine environment

Several studies have found an inverse association between birth weight and the risk of type 2 diabetes in adulthood (Phillips et al. 2006). It has been hypothesized that lower birth weight represents poorer foetal nutrition and that this has a programming effect on aspects of physiology and metabolism. However, there is also evidence for an alternative hypothesis, which is that low birth weight is associated with an increased genetic susceptibility to insulin resistance and type 2 diabetes (Frayling & Hattersley 2001; Hattersley & Tooke 1999). While debate continues on the nature of the relationship, it seems clear that birth weight, and other markers of early life experience, are substantially less important than adult behavioural risk factors (Parker et al. 2003; Boyko 2000).

Biological risk factors

There is a continuous positive relationship between blood glucose level (both fasting and post glucose challenge) and the risk of developing type 2 diabetes—the higher the level, the greater the risk (Unwin et al. 2002). As described above, WHO currently defines two non-diabetic risk categories based on glucose level (see Table 9.6.1): IFG and IGT. The potential benefits of identifying and intervening in people with IGT and IFG are discussed in the section on prevention.

There is a strong tendency for several metabolic and cardiovascular risk factors to cluster within the same individuals. This clustering is strongly associated with abdominal obesity and insulin resistance (Unwin 2006), and has been labelled 'the metabolic syndrome' (Alberti et al. 2005). Core features of the metabolic syndrome include abdominal obesity; raised blood glucose, blood pressure, and triglycerides; and low HDL cholesterol. The presence of the metabolic syndrome in those without diabetes strongly predicts its development (Laaksonen et al. 2002).

Risk scores

Several research groups have derived 'risk scores' based on some of the risk factors described above in order to help predict who is at high risk of developing type 2 diabetes (Glumer et al. 2004; Lindstrom & Tuomilehto 2003; Griffin et al. 2000).

Health consequences

Mortality and life expectancy

People with diabetes have a substantially higher mortality than people without diabetes, and this is found across all age groups. The relative risk of death is 4–6-fold higher at ages 20–29 years, falls with age but is still 40–80 per cent higher at ages 70–79 years (Roglic et al. 2005). Most, but not all, studies have found that the relative risk of death is higher in women (i.e. compared to women without diabetes) than in men (i.e. compared to men without diabetes). It should be noted that the number of good longitudinal studies able to properly compare mortality rates in people with and without diabetes are relatively small and largely limited to wealthier countries. The relative mortality in poorer countries, where diabetes prevalence is increasing rapidly (Wild et al. 2004) but where health care coverage is often wholly inadequate, may be even greater.

The higher mortality rates in people with diabetes across all age groups lead to substantial reductions in life expectancy. For example, in a North of England population, it was estimated that type 2 diabetes at age 40 results in 8 years lost life expectancy in both men and women, and a loss of 4 years at age 60 (Roper et al. 2001).

Recent data on loss of life expectancy in people with type 1 diabetes are hard to find. Widely quoted figures are from a critical review published in 1984 (Panzram 1984) which found that loss of life expectancy was at least 15 years, whatever the age of diagnosis, with some evidence that it may be over 25 years in those diagnosed under the age of 15. However, at least in developed countries, the picture may have improved since then, with some evidence that the difference in mortality between people with type 1 diabetes and those without diabetes, while still substantial, has decreased (Nishimura et al. 2001).

The proportion of deaths attributable to diabetes is not known with accuracy because diabetes is frequently not recorded on death certificates. Estimates of the number of deaths due to diabetes have been made using the relative risk of death in people with diabetes compared to those without, the known prevalence of diabetes and the underlying population mortality. These suggest that in most parts of the world diabetes is responsible for 5–10 per cent of all deaths in adults (Roglic et al. 2005). In the United Kingdom, it is estimated that diabetes accounted for 7.7 per cent of all adult deaths in 2007.

Cardiovascular disease

People with diabetes are at greatly increased risk of diseases of the large arteries, including the coronary and cerebral arteries and those supplying the lower limbs. The risk of cardiovascular disease in people with diabetes is 2–4-fold higher than in people without diabetes (Folsom et al. 1997, 1999; Stamler et al. 1993), and this fact accounts for much of the increased mortality associated with diabetes (Roglic et al. 2005). In most populations, well over 50 per cent of deaths in people with diabetes are from cardiovascular disease. For example, in people with diabetes in Teesside, England, 59 per cent of deaths in men and 74 per cent in women were due to cardiovascular disease (Roper et al. 2002).

Diabetic eye disease

In developed countries, diabetes is the leading cause of blindness in people aged over 25 years (Klein & Klein 1995). Twenty years after diagnosis, virtually 100 per cent of people with type 1 diabetes have diabetic retinopathy (Klein 1997; Roy et al. 2004), and when blood pressure and blood glucose control are poor, it is estimated that 75 per cent will develop proliferative retinopathy, the most severe form, during their lifetime. In type 2 diabetes, between 40 and 60 per cent are expected to develop retinopathy during their lifetime, with around 10 per cent developing proliferative retinopathy (Klein 1997; Eye Diseases Prevalence Research Group et al. 2004).

Diabetes also increases the risk of cataracts and open-angle glaucoma (Klein & Klein 1995).

Diabetic renal disease

Diabetes is the single leading cause of renal failure in developed countries, responsible for 40–50 per cent of all new patients requiring dialysis in North America, and 15–33 per cent in Europe and Australia (Atkins 2005). In cross-sectional surveys in Europe, around 1 in 10 people with type 1 diabetes, and 1 in 7 with type 2 diabetes, have evidence of overt nephropathy (International Diabetes Federation 2006). Approximately 30 per cent of people with diabetes with overt nephropathy will progress to end-stage renal failure (Atkins 2005). Large increases in the number of new cases of end-stage renal failure associated with diabetes have been documented in developed countries such as Australia. These increases largely reflect the increasing prevalence of type 2 diabetes. Figure 9.6.6 shows the year-on-year increase over the past 20 years in the number of people with diabetes and end-stage renal disease in Australia, with virtually all the increase being associated with type 2 diabetes, and not type 1.

Neuropathy and diabetic foot problems

The nerve damage associated with diabetes can affect both peripheral and autonomic nerves and thus affect digestion, urination, heart and blood pressure responses, erectile function, and peripheral sensation and musculature (Little et al. 2007). Diabetic foot problems are a result of peripheral neuropathy, often, but not always, compounded by peripheral vascular disease (Edmonds et al. 1996). In cross-sectional studies, peripheral neuropathy is found in 1 in 5 to more than a third of people with diabetes (International Diabetes Federation 2006). During their life time, roughly 15 per cent of people with diabetes develop a foot ulcer and of these 5–15 per cent go on to amputation (Edmonds et al. 1996). In developed countries, diabetes is the single-most important cause of non-traumatic lower limb amputation, accounting for 40–60 per cent of all

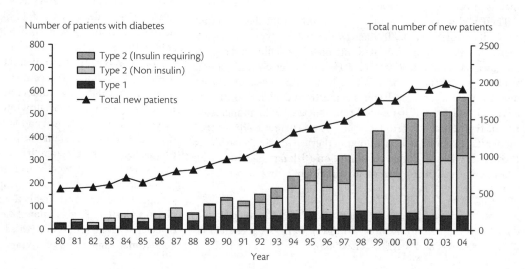

Fig. 9.6.6 Incidence of diabetes-related end-stage renal failure: Australia 1980–2004. *Source*: Atkins (2005).

amputations (Global Lower Extremity Amputation Study Group 2000), and people with diabetes have a 15-fold-risk of amputation compared to people without diabetes (Edmonds *et al.* 1996).

Erectile dysfunction

Diabetes increases the risk of erectile dysfunction in men. A recent study (Bacon *et al.* 2002) found that type 1 diabetes increased the risk threefold, and type 2 diabetes increased the risk by a third. The same study found that the prevalence of erectile dysfunction in men with diabetes was around 50 per cent.

Depression

Depression is more common in people with diabetes than in people without. A recent study reported diagnosed depression in 18 per cent of people with type 2 diabetes compared to 11 per cent in age and sex matched controls (Nichols & Brown 2003). Depression in people with diabetes is associated with more complications and poorer self care (Lin *et al.* 2004).

Economic impact of diabetes

Although there is a lack of robust studies into the economic impact of diabetes, it is clear that the cost of diabetes to individuals and their carers, to health services, and to national economies is substantial. On average, a person with diabetes uses more health care resources than a person without diabetes—around 1.5–3 times more, depending on age (International Diabetes Federation 2006). This fact, along with knowledge of the prevalence of diabetes and the overall health care budget, has been used to derive estimates of the average health care expenditure per person with diabetes and the overall cost to the health care system (Williams 2005; International Diabetes Federation 2006). For example, it has been estimated that, in 2007, the cost of diabetes to the health care system was between 4.4 and 8.8 billion international dollars (ID) in the United Kingdom; 6.1–10.9 billion in India; 14.8–26.9 billion in China; and 119.3–213.8 billion in the United States (International Diabetes Federation 2006). The costs of diabetes care increase dramatically with the presence of complications, being 2–3-fold higher with the presence of either micro- or macro-vascular complications, and 5–6-fold higher with the presence of both micro- and macro-vascular complications than in people with diabetes without complications (Williams 2005).

Diabetes, as with any other chronic illness, may limit employment and impact upon the income of people with it and the people caring for them. A study in the United Kingdom found that, in people with type 2 diabetes aged less than 65 years, 7 per cent lost income because of diabetes. They lost on average £13 800 per year (at 1998 values) and their carers lost £11 000 per year (Holmes *et al.* 2003). A recent study, from the Economist Intelligence Unit, estimated the total economic impact of diabetes, both in terms of costs to the health care system and in terms of lost productivity. The findings suggested that, in 2007, the United Kingdom lost 0.4 per cent of its total gross domestic product to diabetes, the United States 1.2 per cent, and India 2.1 per cent (Economist Intelligence Unit 2007).

Prevention of diabetes and its complications

Prevention of type 1 diabetes

Just as our knowledge of the environmental triggers for type 1 diabetes remains elusive, so does our knowledge of how to prevent it in humans. Interventions that have been evaluated in individuals at high risk of diabetes have included nicotinamide therapy and low-dose insulin, but neither was effective. Other options currently being evaluated include the use of immunosuppressant therapy in individuals at high risk (Gillespie 2006). In those with type 1 diabetes, pancreatic transplantation is of proven benefit, but comes with the drawbacks common to all organ transplantation. At the time of writing, beta cell regeneration is a major area of investigation that holds promise (Gillespie 2006).

Prevention of type 2 diabetes

There is excellent evidence that type 2 diabetes can be prevented, or at least its onset delayed, in individuals at high risk of type 2 diabetes. Interventions aimed at modifying behaviours and pharmacological interventions have both been shown to be effective, and at best to reduce the incidence of type 2 diabetes by 50–60 per cent. The findings of some of the major trials are summarized in Table 9.6.2. Overall, interventions promoting behavioural change were as effective as pharmacological interventions, a conclusion supported by a recent meta-analysis (Gillies *et al.* 2007). Aspects of behavioural change that were promoted included weight loss (in those overweight and obese), increased physical activity, and a low total and saturated fat and high-fibre diet. Follow-up from the Finnish Diabetes Prevention Study suggests, not surprisingly, that the more of the behavioural goals that were achieved, the lower the long-term risk of type 2 diabetes (Lindstrom *et al.* 2006a).

Targeting individuals at high risk of diabetes, based on impaired glucose tolerance or impaired fasting glucose, is unlikely to have a large (e.g. 50 per cent or greater) impact on the overall population incidence of type 2 diabetes. This is because roughly 40–60 per cent of new cases of type 2 diabetes arise in people who had normal glucose tolerance 3–5 years earlier (Unwin *et al.* 2002). Other approaches to identifying and targeting individuals at high risk may improve this, but there seems little doubt that it is only through population-based measures aimed at reducing overweight and obesity and increasing physical activity that a large impact on the incidence of type 2 diabetes will be achieved. The potential impact of population-wide measures was illustrated in an analysis from EPIC-Norfolk, a UK cohort of 24 155 subjects. It assessed the association between the achievement of five 'diabetes healthy behaviour prevention goals' (BMI < 25 kg/m2), fat intake < 30 per cent of energy intake, saturated fat intake < 10 per cent of energy intake, fibre intake ≥ 15 g/1000 kcal, physical activity > 4 hours/week) and the risk of developing diabetes at follow-up (mean 4.6 years). Diabetes incidence was inversely related to the number of goals achieved. None of the participants who met all five of the goals developed diabetes, whereas diabetes incidence was highest in those who did not meet any goals. If the entire population were able to meet one more goal, the total incidence of diabetes would be predicted to fall by 20 per cent (Simmons *et al.* 2006).

As reviewed elsewhere in this Textbook, achieving population-wide changes to reduce the incidence of diabetes and related chronic non-communicable diseases presents major challenges. Despite increasing awareness in many parts of the world amongst both policy makers and the general public of the importance of obesity as a risk factor for diabetes and other adverse health outcomes, there is not yet a single population-wide example where the trend towards increasing levels of obesity has been reversed. This includes high-income countries in which there is a multi-billion-dollar 'diet industry' (Arterburn 2006) ostensibly aiming to help people achieve and

Table 9.6.2 Summary of some of the major prevention trials in people at high risk of type 2 diabetes

Study/authors	Date	Setting	Population	Intervention	Trial groups	Relative risk reduction
Da Qing IGT and Diabetes Study (Pan *et al.* 1997)	1997	China	N=577 Chinese men and women aged over 25 years with IGT	Lifestyle	- Control group - Diet only - Exercise only - Diet and exercise	31% (diet) 46% (exercise) 42% (diet and exercise)
Finnish Diabetes Prevention Study (DPS) (Tuomilehto *et al.* 2001)	2001	Finland	N=552 overweight Finnish men and women aged 40–65 years with IGT	Lifestyle	- Control group - Lifestyle	58% (lifestyle)
Diabetes Prevention Program (DPP) (Knowler *et al.* 2002)	2002	United States	N=3234 overweight American men and women including 45% of African, Hispanic, Asian or Native American descent aged over 25 years with IGT	Lifestyle/ pharmaceutical	- Control group - Metformin (850 mg twice daily) - Lifestyle	31% (metformin) 58% (lifestyle)
STOP-NIDDM Trial (Chiasson *et al.* 2002)	2002	Multi-centre	N=1368 overweight Europid men and women aged 40-70 years with IGT	Pharmaceutical	- Control group - Acarbose (100 mg three times daily)	25%
Troglitazone in Prevention of Diabetes (TRIPOD) (Buchanan *et al.* 2001)	2002	United States	N=266 Hispanic-American women aged ≥18 years with previous gestational diabetes in last 4 years	Pharmaceutical	- Control group - Troglitazone (400 mg daily)	56%
XENical in the Prevention of Diabetes in Obese Subjects (XENDOS) study (Torgerson *et al.* 2004)	2004	Sweden	N=3305 obese Swedish men and women aged 40–60 years with normal glucose tolerance (79%) or IGT (21%)	Pharmaceutical	- Control group (placebo and lifestyle) - Lifestyle and orlistat (120 mg three times daily)	45% (lifestyle and orlistat) in those with IGT
The Indian Diabetes Prevention Program (IDPP-1) (Ramachandran *et al.* 2006)	2006	India	N=531 Asian Indian men and women aged 35–55 years with IGT	Lifestyle/ pharmaceutical	- Control - Lifestyle - Metformin - Metformin and lifestyle	29% (lifestyle) 26% (metformin) 28% (metformin and lifestyle)
Dream trail investigators (DREAM Trial Investigators *et al.* 2006)	2006	Multi-centre	N=5269 men and women, >30 years, with IFG/IGT	Pharmaceutical	Control group Rosiglitazone 8 mg	60% reduction in diabetes incidence or death

(Thanks to Dr R. Simmonds who compiled this table.)

maintain weight loss. This highlights the considerable challenges in achieving population-wide changes in diet and physical activity, and thus reductions in obesity, and it is clear that it will require much more than raising awareness and providing information. This was put succinctly in the 1997 WHO report on obesity (World Health Organization 1997), when it stated that, 'what has been demonstrated . . . is that approaches that are firmly based on the principle of personal education and behaviour change are unlikely to succeed in an environment in which there are plentiful inducements to engage in opposing behaviours'. It went on to suggest that, 'It would therefore seem appropriate to devote resources to programmes which focus on reducing the exposure of the population to obesity promoting agents by addressing the environmental factors such as transportation, urban design, advertising and food pricing'.

The need to change the 'obesogenic environment' (Egger & Swinburn 1997) if the obesity epidemic is to be reversed is now widely accepted. It is the basis for the World Health Organization's Global Strategy on Diet, Physical Activity and Health, which was mandated by the World Health Assembly in 2002 and then accepted in 2004 (World Health Organization 2004). There are some examples to draw on where policy measures have led to, or at least been associated with, improvements in diet and physical activity (Willett *et al.* 2006) although not with declines in obesity. They include community based, multi-faceted approaches, such as undertaken in Finland (Puska *et al.* 1985) and Singapore (Cutter *et al.* 2001), both associated with declines in at least some aspects of CVD risk. Despite such examples, there remains in general a lack of hard evidence on what approaches are effective in achieving population-wide changes in diet and physical activity. In acknowledgement of

- ◆ **Advocacy**
  - ◆ Supporting national associations and non-governmental organizations
  - ◆ Promoting the economic case for prevention
- ◆ **Community support**
  - ◆ Providing education in schools regarding nutrition and physical activity
  - ◆ Promotion opportunities for physical activity through urban design (e.g. to encourage cycling and walking)
- ◆ **Fiscal and legislative measures**
  - ◆ Examining food pricing, labelling, and advertising
  - ◆ Enforcing environmental and infrastructure regulation, e.g. urban planning and transportation policy to enhance physical activity
- ◆ **Engagement of private sector**
  - ◆ Promoting health in the workplace
  - ◆ Ensuring healthy food policies in food industry
- ◆ **Media communication**
  - ◆ Improving level of knowledge and motivation of the population (press, TV, and radio)

Fig. 9.6.7 Recommendations from the International Diabetes Federation for population-wide measures for the prevention of type 2 diabetes.

this, one of the guiding principles of the WHO strategy on Diet, Physical Activity and Health is to seek stronger evidence for what types of policy change are effective in promoting healthier diets and increased levels of physical activity. The strategy aims to use this evidence to advocate for change, supporting countries to develop frameworks for action that are appropriate to their own circumstances. General guidance on a package of measures aimed at producing population-wide changes has been produced by both WHO (World Health Organization 2005) and the IDF (Fig. 9.6. 7) (Alberti *et al.* 2007).

Prevention of diabetes-related complications

There is excellent evidence that the increased morbidity and mortality in people with diabetes, compared to those without, can be significantly reduced (Venkat Narayan *et al.* 2006). This evidence includes approaches to reducing the incidence of complications and to limiting their progression and impact once they exist. A summary of the main interventions and estimates of their effectiveness for preventing diabetes related complications is provided in Table 9.6.3 (Venkat Narayan *et al.* 2006). Control of blood glucose, blood pressure, blood lipids, and the avoidance of smoking are core; with specific measures to reduce the incidence of sight-threatening retinopathy, morbidity and loss of the lower limbs, and progression to end stage renal disease.

A detailed discussion of how to achieve reductions in morbidity and mortality in people with diabetes and the contents of good diabetes care is beyond the scope of this chapter. There are many sources of guidance on this, including the National Service Framework on Diabetes for England (Roberts 2007), the Global Guideline for Type 2 diabetes from the International Diabetes Federation (International Diabetes Federation: Clinical Guidelines Taskforce 2005), and a forthcoming report from the WHO (World Health Organization, forthcoming). However, it is worth making the following points here. People with diabetes play the central role in managing their condition (as with most chronic conditions), and thus core to effective diabetes care is empowering people with diabetes with the knowledge and support they need to do this. Effective health care for diabetes, in common with many other chronic conditions (Epping-Jordan *et al.* 2004), requires a well-functioning health care system, with good communication between many

Table 9.6.3 Examples of treatment strategies and relative reductions in morbidity and mortality in people with diabetes

Strategy	Estimated benefit
Glycaemic control in people with HbA1c greater than 9 per cent	Reduction of 30 per cent in microvascular disease per 1 per cent drop in HbA1c
Glycaemic control in people with HbA1c greater than 8 per cent	Reduction of 30 per cent in microvascular disease per 1 per cent drop in HbA1c
Blood pressure control in people whose pressure is higher than 160/95 mmHg	Reduction of 35 per cent in macrovascular and microvascular disease per 10 mmHg drop in blood pressure
Cholesterol control in people with total cholesterol > 5.2 mmol l^{-1}	Reduction of 25–55 per cent in coronary heart diseases events; 43 per cent fall in death rate
Annual screening for microalbuminuria	Reduction of 50 per cent in nephropathy using ACE inhibitors for identified cases
Annual eye examinations	Reduction of 60 to 70 per cent in serious vision loss
Foot care in people with high risk of ulcers	Reduction of 50 to 60 per cent in serious foot disease
Aspirin use	Reduction of 28 per cent in myocardial infarctions, reduction of 18 per cent in cardiovascular disease
ACE inhibitor use in all people with diabetes	Reduction of 42 per cent in nephropathy; 22 per cent reduction in cardiovascular disease

Source: Based on Venkat Narayan *et al.* (2006).

different specialities and levels of care. Finally, it is an accurate generalization to state that diabetes is care is currently suboptimal the world over (Venkat Narayan *et al.* 2006), in both rich and poor countries. In rich countries, suboptimal care includes inadequate coverage of basic preventive measures, such as regular eye and foot examinations, as well as room for much better control of glucose, blood pressure, and lipids. In poor countries, inadequate care includes no care at all for a large proportion of people with diabetes, including, in many parts of the world, lack of, or intermittent access to, insulin leading to the death of those who require it for survival (Yudkin 2000). It is not hyperbole to state that diabetes presents one of the major public health challenges of the twenty-first century, one that has reached the attention of the United Nations in its call for coordinated global action (Unite for Diabetes 2006).

References

Abu Sayeed, M., ALI, L., Hussain, *et al.* (1997) Effect of socioeconomic risk factors on the difference in prevalence of diabetes between rural and urban populations in Bangladesh. *Diabetes Care*, **20**, 551–5.

Alberti, K.G.M.M., Zimmet, P., and Shaw, J. (2005) The metabolic syndrome: a new worldwide definition. *Lancet*, **366**, 1059–62.

Alberti, K.G.M.M., Zimmet, P., and Shaw, J. (2007) International Diabetes Federation: a consensus on Type 2 diabetes prevention. *Diabetic Medicine*, **24**, 451–63.

Almind, K., Doria, A., and CR., K. (2001) Putting the genes for type II diabetes on the map. *Nature Medicine*, **7**, 277–9.

American Diabetes Association (2004) Diagnosis and classification of diabetes mellitus. *Diabetes Care*, **27**, 5S–10S.

Arterburn, D. (2006) The BBC diet trials. *British Medical Journal*, **332**, 1284–5.

Aspray, T.J., Mugusi, F., Rashid, S., *et al.* & Essential Non-communicable Disease Health Intervention (2000) Rural and urban differences in diabetes prevalence in Tanzania: the role of obesity, physical inactivity and urban living. *Transactions of the Royal Society of Tropical Medicine & Hygiene*, **94**, 637–44.

Atkins, R.C. (2005) The epidemiology of chronic kidney disease. *Kidney International*, **67**, S14–8.

Bacon, C.G., Hu, F. B., Giovannucci, E., *et al.* (2002) Association of type and duration of diabetes with erectile dysfunction in a large cohort of men. *Diabetes Care*, **25**, 1458–63.

Bennett, P., Knowler, W., Pettitt, D., *et al.* (1982) Longitudinal studies of the development of diabetes in the Pima Indians. In *Advances in Diabetes Epidemiology* (ed. E. ESCHWEGE), Amsterdam, Netherlands, Elsevier Biomedical Press.

Berson, S.A. and Yalow, R.S. (1963) Antigens in insulin determinants of specificity of porcine insulin in man. *Science*, **139**, 844–5.

Bornstein, J. and Lawrence, R. D. (1951) Plasma insulin in human diabetes mellitus. *British Medical Journal*, **2**, 1541–4.

Boyko, E.J. (2000) Proportion of type 2 diabetes cases resulting from impaired fetal growth. *Diabetes Care*, **23**, 1260–4.

Buchanan, T., Xiang, A., Peters, R., *et al.*(2001) Protection from type 2 diabetes persists in the TRIPOD cohort eight months after stopping troglitazone. *Diabetes*, **50**, A81.

Buchanan, T.A. & Xiang, A.H. (2005) Gestational diabetes mellitus. *Journal of Clinical Investigation*, **115**, 485–91.

Carlsson, S., Midthjell, K., Grill, V., *et al.* (2004) Smoking is associated with an increased risk of type 2 diabetes but a decreased risk of autoimmune diabetes in adults: an 11-year follow-up of incidence of diabetes in the Nord-Trondelag study. *Diabetologia*, **47**, 1953–6.

Chiasson, J., Josse, R., Gomis, R., *et al.* (2002) Acarbose can prevent the progression of impaired glucose tolerance to type 2 diabetes mellitus: results of a randomised clinical trial, The STOP-NIDDM Trial. *Lancet*, **359**, 2072–7.

Connolly, V., Unwin, N., Sherriff, P., *et al.* (2000) Diabetes prevalence and socioeconomic status: a population based study showing increased prevalence of type 2 diabetes mellitus in deprived areas. *Journal of Epidemiology & Community Health*, **54**, 173–7.

Couper, J.J. (2001) Environmental triggers of type 1 diabetes. *Journal of Paediatrics & Child Health*, **37**, 218–220.

Cutter, J., Tan, B.Y. & Chew, S.K. (2001) Levels of cardiovascular disease risk factors in Singapore following a national intervention programme.[see comment]. *Bulletin of the World Health Organization*, **79**, 908–15.

Decode Study Group (1999) Is fasting glucose sufficient to define diabetes? Epidemiological data from 20 European studies. The DECODE-study group. European Diabetes Epidemiology Group. Diabetes Epidemiology: Collaborative analysis of Diagnostic Criteria in Europe. *Diabetologia*, **42**, 647–654.

Decode Study Group (2001) Glucose tolerance and cardiovascular mortality: comparison of fasting and 2-hour diagnostic criteria. *Archives of Internal Medicine*, **161**, 397–405.

Despres, J.P. (2001) Health consequences of visceral obesity. *Annals of Medicine*, **33**, 534–541.

Diabetes Prevention Trial—type 1 Diabetes Study Group (2002) Effects of insulin in relatives of patients with type 1 diabetes mellitus. *New England Journal of Medicine*, **346**, 1685–91.

Dream Trial Investigators, Gerstein, H.C., Yusuf, S., *et al.* (2006) Effect of rosiglitazone on the frequency of diabetes in patients with impaired glucose tolerance or impaired fasting glucose: a randomised controlled trial. *Lancet*, **368**, 1096–105.

Economist Intelligence Unit (2007) The silent epidemic: an economic study of diabetes in developed and developing countries. London, Economist Intelligence Unit.

Edmonds, M., Boulton, A., Buckenham, T., *et al.* (1996) Report of the diabetic foot and amputation group. **13**, S27–S42.

Egger, G. & Swinburn, B. (1997) An "ecological" approach to the obesity pandemic. *British Medical Journal*, **315**, 477–480.

Epping-Jordan, J.E., Pruitt, S.D., Bengoa, R., *et al.* (2004) Improving the quality of health care for chronic conditions. *Quality & Safety in Health Care*, **13**, 299–305.

Evans, J.M., Newton, R.W., Ruta, D.A., *et al.* (2000) Socio-economic status, obesity and prevalence of Type 1 and Type 2 diabetes mellitus. *Diabetic Medicine*, **17**, 478–80.

Eye Diseases Prevalence Research Group, Kempen, J.H., O'Colmain, B.J., Leske, M.C., *et al.* (2004) The prevalence of diabetic retinopathy among adults in the United States. *Archives of Ophthalmology*, **122**, 552–63.

Folsom, A.R., Rasmussen, M.L., Chambless, L.E., *et al.* (1999) Prospective associations of fasting insulin, body fat distribution, and diabetes with risk of ischemic stroke. The Atherosclerosis Risk in Communities (ARIC) Study Investigators. *Diabetes Care*, **22**, 1077–83.

Folsom, A.R., Szklo, M., Stevens, J., *et al.* (1997) A prospective study of coronary heart disease in relation to fasting insulin, glucose, and diabetes. The Atherosclerosis Risk in Communities (ARIC) Study. *Diabetes Care*, **20**, 935–42.

Foy, C.G., Bell, R.A., Farmer, D.F., *et al.* (2005) Smoking and incidence of diabetes among U.S. adults: findings from the Insulin Resistance Atherosclerosis Study. *Diabetes Care*, **28**, 2501–7.

Frayling, T.M. & Hattersley, A.T. (2001) The role of genetic susceptibility in the association of low birth weight with type 2 diabetes. *British Medical Bulletin*, **60**, 89–101.

Gillespie, K.M. (2006) Type 1 diabetes: pathogenesis and prevention. *CMAJ*, **175**, 165–70.

Gillies, C.L., Abrams, K.R., Lambert, P.C., *et al.* (2007) Pharmacological and lifestyle interventions to prevent or delay type 2 diabetes in people with impaired glucose tolerance: systematic review and meta-analysis. *BMJ*, **334**, 299.

Global Lower Extremity Amputation Study Group (2000) Epidemiology of lower extremity amputation in centres in Europe, North America and East Asia. The Global Lower Extremity Amputation Study Group. *British Journal of Surgery*, **87**, 328–37.

Glumer, C., Carstensen, B., Sandbaek, A., *et al.* (2004) A Danish diabetes risk score for targeted screening: the Inter99 study. *Diabetes Care*, **27**, 727–33.

Gohdes, D. (1995) Diabetes in North American Indians and Alaska Natives. IN NATIONAL DIABETES DATA GROUP (Ed.) *Diabetes in America.* Second ed. Washington, National Institutes of Health.

Griffin, S. J., Little, P. S., Hales, C. N., *et al.* (2000) Diabetes risk score: towards earlier detection of type 2 diabetes in general practice. *Diabetes/Metabolism Research Reviews*, **16**, 164–71.

Harris, M. (1993) Undiagnosed NIDDM: Clinical and public health issues. *Diabetes Care*, **16**, 642–652.

Hartemink, N., Boshuizen, H.C., Nagelkerke, N.J.D., *et al.* (2006) Combining risk estimates from observational studies with different exposure cutpoints: a meta-analysis on body mass index and diabetes type 2. *American Journal of Epidemiology*, **163**, 1042–52.

Hattersley, A.T. & Tooke, J.E. (1999) The fetal insulin hypothesis: an alternative explanation of the association of low birthweight with diabetes and vascular disease. *Lancet*, **353**, 1789–92.

Herman, W.H., Ali, M.A., Aubert, R.E., *et al.* (1995) Diabetes mellitus in Egypt: risk factors and prevalence. *Diabetic Medicine*, **12**, 1126–31.

Himsworth, H.P. (1936) Diabetes mellitus: its differentiation into insulin-sensitive and insulin-insensitive types. *Lancet*, **i**, 127–130.

Hirschhorn, J. N. (2003) Genetic epidemiology of type 1 diabetes. *Pediatric Diabetes*, **4**, 87–100.

Hodge, A.M., English, D.R., O'dea, K., *et al.* (2004) Glycemic index and dietary fiber and the risk of type 2 diabetes. *Diabetes Care*, **27**, 2701–6.

Holmes, J., Gear, E., Bottomley, J., *et al.* (2003) Do people with type 2 diabetes and their carers lose income? (T2ARDIS-4). *Health Policy*, **64**, 291–296.

International Diabetes Federation (2006) Diabetes Atlas: third edition. Brussels, International Diabetes Federation.

International Diabetes Federation: Clinical Guidelines Taskforce (2005) Global Guideline for Type 2 Diabetes. Brussels, International Diabetes Federation.

Jeon, C.Y., Lokken, R.P., Hu, F.B., *et al.* (2007) Physical activity of moderate intensity and risk of type 2 diabetes: a systematic review. *Diabetes Care*, **30**, 744–52.

Karvonen, M., Viik-Kajander, M., Moltchanova, E., *et al.* (2000) Incidence of childhood type 1 diabetes worldwide. *Diabetes Care*, **23**, 1516–1526.

Kenny, S., Aubert, R. & Geiss, L. (1995) Prevalence and Incidence of Non-Insulin-Dependent Diabetes. In National Diabetes Data Group (Ed.) *Diabetes in America.* Second ed. Washington, National Institutes of Health.

Kim, C., Newton, K.M. & Knopp, R.H. (2002) Gestational diabetes and the incidence of type 2 diabetes: a systematic review. *Diabetes Care*, **25**, 1862–8.

Klein, R. (1997) The epidemiology of diabetic retinopathy. In *Textbook of Diabetes* (eds. Pickup, J. and Williams, G.). London, Blackwell Scientific Publications.

Klein, R. & Klein, B. E. (1995) Vision disorders in diabetes. In *Diabetes in America* (ed. National Diabetes Data Group). Second ed. Bethesda, USA, National Institutes of Health.

Knip, M., Veijola, R., Virtanen, S. M., *et al.* (2005) Environmental triggers and determinants of type 1 diabetes. *Diabetes*, **54**, S125–36.

Knowler, W.C., Barrett-Connor, E., Fowler, S.E., *et al.* & Diabetes Prevention Program Research Group (2002) Reduction in the incidence of type 2 diabetes with lifestyle intervention or metformin. *New England Journal of Medicine*, **346**, 393–403.

Kukko, M., Kimpimaki, T., Korhonen, S., *et al.* (2005) Dynamics of diabetes-associated autoantibodies in young children with human leukocyte antigen-conferred risk of type 1 diabetes recruited from the general population. *Journal of Clinical Endocrinology & Metabolism*, **90**, 2712–7.

Kumari, M., Head, J. & Marmot, M. (2004) Prospective study of social and other risk factors for incidence of type 2 diabetes in the Whitehall II study. *Archives of Internal Medicine*, **164**, 1873–80.

Laaksonen, D.E., Lakka, H.-M., Niskanen, L.K., *et al.* (2002) Metabolic syndrome and development of diabetes mellitus: application and validation of recently suggested definitions of the metabolic syndrome

in a prospective cohort study. *American Journal of Epidemiology*, **156**, 1070–7.

Larranaga, I., Arteagoitia, J.M., Rodriguez, J.L., *et al.* & The Sentinel Practice Network Of The Basque Country (2005) Socio-economic inequalities in the prevalence of Type 2 diabetes, cardiovascular risk factors and chronic diabetic complications in the Basque Country, Spain. *Diabetic Medicine*, **22**, 1047–53.

Lin, E.H.B., Katon, W., Von Korff, M., *et al.* (2004) Relationship of depression and diabetes self-care, medication adherence, and preventive care. *Diabetes Care*, **27**, 2154–60.

Lindstrom, J., Ilanne-Parikka, P., Peltonen, M., *et al.* (2006a) Sustained reduction in the incidence of type 2 diabetes by lifestyle intervention: follow-up of the Finnish Diabetes Prevention Study. *The Lancet*, **368**, 1673–9.

Lindstrom, J., Peltonen, M., Eriksson, J.G., *et al.* (2006b) High-fibre, low-fat diet predicts long-term weight loss and decreased type 2 diabetes risk: the Finnish Diabetes Prevention Study. *Diabetologia*, **49**, 912–20.

Lindstrom, J. & Tuomilehto, J. (2003) The diabetes risk score: a practical tool to predict type 2 diabetes risk. *Diabetes Care*, **26**, 725–31.

Little, A.A., Edwards, J.L., & Feldman, E.L. (2007) Diabetic neuropathies. *Practical Neurology*, **7**, 82–92.

Nichols, G.A. & Brown, J.B. (2003) Unadjusted and adjusted prevalence of diagnosed depression in type 2 diabetes. *Diabetes Care*, **26**, 744–9.

Nishimura, R., Laporte, R.E., Dorman, J.S., *et al.* (2001) Mortality trends in type 1 diabetes. The Allegheny County (Pennsylvania) Registry 1965-1999. *Diabetes Care*, **24**, 823–7.

Oldroyd, J., Banerjee, M., Heald, A., *et al.* (2005) Diabetes and ethnic minorities. *Postgraduate Medical Journal*, **81**, 486–90.

Onkamo, P., Vaananen, S., Karvonen, M., *et al.* (1999) Worldwide increase in incidence of Type I diabetes—the analysis of the data on published incidence trends [erratum appears in Diabetologia 2000 May;43(5):685]. *Diabetologia*, **42**, 1395–403.

Palmer, J. P. & Hirsch, I.B. (2003) What's in a Name: Latent autoimmune diabetes of adults, type 1.5, adult-onset, and type 1 diabetes. *Diabetes Care*, **26**, 536–8.

Pan, X., Li, G., Hu, Y.H., *et al.* (1997) Effects of Diet and Exercise in Preventing NIDDM in People With Impaired Glucose Tolerance. The Da Qing IGT and Diabetes Study. *Diabetes Care*, **20**, 537–44.

Panzram, G. (1984) Epidemiologic data on excess mortality and life expectancy in insulin-dependent diabetes mellitus--critical review. *Experimental & Clinical Endocrinology*, **83**, 93–100.

Parillo, M. & Riccardi, G. (2004) Diet composition and the risk of type 2 diabetes: epidemiological and clinical evidence. *British Journal of Nutrition*, **92**, 7–19.

Parker, L., Lamont, D.W., Unwin, N., *et al.* (2003) A lifecourse study of risk for hyperinsulinaemia, dyslipidaemia and obesity (the central metabolic syndrome) at age 49-51 years.[erratum appea rs in *Diabetic Medicine*. 2003 Sep;20(9):781]. *Diabetic Medicine*, **20**, 406–15.

Permutt, M.A., Wasson, J., & Cox, N. (2005) Genetic epidemiology of diabetes *J. Clin. Invest*, **115**, 1431–1439.

Phillips, D.I.W., Jones, A., & Goulden, P.A. (2006) Birth weight, stress, and the metabolic syndrome in adult life. *Annals of the New York Academy of Sciences*, **1083**, 28–36.

Popkin, B.M. (2002) The shift in stages of the nutrition transition in the developing world differs from past experiences! *Public Health Nutrition*, **5**, 205–14.

Popkin, B.M. (2004) The nutrition transition: an overview of world patterns of change. *Nutrition Reviews*, **62**, S140–S143.

Popkin, B.M. & Gordon-Larsen, P. (2004) The nutrition transition: worldwide obesity dynamics and their determinants. *International Journal of Obesity & Related Metabolic Disorders*, **28**, s2–9.

Pozzilli, P. & Buzzetti, R. (2007) A new expression of diabetes: double diabetes. *Trends in Endocrinology & Metabolism*, **18**, 52–7.

Puska, P., Nissinen, A., Tuomilehto, J., *et al.* (1985) The community-based strategy to prevent coronary heart disease: conclusions from the ten years of the North Karelia project. *Annual Review of Public Health*, **6**, 147–93.

Ramachandran, A., Snehalatha, C., Mary, S., *et al.* (2006) The Indian Diabetes Prevention Programme shows that lifestyle modification and metformin prevent type 2 diabetes in Asian Indian subjects with impaired glucose tolerance (IDPP-1). *Diabetologia,* **49,** 289–97.

Rewers, M. & Zimmet, P. (2004) The rising tide of childhood type 1 diabetes—what is the elusive environmental trigger?[comment]. *Lancet,* **364,** 1645–7.

Rimm, E.B., Chan, J., Stampfer, M.J., *et al.* (1995) Prospective study of cigarette smoking, alcohol use, and the risk of diabetes in men. *BMJ,* **310,** 555–9.

Roberts, S. (2007) *Working together for better diabetes care:clinical case for change.* London, Department of Health.

Roglic, G., Unwin, N., Bennett, P.H., *et al.* (2005) The burden of mortality attributable to diabetes: realistic estimates for the year 2000. *Diabetes Care,* **28,** 2130–5.

Roper, N.A., Bilous, R.W., Kelly, W.F., *et al.* (2001) Excess mortality in a population with diabetes and the impact of material deprivation: longitudinal, population based study. *British Medical Journal,* **322,** 1389–1393.

Roper, N.A., Bilous, R.W., Kelly, W.F., *et al.* (2002) Cause-specific mortality in a population with diabetes: South Tees Diabetes Mortality Study. *Diabetes Care.,* **25,** 43–48.

Roy, M.S., Klein, R., O'Colmain, B.J., *et al.* (2004) The prevalence of diabetic retinopathy among adult type 1 diabetic persons in the United States. *Archives of Ophthalmology,* **122,** 546–51.

Salazar-Martinez, E., Willett, W.C., Ascherio, A., *et al.* (2004) Coffee consumption and risk for type 2 diabetes mellitus. *Annals of Internal Medicine,* **140,** 1–8.

Sargeant, L.A., Khaw, K.T., Bingham, S., *et al.* (2001) Cigarette smoking and glycaemia: the EPIC-Norfolk Study. *International Journal of Epidemiology,* **30,** 547–54.

Simmons, R., Harding, A.H., Jakes, R., *et al.* (2006) How much might achievement of diabetes prevention behaviour goals reduce the incidence of diabetes if implemented at the population level? *Diabetologia,* **49,** 905–11.

Sladek, R., Rocheleau, G., Rung, J., *et al.* (2007) A genome-wide association study identifies novel risk loci for type 2 diabetes. *Nature,* **445,** 881–5.

Smith, B., Wingard, D.L., Smith, T.C., *et al.* (2006) Does coffee consumption reduce the risk of type 2 diabetes in individuals with impaired glucose? *Diabetes Care,* **29,** 2385–90.

Stamler, J., Vaccaro, O., Neaton, J.D., *et al.* (1993) Diabetes, other risk factors, and 12-yr cardiovascular mortality for men screened in the Multiple Risk Factor Intervention Trial. *Diabetes Care,* **16,** 434–44.

Tapp, R.J., Zimmet, P.Z., Harper, C.A., *et al.* (2006) Diagnostic thresholds for diabetes: The association of retinopathy and albuminuria with glycaemia. *Diabetes Research and Clinical Practice,* **73,** 315–21.

The Decode Study Group (2003) Age- and Sex-Specific Prevalences of Diabetes and Impaired Glucose Regulation in 13 European Cohorts. *Diabetes Care,* **26,** 61–9.

The Expert Committee on the Diagnosis and Classification of Diabetes Mellitus (1997) Report of the Expert Committee on the Diagnosis and Classification of Diabetes Mellitus. *Diabetes Care,* **20,** 1183–97.

Torgerson, J.S., Hauptman, J., Boldrin, M.N., *et al.* (2004) XENical in the Prevention of Diabetes in Obese Subjects (XENDOS) Study: A randomized study of orlistat as an adjunct to lifestyle changes for the prevention of type 2 diabetes in obese patients. *Diabetes Care,* **27,** 155–61.

Tuomi, T., Groop, L. C., Zimmet, P.Z., *et al.* (1993) Antibodies to glutamic acid decarboxylase reveal latent autoimmune diabetes mellitus in adults with a non-insulin-dependent onset of disease. *Diabetes,* **42,** 359–62.

Tuomilehto, J., Lindstrom, J., Eriksson, J. G., *et al.* & Finnish Diabetes Prevention Study Group (2001) Prevention of type 2 diabetes mellitus by changes in lifestyle among subjects with impaired glucose tolerance. *New England Journal of Medicine,* **344,** 1343–50.

Unite for Diabetes (2006) Resolution adopted by the General Assembly: 61/225. World Diabetes Day.

Unwin, N. (2006) The metabolic syndrome. *Journal of the Royal Society of Medicine,* **99,** 457–62.

Unwin, N. (2007) Diabetes and the good, the bad and the ugly of globalization. *International Diabetes Monitor,* **19,** 5–10.

Unwin, N., Shaw, J., Zimmet, P., *et al.* (2002) Impaired glucose tolerance and impaired fasting glycaemia: the current status on definition and intervention. **19,** 708–23.

Vazquez, G., Duval, S., Jacobs, D.R., JR., *et al.* (2007) Comparison of Body Mass Index, Waist Circumference, and Waist/Hip Ratio in Predicting Incident Diabetes: A Meta-Analysis. *Epidemiol Rev,* **29,** 115–28.

Venkat narayan, K.M., Zhang, P., Kanaya, A.M., *et al.* (2006) Diabetes: The Pandemic and Potential Solutions. In *Disease control priorities in developing countries* (eds. Jamison, D.T., Breman, J.G., Measham, A.R., *et al.*), Second ed. Washington/New York, World Bank/Oxford University Press.

Wannamethee, S.G., Camargo, C.A., JR., Manson, J.E., *et al.* (2003) Alcohol drinking patterns and risk of type 2 diabetes mellitus among younger women. *Archives of Internal Medicine,* **163,** 1329–36.

Whitford, D.L., Griffin, S.J. & Prevost, A.T. (2003) Influences on the variation in prevalence of type 2 diabetes between general practices: practice, patient or socioeconomic factors? *British Journal of General Practice,* **53,** 9–14.

Wild, S., Roglic, G., Green, A., *et al.* (2004) Global prevalence of diabetes: estimates for the year 2000 and projections for 2030. *Diabetes Care,* **27,** 1047–53.

Wilkin, T.J. (2001) The accelerator hypothesis: weight gain as the missing link between Type I and Type II diabetes.[see comment]. *Diabetologia,* **44,** 914–22.

Willett, W.C., Koplan, J.P., Nugent, R., *et al.* (2006) Prevention of Chronic Disease by Means of Diet and Lifestyle Changes. In Jamison, D.T., Breman, J.G., Measham, A.R., *et al.* (Eds.) *Disease control priorities in developing countries.* Second ed. Washington/New York, World Bank/Oxford University Press.

Williams, R. (2005) Medical and economic case for prevention of type 2 diabetes and cardiovascular disease. *Eur Heart J Suppl,* **7,** D14–17.

World Health Organization (1997) Obesity: preventing and managing the global epidemic - Report of a WHO consultation on obesity. Geneva, World Health Organization,.

World Health Organization (1999) Definition, diagnosis, and classification of diabetes mellitus and its complications. Report of a WHO consultation. Part 1: Diagnosis and classification of diabetes mellitus. Geneva.

World Health Organization (2004) Global Strategy on Diet, Physical Activity and Health. Geneva, World Health Organization.

World Health Organization (2005) Preventing chronic diseases: a vital investment: WHO global report. Geneva, World Health Organization.

World Health Organization (2006) Definition and diagnosis of diabetes mellitus and intermediate hyperglycemia: report of a WHO/IDF consultation. Geneva, World Health Organization.

World Health Organization (Forthcoming) Prevention of diabetes mellitus and its complications. Geneva, World Health Organization.

Xu, F., Yin, X.M., Zhang, M., *et al.* (2006) Family average income and diagnosed Type 2 diabetes in urban and rural residents in regional mainland China. *Diabetic Medicine,* **23,** 1239–46.

Yudkin, J. S. (2000) Insulin for the world's poorest countries. *Lancet,* **355,** 919–21.

Zimmet, P. Z. (1992) Kelly West Lecture 1991. Challenges in diabetes epidemiology—from West to the rest. *Diabetes Care,* **15,** 232–52.

Public mental health

Benedetto Saraceno,
Melvyn Freeman, and Michelle Funk

Abstract

Mental health is an integral part of health. Consequently, public mental health is critical to achieving better health in populations. The prevalence of mental disorder is substantial with around 450 million people worldwide suffering from neuropsychiatric conditions. Suicide is among the leading causes of death in 15–45-year-olds. Moreover, mental disorder makes a considerable independent contribution to the burden of disease worldwide—accounting for 13 per cent of the global burden of disease. By 2030, it is estimated that unipolar depression will be the second-highest cause of disability-adjusted life years (DALYs) lost. Globally, the majority of people who need mental health care do not receive it. This 'service gap' is far highest in middle- and low-income countries. There are, however, cost-effective treatments available, and it has been estimated that the benefits of a basic specified package of treatment could lead to a reduction of 2000–3000 DALYs lost per million population. Inadequate and inappropriate mental health systems and services are a major cause of poor mental health outcomes. Decentralization of services and integration of mental health into general health care are critical to improve mental health status in populations. In middle- and low-income countries, additional trained personnel and facilities are required, especially in general health care. Though there are multiple determinants of mental disorder, social and economic factors are fundamental. Poverty, gender discrimination and violence/war are amongst the most important of these. Understanding social determinants is important for planning services; to initiate prevention and promotion; for advocacy and for the information of sectors outside of health that need to assist in improving mental health—such as social development, labour, education, and housing. Finding appropriate and adequate promotive and preventive interventions in mental health is increasing but remains an important area of growth. Given the inextricable connections between mental and physical health, and the importance of mental disorder as a health problem in its own right, this chapter shows that public mental health is central to improved global health.

Introduction

More than 60 years after health was defined in the preamble of the Constitution of the World Health Organization (WHO) as 'a state of complete physical, *mental*, and social well-being, and not merely the absence of disease or infirmity' (WHO 1946), there is still considerable consensus regarding the merit of this definition. Notwithstanding, most countries have not effectively translated this broad conceptualization into health policies and practice. Of particular relevance for this chapter, the 'mental' in the definition has been neglected in public health. This, we maintain, has impeded the realization of better health (both mental and physical) in populations. Nevertheless, public mental health is a rapidly growing discipline and we envisage that it will make a far more substantial contribution to the health status of populations in the future.

There are many reasons for past and current neglect of mental health in health (Saraceno *et al.* 2007). Critical contributory factors include historical deficiencies in information about prevalence, impact, and effective interventions for prevention and treatment and the stigma and discrimination associated with 'abnormalities of the mind'. However, increasing evidence from the study of the epidemiology and burden of mental disorder; mounting knowledge of the relationships between mental and physical health; better understanding of and information on the determinants of mental ill health; increased evidence with regard to prevention and promotion; comprehensive evidence of effective (including cost-effective) interventions for mental disorder and a growing consensus regarding more humane and more efficient ways of organizing mental health systems and services are all contributing to the growing realization that public mental health is vital to improving the health of populations. Though certainly considerably more effort is still needed to 'unblock' various obstacles to the full recognition of mental health as a key public health issue (such as stigma of mental disorder and political commitment to service development in mental health), the reality that mental health interventions are central to health is gaining momentum.

What is mental health, mental disorder, and public mental health?

Developing a consensus around a definition for mental health has proved far more elusive than that attained for health. According to WHO, from a cross-cultural perspective mental health is nearly impossible to define (WHO 2001). Different groups of people value and aspire to different states of well-being and hence mental health is necessarily a matter of ideology. For example, a person who independently achieves great wealth through striving to be better than anyone else and who overcomes all competitors in achieving personal goals may be regarded in one culture as the epitome of success and possibly reflecting superior mental health status. However, in a milieu where collective action and the success of the whole community is valued above individual attainment, the same aspirations and behaviour may be perceived as emotionally astray or even disturbed. Nonetheless, mental health usually includes notions such as subjective well-being, perceived self-efficacy, autonomy, competence, intergenerational dependence, and self-actualizing of one's intellectual and emotional potential (WHO 2001). It has recently been suggested that mental or psychological well-being is part of '. . . an individual's capacity to lead a fulfilling life and that this includes the ability to study, work or pursue leisure interests, and to make day-to-day personal or household decisions about educational, employment, housing and other choices' (WHO 2006b).

Over a number of years, attempts to define and categorize mental and behavioural *disorders* has also proved difficult. However, classification and diagnostic systems such as the International Classification of Mental Disorders (ICD-10) (WHO 1992) and the Diagnostic and Statistical Manual for Mental Disorders DSM -IV-TR (American Psychiatric Association 2000) now allow for a far more scientific categorization of mental disorder and the separation of abnormal or pathological conditions from 'normal' functioning. Mental and behavioural disorders are generally regarded as 'clinically significant conditions characterized by alterations in thinking, mood (emotions) or behaviour associated with personal distress and/or impaired functioning' (WHO 2001). Notwithstanding there is still considerable debate with regard to the impacts of the 'medicalization' of disorder brought about through these instruments, whether diagnostic categories are valid cross-culturally and the importance of the meanings that cultures attribute to symptoms.

Kovel comments that classification and diagnostic instruments such as DSM and ICD encourage the objectification of people. They 'promulgate a structure in which one is simply to observe from the outside . . . and it fosters the discourse of the medical disease in which what is wrong with the person is the disorder that he/she *has*' (Kovel 1988). Thinking about a person in this way is not only 'superficial and instrumental' but encourages the practitioner to forget firstly that the patient has agency and secondly that there are social roots of mental disorder.

While applying diagnostic systems of symptom clusters can be extremely helpful, particularly as this informs treatment, categories may not always have good cultural 'fit' and the treatment required may also be culture specific (see the section 'Brief historical overview of mental health services'). The term 'culture bound syndrome' has been used to describe disturbed behaviour, highly specific to certain cultural systems, which does not conform to Western nosological entities. Given this complexity, diagnosis, especially within cultures that are foreign to individuals, can be fraught with difficulties. Public mental health is concerned with reducing the incidence, prevalence, and impacts of mental disorders and improving the mental health status of populations. In the section 'Mental health as a public health priority', we show that mental and behavioural disorders are indeed a major public health concern. Equally though, optimizing mental health (positive mental health) is an important goal for achieving healthy populations. Furthermore, given the inseparable interrelationship between mental and physical health, public mental health also aims to optimize physical health through mental

and behavioural interventions (see the section 'Treatment efficacy'). The tools of public mental health are no different from other areas of public health; epidemiology, health promotion and prevention, health systems and services development, health economics, and monitoring and evaluation—all play important roles.

Mental health as a public health priority

Different criteria have been used at different times and by different experts in order to decide what health problem is, or should be, regarded as a public health priority. We will show that there is compelling evidence using various criteria and perspectives for prioritizing mental health. These include epidemiological data on mental health, co-morbidity with physical health, treatment efficacy, gaps in current treatment, impacts on individuals and their families, and the ideology of health.

Prevalence of mental disorder

WHO estimates that about 450 million people worldwide suffer from neuropsychiatric conditions (WHO 2001). Mental and behavioural disorders are found in all countries, in women and men at all stages of life, amongst the rich and poor, and amongst rural and urban people.

Surveys to determine the prevalence of mental disorder have been carried out since the end of the World War II; however, the use of a range of different diagnostic instruments and methods have made it difficult to make cross-national comparisons or even assess longitudinal changes within countries. Moreover, different studies have measured 'point prevalence' (people who have a condition at a point in time), 'period prevalence' (presence of disorder in a particular time period such as one year), or 'lifetime prevalence' (having suffered from a disorder at some point in their lives) and, unless it is made very clear in the study what is being measured, and this has not always been the case, comparisons are difficult. Analysis by WHO in 2000 indicated a 10 per cent point prevalence of neuropsychiatric conditions in adults (WHO 2001) and that around 25 per cent of individuals will develop one or more mental or behavioural disorders in their lifetime.

Most studies have found the overall prevalence of mental disorder to be almost the same for men and women. However, almost all studies show a higher prevalence of depression amongst women than men with a ratio of between 1.5:1 and 2:1 as well as higher rates of most anxiety and eating disorders. On the other hand, men have higher rates of attention deficit hyperactivity disorder, autism, and substance abuse disorders (Hyman *et al.* 2006).

In the 1990s, the World Health Organization Composite International Diagnostic Interview (WHO CIDI) was used to determine both prevalence of mental disorder in countries and to assess cross-country differences. While prevalence varied widely, in most countries, more than one third of respondents were found to have had a mental disorder in their lifetime. In 1998, WHO established the World Mental Health (WMH) Survey Consortium to refine the CIDI and conduct mental health surveys around the world. The instrument was modified to measure not only prevalence but also severity, impairment and treatment (WHO 2004). Twenty-eight countries, including both high- and lower-income countries in each region of the world participated in the survey. More than 2 00 000 interviews were conducted. Results of the first 14 countries that had completed the survey were reported in 2004 (WHO World Mental Health Survey

Table 9.7.1 Twelve-month prevalence of WMH CIDI disorders and proportion with mild severity

Country[1]	Percentage prevalence of any mental disorder (95% CI)	Of mild severity[2] (95% CI)
China (Beijing)	9.1 (6–12.1)	5.3 (3.2–7.3)
China (Shanghai)	4.3 (2.7–5.9)	1.8 (0.6–3)
Belgium	12 (9.6–14.3)	6.4 (5–7.7)
Colombia	17.8 (16.1–19.5)	5.9 (5.1–6.8)
France	18.4 (15.3–21.5)	9.7 (7.3–12.1)
Germany	9.1 (7.3–10.8)	4.5 (3.2–5.9)
Italy	8.2 (6.7–9.7)	4.5 (3.2–5.9)
Japan	8.8 (6.4 –11.2)	3.2 (1.7–4.7)
Lebanon	16.9 (13.6–20.2)	6.1 (3.6–8.7)
Mexico	12.2 (10.5–13.8)	4.9 (4–5.8)
Netherlands	14.9 (12.2–17.6)	8.8 (6.1–11.5)
Nigeria	4.7 (3.6–11.2)	3.8 (2.8–4.8)
Spain	9.2 (7.8–10.6)	5.3 (9.4–6.7)
Ukraine	20.5 (17.7–23.2)	8.2 (6.4–10.1)
United States	26.4 (24.7–28)	9.2 (8.1–10.3)

Source: Adapted from World Mental Health Survey Consortium (2004).

[1] Though all sites measured mental disorder in adults there are substantial cross-national differences in age structure between countries with more younger people assessed in developing countries.

[2] Severity was assessed in terms of ability to carry out normal daily activities and rated as severe, moderate, or mild in terms of the Sheehan Disability Scale or the Global Assessment of Functioning.

Table 9.7.2 Mean (95% confidence interval) estimates of the population prevalence (%) of schizophrenia[1]

Point prevalence	0.46 (0.19–1)
12-month prevalence	0.33 (.13–.82)
Lifetime prevalence	0.4 (.16–1.2)
Lifetime morbid risk	0.72 (.31–2.7)

Source: Adapted from Saha et al. (2005)

[1] A systematic review of 188 studies conducted in 46 countries was conducted. All studies that reported primary data on the prevalence of schizophrenia between 1965 and 2002 were included.

No significant differences were found between males and females and between urban, rural, and mixed sites. In terms of economic status, the prevalence estimates from lower-income countries were significantly lower than both 'emerging' and high-income sites.

Not many prevalence studies have been conducted on psychotic disorders other than schizophrenia, though the lifetime prevalence of bipolar disorder, like schizophrenia is often assumed to be about 1 per cent (Perälä *et al.* 2007). A recent comprehensive study of psychotic and bipolar I disorders in Finland found a lifetime prevalence of psychotic disorders of 3.06 per cent. Lifetime prevalence of schizophrenia was 0.87 per cent, schizoaffective disorder 0.32 per cent, schizophreniform disorder 0.07 per cent, delusional disorder 0.18 per cent, bipolar I disorder 0.24 per cent, major depressive disorder with psychotic features 0.35 per cent, substance-induced psychotic disorder 0.42 per cent, and 0.21 per cent for psychotic disorders due to a medical condition (Perälä *et al.* 2007).

Mortality

Causes of mortality are sometimes used to determine priority levels of different disorders. While mental disorders in themselves have relatively low mortality rates, mental disorders, particularly depression and substance abuse, are associated with more than 90 per cent of all cases of suicide (Bertolote *et al.* 2004) and the incidence of suicide is substantial. WHO has reported that in 2000 around 1 million people died from suicide. The 'global' mortality rate was 16 per 1000—or a death through suicide every 40 seconds. Global suicidal rates for 2006 are shown in Fig. 9.7.1. Nearly 20 times this number attempt suicide. Moreover official suicide rates are usually substantially underestimated. In an Indian study using surveillance with validated verbal autopsy, the observed rates exceeded official national estimates tenfold (Aaron *et al.* 2004).

According to WHO, suicide is among the three leading causes of death among 15–45-year-olds (men and women). The numbers of suicides has increased by 60 per cent over a 45-year period. In 2002, it was estimated that self-inflicted injuries were the fourteenth highest cause of all deaths. Projections to 2030 suggest that this will rise to twelfth place in the causes of death (Mathers & Loncar 2006).

Raised non-suicide-related mortality has also been found in, for example, people living with schizophrenia, bipolar disorder, and dementia (Heila *et al.* 2005; Ösby *et al.* 2001; Dewey & Saz 2001). A major investigation by the Disability Rights Commission (England and Wales) found that people with learning disabilities and mental health problems do not live as long as other citizens. Individuals with serious mental health problems were more likely to get strokes and coronary heart disease before 55 years of age and to survive for

Consortium 2004). This included three countries in the Americas, seven in Europe, one in the Middle East, one in Africa, and two in Asia. Six countries were classified by the World Bank as less developed and the others developed.

As seen in Table 9.7.1, the overall prevalence varied from 4.3 per cent in Shanghai, China, to 26.4 per cent in the United States with a 9.1–16.9 per cent inter-quartile range (WHO 2004). The most common disorders found were anxiety and depression (with a high level of co-morbidity). In all but one country, anxiety disorder had the highest prevalence (2.4–18.2 per cent) followed by depression (0.8–9.6). Importantly the proportion of disorders classified as mild is substantial—from 33.1 per cent in Colombia to 80.9 per cent in Nigeria. However in cases of serious mental disorder most respondents reported at least 30 days in the past year where they were totally unable to carry out their usual activities.

It has been recognized by the designers of the WMHS that some of the variation found may be attributable to extraneous factors. For example, perceived stigma is likely to have played an important part in the lower prevalence rate observed in those countries were mental health stigma is highest (Kessler *et al.* 2006).

Determining the prevalence of serious mental disorder, such as schizophrenia, usually requires more specialized and specific studies than the one above and a number have been conducted. A systematic review by Saha and colleagues (Saha *et al.* 2005) identified 188 studies conducted between 1965 and 2002. Table 9.7.2 shows the mean estimates found.

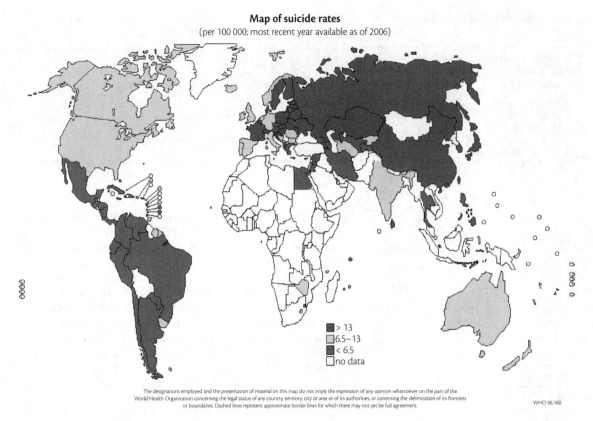

Fig. 9.7.1 Map of suicide rates.
Source: WHO webpage on Suicide Prevention: http://www.who.int/mental_health/prevention/suicide/suicideprevent/en/index.html

less than 5 years thereafter (Disability Rights Commission 2006). Reasons for this include the fact that people with serious mental disorder often live in social deprivation (see the subsection 'Social determinants of mental (ill) health'), but also that the health services discriminate against people with mental health problems. They are less likely to receive medical checks and to be provided with evidence-based treatment.

Burden of disease

While morbidity and mortality are important measures for making health decisions, they fail to take into account important variables necessary for health planning. In response, a joint initiative of the WHO, the World Bank and Harvard University designed and conducted the Global Burden of Disease study. The GBD approach uses a summary measure—DALY—to quantify the burden of disease. DALYs combine the years of life lost due to premature mortality (YLL) in the population and the years lost to due to disability (YLD) for incident cases of the health condition.

The prominence of mental and neurological disorders from the GBD study relative to other disorders was a major revelation to many people and countries. When the DALY figures were first published in 1993, most countries found a major mismatch between the burden of mental health (10.5 per cent of all DALYs lost) and the prominence and attention given it. This was because traditionally only incidence/prevalence and mortality were measured in most international and national statistics. While these indices were well suited to acute diseases that either resulted in death or full recovery, mental and behavioural disorders, which more often cause disability, did not feature prominently. With the loss of 'healthy life' being elevated,

mental and neurological disorders were catapulted into the limelight. Moreover projections showed that the burden due to mental disorders was likely to substantially increase relative to other health conditions. In 2002, mental and substance use disorders accounted for 13 per cent of the GBD (WHO 2004). When taking only the disability component of the burden of disease into account, mental and neurological conditions accounted for 30.8 per cent of all years lived with disability.

In 2006, Mathers and Loncar published an update of earlier DALY figures and projections on the burden of disease (Mathers & Loncar 2006). Estimates are now available up to 2030. Importantly for public mental health, as predicted, the relative burden of mental disorder is rising and is set to rise even further. By far the highest mental health cause of DALYs lost is unipolar depressive disorder and this disorder alone is likely to be the second-highest cause of all DALYs lost by 2030—second only to HIV/AIDS. In high-income countries, depression will become the single-highest cause of DALYs lost.

In Table 9.7.4, the three leading causes of DALYs lost, projected to 2030, by income group, are presented. Crucially unipolar depressive disorder is amongst the top three causes of DALYs lost in high-, middle-, and low-income countries.

Interrelationship between physical and mental health

Over the past 20 years, a fundamental and inseparable interconnection between mental and physical health has been established (WHO 2001) While thoughts, feelings, and behaviour have a major impact on physical health, physical health strongly influences mental health and well-being. There are two key pathways through which the physical and mental interact—firstly through physiological systems such

Table 9.7.3 Changes in ranking for leading causes of DALYs lost, 2002 and 2030—World

Disease or injury	2002 rank	2030 rank	Change in rank
Perinatal conditions	1	5	−4
Lower respiratory infections	2	8	−6
HIV/AIDS	3	1	+2
Unipolar depressive disorder	4	2	+2
Diarrhoeal diseases	5	12	−7
Ischaemic heart disease	6	3	+3
Cerebrovascular disease	7	6	+1
Road traffic accidents	8	4	+4
Malaria	9	15	−6
Tuberculosis	10	25	−15
COPD	11	7	+4
Congenital abnormalities	12	20	−8
Hearing loss, adult onset	13	9	+4
Cataracts	14	10	+4
Violence	15	13	+2
Self-inflicted violence	17	14	+3

Source: Adapted from Mathers *et al.* (2006).

Table 9.7.4 Leading causes of DALYs lost by income group—2030

Income group	Rank	Disease or injury	Per cent total DALYs lost
World	1	HIV/AIDS	12.1
	2	Unipolar depressive disorder	5.7
	3	Ischaemic heart disease	4.7
High-income countries	1	Unipolar depressive disorder	9.8
	2	Ischaemic heart disease	5.9
	3	Alzheimer and other dementias	5.8
Middle-income countries	1	HIV/AIDS	9.8
	2	Unipolar depressive disorder	6.7
	3	Cerebrovascular disease	6.0
Low-income countries	1	HIV/AIDS	14.6
	2	Perinatal conditions	5.8
	3	Unipolar depressive disorder	4.7

Source: Adapted from Mathers *et al.* (2006).

as neuroendocrine and immune functioning, and secondly through health behaviour (WHO 2001). However, these pathways are not independent in that behaviour may affect physiology, while physiological functioning may in turn affect health behaviour.

There are numerous examples of how mental health status may impact on physical health and vice versa. At least one-third of all somatic symptoms remain medically unexplained. Common symptoms include pain, fatigue, and dizziness, while defined syndromes include irritable bowel syndrome, fibromyalgia, chronic fatigue syndrome, chronic pelvic pain, and tempero-mandibular joint dysfunction (Prince *et al.* 2007). Somatization is present in around 15 per cent of patients seen in primary care and is independently associated with poor-health-related quality of life and increased healthcare utilization (Barsky *et al.* 2005).

A review by Prince *et al.* has shown strong evidence from population-based research for moderate to strong prospective associations between depression and anxiety and coronary heart disease outcomes including angina and non-fatal and fatal myocardial infarctions. They also showed strong evidence that depression is an independent risk factor for stroke. Depression is increased after myocardial infarction, mostly in the first month after the event. There is also strong evidence for co-morbidity between mental disorder and diabetes. The prevalence of diabetes among people with schizophrenia has consistently been found to be in the order of 15 per cent compared to a typical community prevalence of 2–3 per cent (Holt *et al.* 2005).

The interrelationships between physical and mental health are highly complex. Here, we illustrate five important mechanisms of this relationship through the example of mental health and HIV/AIDS.

Mental health status increases the risk of infection

In the United States, people with severe mental illness are nearly 20 times more likely to be infected with HIV than the general population

(McKinnon & Rosner 2000). Reasons for this include a lack of appreciation of risk, impaired social interactions, low levels of assertiveness, low use of condoms, injecting drug use, multiple partners, sexual activity within closed environments such as institutions, and homelessness. Though this relationship has not been documented in low- and middle-income countries, and though the ratio would inevitably be lower, the reasons for high-risk sexual behaviour and the chances of transmission within psychiatric institutions pertain at least as much to people in low- and middle-income countries as they do to those in high-income countries. High risk of infection is also not limited to severe mental disorder. In South Africa, depression in youth has been significantly correlated with risky sexual behaviour (Moghraby *et al.* 2005).

HIV infection directly affects the central nervous system functioning

The HIV virus has numerous direct impacts, including on the central nervous system. HIV dementia and minor cognitive disorder are common in people living with HIV/AIDS who are not taking anti-retroviral treatment with between 30 per cent and 50 per cent of HIV-seropositive individuals experiencing cognitive-motor problems (Grant *et al.* 1999). HIV invades the brain early in the infection process and in a certain proportion of people psychotic symptoms manifest—especially in late-stage AIDS. Manic episodes are above the population norm in people with HIV (around 5 per cent), especially at more advanced stages of the disease (Catalan *et al.* 2000). It is clear that a disease that attacks the immune system of the body also has direct 'mental' manifestations.

Psychological impacts

Studies of the mental health status of people infected with HIV have consistently found higher prevalence of mental health problems than is found in community or clinic samples. From the research thus far it has not been possible to reliably separate out people who may have had a pre-existing mental disorder from those that may have developed mental disorder following a positive HIV diagnosis. Moreover the extent to which mood and anxiety disorder may be caused directly by the viral infection itself is not clear. However, we know from qualitative research that receiving a diagnosis of HIV and living with the disease can be highly psychologically distressing.

High levels of major depression, mild depressive disorder, and dysthymia have all been found in seropositive individuals. Bing and his co-researchers found a 36 per cent one-year prevalence of depression among a large national sample of HIV-positive men and women in the United States (Bing *et al.* 2001). This is substantially higher than found in the general population. Ciesla and colleagues conducted a meta-analysis of studies comparing HIV-positive and HIV-negative samples and found that major depressive disorder occurred nearly twice as often among people living with HIV (Ciesla & Roberts 2001). In a review of studies of mental health problems of HIV infected people in developing countries, Collins *et al.* also found a significantly higher prevalence of depressive symptoms among HIV-positive people compared with controls (Collins *et al.* 2006).

Feelings of anxiety and distress are a normal and arguably even a healthy response to a diagnosis of HIV. However anxiety may reach clinical levels and impair overall functioning and people's capacity for adequate self care. The prevalence of anxiety disorders in studies in the United States range from negligible to around 40 per cent. Anxiety can be provoked by the unpredictability of the virus and by certain 'milestones' such as initial diagnosis, first opportunistic infection, declining CD4 count or the onset or progression of an AIDS defining illness.

Influencing the course of the disease

To maintain good health a person living with HIV/AIDS (PLHA) must engage in a number of 'health promoting' behaviours and maintain a 'positive' attitude towards themselves and towards the virus. For example, a PLHA must engage in protected sex to avoid reinfection, they should eat nutritious food, refrain from excessive use of alcohol, not smoke cigarettes, immediately seek treatment for opportunistic infections when needed, and, if they are on antiretroviral treatment (ART), they must adhere to their medication regimen.

A review by Uldall *et al.* (2004) found a number of studies that showed that poor mental health was a barrier to ART adherence. This association was particularly significant in women. At least eight studies have showed that adherence to antiretroviral medication is adversely affected by mood disturbance. In addition, research indicates associations between poor adherence and generalized anxiety disorder, panic disorder, post-traumatic stress disorder (PTSD), recent trauma, and social phobia.

Side effects of medication

Another way that the physical and the mental interact is when medication is given to treat a physical problem and there are mental side effects. (Of course, the opposite is often also true whereby medication given to treat a mental condition has physical side effects such as tardive dyskinesia.) In a minority of patients receiving anti-retroviral therapy, mania and psychosis can occur due to the medication they receive such as AZT, 3TC, efavirenz, abacavir, and nevirapine. Patients who have had multiple episodes of depression are at particular risk of having negative reactions to efavirenz.

Treatment efficacy

Having effective (including cost-effective) treatments available is another crucial component of whether a health condition should be prioritized. Most mental disorders can be effectively treated and at a cost that justifies intervention. Whiteford suggests that the burden of illness on the individual and society combined with treatment efficacy could be used as the basis of decisions to allocate resources (Whiteford 2000). Interventions that demonstrate the greatest health gain for the lowest cost would be the most highly prized. Mental health interventions fall into this category.

A recent analysis by the WHO of the comparative effectiveness and costs of pharmacological and psychosocial interventions for reducing the burden of mental disorders found the following (WHO 2006a):

Pharmacological interventions

Both conventional neuroleptic and newer 'atypical' antipsychotic drugs are effective in treating psychosis. Both types of medication have similar efficacy though the former are less expensive. It is therefore recommended that in countries with limited resources (and until such time as newer drugs come off their patents) conventional neuroleptic drugs should be provided.

Both older tricyclic anti-depressants (TCAs) and selective serotonin reuptake inhibitors (SSRIs) are effective in treating depression. Costs and effectiveness of medication vary in different contexts, and therefore the drug treatment of choice should be driven by patient or clinical preferences and local costs.

Psychosocial interventions

Psychosocial treatment, alongside pharmacological treatment for severe disorders such as schizophrenia and bipolar affective disorder, is expected to result in substantial health gains. A combined strategy is more cost-effective than pharmacotherapy on its own.

Psychotherapy is expected to be as cost-effective as most medication for people with depression or anxiety disorders.

Case management

It is expected that long-term maintenance treatment of depression with pharmacological and psychosocial interventions is a more cost-effective strategy than episodic treatments as it prevents a proportion of recurrent depressive episodes.

The mental health service gap

Another reason to prioritize a condition is if the gap between the existence of a condition and the numbers of people being treated for it (especially if effective treatments are available), or programmes to prevent it, is high. Kohn and colleagues reviewed community-based psychiatric epidemiology studies and calculated the median rates of untreated cases of various mental disorders (Kohn *et al.* 2004). The median treatment gaps are found in Table 9.7.5.

These figures are major underestimates of the gaps globally as most of the data available are from high-income countries that have far greater availability of services. For example, in the only condition where a figure was available for Africa, there was a 67 per cent treatment gap for major depression compared with a 45.4 per cent gap for Europe. In the World Mental Health Survey, 35.5–50.3 per cent of serious cases of mental disorder in high-income countries and 76.3–85.4 per cent in middle- and low-income countries received no treatment in the 12 months before the interview (WHO World Mental Health Survey Consortium 2004).

Table 9.7.5 Treatment gaps for mental disorder—world

Mental disorder	Median treatment gap[1]
Schizophrenia and other non-affective psychotic disorders	32.2%
Depression	56.3%
Dysthymia	56%
Bipolar disorder	50.2%
Panic disorder	55.9%
Generalized anxiety disorder	57.5%
Obsessive compulsive disorder	57.3%
Alcohol abuse and dependence	78.1%

Source: Adapted from Kohn *et al.* (2004)
[1] Treatment gap represents the absolute difference between the true prevalence of a disorder and the treated proportion of individuals over 15 affected by the disorder.

Clearly, the majority of people needing mental health interventions are not receiving it. Some of the reasons for the gap include a lack of identification of mental health problems by health workers; sufferers themselves not seeking treatment due to stigma, fear, or lack of knowledge that they have a treatable condition; lack of or unavailability of resources; seeking assistance elsewhere due to cultural beliefs; affordability; and poor health systems that do not allow or encourage treatment in the community. For many people, the only time they might receive treatment is if they become so disruptive in their families or communities that they are given involuntary treatment.

Personal and family impacts

The GBD study estimated that, in 2000, mental and neurological disorders accounted for 30.8 per cent of all years lived with disability—with depression accounting for 12 per cent of all disability (WHO 2004). This though does not capture the economic and psychological stress to individuals and their families resulting from this disability.

'Days out of role' is a very important measure of the macroeconomic impacts of mental disorder (WHO 2006a); however, for individuals and families, this very often means a direct and personal loss of income (especially where there are no or poor unemployment benefits). Moreover, a family member, often a woman spouse or parent, has to take time off from income-generating activities to care for the person with mental disorder. Income into the family is hence further eroded. Furthermore, due to the person's mental disorder there are additional health care and usually transport costs (to get to a treatment centre) that need to be paid for (Patel & Kleinman 2003). As mental disorder is often chronic, these costs may be ongoing. In addition, in many countries, insurance payouts for mental disorder are limited (even discriminatory relative to other health problems). Thus, health care may become even less accessible and less available with time—and so the condition deteriorates and the need for care increases. The result of this cycle is often a 'drift' into poverty, with little chance for a person to move back to their pre-mental disorder life situation.

Being ill with any condition can be psychologically debilitating. This is exacerbated if one is forced out of work by one's condition and one has to become dependent on others. But when this condition is also quite frightening to oneself and one sometimes feels out of

control, when the condition is shrouded in stigma, where blame is often put on the ill person themselves and where appropriate treatment is not readily available (WHO 2001), the condition can become psychologically devastating to the individual concerned.

For families too, having a person develop and live with mental disorder, can be frightening, extremely disruptive, and a major economic burden. Especially where information and support are not available, family members may be inclined to just want to get rid of the person or to restrain or seclude them. Families too often become the object of discrimination. It has been found that carers who provide someone with substantial support are twice as likely to have mental health problems as those they are caring for (Singleton *et al.* 2007).

In many countries, access to and knowledge of treatment is so poor that it is only when the ill person becomes so disruptive in their family and community and they can no longer be dealt with, that help is sought. At this point, the patient is often unwilling or unable to co-operate and so involuntary care and treatment is required. Poor service accessibility hence results in higher proportions of people receiving care without their consent than would otherwise be the case.

Ideology of health

There is no health without mental health. This seemingly simple assertion, which flows directly from the WHO definition of health, contains a number of important inter-related meanings and has major practical implications for health and health services. Firstly, any reference to health or ill-health or any health condition invariably includes a mental health component. Hence, where a person has developed or contracted a 'physical' disease (communicable or non-communicable), or has even been physically injured, there is usually also a mental aspect that needs consideration. This is important—whether mental health may have been a risk factor of the presenting problem (for example, depression underlying risky sex behaviour resulting in HIV/AIDS or an alcohol problem resulting in a car accident), or is a secondary outcome. Mental health should thus be integral to *all* health assessments and treatment. Secondly, the assertion implies that a state of optimal health also implies a state of optimal mental health. Initiatives directed at attaining good population health should thus include considerations of mental health. Thirdly, if a state of health includes both physical and mental health, then clearly there can be no 'health' if mental disorder is present. Attending to mental health problems should therefore have parity with regard to treatment and prevention of physical conditions. Finally, following from the above points, health policy, health systems, and health service development should always include a mental health component. Hence, there should not only be no health without mental health, but no health *service* that does not provide mental health. Brundtland, a previous Director-General of the WHO, commented that 'talking about health without mental health is a little like tuning an instrument and leaving a few discordant notes' (WHO 2001).

The highly complex nature of human beings involves interacting biological, social, and *mental* components, and to accurately understand and improve human health, all three elements, and the interactions between them, need focus (WHO 2001). Critically, human beings are not mechanical automatons that 'break down' from time to time, but are dynamic and active beings that substantially shape their own state of health and illness. For example, a person's eating habits, the amount of exercise they do, whether they avoid dangerous situations such as drinking and driving or having unsafe sex, and whether they take the medication that is prescribed and in the manner instructed, and whether they seek health care at an early stage of an illness are all fundamental to healthy human states and rely irrevocable on human agency—though decisions are often not taken at a conscious level and are often made without adequate information. People may also be limited in what they can do by their socioeconomic conditions.

Clearly then, mental factors, including personal volition and individual behaviour, are as important to states of health as are biological and social factors. Importantly though, mental states do not have an independent existence from the biological and the social and are in themselves shaped in interaction with these elements. Similarly, the mental states shape the biological and the social components. Hence, while it is useful to theoretically separate out the 'contributors' to health, this is an analytic exercise rather than an empirical one. The interacting process between the components begins at birth and stops only at death. Yet, despite this 'empowering' people to make 'healthy' decisions is seldom seen as an important health intervention (Peterson & Swartz 2002).

In addition to the impacts on health through behaviour, as previously seen, physical and mental states of well-being mutually affect each other (see the section 'Interrelationship between physical and mental health').

Mental disorders, like other health problems, also have physical, psychological, and social components. Hence, in treating and preventing mental disorder, all three components must also be considered. The mental aspect of health probably captures that which is 'most human' in health and without which much of human health care may be likened to veterinary medicine. Considering human health without mental health then is fundamentally flawed, and health policy, systems, and services that neglect the 'mental' side will inevitably be less effectual in improving the health status of populations than those that include mental health.

Cost effectiveness of treatment for mental disorders

The economic costs associated with mental disorder are considerable. Conservative estimates across the 15 countries of the European Union found mental health costs to be at least 3–4 per cent of gross national product. The majority of costs occur outside the health sector, being due to lost employment, absenteeism, poor performance, and premature retirement (McDaid 2005). These costs account for between 60 per cent and 80 per cent of the total economic impact. Millions of working days are lost because of mental health. In France, in 2000, nearly 32 million working days were lost due to depression alone. Though estimates are not available from lower-income countries it is likely that the costs of mental disorders as a proportion of the overall economy are also high (WHO 2001).

Given the high estimates of the burden of mental disorders and cost-effective treatments available (see the subsection 'Treatment efficacy'), Hyman et al. calculated the burden that could be averted by efficacious treatment for schizophrenia, bipolar disorder, depression, and panic disorder. A model was developed that included giving no treatment at all, current treatment, and scaled-up treatment. The model derived the number of additional healthy years gained (equivalent with DALYs averted) each year compared with the outcome of no treatment at all (Hyman et al. 2006). In Table 9.7.6, the estimated costs and effects of a package consisting of a basic mental health

services for the four conditions is outlined. The authors estimate that the benefit of this package would be an annual reduction of 2000–3000 DALYs per million population at a cost of US$3 million to US$9 million (that is US$3–4 per capita in sub-Saharan Africa and South Asia, and US$7–9 per capita in Latin America and the Caribbean). This means that for every US$1 million invested in such a mental health package, 350–700 healthy years of life would be gained over no intervention.

However, even if healthy life years could be gained, how affordable would such mental health interventions be? When set against the gross domestic product per capita, the WHO have found that:

◆ The interventions recommended in the package for depression and anxiety can be considered very cost-effective. Each healthy year gained costs less than one year of average per capita income.

◆ Older anti-psychotic and mood-stabilizing drugs as part of community-based interventions can be considered moderately cost-effective for severe mental disorders. Each healthy year gained costs less than three times average income.

◆ Atypical anti-psychotic drugs at current international prices, especially if delivered in hospital based settings, are not cost-effective in the context of most low- and middle-income countries as each healthy year gained costs significantly more than three times average annual income.

While mental health interventions do not compare favourably in terms of the above affordability criteria with health actions such as vaccinations or tuberculosis control, the WHO estimates that there is just as much economic justification for mental health care as there is for anti-retroviral therapy for AIDS, glycaemic control of diabetes, and cholesterol control with statins (WHO 2006b).

Mental health systems and services

Two critical reasons for poor mental health status of populations is that people do not receive care when they need it (care is not available or accessible) and when treatment is provided it is not given effectively or efficiently. These problems can primarily be attributed to inadequate and inappropriate health systems and services for the delivery of mental health, though personal and social reasons (such as stigma) also inhibit good care.

Brief historical overview of mental health services

Different cultures have viewed mental illness from vastly different perspectives, and hence there has not been one history of mental health care but many highly diverse examples. Still today, the provision of mental health services is often based on misunderstandings about the causes, consequences, and treatment of people with mental disorders. According to Tyrer et al., some of the earliest reports of 'madness' date back to the Anglo-Saxon period where it was generally thought that people exhibiting symptoms of mental disorder were possessed by the devil (Tyrer & Steinberg 1998). Accordingly, the treatment, when available, centred around the practice of exorcism. Those that were not afforded this 'luxury of leniency' were either left to wander aimlessly in a neglected state or were punished by being chained up, beaten, or ultimately burned at stake. In medieval times, in the United Kingdom, there was a shift towards acknowledging that the mad were in fact ill and were treated together with other people who were ill.

Table 9.7.6 Estimated costs and effects of a package consisting of basic mental health services, by region

	Sub-Saharan Africa	Latin America, Caribbean	Middle East, North Africa	Europe, Central Asia	South Asia	East Asia, Asia-Pacific
Total effect (DALYs averted per year per 1 million population)						
Schizophrenia: older antipsychotic drug plus psychosocial treatment	254	373	364	353	300	392
Bipolar; older mood-stabilizing drug plus psychosocial treatment	312	365	322	413	346	422
Depression: proactive care with newer antidepressant drug (SSRI; generic)	1174	1953	1806	1789	1937	1747
Panic disorder: newer antidepressant drug (SSRI; generic)	245	307	287	307	284	330
Total effect of interventions	1985	2998	2779	2862	2867	2891
Total cost (US$ million per year per 1 million population)						
Schizophrenia: older antipsychotic drug plus psychosocial treatment	0.47	1.81	1.61	1.32	0.52	0.75
Bipolar; older mood-stabilizing drug plus psychosocial treatment	0.48	1.80	1.23	1.39	0.62	0.95
Depression: proactive care with newer antidepressant drug (SSRI; generic)	1.80	4.80	3.99	3.56	2.81	2.59
Panic disorder: newer antidepressant drug (SSRI; generic)	0.15	0.27	0.21	0.23	0.16	0.20
Total effect of interventions	2.9	8.7	7	6.5	4.1	4.5
Cost-effectiveness (DALYs averted per US$1 million expenditure)						
Schizophrenia: older antipsychotic drug plus psychosocial treatment	544	206	226	267	574	
Bipolar; older mood-stabilizing drug plus psychosocial treatment	647	203	262	298	560	
Depression: proactive care with newer antidepressant drug (SSRI; generic)	652	407	452	502	690	
Panic disorder: newer antidepressant drug (SSRI; generic)	1588	1155	1339	1350	1765	

Source: Adapted from Hyman *et al.* (2006).

In traditional Chinese medicine, mental disorders were considered, in the same way as physical disorders, to be due to imbalances in the internal organs. The treatment of mental illness was aimed at restoring physiological function and balance (Chang *et al.* 2002). Specialized treatment for the mentally ill was introduced to China by foreign missionaries in the late 1800s, with the establishment of the first asylums. According to Chang *et al.* in the 1950s, the health of the people of China became symbolically intertwined with the health of the new regimen with psychiatric treatment linked with achieving the goals of the 'collective good' and assisting the patient to fulfill his or her prescribed role in society. Unique models have since developed taking into account the cultural, social, political and resource factors in the country. For example the 'Shanghai model' involves inter alia community mental health networks that provide follow-up and rehabilitation in the community. Rehabilitation is implemented through guardianship networks consisting of trained volunteers who supervise individual patients, maintain treatment schedules and provide family support (Chang *et al.* 2002).

Meanings given to behaviour and the resultant intervention is also well illustrated through examination of 'bizarre' behavioural symptoms in isiZulu-speaking communities in South Africa. The syndromes of '*amafufunyana*' and '*ukuthwasa*' are relatively common, and the 'symptoms' of both overlap with ICD 10 and DSM IVTR schizophrenia and other psychotic disorders (Niehaus *et al.* 2004). However, these conditions are understood very differently from allopathic interpretations of mental disorder, and indeed from each other. *Ukuthwasa* is understood as a form of ancestor possession that signifies a calling to become a healer. By removing herself (it is usually a women) to live with a healer/teacher and become a healer herself, the *Thwasa* sufferer is able to overcome the symptoms. On the other hand, *amafufunyana* is caused by spirit possession. Rituals to appease the ancestors usually need to be performed to rid the person of the cause of the usually uncontrollable behaviour exhibited.

The first documented moves to treat people with mental illness in segregated facilities in the United Kingdom was at the turn of the fifteenth century, when the first hospital for the treatment of people with mental illness was set up—Bethlem Hospital. In Europe, during the eighteenth and nineteenth centuries, people with mental illness were moved to large asylums that were built for this purpose. This trend was later exported to Africa, the Americas, and Asia (WHO 2001). The initial aims of these asylums were therapeutic but soon turned into impersonal institutions (Tyrer & Steinberg 1998). At the peak of institutional care in the mid-twentieth century, hundreds of thousands of people were kept in institutions. In the United Kingdom and the United States alone, there were 155000 and 559000 people in asylums, respectively (Hafner & an der Heiden 1989).

In the mid-twentieth century, there was a major ideological and organizational shift away from large institutions towards more community-based care and treatment. Many reasons have been given for this change including the introduction of neuroleptics in the mid-1950s; fiscal considerations (institutional care was seen as expensive); sociological criticisms and an increase in human rights advocacy and the anti-psychiatry movement (Tyrer & Steinberg 1998; Prior 1991; Drew & Funk 2006). It is likely that all of these factors played some role. In any event, in countries that had very high asylum bed to population ratios, significant decreases of bed numbers occurred.

Probably the most radical example of the move away from large mental asylums occurred in Italy. In 1978, 'Psichiatrica Democratica' under the leadership of Franco Basaglia came to fruition through Law 180. The law stated that no patient could be admitted to existing psychiatric asylums and demanded that all chronic patients be gradually discharged from hospital. All existing psychiatric hospitals were to be unlocked and the civil liberties of patients returned to them. Provision was made for 15 beds (maximum) in general hospitals. Importantly, the pressures that brought the changes came predominantly from community groups. The fact that this reform was a social movement towards integrating and accepting the mentally ill into the community distinguishes this experience from any other deinstitutionalization and remains a central ingredient of the Italian success (Scheper-Hughes & Lovell 1986).

All the above examples illustrate how the social and political environment and the cultural meanings ascribed to mental disorder have shaped and continue to shape the treatment and care approach.

Current mental health services

Formal mental health services in many parts of the world, especially in poorer countries, are characterized by poor accessibility, inadequate resources, and far from optimal organization of services. Most people with mental disorders do not have medical care for their conditions (Funk *et al.* 2005). Many people rely on traditional remedies and traditional healers for their mental health care.

Availability of mental health professionals is a major inhibitor to treatment. Table 9.7.7 shows the median number of psychiatrists, psychiatric nurses, and psychologists working in mental health per 100000 population per region (WHO 2005).

People with mental disorders often access health care in large isolated mental health institutions. A disproportionate proportion of most country's mental health budget is spent in these institutions (WHO 2001). However, in Table 9.7.8, it can be seen that despite significant discharge of patients from psychiatric hospitals in

Table 9.7.7 Median number of mental health professionals per 100000 population in WHO regions

Region	Psychiatrists	Psychiatric nurses	Psychologists
Africa	0.04	0.2	0.05
Americas	2	2.6	2.8
Eastern Mediterranean	0.95	1.25	0.6
Europe	9.8	24.8	3.1
Southeast Asia	0.2	0.1	0.03
Western Pacific	0.32	0.5	0.03
World	1.2	2	0.6

Source: WHO Mental Health Atlas 2005 (WHO 2005).

higher-income countries and a concomitant development of community mental health services, there are still far more beds per capita in high-income than in lower-income countries. Hence, though the vast majority of mental health resources in low- and middle-income countries are indeed spent on psychiatric hospitals, these facilities still have far fewer beds per 10000 population than is available in higher-income countries. Though for low- and middle-income countries, moving resources out of psychiatric hospitals is a necessity as additional resources for much needed mental health care in the community is often not available, reduction of bed numbers is from an already very low base.

Accessibility of services

There are a number of reasons why access to services may be limited. Here we consider only two issues: Geographical and financial access.

Geographical accessibility

Primary care is usually the first access point for people needing health care. Many countries have put considerable effort into providing health care as near to people's homes or places of work as possible through initiatives such as community or village health worker programmes and the expansion of health posts and clinics to underserved areas. Health posts or clinics have extended their hours to make it easier for working people to access and to treat people when they fall ill outside of normal working hours. However, many (if not most) of these primary care initiatives have not included mental health.

Table 9.7.8 Hospital beds for mental disorder for WHO regions

Region	Median hospital beds for mental disorder per 10000 population	Per cent of beds in mental hospitals
Africa	0.34	73%
Americas	2.6	80.6%
Eastern Mediterranean	1.07	83%
Europe	8	63.5%
Southeast Asia	0.33	82.7%
Western Pacific	1.06	60.1%
World	1.69	68.6%

Source: WHO Mental Health Atlas 2005 (WHO 2005).

The principle of 'no health without mental health' has not been applied. Some of the reasons put forward regarding why mental health has not been included are that health workers are not trained or supported to do mental health interventions, staff do not have time for mental health and reluctance and fear amongst health workers to see people with mental health problems due to the 'otherness' of mental health. Similarly, most general hospitals do not admit and treat people with mental health problems. Staff at general hospitals are often reluctant to admit people with mental health problems into the general wards as patients with mental disorder are perceived as being disruptive (and sometimes are) and no dedicated psychiatric wards have been set up.

Poor accessibility at primary care and general hospital levels forces people to either not receive care at all or to try and access care at a centralized psychiatric hospital. However, because of the work pressures that people at the psychiatric institutions are under and because the hospital is usually designated as a 'specialist' level, even if the patient does manage to get to the hospital, they are often turned away as the hospital has many more severe cases that have to be dealt with. The outcome of the limited primary care service is that the less severe problems become more severe. When this occurs, the patient may finally receive care at the psychiatric hospital (but by this time often as an involuntary patient). Then, because of the distance of the hospital from the community, family and other community members may not be able to visit the patient, and the patient may lose contact with them. Moreover, if hospitalization has become necessary because the person became disruptive, the family and community often do not want the individual back when they do recover. In many countries, there are no community facilities for the person to be (down) referred to; hence, the progression that started when the person could not access primary or general hospital care continues with the individual becoming a chronic patient in the institution. The alienation of this experience then psychologically 'institutionalizes' them, and

discharge becomes even more difficult. Early and accessible care may have prevented this progression with minimal harm to the person concerned and would have been considerably less expensive to the state!

Financial accessibility

Different countries have different policies on the financing of health care and mental health care in particular. Where mental health services are not free, this has critical consequences for accessibility. It will be shown (see the section 'Understanding the determinants of mental health') that many people who need mental health services are poor, and even if they did not start that way, many drift into poverty. In addition, because many mental health conditions are chronic, health expenses tend to be relatively high. For an individual, ongoing medication and occasional hospitalization may be required.

Moreover, especially where mental health care is not obtainable at a local level (but also then), there may be a number of additional costs for the individual and their family. For example, transport to the facility to get medication and review may be prohibitive. Furthermore, because of their condition, the patient may need to be accompanied to the place they receive care. The accompanying person would then also endure transport costs, they may also have to take leave from their employment to accompany the patient, both the patient and the person accompanying them may need to buy food and so forth. As a result of these expenses, the person may be denied access to mental health care. As in the geographical accessibility scenario, the consequences of not accessing treatment due to no finances is often 'false economy', as the person may land up in expensive and long-term care.

Pyramid of services—an optimal mix for mental health

WHO have put forward a 'pyramid of services' (Fig. 9.7.2) that provides an optimal mix of services required by people with mental disorders (Funk *et al.* 2004). This model is based on the premise that no single service can meet all mental health needs. In fact, without

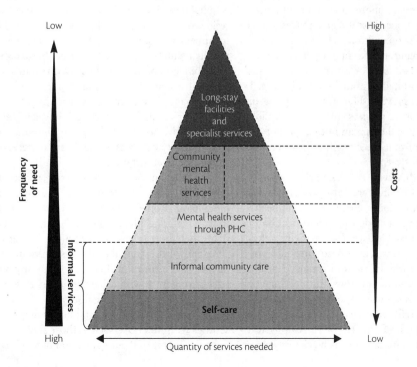

Fig. 9.7.2 Optimal mix of services.
Source: Funk *et al.* (2004).

Box 9.7.1 Examples of providers of informal community mental health services (WHO 2003)

- Traditional healers
- Village of community workers
- Family members
- Self-help and other user groups
- Advocacy services
- Lay volunteers providing parental and youth education on mental health issues and screening for mental disorders (including suicidal tendencies) in clinics and schools
- Religious leaders proving health information on trauma reactions in complex emergencies
- Day care services provided by relatives, neighbours, or retired members of local communities
- Humanitarian aid workers in complex emergencies

any one of these service levels, and referrals up and down the pyramid, the 'system' breaks down, and the other parts are unable to function effectively and efficiently.

At the bottom of the pyramid, and where most care is provided, is *self-care*. Most people can manage their own mental health problems themselves or with help from family or friends. However to facilitate the autonomy and ability of people to care for themselves, the health service or non-governmental organizations need to provide information to people. This should be available and accessible to all people through, for example radio shows or pamphlets that are distributed in languages and literacy levels that people understand.

Informal community mental health services are services provided in the community but that are not part of the formal health and welfare system. Examples of this are traditional healers, professionals in other sectors such as teachers, police, village health workers, services provided by non-governmental organizations, user and family associations, lay-persons, and so forth (see Box 9.7.1). Services at this level are important in preventing people who can effectively be cared for at this level from making demands further up the pyramid, however it is also an extremely important level for 'down referral'. People who may have been treated in a hospital, for example, and discharged, often need informal support to prevent them from relapsing or needing care at a higher level. Informal services are usually accessible and acceptable to the community as they are an integral part of the community. It can be seen then that most mental disorders are dealt with outside of the medical system.

The first 'formal' mental health service is within *primary health care*. The integration of mental health care into primary health services is a critical component of comprehensive mental health care. Essential services at this level include early identification of mental disorders, management of stable psychiatric patients, referral to other levels where required, as well as promotional and prevention activities. Depending on who carries out first-level health care in a particular country, activities and interventions may be carried out by general practitioners, nurses, or other staff that provide assessment, treatment, and referral services.

Mental health services at this level greatly increases physical accessibility as first-level general health care is usually relatively close

to where people live. In addition, the person can be treated as a whole person who may have co-morbid physical and mental health problems. We have previously emphasized the importance of interacting physical and mental health problems. Seeking and receiving treatments part of a general health care is also often less stigmatizing for an individual, especially where having a mental disorder is regarded as shameful. Services are therefore more acceptable to users than having to be treated in a psychiatric facility. From a clinical perspective, it has been found that most common mental disorders can be treated at primary care level. In situations where there are few trained mental health practitioners, an integrated approach substantially increases the chances of being treated for mental disorders.

Integration of mental health into primary health care requires careful training and supervision of staff. Staff needs to be equipped with knowledge and skills that enable them to provide mental health care through training provided as part of initial health worker training as well as ongoing in-service training (WHO 2003). Additionally, they have to be adequately supervised and supported. Health workers often feel ill-equipped and reluctant to undertake mental health in addition to other health care and so ongoing assistance is essential. Critically too, where psychotropic medication is needed, this must be available at this level. This means that these drugs need to become an integral part of the supply, storage, and distribution chain and provision must be made for the prescription of necessary drugs at this level.

Where there is no integrated first-level care, addition pressures are put on the higher levels of care. People are inappropriately referred to levels of care that should be dealing with more complex problems and where there is no early identification of problems, treatment or prevention, and promotion, more people become seriously ill and need to be treated at the higher levels.

The next level of the pyramid has two complementary components, the first is *formal community mental health services* and the second is *mental health services in general hospitals*.

In addition to the informal services that are commonly provided in communities for people with mental disorder, additional formal community services such as day centres, rehabilitation services, hospital diversion programmes, mobile crisis teams, therapeutic and residential supervised services, group homes, home help, assistance to families, and other support services are needed. While not all community mental health services will be able to provide all these services, a combination of some of these, based on needs and requirements, is essential for successful mental health care. Where there are no or highly inadequate community services, it becomes very difficult to discharge patients from psychiatric hospitals, thus 'clogging up' scarce and expensive hospital beds. Others who could avoid hospitalization if community care was available are unnecessarily (though necessary in the circumstances) hospitalized.

Without good community-level care, people often land up either in inhumane institutions or destitute and living on the streets. On the other hand, people receiving good community care have been shown to have better health and mental health outcomes and better quality of life than those treated in institutions (Anderson *et al.* 1993).

As part of the mental health system represented by the pyramid of care, it is important that the community mental health services have strong links with other services such as the primary care and informal and general hospital services.

The development of mental health services in general hospital settings with functions such as those shown in Box 9.7.2 is another critical element of the organization of services. Given the nature of

> **Box 9.7.2 Mental health services offered in general hospitals (WHO 2003)**
>
> ◆ Acute inpatient care
>
> ◆ Crisis stabilization care
>
> ◆ Partial (day/night) hospital programmes
>
> ◆ Consultation/liaison services for general medical patients
>
> ◆ Intensive/planned outpatient programme
>
> ◆ Respite care
>
> ◆ Expert consultation/support/training for primary care services
>
> ◆ Multidisciplinary psychiatric teams linked with other local and provincial sectors (schools, employers, correctional services, welfare) and non-governmental organizations in intersectoral prevention and promotion initiatives
>
> ◆ Specialized units/wards for persons with specific mental disorders and for related rehabilitation programmes

mental disorders, for a number of people some hospitalization at some time (or times) during acute phases of their condition will be necessary. As with integrated primary mental health care, mental health care in general hospitals is more accessible and acceptable than in dedicated psychiatric hospitals. In any country, especially low- and middle-income countries, there are likely to be only a few dedicated psychiatric hospitals and these are usually situated in urban areas—albeit often somewhere out of town. These hospitals are very often not geographically or financially accessible to patients or families wishing to visit them (see the subsection 'Accessibility of services'). There is also often high stigma associated with these facilities which are often the butt of highly discriminatory jokes or references. While clearly the issues of stigma needs to be directly dealt with, until such time as stigma around mental disorder and particularly psychiatric hospitals does change, most people prefer to get treatment in a general hospital. Any co-morbid conditions can also more easily be treated, and special investigations can be conducted.

At the peak of the pyramid, providing services at the highest cost to the least number of people are *long-stay facilities and specialist services.*

A small minority of people with mental disorders require more specialist care than can be provided at general hospital level. Especially in low- and middle-income countries, where there are very few mental health professionals, and certainly not enough highly skilled people to be available in every general hospital, it is necessary to refer people with therapy-resistant or complex presentations to specialized mental health centres—or hospitals where mental health specialists are available. Moreover, a small group of people require ongoing nursing care in a residential facility due to their mental disorder. This, however, is a far cry from 'old style' mental institutions.

Psychiatric institutions have a history of serious human rights violations, poor clinical outcomes, and inadequate rehabilitation programmes. They are also costly and consume a disproportionate proportion of mental health expenditure. The WHO have thus recommended replacing these institutions with a network of services in the community and, for the majority, care in general hospitals where hospitalization is warranted.

Understanding the determinants of mental health

Mental disorders are caused by a combination of biological, psychological and social factors (WHO 2001) and the interactions between them (see the subsection 'Interrelationship between physical and mental health'). Neuroscientists and geneticists have made significant progress regarding biological determinants of mental disorder while psychological research and insight have added substantially to our understanding of mental disorder and human behaviour. For example biochemical and morphological abnormalities of the brain associated with various disorders such as schizophrenia, autism, mood and anxiety disorders are currently being identified through postmortem analysis and noninvasive neuroimaging. Moreover, research identifying risk-conferring genes for mental disorder is underway and it seems that initial results are promising (Hyman *et al.* 2006). Furthermore, improved understanding of the structure and functioning of the brain has led to major advances in psychotropic medications. From a psychological perspective, comprehensive explanations of human dysfunction and behaviour have been translated into effective therapies that improve mental health status.

While all health is determined by biological, psychological, and social factors, in various respects, the aetiology of mental disorder is even more complex than for many physical disorders. The balance between the three domains is often weighted differently for mental health than physical heath with a stronger influence of psychological and social factors. Moreover, cultural differences (including different belief systems regarding the causes of disease and how they can be cured), language, and power relations between provider and patient are also often different when a disorder manifests 'mentally' rather than physically. Stigma is another major public health concern that most disorders do not carry to the same extent as mental disorders do. All these impact on the course and outcome of mental disorders. In the following section, we look primarily at the social determinants of mental (ill) health, as these are of the most specific concern to public mental health.

Social determinants of mental (ill) health

Research in mental health has tended to focus more on the psychological or the biological determinants of mental ill-health than the social determinants. This has led to an imbalanced focus on the use of biomedical interventions and/or a focus on treating the individual to the neglect of altering aspects of the wider social environment. Part of the reason for this imbalance in focus relates to the real difficulties in altering the social environment (especially the macro social environment) since, quite often, these are not within the control of public health practitioners. However, redressing this imbalance can make a highly significant contribution to public health or public mental health and in improving social development.

In this section, we examine four critical ways through which an understanding of the social determinants of mental health can improve public mental health.

1. Careful and scientific documentation of social and economic determinants informs mental health service planning.

Planners of mental health services need to know the extent of mental disorders within a country and whether there are differences between groups of people, but they also need to know what the reasons for these differences are. In addition, they need to be aware of particular 'vulnerable' groups so that they can put in appropriate prevention programmes where possible, identify problems at an early stage and/or allocate resources where they are most needed.

For example, poor and deprived people have a high incidence of mental and behavioural disorders (WHO 2001). Whether this is due to the impacts of poverty on the poor or to a 'drift' of the mentally ill into poverty is often debated, but in all likelihood both are true and in fact they are inextricable.

Patel and Kleinman reviewed 11 studies that examined the relationship between poverty and common mental disorders (Patel & Kleinman 2003). They found that the mean prevalence rates of depression and anxiety disorders varied between 20 per cent and 30 per cent with almost all studies showing a significant relationship between prevalence and various indicators of poverty. The association between poverty and common mental disorders was found to occur in all societies regardless of their levels of development, however they found no 'absolute level' that could be correlated with mental disorder.

Severe mental disorders such as schizophrenia are also highest in people living in lowest socioeconomic circumstances. Saraceno and Barbui showed that people with the lowest SES have eight times higher relative risk for schizophrenia than those in the highest SES groups (Saraceno & Barbui 1997).

Poverty cannot be said to 'cause' mental disorder as most people living in poverty do not have a mental disorder, however it does increase the risk of developing a mental disorder. Poverty and common mental disorders interact with one another in setting up a vicious cycle of poverty and mental illness (Saraceno & Barbui 1997). People are simply more likely to develop mental disorders in conditions of poverty. Moreover the ability of the person to confront or overcome their poverty condition, including getting treatment, is exacerbated if the person has a mental disorder, thus a 'vicious' cycle of poverty/mental health is created.

Access to treatment and rehabilitation is profoundly affected by poverty. People who can afford treatment, whose family members are able to support them financially and emotionally, who can go to rehabilitation therapy, have access to housing, job opportunities, and so forth have a considerable recovery advantage. Where a person has minimal financial means they often put an additional financial and emotional burden on the family. The need to plan services directed at people in poverty is evident.

Another example of how an understanding of social determinants can assist intervention planning is in conflict and post-conflict situations. Wars have significant mental health impacts on both soldier and civilian populations. Baingana et al. report that conflicts cause widespread insecurity due to forced displacement, sudden destitution, the break-up of families and communities, collapsed social structures and breakdown in the rule of law and may last even after the conflicts have ended (Baingana et al. 2005). People in war situations may also have experienced or witnessed killings, injuries, or amputations and gender-based violence. In addition, displaced peoples, whether internally or as refugees in other countries often have difficulties adjusting to losses incurred and the new circumstances they find themselves in. Symptoms of mental dysfunction associated with conflicts include sleeplessness, fear, nervousness, anger, aggression, depression, flashbacks, alcohol and substance abuse, suicide, and domestic and sexual violence (Baingana et al. 2005). Increased rates of PTSD and depression have consistently been found (Murthy & Lakshminarayana 2006). Most recently, Hoge et al. (2004) found that soldiers returning from combat in Afghanistan were more likely to have self-reported alcohol abuse problems than pre-deployment troops, while soldiers serving in Iraq had significantly higher rates of depression, anxiety, and PTSD than either troops that had not been deployed or were deployed in Afghanistan (Hoge et al. 2004). Differences between the troops in Iraq and Afghanistan were attributed to the higher direct combat exposure in Iraq.

Studies examining impacts on non-combatants has increased significantly in the past two decades. Table 9.7.9 summarizes studies that have addressed this issue.

Research has clearly demonstrated that war is a major social determinant of poor mental health. Although there is little that public health experts can do to prevent or stop wars, an important public mental health contribution that can be made is to assist the planning of services for people who require help as a result of the impacts of war.

2. Programmes for prevention of mental disorder and promotion of mental health can be organized around the information and knowledge about social determinants of mental health.

The mental health impacts of major social determinants of mental ill health can, to some extent at least, be mitigated through understanding these causes in a nuanced way and adapting interventions based on evidence from public health research. In their review of mental health and poverty, Patel and Kleinman (2003) showed that mental health was related to income insecurity including fear of losing employment, drop in income, and fear of land loss. High levels of hopelessness mediated by shame, stigma, and the humiliation of poverty were also found to decrease people's psychological ability to cope. Some evidence was also found that social change through changing lifestyles, shifts from rural to urban areas, and lack of social support linked to change played an important role in the development of common mental disorders. The factor that they found had the most consistent relationship with poor mental health was low education. This level of information can be used to prevent mental health problems developing.

Taking the need for social support as an example of risk for the development of common mental disorder, it is highly feasible for public mental health practitioners to identify poor and vulnerable individuals and assist them in accessing support. In situations of rapid urbanization, for instance, many people lose contact with their support systems and often also their cultural roots and practices. Simply organizing get-togethers of people with similar backgrounds and providing transport can be highly cost effective from a mental health perspective but may also enable people who, because of their poor mental health status were unable to become economically productive, to more easily engage in work activities.

Helping people to acquire economic security has been shown to improve psychological well-being. The non-governmental organization BRAC in Bangladesh has developed programmes for poverty alleviation targeting credit facilities, gender equity, basic health care, nutrition, education, and human rights. By, amongst other things, alleviating the stress of being indebted to informal moneylenders, the mental health of many women has been improved (Chowdhury & Bhuiya 2001).

Providing literacy to women is another example where it has been shown that mental health can be promoted through social interventions. Cohen has demonstrated that providing women with information about and ideas from wider worlds, and by empowering them through literacy, it was possible to increase their sense of pride, self-worth, and purpose, and they were more able to exercise greater control of their lives (Cohen 2002).

Table 9.7.9 Impacts of non-combatants of war[†]

Country/territories/areas	Population surveyed	Results
Afghanistan*	Adult household members aged 15 and above. 62% had experienced at least four trauma events in previous 10 years	Depression—67.7% Anxiety—72.2% PTSD—42%
Afghanistan*	Adults 15 and over. Nearly half had experienced traumatic events	Depression—38.5% Anxiety—51.8% PTSD—20.4%
Cambodia*	Adults in displaced persons camp	Depression—55% PTSD—15%
Cambodia*	Young people traumatized at ages 8–12 followed up 3 years later	Depression—41% PTSD—48%
Iraq*	Kurdish families in camps	PTSD in children—87% in caregivers—60%
Israel*	Subjects exposed to war-related trauma	At least one PTSD symptom—76.7% Acute stress disorder—9.4%
Kenya**	Internally displaced people	PTSD—80.2%
Kosovo*	Adults 15 and over	PTSD—17.1%
Lebanon*	Adults 18–65 in communities exposed to war	Major depression—16.3–41.9%
Rwanda*	Community-based sample	PTSD—24.8%
Sri Lanka*	Civilian population	Somatization—41% PTSD—27% Anxiety disorder—26% Major depression—25%
Uganda	Civilian population	Depression—52% Anxiety—60% PTSD—39.9%
West Bank and Gaza Strip*	10–19-year-old children	97.5% had varying levels of PTSD
West Nile region**	Refugees	PTSD—male 31.6% —female 40.1%

* Extracted from Murthy and Lakshminarayana (2006).

** Extracted from Njenga *et al.* (2006).

[†] Neither the methods utilized nor the ages of respondents are standardized across these studies. This figure is thus not intended to give cross-country comparisons, but rather illustrates prevalence found in different studies.

3. Associations and impacts on mental health can be utilized by politicians, economists, and activists to *advocate* for social change.

The evidence for social determinants having negative mental health impacts alone is unlikely to bring about large social changes. However, when considered together with other reasons for change, the evidence for mental health impacts can add significant weight to arguments for change and can be constructively utilized in advocacy for change. A good example to illustrate this is in the field of women's mental health.

Women have around a 1:1.5 or 1:2 times higher levels of depression than men. While some variation is no-doubt attributable to biological factors, for example, in the case of post-natal depression, the social role that women play in most societies is critical. Freeman comments that the traditional role of women as primarily the bearers and rearers of children, inferior and obedient to men (socially and

sexually), whose productive labour has been within the household and without power in social and political decisions, leaves many women feeling disempowered, dehumanized, and without dignity. Without an internal sense of worth, power, and value, many women withdraw into a depressed existence (Freeman 2007). He remarks further that even where there have been changes in labour market roles for women, rather than meaning equality with men it has usually resulted in women having to do 'double work shift'—that is, work both at home and in formal employment. Often without recognition, and even censure from the male partner for not carrying out domestic duties adequately, this often results in severe psychological and physical stress. Given traditional gender roles, working-women may also experience guilt about neglecting their children—leading to further stress and internal conflict. Added to this are high levels of domestic violence. The impacts of abuse, especially in the longer term, are often more sorely experienced on a psychological than a physical level. Undoubtedly, gender discrimination and violence towards women have serious negative impacts on women's mental health.

Analysis of gender discrimination and its consequences reveals numerous economic, social, and health reasons for change. However, the additional fact and evidence for increased prevalence of mental health problems as a result of gender discrimination provides more convincing evidence and reasons which politicians and activists could use in efforts to attain gender equity.

4. Information on social determinants provides the necessary information and impetus for authorities outside of health, that have an indirect responsibility with respect to health, to act accordingly.

Public mental health practitioners do not often have the means to bring about changes to improve mental health; however, they have the information necessary to inform authorities outside of health to make appropriate interventions. For example, because of the high correlation between mental disorder and poverty, special social programmes are usually needed. For example, people may require supported or subsidized housing or to be placed in special skills and job creation programmes or to be supported within the mainstream work environment. Public mental health practitioners have a major responsibility to communicate and persuade officials in departments outside of health to take direct responsibility for providing the necessary social support. Similar to public health practitioners who need to engage authorities involved in water and sanitation supplies to prevent physical diseases, public mental health practitioners too have an important role to play in conveying messages around social actions to be taken to improve people's mental health.

Substance abuse is both a classified disorder in itself and, according to increasing evidence, certain substances such as cannabis may be a direct cause of psychosis (Fergusson *et al.* 2002). Factors that lead individuals to abuse substances include interacting social, psychological, and biological phenomena. Controlling the use of substances and thereby preventing mental disorder thus requires complex intersectoral collaborations involving both supply and demand characteristics. Clearly, while health must care and treat abusers—which also forms part of secondary and tertiary prevention—and must lead in prevention programmes such as media campaigns, the social determinants are linked to issues such as poverty and gangsterism that must be addressed primarily outside of the health system.

Prevention and promotion in mental health

A key part of any public health programme is to prevent disease/disorder wherever possible and to promote good health. This is also true of public mental health. The WHO suggests that it is useful to conceptualize three categories of primary prevention in mental health—i.e. *universal prevention* (targeting the general public or a whole population); *selective prevention* (targeting individuals or subgroups of the population whose risk of developing a mental disorder is significantly higher than that of the rest of the population); and *indicated* prevention (targeting persons at high risk who are identified as having minimal but detectable signs or symptoms foreshadowing mental disorder or biological markers indicating predisposition for mental disorder). In addition, there should be secondary prevention (interventions to reduce the prevalence,

i.e. all specific treatment-related strategies) and tertiary prevention (interventions that reduce disability and includes all forms of rehabilitation as well as prevention of relapses of the illness).

Mental health promotion usually refers to positive mental health, rather than mental ill health, whereas prevention refers to reducing the incidence, prevalence and recurrence of mental disorder. However, there is no clear line between avoiding disease and improving health and well-being. An activity aimed at promoting mental health in a population may also decrease the incidence of disorder or prevent relapse in certain people. As there are numerous determinants of health relating to the actions of individuals as well as social and environmental factors, the objectives of mental health promotion and prevention are to foster the individual, social and environmental qualities that enhance mental health and make sure that factors that may lead to mental health problems are avoided (Herrman 2001; WHO 2004).

Research evidence regarding the impacts and outcomes of promotion and prevention in mental health is somewhat limited but has grown significantly since the early 1980s. While the importance of theory, anecdotes, and personal reports in designing and assessing prevention and promotion programmes cannot be discounted, governments and donors usually need more rigorous evidence to warrant major expenditure and it is important to research, monitor and evaluate preventive interventions. The WHO has collated a number of studies that document successful mental health promotion and disorder prevention strategies (WHO 2002). Some examples of good practice are shown in Box 9.7.3. Up to now, most of the research on prevention and promotion has been conducted in high-income countries, and it is unclear to what extent many of these interventions can be transported into different cultural and economic settings. Some research though is now being conducted in less well-resourced countries. While 'prevention is better than cure' in all situations, in countries with the highest rates of mental disorder and also the least resources for treatment, the need for prevention is even more profound.

Given the close relationships between mental and physical health that have been emphasized in this chapter, not surprisingly prevention programmes can also be combined. For example, the CHAMP (Collaborative HIV/AIDS Adolescent Mental Health Project), adapted in South Africa as the AmaQhawe programme, is a developmentally-timed programme targeting pre-adolescent children and their caregivers that strengthens personal influences (such as assertive and refusal skills) and interpersonal family influences such as caregiver–child communication, caregiver warmth, and active monitoring of children, with the primary aim of reducing risky behaviour in adolescents. Through improved personal well-being and better relationships, including better communication between parents and children around sensitive issues such as sex, transmission of HIV can be reduced (Petersen & Govender 2007).

In 2007, the National Institute for Health and Clinical Excellence in the United Kingdom collated all systematic reviews, syntheses, meta-analyses, and review papers that dealt with non-pharmacological interventions aimed at promoting positive mental health and preventing disorder in adults (Taylor *et al.* 2007). Some of their key findings were:

◆ Following counselling within primary care, people with broad psychological and psychosocial problems showed modest improvements in psychological symptoms in the short term compared with the usual GP care—though recipients of counselling were highly satisfied with the intervention.

Box 9.7.3 Examples of mental health promotion and prevention programmes where scientific evidence of benefit had been found—adapted and selected from the WHO (WHO 2002, 2004)

For mothers during pregnancy and perinatal period

- Home visits during pregnancy and early infancy addressing factors such as maternal smoking, poor social support, parenting skills, and early child–parent interactions has shown positive health, social, and economic outcomes.

- Prenatal and postnatal visits by nurses and community workers to mothers reduced child abuse, led to better vocational adjustment, and better educational achievement in the children.

- Early monitoring of growth development by mothers, along with proper maternal advice by educators and nurses, resulted in better cognitive competence and lower behaviour problems.

- Early stimulation programmes by mothers prevented slow developmental growth in preterm infants and improved growth.

- Breastfeeding, which improves bonding and attachment, has significant benefits to child development.

- Nutrient supplements can prevent neurological impairment (e.g. salt iodization).

For children, adolescents, and schools

- Home visiting programmes for high-risk mothers can prevent child physical abuse and neglect and self-defence for school-aged children can prevent child sexual abuse.

- Self-esteem and life skills can be improved through pro-social behaviour, school based curricula, and improvement of school climate. Training teachers to improve detection of problems and facilitate appropriate intervention provides additional advantages.

- Restructuring the school environment can improve emotional and behavioural functioning of pupils.

- Aggressive behaviour and violence can be reduced through parent training, focused interventions in elementary schools, and comprehensive mental health promotion in primary and middle schools.

- Anxiety disorders can be prevented through individual- and family-based interventions with 'at risk' groups.

- Depression and hopelessness amongst adolescents can be reduced through a resilience-building school-based programme.

- Suicide can be prevented through comprehensive school-based prevention programmes. This includes changing school policy, providing teacher education, parent education, stress management, and providing life skills and a crisis team.

Adults and elderly

- Stress management programmes at work have been found to be effective in preventing adverse mental health outcomes.

- Assistance to individuals who have lost their jobs have been shown to have positive effects on rates of re-employment, quality, and pay of jobs obtained, and to reduce depression and distress.

- Awareness of mental disorder in communities can promote early help seeking behaviour and identification and treatment of severe mental disorder.

- Reducing access to the means to commit suicide is the clearest way for preventing suicide.

- Suicide can be prevented through prescription of psychotropic medicines.

- Head and other injuries can be prevented through legislation around helmets and seat belts.

- Marital and parenting counselling to couples and 'would-be' parents can prevent marital stress and child abuse and promote better parenting.

- Caregivers of people with mental disorder who were taught better coping skills showed reduced incidence of depression and somatic complaints.

- Widowed people who were supported and helped with locating community resources developed relationships quicker and showed fewer depressive symptoms.

- Workplace interventions involving either early referral to occupational health services or group-based information and role play sessions can be effective in reducing sickness absence.

- Stress-reducing interventions in the workplace, focused either on the individual or the organization, can help reduce work-related stress.

- Cognitive behavioural interventions are more effective in improving people's skills for coping than relaxation techniques.

- Family interventions where there is a member with a psychiatric disorder can have a modest positive effect on variables related to the relatives' burden of care.

◆ Cognitive-behavioural parenting programmes are effective in improving measures related to parental psychological health.

◆ Mass media campaigns, particularly those that include community activities, can have beneficial effects on attitudes towards, and knowledge of, mental health issues. They can also impact on an individual's behavioural intentions and support enhancing behaviours to improve their own well-being.

◆ Participation in physical activity is positively associated with mood, emotion, and psychological well-being.

Despite important developments in mental health promotion and the prevention of disorder, this is still a significant growth area for public mental health—both in terms of research that informs focused prevention and promotion programmes and interventions based on existing knowledge.

Stigma: A major public health challenge

One of the principal obstacles to mental health taking its 'rightful' place in health, is the stigma attached to it. Given that a primary goal of public health is to identify and ameliorate the causes of ill health in a population, addressing stigma is undoubtedly a critical public mental health concern. Stigma prevents people from acknowledging any mental health problem and hence seeking care and treatment; providers are reluctant to treat people with mental disorder; people with mental disorder are alienated from and discriminated against by their families and communities and many people experience rampant harassment (Berzins *et al.* 2003). Stigma from communities is an important reason for institutionalization of people with mental disorder. As a result of all these factors, the mental health status of populations is compromised.

The extent of stigma is well illustrated in the following two studies. In the United Kingdom, it was found that community respondents perceived people with schizophrenia as unpredictable (77.3 per cent) and dangerous (71.3 per cent). People with range of mental disorder were perceived as difficult to talk to (Crisp *et al.* 2000). In Nigeria, 96.5 per cent of community respondents believed that people with mental illness are dangerous. Most respondents would not tolerate even basic social contacts with a mentally person with 82.7 per cent saying they would be afraid to have a conversation with a mentally ill person and only 16.9 per cent would even consider marrying a person with mental illness (Gureje *et al.* 2005).

Public mental health has not found adequate solutions to the issue of stigma. Changing media responses, promoting the idea that mental illness is an illness like any other, and community campaigns educating populations about mental disorder have made some headway, but finding innovative ways to redress stigma of mental disorder remains a major challenge for public mental health.

Conclusion: Will greater emphasis on public mental health make a difference to global health?

It is not only conceptually incorrect to consider health without mental health, but there are major practical ramifications in neglecting the 'mental' side of health. Some of the reasons are highlighted in Box 9.7.4, and discussed below:

◆ There is a high prevalence of mental disorder which takes a significant toll on individuals, families, and the economy. Mental disorder

---

Box 9.7.4 Five key points in public mental health

◆ Mental disorder has a high prevalence and burden.

◆ Mental disorders develop through interaction of biological, psychological, and social factors. The social factors are the least studied and understood but are critically important to improving mental health.

◆ Mental and physical health are inextricably linked. Health as a whole will benefit from improved mental health, and particularly public mental health interventions.

◆ Mental health promotion and prevention of disorder show promise, but are areas for further growth and development.

◆ Mental health systems development and economics have the potential to positively and substantially change the lives of people with mental disorder. However, this will require greater use of advocacy and fundamental shifts in people's attitudes (including at a political and health planning level).

---

has been shown to have a very significant burden socially and economically. Unipolar depression is currently ranked as carrying the fourth highest burden of all diseases and by 2030 will become the second-highest cause of all DALYs lost. It is only through concerted public health interventions that a problem of this magnitude can be addressed—especially given major human resource constraints in mental health.

◆ Human behaviour or agency is fundamental to health. Health promoting behaviours are dependent, to some extent at least, on healthy mental states. Moreover, the human behaviour change that is necessary to improve health of populations falls squarely in the realm of public mental health. The development of this area is critical for the health of populations.

◆ There are inextricable links between physical and mental health. Without adequate consideration to improving mental health, physical health is undermined, and vice versa. This applies as much to public health as to clinical health.

◆ Prevention of mental ill-health and prevention of mental disorder is possible. This public health approach is necessary to meaningfully improve mental health status of populations. In addition, prevention of physical diseases can benefit from promoting mental health and preventing mental disorder.

◆ Accessible, affordable, and acceptable mental health care requires mental health systems, and services that take account of culture, available resources, and an optimal mix of levels of care. Public mental health is needed to facilitate this.

◆ From health economics, we know that there are cost-effective interventions for mental health and that these are indeed affordable. This information needs to be incorporated into health care delivery.

Recognition of the role that public mental health can play in improving the health of populations is increasing. However, to fully contribute to improving health of populations, what is already known needs to be much more vigorously promoted, advocated, and implemented, and progress with regard to the many gaps still existing in public mental health research and practice needs to be advanced with some urgency.

References

Aaron R., Joseph A., Abraham S. *et al.* (2004). Suicides in young people in rural southern India. *Lancet,* **363**, 1117–18.

American Psychiatric Association (2000). *Diagnostic and Statistical Manual for Mental Disorders. Fourth edition. Text revision (DSM-IV-TR).* American Psychiatric Association, Washington DC.

Anderson J., Dayson D., Wills W. *et al.* (1993). The TAPS project 13: clinical and social outcomes of long-stay psychiatric patients after one year in the community. *British Journal of Psychiatry,* **162** (suppl), 45–56.

Baingana F., Bannon I., and Thomas R. (2005). *Mental Health and Conflicts: Conceptual Framework and Approaches.* World Bank, Washington.

Barsky A.J., Orav E.J., and Bates D.W. (2005). Somatization increases medical utilization and costs independent of psychiatric and medical comorbidity. *Archives of General Psychiatry,* **62**, 903–10.

Bertolote J.M., Fleischmann A., De Leo D. *et al.* (2004). Psychiatric diagnoses and suicide: revisiting the evidence. *Crisis,* **25**, 147–55.

Berzins K.M., Petch A., and Atkinson J.M. (2003). Prevalence and experience of harassment of people with mental health problems living in the community. *British Journal of Psychiatry,* **183**, 526–33.

Bing E.G., Burnam M.A., Longshore D. *et al.* (2001). Psychiatric disorders and drug use among human immunodeficiency virus-infected adults in the United States. *Archives of General Psychiatry,* **58**, 721–8.

Catalan J., Meadows J., and Douzens A. (2000). The changing pattern of mental health problems in HIV infection: the view from London. *AIDS Care,* **12**, 333–43.

Chang D., Yifeng X., Kleinman A. *et al.* (2002). Rehabilitation of Schizophrenia Patients in China: The Shanghai Model. In Cohen A., Kleinman A. and Saraceno B. *World Mental Health Casebook,* pp. 27–50. Kluwer Academic, New York.

Chowdhury A. and Bhuiya A. (2001). Do poverty alleviation programs reduce inequities in health? The Bangladesh experience. In Leon D., Walt G. eds. *Poverty, Inequality and Health.* Oxford University Press, Oxford.

Ciesla J.A. and Roberts J.E. (2001). Meta analysis of the relationship between HIV infection and risk for depressive disorders. *American Journal of Psychiatry,* **158**, 725–30.

Cohen A. (2002). 'Our Lives were Covered in Darkness': The Work of the National Literacy Mission in Northern India. In Cohen A., Kleinman A. and Saraceno B. *World Mental Health Casebook.* Kluwer Academic, New York.

Collins P., Holman A., Freeman M. *et al.* (2006). What is the relevance of mental health to HIV/AIDS care and treatment programs in developing countries? a review of the literature. *AIDS,* **20**, 1571–82.

Crisp A.H., Gelder M.G., Rix S. *et al.* (2000). Stigmatisation of people with mental illnesses. *British Journal of Psychiatry,* **177**, 4–7.

Dewey M.E. and Saz P. (2001). Dementia, cognitive impairment and mortality in persons aged 65 and over living in the community: a systematic review of the literature. *International Journal of Geriatric Psychiatry,* **16**, 751–61.

Disability Rights Commission (2006). *Equal Treatment: Closing the Gap – A formal investigation into physical health inequalities experienced by people with learning disabilities and/or mental health problems.* Disability Rights Commission, Stratford upon Avon.

Drew N. and Funk M. (2006). Commentary on The Israeli Model of the 'District Psychiatrist' A Fifty-Year Perspective. *Israel Journal of Psychiatry Related Sciences,* **43**, 189–94.

Fergusson D.M., Poulton R., Smith PF. *et al.* (2002). Cannabis and Psychosis. *British Medical Journal,* **332**, 172–5.

Freeman M. (2007). Mental health and social change. In Visser M. *Contextualising Community Psychology in South Africa.* Van Schaik Publishers, Pretoria.

Funk M., Drew N., Saraceno B. *et al.* (2005). A framework for mental health policy, legislation and service development: addressing needs and improving services. *Harvard Health Policy Review,* **6**, 57–69.

Funk M., Saraceno B., Drew N. *et al.* (2004). Mental health policy and plans: promoting an optimal mix of services in developing countries. *International Journal of Mental Health,* **33**, 4–16.

Grant I., Marcotte T.D., and Heaton R.K. (1999). Neurocognitive complications of HIV Disease. *Psychological Science,* **10**, 191–5.

Gureje O., Lasebikan V.O., Ephraim-Oluwanuga O. *et al.* (2005). Community study of knowledge of and attitude to mental illness in Nigeria. *British Journal of Psychiatry,* **186**, 436–41.

Hafner H. and an der Heiden W. (1989). The evaluation of mental health care systems. *British Journal of Psychiatry,* **155**, 12–17.

Heilä H., Haukka J., Suvisaari J. *et al.* (2005). Mortality among patients with schizophrenia and reduced psychiatric hospital care. *Psychological Medicine,* **35**, 725–32.

Herrman H. (2001). The need for mental health promotion. *Australian and New Zealand Journal of Psychiatry,* **35**, 709–15.

Hoge C., Catro C., Messer S.C. *et al.* (2004). Combat duty in Iraq and Afghanistan: mental health problems, and barriers to care. *New England. Journal of Medicine,* **351**, 13–22.

Holt R.I., Bushe C., and Citrome L. (2005). Diabetes and schizophrenia 2005: closer to understanding the link? *Journal of Psychopharmacology,* **19** (6 Suppl), 56–65.

Hyman S., Chisholm D., Kessler R. *et al.* (2006). Mental Disorders. In 2nd ed. *Disease Control Priorities Related to Mental, Neurological, Developmental and Substance Abuse Disorders.* WHO, Geneva.

Kessler R.C., Haro J.M., Heeringa S.G. *et al.* (2006). The World Health Organization World Mental Health Survey Initiative. Editorial. *Epidemiologia e Psichiatria Sociale,* **15**, 161–6.

Kohn R., Saxena S., Levav I. *et al.* (2004). The treatment gap in mental health care. *Bulletin of the World Health Organization,* **82**, 858–66.

Kovel J. (1988). A critique of DSM-111 Research in Law. *Deviance and Social Control,* **9**, 127–46.

Mathers C.D. and Loncar D. (2006). Projections of Global Mortality and Burden of Disease from 2002 to 2030. *PLos Medicine,* **3**, 2011–30.

McDaid D. (2005). *Policy Brief. Mental Health 1. Key issues in the development of policy and practice across Europe.* WHO on behalf of the European Observatory on Health Systems and Policies, Brussels.

McKinnon K. and Rosner J. (2000). Severe mental illness and HIV/AIDS. In Cournos F and Forstein M (Eds) *What Mental Health Practitioners Need to Know About HIV and AIDS.* Jossey-Bass, San Francisco.

Moghraby O., Ferri C., and Prince M. (2005). Risk behaviour in school-based adolescents. Presented at the *Second Annual International Mental Health Conference at the Institute of Psychiatry: Mental Health and the Millennium Development Goals,* August 31st–September 2nd 2005.

Murthy R.S. and Lakshminarayana R. (2006). Mental health consequences of war: a brief review of research findings. *World Psychiatry,* **5**, 25–30.

Niehaus D., Oosthuisen P., Lochner C. *et al.* (2004). A Culture-Bound Syndrome 'Amafufunyana' and a Culture Specific Event 'Ukuthwasa': Differentiated by a Family History of Schizophrenia and other Psychiatric Disorders. *Psychopathology,* **37**, 59–63.

Njenga F., Nguithi A., and Kang'Ethe R. (2006). War and mental disorders in Africa. *World Psychiatry,* **5**, 38–9.

Ösby U., Brandt L., Correia N. *et al.* (2001). Excess Mortality in Bipolar and Unipolar Disorder in Sweden. *Archives of General Psychiatry,* **58**, 844–82.

Patel V. and Kleinman A. (2003). Poverty and common mental disorders in developing countries. *Bulletin of the World Health Organization:* 609–15.

Perälä J., Suvisaari J., Saarni S. *et al.* (2007). Lifetime prevalence of psychotic and bipolar I disorders in a general population. *Archives of General Psychiatry,* **64**, 19–28.

Petersen I. and Govender K. (2007). Health and health promotion. In Visser M. *Contextualising Community Psychology in South Africa.* Van Schaik, Pretoria.

Peterson I. and Swartz L. (2002). Primary health care in the era of HIV/AIDS. Some implications for health systems reform. *Social Science and Medicine*, **55**, 1005–13.

Prince M., Patel V., Rahman A. *et al.* No health without mental health – a slogan with substance. *Lancet* (in press).

Prior L. (1991). Community verses hospital care: the crisis in psychiatric provision. *Social Science and Medicine*, **32**, 483–9.

Saha S., Chant D., Welham J. *et al.* (2005). A Systematic Review of the Prevalence of Schizophrenia. *PloS Medicine*, **2**, 413–33.

Saraceno B. and Barbui C. (1997). Poverty and mental illness. *Canadian Journal of Psychiatry*, **42**, 285–90.

Saraceno B., van Ommeren M., Batniji R. *et al.* Barriers to improving mental health services in low and middle income countries. *Lancet* (in press).

Scheper-Hughes N. and Lovell A.M. (1986). Breaking the circuit of social control: lessons in public psychiatry from Italy and Franco Basaglia. *Social Science and Medicine*, **23**, 159–78.

Singleton N., Maung N.A., Cowie A. *et al.* (2007). Mental Health or Carers. Quoted in Taylor L, Taske N, Swann C and Waller S. *Public Health interventions to promote positive mental health and prevent mental health disorders among adults.* National Institute for Health and Clinical Excellence, London.

Taylor L., Taske N., Swann C. *et al.* (2007). *Public health interventions to promote positive mental health and prevent mental health disorders among adults. Evidence briefing.* National Institute for Health and Clinical Excellence, London.

Tyrer P. and Steinberg D. (1998). *Models for Mental Disorder: Conceptual Models in Psychiatry, 3rd Edition.* John Wiley & Sons Canada, Ltd.

Uldall K., Palmer N., Whetten K. *et al.* (2004). Adherence in people living with HIV/AIDS, mental illness and chemical dependency – a review of the literature. *AIDS Care*, **16** (Suppl. 1), 71–96.

Whiteford H. (2000). Unmet need: a challenge for governments. In Andrews G and Henderson S (Eds) *Unmet need in psychiatry.* Cambridge University Press, Cambridge.

WHO (1946). *Constitution of the World Health Organization*, adopted by the International Health Conference, New York, 19 June to 22 July, and signed on 22 July 1946. WHO, Geneva.

WHO (1992) *The ICD Classification of Mental and Behavioural Disorders.* WHO, Geneva.

WHO (2001). *World Health Report 2001. Mental Health: New Understanding, New Hope.* WHO, Geneva.

WHO (2002). *Prevention and Promotion in Mental Health.* WHO, Geneva.

WHO (2003). *Organization of Services for Mental Health.* WHO, Geneva.

WHO (2004). *World Health Report 2004. Changing History.* WHO, Geneva.

WHO (2005). *Mental health Atlas 2005.* WHO, Geneva.

WHO (2006a) *Dollars, DALYs and Decisions: Economic Aspects of the Mental Health System.* WHO, Geneva.

WHO (2006b). *Economic Aspects of the Mental Health System: Key Messages to Health Planners and Policy Makers.* WHO, Geneva.

WHO World Mental Health Survey Consortium (2004). Prevalence, severity and unmet need for treatment of mental disorders in the World Health Organization World Mental Health Surveys. *Journal of the American Medical Association*, **291**(21), 2581–90.

Dental public health

Zoe Marshman and Peter G. Robinson

Abstract

Dental public health is concerned with preventing oral disease, promoting oral health and improving the quality of life through the organized efforts of society. Oral health is an important public health problem as dental diseases including dental caries, periodontal disease, oral neoplasms, and dento-facial trauma are common, have significant impact on individuals and wider society, and are largely preventable. Individual risk factors for oral disease are largely equivalent to the risk factors for other common diseases namely diet, tobacco, and alcohol use, accidents, ineffective oral hygiene and limited exposure to fluoride. In common with many other diseases, many of these risks are patterned by social and economic factors. Oral health promotion involves a common risk factor approach which may be based on the principles of the Ottawa Charter. Examples include reducing the consumption of sugars through regulation of advertising and labelling of foods, training dental care professionals to give alcohol and tobacco advice, preventing accidents damaging the mouth through promotion of impact-absorbing surfaces for play areas, and the provision of mouthguards for use during contact sports. Good oral hygiene and optimal exposure to fluoride is promoted through provision of low cost fluoride toothpastes and other sources of fluoride including community fluoridation schemes of water, salt, and milk. Dental services are involved in the prevention and treatment of dental disease with the additional aim of improving the quality of life of affected individuals. Opportunities for clinical prevention include sealing the biting surfaces of teeth and the application of fluoride varnishes. Dental services are increasingly expanding the use of dental care professionals other than dentists to improve access to services. Non-specialist personnel can be trained to provide atraumatic restorative techniques, a method of restoring decayed teeth that does not rely on expensive equipment or electricity. To ensure their effectiveness and efficiency, dental services should provide high-quality, evidence-based patient management.

Dental public health: A definition

Dental public health is the science and art of preventing oral disease, promoting oral health, and improving the quality of life through the organized efforts of society. Major areas of dental public health activity include the following:

+ Measures of oral health

+ Determinants of oral health status

+ Prevention and control of oral disease

+ Promotion of oral health

+ Policy and service development and prioritization

+ Evaluation of the effectiveness of oral health services and treatment modalities

+ Evidenced-based commissioning

In some countries, the specialty also involves provision of services to special population subgroups.

These activities may be divided into three broad groups: Oral health needs and demands assessment; oral health promotion; and the planning, commissioning, and evaluation of dental services. All have relevance in both developing and developed countries, although the emphasis will vary according to social conditions, the burden of disease, organization of health services, geographical factors, and the economy.

Oral health needs and demands assessment

This includes improving knowledge of the distribution and determinants of oral disease, identifying those determinants that are amenable to change, and understanding the impacts of oral diseases and conditions.

Oral health promotion

Dental public health focuses on improving oral health by identifying opportunities at community and national levels for evidence-based programmes aimed at improving diet and nutrition, hygiene, tobacco use, and ensuring optimal exposure to fluorides.

Planning, management, and evaluation of dental health services

This area involves using knowledge about disease levels and needs for care to plan and design dental services and to evaluate them to ensure they meet the needs of communities within the constraints of healthcare and political systems.

This chapter describes these three main areas of dental public health activity in relation to the epidemiology, aetiology, and management of the four oral conditions of the greatest public health importance: Dental caries; periodontal diseases; oral cancer; and oro-facial trauma. Approaches to oral health promotion will be outlined within a common risk factor approach. First, we discuss the relevance of oral health for public health.

The importance of oral health

Oral health is often a low priority for individuals, policy makers, and public health specialists. In fact, oral health poses important public health problems because oral diseases have significant impacts on individuals and the community, they are widespread, and the two most common diseases: Tooth decay (dental caries) and gum (periodontal) diseases are almost entirely preventable. The impacts of oral disease range from mortality to effects on general health and quality of life. Oral diseases are associated with a considerable burden to both individuals and the community in terms of lost economic productivity.

Impacts of oral disease

Mortality from oral cancer is related to the site in the mouth and the timing of the diagnosis, but 5-year survival is still less than 50 per cent. In addition to mortality, oral disease affects other aspects of general health. Limited dietary choice and calorific and micronutrient intake are direct consequences of conditions such as xerostomia, poorly fitting dentures, loss of teeth in early childhood caries, and oral developmental disorders.

Oral diseases also directly affect our quality of life and a considerable effort has been made to assess the extent to which oral disorders compromise aspects of daily living (Locker 2004). Dental pain is very common. In the United Kingdom, 40 per cent of dentate adults and 26 per cent of 12-year-olds reported oral pain in the past 12 months (Nuttall & Steele 2001; Nuttall & Harker 2004). Even the appearance of the mouth is hugely important. It affects our self-esteem, our willingness to interact with others, and influences the judgements other people make about us, and good dental appearance is regarded as a requirement for some prestigious occupations.

The economic costs of dental disease are difficult to calculate. As well as the direct costs of disease and treatment there are indirect costs which might include reduced employment or promotion expectations and opportunities, limitation of academic achievement, and the total societal burden through loss of economic productivity. The direct costs are between 0.2 per cent and 1 per cent of the gross national product in developed countries (van Amerongen et al. 1993). The United Kingdom is at the lower end of this range, yet the National Health Service in England and Wales (population 54 million) budget for dentistry is in excess of £2 billion (US$3.9 billion). This sum is all the more surprising when it is considered that only about 50 per cent of the population are registered with an NHS dentist. The cost of treatment provided outside the NHS is not known, but may be an additional £1 billion. Annually, over 20 million work days and 51 million school hours are lost in the United States alone due to oral disease and its treatment (Department of Health and Human Services 2000). These data equate to one and a half hours for each employee annually. Low-income families are more likely to lose time from work and school because of dental disease, and so these impacts of oral disease compound the inequalities that already exist in health, income, and educational attainment.

Frequency of oral disease

Despite decreasing prevalence of dental caries over the last three decades, 40 per cent of 5-year-olds in the United Kingdom have evidence of clinically significant tooth decay (Pitts & Harker 2004). Periodontal diseases are even more common. More than 80 per cent of adults have inflamed gums (gingivitis), and most have evidence of destruction of the attachment between tooth and bone (periodontitis).

Oral cancer is the eighth most common cancer worldwide, and its incidence is increasing particularly in some Western European countries. The highest reported incidence rates are in India and Sri Lanka where the mouth is the most common site comprising up to 40 per cent of all cancers.

Prevention

Finally, the two most common oral diseases are almost entirely preventable. Clinically significant dental caries occurs only in the presence of excess dietary sugar. The incidence of disease is low when the intake of free sugar is less than 15–20 kg/year, which equates to 6–10 per cent of energy intake (Moynihan & Petersen 2004). This dietary control of tooth decay can be supplemented by the use of fluorides, which reduce the disease whether presented in drinking water or in toothpastes. Likewise, the presence of dental plaque is necessary for destructive periodontal disease. Targets for oral cleanliness have been calculated which appear to be compatible with freedom from periodontal disease throughout life (Burt et al. 1985). Slightly higher levels of plaque might be compatible with acceptably low levels of periodontal disease.

Therefore, in terms of prevalence, impact on individuals and society and the possibility of effective interventions, oral health has considerable public health significance.

Dental caries

Dental caries is the demineralization of tooth substance by acid metabolites of oral bacteria. In the very early stages the lesion appears as a chalky white spot on the tooth. If the lesion progresses, the surface of the tooth breaks down leading to cavitation. If the caries reaches the underlying dentine, it can spread more readily through the porous and less mineralized tissue towards the pulp. Infection of the pulp may allow the passage of bacteria along the root canals to the alveolar bone.

The direct consequences of this process are destruction of the tooth, pain, and a possible dental abscess. Dentine is sensitive to physical, thermal, and osmotic stimuli. When it is exposed by cavitation there may be transient pain associated with hot or cold drinks or sweet foods. Later, as the pulp becomes inflamed, the discomfort may be spontaneous, exquisitely painful, and of longer duration. In a dental abscess pressure to the tooth is transmitted to the infected alveolus and the unfortunate person avoids biting or knocking the tooth.

Four factors are necessary for the development of caries: Dietary sugars, a susceptible tooth surface, the microflora of dental plaque, and adequate time.

The evidence implicating sugars in the aetiology of dental caries is convincing. Rugg-Gunn's (1993) encyclopaedic review classifies this evidence methodologically into human observational studies, human interventional studies, animal experiments, enamel slab experiments, plaque pH studies, and incubation experiments. Dietary sugars are essential if the caries is to be of clinical relevance. Dental plaque, a substance that forms on the tooth surface, which is composed mainly of bacteria, particularly *Streptococcus mutans*, metabolize sugars and so produce acids. With each exposure to sugar the plaque pH falls sharply and rises slowly back to normal levels over the following hour. It follows that caries incidence is related to the frequency of intake of sugars.

At high pH, there is remineralization of the tooth, especially in the presence of fluoride. Saliva plays a crucial protective role against caries by simple dilution, by buffering plaque acid and by acting as a source of minerals and chemical and immunological plaque inhibitory factors. For these reasons dental caries is more frequent in the sites less accessible to the saliva: In the pits and fissures of posterior teeth and between these teeth and also in people with restricted salivary flow.

Epidemiology

Caries of the permanent dentition is traditionally measured with the DMF index that records the number of decayed missing and filled teeth. A more precise index records the number of surfaces affected (DMFS). A similar index is used to record the status of the deciduous dentition (DMF). As the index aggregates both disease and treatment experience it is sensitive to the treatment decisions of dentists and so less valid with increasing age. Since each of the categories is equally weighted it is insensitive to both the severity of the disease and outcomes of treatment.

Nonetheless, the DMFT has been used for 60 years and will continue to be so for some years to come. This does not mean that DMF scores of yesteryear are directly comparable with those of today as the criteria for judging a tooth as carious have changed. Previously caries was diagnosed using a sharp dental probe to determine whether there was cavitation of the tooth. If no cavity was judged to be present, the tooth was classed as 'caries free'. More recently, the international convention has become to diagnose caries from much earlier stages, before frank cavitation when caries has visibly progressed into dentine. Sharp probes are no longer used, to prevent damage to the tooth surface. If no caries is visible, the tooth is now judged as having 'no obvious caries'. The changes in the detection thresholds reflect changes of the philosophies of the management of dental caries from an emphasis on early intervention to a more preventive approach.

Although dental caries can be found in the teeth of archaeological remains, dental caries as it is known today did not emerge until sugar became widely available. Disease levels rose during the seventeenth century and reached epidemic proportions in the nineteenth and twentieth centuries in some populations with near universal experience in some generations in many countries. Since systematic data have been collected the typical pattern has been one of high levels of caries in developed countries associated with exposure to sugars. In the mid-1970s, levels in many developed countries began to fall dramatically, for example in the United Kingdom mean DMFT of 12-year-olds decreased from 4.8 to 0.8 between 1973 and 2003 (Pitts & Harker 2004).

This fall in caries prevalence in developed countries appears to have slowed in the early to mid-1980s in the deciduous dentition. The mean dmft of 5-year-olds in England and Wales fell from 4 to 1.8 between 1973 and 1983, but now appears stable at around 1.6 (Pitts & Harker 2004). Nevertheless, children and young adults (that is, under the age of 40 years) have better oral health than preceding generations. As these cohorts age there will be commensurate improvements in adult oral health.

Data on caries levels aggregated at the national level provide useful information, but can mask important trends. The fall in caries prevalence has polarized inequalities in oral health. In times of high disease prevalence, the disease was almost universal and inequalities were manifest merely as differences in the number of teeth affected

in an individual. With lower disease prevalence, a minority of people carry the burden of most of the disease. Data from the United States highlight the difference in proportion of people with at least one untreated, decayed tooth between those above and before the poverty level (Fig. 9.8.1) (Department of Health and Human Services 2000). It is often suggested that 80 per cent of the dental caries in the United Kingdom is concentrated in 20 per cent of the population, particularly those from poor socioeconomic areas. While this statement may be an oversimplification of a more complex picture it serves to illustrate that, as for most important diseases, dental caries and its consequences are increasingly diseases of the poor (Watt 2007).

Although data are scarce, there are concerns of increasing levels of caries in children in some countries undergoing economic growth and nutrition transition while caries levels remain low in countries where a poor economy restricts consumption of sugars. Surveys in Africa show that caries levels in 12-year-olds are still relatively low although aggregated national data may mask local variations, particularly, high caries levels in urban areas. Of particular concern is the fact that 90 per cent of the caries in that continent remains untreated.

Treatment of dental caries

Until the nineteenth century, the only useful treatment for dental caries was extraction of the affected tooth. Since then there has been a transition to restorative care in which the infected parts of the tooth are removed and replaced with an inert obdurating filling. During the latter half of the twentieth century, technology has moved forward, dentists have been keen to make use of innovations, and some patients have been willing to pay for them. The result is that in developed countries operative treatment for adults is increasingly complex and technology intensive. Badly decayed teeth can now be restored with a range of adhesive tooth coloured materials that are either formed in the mouth or prepared in laboratories and then fitted. Originally, missing teeth could only be replaced with removable dentures. Now they can be replaced with bridges that adhere to the remaining teeth or with prostheses supported by osseo-integrated implants that project out through the gingivae.

These treatments provided by dentists might reduce the social impact of dental caries on affected people, but play a very minor role in preventing the disease. Dental services explained 3 per cent of the reduction in caries levels in industrialized countries during the

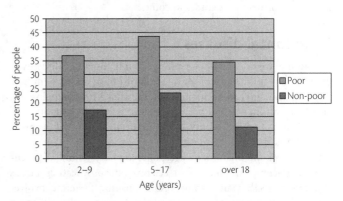

Fig. 9.8.1 Percentage of people above and below the poverty level, with at least one untreated, decayed tooth.
Source: Department of Health and Human Services (2000), United States. Poor is defined as an annual income below the US poverty level.

1970s compared to the 65 per cent contribution made by broader socioeconomic factors and the availability of fluoride toothpastes (Nadanovsky & Sheiham 1994).

In developing countries, the necessary infrastructure is often not available for complex treatment of carious teeth. In some areas the atraumatic restorative technique (ART) is the only sustainable method because the decay is removed only with hand instruments. The cavities are then filled with glass ionomer cements that are hand mixed with water. Upon insertion, the filling adheres to the tooth, gradually leaking fluoride to prevent secondary disease around the cavity. All the instruments can be carried in a small case, and treatment can be provided painlessly, at low cost, without either local anaesthesia, electricity, or expensive dental equipment. Non-dentists can be trained in the technique in a matter of weeks using manuals available from the World Health Organization. The technique is most suitable for exactly the types of cavities found in many developing countries with low caries levels (Yip et al. 2001).

Implications of changes in caries prevalence

The low prevalence of disease experienced in the developed world over the last 15 years has profound implications for the management of dental caries. When the incidence of the disease is low proportionately more caries affects the accessible occlusal surfaces of the teeth. Fissure sealants can be applied to these surfaces to prevent caries and are still cost-effective at low caries levels (Armfield & Spencer 2007). Only simple restorations are needed to treat existing disease at these sites. The disease also progresses more slowly, so allowing deferred operative treatment whilst attempting to prevent the spread of the lesion. Many lesions are detected at an earlier stage so that new dental materials can be used in minimally invasive techniques.

The lower levels of disease mean that the costs of some dental services might be reduced. Increasing the intervals between dental examinations is safe and effective for children and adults with low disease incidence (National Institute for Health and Clinical Excellence 2004). Since most of the restorations required by children are relatively simple, the number and costs of dentists can be reduced by using less highly-trained dental care professionals (DCPs). The reduced burden of disease may allow general dental practitioners to become more involved in health promotion, to place a greater emphasis on prevention and place a greater emphasis on quality. Conversely, there are still many people more than approximately 40 years of age who have suffered the ravages of dental caries and its treatment. These people will continue to need and demand increasingly complex treatment for decades to come.

Periodontal diseases

Periodontal diseases comprise a range of inflammatory diseases of the periodontium categorized by the position of attachment between gingiva and tooth. In gingivitis, the attachment remains in a healthy position, whereas periodontitis is defined by migration of the epithelium which reduces the amount of periodontal ligament and bone supporting the tooth.

Gingivitis is an inflammatory response to plaque. Along with redness and swelling, the gums may bleed on gentle provocation such as cleaning the teeth. Pain is an uncommon feature. Systemic involvement including hormonal changes, skin diseases, and medication use may modify these diseases or cause other gingival changes. The disease is exceedingly common.

In periodontitis, the loss of periodontal attachment is manifest by deepening of the pockets between the gingivae and teeth and by recession of the gingivae. In severe cases, the supporting structures are so depleted that the teeth become loose. The disease is rarely painful unless an acute infection complicates a periodontal pocket ('a lateral periodontal abscess') or if the exposed root surfaces are temperature sensitive.

Mild periodontal pocketing is common. For example, it is seen in half or more of UK and US adults (Department of Health and Human Services 2000; Morris et al. 2001). Severe periodontitis is much less frequent. Lost attachment or pockets of 6 mm or more (thought to be sufficient to threaten tooth survival) are seen in less than 8 per cent of US and UK adults (Department of Health and Human Services 2000; Morris et al. 2001). The disease is more frequent and severe in countries where tooth cleaning practices are less sophisticated.

One other periodontal disease has public health importance. Acute necrotizing ulcerative gingivitis (ANUG, Vincent's infection or 'trenchmouth') causes necrosis, ulceration, soreness and bleeding of the gingivae. The ulcerated papillae may have a grey slough and there may be a characteristic foetor. Lymphadenopathy and mild fever are variable findings. In many developed countries ANUG is a disease of young adults. There are no good incidence data, but anecdotally, it has become less frequent among some developed populations in recent years. A variant of the disease is associated with HIV infection. ANUG is also seen in African children where it can progress in the absence of treatment. In severe cases necrosis may extend over adjacent and contiguous tissues to cause gross destruction of oral and facial tissues (known as cancrum oris or noma).

Pathogenesis

The pathogenesis of periodontitis involves the interaction of plaque pathogens with the host's immune system. Dental plaques are consistently implicated in the aetiology of periodontal diseases. Considerable research is devoted to determining which, if any, specific pathogens are responsible for periodontal destruction (the 'specific plaque hypothesis'). Dental plaque is ubiquitous, but destructive disease occurs only in a minority of people. Plaque is therefore not sufficient cause for periodontitis and technology-intensive research may divert attention from the important determinants of periodontal disease susceptibility.

It is now clear that tobacco exerts an independent deleterious effect. In addition, periodontal treatment is less effective in smokers (Reibel 2003). Stress is also a risk factor in periodontal disease. Greater occupational stress is associated with progression of periodontitis and ANUG has been noted among soldiers on difficult postings, students during exam terms, and people with other negative life events.

Periodontitis often takes decades to become clinically detectable. Accordingly, it is more common and severe with advanced years because age confounds disease duration. Periodontitis is not a consequence of age; it is associated with poor oral hygiene irrespective of age and does not progress in adults with good oral hygiene.

In the last few years periodontal diseases have been linked to a number of other health problems including cardiovascular diseases, stroke, pre-term birth, and low birth weight. A number of authors have gone so far as to suggest that periodontal diseases are independent risk factors for these diseases with many reports focusing on the biological plausibility of these associations. Epidemiological evidence supporting links between periodontal and other diseases suffers from a huge range of possible variables, the potential for misclassification and other sources of bias. Whilst efforts have been made to control for socioeconomic and lifestyle factors, residual confounding resulting from a failure to account fully for these variables seems inevitable. Specific cardiovascular risk factors such as tobacco use, obesity, and lower serum HDL-cholesterol are more common among people with high dental disease experience (Sanders *et al.* 2005). Some of these factors such as tobacco smoking are independent risk factors for both cardiovascular and periodontal diseases, whereas others may be linked less directly.

This area of research is exciting periodontal researchers. Systematic reviews of these possible links have been conducted, yet for the meantime, methodological complexity prevents firm conclusions being drawn (Beck & Offenbacher 2005; Xiong *et al.* 2006).

Treatment

For the majority of people the progression of periodontal destruction is compatible with the retention of a natural dentition into old age. Targets for oral cleanliness have been calculated that appear to be compatible with freedom from periodontal disease throughout life or with acceptably low levels of periodontal disease (Burt *et al.* 1985).

A significant minority of people (perhaps 5–15 per cent) may lose teeth as a result of periodontal diseases and considerable effort is spent by dentists and dental hygienists attempting to prevent and treat them. Both the prevention and treatment of periodontal diseases focus on the mechanical removal of plaque. Dental professionals attempt to bring this about by instructing patients in the use of toothbrushes and dental floss. Adjunctive services provided by dental services include the removal of calcified plaque (calculus) as it may harbour micro-organisms and provide a mechanical barrier to inhibit effective self-care and planning the surfaces of the roots to remove the superficial layers which might be contaminated with bacterial toxins. In some cases the architecture of the periodontium may be surgically adjusted to excise diseased tissue and allow the entry of toothbrush bristles and dental floss into inaccessible areas. In recent times, a technique known as guided tissue regeneration (GTR) has used membranes of synthetic material to prevent epithelial cells proliferating down the root surface after periodontal surgery.

Systematic reviews are beginning to provide an evidence base for periodontal therapy although there may be considerable Hawthorne effects reflecting differences between the effectiveness of treatment provided routinely in primary care and its efficacy in clinical trials conducted in university departments. There are also few long-term studies showing effects on tooth retention.

Interventions aimed at improving oral hygiene produce only short-term changes that are not sustained (Watt & Marinho 2005). Powered toothbrushes with a rotation oscillation action assist self-care although their long-term benefits on periodontal health have yet to be evaluated (Robinson *et al.* 2005). The most common professional procedure to prevent and treat periodontal diseases, the removal of calculus by scaling and polishing, has not been evaluated using contemporary standards of research. Nor is there compelling evidence of benefits from professional mechanical plaque removal alone over simple oral hygiene instruction to prevent periodontal diseases (Needleman *et al.* 2005a).

Another common treatment, subgingival debridement, remains untested in randomized controlled trials, but showed modest short-term reductions in pocket depths in other controlled studies (Van der Weijden & Timmerman 2002) and a systematic review of GTR indicated that the mean level of attachment gained is less than 1 mm with eight sites needing to be treated to regain 2 mm in one site (Needleman *et al.* 2005b).

Oral neoplasms

Benign neoplasms in the oral cavity include papillomas, polyps, and various types of granuloma. This section will deal principally with malignant neoplasms, of which approximately 90 per cent are squamous cell carcinomas. They may occur on the lip, tongue, gingivae, oral floor, or elsewhere in the mouth. The site is often related to the aetiological factors. Lesions may present as swellings, ulcers, or red or white patches and many are painless until they become large. Significantly, survival is related to the stage of the disease at presentation. Five-year survival is less than 50 per cent.

Malignant change is often seen in a number of lesions which precede the development of the tumour. These premalignant lesions present as leukoplakias and erythroplakias of unknown origin. Malignant change is also seen, albeit infrequently, in oral lichen planus and hyperplastic candidiasis.

Overall incidence worldwide for males has been estimated at an age standardized rate of 6.42 per 100 000 population with dramatic variation between and within countries (World Health Organization 2001) (Table 9.8.1). Men are more susceptible than women in almost all populations, independent of the effects of tobacco use.

Variations in the incidence of oral malignancy are largely explained by varying exposure to three major risk factors. Cancer of the lower lip is strongly associated with exposure to sunlight especially in people with fair skin. Tobacco use, whether chewed or smoked, predisposes to intra-oral cancer. The high incidence of oral cancer among southern Asians is largely accounted for by the addition of tobacco to betel quid or 'paan'. There are dose–response relationships for the duration of use and type of tobacco inhaled. Alcohol is also an independent aetiological factor and has a synergistic relationship with tobacco use.

In the past, oral cancer was predominantly a disease of older people (over 60 years). However, there is now evidence of an increased incidence in those less than 45 years with a suggestion that oral cancer in this younger age-group may be a distinct and more aggressive disease entity (Conway 2006).

Because early intervention determines survival in oral cancer, and many cases are preceded by premalignant lesions, there is a strong argument for case finding as a method of disease control.

Table 9.8.1 Oral cancer in males—age standardized rate per 100 000 population

	Rate per 100 000
Worldwide	6.42
India	12.6
Thailand	4.6
China	0.7

Source: World Health Organization (2001).

However, active screening does not appear to be justified in part because of the low incidence of the disease (Downer *et al.* 2006). Opportunistic screening, when patients may already visit the dentist for a dental check up, may be viable.

Dento-facial trauma

Trauma to the teeth is common and frequently causes fracture of the tooth or supporting bone or bodily movement of the tooth including complete avulsion. In many cases the long-term survival of the tooth is threatened. As the anterior and most visible teeth are most often involved the result is disfiguring. Worldwide the prevalence of dento-facial trauma is approximately 10–15 per cent. Risk factors include contact sports, bicycle/skateboard accidents, falls, violence and poor environments such as overcrowding. Clinical features of protruding upper front teeth and inadequate lip coverage also put individuals at risk. The peak age for trauma is early adolescence with boys experiencing more injuries than girls.

Trauma to deciduous teeth is managed by monitoring in case any consequent infection threatens the permanent tooth developing beneath it. In permanent teeth, adhesive fillings can be used to protect sensitive fractured teeth and calcium hydroxide dressings may be placed to allow continued root development in immature teeth. For permanent teeth that have been knocked out, timely first-aid is crucial. They should be replaced in the socket as soon as possible or else placed in a suitable container of milk or normal saline. Dental care should be sought immediately as the long term survival rates of avulsed teeth are greatest if the tooth is replanted within 30 minutes. The tooth should be held in place by non-rigid splint to adjacent teeth for 7–10 days. Systemic antibiotic and anti-tetanus treatments are required. The need for almost immediate care means that skilled emergency dental services should be available wherever possible. Unfortunately dento-facial trauma is not limited to office hours.

The cost of treating dento-facial trauma has been estimated at US$3.2–3.5 million per million subjects (Andreasen 1997) and in the United Kingdom the average total cost of treating one patient with a dental traumatic injury has been estimated at £856 (US$1665) (Wong & Kolokotsa 2004).

Oral health promotion

Because oral diseases are brought about by people's behaviours, dentistry has traditionally adopted health education as the central thrust of prevention. Toothbrushing and sugar reduction messages have been repeated *ad nauseam* in both chairside and public education campaigns. But dental educators became disillusioned with the recognition that health education cannot readily change these behaviours which are largely determined by our social and cultural environment. Indeed, health education carries its own dangers of disempowerment and victim-blaming and may increase inequalities in oral health (Watt 2007).

Closer examination of the causes of oral disorders reveal the potential value of community-based approaches to maintain oral health by acting on the wider determinants of health. Oral disease is brought about by the consumption of sugars, ineffective oral cleaning, tobacco and alcohol use, limited exposure to fluoride, and stress. The determinants of oral health are largely equivalent to the determinants of health in general, and there are many opportunities for wider social and environmental action to play an invaluable role in promoting oral health. There is an increasing recognition that a 'common-risk factor' approach is fundamental to the integrated approach to oral health promotion (Sheiham & Watt 2000). The key principle behind this approach is that controlling a number of risk factors through multidisciplinary action can have a major impact on a large number of chronic diseases. This approach then reduces duplication, saves resources, and improves effectiveness.

An additional consideration is that preventive strategies that focus on individuals does not appear to be suitable for dental caries and periodontal diseases since there are, as yet, no effective ways of identifying which individuals are at high risk of developing the diseases (Rose 1992; Watt 2007). Whilst individuals at high risk for dental disease cannot be identified with adequate sensitivity and specificity, it is possible to identify at risk populations. In these situations, it can be cost-effective to target preventive interventions at people in specific socioeconomic groups, attending particular schools or living in an area with high disease incidence (Burt 1998). However, a strategy of targeted interventions should take place within a common risk factor approach that addresses general health conditions for the whole population. Such an approach will reduce social inequalities and will provide a multiplicity of benefits, especially as risk factors for oral and general health tend to be clustered in the same groups (Sanders *et al.* 2005). It also avoids the limitations inherent in attempting to identify and treat differently those individuals at high risk for disease. Finally, a recognition of the social context in which personal choices are made avoids the social iatrogenesis of describing oral heath in individual terms (Dickson 1995). Dentistry has been quick to adopt approaches which would now be recognized as health promoting. For example, fluoride levels in water supplies were adjusted to prevent dental caries as early as 1945 (Dean *et al.* 1950).

Health promotion, the process of enabling people to take control over and to improve their health', has five broad actions as outlined in the Ottawa Charter: Creating supportive environments, building healthy public policy, strengthening community action, developing personal skills and reorienting health services (World Health Organization 1984, 1986). Within this approach Sheiham (1995) suggested six policy areas relevant to oral health that are used in this review (Box 9.8.1).

With the growing emphasis on evidence-based healthcare oral health promotion must increasingly demonstrate its effectiveness. Repeated systematic reviews have aimed to identify oral health promotion practices which yield demonstrable health gains or modified knowledge or behaviours (Sprod *et al.* 1996; Kay & Locker 1997). These reviews reveal a paucity of evidence with few reports of well-designed studies in which the intended outcome was health gain. The most robust studies tended to focus on programmes in which the intended outcome was improved knowledge or modification of the behaviours of individuals. Even these studies, which might be termed 'health education' usually involved a relatively short follow-up. The main finding from meta-analysis was the effectiveness of fluoride to prevent caries (Kay & Locker 1997). A less rigorous approach adopted by Sprod and colleagues (1996) allowed exploration of other avenues of activity and research, but still concluded there was little evaluative literature on broader approaches to health promotion.

Other chapters in this text will consider the evaluation of health promotion in some detail, but it needs to be stressed that key features of broader approaches to health promotion may render them

Box 9.8.1 Policy areas relevant to oral health promotion (Sheiham 1995)

1. Use of fluoride
   - Including water, milk, salt, tablets/drops, toothpaste, mouthrinses, and varnishes/gels

2. Food and health policies to reduce sugars consumption
   - National policies recommending proportion of energy intake from sugars and frequency of intake
   - Regulation of advertising and labelling of foods

3. Community approaches to improve body hygiene including oral cleaning
   - Emphasis on toothbrushing with fluoride toothpaste

4. Smoking cessation
   - Advice and support from dental team members

5. Policies on reducing accidents
   - Use of impact-absorbing materials
   - Mouthguards for contact sports

6. Ensuring access to appropriate preventive care
   - Ensuring clinical effectiveness
   - Equity of access
   - Appropriate skill mix

unsuitable for evaluation by randomized controlled trials. Health promotion inevitably takes place in 'real world' settings rather than the strictly controlled environment of randomized controlled trials, many other factors and considerable time often intervene between the intervention and a health outcome and the need for strictly specified outcomes in trials mitigates against the ethos of a common risk factor approach. These factors have led the World Health Organization (1998) to conclude that: 'The use of RCTs to evaluate health promotion initiatives is, in most cases, inappropriate, misleading and unnecessarily expensive'. Even the keenest advocates of RCTs acknowledge that they are unsuitable for evaluating legislative and policy changes (Rosen *et al.* 2006). Other approaches to evaluating health promotion involve other research designs and the use of underlying theory to guide the design of evaluations and the selection of intermediate indicators as proxies of health outcomes (Tones & Tilford 2001).

The use of fluoride

The presence of fluoride at the interface between plaque and dental enamel inhibits the development of caries. To be most effective fluoride should be present both before the teeth start to develop and then continuously throughout life. These findings suggest its effect is derived from a combination of modes of action. Three modes currently receive the most attention: The effect of fluoride on plaque metabolism; the effect of its incorporation during tooth development and its effect on the dynamics of demineralization and remineralization after tooth development.

Water fluoridation

Beneficial effects of fluoride on dental health were discovered as a consequence of investigations of endemic developmental defects of the teeth in Colorado. McKay implicated the water supplies in the aetiology of the staining and pits and discovered that the teeth with defects were less susceptible to dental caries than those without (McKay 1933). The staining was shown to be due to fluoride which existed in some of McKay's samples at levels as high as 14 parts per million (ppm). This staining (now known as dental fluorosis) is hypomaturation or hypomineralization of the teeth caused by chronic ingestion of fluoride during tooth development. It has a variety of presentations from small white flecks on the tooth to larger yellow/brown defects.

Dean and colleagues went on to demonstrate an inverse relationship between dental caries and the fluoride concentration of drinking water (and the associated fluorosis) in two cross-sectional ecological studies (now called the '21 cities studies'). The first intervention trial of fluoridation started in Grand Rapids in 1945 (Dean *et al.* 1950). Since then, similar studies have taken place in many countries including the United Kingdom, the Netherlands and Australia. Worldwide around 400 million people now receive water from a fluoridated water supply and water fluoridation has been designated one of the ten most important public health measures currently available (Centers for Disease Control and Prevention 1999). Dean originally suggested that the optimal concentration for water fluoridation was 1 ppm (1 mg/l), the recommended optimal range of fluoride is now 0.6–1 ppm F.

A systematic review of the effectiveness and safety of water fluoridation included the results of 88 studies (83 of which were cross-sectional) from 30 different countries. Study areas above 5 ppm F were excluded (McDonagh *et al.* 2000). Overall, the included studies were judged to be of low to moderate quality, mainly because of the lack of appropriate adjustment for the effect of confounding factors. Bearing in mind the concerns about the quality of the included studies, water fluoridation was associated with a median increase of 14.6 per cent in the proportion of children without caries experience and a median reduction in dmft/DMFT of 2.25 teeth. For one extra child to be 'caries-free', six children would need to be exposed to water fluoridated at 1 ppm F. Water fluoridation was also found to have an effect over and above that of other sources of fluoride, particularly toothpaste.

A direct dose–response relationship was found between water fluoridation and dental fluorosis. At 1 ppm F, the prevalence of fluorosis was estimated to be 48 per cent and for fluorosis of aesthetic concern 12.5 per cent. The number of additional people who would have to be exposed to water fluoridation at this level for one additional person to develop fluorosis of any level was six. Other possible negative effects considered included bone fracture, cancer, Down syndrome, senile dementia, and goitre. No clear evidence of these potential effects was found, but interpretation of the results of these studies was difficult due to the quality of the primary data.

The cost-effectiveness of water fluoridation depends on the baseline level of caries and the capital costs of the necessary equipment. In areas where water is supplied to large numbers of people via a single source, fluoridation is more cost-effective than in areas supplied by many smaller water sources. In the United Kingdom, water fluoridation is recommended for those areas where the mean DMFT of 5-year-olds is greater than 2 and where water schemes cover approximately 200 000 residents (Sanderson 1998).

Further high-quality research into the safety, efficacy, cost-effectiveness (McDonagh *et al.* 2000), and impact of fluoridation on quality of life has been recommended (Medical Research Council 2002).

The introduction of water fluoridation schemes has been opposed by active antifluoridationist lobbies. Such groups tend to be small, but very enthusiastic and vociferous, with an impact which is often disproportionate to their size or the support they garner. The main arguments against water fluoridation include the safety concerns investigated in the York Review together with ethical objections concerning infringement of individual liberties.

Those against fluoridation argue that it is unethical to fluoridate water supplies as this infringes on the individual's freedom of choice and removes the rights of adults to refuse medical treatment. The claim of fluoridation being an attempt at 'mass medication' is made frequently. The ethical objections to water fluoridation have been discussed by applying the four principles that encompass most of the moral aspects of healthcare, that is; respect for autonomy, beneficence, non-maleficence and justice (Jones & Lennon 1997) (Table 9.8.2).

Opponents claim water fluoridation represents a loss of autonomy, but those proposing fluoridation suggest that in society, some reduction of individual freedom is accepted for the overall good of the community. Anti-fluoridationists argue the only members of society to potentially benefit from water fluoridation are dentate individuals particularly children. Those in favour of fluoridation acknowledge that edentulous people will not benefit, but fluoridation will 'do no harm' to any members of society. On the principle of justice, some claim that imposing water fluoridation is not fair on those against it. Proponents counter this argument by suggesting that the reduction in inequalities in dental health that fluoridation potentially provides is a just way of helping those least able to help themselves.

The debate about fluoridation is an interesting one. Anti-fluoridationists tend to come from relatively healthy middle-class groups. Because children in these groups have the lowest caries experience they have the least to benefit from the intervention. Unfortunately, their effect is to maintain social inequalities in health. Anti-fluoridationist arguments are often alarmist and sometimes unorthodox from the viewpoint of scientists. Unfortunately, public debates between pro- and anti-fluoridationists often end in pro-fluoridationists attempting to refute, in detailed scientific terms, an extensive list of claims. With the current mistrust of science it can be difficult to make such a position attractive in the face of very emotional arguments. Some proponents of fluoridation avoid open debate with anti-fluoridationists for this reason.

Other vehicles for administering fluoride
Fluoride milk
Fluoride has been added to milk as an alternative to water since the 1950s in many countries worldwide. These schemes vary in the age at which children start drinking the milk, the number of years over which it is consumed, the number of days a year the milk is consumed, and the concentration of fluoride added (Marino *et al.* 2006). A systematic review to determine the effectiveness of fluoridated milk for preventing caries on a community basis found insufficient studies of good quality to make a definitive conclusion, but stated fluoridated milk may be beneficial for the permanent dentition (Yeung *et al.* 2005).

Fluoride salt
Salt fluoridation was first used in Switzerland in the 1950s. In certain cantons and in some Latin American countries, all salt for human consumption is fluoridated. Other European countries including France only sell fluoridated salt for domestic use. The typical concentration is 250 ppm F. Several cross-sectional studies report fluoride salt to be effective at reducing caries (Jones *et al.* 2005).

Fluoride tablets/drops
Fluoride tablets/drops use also began in the 1950s. They have been used as dietary supplements with different countries having different dosing regimens (based on child's age, weight, caries-risk, fluoride in the water). Their effectiveness has not been confirmed by any well-designed trials or systematic reviews and the available studies fail to account for confounding factors. There is some evidence that when sucked to maximize the topical dose a preventive effect is observed in deciduous teeth.

Others problem with fluoride supplementation include compliance of individuals and their families and risk of fluorosis. Many of the people most susceptible to caries find the dosing schedules difficult to maintain and taken as a daily bolus fluoride supplements increase the risk of fluorosis (Ismail & Bandekar 1999). These concerns have led to a reduction in the use of tablets/drops as a public health measure.

Topical fluorides
Topically applied fluoride includes delivery systems where fluoride is applied to tooth surfaces at high concentrations for a local protective effect. A series of systematic reviews of trials have investigated the effectiveness of various topical fluorides expressing the effectiveness in terms of the preventive fraction (the difference in caries increments between the intervention and control groups expressed as a percentage of the increment in the control group) (Table 9.8.3).

Fluoride toothpaste
Toothpaste is the most widespread source of fluoride and the decline in caries experience in children in some countries has been attributed to its regular use. The fluoride compounds and concentrations found in toothpastes vary between brands and between countries. The usual concentration is 1000–1500 ppm F with higher (over 2000 ppm F) and lower (less than 600 ppm F) formulations available. They present a good vehicle for the frequent low dose

Table 9.8.2 Summary of ethical arguments about water fluoridation

	For	Against
Autonomy	Some reduction of individual freedom accepted for overall good of the community	Loss of autonomy
Beneficence	Those most in need gain benefit	Only dentate individuals benefit
Non-maleficence	Fluoridation 'does no harm'	Fluoridation causes adverse health effects
Justice	Fluoridation reduces inequalities	Fluoridation is not fair

Source: Jones & Lennon (1997).

application of fluoride and their effectiveness of fluoride toothpaste in reducing caries in children has been confirmed with a PF of 24 per cent (Marinho et al. 2003a). The risk of fluorosis from toothpaste can be minimized by using a smear of paste and supervising children under 6 years of age.

The use of fluoride toothpaste has a distinct disadvantage over water fluoridation as a broad preventive strategy. It relies on people brushing their teeth. In developed countries, poor oral hygiene and high caries incidence are *associated* (although not necessarily causally) and so the people who have most to benefit from the use of fluoride toothpastes are less likely to use them frequently. In developing countries there may not be a tradition of tooth cleaning with toothpastes and western proprietary brands are likely to be expensive. However, cheap locally made pastes can be profoundly effective (Yee et al. 2003).

Fluoride mouthrinses

Fluoride mouthrinses have been used extensively for the past 30 years. School-based programmes were common in certain countries although individual home use now predominates. Mouthrinsing is not recommended for children under 6 years of age, due to the risk of fluoride ingestion. The two main concentrations available are 0.05 per cent (230 ppm F) sodium fluoride used daily and 0.2 per cent (900 ppm F) sodium fluoride weekly. The effectiveness of mouthrinses in children has also been confirmed with a PF of 26 per cent (Marinho et al. 2003b).

Fluoride varnishes/gels

Topically applied fluoride varnishes and gels have been used widely for over two decades both as part of community-based programmes and on an individual basis. Fluoride varnishes are professionally applied with the two most commonly used varnishes containing 22 600 ppm F or 7000 ppm F. A systematic review of trials has confirmed the effectiveness of topical varnishes although the included studies were of poor quality. The PF in permanent teeth was 46 per cent (Marinho et al. 2002a).

Fluoride gels can be professionally or self-applied under supervision. The most commonly used gel is a professionally applied 12 300 ppm F acidulated phosphate fluoride (APF). Due to the risk of excessive ingestion this gel is not recommended for young children. The effectiveness of professionally-applied and self-applied gels have been reviewed with a prevented fraction of 28 per cent (Marinho et al. 2002b).

Diet

Dietary sugars are a necessary cause of clinically significant decay. However, evidence that health education can reduce their intake and so reduce the incidence of caries is lacking (Kay & Locker 1997). Many studies of health education interventions have used self-reported sugar consumption as the primary outcome with the obvious danger of ascertainment bias. Studies that have measured clinical outcomes have combined health education approaches with the use of fluorides and thus the independent effect of the health education cannot be assessed.

Some of the data that implicate sugars in the aetiology of caries suggest that restriction of dietary sugar is preventive. For example, per capita sugar supplies and caries experience data correlate significantly in simple national ecological comparisons. A children's home in Australia had a dietary regimen with almost no sugar and the children had very low caries levels until they were allowed to

Table 9.8.3 Relative effectiveness of sources of topical fluoride

Source	ppm F	Prevented fraction (%)
Toothpaste	500–1500	24
Mouthrinse	230–900	26
Varnish	7000–22 000	46 (permanent)
		33 (deciduous)
Gel	12 300	28

Source: Marinho et al. (2002a, 2002b, 2003a, 2003b).

make their own food choices at the age of 12. Likewise, caries levels fell in parallel with the availability of sugar during World War II (Rugg-Gunn 1993).

Whether these findings can be translated into effective public health strategies remains uncertain. A health-directed food policy seems logical. A common risk factor approach might impact on dental diseases as well as obesity, diabetes and cardiovascular diseases. Possible strategies fall within the framework of education, substitution, regulation, pricing, or provision (Sanderson 1984). However, few countries have such policies in place, and the resources of health advocates are very limited in comparison to those of the affluent and powerful lobby of the commercial food industry. Despite these difficulties, it is by operating at this level that public health might have its greatest impact.

In addition to approaches aimed at individuals, education can take the form of authoritative dietary guidelines to inform national policies, community initiatives, and caterers. The World Health Organization recommends countries to formulate their own specific goals to reduce the amount of free sugars, recommending a maximum of no more than 10 per cent of energy intake. In addition, the frequency of consumption of foods containing free sugars should be limited to a maximum of four times per day (Moynihan & Petersen 2004).

Dietary sugars can be substituted with artificial sweeteners to reduce caries increments. Sales of sugar-free carbonated drinks in Europe and North America demonstrate the compatibility of this tactic with commercial interests. However, substitution of dietary sugars has only limited potential in oral health promotion. The manufacture of many food stuffs relies on the bulk and other specific properties of sugars. In addition, some sweeteners have side effects and resistance to the extended use of artificial sweeteners persists.

Regulation of advertising and labelling of foods in tandem with the effective use substitution is illustrated by a partnership between dentists and the confectionery industry in Switzerland. The *Zahnfreundlich* (toothfriendly) logo is used to label non-acidogenic confectionery (Rugg-Gunn 1997). The label is well recognized by children, is commonly seen on confectionery, and is thought to have been effective in reducing levels of decay (Marthaler 1990). Fiscal policies might be used to discourage manufacture and sale of sugar-containing products. All of the above approaches and direct consumer pressure can be brought to bear on caterers and retail outlets to provide food in a way that makes the healthy choices the easier choices. There are numerous other examples of approaches which may reduce sugars consumption and an exhaustive list is presented by Sheiham (1995).

Oral cleaning

Plaque is a necessary cause of periodontal diseases and so it seems logical that tooth cleaning should be the cornerstone of their management and prevention. Interventions aimed at improving oral hygiene can be successful and achieve a commensurate reduction in gingival inflammation (Kay & Locker 1997; Watt & Marinho 2005). Interestingly, interventions carried out in dental surgeries have been more effective than school-based interventions. However, most studies have had short follow-up periods and the effectiveness of even the best interventions diminishes with time. Therefore, few data show that attempts to improve oral hygiene to prevent destructive disease are effective. Nonetheless, there remains a consensus that the best public health approach to improve periodontal health remains with improved oral hygiene.

The relationship between plaque removal and tooth decay is much more contentious. In a carefully designed trial, professional oral cleaning did not demonstrate any additional preventive effect above a standard preventive programme of fissure sealants and locally applied topical fluoride received by the control groups (Arrow 1997). Sutcliffe's (1996) traditional review considered the effect of research methods on the observed relationship between oral cleaning and dental caries and concluded that there was 'no unequivocal evidence that good oral cleanliness reduces caries experience'. This area of research is fraught with difficulty. As well as the difficulties of measuring dental disease, studies are susceptible to selection bias, leakage of intervention, and the likely confounding effects between self-reported behaviours, diet and oral hygiene. Studies where professional cleaning has been effective have used pastes containing fluoride.

What is known is that brushing with a *fluoride* toothpaste is effective in preventing caries. Therefore, brushing as it is currently practised in most developed countries combats both caries and periodontal diseases, and is to be encouraged.

The systematic reviews cited earlier demonstrated that it is difficult to achieve sustainable changes in oral hygiene behaviour. A study of teenagers found good oral hygiene to be associated with not smoking, exercise, healthy eating, managing in school, and having confidence in one's family (Schou 1998). These types of findings invite the common risk factor approach in which oral cleanliness is promoted as both a health related and health directed behaviour where cleaning ones teeth makes one feel and look nice and is part of a part positive and healthy lifestyle. Toothbrushing is a habit learnt as a young child and is therefore difficult to change later in life. This behaviour is often an established routine before the child has seen a dentist, and interventions via healthcare workers and social agencies working with young children and their mothers may be useful.

Smoking cessation

The role of smoking in the aetiology of oral cancers and periodontal diseases has already been discussed. Johnson has listed 20 oral conditions either directly or indirectly associated with tobacco smoking (Johnson 1997). In addition to the well-known benefits to cardiovascular and respiratory health, cessation of smoking almost eliminates the increased risk of oral cancer within 5–10 years.

Many of the oral conditions such as stained teeth, receding gums, and altered taste are readily perceptible to the individual and may encourage or reinforce the desire to stop smoking. The dental team are also often aware of the personal and social circumstances (e.g. pregnancy or a new job) that prompt people to give up. Therefore, smoking cessation is another area where it is particularly appropriate for dentistry to become integrated into a common risk factor approach. As clinicians, the dental team can be effective in supporting smoking cessation by providing advice (Carr & Ebbert 2006).

Prevention of accidents

Several strategies can be used to reduce trauma to teeth. Playground surfaces can be made of impact-absorbing materials which cushion against trauma. The use of mouthguards is compulsory for some sports in some countries. Mouthguards not only prevent dental injuries, but also prevent laceration of the facial soft tissues against the teeth, reduce the risk of mandibular fracture and may protect the cranial cavity. Mouthguards are usually made of a copolymer of polyvinyl acetate and polyethylene. The most basic type may be obtained prefabricated in a range of sizes. A more sophisticated type may be adapted to fit the mouth, typically by softening it in hot water first. Custom-made devices constructed on models made from impressions of the teeth are the most comfortable and can be made to support the lower teeth and mandible during trauma.

As immediate first-aid for dental trauma, particularly avulsed teeth, is so important for the long-term survival of the traumatized teeth, informing athletes and their teachers and trainers of the need for immediate action can reduce the impact of the trauma.

Unfortunately, orthodontic treatment of protruding front teeth is complex and prolonged, but can be justified in children of 8 or 9 years to reduce the risk of trauma (Welbury 1996).

Ensuring access to appropriate preventive care

There has been disillusionment with the biomedical model of healthcare. By focusing on the diseases of individuals, it was criticized for emphasizing the hierarchy of professionals over lay people and treatments rather than prevention. All of these things have taken place with substantial economic and social costs and yet medical care was said to make a relatively small contribution to health (McKeown 1976; Illich 1976).

Within this view, the biomedical approach distracts attention from the wider social, political, and economic determinants of health. The Primary Health Care Approach (PHCA) recognized that these determinants are more important than medical interventions (World Health Organization 1978).

Whilst dental services are rarely designed to deliver benefits at the public health level, they are just as susceptible to the criticisms of the medical model of healthcare. Dental treatment has made a relatively small contribution to aspects of oral health. For example, orthodontic treatment is often advocated on the basis of social and psychological benefit; however, a recent 20-year follow-up study of orthodontic treatment was unable to find evidence to support such a benefit (Kenealy et al. 2007). Data from the 1970s show that dental services explain 3 per cent of the variation in oral health of 12-year-olds in developed countries, compared to the 65 per cent contribution made by broader socioeconomic factors (Nadanovsky & Sheiham 1994, 1995). Furthermore, the interventions used in dentistry may also be clinically inappropriate. Dentistry has adopted a surgical approach to treatment with a cycle of placing and replacing fillings. It has long been recognized that the quality of many fillings is not high and that even the decisions to place fillings are idiosyncratic (Elderton & Nuttall 1983). Since fillings are often replaced several times over a lifetime, the remaining tooth is increasingly damaged with each new filling.

Clinical dental services also neglect the determinants of disease. With its emphasis on personal behaviour and even with the search for specific periodontal pathogens, clinical dentistry and some dental research diverts attention from the factors that determine oral health and disease.

Dental services are also costly. National Health Service dentistry costs £2 billion per year for the 54 million people living in England and Wales. Compared to the potential costs of treatment the resources available are few and are likely to reduce in future. Curative services serve those who can afford them. In addition to creating dependence on professionals, the services become focused on those with least health problems.

The problems of medical and dental care exist in parallel; therefore, the same kinds of changes are applicable to both. There are too few resources, the resources that are available are still poorly allocated, services still congregate around the wealthy people, ordinary people have little control over own health, and health professionals still do not trust people to make good decisions about their health. All of these points apply to dentistry. In every country of the world, there are people who cannot attend and or cannot afford dental treatment in its current guise. Even in countries with well-developed socialized systems of dental care, there are major inequalities in oral health (Watt & Sheiham 1999).

Views about the relative role of health services remain polarized. From one perspective, too narrow a focus on 'health service issues' contributes to the failure of public health to improve population health (Holland 2002; Beaglehole & Bonita 2004). The 'post-new public health' view argues that preventive and curative measures prolong life expectancy and maintain and improve the quality of life. Bunker (2001) estimated the increases in life expectancy attributable to clinical care by calculating increases resulting from declines in disease-specific death rates and from specific treatments. His conclusions may have been optimistic in both generalizing from results achieved in research trials to routine practice with patients with complex problems and in underestimating the continuing role of social and other environmental factors in health (Frankel 2001; Tudor Hart 2001).

At a population level, it remains exceedingly difficult to distinguish the effects of medical care from those of other health determinants. In addition, clinical services offer advantages other than those of life expectancy (or tooth survival). As we gain greater knowledge of the effects of specific clinical and public health interventions, we can regard the direct opposition of the two approaches as a false dichotomy (Frankel 2001). The key decisions are to select which interventions can improve the health of the population.

Unfortunately, as this review has shown, when compared to medicine, the benefits and costs of clinical dentistry at either an individual or population level are relatively unknown. Some check is required to counter the assumption that the principle way to improve the oral health of a population is via the provision of more dental treatment. Dental services remain overdue for an evaluation and reorientation. A more holistic practice of dentistry will also ensure that services are more equitable and appropriate.

Public health specialists can contribute to increasing the effectiveness of services and facilitating equity of access to services when needed. For example, clinical dentistry can have a role in reducing the psycho-social impacts of oral disease (Awad et al. 2000;

Robinson et al. 2005). For this reason, it is essential that we generate a greater understanding within dentistry of the nature of oral health. The movement to identify more relevant measures of oral health to assess treatment need and the outcomes of care should be encouraged. The evidence-based approach, the use of clinical governance, and managed care should provide both the impetus and the means to ensure that only effective and efficient interventions are used.

Dental surgeries are a natural health-related setting for health promotion. Practice-based oral health promotion activities provide an opportunity to increase knowledge and promote self-esteem and empowerment. Their role could be expanded by adopting a common risk factor approach. However, practice-based health promotion is only useful for those who attend the services and may exclude those people with the greatest need who do not. In addition, there needs to be a change in emphasis in health education from the prescriptive approaches that ignore the needs of people they serve and so blame the victims. Patients should not feel they are being chastised or told to do things. A more effective approach would be a patient-centred model which respects patients' autonomy and seeks their active participation in defining their needs (Croucher 1989).

Specific changes that could be made to ensure access to dental services can still be categorized in the framework used by Penchansky and Thomas (1981). Services must be available, accessible, affordable, acceptable, and accommodating. This framework is broadly compatible with the characteristics of dental services as seen within Andersen's (1995) behavioural model of access.

Clearly people cannot use services that do not exist, so increasing their availability has a direct effect on service use. One way of making dental services more available at limited cost is to delegate care to other DCPs. In developed countries the majority of treatment required falls within the remit of DCPs. It is therefore not cost-effective to employ highly trained and highly paid dentists to undertake this less demanding and repetitive work. A number of countries including Australia, New Zealand, Canada, and the United Kingdom employ dental care professionals with a limited repertoire of treatment options (variously called school dental nurses, dental auxiliaries, and dental therapists) who provide high quality care at lower cost. Similar data exist for dental hygienists. DCPs work under the supervision of a dentist. By reducing the level of supervision required and expanding there role, the availability of care can be increased whilst limiting costs. Dental hygienists can work independently without reducing either the quality of treatment or patients' satisfaction with it. Likewise, hygienists can be trained to conduct clinical examinations in dental surveys with no compromise to the quality of the data (Kwan et al. 1996).

Clearly the expanded use of DCPs threatens the monopoly on the provision of dental treatment held by dentists and the profession has been a frequent barrier to their wider use. For example, executives of the American Dental Association have recently advocated a free market dental system with subsidized treatment for disadvantaged families rather than a needs-based system using DCPs in areas with an undersupply of care (Bramson & Guay 2005).

One particular aspect of dentistry in many countries that could be revised is the system of payment of fees to dentists for each item of service provided. Fee-per-item service payments encourage dentists to work quickly and have been associated (in the past at least) with over-treatment. This system of payment tends to encourage the curative technical approach to treatment, unless there is a specific fee for prevention. On the other hand, services based on capitation per patient enrolled reduce restorative treatment, increase preventive care with no evidence of 'supervised neglect' (Johansson *et al.* 2007).

The acceptability of dental services was highlighted in a qualitative study of people who did not go to the dentist (Gregory *et al.* 2007). As well as being influenced by the perceived accessibility of care, participants were swayed by their trust in dentistry and their perceptions of oral health as a commodity. For these people at least, greater marketing may have been counter-productive in encouraging use of dental services.

Middle- and low-income countries

Whilst the prevalence of dental caries in many developing countries is still low, other diseases such as oral cancer and dental fluorosis are more common than in most developed countries. Non-industrialized countries also suffer from a shortage of resources including workforce, appropriate technology and universally available power supplies. For example, the dentist: Population ratio in many countries in Africa is less than 1 to 100 000 population compared to 1 to 1100 population in many Scandinavian countries. Over the last two decades, the additional burden of meeting the costs of the infection control implications of the HIV epidemic have exacerbated any deficiencies in resources.

The traditional curative approach to dental health is limited in any setting but these limitations are more extreme when they are exported to the developing world. The surgical approach to dentistry used in industrialized countries is technology intensive and requires an infrastructure of continuous power and water supply. It involves expensive equipment that is difficult to use and maintain. Dentists, therefore, need to treat patients who can help them recoup their costs. These pressures limit the availability of services and contribute to the inequalities in their provision. Hobdell (1993) described this situation as 'trying to implement a type of oral healthcare developed mainly in the last century in another part of the world using equipment and materials developed for use in an entirely different socioeconomic and political setting'. Large parts of the western model of dental care may be inappropriate in developing countries, including an over-emphasis of clinical surveys in healthcare planning. Services based on normative assessment limit community participation in healthcare and ignore the sociodental implications of oral disease. They may also over complicate healthcare. In one notorious example, survey data were used to calculate the periodontal treatment needs of children in Kenya (Manji & Sheiham 1986). Using the World Health Organization model the treatment proposed would have used the entire dental workforce of Kenya for up to 21 years, allowing for no other care. Services could concentrate on the relatively few conditions that comprise the bulk of oral health problems: Toothache (not *tooth decay*), trauma, oral infections, and neoplasms (Hobdell 1993).

The primary healthcare approach is still relevant to oral healthcare in all countries but it is particularly applicable to the developing world. It has five principles: An equitable distribution of services; community involvement in health; a focus on prevention; the use of appropriate technology and a multi-sectoral approach. *The Berlin Declaration on Oral Health and Oral Health Services in Deprived Communities* provides comprehensive guidelines for planning, implementing and evaluating oral health

projects within this framework (Mautsch & Sheiham 1995). It was conceived by the Oral Health Alliance: An international network which provides support and information to colleagues working in this field. Specific examples of activities within this framework are presented below.

Equitable distribution

Tudor Hart's (1971) 'Inverse care law' between the availability of services and the need for them also occurs in dentistry. It is particularly extreme in countries where there are wide disparities between rich and poor. In Africa 80 per cent of the trained professional personnel live and work in affluent neighbourhoods in cities although the same proportion of the population lives in rural areas (Thorpe 1993). The scope for other dental care professionals in developing countries may be greater since advocates of their use may not have to compete with the well established political lobbies of dentists which exist in industrialized nations. DCPs can be used to provide simple, but essential treatments to extend the availability of services and reduce inequalities in access.

Models exist for identifying the types of personnel needed for oral healthcare in deprived communities along with training and evaluation methods (Samarawikrama 1995). Such models consider the frequency of problems, the difficulties encountered in undertaking the different roles and the identification of the difficulties themselves.

Community development

Community involvement means that people are allowed to take control of their own health and is necessary if programmes are to thrive. It is perhaps the most difficult aspect of the PHCA since it requires that health professionals must relinquish their traditional hierarchical role. In addition, individuals and communities often regard health as beyond their control and may not regard oral health as a priority. There are isolated examples of wide involvement in oral health. In Glasgow, Scotland, community-based Oral Health Action Teams—partnerships of parents, teachers, nursery nurses, health visitors and dentists—have reduced levels of caries in young children in deprived areas of the city (Blair 2004).

Focus on prevention

Prevention is universally accepted as an essential component of healthcare. However, if prevention is to avoid the existing system in which people are passive recipients of information and preventive therapies, it must adopt the principles of health promotion.

Appropriate technology

'Appropriate technology' is sometimes taken to mean 'cheap' and 'second rate'. It is neither of these things, but is an approach which recognizes the needs and resources of the local community. For example, the ART referred to earlier combines these requirements with new knowledge of the process of dental caries and developments in dental materials science (Frencken *et al.* 1966).

Multisectoral approach

We have seen how an effective health strategy might involve a number of departments of both national and local governments, water providers, the educational system, community members, and healthcare workers. All of the approaches to health promotion outlined in the second part of this essay must be integrated. However, integration should mean more than using the resources of other sectors to promote oral health. Such an approach often means that dentists simply get teachers to provide dental health education which carries the risk of not truly involving the other sectors (Mautsch & Sheiham 1995).

Conclusions and future developments in dental public health

Our understanding of the importance of oral health and its significance as a public health concern continues to grow. There is a greater knowledge than ever before of the nature of the oral diseases that threaten health (dental caries, periodontal diseases, oral cancer, and dento-facial trauma), the epidemiology of those diseases, and the factors that determine them. Moreover, we are starting to accumulate a body of evidence on the effectiveness of health promotion and treatment strategies. Those strategies include the use of fluoride; food and health policies to reduce sugar consumption; and community approaches to improve body hygiene including oral cleaning, smoking cessation, policies on reducing accidents, and ensuring access to appropriate preventive care. Many of these strategies could work in common with approaches to the promotion of general health.

Many oral health strategies discussed in this review do not involve clinical dental services. Dentistry lags behind medicine in recognizing the relative impotence of clinical dentistry to bring about oral health for populations and a greater awareness of its potential harm. The evidence of effectiveness should be used to identify beneficial interventions and should help re-orientate dentistry from its traditional curative approach that focuses on the responsibility of clinicians and their individual patients. In so doing we may be able to move toward a more shared responsibility in which all participate.

It is important that all these strands of information are combined. Perhaps most important of all, we need a more universal understanding of what is meant by 'oral health' and its relationship with oral disease. The ways we measure health and the outcomes of interventions will determine not only which interventions we choose but whether we choose to intervene at all.

Future developments in dental public health can be considered in four areas: Trends in oral health, the deprofessionalization of dentistry, technological developments, and relationships between oral and general healthcare delivery.

Two trends in oral health have been observed. Some countries, particularly developing countries, may be experiencing increases in dental caries. Any increases are related to the adoption of western dietary patterns high in sugars. Even if these trends are currently limited to more affluent city dwellers, they represent worrying concerns for the future. The increase in treatment needs created by these trends is likely to place an unaffordably high burden on developing economies. To some extent, this burden will be moderated by the low levels of perceived need in communities unused to receiving dental treatment. However, if disability and handicap brought about by oral disease is to be minimized, then appropriate methods of treating it will be required. Numerous examples now exist of dental care professionals being used to provide a limited range of treatments in both the developed and developing world. DCPs can be trained quicker to provide care to similar standards to dentists, but at greatly reduced costs. Food and health policies could also be used in countries with rising caries levels to control imports, the production and sale of cariogenic foods and drinks while encouraging the use of traditional foods.

In many developed countries, the decreased caries incidence witnessed over the last two decades appears to have stabilized in young children. The trend may have stabilized but its effects will continue to change dentistry for decades to come. When coupled with demographic changes, changed attitudes towards oral health and the preservation of teeth seen in developing countries over the last 50 years, this trend produces an interesting pattern. On the one hand, there is a growing and ageing group of younger people whose treatment needs will remain lower in terms of volume and complexity than preceding generations. On the other hand, there is a large group of older people who will live for longer and retain many heavily restored teeth. These people will require more care, some of it more complex, than the generations that preceded them. It is difficult to predict whether there will be a net change in the need for dental care or in which direction such a change would be. One likely change will be a greater emphasis on specialization within dentistry. The majority of the young people's needs will comprise simple one surface fillings that could be placed by DCPs. However, this change could be offset by the more complex demands of older people seeking dental implants and treatment for root caries and tooth wear that may remain in the domain of specialists.

A dominant political direction over recent years has been the deprofessionalization of dentistry. This trend is manifest in several different forms. In many developed countries, patients are demanding 'rights' as consumers of care. These demands are complemented by the application of marketing theory to dentistry, which places consumer satisfaction as an essential criterion in business success. Thus, patients have been directly and indirectly implicated in moves to regulate the way in which dentists market themselves and have ensured that patient satisfaction is an active concern of dentists. Similar principles are cornerstones of new public health. Health promotion takes public involvement in oral health well beyond clinical dentistry. Even within clinical care, satisfaction is an integral part of the process of care rather than just an outcome. Other agencies, such as governments and insurance companies, are increasingly involved in healthcare. Externally applied measures to minimize the costs of care and increase the accountability of healthcare organizations whilst assuring the quality of care all serve to reduce professional power within dentistry.

This trend of deprofessionalization is likely to continue and may help to make oral care more relevant to the needs of the people it serves. Professions resist any tendency to undermine their power. This reaction could present an opportunity for dental public health to facilitate and manage the deprofessionalization of dentistry.

A number of technological developments may also influence oral health and care. The ART shows considerable potential for providing simple, inexpensive, and effective treatment for the type of minimal caries seen in developing countries. Because the technique requires minimal training and equipment, it will allow services to be provided in relatively small and isolated communities. If the technique is used by partially skilled staff it may also contribute to the deprofessionalization of dentistry in these countries; it will certainly reduce the cost.

In developed countries, osseo-integrated implants are increasingly used to support dental prostheses. By providing a stable and retentive base for both single and multiple tooth prostheses, implants show great potential for reducing the handicap brought about by oral disease (Awad et al. 2000). One disadvantage is that, for the time being at least, implant treatment demands considerable specialist expertise, and is costly. Implants may therefore become a treatment limited to those who can afford them and thus contribute to inequalities in oral health.

Oral healthcare is becoming increasingly integrated with the delivery of other services. In policy terms greater integration can be seen as part of a multidisciplinary approach (World Health Organization 1978). There are many examples of integration at the level of clinical service provision. Dental surgeries may be linked with other clinical services in health centres. In some cases, dentists invite other types of healthcare workers into their practices to provide services. At a broader level of health promotion, integration is particularly compatible with a common risk factor approach to disease. Health educators and health promoters recognize the value of involving other healthcare workers, teachers, and other community workers, either as original deliverers or reinforcers of their messages. Oral health also becomes a consideration of local and national governments with debates about fluoridation of water supplies and whether agricultural and fiscal policy are used to promote oral health. It is the role of specialists in dental public health to act as advocates at all these levels.

References

Andersen, R.M. (1995) Revisiting the behavioral model and access to medical care: Does it matter? *Journal of Health and Social Behavior*, **36**, 1–10.

Andreasen, J.O. and Andreasen, F.M. (1997) *Textbook and Color Atlas of Traumatic Injuries to the Teeth*. Munksgaard, Copenhagen.

Armfield, J.M. and Spencer, A.J. (2007) Community effectiveness of fissure sealants and the effect of fluoridated water consumption. *Community Dental Health*, **24**, 4–11.

Arrow, P. (1997) Control of occlusal caries in the first permanent molars by oral hygiene. *Community Dentistry and Oral Epidemiology*, **25**, 278–83.

Awad, M.A., Locker, D., Korner-Bitensky, N., *et al.* (2000) Measuring the effect of intraoral implant rehabilitation on health related quality of life in a randomised controlled clinical trial. *Journal of Dental Research*, **79**, 1659–63.

Beck, J.D., Offenbacher, S. (2005) Systemic effects of periodontitis: epidemiology of periodontal disease and cardiovascular disease. *Journal of Periodontology*, **76** (Suppl.), 2089–100.

Beaglehole, R., Bonita, R. (2004) *Public Health at the Crossroads*. Cambridge University Press, Cambridge.

Blair, Y., Macpherson, L.M., McCall, D.R., *et al.* (2004) Glasgow nursery-based caries experience, before and after a community development-based oral health programme's implementation. *Community Dental Health*, **21**, 291–8.

Bramson, J.B., Guay, A.H. (2005) Comments on the proposed pediatric oral health therapist. *Journal of Public Health Dentistry*, **65**, 123–27.

Bunker, J.P. (2001) The role of medical care in contributing to health improvements within societies. *International Journal of Epidemiology*, **30**, 1260–1263.

Burt, B.A. (1998) Prevention policies in the light of the changed distribution of dental caries. *Acta Odontologica Scandinavia*, **56**, 179–86.

Burt, B.A., Ismail, A.I., and Eklund, S.A. (1985) Periodontal disease, tooth loss, and oral hygiene among older Americans. *Community Dentistry and Oral Epidemiology*, **13**, 93–6.

Carr, A.B., Ebbert, J.O. Interventions for tobacco cessation in the dental setting. *Cochrane Database of Systematic Reviews* 2006, Issue 1. Art. No.: CD005084. DOI: 10.1002/14651858.CD005084.pub2.

Centers for Disease Control and Prevention. (1999) Ten Great Public Health Achievements - United States, 1900-1999. *MMWR CDC Surveillance Summaries*, **48**, 241–243.

Conway, D.I., Stockton, D.L., Warnakulasuriya, K.A., *et al.* (2006) Incidence of oral and oropharyngeal cancer in United Kingdom (1990-1999) - recent trends and regional variation. *Oral Oncology*, **42**, 586–92.

Croucher, R. (1989) *The Performance Gap*. Health Education Authority, London.

Dean, H.T., Arnold, F.A. Jr., Jay, P., *et al.* (1950) Studies on mass control of dental caries through fluoridation of the public water supply. *Public Health Reports*, **65**, 1403–8.

Department of Health and Human Services (2000) *Oral Health in America: A report of the Surgeon General*. Washington: Department of Health and Human Services.

Dickson, M. (1995) Oral Health Promotion In *Promoting oral health in deprived communities* (ed. Mautsch, W. and Sheiham, A.), pp. 175–86. Deusche Stiftungfur Internationale Entwicklung, Berlin.

Downer, M.C., Moles, D.R., Palmer, S., *et al.* (2006) A systematic review of measures of the effectiveness of screening for oral cancer and precancer. *Oral Oncology*, **42**, 551–60.

Elderton, R.J. and Nuttall, N.M. (1983) Variation among dentists in planning treatment. *British Dental Journal*, **154**, 201–6.

Frankel, S. (2001) Commentary: Medical care and the wider influences upon population health: a false dichotomy. *International Journal of Epidemiology*, **30**, 1267–8.

Frencken, J.E., Pilot, T., Songpaisan, Y., *et al.* (1996) Atraumatic restorative treatment (ART): rationale, technique, and development. *Journal of Public Health Dentistry*, **56**, 135–40.

Gregg, T.A. and Boyd, T.H (1998) Treatment of avulsed permanent teeth in children. *International Journal of Paediatric Dentistry*, **8**, 75–81.

Gregory, J., Gibson, B., Robinson, P.G. (2007) The relevance of oral health for attenders and non-attenders: a qualitative study. *British Dental Journal*, **202**, E 18.

Hobdell, M.H. (1993) Essential elements of a primary oral health care model. In *Promotion of Oral Health in the African Region. Proceedings of Workshop held in Nairobi, Kenya, 2–6 August 1993* (ed. Akpabio, S.P.), pp. 99–108. Commonwealth Dental Association, London.

Holliser, M.C. and Weintraub, J.A. (1993) The association of oral status with systemic health, quality of life, and economic productivity. *Journal of Dental Education*, **57**, 901–12.

Holland, W.W. (2002) A dubious future for public health? *Journal of the Royal Society of Medicine*, **95**, 182–8.

Illich I. (1976) *Limits to Medicine*. Penguin, London.

Ismail, A.I. and Bandekar, R.R. (1999) Fluoride supplements and fluorosis: a meta-analysis. *Community Dentistry and Oral Epidemiology*, **27**, 48–56.

Johansson, V. Axtelius, B., Soderfeldt, B., *et al.* (2007) Financial systems' impact on dental care: a review of fee-for-service and capitation systems. *Community Dental Health*, **24**, 12–20.

Johnson, N.W. (1997) Oral cancer: practical prevention. *FDI World*, **6**, 6–13.

Jones, S., Burt, B. A., Petersen, P. E., *et al.* (2005) The effective use of fluorides in public health. *Bulletin of World Health Organization*, **83**, 670–6.

Jones, S. and Lennon, M. A. (Eds.) (1997) Fluoridation. Community Oral Health. Bath, Wright.

Kay, E.J. and Locker, D. (1997) *Effectiveness of oral health promotion: a review*. Health Education Authority, London.

Kenealy, P.M., Kingdon, A., Richmond, S., *et al.* (2007) The Cardiff dental study: A 20-year critical evaluation of the psychological health gain from orthodontic treatment. *British Psychological Society*, **12**, 17–49.

Kwan, S.Y., Prendergast, M.J., and Williams, S.A. (1996) The diagnostic reliability of clinical dental auxiliaries in caries prevalence surveys – a pilot study. *Community Dental Health*, **13**, 145–49.

Locker, D. (2004) Oral health and quality of life. *Oral Health & Preventive Dentistry*, **2** (Suppl.), 247–53.

Manji, F. and Sheiham, A. (1986) CPITN findings and the manpower implications of periodontal treatment needs for Kenyan children. *Community Dental Health*, **3**, 143–51.

Marino, R., Villa A., and Weitz, A. (2006) Dental Caries Prevention using Milk as the vehicle for Fluorides: The Chilean Experiences. Melbourne, Australia: School of Dental Science, The University of Melbourne.

Marinho, V.C.C., Higgins, J.P.T., Logan, S., *et al.* (2002a) Fluoride varnishes for preventing dental caries in children and adolescents. *Cochrane Database of Systematic Reviews*. Issue 1. Art. No.: CD002279. DOI: 10.1002/14651858.CD002279.

Marinho, V.C.C., Higgins, J.P.T., Logan, S., *et al.* (2002b) Fluoride gels for preventing dental caries in children and adolescents. *Cochrane Database of Systematic Reviews*. Issue 1. Art. No.: CD002280. DOI: 10.1002/14651858.CD002280

Marinho, V.C.C., Higgins, J.P.T., Logan, S., *et al.* (2003a) Fluoride toothpastes for preventing dental caries in children and adolescents. *Cochrane Database of Systematic Reviews*. Issue 1. Art. No.: CD002278. DOI: 10.1002/14651858.CD002278.

Marinho, V.C.C., Higgins, J.P.T., Logan, S., *et al.* (2003b) Fluoride mouthrinses for preventing dental caries in children and adolescents. *Cochrane Database of Systematic Reviews*. Issue 3. Art.No.: CD002284. DOI: 10.1002/14651858.CD002284.

Marthaler, T.M. (1990) Changes in the prevalence of dental caries: How much can be attributed to changes in diet. *Caries Research*, **24**, 212–23.

Mautsch, W. and Sheiham, A. (1995) *Promoting Oral Health in Deprived Communities*. Zahnmedizinische Entwicklungshilfe e.V., Berlin.

McDonagh, M., Whiting, P., Bradley, M., *et al.* (2000) *A Systematic Review of Public Water Fluoridation*. York: Publications Office, NHS Centre for Reviews and Dissemination, University of York.

McKay, F.S. (1933) Mottled enamel: The prevention of its further production through a change of water supply at Oakley, Idaho. *Journal of the American Dental Association*, **20**, 1137–49.

McKeown, T. (1976) *The Role of Medicine: Dream, Mirage or Nemesis?* The Nuffield Provincial Hospitals Trust, London.

Medical Research Council. (2002) *Water Fluoridation and Health*. Medical Research Council, London.

Moynihan, P. and Petersen, P.E. (2004) Diet, nutrition and the prevention of dental diseases. *Public Health Nutrition*, **7**, 201–26.

Morris, A.J., Steele, J., and White, D.A. (2001) The oral cleanliness and periodontal health of UK adults in 1998. *British Dental Journal*, **191**, 186–92.

Nadanovsky, P. and Sheiham, A. (1994) The relative contribution of dental services to the changes and geographical variations in caries status of 5- and 12-year-old children in England and Wales in the 1980s. *Community Dental Health*, **11**, 215–23.

Nadanovsky, P. and Sheiham, A. (1995) Relative contribution of dental services to the changes in caries levels of 12-year-old children in 18 industrialized countries in the 1970s and early 1980s. *Community Dentistry and Oral Epidemiology*, **23**, 331–9.

National Institute for Health and Clinical Excellence (2004) *Dental recall- recall interval between routine dental examinations*. National Institute for Health and Clinical Excellence, London.

Needleman, I., Suvan, J., Moles, D.R., *et al.* (2005a) A systematic review of professional mechanical plaque removal for prevention of periodontal diseases. *Journal of Clinical Periodontology*, **32** (Supplement), 229–82.

Needleman, I., Tucker, R., Giedry-Leeper, E., *et al.* (2005b) Guided tissue regeneration for periodontal intrabony defects - a Cochrane Systematic Review. *Periodontology 2000*, **37**, 106–123. doi:10.1111/j.1600-0757.2004.37101.x

Nuttall, N., Steele, J.G., Pine, C.M., *et al.* (2001) The impact of oral health on people in the UK in 1998. *British Dental Journal*, **190**, 121–126.

Nuttall, N. and Harker, R. (2004) *Impact of oral health- Children's Dental Health in the United Kingdom 2003*. http://www.statistics.gov.uk/ downloads/cdh5_Impact_of_oral_health.pdf Accessed 19th March 2007.

Penchansky, R. and Thomas, J.W. (1981) The concept of access. Definition and relationship to consumer satisfaction. *Medical Care*, **19**, 127–40.

Pitts. N. and Harker, R. (2004) *Obvious decay experience. Children's Dental Health in the United Kingdom 2003*. http://www.statistics.gov.uk/ children/dentalhealth/downloads/cdh_dentinal_decay.pdf. Accessed 19th March 2007.

Reibel, J. (2003) Tobacco and oral diseases. Update on the evidence, with recommendations. *Medical Principles and Practice*, **12** (Suppl. 1), 22–32

Robinson, P.G., Deacon, S.A., Deery, C., *et al.* Manual versus powered toothbrushing for oral health. *The Cochrane Database of Systematic Reviews* 2005, Issue 2. Art. No.: CD002281.pub2. DOI: 10.1002/14651858.CD002281.pub2.

Robinson, P.G., Pankhurst, C.L., Garrett, E.J. (2005) Randomized-controlled trial: effect of a reservoir biteguard on quality of life in xerostomia. *Journal of Oral Pathology and Medicine*, **34**, 193–7.

Rose, G. (1992) *The Strategy of Preventive Medicine*. Oxford University Press, Oxford.

Rosen, L., Manor, D., Engelhard, D., *et al.* (2006) In defense of the randomized controlled trial for health promotion research. *American Journal of Public Health*, **96**, 1181–6.

Rugg-Gunn, A. (1997) Nutrition, dietary guidelines and food policy in oral health. In *Community Oral Health* (ed. Pine, C.), pp. 206–20. Wright, Oxford.

Rugg-Gunn, A.J. (1993) *Nutrition and Dental Health*. Oxford University Press, Oxford.

Samarawikrama, D.Y.D. (1995) Appropriate technology, personnel and training. In *Promoting Oral Health in Deprived communities* (ed. Mautsch, W. and Sheiham, A.), pp. 347–61. Deusche Stiftungfur Internationale Entwicklung, Berlin.

Sanders, A.E., Spencer, A.J., and Stewart, J.F. (2005) Clustering of risk behaviours for oral and general health. *Community Dental Health*, **22**, 133–40.

Sanderson, M.E. (1984) Strategies for implementing NACNE recommendations. *Lancet*, **10**, 1352–6.

Sanderson, D. (1998) *Water fluoridation - an economics perspective*. York: York Health Economics Consortium. University of York.

Schou, L. (1998) Behavioural aspects of dental plaque control measures: an oral health promotion perspective. In *European workshop on mechanical plaque control* (eds Lang, N.P., Attstrom, R., and Loe, H.), pp. 287–99. Quintessence, Chicago.

Sheiham, A. (1995) Development of oral health promotion strategies In *Turning Strategy into Action* (ed. Kay, E.), pp. 9–46. Eden Bianchi Press, Manchester.

Sheiham, A. and Watt, R.G. (2000) The common risk factor approach: a rational basis for promoting oral health. *Community Dentistry and Oral Epidemiology*, **28**, 399–406.

Smith, S.E., Warnakulasuriya, K.A., Feyerabend, C., *et al.* (1998) A smoking cessation programme conducted through dental practices in the UK. *British Dental Journal*, **185**, 299–303.

Sprod, A., Anderson, R., and Treasure, E.T. (1996) *Effective Oral Health Promotion: Literature Review*. Health Promotion Wales, Cardiff.

Sutcliffe, P. (1996) Oral cleanliness and dental caries In *Prevention of oral disease* (ed. Murray, J.J.), pp. 68–77. Oxford University Press, Oxford.

Thorpe, S.J. (1993) Oral health status and trends in Africa – A WHO overview. In *Promotion of oral health in the African region. Proceedings of workshop held Nairobi, Kenya, 2–6 August 1993* (ed. Akpabio, S.P.), pp. 72–6. Commonwealth Dental Association, London.

Tones, K. and Tilford, S. (2001) *Health Promotion. Effectiveness, Efficiency and Equity*. Nelson Thornes Ltd, Cheltenham.

Tudor Hart, J. (1971) The inverse care law. *Lancet*, **1**, 405–12.

Tudor Hart, J. (2001) Commentary: Can health outputs of routine practice approach those of clinical trials? *International Journal of Epidemiology*, **30**, 1263–7.

van Amerongen B.M., Schutte G.J.B. and Alpherts W.C.J. (1993) *International dental key figures: A dynamic and relational data base analyzing oral health care*. Key Figure, Amsterdam.

Van der Weijden, G.A. and Timmerman, M.F. (2002) A systematic review on the clinical efficacy of subgingival debridement in the treatment of chronic periodontitis. *Journal of Clinical Periodontology*, **29** (Suppl. 3), 55–71.

Watt, R. and Marinho, V.C. (2005) Does oral health promotion improve oral hygiene and gingival health? *Periodontology 2000*, **37**, 35–47.

Watt, R. and Sheiham, A. (1999) Inequalities in Oral Health: A review of the evidence and recommendations for action. *British Dental Journal*, **187**, 6–12.

Watt, R. (2007) From victim blaming to upstream action: tackling the social determinants of oral health inequalities. *Community Dentistry and Oral Epidemiology*, **35**, 1–11.

Welbury, R.R. (1996) The prevention of dental trauma. In *The prevention of oral disease* (ed. Murray, J.J.), pp. 147–52. Oxford University Press, Oxford.

WHO/UNICEF (1978) *Primary Health Care, Alma-Ata 1978*. World Health Organization, Geneva.

Wong, F.S. and Kolokotsa, K. (2004) The cost of treating children and adolescents with injuries to their permanent incisors at a dental hospital in the United Kingdom. *Dental Traumatology*, **20**, 327–33.

World Health Organization (1984) *Health Promotion: A Discussion Document on the Concepts and Principles*. World Health Organisation Regional Office for Europe, Copenhagen.

World Health Organization (1986) *Ottawa Charter for Health Promotion*. World Health Organisation, Geneva.

World Health Organization (1998) *Health Promotion Evaluation: Recommendations to policy makers*. World Health Organisation, Geneva.

World Health Organization (2001) *Global Oral Health Data Bank*. Geneva: World Health Organization.

World Health Organization (1980) *Risk factors and comprehensive control of chronic diseases. Report ICP/CVD 020(2)*. Geneva: World Health Organization.

Xiong, X., Buekens, P., Fraser, W.D., *et al.* (2006) Periodontal disease and adverse pregnancy outcomes: a systematic review. *British Journal of Obstetrics and Gynaecology*, **113**, 135–43.

Yee, R., McDonald, N., and Walker, D. (2003) An advocacy project to fluoridate toothpastes in Nepal. *International Dental Journal*, **53**, 220–30.

Yeung, C.A., Hitchings, J.L., Macfarlane, T.V., *et al.* (2005) Fluoridated milk for preventing dental caries. *Cochrane Database of Systematic Reviews*. Issue 3. Art. No.: CD003876. DOI: 10.1002/14651858. CD003876.pub2.

Yip HK, Smales RJ, Ngo HC, Tay FR, Chu FC. (2001) Selection of restorative materials for the atraumatic restorative treatment (ART) approach: a review. *Special Care Dentistry*, **21**, 216–21.

9.9

Musculoskeletal diseases

Jennifer L. Kelsey and Marian T. Hannan

Abstract

Musculoskeletal conditions are a major cause of impairment, disability, health care utilization, and loss of economic productivity throughout the world. Among adults, *osteoarthritis* is one of the leading causes of disability worldwide. Risk factors include increasing age and the female sex, as well as obesity, malalignment and repetitive loading of joints, and previous congenital and developmental conditions and injuries involving joints. Reduction of exposure to these factors, when possible, should retard the development and progression of osteoarthritis. *Rheumatoid arthritis*, although less common, often results in significant disability. It is considered to be of autoimmune aetiology, with a strong genetic component. The incidence and severity are associated with a specific amino acid sequence on several human leukocyte antigen (HLA) DRB1 alleles. New drugs are helping to alleviate symptoms and inhibit structural damage.

Osteoporosis, a common condition in older people, predisposes to fractures. Among the risk factors are increasing age, the female sex, thinness, low oestrogen concentrations, frailty and poor health, and to a lesser extent, low calcium and vitamin D intake, and lack of physical activity. Prevention of falls in older people can reduce the frequency of osteoporosis-associated fractures. *Low back and neck pain* affect the majority of the people throughout the world at some time during their lives. Heavy manual labour and exposure to whole-body vibration are major risk factors, and reduction in these activities should reduce the frequency of low back and neck pain. *Foot disorders* represent a variety of structural, biomechanical, skin, and sensory conditions as well as manifestations of systemic diseases such as arthritis, diabetes mellitus, and peripheral vascular disease. Wearing appropriate shoes and weight reduction are possible preventive measures for some common structural foot problems.

Disorders of adolescents and children include conditions associated with the adolescent growth spurt such as scoliosis and slipped epiphysis, injuries such as childhood fractures, and conditions of infants such as developmental dislocation of the hip.

Musculoskeletal conditions are common in all age groups, but their greatest impact is on the elderly. The number of elderly persons is rapidly increasing worldwide, especially in developing countries. Thus, the burden of musculoskeletal conditions will become substantially greater over the next several decades.

Application of known methods of prevention at all levels and development of new preventive methods are urgently needed.

Magnitude of the problem

Musculoskeletal diseases are common, affect both sexes and all age groups, and are responsible for a substantial amount of impairment, disability, and economic burden throughout the world. These disorders range from minor aches and pains to chronic disabling conditions. Although they are occasionally fatal, their main effects are on the quality of life and economic productivity.

The World Health Organization (WHO) uses disability-adjusted life years (DALYs), which are the sum of the years of life lost from premature mortality and the years of life lived with disability, as an indicator of the burden of disease. Table 9.9.1 shows that throughout the world musculoskeletal diseases account for a large number of DALYs, including almost 9 000 000 in developed regions and about 21 000 000 in developing regions in 2001 (Brooks 2006). These estimates do not include fractures and other injuries, which are classified separately by the WHO under trauma.

High-income countries

In high-income countries, musculoskeletal conditions affect almost all people at some time during their lives. In the United States, musculoskeletal conditions are the most frequently reported impairment, defined as a chronic or permanent defect representing a decrease or loss of ability to perform various functions. Each year,

Table 9.9.1 Estimated number of disability-adjusted life years (DALYs) in the developing and developed regions of the world, 2001

Region	Number of DALYs[a]
Developing regions	21 076 000
Developed regions	8 723 000
Total	29 798 000

[a] DALYs are the sum of the years of life lost from premature mortality and the years of life lived with disability.

Source: Modified from Brooks P.M. The burden of musculoskeletal disease—a global perspective. *Clinical Rheumatology* 2006;**25**:778–81.

about 14 per cent of the population of all ages reports a musculoskeletal impairment (Praemer *et al.* 1999). The prevalence of musculoskeletal impairments increases with age. Among those aged 85 years and older, the annual prevalence is 20 per cent, with impairments of the back or spine and lower extremity or hip accounting for slightly more than half of the musculoskeletal impairments. Among impairments, musculoskeletal disorders are the leading cause of days of restricted activity and days in bed.

A survey in the United Kingdom found that 17 per cent of adults report a long-standing musculoskeletal disorder (Bowling 1996). The most important areas of life affected by long-standing disorders of the musculoskeletal system are ability to move around, stand, walk, and go shopping (24 per cent), and to participate in social and leisure-time activities (24 per cent). The ability to work is also a major issue (17 per cent), particularly for those of working age.

Acute injuries of the musculoskeletal system, including fractures, dislocations, sprains, and strains, are also common. According to the US Health Interview Survey (Praemer *et al.* 1999), 14.5 musculoskeletal injuries occur per 100 people per year of sufficient severity to warrant medical care or at least one half day of restricted activity.

Musculoskeletal conditions generate substantial health care utilization. About 11 per cent of all hospitalizations in short-stay hospitals in the United States are attributed to musculoskeletal conditions (Praemer *et al.* 1999). Fractures, arthritis, intervertebral disc disorders, and other back problems are responsible for the greatest number of hospitalizations. The population aged 65 years and older accounts for 44 per cent of the hospitalizations for musculoskeletal conditions. Among visits to physicians in office-based practice, musculoskeletal conditions rank first, accounting for 17 per cent of all office visits. Fifteen per cent of the visits to hospital outpatient departments and 26 per cent of the visits to emergency departments are attributable to musculoskeletal conditions.

In addition, a significant and increasing number of people throughout the industrialized world are using complementary and alternative medicine. In a national sample of adults in the United States, 48 per cent of those with back pain, 27 per cent of those with arthritis, 57 per cent of those with neck problems, and 24 per cent of those with sprains and strains had used complementary and alternative medicine for their condition in the past year (Eisenberg *et al.* 1998).

The monetary cost of these diseases to society is substantial, especially because of the decreased productivity of those affected. Felts and Yelin (1989) reported that costs of musculoskeletal diseases accounted for 1 per cent of the gross national product in the United States. Badley (1995) noted that musculoskeletal diseases account for 32 per cent of all chronic disability costs in Canada.

Middle- and low-income countries

The impact of musculoskeletal diseases on the work and personal lives of people in middle- and low-income countries is also enormous, but only limited data are currently available on this impact. As in industrialized countries, pain, disability, and loss of employment are major problems. In Bangladesh, for instance, 26 per cent of those surveyed had musculoskeletal pain at the time of the survey, most commonly in the low back, knees, hips, and shoulders (Haq *et al.* 2005). The two most common musculoskeletal disorders were osteoarthritis of the knees and non-specific low back pain. In an urban area of Indonesia, the prevalence of pain in the joints, back, or neck was 31 per cent, and in a rural area, 24 per cent.

Among those with pain, 78 per cent in the urban area and 75 per cent in the rural area had to discontinue work because of the pain; these high percentages reflect the preponderance of jobs requiring manual labour in both urban and rural areas (Darmawan *et al.* 1992). Work-related problems, many of which can be prevented with proper ergonomic techniques, are particularly common in developing countries (Ahasan *et al.* 1999). In a survey in Thailand, about 50 per cent of the female workers in five industries (garment, fertilizer, pharmaceutical, textile, and cigarettes) reported low back symptoms, most of which could be attributed to the work environment (Chavalitsakulchai & Shahnavaz 1993).

In addition, because common musculoskeletal conditions such as osteoarthritis and osteoporosis are most prevalent at older ages and because the numbers of elderly in developing countries are rapidly increasing, the burden of musculoskeletal conditions in these areas will become even greater. For instance, in the early 1990s it was estimated that about half of the estimated 1 660 000 hip fractures worldwide occurred in Europe and North America, but by 2050 it is predicted that three quarters of the 6 260 000 hip fractures will occur in other parts of the world, with almost two thirds occurring in Asia and Latin America (Cooper *et al.* 1992). In younger age groups, the increasing frequency of accidents related to motor vehicles in low- and middle-income countries is resulting in a steep increase in the number of severe injuries, many of which involve the musculoskeletal system (Beveridge & Howard 2004). Thus, the burden of musculoskeletal conditions will continue to rise substantially over the next few decades in these countries.

Some common problems in epidemiologic studies of musculoskeletal conditions

Conducting epidemiologic studies of musculoskeletal conditions even in high-income countries presents several difficulties not experienced to the same extent in studies of other important chronic diseases such as cancer and coronary heart disease. First, because many musculoskeletal conditions are not fatal, have a gradual onset, and often do not even come to medical attention, ascertainment of representative cases for epidemiologic study may be difficult. Consequently, many studies of musculoskeletal diseases are based on the experiences of particular clinics or hospitals. However, cases representative of those occurring in the general population are needed in order to provide an accurate description of disease occurrence, aetiology, and progression in the community.

Even if all cases coming to medical attention within a defined geographic area are included in a study, unless the disease under study almost invariably comes to medical attention, the factors that bring persons with a given condition to medical attention often cannot be separated from factors that may be related to disease aetiology. For instance, it may be difficult to know whether psychological characteristics of persons seeking care for low back pain are involved in the aetiology of low back pain or if they are related to the care-seeking behaviour among those with low back pain. A person may also report low back pain only in order to obtain worker's compensation. A person may say that he or she has low back pain, but the researcher or practitioner cannot know with certainty when no radiographic or other signs are apparent. Even if objective evidence of an abnormality is present, interpretation may be difficult. For instance, as the majority of the asymptomatic people in the general population show evidence of bulging or protruding intervertebral discs on magnetic resonance imaging, even such imaging may be of limited value without clinical evidence of pathology.

Sometimes, a condition for which medical care is virtually always sought, and for which case ascertainment is therefore relatively easy, is used as a surrogate for a disease for which medical care is not necessarily sought. For instance, hip fracture, which is almost always seen in a hospital, is used as a surrogate for osteoporosis. Hip fracture, however, usually depends not only on whether a person has poor bone quality, but also on whether the person falls and how he or she falls. Thus, the risk factors for osteoporosis and hip fracture will overlap, but they also differ in some respects.

The diagnostic criteria used for a disease may differ from one study to another, making it difficult to compare results. To address this problem for major arthritic disorders, expert committees were established to develop and then periodically revise diagnostic criteria for several diseases. The comparability of cases from one study to another increases when the diagnostic criteria are uniformly applied; however, this is not always the case, and as the criteria change over time, it may not be possible to examine corresponding changes in disease frequency.

Diseases that constitute one end of a continuous distribution, such as osteoporosis and scoliosis, present other problems. To define cases of these conditions, relatively arbitrary cut-off points aimed at classifying individuals as 'diseased' and 'normal' are employed, which has made comparisons of prevalence among countries more meaningful. Nevertheless, some investigators may choose different cut-off points, precluding comparison. In addition, people with values just above or just below the cut-off point are actually quite similar to each other, yet one group is considered diseased and the other is not.

Labels for diseases once considered a single entity may become irrelevant when subcategories of the disease are more clearly delineated. For instance, what was once called 'juvenile rheumatoid arthritis' is now known to comprise several subtypes, each with its own aetiology. Much information may be lost when several distinct entities are considered as one disease, as exemplified by studies of low back pain that do not consider the contribution of many different disease processes, such as sprains and strains, intervertebral disc herniations, osteoarthritis, and osteoporosis.

Another concern relates to study design. Cross-sectional studies are often undertaken, such as of the relation between neuromuscular abnormalities and scoliosis. Results from such studies, however, are difficult to interpret because it is not known whether the neuromuscular abnormalities lead to curvature of the spine, whether curvature of the spine leads to neuromuscular defects, or whether some other factor leads to both. Cross-sectional studies of psychological symptoms and low back pain and of obesity and osteoarthritis present similar difficulties in interpretation. In such situations, longitudinal studies, despite their great expense, are needed.

Problems in conducting epidemiologic studies of musculoskeletal diseases are considerably magnified in low-income countries. Because of money and staff shortages, many studies are based in hospitals or clinics. However, in many developing countries, most people do not seek care from a physician or in a hospital unless the disease is quite severe; instead, care may be obtained from community-based nurses. In a survey in the Philippines it was found that most people who sought treatment for rheumatic complaints were seen by someone other than a physician. Only 23 per cent had seen a general practitioner, and 2 per cent saw a rheumatologist.

Care from a physician is frequently not available, accessible, or affordable (Dans *et al.* 1997). Some countries have no rheumatologists at all. Patriarchal societies may limit access to medical care for women, and relatively few women survive to old age. Consequently, both comparisons of disease frequency in men and women within such countries and comparisons with other countries may be difficult to interpret (Hameed *et al.* 1995; Farooqi & Gibson 1998). In addition, even when affected individuals are seen by qualified medical personnel, the diagnostic criteria vary considerably (Ferraz 1995).

If community surveys are undertaken in low-income countries, many difficulties are likely to be encountered. Poor training of personnel, inadequate facilities, limited ability to reach populations for study, a low level of public support, political instability, and bureaucratic rigidity are often encumbrances to epidemiologic studies (Ferraz 1995). The diagnostic tests used in such surveys must be simple and inexpensive. If the study is being conducted in a tropical region, reagents and tests used in other geographic areas may not work because of the heat. In addition, pain, complaints, and manifestations of disability may vary cross-culturally, and measures of disability often require modification. Risk factors may also be quite different in low-income countries.

Finally, great variation in disease frequency and risk factor prevalence occurs among and within developing countries. In north Pakistan, for instance, osteoarthritis of the knee is an especially common complaint; fibromyalgia, low back pain, and soft-tissue rheumatism are the next most common, mainly among the urban poor (Farooqi & Gibson 1998). Thus, not only should one avoid generalizing from one country to another, but frequently one cannot generalize from one part of the same country to another part.

Selected musculoskeletal disorders of adults

Osteoarthritis

Osteoarthritis, also known as degenerative joint disease, is a gradual deterioration of the joint cartilage with proliferation and remodelling of subchondral bone. Any of the joint tissues may be involved, including synovium, joint capsule, periarticular muscles, sensory nerve endings, and ligaments. The usual symptoms are pain and stiffness, followed by loss of function. The typical radiographic appearance of the joint includes osteophyte formation, joint space narrowing, and subchondral sclerosis. Single joints may be affected, with the hands, knees, feet, hips, and spine most commonly involved. Generalized osteoarthritis is defined as having three or more affected joint groups.

Several pathologic features of osteoarthritis, including the proliferative bone changes, may represent attempted repair responses in an injured joint. Osteophytes, for example, may result from a reactive response of cartilage and bone to abnormal mechanical loading, conferring protection to a damaged joint by reducing instability (Arden & Nevitt 2006).

Estimates of osteoarthritis prevalence have generally used an individual's report of pain or decreased articular movement in the joint and/or radiographs of the joint. According to the United States Health Interview Survey, an estimated 22 per cent of adults have osteoarthritis (Centers for Disease Control and Prevention 2006). The proportions affected in Caucasian populations in various high-income countries are quite similar, but hip osteoarthritis may be less common in Africa and Asia than in the Western countries. Knee osteoarthritis shows less geographical variation than hip and hand osteoarthritis, possibly reflecting the importance of injury as a cause of knee disease. Most studies of osteoarthritis have been conducted in developed countries. Worldwide symptom-based prevalence is estimated at 10 per cent among men and 18 per cent among women aged 60 years and older (Woolf & Pfleger 2003). The prevalence of symptomatic osteoarthritis in Turkey is 15 per cent among adults aged 50 years and older (Kacar *et al.* 2005).

Osteoarthritis is the leading cause of disability in the United States (Centers for Disease Control and Prevention 2001). As the populations of low-income countries age, osteoarthritis will become an increasing burden in these populations as well. The WHO has predicted that osteoarthritis will become the fourth leading cause of disability worldwide by the year 2020 (Woolf & Pfleger 2003).

Many individuals with radiographic evidence of osteoarthritis are asymptomatic. In the United States, European, and Asian populations, roughly 50 per cent of the adults with radiographic evidence of knee osteoarthritis report knee pain; discrepancy between radiographic evidence of osteoarthritis and pain has been noted for the hands and hips as well (World Health Organization 2003).

Risk factors

Prevalence increases steeply with age in all populations, especially after 50 years. On autopsy, almost everyone 65 years or older has at least one joint with features of osteoarthritis. Individual joints show the same age-related rise in osteoarthritis prevalence, with the hip showing a later rise than the knee. Women are at least twice as likely to be affected as men, especially for hand and knee osteoarthritis, and particularly after age 50 years.

Overweight persons are at increased risk for osteoarthritis of several sites, most notably the knees and hands. In the United States, obese persons have double the prevalence of osteoarthritis at most sites compared with persons of normal weight, especially at the knee (Centers for Disease Control and Prevention 2006); the higher prevalence exists whether osteoarthritis is defined by symptom or radiograph. Longitudinal studies show that increased weight precedes the occurrence of hand or knee osteoarthritis and is not merely a consequence of it. Furthermore, overweight persons with knee osteoarthritis are at higher risk of experiencing progressive disease than persons who are not overweight. Weight loss reduces the risk of symptomatic knee disease (Centers for Disease Control and Prevention 2006).

Repetitive loading of joints, particularly in certain occupations and sports, is a strong risk factor for osteoarthritis. It has long been noted that miners often develop osteoarthritis of the elbows and knees, cotton pickers of particular joints in the fingers, farmers of the hips, and dockworkers of the fingers, elbows, and knees. Specific on-the-job activities that predispose to knee and hip osteoarthritis are knee bending, squatting, kneeling, stair climbing, heavy lifting, and carrying heavy loads (Cooper *et al.* 1994). In high- and low-income countries, hip osteoarthritis is more frequent among farmers than among persons in non-farming occupations. These risks are cumulative, and evidence indicates increasing risk with greater number of years spent in such occupations.

Studies of recreational and competitive athletes suggest that frequent exercise, including jogging or moderate low-impact running, is not a detectable risk factor for hip and knee osteoarthritis in those with normal joints. However, these activities may increase the risk in those with previous joint injuries or developmentally defective joints. Prolonged decreased joint use and decreased loading generate changes that make cartilage more vulnerable to injury.

Congenital and developmental disorders and injuries involving joints, particularly if not treated early, greatly increase the likelihood of developing osteoarthritis in the affected joint. Prior inflammatory joint disease is also a risk factor. Greater grip strength appears to increase the risk for osteoarthritis of the hands, whereas muscle weakness may be a risk factor for other sites such as the knees and hips. Nutritional factors, high bone mineral density, and low concentrations of serum oestradiol have been linked to osteoarthritis in some studies, but the evidence is not conclusive (Arden & Nevitt 2006).

Genetic susceptibility is considered to be important (Arden & Nevitt 2006); multiple genes are likely to be involved in the aetiology of osteoarthritis. Polymorphisms of the type II collagen gene (Col2A1) are of particular interest because type II collagen is a major constituent of the articular cartilage. The vitamin D and oestrogen receptor genes may contribute as well. Genes encoding other structural proteins of the cartilage matrix and bone as well as cartilage growth factors are under study.

Prevention

Preventive measures include weight loss, reduction of repetitive biomechanical stress on the joints, and prevention and early treatment of congenital, developmental, and adult diseases involving the joints. Techniques for avoiding sports-related joint trauma include providing appropriate protection and padding for contact sports and modifying game rules to minimize contact that is associated with joint trauma. Developing and maintaining adequate muscle strength is an important mechanism to minimize joint stress.

To decrease pain and stiffness and reduce functional limitations, several steps may be taken, depending on the severity of the disease (Bartlett *et al.* 2006). Self-management, which incorporates self-care and self-treatment, is one of the first-line non-pharmacologic treatment options for management of osteoarthritis. Self-care and self-treatment may include education, exercise, healthy eating, and over-the-counter remedies, as well as pain coping skills. Studies in the United States, United Kingdom, and China show that arthritis self-management programmes improve health behaviours and health status. Weight reduction has been shown to protect against both the development and progression of osteoarthritis. Therapy can involve the use of analgesics, nutriceuticals, and/or non-steroidal anti-inflammatory drugs to control symptoms of pain, combined with physical and occupational therapy to maintain joint range of motion, muscle strength, and an individual's ability to perform everyday activities. Other steps may include steroid injections into joints or minor surgery. Finally, joint replacement surgery of the hips and knees has been highly successful for those with severe osteoarthritis.

Rheumatoid arthritis

Rheumatoid arthritis is a chronic inflammatory joint disorder characterized by proliferative synovitis leading to destruction of the articular cartilage and bony erosions. Symptoms typically include pain and stiffness of multiple joints (particularly the small joints of the hands and feet), soft-tissue swelling, increased temperature of affected joints, decreased range of motion, weakness, and fatigue. Systemic manifestations of rheumatoid arthritis include vascular, renal, and eye complications. The diagnostic classification system generally used is the 1987 American College of Rheumatology revised criteria (Bartlett *et al.* 2006).

Rheumatoid arthritis is usually not a fatal disorder. The clinical course is variable, but as the disease progresses, most people with rheumatoid arthritis develop functional limitations, physical disabilities, and sometimes early mortality.

The prevalence of rheumatoid arthritis in the United States and Western Europe ranges from 0.5 to 1 per cent. There is evidence of a decline in rheumatoid arthritis incidence over the last few decades in US and European populations (Bartlett *et al.* 2006). The prevalence is similar among African-Americans and Caucasian Americans, but greater prevalence of rheumatoid arthritis has been reported among several Native American tribes. Lower prevalence has been reported among some Asian populations, and Asians may also have milder disease compared to Caucasians (Lau *et al.* 1996).

Risk factors

Overall, the incidence among females is about twice that of males, although this gender gap decreases with age. Over the age of 60 years, women are affected about 1.5 times more often than men (Rasch *et al.* 2003).

Rheumatoid arthritis is considered to be of autoimmune aetiology, and genetic factors are important. Genetic studies have focused primarily on autoimmune aspects of the disease, especially the role of the human leukocyte antigen (HLA) alleles. HLA-DR4 was the first allele to be associated with rheumatoid arthritis, and it is now known that the incidence and severity of rheumatoid arthritis are associated with a specific amino acid sequence on several HLA-DRB1 alleles called the *rheumatoid arthritis shared epitope* (Bartlett *et al.* 2006).

Although the potential contribution of genetic susceptibility is widely recognized, questions remain regarding the triggering events that lead to rheumatoid arthritis and its patterns of expression. Infectious agents have been proposed but none have been definitively linked with rheumatoid arthritis. Oral contraceptives may retard the progression from mild to severe disease. Previous blood transfusion, obesity, and cigarette smoking may be associated with increased risks (Bartlett *et al.* 2006).

Prevention

No viable primary or secondary prevention measures are available for rheumatoid arthritis. Treatment includes the use of analgesics and/or non-steroidal anti-inflammatory drugs to control pain and stiffness, physical therapy to maintain and improve joint range of motion, and occupational therapy to maximize the individual's ability to perform daily activities. Disease-modifying drugs, including gold, penicillamine, and sulfasalazine, are believed to inhibit cytokines. These drugs produce a slow response and a high level of toxicity, and thus typically have not been taken for long periods of time. Methotrexate has somewhat better properties, but is still not used for lengthy periods. Nevertheless, use of these drugs early in the disease course and aggressive escalation of therapy based on objective evidence of continued disease activity have greatly improved the course of the disease (Emery 2006).

In addition, the discovery that the pro-inflammatory cytokine tumour necrosis factor α (TNF-α) plays a major role in pathogenesis has led to the use of TNF-α antagonists in the treatment of rheumatoid arthritis. These agents have been shown to be highly effective in reducing symptoms and signs and in inhibiting structural damage in patients who have not responded to disease-modifying anti-rheumatic drugs, including methotrexate. Cases of severe and disabling rheumatoid arthritis require careful and integrated health care delivery, as many of these drugs have significant toxicity and the potential for serious side effects. In addition, patients with severe disease may require more support services, assistive devices, and possibly surgical interventions at relatively young ages.

Osteoporosis and associated fractures

Osteoporosis is a skeletal disorder characterized by compromised bone strength, predisposing to an increased risk of fracture. Fractures of the hip, vertebrae, and distal radius are particularly common. The WHO has defined osteoporosis as bone mineral density more than 2.5 standard deviations below the mean value of peak bone mass in young adults of the same sex. Using the WHO definition, the estimated prevalence of osteoporosis in the femoral neck among women aged 50 years and older was found to be 18 per cent in the United States (Looker *et al.* 1997), from 8 to 22 per cent in various Latin American countries (Morales-Torres & Gutiérrez-UrenÞa 2004), 44 per cent in Saudi Arabia (Sadat-Ali *et al.* 2004), and 29 per cent for low-income Indian women (Shatrugna *et al.* 2005). As discussed later in this subsection, different lifestyle characteristics in these various regions are believed to contribute to the variations in prevalence.

In addition to low bone mass, other aspects of bone quality that affect fracture risk include structural properties such as the size and shape of bone, microarchitectural properties such as trabecular thickness and connectivity, cortical thickness and porosity, material properties such as mineralization, collagen composition, and damage accumulation (Seeman & Delmas 2006).

Osteoporosis-associated hip fractures in older people are particularly common and disabling. Globally, hip fracture incidence rates vary considerably and are highest among whites in northern Europe and North America, slightly lower among Asians living in economically developed areas such as Hong Kong and the United States, still lower among Hispanics and Blacks in the United States and in South America, and the lowest in less developed areas of Asia such as China as well as in Africa. In general, the ratio of female to male incidence rates is greater in the areas with the highest incidence rates. Table 9.9.2 shows age-adjusted incidence rates for females and males in selected countries among people of age 50 years and

Table 9.9.2 Age-adjusted incidence rates per 100 000 of hip fracture among females and males aged 50 years and older in selected localities

Locality	Females	Males
Beijing, China	96	107
Porto Alegre, Brazil	202–327.2	104.7–169.6
Budapest, Hungary	316	251
Hong Kong	428.3	269.6
Reykjavik, Iceland	696.6	348.7

Age adjusted to the 1990 non-Hispanic white US population.
Source: Modified from Schwartz A.V., Kelsey J.L., Maggi S., *et al.* International variation in the incidence of hip fractures: cross-national project on osteoporosis for the World Health Organization Program for Research on Aging. *Osteoporosis International* 1999;**9**:242–53.

older (Schwartz *et al.* 1999). Hip fracture incidence rates in Beijing, China, are among the lowest in the world. However, in China and other developing countries (World Health Organization 2003), age-adjusted hip fracture incidence rates appear to be rising. With the increasing numbers of elderly in these countries, the numbers of hip fractures will be dramatically increasing.

Risk factors

In most areas, osteoporosis is much more common among females than males. In both sexes, prevalence increases markedly with age, but the increase in prevalence occurs about 10 years earlier for females than males. Table 9.9.3 shows prevalence by age among females in the United States (Melton 1995). A particularly rapid decrease in bone mass occurs in females in the years immediately following menopause, suggesting that loss of oestrogen is an important aetiological factor in women.

Bone mass in later adulthood, when fracture risk is the greatest, depends on bone mass in young adulthood, when bone mass is at its peak, and the rate of loss of bone mass after the peak is reached. Heredity is an important determinant of bone mass in childhood, adolescence, and early adulthood, but the role of genetics in loss of bone mass at older age is less certain; multiple genes are probably involved, each with a small effect. Although results of studies are not entirely consistent, it appears that modifiable risk factors such as weight, calcium intake, and physical activity also affect premenopausal bone mass, but to a lesser extent than heredity. Premenopausal oophorectomy results in loss of bone mass if menopausal hormone therapy is not used.

In postmenopausal women, the evidence is strong that the risk for low bone mass or hip fracture is increased by prolonged immobility, prolonged corticosteroid use, a history of a previous fracture, a history of falls, maternal history of an osteoporotic fracture, very low concentrations of endogenous oestradiol, poor self-rated health, poor vision, use of psychotropic drugs, and cigarette smoking. Probable risk factors include tallness, a recent increase in the frequency of falls, high alcohol consumption, and high caffeine consumption. Strong protective factors include obesity and menopausal hormone therapy, and to a lesser extent, calcium supplements, adequate dietary calcium consumption, adequate vitamin D intake, adequate vitamin D metabolism, physical activity, and use of thiazide diuretics.

Risk factors appear to be similar in low- and middle-income countries, but special circumstances make certain risk factors of particular importance in some areas. In Middle Eastern countries such as Saudi Arabia and Turkey, inadequate levels of vitamin D are found in most postmenopausal women, probably because of their clothing and a reclusive lifestyle. In other regions, such as low-income areas of India, poor nutrition and failure to maintain adequate body weight may increase the risk for osteoporosis and fractures (Shatrugna *et al.* 2005; Morales-Torres 2007). On the other hand, lack of physical activity may not be an important risk factor in areas where levels of physical activity are high.

Most fractures of sites other than the spine depend on whether a person falls and how the person falls. Among the risk factors for falls in older adults are problems with balance and gait, limited muscle strength, deficiencies in vision, arthritis, depressive symptoms, orthostasis, cognitive impairment, and the use of multiple prescription medications. As the number of these risk factors increases, so does the risk of falling (Tinetti 2003). How a person falls also affects the likelihood that a fracture will occur and which skeletal site is fractured. Falling sideways or straight down and landing on the hip or leg, for instance, greatly increase the risk of a hip fracture. Breaking the fall with a hand decreases the risk of hip fracture, but increases the risk of lower forearm fracture (Nevitt & Cummings 1993). Frail women are more likely to fracture their hip whereas healthier active women are more likely to fracture their lower forearm. Falls from heights or on hard surfaces increase the risk for fracture.

Prevention

Primary prevention includes trying to achieve high bone mass at younger ages by having a diet adequate in calcium and vitamin D and engaging in sufficient physical activity. Once loss of bone mass has begun, calcium supplementation can provide a small amount of protection, especially in those with low dietary calcium intake (Jackson *et al.* 2006). Moderate physical activity, such as brisk walking, is often recommended for older people to reduce loss of bone mass, but at most this probably has a modest beneficial effect.

Because only a small amount of protection is provided by increased dietary calcium consumption, calcium supplementation, and physical activity, much attention has been focused on the use of pharmaceutical agents to retard loss of bone mass and to reduce the risk of fractures in older adults. Menopausal hormone therapy, once used effectively for this purpose, is no longer recommended because of its association with an increased risk for other major diseases such as breast cancer, coronary heart disease, and pulmonary embolism. Other agents commonly used for retarding loss of bone mass and possibly reducing the risk for fractures are bisphosphonates, the selective oestrogen receptor modulator raloxifene, and for severe osteoporosis, parathyroid hormone.

Although bisphosphonates, including alendronate, ibandronate, and risedronate, have been shown to reduce loss of bone mass in the hip and spine, randomized trials among women have shown that bisphosphonates protect against fracture only in those who already have very low bone mass (Cummings *et al.* 1998). A recent extension of an earlier randomized trial (Black *et al.* 2006) suggests that little additional benefit on bone mineral density and fracture risk is gained from using alendronate for an additional five years after the first five years of treatment in most women. In addition, compliance is a problem because alendronate has to be taken in a rather strict manner to achieve maximal absorption and avoid unpleasant upper gastrointestinal effects.

Table 9.9.3 Percentage of Rochester, Minnesota, women with bone mineral measurements in the spine, hip, or mid-radius more than 2.5 standard deviations below the mean for young normal women

Age group (years)	Percentage
50–59	14.8
60–69	21.6
70–79	38.5
≥80	70
Total[a]	30.3

[a] Age adjusted to the 1990 US white women population aged 50 years or older.
Source: Modified from Melton L.J. III. How many women have osteoporosis now? *Journal of Bone and Mineral Research* 1995;**10**:175–7.

The selective oestrogen receptor modulator raloxifene has been shown to reduce loss of bone mass in the hip and spine and to protect against vertebral fractures in women regardless of their baseline bone mass, but not against non-vertebral fractures, including hip fracture (Ettinger *et al.* 1999). Teriparatide, a recombinant human parathyroid hormone that acts through increasing bone formation, may be useful in reducing risk for vertebral and non-vertebral fractures in those with severe osteoporosis, but its use is approved for a maximum of only two years because its long-term effects are not known. Thus, available evidence suggests that none of these agents is useful in the primary prevention of osteoporosis, although each has utility as a therapeutic agent.

In low- and middle-income countries, the cost of these pharmaceutical agents precludes their widespread use for treatment. Rather, inexpensive primary prevention measures such as supplemental calcium and vitamin D, attainment of adequate body weight, exercise, avoidance of smoking and alcohol abuse, and fall prevention programmes could be useful preventive measures, but extensive education of high-risk populations is needed (Morales-Torres 2007).

Regarding secondary prevention, in high-income countries screening women in the perimenopausal and postmenopausal years for high fracture risk by measuring their bone mass, usually with dual-energy X-ray absorptiometry, has achieved some popularity in recent years. However, many questions have been raised about the usefulness of such screening, such as who should be screened, whether multiple measurements over time are needed, what other information on risk should be obtained along with the measure of bone mass, and what therapy should be used in those with various degrees of low bone mass. Ultrasonography, usually of the heel bone, provides information about bone architecture and elasticity as well as bone mineral density, and has been found to predict fracture (Hans *et al.* 1996). As ultrasound is less expensive and radiation-free compared to other methods of measuring bone mass, it is possible that it will be used more widely for screening in the future. At present, however, there is no consensus that any screening method should be used for healthy women in the general population.

Finally, reducing the frequency and impact of falls among those with osteoporosis is another potential means of reducing the incidence of fracture. Table 9.9.4 shows strategies demonstrated in randomized trials to be effective in reducing the occurrence of falls among elderly persons living in the community (Tinetti 2003). Preventive measures may differ somewhat from one country to another. For instance, in countries such as Iran (Abolhassani *et al.* 2006) where older people and particularly women spend little time outdoors, preventive efforts should focus on indoor rather than outdoor risk factors for falls.

Low back pain

About 75–85 per cent of adults in Western countries have low back pain during their lifetime. In the United States, around 15–20 per cent of adults experience low back pain during the course of a year, about 1 per cent are chronically disabled because of low back pain, and another 1 per cent are temporarily disabled. About 5 per cent of workers lose one or more workdays because of low back pain and 2 per cent have compensable back injuries each year. Back pain is the most frequently reported reason for a physician visit in the United States (Andersson 1998).

Table 9.9.4 Strategies found in randomized trials to be effective in decreasing the number of falls among the elderly living in the community

Strategy	Estimated risk reduction (per cent)
Health care based	
Balance and gait training and strengthening exercise	14–27
Reduction in home hazards after hospitalization	19
Discontinuation of psychotropic medication	39
Multifactorial risk assessment with targeted management	25–39
Community-based	
Specific balance or strength exercise programmes	25–49

Source: Modified from Tinetti M.E. Preventing falls in elderly persons. *New England Journal of Medicine* 2003;**348**:42–9.

Most low back problems resolve within 2–4 weeks, and almost 90 per cent resolve within 12 weeks (Andersson 1998). Recurrences are common, however, and low back pain often becomes a chronic problem with intermittent, usually mild exacerbations. In a study of English patients seen by general practitioners for low back pain, after one year only 25 per cent had no disability even though most were no longer seeking care for their problem from their practitioner (Croft *et al.* 1998). In a small proportion of cases, the pain becomes constant and severe.

The prevalence of low back pain is also high in low-income areas of the world. In a community-based study in rural China, the percentage having low back pain during the course of a year was 65 per cent (Barrero *et al.* 2006); it was 61 per cent for tannery workers in India (Öry *et al.* 1997), 56 per cent in a steel industry in South Africa (Van Vuuren *et al.* 2005), and 36 per cent in an urban population in Turkey (Gilgil *et al.* 2005).

As noted earlier, the category low back pain consists of a variety of entities with somewhat different aetiologies. However, almost all studies have considered low back pain as a whole, so the general category is considered here unless otherwise mentioned.

Risk factors

The best predictor of low back pain is a history of low back pain. First episodes of low back pain most frequently occur among persons in the age range 20–39 years, but the proportion of the population reporting low back pain (either old or new) is relatively uniform across the working years. If only cases seeking medical care or compensation are considered, low back pain is seen more frequently among males than females in Western countries, but in surveys in the general population, males and females are affected with approximately equal frequency (Biering-Sorenson 1982). Persons in lower social classes are more likely to report low back pain than those in higher classes, probably because of their tendency to have jobs requiring heavy physical labour.

In Western countries, people who do heavy manual labour are at increased risk for low back pain. Lifting objects of 25 lb or more appears to be particularly detrimental. Specific activities that probably further increase the risk are frequent lifting of heavy objects while bending and twisting the body, holding heavy objects away from the body while lifting, and failing to bend the knees while lifting (Andersson 1981; Kelsey *et al.* 1984). Driving motor vehicles either on or off the job and exposure to whole-body vibration increase the risk for low back pain (Pope *et al.* 1998). A recent review (Lis *et al.* 2007) indicates that sitting by itself does not increase the risk for low back pain, but sitting in combination with other exposures such as whole-body vibration and awkward posture increases the risk. Cigarette smoking has been found in many studies to be associated with an increased risk. Psychological attributes such as low social support in the workplace and low job satisfaction may increase risk (Hoogendoorn & van Poppel 2000).

Many risk factors in middle- and low-income countries are similar to those in high-income countries. In rural China, having been a farmer, reporting moderate or heavy physical stress, and being exposed to vibration were associated with low back pain (Barrero *et al.* 2006). In urban Turkey, cigarette smoking was related to the occurrence of low back pain (Gilgil *et al.* 2005). Among steel workers in a factory in South Africa, carrying heavy loads, bulky manual handling, twisting and bending, kneeling and squatting, prolonged sitting, and working on slippery and uneven surfaces conferred increased risks (Van Vuuren *et al.* 2005). Heavy manual lifting was also a risk factor among tannery workers in India (Öry *et al.* 1997). Within low-income countries, back pain is particularly prevalent in various types of workshops, factories, and storage facilities, which have been referred to as 'enclosed workshops' (Volinn 1997). As indicated earlier, in a survey in Thailand about 50 per cent of the female workers in the garment, fertilizer, pharmaceutical, textile, and cigarette industries reported low back symptoms (Chavalitsakulchai & Shahnavaz 1993). Worldwide, at least 37 per cent of low back pain has been attributed to occupational factors; Table 9.9.5 presents the relative risks upon which this estimate is based (Punnett *et al.* 2005).

In Western countries, predictors of disability from low back pain include previous episodes of law back pain, long duration of pain, a history of past disability and hospitalizations, an onset of pain attributable to trauma, lack of recognition and respect at work, low supervisory support, unemployment, other disabilities, self-reported poor health, low educational level, heavy physical demands on the job, dissatisfaction with the job, whether insurance payments are being received, the perception of fault, and whether a lawyer has

been retained (Deyo & Diehl 1988; Cats-Baril & Frymoyer 1991; Wickstrom & Pentti 1998). Little information is available on predictors of disability in low-income countries, but in the South-African steel factory mentioned previously, heavy manual handling, kneeling and squatting, and working on slippery and uneven surfaces were associated with disability from low back pain (Van Vuuren *et al.* 2005).

Prevention

Various approaches have been used for the primary prevention of low back pain in the workplace, and these measures are applicable to high-, middle-, and low-income countries. Low back X-rays and medical examinations have not proved useful as predictors of who will develop back pain on the job. However, careful selection of workers for jobs involving heavy manual work by strength testing may be helpful (Keyserling *et al.* 1980). It has been found that training workers to bend their knees while lifting does not reduce the likelihood of low back injuries, in part because of poor compliance. A better approach may be to redesign jobs to minimize bending and twisting motions while lifting and to reduce the amount of weight that must be lifted (Snook 1988). Redesigning jobs in these ways may also allow injured workers to return to work sooner. Other ways of reducing the frequency of back pain may include smoking cessation, improved physical fitness, moving around from time to time in situations requiring prolonged exposure to one position, vibration dampening, and use of motor vehicles with good lumbar support and positioning.

To reduce the likelihood of acute back pain progressing to chronic back pain, it is important for those affected to continue their normal activity to the extent that they are able (Malmivaara *et al.* 1995). Upon return to work, however, the worker should avoid activities that may exacerbate the problem, such as heavy lifting or staying in one position for long periods of time.

Neck pain

Neck pain has been less well studied than low back pain, and as with low back pain, a variety of conditions can result in neck pain. In high-income countries, about 60–70 per cent of the adults report having experienced neck pain at some time during their lives (Côté *et al.* 1998). Most neck pain is mild, but as with low back pain, episodes may be recurrent, and about 5 per cent of the cases result in disability. Little information is available from middle- and low-income countries.

Risk factors

Some studies report that males and females are affected with approximately equal frequency, whereas others show a female excess. Chronic neck pain and disability from neck pain occur more often in females than males. Neck pain occurs most frequently in young adulthood, and some evidence suggests that its prevalence decreases with age (Côté *et al.* 1998; Leclerc *et al.* 1999).

Only a few studies have been undertaken to identify other risk factors for neck pain, and many of the risk factors appear to be similar to those for low back pain. Prolonged exposure to awkward postures may be associated with mild neck pain. For instance, in Hong Kong, frequent use of video display units with a fixed keyboard height requiring a bent neck was found to result in neck pain (Yu & Wong 1996). Other risk factors for either general neck pain or herniated cervical disc found in one or more studies (Kelsey *et al.* 1984; Magnusson *et al.* 1996; Krause *et al.* 1997) include heavy lifting,

Table 9.9.5 Relative risk for low back pain by selected occupational category

Occupational category	Relative risk
Managers and professionals	1 (referent)
Clerical and sales workers	1.38
Production workers	2.39
Service workers	2.67
Farmers	5.17

Source: Modified from Punnett L., Prüss-Üstün A., Nelson D.I., *et al.* Estimating the global burden of low back pain attributable to combined occupational exposures. *American Journal of Industrial Medicine* 2005;**48**:459-69

cigarette smoking, driving motor vehicles, exposure to whole-body vibration, and psychological distress, psychosomatic problems, and headaches (Leclerc *et al.* 1999). One study (Krause *et al.* 1997) found that particularly detrimental were vehicles in which seat adjustment was difficult.

Prevention

Little research has been undertaken on predictors of disability from neck pain and on primary prevention. However, it would appear that reduction in the amount of heavy lifting, cigarette smoking, awkward positions (especially at video display units), prolonged driving in motor vehicles, and exposure to other sources of whole-body vibration should reduce the incidence.

Foot disorders

Foot disorders represent a number of structural or biomechanical conditions, skin conditions, manifestations of systemic disease, and sensory conditions. Structural problems include bunions, flat feet, hammer toes, overlapping toes, and high arches. Systemic diseases often seen with foot symptoms include arthritis, diabetes mellitus, and peripheral vascular disease. Foot complications of diabetes may be caused by ischaemia, neuropathy, and susceptibility to infection. Foot ulcers are common in persons with peripheral vascular disease, vascular insufficiency, or trauma. Peripheral vascular disease is associated with colour changes and oedema, and may cause inadequate blood flow with symptoms of pain or numbness (Karpman 1995).

In the United States, foot and toe symptoms are among the top twenty reasons for physician office visits among persons aged 65–74 years (US Department of Health and Human Services 1997). Karpman (1995) has reported that up to 80 per cent of elderly patients are afflicted with a bunion, hammer toe deformity, callus, or other structural deformity. A population-based study (Clarke 1969) of adults 18–90 years of age in the United Kingdom found that 60 per cent of those surveyed reported a painful foot problem, yet a podiatric examination found 85 per cent to have some foot condition. The most frequent foot disorders were bunions, arthritis, claw toes, hammer toes, overlapping toes, and aching, swollen feet that might have arisen from a general condition such as peripheral vascular disease. In this study, women reported foot pain (71 per cent) more often than men (53 per cent). Of those reporting foot disorders, about half reported foot pain and approximately 10 per cent reported that their foot condition limited at least one of their daily activities. Another US population-based study (Dunn *et al.* 2004) noted that the most prevalent foot conditions were toe deformities, bunions, and toe infection or maceration. A study of geriatric patients in Hong Kong found that half had foot deformities (Hung *et al.* 1985).

In an Australian study of older adults (Menz & Lord 2001), foot problems were associated with slower walking speed and poor balance. A British study (Clarke 1969) found that 40 per cent of adults aged 65 years and older reported difficulty walking, and 16 per cent stated that their difficulty in walking was due to trouble with their feet. Studies in other localities (Benvenuti *et al.* 1995; Leveille *et al.* 1998) also report that older people with foot problems have difficulty walking, standing, and with everyday activities. A study in Beijing (Cummings *et al.* 1997) found that 38 per cent of women aged 80 years and older and 18 per cent of women aged 70–79 years were affected by deformities resulting from previous

foot binding and that these deformities caused substantial disability in standing and balance. There are few, if any, other studies of the prevalence of or disability from foot disorders in low- or middle-income countries.

Risk factors

Women are more likely to have foot pain than men, but it is not known whether this is because of a higher prevalence of primary foot deformities or underlying disease. An Italian study (Benvenuti *et al.* 1995) reported that 56 per cent of women over 65 years of age had foot pain compared to 24 per cent of older men. The Third National Health and Nutrition Examination Survey in the United States (US Department of Health and Human Services 1996) reported that 60 per cent of women over age 65 years had bunions compared to 40 per cent of men. Additionally, older women are more likely to have arthritis than men, and the foot is the fourth most commonly affected site in those with osteoarthritis.

Structural foot deformities are thought often to be caused by long-term use of ill-fitting shoes. Shoes with an improper fit worn over years, or other stress to the feet, can result in various deformities including bunions, hammer toes, and claw toes, in turn leading to muscle maladaption and progression of the deformity (Karpman 1995).

The only other risk factor consistently linked with painful foot disorders is obesity. Obesity has a major effect on soft-tissue structures such as tendon and cartilage.

Little is known of how the foot might affect physical functioning of the lower extremity in adults. Extrapolating from clinical studies of patients with diabetes, it is thought that even slight deformities of the feet can lead to impaired balance, changes in gait, and pain. Foot disorders may often be overlooked as an important cause of falls, poor balance, and walking problems.

Prevention

Primary prevention measures include appropriate footwear that protects and supports the foot without confining the toes, as well as weight loss in those who are obese to reduce biomechanical stress on the foot. These aspects become even more important in those whose health is compromised by diabetes, arthritis, vascular disease, or other chronic systemic disease.

Once people have foot pain, interventions should be directed to both the location of the pain and underlying muscle, tendons, or ligaments. These interventions vary by foot disorder and may include heel lifts, gel inserts, injection with pain-relieving medications, orthotic devices, and avoidance of activity that irritates the tenderness. Other tertiary prevention measures are aimed at reduction of pain, inflammation, and maladaptive response and include use of foot inserts, stretching and strengthening exercises, nonsteroidal anti-inflammatory drugs, short-term cast immobilization, joint injection, reduction of weight bearing, and other measures to reduce symptoms. Finally, adaptive shoes as well as surgical options may be considered for long-term foot disorders. Prompt diagnosis and early treatment may lessen the possible long-term maladaption and structural disability seen with many foot disorders.

Selected musculoskeletal disorders of adolescents and children

Adolescent idiopathic scoliosis

The Scoliosis Research Society defines scoliosis as a lateral spinal curve of greater than 10 degrees as measured by the Cobb angle on a radiograph taken with the person standing. The curvature is usually associated with rotation of the vertebrae. In Western countries, about 2–3 per cent of the adolescents develop curves of 10 degrees of more before growth ceases, and 2 per 1000 children develop curves of 30 degrees or more (Miller 1999). Prevalence estimates of 1 per cent in Nigeria (Jenyo & Asekun-Olarinmoye 2005) and 3 per cent in Mostar, Bosnia, and Herzegovina (Ostojic et al. 2006) have been reported. Those with large curvature usually develop spinal osteoarthritis in their adult years. Lung and heart complications may also occur. Additional progression of curves sometimes takes place in adults with scoliosis.

Risk factors

The ages at which adolescent idiopathic scoliosis is most frequently diagnosed are 11–14 years in girls and 14–16 years in boys, the difference in ages reflecting the earlier onset of the adolescent growth spurt in females. The ratio of females to males among the more severe cases seen at surgery is around 4–5 to 1, but curves of less than 15 degrees are seen with about equal frequency in females and males. Reports from surgical case series indicate that curves occur most frequently at the thoracic level, but school screening programmes that identify mild as well as severe cases have found curves to be most common at the thoracolumbar level.

The risk of scoliosis in first-degree relatives of cases is about three to four times that in children from the general population, but the mode of inheritance is unclear. A prospective study in Finland (Nissinen et al. 1993) identified several factors that may predict the development of scoliosis, including the female sex, trunk asymmetry as indicated by large rip humps on the forward-bend test (see Prevention for a description), the degree of thoracic kyphosis, the degree of lumbar lordosis in boys, and probably standing height, sitting height, recent increase in sitting height, and early age at gain in sitting height. Once girls reach menarche, their risk is considerably reduced.

Specific mechanisms hypothesized to be involved in the development of scoliosis, but for which the evidence is not conclusive, include connective tissue abnormalities, particularly of collagen, proteoglycan, and elastic fibres; a growth or functional defect within skeletal muscle; neuromuscular abnormalities including of proprioception, postural equilibrium, oculovestibular function, and vibratory sensation; central nervous system asymmetries; hormonal characteristics involving growth hormone and melatonin; and biomechanical imbalances and abnormalities in vertebral bodies, muscles of the ribs and trunk, ligaments, and intervertebral discs (Miller 1999).

Once a curve has developed, several risk factors for progression have been identified, including double curves as opposed to single curves, thoracic curves, larger curves, the female sex, skeletal immaturity, the absence of a sacral tilt, leg length inequality, early chronological age, and low bone mass (Hung et al. 2005).

Prevention

No means of primary prevention are known. Therefore, secondary prevention by screening in schools has become widespread and is in fact required by law in many localities in the United States. The assumption of the screening programme is that if cases of scoliosis are detected early, they can be treated conservatively and surgery can be avoided.

The forward-bend test has been used for screening for many years in high-income countries. It is simple and affordable in developing countries such as Nigeria (Jenyo & Asekun-Olarinmoye 2005) as well as in high-income countries. In the forward-bend test, the child's back is examined while the child bends forward from the waist. In scoliosis, the rotation of vertebrae that is often associated with the lateral curvature results in prominent ribs on the concave side of the curve. Accordingly, in this test, evidence of a 'rib hump' is considered positive for scoliosis. Recently, the scoliometer, an inclinometer used to measure axial trunk rotation during forward bending, has been introduced as a screening test and to monitor curve progression, but only limited evaluation has been undertaken to date.

School screening programmes identify relatively large numbers of children with possible curvature in their spine. Positive tests are followed by X-ray examination for a more definitive diagnosis. Curves of 5–19 degrees are generally monitored by subsequent X-rays every few months. If a curve progresses to 20–25 degrees or more, treatment is usually started to prevent further progression. Methods of treatment include exercises, braces, external or internal muscle stimulators, and especially for curves of greater than 40 degrees, surgery.

Despite the widespread acceptance of screening for scoliosis, its effectiveness has been questioned (US Preventive Services Task Force 1993; Goldberg et al. 1995). Many children screened as positive are not followed up for definitive diagnosis. Many false positives occur even with the forward-bend test, resulting in an excess of X-ray examinations and considerable expense and anxiety. A report from a screening programme in Ireland (Goldberg et al. 1995) indicates that the positive predictive value of the forward-bend test is only 8 per cent; that is, of every 100 forward-bend tests classified as positive, only 8 develop clinically significant scoliosis. It is uncertain whether school screening programmes have actually caused a reduction in the number of cases of severe curvature that require surgery. Disagreement exists about the optimal ages for screening and about whether males should be screened at all. Criteria for referral for diagnosis and treatment need to be better specified, and improved training and evaluation of the nurses who do the screening is needed. In view of all these uncertainties, the US Preventive Services Task Force (US Preventive Services Task Force 1993) did not recommend either for or against routine screening for scoliosis in adolescents, and routine screening is not recommended by the United Kingdom National Screening Committee.

Slipped capital femoral epiphysis

In slipped capital femoral epiphysis, the head of the femur is displaced backward and downward off the diaphysis. The actual separation takes place through the layer of hypertrophied cartilage next to the zone of calcified cartilage of the epiphyseal plate. The usual symptoms are pain, stiffness, limp, and a limited range of motion of the hip joint. Slipped epiphysis usually occurs during the adolescent growth spurt, and does not occur once the epiphysis is fused to the shaft of the femur. In northern urbanized areas, about 1 in 1000 males and 1 in 1800 females are diagnosed with a slipped epiphysis over the age range at risk (Jerre et al. 1996).

Risk factors

Most cases occur between the ages of 10–17 years in males and 8–15 years in females. The median age at diagnosis is 13 for males and 11–12 for females, the earlier age in females corresponding to their earlier onset of puberty. Males are affected more frequently than females, although the male to female ratio appears to have decreased over time and varies from one geographic area to another. In males, the left hip is affected about twice as frequently as the right, whereas in females the left and right hips are affected with approximately equal frequency. In both sexes, about 20–25 per cent of the cases are bilateral.

Slipped epiphysis appears to be particularly common among the Maori of New Zealand (Stott & Bidwell 2003). Worldwide, Polynesian and Black children have higher incidence rates than White children, whereas residents of Asia (including the Indian subcontinent), the Near East, and north Africa have lower rates (Loder 1996). The incidence in Japan is reported to have increased considerably in the past 25 years, a trend in all likelihood attributable to the increased prevalence of childhood and adolescent obesity (Noguchi *et al.* 2002).

About half of those with slipped epiphysis have weights at or above the 95th percentile for their age (Loder 1996). Children with slipped epiphysis tend to have undergone slower skeletal maturation than average for their age (Sorenson 1968). They tend to be tall for their age at the time of diagnosis, but at maturity their heights are almost normal for their chronological age (Hansson *et al.* 1987). Familial aggregation of cases has been noted by several investigators.

Most of the established risk factors for slipped epiphysis are related either to a weakening of the epiphyseal plate or to an increase in the shearing stress on the plate. The epiphyseal plate is weaker during periods of rapid growth, such as during the adolescent growth spurt. The growth spurt in males is of greater magnitude and of longer duration than that in females, and the male growth spurt is more likely to have periods of acceleration and deceleration

A deficit of sex hormones relative to the growth hormone brings about a widening of the epiphyseal plate and a reduction in the shearing force needed to displace the epiphysis. Oestrogens protect against slipped epiphysis, whereas androgens are protective only in large doses after prolonged exposure. Slowly maturing children are exposed for a longer period to high levels of growth hormone relative to sex hormones than are children who mature faster. Tall children also have a longer exposure to growth hormone relative to sex hormones (Morscher 1968).

During adolescence the epiphyseal plate changes from a horizontal to an oblique plane, so that it becomes more vulnerable to stress from superincumbent weight. Children who are overweight put more stress on their plate than lighter children.

Prevention

Reducing the prevalence of adolescent obesity would have a large impact on the number of cases of slipped epiphysis. No screening tests are available, but slipped epiphysis should be considered in adolescents who have a limp and hip or knee pain or restriction of motion in the hip. The contralateral hip in children with slipped epiphysis in one hip needs to be carefully monitored, especially if the first slipped epiphysis occurred at an early age (Loder 1996). Early diagnosis is important, as slight displacement treated early by pinning the hip has a favourable prognosis, whereas cases that are diagnosed late and that have severe displacement usually have early onset of osteoarthritis of the hip and permanent disability.

Childhood fractures

In the United States, about 1 in 36 persons of age 18 years or younger fractures a bone each year (Praemer *et al.* 1999). In South Wales,

about 64 per cent of boys and 39 per cent of girls can expect to fracture a bone by 15 years of age (Lyons *et al.* 1999). Except when rare complications occur, most fractures heal quickly in children, and the younger the age, the more rapid the healing.

Risk factors

Among children, incidence rates of fracture peak at about age 14 years in boys and age 11 years in girls (Cooper *et al.* 2004). Throughout childhood, incidence rates are higher in males than females. In one study (Brudvik & Hove 2003), the ratio of male to female fracture cases rose from 1.1 among children less than age 6 years to 2.1 in those of ages 13–15 years. Most forms of trauma associated with fractures are more common in boys than girls.

Fractures of the radius and ulna are the most frequent of the childhood fractures. Other common sites are the carpals, hands, feet, humerus, and clavicle (Cooper *et al.* 2004; Brudvik & Hove 2003). Children who have one fracture are at increased risk of having an additional fracture.

In a series of childhood fracture cases in Wales, sports and leisure-time activities accounted for 36 per cent of fractures, assaults for 3.5 per cent, and road traffic accidents for 1.4 per cent (Lyons *et al.* 1999). In a study in Norway (Brudvik & Hove 2003), fractures in children under 6 years of age most commonly occurred indoors at home (32 per cent), outdoors near the home (23 per cent), and outdoors in kindergarten (17 per cent). Among school children, fractures were most common outdoors near the home (23 per cent), outdoors at school (20 per cent), and indoors at school (10 per cent), mainly in school gymnastics. The activities associated with fractures included soccer, bicycling, handball, volleyball, basketball, and rollerblading or skateboarding. Over time, rollerblading and skateboarding, along with snowboarding, have been accounting for increasing proportions of fractures, and a high proportion of the injuries associated with these sports are fractures (Brudvik & Hove 2003).

Little information is available from low- and middle-income countries, but injuries from falls and road traffic incidents are the leading causes of disease burden among children of ages 5–14 years in these countries (Beveridge & Howard 2004). In a study that included children from Ethiopia, Peru, Vietnam, and India (Howe *et al.* 2006), fractures in very young children were found to be associated with chronic mental disease in the caregiver, the father not living in the household, and a long-term health problem in the child.

Prevention

Preventing accidents and reducing the impact on bones when accidents do occur are key to decreasing the number of fractures in children, including decreasing the number of sports and recreational injuries; falls; bicycle, motorcycle, and automobile accidents; child-battering injuries; and other childhood traumas. Many fractures resulting from falls on hard surfaces could be reduced by the use of impact-absorbing surfaces in playgrounds. Many distal forearm fractures, the most common fracture site in children, could be prevented by the use of wrist guards while engaging in such activities as soccer, rollerblading, skateboarding, and snowboarding, although some evidence indicates that the number of fractures in the forearm just above the brace might be increased (Lyons *et al.* 1999; Brudvik & Hove 2003).

Developmental dysplasia of the hip

Developmental dysplasia of the hip includes a spectrum of abnormalities in which the femoral head and the acetabulum are either in improper alignment or grow abnormally. Long-term complications include osteoarthritis, difficulty walking, and chronic pain.

The diagnosis is made shortly after birth in about 80 per cent of cases, whereas about 20 per cent of cases are diagnosed later, especially when the child starts to walk. From 60 to 80 per cent of hips identified as abnormal or suspicious for developmental dysplasia by physical examination and over 90 per cent of those identified with mild dysplasia by ultrasound in the newborn period resolve spontaneously and require no intervention (US Preventive Services Task Force 2006).

Considerable variation occurs in the frequency of developmental dysplasia of the hip from one geographic area to another and from one racial or ethnic group to another. Using data collected before screening at birth became widespread, in most North American and western European countries as well as in Australia, New Zealand, and Israel, prevalence rates of around 1 per 1000 to 10 per 1000 births were found. In the Navajo, Apache, and Cree-Ojibwa of North America, and the Lapps, as well as in Hungary, northern Italy, Brittany, and the Faroe Islands, rates from 10 per 1000 to 100 per 1000 births were reported. On the other hand, developmental dysplasia of the hip was rare among blacks in South Africa, the West Indies, and Uganda, and among Chinese living in Hong Kong (reviewed in Kelsey (Kelsey 1982)). It must be kept in mind that the nature of the neonatal examination of the infant, the experience of the examiner, the timing of the examination, and the criteria for developmental dysplasia of the hip could all affect these figures.

Risk factors

Risk factors for developmental dysplasia of the hip have been reviewed (Storer & Skaggs 2006). Females are affected about four to six times more frequently than males. In the United States, whites are affected more often than blacks. First-born children are at higher risk than later-born children; in pregnancies after the first, the ligaments and other tissues in and around the maternal uterus have already been stretched during previous pregnancies, allowing more foetal movement. In unilateral cases, the left hip is affected more frequently than the right, probably because the left hip is positioned against the maternal spine more often than is the right hip.

Familial aggregation occurs, and both hereditary and environmental factors are believed to contribute to the familial excess. Infants with developmental dysplasia of the hip are considerably more likely to have been born by breech delivery than other infants. *In utero* postural deformities and oligohydramnios are also associated with an increased risk.

Prevention

No means of primary prevention are known, but screening of newborns either by serial physical examination using the Ortolani or Barlow procedures or by ultrasonography is now widely used. In the Ortolani test, the hip is placed in flexion and gently adducted and then abducted. The Ortolani test is considered positive if a palpable jerk and an audible click are heard as the head of the femur returns to the acetabulum. Some physicians consider just an audible click to be a positive test. The Barlow test involves exerting gentle downward pressure over the lesser trochanter with the hip in flexion and adduction; an unstable hip will shift from the acetabulum and a sensation similar to the Ortolani sign is produced. When the leg is allowed to abduct, the hip is reduced. Because many hips noted to be unstable at birth soon become stable spontaneously, these tests are often repeated at around three weeks. Infants who

are positive by either the Ortolani or Barlow test are generally treated with braces, splints, or harness for 2–4 months. Routine checks of the hips of these infants should be performed until they are walking well. If diagnosis is delayed until after the neonatal period, surgery is usually required and the prognosis is poorer.

Although screening for developmental dysplasia of the hip by the Ortolani or Barlow tests is routine in many localities, the US Preventive Services Task Force (US Preventive Services Task Force 2006) concluded that the evidence for the effectiveness of these tests is insufficient to recommend their use for routine screening. First, the Task Force could find no direct evidence that screening leads to a reduced need for surgery or improved functional outcomes. Second, because the majority of hips that are abnormal at birth resolve spontaneously within 2–8 weeks, intervention is not needed for most of those screened as positive. Third, the accuracy of the screening tests is difficult to assess because of variable definitions of a positive test and the lack of a practical confirmatory gold standard for a positive result. Fourth, the effectiveness of both surgical and non-surgical interventions is uncertain because of the high rate of spontaneous resolution and various deficiencies in the studies examining the effectiveness of surgery. Fifth, the potential harm from screening has not been well evaluated, such as the possibility that the procedures themselves could dislocate a hip, the radiation exposure from follow-up radiography, parental psychosocial stress, and false-positive tests that result in unnecessary and possibly harmful follow-up and treatment, including the risks associated with surgery. The training and experience of physicians performing the tests and interventions vary considerably.

Ultrasound, in which a defined image of the bony and cartilaginous hip can be examined, has become widely available for screening for developmental dysplasia of the hip. Ultrasound may be of value in following up infants who have shown hip instability on clinical examination (Elbourne *et al.* 2002), but its use for routine screening and even its use in high-risk infants are controversial. Some of the problems are that ultrasound is expensive, cases developing after the neonatal period will not be detected if ultrasound is done only in newborns, and the vast majority of hips classified as positive on ultrasound develop normally. It is unclear how an infant with a normal clinical examination but with abnormal ultrasonogram should be treated. In addition, better training is needed to improve the scans and their interpretation.

Conclusion

The global impact of musculoskeletal diseases, though now substantial, will become much greater over the next several decades. Musculoskeletal diseases are common at all ages, but their greatest impact is on the elderly. The number of people aged 65 years or older in the world is expected to more than double between 2007 and 2035, for a total of about 1.16 billion people of age 65 years and older in 2035 (US Census Bureau 2007). Thus, musculoskeletal diseases will account for an increasing portion of health care costs. In addition to the development and application of better methods of primary prevention, much more needs to be done to limit the pain and disability among the large number of those already affected and to help people learn how best to cope with these frequently lifelong disabilities. Musculoskeletal disorders are often not given high priority in developing countries, despite the large amount of disability they cause and their high monetary cost to the community.

Several measures could be undertaken on the basis of current knowledge. For instance, total joint replacements of the hip and knee are highly successful and cost-effective operations for disabled people in high-income countries, but are not widely used in low-income countries because of cost and limited resources (Brooks 2006). Ergonomic improvements and better training in the workplace could now be instituted in many regions. In addition, more information on the most important musculoskeletal problems and risk factors in specific geographic areas is needed if limited funds are to be used wisely. Thus, we are at a time when more epidemiologic and clinical research is needed and when current knowledge could be much more widely applied to reduce the frequency and burden of musculoskeletal diseases throughout the world.

References

Abolhassani F., Moayyeri A., Naghavi M. *et al.* Incidence and characteristics of falls leading to hip fracture in Iranian population. *Bone* 2006;**39**:408–13.

Ahasan M.R., Mohiuddin G., Vayrynen S. *et al.* Work-related problems in metal handling tasks in Bangladesh: obstacles to the development of safety and health measures. *Ergonomics* 1999;**42**:385–96.

Andersson G.B.J. Epidemiologic aspects of low-back pain in industry. *Spine* 1981;**6**:53–60.

Andersson G.B.J. Epidemiology of low-back pain. *Acta Orthopaedica Scandinavica Supplement* 1998;**281**:28–31.

Arden N., Nevitt M.C. Osteoarthritis: epidemiology. *Best Practice and Research Clinical Rheumatology* 2006;**20**:3–25.

Badley E.M. The economic burden of musculoskeletal disorders in Canada is similar to that for cancer, and may be higher [Editorial]. *Journal of Rheumatology* 1995;**22**:204–6.

Barrero L.H., Hsu Y.H., Terwedow H. *et al.* Prevalence and physical determinants of low back pain in a rural Chinese population. *Spine* 2006;**31**:2728–34.

Bartlett S.J., Bingham C.O., Maricic M.J. III *et al. Clinical care in the rheumatic diseases.* 3rd ed. Atlanta (GA): Association of Rheumatology Health Professionals; 2006.

Benvenuti F., Ferrucci L., Guralnik J.M. *et al.* Foot pain and disability in older persons: an epidemiologic survey. *Journal of the American Geriatrics Society* 1995;**43**:479–84.

Beveridge M., Howard A. The burden of orthopaedic disease in developing countries. *Journal of Bone and Joint Surgery* 2004;**86**A:1819–22.

Biering-Sorenson F. Low back trouble in a general population of 30-, 40-, 50-, and 60-year-old men and women. *Study design, representativeness, and basic results. Danish Medical Bulletin* 1982;**29**:289–99.

Black D.M., Schwartz A.V., Ensrud K.E. *et al.* Effects of continuing or stopping alendronate after 5 years of treatment. The Fracture Intervention Trial Long-term Extension (FLEX): a randomized trial. *Journal of the American Medical Association* 2006;**296**:2927–38.

Bowling A. The effects of illness on quality of life: findings from a survey of households in Great Britain. *Journal of Epidemiology and Community Health* 1996;**50**:149–55.

Brooks P.M. The burden of musculoskeletal disease—a global perspective. *Clinical Rheumatology* 2006;**25**:778–81.

Brudvik C., Hove L.M. Childhood fractures in Bergen, Norway: identifying high-risk groups and activities. *Journal of Paediatric Orthopaedics* 2003;**23**:629–34.

Cats-Baril W.L., Frymoyer J.W. Identifying patients at risk of becoming disabled because of low-back pain. The Vermont Rehabilitation Engineering Center predictive model. *Spine* 1991;**16**:605–7.

Centers for Disease Control and Prevention. Prevalence of disabilities and associated health conditions among adults—United States, 1999. *Morbidity and Mortality Weekly Report* 2001;**50**:120–5.

Centers for Disease Control and Prevention. Prevalence of doctor-diagnosed arthritis and arthritis-attributable activity limitation–United States, 2003–2005. *Journal of the American Medical Association* 2006;**296**:2671–2.

Chavalitsakulchai P., Shahnavaz H. Musculoskeletal disorders of female workers and ergonomics problems in five different industries of a developing country. *Journal of Human Ergology (Tokyo)* 1993;**22**:29–43.

Clarke M. Trouble with feet. In: Titmuss RM, editor. *Occasional papers on social administration.* London: Bell G and Sons; 1969. vol 29. p.1–182.

Cooper C., Campion G., Melton L.J. III. Hip fractures in the elderly: a worldwide projection. *Osteoporosis International* 1992;**2**:285–9.

Cooper C., Dennison E.M., Leufkens H.G. *et al.* Epidemiology of childhood fractures in Britain: a study using the general practice research database. *Journal of Bone and Mineral Research* 2004;**19**:1976–81.

Cooper C., McAlindon T., Coggon D. *et al.* Occupational activity and osteoarthritis of the knee. *Annals of the Rheumatic Diseases* 1994;**53**:90–3.

Côté P., Cassidy J.D., Carroll L. The Saskatchewan Health and Back Pain Survey. The prevalence of neck pain and related disability in Saskatchewan adults. *Spine* 1998;**23**:1689–98.

Croft P.R., Macfarlane G.J., Papageorgiou A.C. *et al.* Outcome of low back pain in general practice: a prospective study. *British Medical Journal* 1998;**316**:1356–9.

Cummings S.R., Black D.M., Thompson D.E. *et al.* Effect of alendronate on risk of fracture in women with low bone density but without vertebral fractures: results from the Fracture Intervention Trial. *Journal of the American Medical Association* 1998;**280**:2077–82.

Cummings S.R., Ling X., Stone K. Consequences of foot binding among older women in Beijing, China. *American Journal of Public Health* 1997;**87**:1677–9.

Dans L.F., Tankeh-Torres S., Amante C.M. *et al.* The prevalence of rheumatic diseases in a Filipino urban population: a WHO-ILAR COPCORD Study. *Journal of Rheumatology* 1997;**24**:1814–9.

Darmawan J., Valkenburg H.A., Muirden K.D. *et al.* Epidemiology of rheumatic diseases in rural and urban populations in Indonesia: a World Health Organisation-International League Against Rheumatism COPCORD study, stage 1, phase 2. *Annals of the Rheumatic Diseases* 1992;**51**:525–8.

Deyo R.A., Diehl A.K. Psychosocial predictors of disability in patients with low back pain. *Journal of Rheumatology* 1988;**15**:1557–64.

Dunn J.E., Link C.L., Felson D.T. *et al.* Prevalence of foot and ankle conditions in a multiethnic community sample of older adults. *American Journal of Epidemiology* 2004;**491**–8.

Eisenberg D.M., Davis R.B., Ettner S.L. *et al.* Trends in alternative medicine use in the United States, 1990–1997. Journal of the American Medical Association 1998;**280**1569–75.

Elbourne D., Dezateux C., Arthur R. *et al.* Ultrasonography in the diagnosis and management of developmental hip dysplasia (UK Hip Trial): clinical and economic results of a multicentre randomised controlled trial. *Lancet* 2002;**360**:2009–17.

Emery P. Treatment of rheumatoid arthritis. *British Medical Journal* 2006;**332**:152–5.

Ettinger B., Black D.M., Mitlak B.H. *et al.* Reduction of vertebral fracture risk in postmenopausal women with osteoporosis treated with raloxifene. Results from a 3-year randomized clinical trial. *Journal of the American Medical Association* 1999;**282**:637–45.

Farooqi A., Gibson T. Prevalence of major rheumatic disorders in the adult population of north Pakistan. *British Journal of Rheumatology* 1998;**37**:491–5.

Felts W., Yelin E. The economic impact of the rheumatic diseases in the United States. *Journal of Rheumatology* 1989;**16**:867–84.

Ferraz M.B. Tropical rheumatology. Epidemiology and community studies: Latin America. *Baillieres Clinical Rheumatology* 1995;**9**:1–9.

Gilgil E., Kaçar C., Bütün B. *et al.* Prevalence of low back pain in a developing urban setting. *Spine* 2005;**30**:1093–8.

Goldberg C.J., Dowling F.E., Fogarty E.E. *et al.* School scoliosis screening and the United States Preventive Services Task Force. *Spine* 1995;**20**:1368–74.

Hameed K., Gibson T., Kadir M. *et al.* The prevalence of rheumatoid arthritis in affluent and poor urban communities of Pakistan. *British Journal of Rheumatology* 1995;**34**:252–6.

Hans D., Dargent-Molina P., Schott A.M. *et al.* Ultrasonographic heel measurements to predict hip fracture in elderly women: the EPIDOS prospective study. *Lancet* 1996;**348**:511–4.

Hansson L.I., Hagglund G., Ordeberg G. Slipped capital femoral epiphysis in southern Sweden, 1910–1982. *Acta Orthopaedia Scandinavica* 1987;**226**:1–67.

Haq S.A., Darmawan J., Islam M.N. *et al.* Prevalence of rheumatic diseases and associated outcomes in rural and urban communities in Bangladesh: a COPCORD study. *Journal of Rheumatology* 2005;**32**: 348–53.

Hoogendoorn W.E., van Poppel M.N., Bongers P.M. *et al.* Systematic review of psychosocial factors at work and private life as risk factors for back pain. *Spine* 2000;**25**:2114–25.

Howe L.D., Huttly S.R.A., Abramsky T. Risk factors for injuries in young children in four developing countries: the Young Lives Study. *Tropical Medicine and International Health* 2006;**11**:1557–66.

Hung L.K., Ho Y.F., Leung P.C. Survey of foot deformities among 166 geriatric inpatients. *Foot and Ankle* 1985;**5**:156–64.

Hung V.W.Y., Qin L., Cheung C.S.K. *et al.* Osteopenia: a new prognostic factor of curve progression in adolescent idiopathic scoliosis. *Journal of Bone and Joint Surgery* 2005;**87**A:2709–16.

Jackson R.D., LaCroix A.Z., Gass M. *et al.* Calcium plus vitamin D supplementation and the risk of fractures. *New England Journal of Medicine* 2006;**354**:669–83.

Jenyo M.S., Asekun-Olarinmoye E.O. Prevalence of scoliosis in secondary school children in Osogbo, Osun State, Nigeria. *African Journal of Medicine and Medical Sciences* 2005;**34**:361–4.

Jerre R., Karlsson J., Henrikson B. The incidence of physiolysis of the hip. A population-based study of 175 patients. *Acta Orthopaedica Scandinavica* 1996;**67**:53–6.

Kacar C., Gilgil E., Urhan S. *et al.* The prevalence of symptomatic knee and distal interphalangeal joint osteoarthritis in the urban population of Antalya, Turkey. *Rheumatology International* 2005;**25**:201–4.

Karpman R.R. Foot problems in the geriatric patient. *Clinical Orthopedics* 1995;**316**:59–62.

Kelsey J.L., Githens P.B., Walter S.D. *et al.* An epidemiologic study of acute prolapsed cervical intervertebral disc. *Journal of Bone and Joint Surgery* 1984;**66**A:907–14.

Kelsey J.L., Githens P.B., White A.A. III *et al.* An epidemiological study of lifting and twisting on the job and risk for acute prolapsed lumbar intervertebral disc. *Journal of Orthopaedic Research* 1984;**2**:61–6.

Kelsey J.L. *Epidemiology of musculoskeletal disorders.* New York (NY): Oxford University Press; 1982.

Keyserling W.M., Herrin G.D., Chaffin D.B. Establishing an industrial strength testing program. *American Industrial Hygiene Association Journal* 1980;**41**:730–6.

Krause N., Ragland D.R., Greiner B.A. *et al.* Physical workload and ergonomic factors associated with prevalence of back and neck pain in urban transit operators. *Spine* 1997;**22**:2117–26.

Lau E.M.C., Symmons D.P.M., Croft P. The epidemiology of hip osteoarthritis and rheumatoid arthritis in the Orient. *Clinical Orthopaedics and Related Research* 1996;**323**:81–90.

Leclerc A., Niedhammer I., Landre M.F. *et al.* One-year predictive factors for various aspects of neck disorders. *Spine* 1999;**24**:1455–62.

Leveille S.G., Guralnik J.M., Ferrucci L. *et al.* Foot pain and disability in older women. *American Journal of Epidemiology* 1998;**148**:657–65.

Lis A.M., Black K.M., Korn H. *et al.* Association between sitting and occupational LBP. *European Spine Journal* 2007;**16**:283–98.

Loder R.T. The demographics of slipped capital femoral epiphysis. An international multicenter study. *Clinical Orthopaedics and Related Research* 1996;**322**:8–27.

Looker A.C., Orwoll E.D., Johnston C.C. Jr. *et al.* Prevalence of low femoral bone density in older U. S. adults from HNANES III. *Journal of Bone and Mineral Research* 1997;**12**:1761–8.

Lyons R.A., Delahunty A.M., Kraus D. *et al.* Children's fractures: a population based study. *Injury Prevention* 1999;**5**:129–32.

Magnusson M.L., Pope M.H., Wilder D.G. *et al.* Are occupational drivers at an increased risk for developing musculoskeletal disorders? *Spine* 1996;**21**:710–7.

Malmivaara A., Häkkinen U., Aro T. *et al.* The treatment of acute low back pain—bed rest, exercises, or ordinary activity? *New England Journal of Medicine* 1995;**332**:351–5.

Melton L.J. III. How many women have osteoporosis now? *Journal of Bone and Mineral Research* 1995;**10**:175–7.

Menz H.B., Lord S.R. The contribution of foot problems to mobility impairment and falls in community-dwelling older people. *Journal of the American Geriatrics Society* 2001;**49**:1651–6.

Miller N.H. Cause and natural history of adolescent idiopathic scoliosis. *Orthopedic Clinics of North America* 1999;**30**:343–52.

Morales-Torres J., Gutiérrez-Urenþa S. The burden of osteoporosis in Latin America. *Osteoporosis International* 2004;**15**:625–32.

Morales-Torres J. Strategies for the prevention and control of osteoporosis in developing countries. *Clinical Rheumatology* 2007;**26**:139–43.

Morscher E. Strength and morphology of growth cartilage under hormonal influence of puberty. *Reconstructive Surgery and Traumatology* 1968;**10**:3–104.

Nevitt M.C., Cummings S.R. Type of fall and risk of hip and wrist fractures: the Study of Osteoporotic Fractures. *Journal of the American Geriatrics Society* 1993;**41**:1226–34.

Nissinen M., Heliövaara M., Seitsamo J. *et al.* Trunk asymmetry, posture, growth, and risk of scoliosis. A three-year follow-up of Finnish prepubertal school children. *Spine* 1993;**18**:8–13.

Noguchi Y., Sakamaki T., the Multi-center Study Committee of the Japanese Pediatric Orthopaedic Association. Epidemiology and demographics of slipped capital femoral epiphysis in Japan: a multicenter study by the Japanese Paediatric Orthopaedic Association. *Journal of Orthopaedic Sciences* 2002;**7**:610–7.

Öry F.G., Rahman F.U., Katagade V. *et al.* Respiratory disorders, skin complaints, and low-back trouble among tannery workers in Kanpur, India. *American Industrial Hygiene Association Journal* 1997;**58**:740–6.

Ostojic Z., Kristo T., Ostojic L. *et al.* Prevalence of scoliosis in school-children from Mostar, Bosnia and Herzegovina. *Collegium Antropologicum* 2006;**30**:59–64.

Pope M.H., Magnusson M., Wilder D.G. Low back pain and whole body vibration. *Clinical Orthopaedics and Related Research* 1998;**354**:241–8.

Praemer A., Furner S., Rice D.P. *Musculoskeletal conditions in the United States.* Rosemont (IL): American Academy of Orthopaedic Surgeons; 1999.

Punnett L., Prüss-Üstün A., Nelson D.I. *et al.* Estimating the global burden of low back pain attributable to combined occupational exposures. *American Journal of Industrial Medicine* 2005;**48**:459–69.

Rasch E.K., Hirsch R., Paulose-Ram R. *et al.* Prevalence of rheumatoid arthritis in persons 60 years of age and older in the United States: effect of different methods of case classification. *Arthritis and Rheumatism* 2003;**48**:917–26.

Sadat-Ali M., Al-Habdan I.M., Al-Mulhim F.A. *et al.* Bone mineral density among postmenopausal Saudi women. *Saudi Medical Journal* 2004;**25**:1623–5.

Schwartz A.V., Kelsey J.L., Maggi S. *et al.* International variation in the incidence of hip fractures: cross-national project on osteoporosis for the World Health Organization Program for Research on Aging. *Osteoporosis International* 1999;**9**:242–53.

Seeman E., Delmas P.D. Bone quality—the material and structural basis of bone strength and fragility. *New England Journal of Medicine* 2006;**354**:2250–61.

Shatrugna V., Kulkarni B., Kumar P.A. *et al.* Bone status of Indian women from a low-income group and its relationship to the nutritional status. *Osteoporosis International* 2005;**16**:1827–35.

Snook S.H. Approaches to the control of back pain in industry: job design, job placement, and education/testing. Spine: State of the Art Reviews. *Occupational Back Pain* 1988;**2**:45–59.

Sorenson K.H. Slipped upper femoral epiphysis. *Acta Orthopaedica Scandinavica* 1968;**39**:499–517.

Storer S.K., Skaggs D.A. Developmental dysplasia of the hip. *American Family Physician* 2006;**74**:1310–6.

Stott S., Bidwell T. Epidemiology of slipped capital femoral epiphysis in a population with a high proportion of New Zealand Maori and Pacific children. New Zealand Medical Journal 2003;**116**:U647.

Tinetti M.E. Preventing falls in elderly persons. *New England Journal of Medicine* 2003;**348**:42–9.

US Census Bureau. International database [Online]. 2007.

US Department of Health and Human Services, National Center for Health Statistics. *National Ambulatory Medical Care Survey, 1995 summary.* Hyattsville (MD): Centers for Disease Control and Prevention; 1997.

US Department of Health and Human Services, National Center for Health Statistics. *Third National Health and Nutrition Examination Survey, 1988–94* [NHANES III Examination Data File, CD-ROM]. Public Use Data File Documentation Number 76200. Hyattsville (MD): Centers for Disease Control and Prevention; 1996.

US Preventive Services Task Force. Screening for adolescent idiopathic scoliosis: review article. *Journal of the American Medical Association* 1993;**269**:2667–72.

US Preventive Services Task Force. Screening for adolescent idiopathic scoliosis: policy statement. *Journal of the American Medical Association* 1993;**269**:2664–6.

US Preventive Services Task Force. Screening for developmental dysplasia of the hip: recommendation statement. *Pediatrics* 2006;**117**:898–902.

Van Vuuren B.J., Becker P.J., van Heerden H.J. *et al.* Lower back problems and occupational risk factors in a South African steel industry. *American Journal of Industrial Medicine* 2005;**47**:451–7.

Volinn E. The epidemiology of low back pain in the rest of the world: a review of surveys in low-and middle-income countries. *Spine* 1997;**22**:1747–54.

Wickstrom G.J., Pentti J. Occupational factors affecting sick leave attributed to low-back pain. *Scandinavian Journal of Work, Environment and Health* 1998;**24**:145–52.

Woolf A.D., Pfleger B. Burden of major musculoskeletal conditions. *Bulletin of the World Health Organization* 2003;**81**:646–56.

World Health Organization. *Prevention and management of osteoporosis.* WHO technical report series 921. Geneva: World Health Organization; 2003.

World Health Organization. *The burden of musculoskeletal conditions at the start of the new millennium.* WHO technical report series 919. Geneva: World Health Organization; 2003.

Yu I.T.S., Wong T.W. Musculoskeletal problems among VDU workers in a Hong Kong bank. *Occupational Medicine* 1996;**46**:275–80.

Neurologic diseases, epidemiology, and public health

Walter A. Kukull and James Bowen

Abstract

This chapter presents information for selected neurological conditions by referring to current or classic research papers. Conditions such as headache have substantial public health impact because of the age groups affected, the prevalence, and the associated lost economic productivity. Multiple sclerosis (MS), a relatively common neurologic disease, can affect individuals in young adulthood, decrease their productivity and ultimately make them dependent on others. Traumatic brain injury occurring in youth or young adulthood can cause years of extra medical care in addition to lost productivity among those who survive the immediate event. Epilepsy may have onset throughout the life course, it may result from trauma or may be caused by specific genes, among other causes. While there are intractable forms of epilepsy, great strides have been made in seizure control enabling patients to lead relatively full and normal lives. Neurodegenerative diseases, such as Parkinson's disease (PD) and Alzheimer's disease (AD), rob productivity, functional ability, and independence from older individuals; they also force huge increases in health care costs. Without question neurologic diseases have substantial public health impacts.

Introduction

Included in this chapter are brief descriptions of some selected neurological disorders along with a discussion of their general epidemiology. Several themes cut across all of the sections. Case diagnosis is critical to epidemiologic study of neurological diseases and disorders. Diagnosis is, however, difficult for many neurological diseases because specific histologic evidence or antemortem biologic markers may not exist and clinical diagnosis must be relied upon. Variation in clinical criteria can lead to misclassification of disease. As a case series includes more misclassification of disease diagnoses, the ability to recognize risk factors becomes reduced. Standardization of clinical criteria is one method to reduce the amount of misclassification; in practice, standardization across unrelated sites is difficult to achieve, however.

Case ascertainment and selection for inclusion are more substantial problems for the validity of most epidemiologic studies.

If an incidence study must rely on death certificates in order to count new cases, and the course of disease is long, the characteristics of cases identified in that way are likely to be skewed and will reflect factors associated with survival. The method of identifying and including cases in a case–control study is important because if identification is associated with exposure history, selection bias could result and the findings could then be spurious. Can all cases identified from a particular study base be enrolled in the study at hand? Usually not; many persons decline to participate in studies. Frailty, age, ethnicity, gender, education, and a host of other factors influence participation. If any of those participation factors are systematically related to exposure status, an uncontrolled bias may result, also. Case identification methods are critical to cohort studies (and intervention trials) as well. Failure to start with a cohort that is free of the disease of interest will potentially bias results. Lack of, or differential sensitivity or specificity in screening or diagnosing disease during cohort follow-up will lead to miss-estimated incidence and to distorted risk factor relationships. The choice of controls in a case–control study also determines the size of the measure of effect. Selection of appropriate controls is even more difficult than selection of cases. Controls should be selected from the same study base that gave rise to the cases. In fact, if persons we would have available to select controls from were to contract the disease under study we would expect that they would be included as cases in our study. Briefly, that is how case and control definition may be used to define the underlying study base, as well.

Obtaining valid estimates of exposures for analytic risk factor studies is of great importance. For most neurological diseases, exposure determination is complicated by insidious and indeterminate onset of disease, obscuring the temporal relationship between exposure and disease. Long past exposure histories are difficult to construct and validate, especially in diseases that affect memory. Self report histories and those obtained from proxies are often the basis for risk factor inference, but may be flawed by distorted recollection or recall bias. Actual records, for example of medication history or occupational exposures, are seldom available. Biological markers of exposure (except for genotype) are difficult to obtain; and some may be affected by disease. Peripheral markers, if available may not correspond to exposure levels in neuronal tissue. Biopsy may not be feasible or possible and autopsy, while often the gold standard for diagnosis, may reflect cumulative disease processes, leaving the picture additionally confusing.

As one leaves major research institutions or attempts to begin epidemiologic research studies in less developed countries, the problems grow in magnitude. Differences in available facilities and local practices are likely the easiest to overcome. Addressing political concerns and suspicions to gain cooperation necessary to begin a study may take additional time and preparation. Case detection, acquisition and exposure measurement still remain critical but the difficulty in obtaining acceptable levels of each is increased by an order of magnitude.

In following sections, we discuss the current descriptive and analytic research for a number of neurological disorders. We also provide a brief appraisal of the public health burden for these conditions.

Headache

Clinical overview

The pathogenesis of most headaches is poorly understood. Therefore, the nosology of headaches is based on the cause of headaches in those types that the cause is known, and the clinical picture in those in which the cause is unknown. The International Headache Society (IHS) classification, second edition, is currently the most commonly used system of classifying headaches (Table 9.10.1) (..2004a) It is important to realize that this system is used to classify individual headaches. Patients may suffer from more than one type of headache with each headache type fulfilling one of the IHS classifications. In fact, most headache patients have more than one type of headache. The IHS classification contains a large number of conditions in which the headaches are symptomatic of neurologic or systemic diseases. Headaches associated with these conditions

Table 9.10.1 International Headache Society, abbreviated classification of headache

1. Migraine
1.1 Migraine without aura
1.2 Migraine with aura
2. Tension-type headache
3. Cluster headache and chronic paroxysmal hemicrania
4. Miscellaneous headaches unassociated with structural lesion
5. Headache associated with head trauma
6. Headache associated with vascular disorders
7. Headache associated with nonvascular intracranial disorder
8. Headache associated with substances or their withdrawal
9. Headache associated with noncephalic infection
10. Headache associated with metabolic disorder
11. Headache or facial pain associated with disorder of cranium, neck, eyes, ears, nose, sinuses, teeth, mouth, or other facial or cranial structures
12. Cranial neuralgias, nerve trunk pain, and deafferentation pain
13. Headache not classifiable

are comparatively rare. Idiopathic conditions are far more common and include migraine (with or without aura), tension-type headaches and cluster headaches. Because these idiopathic headaches are the overwhelming majority, they have the greatest impact on epidemiologic studies.

Migraine without aura was previously named common migraine. It is an episodic headache that, as its name suggests, has no aura. The headache may be unilateral or bilateral. Some have throbbing pain while others have constant non-throbbing pain. Nausea, vomiting, or diarrhoea may occur. The pain often builds over a few hours. The typical length of the headache is 4–72 h.

Migraine with aura was previously named classic migraine. The identifying feature of this type of headache is the aura. This consists of an alteration of neurologic function that usually precedes the headache. The aura most commonly consists of changes in vision with a central area of visual loss surrounded by a rim of shimmering light (the scintillating scotoma). Non-visual auras may also occur including paresthesias, numbness, weakness, aphasia, or vertigo. Auras usually precede the headache by about 20 min, though the timing may vary. The headache resembles that seen in migraine without aura. It is most commonly, though not always, unilateral. It is most often throbbing and often associated with nausea and vomiting. It typically lasts a few hours. It is episodic and may have premonitory symptoms preceding the headache and aura.

Tension-type headaches, the most common type of headache, are usually bilateral and have a sensation of pressure or a tight band around the head. They are less likely to have premonitory symptoms and less likely to have nausea or vomiting. They do not have auras. They usually last longer than migraine headaches and typically last an entire day or even several days. They build up more slowly than migraine headaches. Episodic and chronic subtypes are recognized.

Cluster headaches are named after the tendency to occur in clusters lasting weeks to months. However, other types of headaches may also occur in clusters and the diagnosis is made based on the characteristics of the headache rather than the clustering. The headache develops abruptly. During a cluster, it usually occurs between one and eight times a day, often at the same time of day. The pain is more short-lived than that of other idiopathic headaches and generally subsides within 3 h. The pain is often more severe than that seen with migraine and patients are often agitated during the attack.

As previously noted, patients often suffer from more than one type of headache. In a single patient, less severe headaches tend to be tension-type while more severe headaches are migraine. There is also a tendency for patient's headaches to change over time with the headache pattern being classic migraine in youth but more closely matching that of tension-type headaches with time. These headaches may increase in frequency with age and become chronic daily headaches. Some term these headaches as 'transitioned migraines'. This term is not included in the International Headache Classification and many of these cases are actually due to medication overuse.

Prevalence

Recent studies have assessed the prevalence of headache and migraine in many countries. Most recent studies have used the IHS criteria to determine probable diagnosis. Characteristics of the samples selected and analytic designs have differed, sometimes substantially, raising questions of comparability.

The 1-year prevalence of all types of headache varies widely between different studies, from 20 to 90 per cent (Stovner *et al.* 2007). Migraine varied from 3 to 24.6 per cent, tension-type headache from 9.8 to 72.3 per cent, and chronic headache from 0.5 to 7.3 per cent. Much of this variability can be attributed to differences in methodology including survey methods, case definition, and the study population involved. Several large population-based studies have been completed. A survey of 5000 adults in the United Kingdom (Boardman *et al.* 2006) found that 71 per cent had suffered a headache in the past 3 months, with 76 per cent having headaches over a 1-year period. In a Spanish study, a mail-in survey followed by clinical evaluations found that 77 per cent had headaches, with 4.7 per cent having headaches 15 or more days per month (Castillo *et al.* 1999). The head-HUNT study began with all people 20 years of age or older, who resided in a single county in Norway. Of 51 383 respondents, the 1-year prevalence of all headaches was 38 per cent and of migraine was 12 per cent (Hagen *et al.* 2000).

Several studies have evaluated the prevalence of migraine. This reflects the availability of survey instruments that have been validated to identify migraine in study populations. The 1-year period prevalence of migraine is approximately 12 per cent (Rasmussen 1995). The American Migraine Prevalence and Prevention study assessed 162 576 individuals by mail survey (Lipton *et al.* 2007). It found a 1-year prevalence rate of migraine in men of 5.6 per cent and in women of 17.1 per cent. Prevalence peaked at 30–39 years of age, and was higher in whites and in those with lower incomes. Only 68 per cent of women and 57 per cent of men reported their migraines to a physician. Of those that did, approximately 40 per cent did not receive a correct diagnosis of migraine (Lipton *et al.* 1998). These estimates compare favourably with other studies that included both treated and untreated, self-reported headache. Gobel *et al.* (1994) selected a representative sample of 5000 persons from among 30 000 households in Germany. Using IHS criteria, approximately 71 per cent of the subjects reported any history of headache. The lifetime prevalence of migraine was 27.5 per cent. This survey did not rely on access to medical care and so may estimate the underlying lifetime prevalence of both treated and untreated migraine. Merikangas *et al.* (1994) studied the prevalence of headache in persons aged 29–30 in Zurich, Switzerland, again using the IHS criteria. Migraine with aura had a 1-year prevalence of 3.3 per cent and migraine without aura showed a 1-year prevalence of 21.3 per cent. Franceschi *et al.* (1997) studied an elderly population (mean age 73 years) in Italy to determine whether increasing age would affect reported prevalence. Although 18 per cent of subjects admitted to 'troublesome' headaches in the past, only 6 per cent were currently bothered by headache and 1 per cent met HIS criteria for current migraine. These results leave the impression that headache problems in young adulthood, may not persist into old age. However, in order to adequately evaluate change in the frequency of headache events with age would require a cohort study design instead of a cross-sectional one. O'Brien *et al.* (1994) drew a stratified sample in Canada, selecting 2922 subjects for a telephone interview based on IHS criteria. The prevalence of migraine was 7.8 per cent in male and 24.9 per cent in females; only about 46 per cent of those with migraine were reported to have ever contacted a physician for their problem. Within women, the peak prevalence was seen in the 40–44-year age group. A recent meta-analysis included 24 population-based studies of migraine (Stewart *et al.* 1995). Most of the variation in prevalence estimates, among the studies included, was accounted

for by age and gender differences along with case definition. Stewart concluded that after accounting for age gender and case definition, migraine prevalence estimates were stable across the studies included in the meta-analysis. Thus, despite variations in design and case ascertainment methods, there appears to be a gender difference and age-related differences that appear with some consistency in a number of countries. Many people apparently do not mention their headaches to physicians, and physicians often do not correctly identify headache subtypes.

Osuntokun *et al.* (1992) applied a screening questionnaire to more than 18 000 persons in Nigeria. The questionnaire was not strictly the IHS criteria but reportedly showed high sensitivity and specificity when compared to the gold standard neurologist examination for headache. Much lower lifetime prevalence of migraine (5.3%) was reported in this study than in those primarily comprised of Caucasians. No gender difference was noted, also in contrast to the studies reported above. Stewart *et al.* (1996a) compared migraine prevalence in Caucasians, African Americans, and Asian Americans living in the United States. The study involved about 12 000 persons aged 18–65 selected from Baltimore County, Maryland, selected by random digit dialling, and interviewed by telephone. Observed prevalence of migraine in Caucasians was 20.4 per cent for women and 8.6 per cent for men; among African Americans: 6.2 per cent in women and 7.2 per cent in men; and among Asian-Americans: 9.2 per cent in women and 4.2 per cent in men. Despite obvious geographic, and sociodemographic differences as well as methodologic differences between the two studies (Stewart *et al.* 1996a; Osuntokun *et al.* 1992), there appears to be a suggestion that susceptibility to migraine may be affected by ethnicity.

There are far fewer studies on tension-type headaches. Up to 89 per cent of people suffer tension-type headaches at some point in their lives, but for most, this is infrequent. About 25 per cent have tension-type headaches weekly while only 2–3 per cent of the population has chronic tension-type headaches (Lyngberg *et al.* 2005a). The 1-year prevalence appears to be increasing, though the factors leading to this increase are not entirely clear. About half of people with tension-type headaches improve within a decade (Lyngberg *et al.* 2005b).

Cluster headaches are the least common of the idiopathic headache disorders. In Germany, the 1-year prevalence of cluster headache was 0.119 per cent (Katsarava *et al.* 2007). However, an Italian survey found a higher rate of cluster headache of 0.279 per cent overall, 0.227 per cent in women and 0.338 per cent in men (Torelli *et al.* 2005). In San Marino, a point prevalence rate of 0.056 per cent was found in 1999. A previous survey in 1985 found a rate of 0.069 per cent indicating the rates remained approximately stable over the time interval (Tonon *et al.* 2002).

Familial and genetic risks

The influence of genetic constitution on the occurrence of migraine has been investigated principally by studies of familial aggregation and by twin studies. While these classic methods provide general clues concerning whether a genetic component to the disease may exist, their lens is generally not of sufficient resolution to identify specific genes or linked markers. Progress in molecular genetics is providing remarkable discoveries for many diseases. Preliminary reports of rare mutations in the mitochondrial genome and associations with polymorphic forms of serotonergic and dopaminergic genes and migraine are as yet unsubstantiated, but may be more carefully evaluated and tested in the future.

Two recent twin studies based in the Danish Twin Registry (Gervil et al. 1999; Ulrich et al. 1999) compared concordance rates of migraine without aura and migraine with aura, respectively. Twin pairs with one member affected by a specific type of migraine were selected from the registry. Both monozygotic (MZ) and dizygotic (DZ) twins (same sex) were selected for study and the occurrence of migraine was determined by interview and/or examination. The overall lifetime prevalence of migraine with aura for MZ and DZ twins was 7 per cent, similar to population surveys. The concordance in MZ twins was 34 per cent compared to 12 per cent for DZ twins. For migraine without aura the pairwise concordance for MZ twins was 28 per cent, compared with 18 per cent for DZ. This indicates a potential genetic contribution to migraine. But, because there is substantially less than 100 per cent concordance among MZ twins the modifying influence of environmental factors may also be important in migraine aetiology. Ziegler et al. (1998) studied MZ and DZ, female twin pairs, raised together ($n = 154$) and apart ($n = 43$). This classical twin study design showed that concordance was higher for MZ than DZ twins whether raised together or raised apart. Zeigler et al. concluded that about 50 per cent of the variance was explained by genetic factors and the remaining half was due to 'nonshared environmental factors', and measurement error. This conclusion was confirmed in a recent update to this study (Russell et al. 2007).

Stewart et al. (2006) examined familial aggregation in first degree relatives of migraine probands and first-degree relatives of unaffected control subjects. The relative risk (RR) of migraine in first degree relatives of migraineurs was 1.88 (95 per cent confidence interval [CI] 1.30–2.72] compared to relatives of a control group. The relative risk was higher in relatives of those whose headaches began before 16 years of age (RR = 2.50; 95% CI 1.65–3.79) than those whose headaches began later (RR = 1.44; 95% CI 0.93–2.23). The risk in relatives of those with severe headaches had a relative risk of 2.38 (95% CI 1.56–3.62) while relatives of those with less severe pain had a relative risk of 1.52 (0.99–2.34).

Recently, individual genetic alleles have been linked to various types of headache. Though each of these account for only a small proportion of headaches, they serve as important models for understanding the pathogenesis of these disorders. A study by Nyholt et al. (..1998) was based on three large multigenerational families. It shows linkage between headaches and a locus on the X-chromosome (Xq) (Nyholt et al. 1998). Some polymorphisms of the angiotensin-converting enzyme (ACE) and matrix metalloproteinase (MMP) genes may increase the risk of headache, while other polymorphisms decrease the risk (Kara et al. 2007). Polymorphisms of the 5,10-methylenetetrahydrofolate reductase gene have been reported to increase the risk of headaches, migraine with aura, migraine without aura, and tension-type headache (Kara et al. 2003). Alleles of the dopamine b-hydroxylase gene have also been linked to migraine (Lea et al. 2000). It is expected that rapid progress will be made in understanding the genetic underpinnings of this group of diseases and that this will influence future treatment strategies.

Risk factors for headaches

Stress or psychological factors are often cited as contributing to tension-type headaches. However, the frequency of these factors is similar in patients with migraine and tension-type headaches. With chronicity, psychological changes increase in frequency, suggesting that psychological issues are secondary to chronic headaches rather than causative.

Breslau and Davis (1993) and Breslau et al. (1994) conducted a longitudinal study in 1007 young adults to observe the association between migraine and major depression. She reported a significant threefold increased risk of major depression among those with a history of migraine and also a threefold increased risk for migraine among those with prior depression. This finding raised the possibility that the two disorders may have mechanisms in common. Pine et al. (1996) reported a similar longitudinal study that followed 776 persons aged 9–18 (in 1983) for up to 9 years. They reported that in subjects with no history of 'chronic impairing headache', those with major depression at baseline had a tenfold risk of developing such headaches during follow-up. Breslau et al. (2000) conducted another study to clarify the association between severe headache or migraine and depression. In this longitudinal study, persons with severe headache experienced approximately a threefold increased risk of first onset depression but those with major depression at baseline experienced no significantly increased risk of severe headache. However, the previously reported 'bi-directional' association between migraine and depression was replicated. The issues of migraine and depression have recently been reviewed (Frediani & Villani 2007).

In a case–control study, Scher found that chronic daily headaches were more common in women, whites, and those with less education. An improvement in headache frequency after 1 year was more common in those with higher education, non-whites, and those who were married (Scher et al. 2003). Migraine is higher in those with lower education and socioeconomic levels, though it is not known whether this is a cause or an effect of the headaches (Hagen et al. 2002a). However, in adolescents with a family history of migraine, the prevalence of migraine is the same in low- vs. high-income groups (OR 0.97, 95% CI 0.81–1.15) suggesting that genetic factors overwhelm environmental risk factors in those genetically susceptible. In contrast, those without a family history of migraine have a lower prevalence of headaches within those from the higher-income group (OR –0.49, 95% CI 0.38–0.63) suggesting a socioeconomic contribution in those who are not genetically predisposed to the disease (Bigal et al. 2007). One of the strongest risk factors for headaches is prior headaches (RR = 4.15), but difficulty sleeping (did not reach significance) and caffeine intake (NS) are also factors (Boardman et al. 2006). Pain in other areas of the body are associated with headache (RR = 1.43, 95% CI 1–2)

Stroke and migraine

Data from the Physicians Health Study (Buring et al. 1995) and from the National Health and Nutrition Examination Survey (Merikangas et al. 1997) support a significantly increased risk of stroke in persons with a history of migraine. Because of the relatively high prevalence of migraine among young women the occurrence of stroke in that population is of some concern. In a World Health Organization case–control study sample, Chang et al. (1999) reported an approximately threefold increased odds ratio for history of migraine in young women with ischaemic stroke as compared to controls. Tietjen (2000) cautions that the relationship between migraine and stroke may be complicated by the contribution of additional risk factors, such as cigarette smoking and oral contraceptives, and possibly by genetic factors as well. In the Stroke Prevention in Young Women study, a case–control investigation of migraine and stroke was undertaken (MacClellan et al. 2007). Women who had migraine with visual aura had a relative risk of having an ischaemic stroke of 1.5 (95% CI 1.1–2), but there was no increased risk in those with migraine without aura. The odds ratio for those with more than 12 headaches per year was 1.7 (95% CI, 1.1–2.8) and 1.3 (95% CI, 0.8–1.9) in those requiring bedrest or absence from work. In the Women's Health Study, those having a history of migraine with aura had a hazard ratio of 1.53 (95% CI 1.02–2.31) for all strokes and 1.71 (95% CI 1.11–2.66) for ischaemic strokes (Kurth et al. 2005). There was no increase in risk for those having migraine without aura. Additional study may be needed to adequately describe the true relationship between migraine and stroke.

Costs and public health impact

The estimated 23 million persons with migraines in the United States may miss 150 million workdays each year with an associated cost of up to US$17 billion (Cady 1999; Hu et al. 1999). Many more persons suffer with decreased effectiveness at work than actually miss work days; this results in additional hidden loss of productivity due to migraine (Schwartz et al. 1997). Estimates of costs are challenging because of differences in the methodology used to determine prevalence and indirect costs of lost wages, decreased productivity while at work with a headache, and related factors. Insufficient data exists to calculate results for tension-type headache in Europe, but an estimate of migraine costs has been performed. This found a range of direct costs over 1 year from €12 in the United Kingdom, to 68 in the Netherlands, using 2004 prices. Indirect costs ranged from €80 in Sweden to €850 in Germany. Indirect costs included lost wages and decreased productivity on days worked with headache. Only migraine was evaluated. Workers lost on average 2.5 workday/patient/year due to HA and had a reduced work efficiency of 65 per cent during 4.1 additional days (Berg & Stovner 2005). New treatments are relatively effective but only a minority of persons consult physicians for their problem or receive the effective medications (Lipton 1998). Early recognition and treatment of migraine may significantly limit societal and personal costs (Cady 1999).

Health-related quality of life is lower in those with migraine, and this is related to the frequency of attacks (Wang et al. 2001). There are many challenges in making cost determinations due to limits on available epidemiological data (Leonardi et al. 2005). However, the best estimate suggests that migraine accounts for 1.4 per cent of all years of healthy life lost worldwide. It is the nineteenth leading cause of years of healthy life lost in men and twelfth in women. This major public health issue deserves continued attention.

Traumatic brain injury

Clinical overview

Traumatic brain injury (TBI) is commonly divided into categories by mechanism of action: Penetrating or closed head injuries. These also may be characterized as resulting from direct contact injuries or from concussive 'acceleration deceleration' types of injuries (Werner & Engelhard 2007). Among penetrating injuries, greater tissue damage is caused by high velocity penetrating objects than by lower velocity ones. Both penetrating and closed injuries may perturb or impair cerebral blood flow (CBF) leading to ischaemia

and altered cerebral metabolism. Impaired CBF resulting from cerebral vasospasm predicts poorer outcome and may occur in approximately 30 per cent of TBI cases (Werner & Engelhard 2007). Brain contusions may lead to both blood vessel and cell membrane injury resulting in vasogenic or cytotoxic edema. Hydrocephalus may develop due to blockage of the routes of normal cerebrospinal fluid flow. Finally, closed head injuries may lead to diffuse axonal injury. Diffuse axonal injury results in balls of axonal material occurring at axon transection sites or sites of altered axonal flow. Therefore, much of the neurological damage due to TBI does not occur at the time of impact but grows with impaired cerebral perfusion and other factors in the hours and days after the injury itself. Treatment or prevention of the insults that are the physiological result of the injury may ultimately decrease morbidity and mortality.

The symptoms of focal head injuries have been thought to be determined by the site of injury. However, Power et al. (2007) have shown that among children aged 6–14 the severity of the injury is a better predictor of neurobehavioural outcome than is location.

For mild head injuries, including skull fracture, concussion, and unspecified intracranial or head injury (Bazarian et al. 2005), the severity of the injury is usually measured by the degree of post-traumatic amnesia. Amnesia lasting less than 5 min is classified as very mild, less than 1 h is mild, 1–24 h is moderate, 1–7 days is severe, more than 7 days is very severe and more than 4 weeks is extremely severe. Mild and severe head injuries are usually classified by the Glasgow Coma Scale: Scores of 13–15 are minor, 9–12 are moderate, 5–8 are severe, and 4 or less are very severe; and by length of coma (Sherer et al. 2007).

Incidence and prevalence

The CDC estimates that 1.57 million persons (95% CI = 1.37–1.77 million) suffered a TBI in 2003 in the United States (538.2 per 100 000 population), approximately 51 000 of those resulted in death (TBI mortality 17.5 per 100 000 population) based on all reported emergency department visits, hospitalizations and deaths. The numbers of TBIs reported during each of the previous 5 years were not statistically significantly different. TBI incidence among children aged 0–4 was the highest of all age groups at 1188.5 per 100 000, while hospitalization and death rates were highest among those aged 65 and older. Falls accounted for 32 per cent of TBIs, motor vehicle traffic for 19 per cent, struck by/against events 18 per cent and assaults 10 per cent. Men experienced about 1.5 times greater rate of TBI than women (Rutland-Brown et al. 2006). Cassidy et al. (2004) compiled a review of more than 160 published studies to estimate the occurrence of mild TBI. They found that approximately 70–90 per cent of all treated TBIs are likely to be mild and which results in an expected rate for treated mild TBI of 100–300 per 100 000 population. Because most mild TBIs are not hospitalized however, Cassidy et al. further estimate that overall population rate for mild TBI might approach 600 per 100 000 population. This may have implications for the occurrence of post traumatic epilepsy also, as a related neurological public health problem.

Incidence of TBI in Europe was the subject of a recent review (Tagliaferri et al. 2006); the authors compared 23 European studies and noted that the incidence varied from about 546 per 100 000 to about 91 per 100 000. Reasons for the reported wide variation in incidence were thought to depend at least in part on case definition, inclusion criteria and methodological differences between the studies. Generally speaking, most of the incidence rates ranged between 150/100 000 and 300/100 000 with a mean value of 243/100 000. The mean incidence changed only modestly if the two most extreme observed rates were excluded from the calculation, to 235/100 000 (Tagliaferri *et al.* 2006). Based on that conservative estimate of hospitalized TBI incidence and a European population of 330 million, then 775 500 new TBI cases would occur each year. If for these cases injury-related morbidity remained active for 10 years then about 7.8 million prevalent TBI cases would be expected in Europe (Tagliaferri *et al.* 2006).

Reports from investigators associated with the CDC have focused on the incidence of TBI hospitalizations (only), based on a 15-State surveillance system (..2006). During 2002, the age-adjusted annual TBI hospitalization incidence rate (also adjusted for false-positives) was 79 per 100 000 population. Age-specific rates varied substantially from 264.4 per 100 000 among those aged 75 years or older to 103.3 among those aged 15–24, the next highest incidence age group. Unintentional falls accounted for 203.9 per 100 000 of the TBI hospitalizations among person aged 75 of more. Motor Vehicle Traffic incidents were also a prominent cause of TBI hospitalization among those aged 75+, but the rate for 15–24-year olds was approximately double that of any other age group. TBI hospitalization associated with assault was nearly six times higher for males than females across all age groups 15–64. Sadly, females aged 0–4 years showed approximately twice the TBI hospitalization rate due to assault as any other female age group. The proportion of in-hospital deaths (13%) and the proportion needing continuing health-care assistance after discharge (68%) were greatest among those aged 75 years or greater (..2006).

Risk factors

Falls

Falls are either the first or second most common cause of TBI, depending in part of the age group chosen for comparison. The incidence of TBI resulting from falls increases dramatically with advanced age. An analysis of hospitalizations resulting from nonfatal TBI showed that while the all ages incidence of these events was approximately 21 per 100 000 population (in California, 1996–99), age-specific rates ranged from about 13.6 per 100 000 in persons aged less that 65 years, to 41.8 in those aged 65–74, to 104 in those aged 75–84 and then more than doubled to 223 per 100 000 among those aged 85 years or older (..2003). Among the elderly, who suffer TBI as a result of falls co-morbidity with several other conditions is relatively common (Coronado *et al.* 2005). Use of four or more medications may significantly increase of TBI from falling.

Falls are an important cause of TBI among very young also. The 15-State CDC surveillance system allowed calculation of TBI hospitalization rates due to unintentional falls for children aged 0–11 months compared to those aged 12–23 months. Fall-related TBI hospitalizations were 71.5 per 100 000 person-years in the younger group as compared to 36.5 per 100 000 person-years in the older group. Skull fracture with or without intracranial injury predominated in those aged less than 1 year while nonspecific concussion injuries were most common in the older group (Eisele *et al.* 2006). Careful examination of the consistency of reported mechanisms of the injury with the resulting pathology is often necessary to discriminate whether the TBI may have been due to an unintentional falls or inflicted trauma. Among toddlers and older young children. falls from stairs, furniture and playground equipment become more common; however, these are more often associated with hospitalization than with mortality. Among older children, motor vehicle accidents contribute substantially more to TBI than falls do (Keenan & Bratton 2006).

Vehicle accidents

A report constructed by the CDC based on TBI which led to an emergency department visit, hospitalization or death in 2003, showed that overall motor vehicle accidents (19%) were second only to falls (32%) as a cause of TBI based on a total overall estimate of TBI of between 1.37 million and 1.77 million events (Rutland-Brown *et al.* 2006). Injuries resulting from motor vehicle accidents whether occurring to occupants or as pedestrian or cyclist vs. motor vehicle, result in many of the more severe TBIs. Mandatory seatbelt and child seat laws could have an effect on reducing occupant injuries, while bicycle and motorcycle helmet use may reduce the occurrence of TBI in those constituent categories (Rezendes 2006). In the United States, between 1975 and 2004, states which have repealed motorcycle helmet laws have shown a 12 per cent increase in motorcycle fatalities while those that have instituted such laws have experienced an 11 per cent reduction in motorcycle fatalities (Houston & Richardson 2007). Elderly individuals generally appear to be at higher risk of poor outcome or more severe TBI resulting from motor vehicle traffic (Thompson *et al.* 2006).

Violence

Assaults are estimated to have accounted for approximately 10 per cent of the TBIs occurring in the United States in 2003 or roughly 160 000 TBIs (Rutland-Brown *et al.* 2006). As much as 20 per cent of TBI may be the result of violence, roughly half of these are due to firearms. The age group at highest risk is 15–24 years. While males appear to be more likely to sustain an injury due to violence, women may be more likely to die as a result. Generally, community violence indicates an increased opportunity that TBI will be involved. Durkin *et al.* (1996) describes the incidence of paediatric severe nonfatal assault in North Manhattan (NYC) as approximately 60 per 100 000 (about 30 per 100 000 due to firearms). Among adolescents, firearms were the most common method of serious assault and carried more than a tenfold increased fatality risk. A similar study of general trauma was conducted in Los Angeles County (Demetriades *et al.* 1998). In that study, homicides accounted for 45 per cent of traumatic deaths compared to 32 per cent resulting from traffic accidents. The incidence of firearm-related injury or death was 42 per 100 000. The homicide rate varied dramatically by age and ethnic group. Overall it was about 14 per 100 000, but rose to 73 per 100 000 in African-American males and further to 164.2 per 100 000 among 15–34-year-old African American males. While this study speaks to trauma and homicide generally, Lam and MacKersie (1999) states that among children admitted to hospitals 75 per cent are admitted because of trauma and as many as 70 per cent of paediatric trauma deaths are due to head injury. Also, firearms may be involved in a substantial proportion of TBI, hence, the relevance of these statistics.

Abuse and domestic violence are important causes of TBI among women and among children (Monahan & O'Leary 1999). Monahan estimates that about 35 per cent of the 2–3 million women battered each year by their domestic partner sustain TBI as a result. The sequellae of these injuries may be difficult to document because they may include behavioural and cognitive deficits as well as the acute physical problems. Abusive head trauma may also be an under-recognized problem among very young children. Keenan *et al.* (2003) found that physical abuse may be the most frequent cause of TBI in children aged less than 2 years with an estimated incidence rate of approximately 17 per 100 000 person-years; infants had a higher incidence that older children and boys were at somewhat greater risk than girls. Children born to younger mothers or who were part of multiple births also showed greater risk (Keenan *et al.* 2003). So-called 'shaken baby syndrome' and other forms of physical abuse may result in TBI as well as in spinal cord injury.

Sports injuries account for a relatively small proportion of serious TBI. Between 2001 and 2005, approximately 208 000 emergency department visits each year in the United States were the result of sports and recreational activities (..2007b). The majority of these injuries occurred among children aged 10–14 years, closely followed by those aged 15–19 years. Hospital admission resulted in approximately 10 per cent of these incidents. Among the more frequent causes were riding horses, bicycles or motorized bikes, and all terrain vehicles along with ice skating and sledding (..2007b). However, many mild head injuries may go unreported, and it is unclear what the long-term risk of such injuries may be.

A comprehensive review of mild TBI was accomplished by Holm *et al.* (2005) for the World Health Organization Task Force on Mild TBI. Mild TBI resulting from most sports injuries resolve relatively spontaneously with 'no objective evidence' of cognitive deficits remaining longer that several months. However, Holm *et al.* (2005) caution that better designed and more objective studies are needed to adequately characterize the outcomes.

War and sociopolitically directed violence

By the end of 2007, over a million US and UK men and women have served in the wars in Iraq and Afghanistan, resulting in thousands of deaths and tens of thousands of severe injuries. The local populations of those countries have suffered perhaps several orders of magnitude greater numbers of casualties. Similarly, around the world, there are almost daily, similar situations involving sociopolitical violence which may also affect large numbers. Injuries related to explosive blasts may account for many or most of these (Warden 2006) and lasting results of these types of injuries could have important individual and public health consequences for many years to come. Not only do blasts account for much of the observable and immediate injuries, but they may also lead to more mild or unreported TBI that can be coupled with post-traumatic stress disorder (PTSD) (Okie 2005). In addition, manifestation of sequellae may be dependent upon the age at which the injury occurred, with younger people tending to develop psychotic symptoms, middle aged developing anxiety and depression and older individuals developing cognitive deficits (Keltner & Cooke 2007). It is not clear whether the younger and middle-aged persons who may have experienced TBI or blast-related TBI will ultimately be at higher risk for dementia and developing cognitive impairment as they enter ages 60–80, for example, but it would be consistent with head trauma as a risk factor for dementia (Mehta *et al.* 1999). Of course, there is also the potential for developing epilepsy as a result of TBI possibly due to blast, though it may be more commonly due to other mechanisms.

Implications for public health

Both mild and severe TBI impact the public health. Severe TBI may frequently result in death or long-term disability. The potential years of productive life lost, due to TBI varies with its cause, and causes are differentially age-related. Personal costs experienced by victims of TBI have no monetary cost estimate; lost opportunities for education and employment, changed or foregone personal relationships, psychological distress may all result from TBI (Colantonio *et al.* 1998). Further, the risk of seizures following TBI is increased up to seventeen-fold in patients with severe injuries (Annegers *et al.* 1998). While injuries related to motor vehicles and falls are the most common, those who are most severely affected, have the poorest outcomes and require the most continuing care, tend to be the very young and the elderly. Sports injuries despite their public visibility, especially when severe, and because of their occurrence in active and otherwise healthy individuals, tend to be mild, resolving and carry few sequellae. Sociopolitically related TBIs could be source of unexpected public health burden in the future with the potential long-term development of PTSD, psychiatric symptoms, cognitive deficits and degenerative dementias or other neurological disorders. While the actual short-term case fatality rate for TBI may be high, that in itself does not describe the major cost.

Epilepsy

Clinical overview

The International League Against Epilepsy (ILAE) classification system for epilepsy, proposed in 1985 and revised in 1989 (Table 9.10.2), is currently the most commonly used classification for epileptic syndromes (..1989). Syndromes may be classified according to the characteristics of the individual seizures. They are divided into location-related seizures (formerly named partial or local seizures) that begin in a localized part of the brain, and generalized epilepsies that begin diffusely in the brain. The areas of brain initially involved determine the symptoms of location-related seizures. Location-related seizures may (simple partial) or may not (complex partial seizures) be associated with altered consciousness. They may secondarily generalize after a focal onset.

Generalized seizures are those that begin in widespread areas of the brain. The most common type of generalized seizure is noted for muscle stiffening followed by jerking (tonic–clonic). Generalized seizures were formerly called *grand mal* seizures. Absence seizures (formerly *petit mal*) consist of brief episodes of staring and lack of responsiveness. Myoclonic seizures involve brief jerks of muscles rather than repetitive clonic movements. Tonic seizures involve a generalized muscle stiffening. Atonic seizures involve sudden loss of muscle tone.

9.10.2 The international league against epilepsy classification of epileptic seizures

I. Partial (focal, local) seizures
A. Simple partial seizures
B. Complex partial seizure (with impairment of consciousness)
C. With impairment of consciousness at onset
D. Partial seizures evolving to secondarily generalized seizures
II. Generalized seizures
A. Absence seizures
B. Myoclonic seizures
C. Clonic seizures
D. Tonic seizures
E. Tonic–clonic seizures
F. Atonic seizures
III. Unclassified epileptic seizures

Recently, a diagnostic scheme has been proposed that emphasizes different ways (or axes) of classifying seizure and epileptic syndromes. Axis 1 describes the ictal semiology, axis 2 the seizure type, axis 3 the syndromic diagnosis, axis 4 the aetiology, and axis 5 the degree of impairment (Engel 2001). The terminology in this scheme has changed to focal seizures and generalized seizures.

Incidence and prevalence

Aspects of epilepsy epidemiology have been reviewed by a number of contemporary authors (e.g. Jallon & Latour 2005). Epidemiological studies of epilepsy are challenged by the difficulty in making a correct diagnosis and the sophisticated technology required for proper diagnosis and classification. For example, Uldall et al. studied all cases of paediatric epilepsy admitted to a tertiary centre in Denmark (Uldall et al. 2006). Of 223 children admitted, 87 (39%) did not have epilepsy on sophisticated EEG monitoring. Of the 184 cases in which there was no doubt expressed about the diagnosis of epilepsy on admission, 30 per cent were found to not have epilepsy. There is also difficulty with standardizing case ascertainment. For example, a recent study found a mean prevalence of 8.2/1000 for active epilepsy defined as those having a seizure within the past 5 years or on antiepileptic drugs (Svendsen et al. 2007). This rate fell to 5.3/1000 if the definition was changed to having a seizure within the past 5 years regardless of medication status. Nevertheless, the incidence of epilepsy has been estimated to be 46/100 000/year (range 32–71) (Hirtz et al. 2007). This rises to 57/100 000/year in children (range 41–65 per 100 000). The prevalence is estimated to be 7.1/1000 (range 4–8.9). Below, we present several studies that focus on the incidence and prevalence of epilepsy.

Hauser et al. (1996) reported the age-adjusted incidence of epilepsy as 44 per 100 000 person-years, based on data from the Rochester Epidemiology Project spanning approximately a 50-year period up to 1980. Reassessment in that same population in 1980–84 yielded a consistent though slightly higher estimate of epilepsy incidence (Zarrelli et al. 1999). Importantly, Hauser noted that the incidence and prevalence of epilepsy and unprovoked seizures decreased with calendar time among children and increased among the elderly. The prevalence of active epilepsy among those aged 75 or older was reported as 1.5 per cent (as of January 1980). About 1 per cent of persons under age 20 experienced epilepsy (Hauser 1995), and their prognosis was generally favourable with most achieving control within 2 years. Kramer et al. (1998) reported the distribution of different seizure types, among 440 children with two or more unprovoked seizures, attending the paediatric neurology clinic in Tel Aviv. Partial seizures accounted for 52 per cent and primary generalized seizures 33 per cent. This is in general agreement with a prospective German study where an annual incidence of 60.3/100 000 was seen in children aged 1 month to 15 years (Freitag et al. 2001). Focal (partial) seizures accounted for 58 per cent of these.

Olafsson and Hauser (1999) conducted a survey in rural Iceland, determining the prevalence of recurrent unprovoked seizures. Records of primary care physicians and neurologists were used for case identification. The crude age adjusted prevalence was 4.8 per 1000 population. The British national child development study followed all 17 733 children who were born during a single week in 1958 in England, Scotland, and Wales (Kurtz et al. 1998). A screening survey asking about symptoms consistent with seizures was supplemented by medical records. The cumulative incidence by age 23 was 8.4/1000 (95% CI 6.8–10). The prevalence of 'active' epilepsy, defined as having a seizure within the past 2 years or currently taking anticonvulsant medications, at age 23 was 6.3/1000 (95% CI 4.9–7.7). Christensen et al. studied cases through the Danish Civil Registration System (Christensen et al. 2007). This system identifies patients who were inpatients or outpatients in Danish hospitals, but not those in private practitioner's offices. The diagnosis was determined by the International Classification of Disease (ICD-10) coding, which depended on the diagnosis of the admitting physician. In recent years, this study found an incidence of epilepsy of 83.3/100 000/year.

Another method of case ascertainment was used by Nicoletti et al. (1998, 1999) to study epilepsy and other neurologic conditions in Bolivia. For this study a 'door-to-door survey' was conducted; 10 000 persons were screened, approximately 1000 were referred to neurologists and of those 112 were determined to have active epilepsy, leading to a prevalence estimate of 11.1 per 1000. In contrast to studies reported above (Hauser et al. 1996), the highest prevalence occurred in the 15–24-year age group (20.4 per 1000). Regardless of the shift in peak occurrence the prevalence appears dramatically higher than in other studies. A telephone survey of random households was conducted in a minority community of New York City (Kelvin et al. 2007). The age-adjusted prevalence of active epilepsy was 5/1000. Differences in racial groups were noted with rates of 5.2 in Blacks, 5.9 in Whites and 6.3 in Hispanics. These rates contrast with those found in other regions. In Southern Italy a survey of physician's records found a point prevalence rate of 3.13 (95% CI 2.2–4.2) (Gallitto et al. 2005). These researchers speculated that the low rate may, in part, be due to a cultural prejudice regarding epilepsy. Differences in study methodology, survey methods, case definition, the availability of sophisticated medical technology in a community, and cultural differences make epilepsy studies particularly challenging.

Mortality

Persons with epilepsy may experience two to three times the risk of death as their unaffected counterparts, Sperling et al. (1999) examined the relationship between recurrent seizure and risk of death; they compared persons whose seizures had been eliminated by surgery to those with recurrent seizures. The standardized mortality ratio (SMR) for persons with recurrent seizure was approximately fourfold higher than expected. A longitudinal study conducted in the Netherlands (Shackleton et al. 1999) enrolled newly diagnosed epilepsy patients (n=1355) who were followed a mean of 28 years. Overall they observed a threefold excess in all cause mortality, and a sevenfold increase among those under age 20. Loiseau et al. (1999) studied short-term mortality after first afebrile, provoked, or unprovoked seizure (n=804). After 1 year of follow-up, no deaths had occurred among patients with idiopathic seizures. Increased SMRs were observed for those with provoked seizures or seizures related to other CNS disorders. Some of the risk of death in epilepsy reflects underlying diseases like brain neoplasms and cerebrovascular disease. However, there is also an increased mortality compared to the non-epileptic population due to accidents (often drowning and burns) and suicide (Lhatoo & Sander 2005).

Sudden unexplained death in persons with epilepsy (SUDEP) (Annegers & Coan 1999) is a substantial risk in younger aged persons as compared to people without epilepsy. Much of the excess risk may be associated with seizure severity with greater severity leading to greater risk of death (Annegers & Coan 1999). Careful definition of SUDEP is necessary as is attention to methodologic detail; early findings may have been the result of selection bias and similar problems,. The incidence of SUDEP varies between 0.9 and 1.5/1000 person-years for people with epilepsy (Tomson et al. 2005) In a population-based study in Rochester, Minnesota, all persons diagnosed with epilepsy between 1935 and 1994 were followed to determine cause of death. SUDEP rates were compared to the rate of sudden unexplained death in the general population for ages 20–40. Although the SUDEP death rate exceeded the expected by 23.7 times, it was still a rare cause of death accounting for only 1.7 per cent of the deaths in the epilepsy cohort. Nilsson et al. (1999) investigated SUDEP in Sweden focusing on risk factors. They found that patients with 50 seizures per year were about 10 times more likely to succumb to SUDEP than patients with 2 or fewer seizures. Risk of SUDEP was also substantially increased with the number of concomitant antiepileptic drugs, and among those who had frequent medication changes. Compared to the general population the cohort of epilepsy patients experienced an all-cause mortality approximately 3.6 times greater than the general population with the majority of the excess mortality due to malignant neoplasms; diseases of the circulatory, respiratory, and digestive systems; injury; and poisoning (Nilsson et al. 1997). Though seizure severity has been linked to SUDEP, other factors are also associated with it including prone positioning, respiratory factors, and cardiac factors (Nashef et al. 2007). Genetic risks including mutations in ion channel genes have been postulated as risk factors, but to date clear links with SUDEP have not been made (Nashef et al. 2007). Tomson et al. provides a current review (Tomson et al. 2005).

Infectious causes of epilepsy

In developing countries, infections are a much more important cause of epilepsy than in the United States and Europe (Senanayake & Roman 1993), and the overall prevalence of epilepsy may approach 57 per 1000 population. Parasitic, bacterial, and viral infections contribute substantially to the prevalence, but hereditary factors, perinatal damage, head trauma, and toxic exposures also play important aetiologic roles. From a public health view, the excess risk attributable to many of these exposures is potentially preventable (Senanayake & Roman 1993).

An example of an important infectious risk factor is *Taenia solium* cysticercosis (from pork tapeworm) which can lead to neurocysticercosis. Palacio et al. (1998) examined a series of 643 epilepsy patients in Columbia, of those 376 had serologic tests for cysticercosis. The prevalence of antibody was 17.5 per cent among late onset epilepsy patients. Among patients with no CT-scan evidence of neurocysticercosis only 2.7 per cent had antibody. However, a similar study conducted in Honduras (Sanchez et al. 1999) raises questions as to the validity of the serology antibody tests in predicting neurocysticercosis. Sanchez et al. conclude CT-scan findings of neurocycticercosis are necessary for diagnosis. Even though *T. solium* is a frequent exposure in the population as indicated by serology, neurocystericosis is not always the result. A different view is presented by Bern et al. (1999). They combined data from 12 population-based community studies in Peru and showed a seroprevalence of 6–24 per cent. The high seroprevalence was presented as evidence for the prevalence of neurocysticercosis.

Bern et al. estimated a burden of 23000 to 39000 symptomatic neurocysticercosis cases in Peru. Extrapolating from these data, Bern et al. concluded that cysticercosis is a formidable cause of neurologic disease in Latin America. Whether seropositivity is synonymous with neurocysticercosis appears controversial. The common occurrence of the *T. solium* cyst may account for an important fraction of epilepsy in Latin American countries. Though serological testing may not firmly establish the role of *T. solium* in epilepsy, it is believed to be an important cause of epilepsy, particularly in developing countries.

Genetics

Rapid progress is being made in determining the genetic contributions to epileptic disorders. Several authors have recently reviewed this field (Crino 2007). A number of types of epilepsy have now been explained as genetic disorders. However, these are rare forms of epilepsy and the genetic contribution to the majority of cases remains unexplained. There is some degree of consensus, however, that idiopathic generalized epilepsies are likely to have a genetic aetiology (Steinlein 1999). First-degree relatives of people with epilepsy have a two- to fourfold increase in epilepsy risk (Annegers et al. 1982). However, the absence of clear genetic contributions to many forms of epilepsy, and the presence of differing phenotypes resulting from a given genotype emphasizes the importance of environmental factors in epilepsy. Most of the study of genetics in epilepsy has been directed towards primary generalized epilepsies. This reflects the belief that primary generalized epilepsy is often due to some 'brainwide' disorder that would be more likely due to a genetic disorder. Localized seizures more often reflect focal brain disease that is less likely to be due to a genetic mutation. However, it should be kept in mind that in some cases genes may have focal influences on the brain (Dobyns et al. 1999). A number of epilepsies have now been shown to be due to channelopathies, mutations in ion channels (Avanzini et al. 2007). It is expected that additional genes will soon be identified that cause epilepsy, or that influence environmental epileptic factors.

Costs and public health burden

The costs of epilepsy are often categorized as direct and indirect (Begley et al. 2000). The direct costs refer to those specifically involved with epilepsy treatment; the indirect costs include lost work days and unrealized earnings. Begley et al. (2000) estimates that 181000 new cases of epilepsy in the United States in 1995 will result in a lifetime cost of US$11.1 billion. The 2.3 million prevalent cases, in 1995, resulted in an annual cost of US$12.5 billion. Indirect costs may account for 85 per cent of the total, and the largest share of direct costs is attributable to patients with intractable epilepsy (Begley et al. 2000). Annegers et al. cautions that cost figures may derive from different methodologies between United States and Europe, which may influence the degree of comparability (Annegers et al. 1999). With regard to the quality of life reported by persons with epilepsy, Leidy et al. (1999) report that seizure frequency is inversely associated with health-related quality of life. Seizure-free individuals report a quality of life similar to the general population; however more seizures lead to a poorer quality of life, regardless of additional comorbidity, and irrespective of gender. Effective seizure control appears to be important in reducing costs as well as increasing patient quality of life.

Dementia

Clinical overview

Dementia presents with a progressive loss of a person's usual and customary cognitive function from any of several domains. This often begins with memory problems in AD but could also begin with language deficits or disinhibition in frontotemporal lobar degeneration, or with deficits in executive function in vascular cognitive impairment, or with sleep disorders or hallucinations in Lewy body disease, additional symptoms may initially predominate where other dementias may be the underlying cause. Regardless of the beginning domain, initial cognitive impairment associated with dementia tends to progress and affect other cognitive domains with time. Behavioural changes may be prominent, including agitation, wandering, personality change or depression, as well as sleep disturbances and psychiatric symptoms. In late stages of dementia, patients frequently become completely dependent on others. Various definitions of dementia have been used in past research studies, but the Diagnostic and Statistical Manual, Edition IV (DSM-IV) is one of the most commonly used now (APA & AMA Task Force on DSM-IV 1994). The DSM-IV criteria for dementia require memory impairment and one or more additional cognitive disturbance, because of the memory predominance, it is often criticized as being too specific for AD, despite the other domains involved. These other domains involve aphasia (language disturbance), apraxia (impaired ability to carry out motor activities despite intact motor function), agnosia (failure to recognize or identify objects despite intact sensory function) and disturbances in executive functioning (i.e. planning, organizing, sequencing, abstracting). The cognitive deficits must be severe enough to cause significant impairment in social or occupational functioning and represent a significant decline from a previously attained level of functioning. The DSM criteria were originally constructed to provide for mutually exclusive diagnostic subgroups, but that schema is becoming more problematic as the research community now understands that more than one underlying dementia causes may coexist and the location of the specific pathologies in the brain may determine the clinical picture expressed. Furthermore, the clinical diagnosis of AD was originally conceptualized within the DSM criteria as a diagnosis of exclusion, however that view now, is becoming rapidly obsolete.

Dementia represents the severe decline from a usual or customary degree of cognitive function enjoyed in a person's adult life; it may have many causes including neurodegenerative, vascular, infectious, and traumatic, to name a few. Among the neurodegenerative dementias that predominate with aging are AD, Lewy body disease (dementia with Lewy bodies [DLB] or PD dementia), and frontotemporal lobar degeneration (FTLD) dementias. Cerebrovascular disease may co-exist with and contribute to any of these or may be a primary cause on its own as vascular dementia, still considered to be the second most frequent cause of dementia. Prion disease, and associated spongiform encephalopathies (e.g. Creutzfeldt–Jakob disease [CJD] and variant CJD) are potentially transmissible from ingestion of animal tissue or from contact or transplantation of human tissue. HIV infection and other infections causing encephalitis may affect wider age groups and specific populations or exposure groups. Though AD, vascular dementia, Lewy body disease, and FTLD are likely to be the most common and well known, there are many other disorders and insults which can result in dementia including drug-induced conditions, alcoholism, Huntington's disease, amyotrophic lateral sclerosis, subdural hematoma, brain tumours, hydrocephalus, B_{12} deficiency, multiple medical conditions, hypothyroidism, and neurosyphilis.

Current criteria for the clinical diagnosis of dementia and AD, specifically, are applied relatively consistently by research studies and have been active for some time (American Psychiatric Association and American Psychiatric Association Task Force on DSM-IV). Neuropathological criteria for the diagnosis of AD are currently accepted as those of the NIA-Reagan consensus working group (..1997a). However, possibly because of the increasing understanding that underlying causes or pathologies may co-exist and initial cognitive changes may be noted earlier in the course of disease, the primary AD criteria may soon be considered for revision (Morris 2006). Accurate identification of preclinical or asymptomatic disease is thought to provide the best opportunity to intervene with disease modifying therapies—if such effective therapies can be developed.

Mild cognitive impairment

Determination of when a particular disease is clinically evident and diagnosable is of great interest to epidemiologists as well as to those involved with clinical medicine. Certainly the principles of early detection and potential early treatment lead us to expect a better prognosis, in most conditions, if there are effective treatments. The usually gradual and insidious nature of symptom onset for AD and some other dementias, and the current practical absence of adequate asymptomatic disease pathology detection (by biologic test or neuroimaging) has forced investigators to attempt to characterize the earliest clinical features of cognitive impairment, in order to approach an earlier diagnostic threshold. For epidemiologists searching for risk factor associations this earlier threshold is somewhat of a double edged sword. If diagnosis cannot be made with certainty at the earlier point: (a) diagnostic misclassification may distort risk factor associations, (b) earlier detection may allow better determination of the critical exposure period, prior to pathological onset, when the putative risk factor could have had an initiating or promoting effect. Thus, mild cognitive impairment is often characterized as a segment of the overall, underlying disease development trajectory by some, or as a diagnostic entity representing the transitional phase from cognitively normal to demented by others.

Efforts to observe and characterize the spectrum of observable cognitive decline from mild to severe cases of dementia have been with us at least since more intense studies of the dementias developed in the late 1970s and 1980s. Those efforts began to focus on and more carefully describe the early clinical presentation of dementia in the late 1980s and 1990s, for example, Bowen et al. (1997). While mild impairment was well recognized, it carried many names and definitions: Age associated memory impairment, age associated cognitive decline, cognitive impairment no dementia, benign senescent forgetfulness, questionable dementia. The concept of Mild Cognitive Impairment (MCI) emerged from careful consideration of much of this prior information but also included additional intellectual structure and definition (Petersen et al. 1999). The original criteria for MCI included: (1) memory complaint, preferably qualified by an informant; (2) memory

Table 9.10.3 Causes of dementia

Idiopathic	**Systemic disease**
Alzheimer's disease	Cardiac
Frontotemporal lobar degeneration (tauopathies and	Pulmonary
non-tau ubiquitin positive)	Renal
Lewy body disease	Renal failure
Amyotrophic lateral sclerosis	Dialysis dementia
Focal CNS pathology	Hepatic
Vascular dementia	Hepatic failure
Binswanger's disease	Hepatocerebral degeneration
Multiple sclerosis	Wilson's disease
Mass lesions	**Endocrine**
Tumours, multiple sites	Hyper/hypo thyroid
Tumours, single site	Hyper/hypo parathyroid
Gliomatosis cerebri	Hyper/hypo adrenalism
Abscess	SIADH
Subdural malformation	Rheumatologic
Hydrocephalus	Vasculitis (including SLE)
Infections	Giant cell arteritis
AIDS (HIV)	Sarcoid
Chronic meningitis	Amyloid
Encephalitis	Neoplastic
Progressive multifocal leukoencephalopathy	Metastasis
Subacute sclerosing panencephalitis	Carcinomatous meningitis
Syphilis	Paraneoplastic (limbic encephalitis)
Lyme disease	**Associated movement disorder**
Prion disease (kuru, Creutzfeldt–Jacob, vCJD)	Huntington's disease
Toxins	Parkinsonian diseases
Drugs	Parkinson's disease
Alcohol	Progressive supranuclear palsy
Heavy metals	Postencephalitic dementia
Industrial toxins	Post-traumatic (dementia pugilistica)
Domoic acid	Diffuse Lewy body disease
Inherited disease	Multiple-system atrophy
Huntington's disease	Myoclonus
Gerstmann–Straussler syndrome	Creutzfeldt–Jakob disease
Porphyria	Alzheimer's
Propionic aciduria	Metabolic derangement
Adult onset lysosomal storage diseases	Other movement disorder
Hexosaminidase	Hereditary ataxias
Arylsulfatase (MLD)	Hereditary spastic paraplegia
Kuf disease	Kuru
Adrenoleukodystrophy	Wilson's disease
Others	Seizures
Myotonic muscular dystrophy	Kuf disease
Down's syndrome	**Deficiency**
Hereditary ataxias	B$_{12}$ deficiency
Hereditary spastic paraplegias	Thiamine
Cerebrotendinous Xanthomatosis	Niacin (Pellagra)

impairment for age and education; (3) preserved general cognitive function; (4) intact activities of daily living; (5) not demented (Petersen *et al.* 1999). These criteria were later revised to include both memory and non-memory affected groups allowing for 'amnestic' with single and multiple cognitive domains affected and 'non-amnestic' with single or multiple cognitive domains affected (Petersen 2007). The Petersen schema allowed for MCI to represent a variety of aetiologies in addition to AD. On the non-amnestic side, it could easily include vascular cognitive impairment) as well

as cognitive impairment due to frontotemporal lobar degeneration or Lewy body disease. However, the amnestic side of MCI is regarded by many to represent primarily early AD (Morris 2006). Persons diagnosed with MCI also are known to recover and not go on to develop dementia. For example, in the Cardiovascular Health Study approximately 18 per cent of those initially diagnosed with amnestic MCI recovered (Lopez *et al.* 2007).

Since the concept was solidified by Petersen *et al.* (1999), literally thousands of research papers have been generated on the topic and with the effort a good deal of controversy has ensued, as well. In part because some of the controversy was becoming counterproductive to understanding, Winblad *et al.* (2004) hosted an international working group to arrive at a consensus understanding of MCI for the international research community. The resulting comprehensive recommendations allowed for self and informant report of deficits, as well as for more objective testing to be considered. The consensus recommendation also encouraged that the potential underlying cause of the impairment might be specified, if clinical judgment would allow. Age and educational status are also important in the determination of whether current performance represents cognitive decline, but to most carefully evaluate whether decline has taken place there should also be consideration of the intra-individual change. Despite comparison of individual performance with group test norms, for example, one should also evaluate whether the individual's performance represents a change in his/her usual and customary functioning, in order to determine whether cognitive decline has taken place.

Dementia and Alzheimer's disease

Prevalence and incidence

Almost two decades ago, Evans reported prevalence estimates for dementia and AD based on a community study in East Boston (Evans *et al.* 1989). The results of this study seemed controversial because of their magnitude but they placed an heuristic upper bound on estimated prevalence of dementia in United States' communities. Prevalence rose from 3 per cent among those 65–74 years of age to 47 per cent in those over age 85. Over 80 per cent of the observed dementia was classified as AD. Evans later applied the observed rates to census data projecting that 10.3 million persons would have AD in the year 2050. Meta-analyses of prevalence studies worldwide (Fratiglioni *et al.* 1999); and individual prevalence studies seemed to show consistency within geographical regions except for some variation due to methodological differences. Generally, the prevalence proportion was reported to rise from about 0.3–1 per cent in 60–64-year-olds to 43–68 per cent in persons aged 95 or older, or often reported as a summary figure of 6 per cent to 10 per cent among persons aged 65 or older in North America (Hendrie 1998). Based on estimates like these, Brookmeyer *et al.* estimated that if disease onset could be delayed 2 years the future disease burden would be reduced by 2 million cases (Brookmeyer *et al.* 1998).

More recently, Ferri *et al.* (2005) conducted a systematic review of published studies to estimate dementia prevalence in 14 world regions, as designated by the World Health Organization. They assembled a panel of 12 experts to arrive at individual estimates for each region based on the accumulated published studies resulting from the literature search. A 'Delphi' technique was implemented and agreement between experts within region was estimated. The mean prevalence estimates for each of the 14 world regions were then used to project numbers of cases in the future, also taking into account population and mortality changes, but maintaining the agreed upon prevalence estimates, and arriving at an estimated incidence rate through the use of standard software. Given the derived incidence rates, Ferri *et al.* estimated approximately 4.6 million new cases of dementia would occur each year in the world and this would cause the number of prevalent dementia cases to double about every 20 years. However, the increase is not expected to be constant across regions. Developed regions similar to Europe and North

America are expected to increase their number of prevalent cases about 100 per cent by 2040, while Latin America and Africa are expected to increase 235–393 per cent, and India, China, and the South Asia/Western Pacific regions' numbers are expected to increase 314–336 per cent. As a result, the China, South Asia, and Western Pacific regions are projected by 2040 to have three times more prevalent cases of dementia than Western Europe will have and Latin America will have as many persons living with dementia as North America will have (Ferri *et al.* 2005). These projection are for all dementias rather than being limited to a particular subtype such as AD. However, there is increasing evidence that treatable factors associated with cardiovascular disease, such as hypertension or cholesterol level or those related to diabetes may play a role not only in vascular dementia, but also in the aetiology or progression of AD (Kukull 2006). Though there remains some controversy as to the nature of these putative associations, such an association, if causal, could allow existing treatments to potentially reduce the incidence of dementia or delay its onset for some number of years as suggested by Brookmeyer *et al.* (1998) and therefore could reduce the global dementia health care burden substantially. The health care burden of dementia is represented primarily by the prevalence proportion, which is a function of disease incidence and subsequent duration of survival.

In contrast to prevalence, incidence provides a means to estimate the risk of disease and the identification of risk factors (not directly possible with prevalence data alone). Jorm and Jolley (1998) gathered data from 23 studies and produced a meta-analysis of dementia incidence. Incidence was estimated for Europe, the United States, and East Asia; dementia, AD, and vascular dementia rates were computed. Incidence rates for the United States and Europe were quite similar: 'moderate' dementia incidence rose from 3.6 per 1000 person-years (65–69 ages) to 37.7 per 1000 person-years (85–89 ages) in Europe and from 2.4 to 27.5 per 1000 person years for the same age groups in the United States. 'Mild' AD incidence was also computed ranging from 2.5 per 1000 person years (65–69 ages) to 46.1 per 1000 person-years, for Europe, compared with 6.1– 74.5 for the United States, and, 0.7– 39.7 for East Asia.

The unique character of the Rochester Epidemiology Project at Mayo Clinic has allowed for the estimation of AD and dementia incidence over an extended period. While this project did not constitute an 'active' cohort study per se, the nature of the health care system and its nearly exclusive use by the surrounding population allowed for the observation and estimation of incident cases of disease through the review of medical records. These data provide some of the few estimates of secular trends for dementia incidence in the United States. Rocca *et al.* (1998) re-analysed dementia and AD incidence data for 1975 through 1984, from the Rochester Epidemiology Project at Mayo Clinic. The results showed dementia incidence overall as 2.2 per 1000 person-years in 65–69-year-olds rising to 40.8 per 1000 person-years in those aged 90 or more. Similarly for AD, rates rose from 1.2 to 33.9 per 1000 person-years. Because of the remarkable consistency of these incidence rates with more recent active cohort studies in Europe and North America one might also have some degree of confidence in Rocca's observation that annual age-specific incidence rates have appeared to stay quite stable with time stable during the 1975–1984 time interval. After disaggregating the data for the oldest old Rocca also reported that rates appeared to continue to rise with age after age 84; they also noted that rates were similar for men and women. As data continue to accumulate with time, it will be interesting to note if the effects of, for example, anti-hypertensive and lipid-lowering agents may be seen to alter the incidence, or perhaps whether potential gains there might be offset by increases in population obesity or diabetes.

Still one of the better estimates of dementia incidence for Europe comes from the combined analysis of four large, ongoing European cohort studies of dementia and AD as reported by Launer et al. (1999). Cohorts enrolled in Denmark, France, the Netherlands, and the United Kingdom summed to more than 16 000 members age 65 or older at enrolment. After a mean follow-up of 2.2 years (comprising approximately 28 600 person-years), the overall incidence of dementia was 14.6 per 1000 person-years, about two-thirds of these cases were due to AD. Incidence of dementia was 2.5 per 1000 person-years at age 65–69 an rose to 85.6 per 1000 person-years in those age 90 and older. Similarly AD rose from 1.2 per 1000 person-years to 63.5 per 1000 person-years across the same age groups. Launer's report was one of the first to include combined data from large cohort studies in Europe. Over the last 5 years more cohort studies begun to report incidence figures which are consistent, generally, with the estimates above. Among the more recent well-designed cohort studies that have reported comparable incidence rates within various population groups are Kukull et al. 2002, Lopez et al. 2007, Newman et al. 2005, Tyas et al. 2006, Brayne 2006, and Ganguli et al. 2000. The long-standing Framingham Study, the population-based approaches of the Mayo Clinic, studies of specific religious groups and orders, and other population-based cohorts are also of tremendous importance, in addition to those mentioned earlier.

While the tendency has been to attempt to count primary cause or pathologically 'pure' cases of dementia subtypes those single aetiology cases may be less frequent than previously suspected. In studies conducted in communities, dementia aetiologies (e.g. AD, vascular, Lewy body, tauopathy) appear to comingle frequently in community dwelling cases (Schneider et al. 2007). This co-mingling is consistent with the view that features of AD, Lewy body disease and frontotemporal lobar degeneration may exist as a multiple amyloidoses resulting from aggregation of amyloid-beta (neuritic plaques), tau (neurofibrillary tangles), alpha-synuclein (Lewy bodies) and other proteins (Morimoto 2006; Trojanowski & Mattson 2003; Trojanowski & Lee 2002; Lippa et al. 2007).

Because identification of late stage dementia and AD holds little hope for curative or restorative treatment applications or for identification of consistent risk factors, interest has begun to focus on early identification of disease through mild cognitive impairment or simply early identification of the aetiologic cause of decline prior to the criteria-based diagnosis of dementia, as discussed in detail above. Early forms of pre-AD or dementia are difficult to distinguish from relatively benign, cognitive decline associated with aging. Distinguishing between normal persons, those with mild cognitive impairment and those asymptomatic persons with incipient, occult dementia-related pathology, now possible to some degree with newly developed neuroimaging techniques, may provide important clues about pathological onset of disease as well as inform the study of risk factors and critical periods of exposure prior to disease onset (Rowe et al. 2007).

Risk (and protective) factors for AD

Until the mid-1990s, most analytic observational epidemiologic studies of AD were based on a case–control design. In this design,

cases of disease were identified and their exposure histories were compared to those of persons without the disease. The design itself is well accepted as a method of study. However, in the study of AD (and other dementias), problems with case ascertainment, case selection, and misclassification of disease and exposure may have caused at least some results to be biased or spurious. Now, as cohort studies of AD and dementia are beginning to emerge, findings which were viewed as consistent in case–control studies are being questioned or refuted. One example of incompatible conclusions concerns the observation of a potential protective effect for AD associated with cigarette smoking. A meta-analysis of smoking–AD studies showed a consistent decreased risk associated with smoking (Lee 1994). The majority of these studies were of the case–control design. When case–control studies rely on cross-sectional samples to obtain cases, they are most likely to encounter those cases with the longest survival after diagnosis (Rothman & Greenland 1998). Also, when decreased post diagnosis survival among cases is associated with the exposure of interest (e.g. smoking) a potential spurious excess of exposure among controls may be observed. Cohort studies, where this selection bias is eliminated (essentially) now report either 'no association' or a potential *increased* risk of AD associated with smoking. A recent and comprehensive meta-analysis of prospective studies investigating smoking as a risk factor for dementia and AD involving more than 26 000 persons followed for 2–30 years showed a significantly increased risk of AD in smokers as compared to non-smokers, relative risk = 1.79 (95% CI 1.43–2.23) (Anstey et al. 2007).

Head trauma has also been shown to be a relatively consistent risk factor for AD, primarily based on case–control studies. Here, selective recall or recall bias may be more important than the effect of survival, even though risk of death and/or continued cognitive impairment immediately resulting from the injury is substantial (..1998). Several longitudinal studies now show negligible risk of AD associated with head injury (Nee & Lippa 1999) though others still find some potentially increased risk sometimes modified by other factors (e.g. Schofield et al. 1997). Many studies of head trauma focus on injuries severe enough to cause loss of consciousness. There is little rigorous analytic investigation of mild traumatic brain injury as a potential risk factor. TBI due to blast injuries, suffered in war, provide an important cohort in which to study the future incidence of dementia and AD.

Higher educational level has been proposed as influencing decreased risk of AD, but the relationship between education and AD may be quite complex (e.g. Koepsell et al. 2007). Educational level influences subject's likelihood of participation in epidemiologic studies, and may do so differentially between cases and controls. Educational level influences the diagnostic process, at least in the early stages of disease, because of the individual's ability to respond correctly in testing situations. Education may influence health care usage and may result in greater income or higher occupational level. The idea that higher education confers greater 'cognitive reserve' to be accessed when disease strikes is tantalizing, though biologically unsubstantiated. Koepsell et al. in a clinico-pathologic study found that there was 'no evidence of larger education-related differences in cognitive function when AD neuropathology was more advanced', and concluded further that 'higher Mini-Mental State Examination scores among more educated persons with mild or no AD may reflect better test-taking skills or cognitive reserve, but these advantages may ultimately be overwhelmed by

AD neuropathology' (Koepsell *et al.* 2007). Quality of early life environment, as measured by number of siblings, area of residence was associated with developing AD in late life, but educational level was not significantly associated with risk of AD (Moceri *et al.* 2000).

Anti-inflammatory medications have been studied for their potential protective effect on AD. Even though the quality of the studies has varied with respect to determination of exposure, the results appear to have been quite consistent in showing significant associations, which if causal could be interpreted as protective (e.g. Hayden *et al.* 2007). Because of this evidence and the potential biological plausibility related to the role of inflammation in the aetiology of AD, a randomized placebo controlled prevention trial was launched, known as the AD anti-inflammatory prevention trial (ADAPT), enrolment began in 2001. The trial planned to enrolled 2625 subjects, aged 70 years or older, who had a family history of dementia and randomized them to placebo, celecoxib, or naproxsyn sodium treatment arms. The plan was to follow the enrollees for approximately 7 years; however, the trial was stopped in December 2004 because of concerns that adverse cardiovascular events which were related to use of similar anti-inflammatory drugs might also apply to the trial treatments. A preliminary analysis based on the small amount of accumulated data available following trial closure showed no significant effect of either celecoxib or naproxsyn as compared to placebo for the prevention of AD.

Oestrogen replacement therapy as a protective factor has shown a remarkably similar checkered research results history as anti-inflammatory medications, with the bulk of epidemiologic evidence favouring protection and a fair amount of biological plausibility also marshalled in its support (e.g. Henderson *et al.* 2000). Despite this large accumulation of epidemiologic and laboratory evidence supporting the potential protective effect of oestrogen against the onset of AD, the Women's Health Initiative Memory Study (a randomized controlled trial of oestrogen and oestrogen plus progestin v. placebo) showed a statistically significant increased risk of dementia among those given the active treatments (Shumaker *et al.* 2004). In the case of oestrogen as a potential treatment for AD, results also have shown no indication that oestrogen replacement therapy is an effective treatment for AD (Henderson *et al.* 2000).

Few environmental risk or protective factors for AD have been consistently described. There is much current interest in the potential for factors related to cardiovascular disease and metabolic syndrome (including diabetes) having an influence on AD and other dementias even though the exact mechanisms of interaction may not yet have been shown beyond reasonable doubt, nor have they in most cases yet reached the bar for clear and convincing evidence (Whitmer *et al.* 2007). The rationale for this approach appears to be that it is sound medical practice to treat hypertension, high cholesterol, diabetes and obesity, and if more complete and effective treatment can be accomplished it may also, secondarily, serve to reduce the occurrence of dementia.

Elevated homocysteine levels, also associated with cardiovascular disease, have been reported to increase risk of AD (Haan *et al.* 2007). Whether hyperhomocysteinemia may be related to mutations in the methylenetetrahydrofolate reductase gene or to dietary intake or to other factors is unclear. However, homocysteine levels can reportedly be modified with vitamin B_{12} and folate intake, so there may be a potentially safe, intervention to evaluate in that regard, though it seems unlikely a formal prevention trial would be mounted unless the strength and specificity of the effect might be better described along with the potential attributable fraction.

AD is likely to be heterogeneous both diagnostically and aetiologically. What results in the AD phenotype may be the sum or product of aging, environmental factors, genetic constitution, and sociodemographic experiences. Aside from the observable effect of aging dramatically increasing the risk of dementia and AD, success in finding environmental risk factors has been limited and potentially related to design and selection factors. At this point disease modifying therapies and drug targets are being developed primarily from basic science research.

Genetics and AD

Great progress was made in the genetics of AD during the late 1980s and 1990s. Since then, despite lots of activity, it has been in the doldrums regarding consistent and important results. Most of the strict genetic 'causes' of disease have been limited to so-called 'familial' AD. Familial AD behaves similar to an autosomal dominant genetic pattern and tends to affect predominantly, persons less than age 60. Familial AD, so defined appears to account for less than 5 per cent of all AD, but important clues may be learned from study of Familial disease which will apply to the more common forms of primarily late onset AD (often called sporadic—but it too may have undiscovered genetic causes). Several reviews of AD genetics describing this period of growth in greater detail include St George-Hyslop (2000).

The largest proportion of familial AD is attributed to mutations in the Presenilin 1 gene (chromosome 14) and the next largest known contribution is due to mutations in a homologous gene on chromosome 1, Presenilin 2. Very small proportion of cases is due to specific mutations in the amyloid precursor protein gene (chromosome 21). It is abnormal cleavage of the amyloid precursor protein, which results in the formation of amyloid beta (1–42) protein. Amyloid beta protein aggregates in the brain forming the characteristic plaques of AD. Important work has been published concerning identification of enzymes (for example, BACE and PS1, itself), which cleave the precursor protein abnormally forming the amyloid beta 1–42 protein (Zhao *et al.* 2007; Multhaup 2006). This work may ultimately help to identify sites for drug intervention, not only for Familial but also for non-familial AD (Octave *et al.* 2000). Perhaps one quarter to one half of familial AD is still of unknown genetic cause (Shastry & Giblin 1999).

The strongest and most consistent genetic risk factor for non-familial AD today is apolipoprotein E (APOE) genotype. The association was first described from Dr Allen Roses' laboratory (Roses 1994). APOE naturally occurs as three different alleles (epsilon 2, epsilon 3 and epsilon 4) which pair to form one of six genotypes for each individual. Genotypes containing the epsilon 4 allele are associated with increased risk of AD; homozygous epsilon 4 greatly increases risk (e.g. >eightfold). Since the initial description of increased risk associated with the epsilon 4 allele, many investigators have observed the association. Discussion of APOE genotype is now included in most risk factor studies of AD, either as a focus or as a potential confounder/effect modifier of an association. Despite the huge volume of studies including APOE genotype relatively little is known concerning how the e2, e3, and e4 alleles actually work to influence the risk of AD.

Since the discovery of the association between APOE and AD a huge number of other candidate genes, single nucleotide polymorphisms and other mutations have been examined by a variety of methods. An up-to-date meta-analysis of the studies related to most of these published associations is available through AlzGene (Bertram *et al.* 2007) (http://www.alzgene.org). It is safe to say that none of the other candidates have shown the strength or consistency of APOE.

Vascular dementia

Vascular dementia is difficult to describe clinically and neuropathologically. This may be due in part to the rather common coexistence of vascular features with AD in the elderly. The more sophisticated the search for stroke and cerebrovascular disease becomes, for example, by identifying white matter hyperintensities (WMH) through magnetic resonance imaging (MRI), the more likely such evidence will be found (Au *et al.* 2006). The clinical identification of stroke is surpassed and augmented by CT, which, in turn, has been surpassed by MRI; other specialized neuroimaging techniques may continue this progression. Hopefully, as the resolution provided by the progression from clinical to detailed imaging evidence increases, the false positive identification of stroke and cerebrovascular disease should decrease. Several different criteria have been developed to diagnose vascular dementia (American Psychiatric Association and American Psychiatric Association Task Force on DSM-IV 1994; Roman *et al.* 1993). Much of the pioneering work in the definition and recognition of vascular dementia can be attributed to Hachinski and colleagues, and the Hachinski Ischemic Score continues to be used in many research settings to indicate the extent of cerebrovascular involvement in cognitive decline (Rockwood *et al.* 2000).

Despite clinical diagnostic criteria for vascular dementia (Roman *et al.* 1993), this syndrome remains an area of controversy and uncertainty. Pathologically, vascular dementia also represents somewhat of an enigma, reportedly because of the lack of clear definitional thresholds for white matter damage, infarcts, and lesion location especially in strategic areas of the brain—vascular dementia, in effect, lacks a pathological gold standard against which to compare the clinical diagnosis or clinical criteria and measure their effectiveness (Murray *et al.* 2007). In part because of this problem application of the clinical diagnostic criteria has been shown to be difficult and potentially unreliable in practice, even when applied by well-experienced research investigators (Chui *et al.* 2000). Some of the reliability and validity problems experienced by investigators in classifying a case as 'vascular' or AD may stem from the mutual exclusion of the two conditions, imposed by the various criteria, when the conditions frequently co-exist.

Lewy body disease and frontotemporal lobar degeneration

Two additional types of dementia, Lewy body disease (McKeith 2006) and frontotemporal dementia (Cairns *et al.* 2007a) have been separated from AD based on their clinical presentations and pathology. Lewy body disease or DLB may be more common than originally thought, potentially diagnosable in up to 30 per cent of dementia cases (Tsuang *et al.* 2006). Lewy body disease often presents with fluctuating cognitive performance, visual hallucinations, REM sleep behaviour disorder and/or Parkinsonism. Memory impairment may not be as prominent in the early stages of the disease as deficits in attention, frontal sub-cortical skills and visuospatial ability.

Frontotemporal lobar degeneration includes specific disease subtypes and may be the most frequently occurring dementia in persons under age 65 (Mackenzie & Rademakers 2007).

Frontotemporal dementia (FTD) represents a behavioural subtype where changes may include loss of personal awareness, loss of social graces, disinhibition, overactivity, restlessness, impulsivity, distractibility, hyperorality, withdrawal from social contact, apathy or inertia, and stereotyped or perseverative behaviours. The memory loss is variable and often appears to be due to lack of concern or effort. Frontal lobe impairments are notable including abstraction, planning, and self-regulation of behaviour. FTLD may also be associated with Parkinsonism or motor neuron disease. Pathologically, approximately 40 per cent of FTLDs are related to mutations in the microtubule associated protein tau gene (MAPT) on chromosome 17 and are therefore 'tauopathies', these include Pick's disease, corticobasal degeneration and progressive supranuclear palsy (Rademakers & Hutton 2007; Tolnay & Frank 2007). About 50 per cent of FTLDs are not tauopathies but are reactive to ubiquitin (FTLD-U) rather than mutations in MAPT (Mackenzie & Rademakers 2007). Recently, it was discovered that mutations in the progranulin gene, also on chromosome 17, were an important cause of FTLD-U disorders (Cruts *et al.* 2006; Gass *et al.* 2006) including primary progressive aphasia (Mesulam *et al.* 2007). The pathological protein involved in these disorders as well as in motor neuron disease is TDP-43 (Kwong *et al.* 2007; Cairns *et al.* 2007b). Especially in the FTLDs, location of the pathology appears to determine the clinical dementia syndrome expressed. This question of pathology and location is certainly an important focus for future elucidation. The progranulin and TDP-43 discoveries were arguably the most exciting and important findings for dementia and FTLD in recent times.

Peripheral neuropathy

Clinical overview

Though the term 'peripheral neuropathy' may refer to any disease of the peripheral nerves, it generally is used to describe a group of systemic diseases that affect the peripheral nerves rather than focal diseases affecting an isolated nerve. Most of these diseases affect longer nerves first with symptoms developing first in the feet and progressing up the legs. There are a few peripheral neuropathies that affect the shorter proximal nerves first. By the time the symptoms have reached the knees, the hands become symptomatic followed by the anterior trunk and crown of the head. The symptoms that develop depend on the type of nerve fibre involved. Involvement of motor fibres leads to weakness, muscle wasting, and hyporeflexia. If longstanding, motor neuropathies may lead to high arches (pes cavus) or hammer toes. Sensory nerve involvement leads to loss of sensation, distorted sensation (dysesthesias), or spontaneous unpleasant sensations (paresthesias). Autonomic neuropathies most commonly lead to postural hypotension but may also include sexual dysfunction, bowel dysfunction, bladder dysfunction, disorders of gastroparesis. The size of the affected nerve fibre can often be suggested by the history with disease of large fibre causing reflex loss, vibration loss, and joint position loss. Small fibre disease often leads to autonomic dysfunction, dysesthesias, loss of pain sensation, and loss of temperature sensation.

Electrodiagnostic testing is often performed to diagnose and further classify peripheral neuropathies. Nerve conduction velocities can be used to classify peripheral neuropathies into those that are demyelinating and those that are axonal. Demyelinating neuropathies lead to disproportionate slowing of nerve conduction speeds and increases in latency of responses. Axonal diseases cause disproportional loss of amplitude with relative preservation of conduction speed. Nerve conduction studies measure only the fast-conducting large diameter fibres. Electromyography (EMG) measures the electrical activity of muscle fibres. It is useful in diagnosing a number of muscle and myoneural junction diseases. The use of EMG in the diagnosis of peripheral neuropathy is primarily in recognizing the loss of innervation of muscle fibres by large myelinated neurons. Loss of innervation leads to increased insertional activity, positive waves, fibrillation potentials, polyphasic motor unit potentials, and decreased recruitment patterns. Occasionally, electrodiagnostic studies are supplemented with nerve or muscle biopsy.

Generally, polyneuropathies are the result of lesions involving many peripheral nerves and result in autonomic neuropathies, sensory loss or weakness. Mononeuropathies, as the name implies, involve a single nerve injury or entrapment. Carpal tunnel syndrome and Bell's palsy are common examples of mononeuropathies. Peripheral nerve disorders are, also, often classified as either hereditary or acquired. Charcot–Marie–Tooth syndrome is perhaps the most well-known hereditary form. Acquired nerve disorders are commonly associated with trauma or compression, diabetes, alcoholism and other nutritional and metabolic problems. They may also be related to infectious causes such as, Guillian–Barré syndrome, leprosy, Lyme disease or, HIV-infection; or, they may be caused by toxic exposures to metals (e.g. lead, mercury) or industrial chemicals or even by therapeutic drugs (e.g. anti-neoplastic agents) (Rowland & Merritt 1995).

Little is known about the epidemiology of peripheral neuropathies, though they appear to be common. Few studies have been conducted on the prevalence of these diseases, but what scant data exists finds prevalence to range from 2.4 to 8 per cent (Martyn & Hughes 1997). Prevalence increases considerably with age. Mold reported that 54 per cent of those aged 85 and older seen in practices of family practitioners had evidence of peripheral neuropathy on physician examination (Mold et al. 2004).

Carpal tunnel syndrome

First characterized in 1880 by James J. Putnam, carpal tunnel syndrome is probably the most common neuropathy. Carpal tunnel release surgery is also one of the most common hand surgeries performed in the United States (Rayan 1999). Franklin et al. reported that 'occupational' carpal tunnel syndrome (CTS) resulting from repetitive, higher impact actions may differ from CTS occurring in a non-occupational setting (Franklin et al. 1991). Specifically, occupational CTS appeared to occur nearly equally among men and women and at a substantially lower mean age than had been reported for non-occupational CTS (37 vs. 51 years). Based on workman's compensation records in 1984–88, an incidence of 1.74 per 1000 full-time equivalent jobs was observed (Franklin et al. 1991). Abbas et al. (1998) conducted a meta-analysis of work-related CTS. They showed that force and repetitive motion were important predictors of CTS after adjusting for study population and country of origin.

A general population estimate of CTS incidence was reported by Nordstrom et al. (1998). Medical records of all cases occurring in 2 years, in a defined population were reviewed and classified as definite or probable CTS. In contrast to the occupational CTS incidence observed by Franklin, as well as other previous incidence estimates Nordstrom et al. reported a CTS incidence of 3.46 per

1000 person-years. The apparent increase in incidence may reflect a true change in incidence or may be partially due to popular knowledge of the condition and diagnostic suspicion. Prevalence of symptoms in relation to true disease prevalence is also an important consideration (Atroshi et al. 1999). Reported CTS symptoms of tingling, pain, and numbness have a prevalence of about 14 per cent, whereas CTS was clinically and electrophysiologically confirmed in less than 3 per cent. Atroshi concludes that symptoms of CTS are common but only about 1 in 5 of the persons complaining of symptom is likely to actually have confirmed CTS (Atroshi et al. 1999).

Non-occupational factors related to the occurrence and treatment of CTS were studied by Solomon et al. (1999) and Stallings et al. (1997). Solomon found that CTS patients with inflammatory arthritis were about 3 times more likely to undergo carpal tunnel release surgery; patients with diabetes and hypothyroidism were also significantly more likely to receive surgery. Using data from a United Kingdom twin study, Hakim et al. reported that heredity was the single strongest predictor of CTS (Hakim et al. 2002). The overall prevalence was 14.2 per cent among the 4488 women. Using monozygotic and dizygotic twins, the heritability was estimated to be 0.46 (95% CI 0.34–0.58) indicating that half of the risk of CTS is due to genetic factors. Age is also related to the development of CTS. Bland found that there was a bimodal age distribution with peaks at 50–54 and 75–84 years of age (Bland & Rudolfer 2003). Obesity has been reported as a risk factor for the occurrence of CTS (Bland 2005) This association was addressed in a case–control study by Stallings et al. (1997). Results indicated that obesity, as determined by body mass index, was significantly more common among cases than among control subjects.

Diabetes mellitus

Diabetes is a common, yet complex cause of both mono- and polyneuropathies. Diabetes may affect up to 7 per cent of the US population, and peripheral neuropathy may affect 26–47 per cent of these (Barrett et al. 2007). More effective glucose control could reduce the risk to some extent (Boulton 1998a). Patients with diabetes have a higher hospital admission rate, length of stay and mortality than non-diabetics (Currie et al. 1998) indicating the potential human and economic cost of the disease. The cost of diabetic peripheral neuropathy, particularly in those with pain, can be substantial (Barrett et al. 2007).

Dyck et al. (1999) developed a composite score for assessing the degree of diabetic polyneuropathy, then conducted a longitudinal study of 264 diabetics to determine how hyperglycaemia related to diabetic polyneuropathy. Microvessel disease, chronic hyperglycaemia and type of diabetes were the most important predictors of polyneuropathy. Orchard et al. (1996) has also shown that among patients with insulin dependent diabetic, autonomic neuropathy is strongly influenced by chronic hyperglycaemia and is associated with increased mortality. A study of diabetic peripheral neuropathy in 16 European countries identified several additional risk factors: Elevated diastolic blood pressure, ketoacidosis, elevated fasting triglyceride level, and microabuminuria (Tesfaye et al. 1996). It is now recognized that a substantial number of patients with peripheral neuropathy of unknown cause have prediabetes with impaired fasting glucose or glucose tolerance tests (Smith & Singleton 2006). Improved diabetes control may minimize the impact of diabetic peripheral neuropathy.

Nutritional neuropathies

A number of nutritional deficiencies can lead to peripheral neuropathies. The most common is vitamin B_{12} deficiency. An epidemic of peripheral neuropathy was reported in Cuba during 1992–1993 (Roman 1994). That epidemic was said to affect over 50 000 Cubans and achieved a cumulative incidence rate of 461 per 100 000. An optic form and a peripheral form of the disease were observed. Extensive search for toxic exposures and a variety of other risk factors eventually lead to nutritional deficiency as the principal explanation for the outbreak (Roman 1994). Intervention and treatment with multivitamins, in particular B-vitamins, acted to stop the outbreak.

Peripheral neuropathy due to infection

Infection with HIV is emerging as an increasing source of a number of neurological conditions including peripheral neuropathies. There are many different types of peripheral neuropathy associated with HIV infections including diffuse peripheral neuropathy, Guillain–Barré syndrome, mononeuropathies, neuropathies due to secondary infections and neuropathies due to medications (Brew 2003). The prevalence of peripheral neuropathy reached 44 per cent in one African HIV study (Parry et al. 1997). Distal symmetrical polyneuropathy affects about 30 per cent of people with HIV who have CD4 counts less than 200 per μl (Tagliati et al. 1999). The cause of this peripheral neuropathy is uncertain, but one potential cause may be the AIDS therapy itself. Specifically, nucleosides may act, in about 15–40 per cent of patients to promote neuropathy (Brew 2003). The severity of the neuropathy may then cause patients to discontinue the needed therapy.

Guillain–Barré syndrome is due to an autoimmune attack on the peripheral nerve myelin. Previously considered an idiopathic disease, it is now recognized that a significant proportion of cases are associated with prior infections. The best documented of these infections is *Campylobacter jejuni* (Yuki 2007). Other infectious organisms have also been implicated. There appears to be molecular mimicry between gangliocides found in the organism and gangliocides found in myelin (Yuki 2007).

Though the prevalence of leprosy is declining, it remains one of the most important causes of peripheral neuropathy in the developing world (Ooi & Srinivasan 2004). Fortunately, early treatment can prevent many of the disabling and disfiguring effects of the disease. However, as the disease becomes less common, healthcare providers become increasingly unfamiliar with its early manifestations.

Parkinsonism

The Parkinson's research community is experiencing considerable controversy related to the conceptual description of idiopathic PD. Whether, as in the past the definition should be confined to the clinical motor phenotype and the pathological description of loss of dopaminergic neurons in the substantia nigra along with the occurrence there of alpha-synuclein deposits in the form of Lewy bodies or neurites, or, whether because of the widespread occurrence of these misfolded proteins throughout the body, PD should be viewed and studied more systemically (Langston 2006). The argument for expanding the view of PD continues that limiting the clinical and pathologic view of the disease itself limits the potential for research progress (Langston 2006).

Clinical overview

There are four cardinal features of Parkinsonism: Tremor, rigidity, bradykinesia, and postural gait changes. Though there are no established criteria, the diagnosis of Parkinsonism usually requires two or more of these symptoms In severe cases, patients may be unable to move (freezing) when they encounter minor obstacles such as doorways or cracks. While movement disorder specialists make the diagnosis of Parkinsonism with some degree of confidence, PD usually requires histopathologic confirmation. In an attempt to increase the accuracy and validity of clinical diagnosis, improvements in clinical diagnostic criteria have been proposed (Jankovic et al. 2000).

Parkinsonism includes several major subclasses: Idiopathic Parkinsonism (PD), symptomatic Parkinsonism (e.g. drug-induced, toxin-induced, and other specific causes), 'Parkinson's-plus' syndromes (e.g. multiple system atrophy; MSA), progressive supranuclear palsy), and hereditary degenerative diseases (e.g. Hallervorden–Spatz disease, Huntington disease). PD or idiopathic Parkinsonism comprises approximately 80 per cent of Parkinsonism.

Multiple System Atrophy is sometimes misdiagnosed as PD; it is a relatively rare and very debilitating condition usually involving progressive autonomic failure plus poor responsiveness to levodopa or cerebellar ataxia. The is some evidence that MSA is a synucleinopathy (Armstrong et al. 2006). There role of environmental toxins such as pesticides, in the pathogenesis of MSA has also been discussed but little evidence for such an association has been established to date.

Incidence and prevalence of PD

Parkinson's disease prevalence has been reported with dramatic inconsistency. Case ascertainment, age structure of the population and study design may account for some part of the variability. Certainly door-to-door screening may find more disease that relying on medical records or death certificates. Decisions regarding the inclusion of institutionalized subjects in a screening effort may also impact obtained prevalence.

Consider that PD prevalence typically has been reported in the range of about 50 per 100 000 to 200 per 100 000 population, with a maximum of about 350 per 100 000. Morgante conducted a study in Sicily and found 63 PD cases among 24 496 persons in the population base which results in a prevalence proportion of 257.2 per 100 000 (or 0.257%) (Morgante et al. 1992). The Rotterdam Study (de Rijk et al. 1995) reported identifying a total of 97 PD cases from among 6969 enrolled subjects *age 55 or older* for a crude prevalence of 1.39 per cent or 1392 per 100 000. Recently, combined results of five European studies were published (de Rijk et al. 1997). The combined studies included 14 636 persons *age 65 or older*; after age adjusting to the European 1991 standard population the prevalence of PD was reported as 1.6 per 100 population (presumably age 65 or older), this translates to about 1600 per 100 000. In addition, the age-specific prevalence of PD was reported to increase from 0.6 per cent in 65–69-year-olds to 3.5 per cent in 85–89-year-olds (or 600 per 100 000 to 3500 per 100 000) (de Rijk et al. 1997). The example above is instructive. Not only must the reader attend to differences in case ascertainment when evaluating reported prevalence estimates, but also attention should be directed to the base from which the prevalence proportion is calculated.

Incidence rates for PD and Parkinsonism carry many of the same caveats as raised (above) for prevalence. In addition, confusion is added by choosing to report incidence in terms of person-years, or per population per year, or perhaps as projected cumulative lifetime incidence. With some effort, or with some assumptions, conversions can be made, but such may not be obvious to the reader. Bower et al. (1999) studied the incidence of Parkinsonism and PD in Rochester, Minnesota, during 1976–1990. The overall figures for PD showed an incidence rate of 10.8 per 100 000 person-years (i.e. based on the entire age distribution population). The age-specific incidence for the 50–59 age group was 17.4 per 100 000 person-years, rising to 52.5 for 60–69 ages and peaking at 93.1 for 70–79 age group and 79.1 for 80–99-year-olds. Parkinsonism showed an overall incidence rate of 25.6 per 100 000 person years and rose from 26.5 at ages 50–59 to 304.8 per 100 000 person-years in those aged 80–99 (Bower et al. 1999).

Age-specific incidence rates provide critical information not available from summary rates. The strong influence of age on the disease process is evident from the Rochester, Minnesota, data: The incidence among those aged 0–29 is practically nil; while the incidence triples from 50–59 to 60–69, then nearly doubles again in the 70–79 age group (Bower et al. 1999). How aging contributes to the degenerative process of PD or how aging increases susceptibility to genetic and environmental risk factors is important to describe the epidemiology of Parkinsonism and PD.

Risk factors

Clear and consistent evidence of specific, strong, environmental risk factors has been evasive. However, the possibility of environmental causes was increased by the observation that 1-methyl-4-phenyl-1,2,3,6-tetrahydropyridine (MPTP), a 'designer' street drug, was observed to cause acute PD shortly after ingestion (Langston et al. 1983). Because the structure of MPTP and its metabolism products are somewhat similar to some pesticides and herbicides there was and is great interest in exploring the potential for those types of exposures as risk factors or causes of PD. Observations focusing on family history and familial cases, along with the rapid increase in information available on the human genome, has led to new interest in describing the genetics of PD.

Rural living, well-water consumption, and pesticide/herbicide exposure are reported relatively frequently as potential risk factors for PD, although, neither critical time periods nor duration for these exposures necessary to influence onset, nor specific mechanisms have been identified. For example, a case–control study conducted by Gorell et al. (1998) found about a fourfold increase in risk of PD for exposure to herbicides and insecticides and nearly a three time the risk of PD for those who had a farming occupation (but no increase for rural or farm residence, nor well-water use). Firestone et al. reported consistently elevated, though not statistically significant risks due to pesticide exposure raising some doubts as to the role of pesticides in PD (Firestone et al. 2005). Petrovitch et al. also have shown, in the Honolulu Asia Aging Study that the risk of PD increased significantly for long-term plantation workers as compared to those who worked on plantations 10 years or less, to approach a dose–response relationship (Petrovitch et al. 2002). Marder et al. (1998) found an association between farming, rural living and well-water in multi-ethnic case–control study, but that association held only for African Americans and not for Hispanics. Kuopio et al. (1999) conducted a population-based case–control study in Finland and found no association between farming, drinking water, pesticide/herbicide use, and PD.

An association between exposure to metals and PD has been described by Gorell et al. (1999a,b). An association was noted with manganese exposure and with copper, also with combinations of lead and iron or copper. While this association is interesting, it raises the question of whether the manganese association represented manganism rather than PD.

Smoking has been rather consistently associated with decreased risk of PD in reported reviews and in individual studies (Ritz et al. 2007). Reasons for the plausibility of such an association revolve around the potential action of nicotine on neurons. Although this is one of the more consistent findings, it is not completely without alternative explanations. Most epidemiologic studies of PD use 'prevalent' or existing cases in their studies. The low incidence of PD effectively precludes concentrating on only newly diagnosed cases in all but the largest of studies (or in very large cohort studies). When attempting to identify a cross-sectional sample of cases for enrolment into a case–control study, it can be shown that those patients who have had the disease the longest are the most likely to be included. The most severe, short duration or rapidly declining cases tend to be missed. If PD cases who had a history of smoking were much more likely to die than non-smoking PD cases; and at the same time if the smoking–non-smoking mortality differential was somewhat less among the controls, then, the cross-sectional sampling of cases and controls could give the spurious impression of an excess of smoking among controls. The excess numbers of smokers among controls might then be misinterpreted as a causal, protective effect. At this point, however, the PD research community appears to be relatively confident in the potential protective effect of smoking (Ritz et al. 2007). Because DLB represents similar molecular pathology (i.e. alpha-synuclein, Lewy bodies) which develops primarily in a different brain location, it would be interesting to test whether the apparent protective effect of smoking seen in PD could also be observed in DLB and similar Lewy body diseases.

Dietary-related factors have been shown in some studies to affect risk of PD, with more fish and vegetables appearing to protect (Gao et al. 2007). Coffee and caffeine intake appears to lower risk of PD even after adjusting for smoking (Ross et al. 2000). Dietary folate and vitamin B_{12} intake were reported as potentially protective for PD in the Rotterdam study (de Lau et al. 2006). The relation to dietary folate and B_{12} is somewhat consistent to similar reports concerning high homocystiene as a risk factor for AD. Also, consistent with work in AD, body mass index has been reported by researchers in Finland to increase the risk of PD (Hu et al. 2006). Coincidently, the occurrence of gout and hyperuricemia has been reported to protect against PD through an hypothesized link to the antioxidant properties of uric acid (de Lau et al. 2005; Alonso et al. 2007). It is not clear whether the pathway might be different for persons who are overproducers of uric acid due to one type of genetic defect, as compared to those who simply indulge in large quantities of high urate generating foods, or those whose serum uric acid levels are raised because of the use of diuretics.

Interest in pesticide exposure as a potential cause, led to a biotransformation gene approach for evaluating the occurrence of susceptible persons. Specifically, some persons may be more, or less, able to metabolize environmental toxins because of polymorphic genes involved in metabolism. One of the family of cytochrome P-450 biotransformation genes, CYP2D6 is involved in metabolism of debrisoquine (structurally similar to pesticides); some polymorphic forms are 'poor' metabolizers and others are normal or rapid metabolizers of debrisoquine. Initial studies appeared to show that poor metabolizers were at increased risk of PD but later studies and meta analyses fail to support this conclusion (Scordo et al. 2006; Maraganore et al. 2000).

A similar approach has been taken to identify susceptibles focusing on polymorphic forms of glutathione transferases (GST) which are involved in the metabolism of pesticides and other xenobiotics

Table 9.10.4 Genes associated with PD aetiology

Gene	a.k.a.	Chromosome	Occurrence
SNCA (α-Synuclein)	PARK1 or PARK4	4q21	Lewy body component Sporadic PD
PARK2 (Parkin)	PARK2	6q25–q27	Recessive; juvenile/ early onset
UCHL1	PARK5	4p14	Sporadic PD
PINK1	PARK6	1p35–p36	Recessive; rare, slowly progressive
DJ1	PARK7	1p36	Recessive; rare; early onset
LRRK2	PARK8	12p12	Sporadic PD; LBs or NFTs

(Menegon *et al.* 1998). Continued effort to identify gene environment interaction in this way may eventually prove fruitful, but success is rather limited to date.

As recently as two decades ago, it was commonly taught that PD had little genetic basis. With the explosion of genetic knowledge and technology and an understanding of some of the proteins potentially involved in pathogenesis, the picture has changed dramatically. Table 9.10.4 shows genes most commonly agreed to be involved with PD aetiology (Farrer 2006). The number of genes associated with PD will almost certainly have increased by the time this current chapter is published. Genome-wide association studies are also beginning to be mounted by investigators to further elucidate the potential genetic relationships that influence the occurrence of PD and Parkinsonism (Evangelou *et al.* 2007).

Public health impact

PD is progressive and debilitating. While initial treatments with levodopa and similar medications effectively quell most motor symptoms, their effectiveness begins to subside in about 50 per cent of patients after 3–5 years. With increasing motor problem comes increased health care cost and decreased quality of life (de Boer *et al.* 1999). For many patients, dementia also ensues as PD progresses (Marder *et al.* 1999), leading to the need for long-term care in many instances. The overlap between PD dementia and DLB is of great interest because of the potential underlying synuclein pathology and there for the potential genetic relationships as well (Rocca *et al.* 2007).

Multiple sclerosis

Clinical overview

Although multiple sclerosis (MS) is not as common as most of the neurological diseases previously discussed, it is an important cause of disability in young adults in developed countries, and is thus worthy of at least brief discussion here. The impact of this disease on society is disproportionately large because it strikes people 20–50 years of age. The impact of MS on wage earning is notable with only 21 per cent of MS patients having no work limitations and only 29 per cent remaining in the work force (Minden *et al.* 2004). In addition to the stresses the disease places on home life and employment, MS patients have substantial increases in medical costs compared to the general population (Minden *et al.* 2004). Because of lost earnings and increased healthcare costs, MS is the third leading cause of significant disability in the 20–50-year age range (LaRocca *et al.* 1984).

Clinically, MS is characterized by demyelination of central nervous system white matter tracts including motor, sensory, cerebellar, visual, brainstem, autonomic, and spinal cord pathways (Noseworthy *et al.* 2000). The symptoms may be episodic, with exacerbations and remissions, with symptoms remaining stable between exacerbations (relapsing/remitting disease) (Lublin & Reingold 1996). Alternatively, symptoms may slowly progress in the absence of exacerbations (primary progressive disease). Relapsing/remitting cases may change to include slow deterioration of the baseline in between attacks (secondary progressive disease). When the disease results in death, the immediate cause is usually infectious, secondary to urinary tract involvement or pneumonia.

At present, corticosteroids are used to shorten the length of acute relapses. Interferon beta 1a, interferon beta 1b, glateramer acetate, mitoxantrone, and natalizumab have all been shown to slow the progression of the disease. In addition to disease-modifying therapy, symptomatic treatments are often required. A multitude of new immunosuppressive and immunomodulating treatments are being tested, giving hope for more effective treatments in the future.

Definition

The criteria developed by Schumacher *et al.* (1966) and revised by Poser and Kurtzke (1991) were previously used for diagnosis. These have recently been replaced by the McDonald criteria (McDonald *et al.* 2001; Polman *et al.* 2005). These new criteria for MS retain the previous requirements for two or more episodes of neurologic deficit at different times and different locations within the nervous system. For those MS attacks used to fulfil the criteria, symptoms must be typical of those seen with MS and objective findings on examination or paraclinical tests must be present. The new criteria allow diagnosis by clinical presentation alone, but also allow MRI findings to be used to demonstrate dissemination in time or locations within the nervous system. The revised McDonald criteria have allowed the disease to be diagnosed at an earlier stage than previous criteria.

Case ascertainment

Because of the necessity for neurological expertise and special studies to make reliable diagnoses, reported worldwide prevalences may not be completely comparable, especially where differences in the availability and quality of health care exist. This is especially true in light of the highly variable clinical presentation of the disease, and the variable course. The requirement for repeated attacks before a diagnosis is made and the often vague nature of the initial clinical symptoms leads to difficulties in determining exact incidence figures in a timely manner.

Prevalence

Disease prevalence is easier to determine than incidence, particularly considering the difficulty in determining the time of onset of the disease. With the new McDonald criteria, MRI availability and increasing awareness of the disease, the time from symptom onset until diagnosis is rapidly shortening in regions with ready access to sophisticated neurological care (Marrie et al. 2005). The reported prevalence of MS varies widely with latitude, from one per 100 000 or less near the equator, to over 150 per 100 000 in some high latitude areas. In the Southern Hemisphere less data are available, but studies in Australia and New Zealand support a similar gradient in prevalence (Skegg et al. 1987). Persons who migrate in childhood from high risk to lower risk areas seem to lower their risk of MS, while migrants over age 15 retain the risk associated with their areas of origin (Alter et al. 1966a,b). However, the prevalence and incidence of MS in relation to latitude appears to be changing rapidly over the past few years. In the United States, nurses born in the North before 1946 had a threefold greater risk of developing MS than their Southern counterparts. In those born after 1946, there was no difference in risk between those born in the North or the South (Hernan et al. 1999). In a study of US veterans, the relative risk of developing MS in white men born in the North compared to those born in the South was 2.47 among World War II and Korean veterans compared to 1.97 in Vietman era veterans (Wallin et al. 2004) Among white women veterans, the rates fell from 3.46 to 1.52 during the same time period. The study of veterans minimizes regional and socioeconomic differences in access to healthcare. It appears that this change is due primarily to an increase in MS in the South rather than to a decrease in the North.

The prevalence of MS also appears to be changing in Europe. The North–South gradient is now less pronounced and areas that previously had low incidence rates are now increasing (Pugliatti et al. 2006). This is particularly notable for areas around the Mediterranean and the far North. Previously, the Middle East was considered a region of low risk for developing MS. Like low-prevalence regions in North America and Europe, this risk also appears to be changing. The prevalence of MS in Kuwait increased from 6.68/100 000 in 1993 to 14.77/100 000 in 2000 (Alshubaili et al. 2005). Most of this increase was due to an increase in native Kuwaitis where the prevalence was 31.15/100 000. In Asia, the prevalence of MS remains low, but this rate appears to be increasing in some regions including China (Cheng et al. 2007). The leveling of MS rates with latitude may reflect an improvement in case ascertainment, but it likely also reflects a true increase in MS in areas in which it was previously rare.

Risk factors

Gender

Multiple sclerois is more common in females. Approximately 75 per cent of people with MS are female. However, the increased incidence among females has not always been a feature of the disease. In the first half of the twentieth century, males predominated (Kurtzke 2005). Some of the male preponderance may be related to a tendency to misdiagnose females as hysterical during that period of time. However, most believe that there was truly a male preponderance. The gender rates of MS gradually changed to a female preponderance during the middle of the century. In a longitudinal population-based cohort of 27 074 people with MS, the proportion of cases that are female has been slowly increasing over the past 50 years (Orton et al. 2006). The disease is less active during pregnancy and more active during the three months immediately postpartum (Confavreux et al. 1998). In a case–control study of 242 MS cases nested within a large British primary care database, the incidence of MS was lower in those taking oral contraceptives during the past 3 years (OR 0.6, 95% CI 0.4–1) (Alonso et al. 2005). The changes in MS activity with hormones and pregnancy may be due to alterations in immune system function, but the temporal changes in gender ratios remain unexplained.

Ethnic background

In general, MS occurs with greater frequency in whites, particularly those of northern European ancestry. Other ethnic groups have a lower incidence and prevalence of MS. However, the ethnic contributions to MS risk appear to be changing also. In a study of Canadian First Nations people, the prevalence of MS has increased from 56.3/100 000 in 1994 to 99.9/100 000 in 2002 (Svenson et al. 2007). The prevalence of MS in blacks has increased dramatically. The relative risk of MS in black compared with white males increasing from 0.44 in World War II/Korean conflict veterans to 0.67 in Vietnam era veterans (Wallin et al. 2004). The relative risk among black females compared to white males increased from 1.28 to 2.86 during the same time period, essentially catching up to the risk of white females.

Genetic susceptibility

There are several types of evidence for genetic influences on susceptibility. Asian, African, and aboriginal groups seem to have lower prevalence than Caucasians, regardless of latitude of residence. In Caucasians, it has been shown that some alleles of the HLA complex are associated with MS susceptibility, particularly the HLA-DRB1.1501 locus (Haines et al. 1996). In addition, other groups of genes that influence the immune response or myelin structure have been investigated (Sadovnick et al. 1991). A study by the International MS Genetics Consortium looked at 500 000 single nucleotide polymorphisms in 12 360 subjects (Hafler et al. 2007). In addition to the known HLA genes, only two additional alleles, IL2RA and IL7RA, were found to be risk factors for MS. Both of these genes are involved in T cell immunity, but each accounts for only 0.2 per cent of the variance in the risk of MS.

The hereditability of MS may also be instructive. There is an extremely high rate of concordance in monozygotic twins, supporting a genetic contribution to the disease. In the Danish twin study, there was concordance for MS in 24 per cent of monozygotic twins and 3 per cent of dizygotic twins (Hansen et al. 2005). The standardized incidence ratio for monozygotic twins compared to nontwins was 1.23 (Hansen et al. 2005). This contrasts with the standardized incidence ratio of 0.78 for dizygotic twins. However, areas with a lower prevalence of MS appear to have lower concordance rates for MS in monozygotic twins (..1992). In addition to the risk in twins, there is an increased risk of MS in other first degree relatives of people with MS. In a Danish study, the relative risk of MS in first degree relatives of people with MS was 7.1 (95% CI 5.8–8.8) (Nielsen et al. 2005). The lifetime risk was calculated to be 2.8 per cent for male and 2.9 per cent for female first degree relatives. Some have found that the risk of MS is higher in children of MS fathers than MS mothers (OR 1.99, 95% CI 1.05–3.77) (Kantarci et al. 2006).

This increased rate of transmission to offspring by a subgroup in which the disease is less common (men) suggests a genetic contribution in which genes are concentrated in men with the disease. However, others have reported that the risk of MS in children whose parents have MS is similar regardless of whether the affected parent was the father or mother (Herrera *et al.* 2007). A Canadian study found that the age-adjusted risk of MS in siblings was 3.11 per cent (95% CI 2.39–3.83) (Ebers *et al.* 2004). In half siblings, the risk was 1.89 per cent (95% CI 1.36–2.41). This risk was greater for maternal half siblings (2.35%, 95% CI 1.57–3.13) than paternal half siblings (1.31%, 95% CI 0.65–1.96). These genetic studies indicate that there is an important genetic contribution to the disease, but that environmental factors also play a major role.

Environmental factors

In the presence of inherent susceptibility, some external factors seem to be associated with MS. People with MS have a later age of exposure to common childhood exanthematous diseases, and lower birth orders though not all studies have supported this finding (Bager *et al.* 2006). There have been reports of clusters of disease, thought to have been related to environmental exposures, but on investigation these supposed clusters have generally not been beyond expected variability.

The strong relationship between MS and latitude has led some to postulate that areas with less sun exposure, and thus lower levels of vitamin D, may be responsible for the disease. A North American study of monozygotic twins who were discordant for MS found that childhood activities involving sun exposure decreased the risk of MS. Nine sun-related activities were investigated (Islam *et al.* 2007). The odds ratio of developing MS ranged from 0.25 to 0.57, indicating that sun-related activities in childhood decreased the risk of developing MS in later life. Each unit increase in a sun exposure index decreased the relative risk of MS by 25 per cent. In a study of US military recruits, blood samples were obtained at entry into the military (Munger *et al.* 2006). A case–control study was then performed to evaluate premorbid vitamin D levels in those who subsequently developed MS. The odds ratio for a 50 nmol/l increase in 25-hydroxyvitamin D was 0.59 (95% CI 0.36–0.97). Thus far, it has been impossible to determine whether vitamin D deficiency causes or worsens MS, or whether MS patients develop vitamin D deficiency by avoidance of the sun. This issue is further complicated by the fact that many MS patients avoid overheating because it worsens their symptoms. Also, since the disease may be present for many years before it is diagnosed the occurrence of vitamin D deficiency prior to diagnosis cannot be taken as proof that the deficiency preceded the disease.

The relationship between MS prevalence, latitude, migration, and socioeconomic factors has led some to suggest that MS is related to the degree and timing of exposure to various infectious organisms (Fleming & Cook 2006). This hygiene hypothesis states that exposure to one or more infectious agents later in life (due to high levels of hygiene) leads to changes in the immune system that eventually lead to MS. A number of infectious agents have been postulated to cause MS. Epstein–Barr virus (EBV) is associated with MS (Ascherio & Munger 2007). MS is extremely rare in people who have never had EBV. Furthermore, those exposed to EBV later in childhood have a two- to threefold increase in risk relative to those who acquire EBV in early childhood. Antibody titres to EBV are increased in MS, often years before recognition of the disease, but this may reflect a general upregulation of the immune system. Chlamydia pneumoniae has also been suspected as a cause of MS. A case–control study within the Nurses Health Study found an odds ratio of 1.7 (95% CI 1.1–2.7) in those who were seropositive for antibodies to the organism (Munger *et al.* 2003). Human herpes virus-6 (HHV6) has also been associated with MS. Human endogenous retroviruses have also been implicated in the disease (Sotgiu *et al.* 2006). Despite these associations, to date the relationship between specific viruses and MS remains uncertain.

Trauma does not appear to explain the onset of disease (Goldacre *et al.* 2006) or exacerbations of the disease (Sibley *et al.* 1991). Smoking prior to disease onset increases the risk of MS (OR 1.22–1.51) (Hawkes 2007). However, children exposed to cigarette smoke have a higher risk of developing MS (Mikaeloff *et al.* 2007). The environmental factors that contribute to MS remain uncertain.

Overview

The risk of MS appears to be due to environmental factors acting on genetically predisposed people. Eventually, these factors lead to an immune attack on the central nervous system, resulting is symptoms. The genetic factors appear to be polygenetic. The environmental factors remain uncertain. Immunomodulating treatments have played an important role in slowing the disease, but their benefits are only partial. Much remains to be clarified about the mechanisms of the disease process, and it is hoped that a better knowledge of these mechanisms will lead to improved treatments.

Epilogue

Presenting current and useful research information on a number of neurologic conditions is a difficult task. This chapter has attempted to address that challenge, for some selected neurologic conditions . We have attempted to cite important current or classic research papers, but many potentially important references included in earlier drafts became merely stubble for Occam's razor, as wielded by the editor. Conditions such as headache and TBI have substantial public health impact because of the age groups affected, their prevalence and the lost productivity (or economic loss) related to them. Multiple sclerosis, a relatively common neurologic disease, can affect individuals in young adulthood, decrease their productivity and ultimately make them dependent on others. Traumatic brain injury occurring in youth or young adulthood can cause years of extra medical care in addition to lost productivity among those who survive the immediate event. Epilepsy may have onset throughout the life course, it may result from trauma or may be caused by specific genes, among other causes. While there are intractable forms of epilepsy, great strides have been made in seizure control enabling patients to lead relatively full and normal lives. Neurodegenerative diseases, such as PD and AD, rob productivity, functional ability and independence from older individuals; they also force huge increases in health care costs. Without question neurologic diseases have substantial public health effects.

Determining the incidence and prevalence for most of the diseases and conditions in this chapter is quite an inexact science. The conditions are often difficult to define and detect in the population and for the most part they are not regarded as 'reportable' conditions. Therefore we gain insight as to disease occurrence primarily from limited but (hopefully) well-designed and conducted studies. As mentioned in the introduction to this chapter, the epidemiologic study of neurologic conditions is a complicated matter. Problems with diagnostic inaccuracy and insidious disease onset influence our ability to observe risk factor associations; factors related to survival may be mistaken for risk/protective factors.

The recent work of the Human Genome Project and the HapMap Project has greatly influenced technology and has now made possible genome-wide studies that could not have been imagined a decade ago. The contribution to disease incidence of genes, that in and of themselves cause disease may be smaller than that of genes which act together with other genes in complex ways, or act to metabolize or potentiate environmental exposures. The interaction between genes and environment will be increasingly well studied in the future. Description of gene products and functions may lead to specific drug therapies never before possible. The genetic information presented in this chapter, while relatively current, may become obsolete quickly. The fields of genetics and molecular biology are moving rapidly. It is a challenge also for epidemiologists to apply the knowledge gained by the genetic researchers to the design and analysis of epidemiologic studies. The diagnosis of neurologic conditions may ultimately be made more accurately and earlier by incorporating as yet undiscovered genetic information. Science and the public health will benefit beyond even our current grand expectations.

Epidemiology must take advantage of these molecular advances. Many scholars have written on pros and cons of reductionism in science. Much of epidemiology lies in its public health context, and the same is likely to be true for genetic influences on neurologic diseases. Arrays of genes may identify susceptible individuals however those individuals may avoid disease unless met with specific environmental or behavioural exposures. The tasks of public health and epidemiology will still involve prevention, the non-random occurrence of disease and its environmental context—in addition to heredity. The tools to address those tasks will continue to be refined.

References

(..1989) Proposal for revised classification of epilepsies and epileptic syndromes. Commission on Classification and Terminology of the International League Against Epilepsy. *Epilepsia*, **30**, 389–99.

(..1992) Multiple sclerosis in 54 twinships: concordance rate is independent of zygosity. French Research Group on Multiple Sclerosis. *Ann Neurol*, **32**, 724–7.

(..1997a) Consensus recommendations for the postmortem diagnosis of Alzheimer's disease. The National Institute on Aging, and Reagan Institute Working Group on Diagnostic Criteria for the Neuropathological Assessment of Alzheimer's Disease. *Neurobiol Aging*, **18**, S1–2.

(..1998) Rehabilitation of persons with traumatic brain injury. NIH Consensus Statement 1998 Oct 26–28, **16**, 1–41.

(..2003) Nonfatal fall-related traumatic brain injury among older adults—California, 1996–1999. *MMWR Morb Mortal Wkly Rep*, **52**, 276–8.

(..2004a) The International Classification of Headache Disorders: 2nd edition. *Cephalalgia*, 24 Suppl 1, 9–160.

(..2006) Incidence rates of hospitalization related to traumatic brain injury—12 states, 2002. *MMWR Morb Mortal Wkly Rep*, **55**, 201–4.

(..2007a) Introduction. Guidelines for the management of severe traumatic brain injury. *J Neurotrauma*, 24 Suppl 1, S1–2.

(..2007b) Nonfatal traumatic brain injuries from sports and recreation activities—United States, 2001–2005. *MMWR Morb Mortal Wkly Rep*, **56**, 733–7.

Abbas, M.A., Afifi, A.A., Zhang, Z.W., *et al.* (1998) Meta-analysis of published studies of work-related carpal tunnel syndrome. *Int J Occup Environ Health*, **4**, 160–7.

Aisen, P.S., Schafer, K.A., Grundman, M., *et al.* (2003) Effects of rofecoxib or naproxen vs placebo on Alzheimer disease progression: a randomized controlled trial. *JAMA*, **289**, 2819–26.

Alonso, A., Jick, SS., OLEK, M. J., *et al.* (2005) Recent use of oral contraceptives and the risk of multiple sclerosis. *Arch Neurol*, **62**, 1362–5.

Alonso, A., Rodriguez, L.A., Logroscino, G., *et al.* (2007) Gout and risk of Parkinson disease: a prospective study. *Neurology*, **69**, 1696–700.

Alshubaili, A.F., Alramzy, K., Ayyad, Y. M., *et al.* (2005) Epidemiology of multiple sclerosis in Kuwait: new trends in incidence and prevalence. *Eur Neurol*, **53**, 125–31.

Alter, M., Leibowitz, U. and Halpern, L. (1966a) Multiple sclerosis in European & Afro-Asian populations of Israel. *A clinical appraisal. Acta Neurol Scand*, **42**, Suppl 19:47–54.

Alter, M., Leibowitz, U. and Speer, J. (1966b) Risk of multiple sclerosis related to age at immigration to Israel. *Arch Neurol*, **15**, 234–7.

American Psychiatric Association & American Psychiatric Association (APA & AMA) Task Force on DSM-IV (1994) Diagnostic and statistical manual of mental disorders: DSM-IV, Washington, American Psychiatric Association.

Annegers, J.F., Beghi, E. & Begley, C.E. (1999) Cost of epilepsy: contrast of methodologies in United States and European studies. *Epilepsia*, **40**, 14–8.

Annegers, J.F. and Coan, S.P. (1999) SUDEP: overview of definitions and review of incidence data. *Seizure*, **8**, 347–52.

Annegers, J.F., Hauser, W.A., Anderson, V. E., *et al.* (1982) The risks of seizure disorders among relatives of patients with childhood onset epilepsy. *Neurology*, **32**, 174–9.

Annegers, J.F., Hauser, W.A., Coan, S. P., *et al.* (1998) A population-based study of seizures after traumatic brain injuries. *N Engl J Med*, **338**, 20–4.

Anstey, K.J., Von sanden, C., Salim, A., *et al.* (2007) Smoking as a risk factor for dementia and cognitive decline: a meta-analysis of prospective studies. *Am J Epidemiol*, **166**, 367–78.

Armstrong, R.A., Cairns, N.J. and Lantos, P.L. (2006) Multiple system atrophy (MSA): topographic distribution of the alpha-synuclein-associated pathological changes. *Parkinsonism Relat Disord*, **12**, 356–62.

Ascherio, A. and Munger, K. L. (2007) Environmental risk factors for multiple sclerosis. Part I: the role of infection. *Ann Neurol*, **61**, 288–99.

Atroshi, I., Gummesson, C., Johnsson, R., Ornstein, E., Ranstam, J. & Rosen, I. (1999) Prevalence of carpal tunnel syndrome in a general population [see comments]. *JAMA*, **282**, 153–8.

AU, R., Massaro, J.M., Wolf, P.A., *et al.* (2006) Association of white matter hyperintensity volume with decreased cognitive functioning: the Framingham Heart Study. *Arch Neurol*, **63**, 246–50.

Avanzini, G., Franceschetti, S. and Mantegazza, M. (2007) Epileptogenic channelopathies: experimental models of human pathologies. *Epilepsia*, **48** Suppl 2, 51–64.

Bager, P., Nielsen, N.M., Bihrmann, K., *et al.* (2006) Sibship characteristics and risk of multiple sclerosis: a nationwide cohort study in Denmark. *Am J Epidemiol*, **163**, 1112–7.

Barrett, A.M., Lucero, M.A., LE, T., *et al.* (2007) Epidemiology, public health burden, and treatment of diabetic peripheral neuropathic pain: a review. *Pain Med*, **8** Suppl 2, S50–62.

Bazarian, J.J., Mcclung, J., Shah, M.N., *et al.* (2005) Mild traumatic brain injury in the United States, 1998–2000. *Brain Inj*, **19**, 85–91.

Begley, C.E., Famulari, M., Annegers, J.F., *et al.* (2000) The cost of epilepsy in the United States: an estimate from population-based clinical and survey data. *Epilepsia*, **41**, 342–51.

Berg, J. and Stovner, L.J. (2005) Cost of migraine and other headaches in Europe. *Eur J Neurol*, **12** Suppl 1, 59–62.

Bern, C., Garcia, H.H., Evans, C., *et al.* (1999) Magnitude of the disease burden from neurocysticercosis in a developing country. *Clin Infect Dis*, **29**, 1203–9.

Bertram, L., Mcqueen, M.B., Mullin, K., *et al.* (2007) Systematic meta-analyses of Alzheimer disease genetic association studies: the AlzGene database. *Nat Genet*, **39**, 17–23.

Bigal, M., Rapoport, A., Aurora, S., *et al.* (2007) Satisfaction with current migraine therapy: experience from 3 centers in US and Sweden. *Headache*, **47**, 475–9.

Bland, J.D. (2005) The relationship of obesity, age, and carpal tunnel syndrome: more complex than was thought? *Muscle Nerve*, **32**, 527–32.

Bland, J.D. and Rudolfer, S.M. (2003) Clinical surveillance of carpal tunnel syndrome in two areas of the United Kingdom, 1991–2001. *J Neurol Neurosurg Psychiatry*, **74**, 1674–9.

Boardman, H.F., Thomas, E., Millson, D.S., *et al.* (2006) The natural history of headache: predictors of onset and recovery. *Cephalalgia*, **26**, 1080–8.

Boeve, B.F., Silber, M.H., Parisi, J.E., *et al.* (2003) Synucleinopathy pathology and REM sleep behavior disorder plus dementia or Parkinsonism. *Neurology*, **61**, 40–5.

Boulton, A. J. (1998a) Guidelines for diagnosis and outpatient management of diabetic peripheral neuropathy.European Association for the Study of Diabetes, Neurodiab. *Diabetes Metab*, **24** Suppl 3, 55–65.

Bowen, J., Teri, L., Kukull, W., *et al.* (1997) Progression to dementia in patients with isolated memory loss. *Lancet*, **349**, 763–5.

Bower, J.H., Maraganore, D.M., Mcdonnell, S.K., *et al.* (1999) Incidence and distribution of Parkinsonism in Olmsted County, Minnesota, 1976–1990. *Neurology*, **52**, 1214–20.

Braak, H., Del tredici, K., Rub, U., *et al.* (2003) Staging of brain pathology related to sporadic Parkinson's disease. *Neurobiol Aging*, **24**, 197–211.

Brayne, C. (2006) Incidence of dementia in England and Wales: the MRC Cognitive Function and Ageing Study. *Alzheimer Dis Assoc Disord*, **20**, S47–51.

Breitner, J.C., Martin, B.K. and Meinert, C.L. (2006) The suspension of treatments in ADAPT: concerns beyond the cardiovascular safety of celecoxib or naproxen. PLoS Clin Trials, 1, e41.

Breslau, N. and Davis, G. C. (1993) Migraine, physical health and psychiatric disorder: a prospective epidemiologic study in young adults. *J Psychiatr Res*, **27**, 211–21.

Breslau, N., Davis, G.C., Schultz, L.R., *et al.* (1994) Joint 1994 Wolff Award Presentation. Migraine and major depression: a longitudinal study. *Headache*, **34**, 387–93.

Breslau, N., Schultz, L.R., Stewart, W. F., *et al.* (2000) Headache and major depression: is the association specific to migraine? *Neurology*, **54**, 308–13.

Brew, B.J. (2003) The peripheral nerve complications of human immunodeficiency virus (HIV) infection. *Muscle Nerve*, **28**, 542–52.

Brookmeyer, R., Gray, S. and Kawas, C. (1998) Projections of Alzheimer's disease in the United States and the public health impact of delaying disease onset. *Am J Public Health*, **88**, 1337–42.

Bruns, J., JR. and Hauser, W.A. (2003) The epidemiology of traumatic brain injury: a review. *Epilepsia*, **44** Suppl 10, 2–10.

Buring, J.E., Hebert, P., Romero, J., *et al.* (1995) Migraine and subsequent risk of stroke in the Physicians' Health Study. *Arch Neurol*, **52**, 129–34.

Cady, R.K. (1999) Diagnosis and treatment of migraine. Clin Cornerstone, **1**, 21–32.

Cairns, N.J., Bigio, E.H., Mackenzie, I.R., *et al.* (2007a) Neuropathologic diagnostic and nosologic criteria for frontotemporal lobar degeneration: consensus of the Consortium for Frontotemporal Lobar Degeneration. *Acta Neuropathol*, **114**, 5–22.

Cairns, N.J., Neumann, M., Bigio, E.H., *et al.* (2007b) TDP-43 in familial and sporadic frontotemporal lobar degeneration with ubiquitin inclusions. *Am J Pathol*, **171**, 227–40.

Cassidy, J.D., Carroll, L.J., Peloso, P.M.,*et al.* (2004) Incidence, risk factors and prevention of mild traumatic brain injury: results of the WHO Collaborating Centre Task Force on Mild Traumatic Brain Injury. *J Rehabil Med*, 28–60.

Castillo, J., Munoz, P., Guitera, V., *et al.* (1999) Epidemiology of chronic daily headache in the general population. *Headache*, **39**, 190–6.

Chang, C.L., Donaghy, M. and Poulter, N. (1999) Migraine and stroke in young women: case–control study. The World Health Organisation Collaborative Study of Cardiovascular Disease and Steroid Hormone Contraception [see comments]. *BMJ*, **318**, 13–8.

Cheng, Q., Miao, L., Zhang, J., *et al.* (2007) A population-based survey of multiple sclerosis in Shanghai, China. *Neurology*, **68**, 1495–500.

Christensen, J., Vestergaard, M., Pedersen, M.G., *et al.* (2007) Incidence and prevalence of epilepsy in Denmark. *Epilepsy Res*, **76**, 60–5.

Chui, H.C., Mack, W., Jackson, J.E., *et al.* (2000) Clinical criteria for the diagnosis of vascular dementia: a multicenter study of comparability and interrater reliability [see comments]. *Arch Neurol*, **57**, 191–6.

Colantonio, A., Dawson, D.R. and Mclellan, B.A. (1998) Head injury in young adults: long-term outcome. *Arch Phys Med Rehabil*, **79**, 550–8.

Confavreux, C., Hutchinson, M., Hours, M.M., *et al.* (1998) Rate of pregnancy-related relapse in multiple sclerosis. Pregnancy in Multiple Sclerosis Group. *N Engl J Med*, **339**, 285–91.

Coronado, V.G., Thomas, K.E., Sattin, R.W., *et al.* (2005) The CDC traumatic brain injury surveillance system: characteristics of persons aged 65 years and older hospitalized with a TBI. *J Head Trauma Rehabil*, **20**, 215–28.

Crino, P.B. (2007) Gene expression, genetics, and genomics in epilepsy: some answers, more questions. *Epilepsia*, **48** Suppl 2, 42–50.

Cruts, M., Gijselinck, I., Van der zee, J., *et al.* (2006) Null mutations in progranulin cause ubiquitin-positive frontotemporal dementia linked to chromosome 17q21. *Nature*, **442**, 920–4.

Currie, C.J., Morgan, C.L. and Peters, J.R. (1998) The epidemiology and cost of inpatient care for peripheral vascular disease, infection, neuropathy, and ulceration in diabetes. *Diabetes Care*, **21**, 42–8.

Dahlof, C. and Linde, M. (2001) One-year prevalence of migraine in Sweden: a population-based study in adults. *Cephalalgia*, **21**, 664–71.

De boer, A.G., Sprangers, M.A., Speelman, H.D. and De haes, H.C. (1999) Predictors of health care use in patients with Parkinson's disease: a longitudinal study. *Mov Disord*, **14**, 772–9.

De lau, L.M., Koudstaal, P.J., Witteman, J.C., *et al.* (2006) Dietary folate, vitamin B_{12}, and vitamin B6 and the risk of Parkinson disease. *Neurology*, **67**, 315–8.

De rijk, M.C., Breteler, M.M., Graveland, G.A., *et al.* (1995) Prevalence of Parkinson's disease in the elderly: the Rotterdam Study. *Neurology*, **45**, 2143–6.

De rijk, M.C., Tzourio, C., Breteler, M.M., *et al.* (1997) Prevalence of Parkinsonism and Parkinson's disease in Europe: the EUROPARKINSON Collaborative Study. European Community Concerted Action on the Epidemiology of Parkinson's disease. *J Neurol Neurosurg Psychiatry*, **62**, 10–5.

Demetriades, D., Murray, J., Sinz, B., *et al.* (1998) Epidemiology of major trauma and trauma deaths in Los Angeles County. *J Am Coll Surg*, **187**, 373–83.

Dobyns, W.B., Truwit, C.L., Ross, M.E., *et al.* (1999) Differences in the gyral pattern distinguish chromosome 17-linked and X-linked lissencephaly. *Neurology*, **53**, 270–7.

Durkin, M.S., Kuhn, L., Davidson, L.L., *et al.* (1996) Epidemiology and prevention of severe assault and gun injuries to children in an urban community. *J Trauma*, **41**, 667–73.

Dyck, P.J., Davies, J.L., Wilson, D.M., *et al.* (1999) Risk factors for severity of diabetic polyneuropathy: intensive longitudinal assessment of the Rochester Diabetic Neuropathy Study cohort. *Diabetes Care*, **22**, 1479–86.

Ebers, G.C., Sadovnick, A.D., Dyment, D.A., *et al.* (2004) Parent-of-origin effect in multiple sclerosis: observations in half-siblings. *Lancet*, **363**, 1773–4.

Eisele, J.A., Kegler, S.R., Trent, R.B., *et al.* (2006) Nonfatal traumatic brain injury-related hospitalization in very young children-15 states, 1999. *J Head Trauma Rehabil*, **21**, 537–43.

Elias, M.F., Sullivan, L.M., D'agostino, R.B., *et al.* (2005) Homocysteine and cognitive performance in the Framingham offspring study: age is important. *Am J Epidemiol*, **162**, 644–53.

Engel, J., JR. (2001) A proposed diagnostic scheme for people with epileptic seizures and with epilepsy: report of the ILAE Task Force on Classification and Terminology. *Epilepsia*, **42**, 796–803.

Evangelou, E., Maraganore, D.M. and Ioannidis, J.P. (2007) Meta-analysis in genome-wide association datasets: strategies and application in Parkinson disease. *PLoS ONE*, 2, e196.

Evans, D.A., Funkenstein, H.H., Albert, M.S., *et al.* (1989) Prevalence of Alzheimer's disease in a community population of older persons. Higher than previously reported [see comments]. *JAMA*, **262**, 2551–6.

Farrer, M.J. (2006) Genetics of Parkinson disease: paradigm shifts and future prospects. *Nat Rev Genet*, **7**, 306–18.

Ferri, C.P., Prince, M., Brayne, C., *et al.* (2005) Global prevalence of dementia: a Delphi consensus study. *Lancet*, **366**, 2112–7.

Firestone, J.A., Smith-Weller, T., Franklin, G., *et al.* (2005) Pesticides and risk of Parkinson disease: a population-based case–control study. *Arch Neurol*, **62**, 91–5.

Fleming, J.O. and Cook, T.D. (2006) Multiple sclerosis and the hygiene hypothesis. *Neurology*, **67**, 2085–6.

Franceschi, M., Colombo, B., Rossi, P., *et al.* (1997) Headache in a population-based elderly cohort. An ancillary study to the Italian Longitudinal Study of Aging (ILSA). *Headache*, **37**, 79–82.

Franklin, G.M., Haug, J., Heyer, N., *et al.* (1991) Occupational carpal tunnel syndrome in Washington State, 1984–1988. *Am J Public Health*, **81**, 741–6.

Fratiglioni, L., De Ronchi, D. and Aguero-Torres, H. (1999) Worldwide prevalence and incidence of dementia. *Drugs Aging*, **15**, 365–75.

Frediani, F. and Villani, V. (2007) Migraine and depression. *Neurol Sci*, **28** Suppl 2, S161–5.

Freitag, C.M., May, T.W., Pfafflin, M., *et al.* (2001) Incidence of epilepsies and epileptic syndromes in children and adolescents: a population-based prospective study in Germany. *Epilepsia*, **42**, 979–85.

Gallitto, G., Serra, S., La Spina, P., *et al.* (2005) Prevalence and characteristics of epilepsy in the Aeolian islands. *Epilepsia*, **46**, 1828–35.

Ganguli, M., Dodge, H.H., Chen, P., *et al.* (2000) Ten-year incidence of dementia in a rural elderly US community population: the Movies Project [In Process Citation]. *Neurology*, **54**, 1109–16.

Gao, X., Chen, H., Fung, T.T., *et al.* (2007) Prospective study of dietary pattern and risk of Parkinson disease. *Am J Clin Nutr*, **86**, 1486–94.

Gass, J., Cannon, A., Mackenzie, I.R., *et al.* (2006) Mutations in progranulin are a major cause of ubiquitin-positive frontotemporal lobar degeneration. *Hum Mol Genet*, **15**, 2988–3001.

Gervil, M., Ulrich, V., Kyvik, K.O., *et al.* (1999) Migraine without aura: a population-based twin study. *Ann Neurol*, **46**, 606–11.

Gobel, H., Petersen-Braun, M. and Soyka, D. (1994) The epidemiology of headache in Germany: a nationwide survey of a representative sample on the basis of the headache classification of the International Headache Society [see comments]. *Cephalalgia*, 14, 97–106.

Goldacre, M.J., Abisgold, J.D., Yeates, D.G., *et al.* (2006) Risk of multiple sclerosis after head injury: record linkage study. *J Neurol Neurosurg Psychiatry*, **77**, 351–3.

Gordon Smith, A. and Robinson Singleton, J. (2006) Idiopathic neuropathy, prediabetes and the metabolic syndrome. *J Neurol Sci*, **242**, 9–14.

Gorell, J.M., JOHNSON, C. C., RYBICKI, B. A., *et al.* (1999a) Occupational exposure to manganese, copper, lead, iron, mercury and zinc and the risk of Parkinson's disease. *Neurotoxicology*, **20**, 239–47.

Gorell, J.M., Johnson, C.C., Rybicki, B.A., *et al.* (1998) The risk of Parkinson's disease with exposure to pesticides, farming, well water, and rural living. *Neurology*, **50**, 1346–50.

Gorell, J.M., Rybicki, B.A., Cole Johnson, C., *et al.* (1999b) Occupational metal exposures and the risk of Parkinson's disease. *Neuroepidemiology*, **18**, 303–8.

Haan, M.N., Miller, J.W., Aiello, A.E., *et al.* (2007) Homocysteine, B vitamins, and the incidence of dementia and cognitive impairment: results from the Sacramento Area Latino Study on Aging. *Am J Clin Nutr*, **85**, 511–7.

Hafler, D.A., Compston, A., Sawcer, S. *et al.* (2007) Risk alleles for multiple sclerosis identified by a genomewide study. *N Engl J Med*, **357**, 851–62.

Hagen, K., Vatten, L., Stovner, L. J., *et al.* (2002a) Low socio-economic status is associated with increased risk of frequent headache: a prospective study of 22718 adults in Norway. *Cephalalgia*, **22**, 672–9.

Hagen, K., Zwart, J.A., Vatten, L., *et al.* (2000) Prevalence of migraine and non-migrainous headache—head-HUNT, a large population-based study. *Cephalalgia*, **20**, 900–6.

Haines, J.L., Ter-Minassian, M., Bazyk, A., *et al.* (1996) A complete genomic screen for multiple sclerosis underscores a role for the major histocompatibility complex. The Multiple Sclerosis Genetics Group. *Nat Genet*, **13**, 469–71.

Hakim, A. J., Cherkas, L., El Zayat, S., *et al.* (2002) The genetic contribution to carpal tunnel syndrome in women: a twin study. *Arthritis Rheum*, **47**, 275–9.

Hansen, T., Skytthe, A., Stenager, E., *et al.* (2005) Concordance for multiple sclerosis in Danish twins: an update of a nationwide study. *Mult Scler*, **11**, 504–10.

Hauser, W.A. (1995) Epidemiology of epilepsy in children. *Neurosurg Clin N Am*, **6**, 419–29.

Hauser, W.A., Annegers, J.F. and Rocca, W.A. (1996) Descriptive epidemiology of epilepsy: contributions of population-based studies from Rochester, Minnesota. *Mayo Clin Proc*, **71**, 576–86.

Hawkes, C.H. (2007) Smoking is a risk factor for multiple sclerosis: a metanalysis. *Mult Scler*, **13**, 610–5.

Hayden, K.M., Zandi, P.P., Khachaturian, A.S., *et al.* (2007) Does NSAID use modify cognitive trajectories in the elderly? The Cache County study. *Neurology*, **69**, 275–82.

Henderson, V.W., Paganini-Hill, A., Miller, B. L., *et al.* (2000) Estrogen for Alzheimer's disease in women: randomized, double-blind, placebo-controlled trial. *Neurology*, **54**, 295–301.

Hendrie, H.C. (1998) Epidemiology of dementia and Alzheimer's disease. *Am J Geriatr Psychiatry*, **6**, S3–18.

Hernan, M.A., Olek, M.J. and Ascherio, A. (1999) Geographic variation of MS incidence in two prospective studies of US women. *Neurology*, **53**, 1711–8.

Herrera, B.M., Ramagopalan, S.V., Orton, S., *et al.* (2007) Parental transmission of MS in a population-based Canadian cohort. *Neurology*, **69**, 1208–12.

Hirtz, D., Thurman, D.J., Gwinn-Hardy, K., *et al.* (2007) How common are the 'common' neurologic disorders? *Neurology*, **68**, 326–37.

Holm, L., Cassidy, J.D., Carroll, L.J. and Borg, J. (2005) Summary of the WHO Collaborating Centre for Neurotrauma Task Force on Mild Traumatic Brain Injury. *J Rehabil Med*, **37**, 137–41.

Houston, D.J. and Richardson, L.E., JR. (2007) Motorcycle safety and the repeal of universal helmet laws. *Am J Public Health*, **97**, 2063–9.

Hu, G., Jousilahti, P., Nissinen, A., *et al.* (2006) Body mass index and the risk of Parkinson disease. *Neurology*, **67**, 1955–9.

Hu, X.H., Markson, L.E., Lipton, R.B., *et al.* (1999) Burden of migraine in the United States: disability and economic costs. *Arch Intern Med*, **159**, 813–8.

Islam, T., Gauderman, W.J., Cozen, W. *et al.* (2007) Childhood sun exposure influences risk of multiple sclerosis in monozygotic twins. *Neurology*, **69**, 381–8.

Jallon, P. and Latour, P. (2005) Epidemiology of idiopathic generalized epilepsies. *Epilepsia*, **46** Suppl 9, 10–4.

Jankovic, J., Rajput, A.H., Mcdermott, M.P., *et al.* (2000) The evolution of diagnosis in early Parkinson disease. Parkinson Study Group. *Arch Neurol*, **57**, 369–72.

Jorm, A.F. and Jolley, D. (1998) The incidence of dementia: a meta-analysis. *Neurology*, **51**, 728–33.

Kantarci, O.H., Barcellos, L.F., Atkinson, E.J., *et al.* (2006) Men transmit MS more often to their children vs women: the Carter effect. *Neurology*, **67**, 305–10.

Kara, I., Ozkok, E., Aydin, M., *et al.* (2007) Combined effects of ACE and MMP-3 polymorphisms on migraine development. *Cephalalgia*, **27**, 235–43.

Kara, I., Sazci, A., Ergul, E., *et al.* (2003) Association of the C677T and A1298C polymorphisms in the 5,10 methylenetetrahydrofolate reductase gene in patients with migraine risk. *Brain Res Mol Brain Res*, **111**, 84–90.

Katsarava, Z., Obermann, M., Yoon, M.S., *et al.* (2007) Prevalence of cluster headache in a population-based sample in Germany. *Cephalalgia*, **27**, 1014–9.

Keenan, H.T. and Bratton, S.L. (2006) Epidemiology and outcomes of pediatric traumatic brain injury. *Dev Neurosci*, **28**, 256–63.

Keenan, H.T., Runyan, D.K., Marshall, S.W., *et al.* (2003) A Population-Based Study of Inflicted Traumatic Brain Injury in Young Children. *JAMA*, **290**, 621–626.

Kegler, S.R., Coronado, V.G., Annest, J.L., *et al.* (2003) Estimating nonfatal traumatic brain injury hospitalizations using an urban/rural index. *J Head Trauma Rehabil*, **18**, 469–78.

Keltner, N.L. and Cooke, B.B. (2007) Biological perspectives: traumatic brain injury-war related. *Perspect Psychiatr Care*, **43**, 223–6.

Kelvin, E.A., Hesdorffer, D.C., Bagiella, E., *et al.* (2007) Prevalence of self-reported epilepsy in a multiracial and multiethnic community in New York City. *Epilepsy Res*, **77**, 141–50.

Koepsell, T.D., Kurland, B.F., Harel, O., *et al.* (2008) Education, cognitive function, and severity of neuropathology in Alzheimer disease. *Neurology*, **70**, 1725–7.

Kramer, U., Nevo, Y., Neufeld, M.Y., *et al.* (1998) Epidemiology of epilepsy in childhood: a cohort of 440 consecutive patients. *Pediatr Neurol*, **18**, 46–50.

Kukull, W.A. (2006) The growing global burden of dementia. *Lancet Neurol*, **5**, 199–200.

Kukull, W.A., Higdon, R., Bowen, J.D., *et al.* (2002) Dementia and Alzheimer disease incidence: a prospective cohort study. *Arch Neurol*, **59**, 1737–46.

Kuopio, A.M., Marttila, R.J., Helenius, H., *et al.* (1999) Environmental risk factors in Parkinson's disease. *Mov Disord*, **14**, 928–39.

Kurth, T., Slomke, M.A., Kase, C.S., *et al.* (2005) Migraine, headache, and the risk of stroke in women: a prospective study. *Neurology*, **64**, 1020–6.

Kurtz, Z., Tookey, P. and Ross, E. (1998) Epilepsy in young people: 23 year follow up of the British national child development study. *Bmj*, **316**, 339–42.

Kurtzke, J.F. (2005) Epidemiology and etiology of multiple sclerosis. *Phys Med Rehabil Clin N Am*, **16**, 327–49.

Kurtzke, J.F. and Heltberg, A. (2001) Multiple sclerosis in the Faroe Islands: an epitome. *J Clin Epidemiol*, **54**, 1–22.

Kwong, L.K., Neumann, M., Sampathu, D.M., *et al.* (2007) TDP-43 proteinopathy: the neuropathology underlying major forms of sporadic and familial frontotemporal lobar degeneration and motor neuron disease. *Acta Neuropathol*, **114**, 63–70.

Lam, W.H. and Mackersie, A. (1999) Paediatric head injury: incidence, aetiology and management. *Paediatr Anaesth*, **9**, 377–85.

Langston, J.W. (2006) The Parkinson's complex: Parkinsonism is just the tip of the iceberg. *Ann Neurol*, **59**, 591–6.

Langston, J.W., Ballard, P., Tetrud, J.W., *et al.* (1983) Chronic Parkinsonism in humans due to a product of meperidine-analog synthesis. *Science*, **219**, 979–80.

Larocca, N.G., Scheinberg, L.C., Slater, R.J., *et al.* (1984) Field testing of a minimal record of disability in multiple sclerosis: the United States and Canada. *Acta Neurol Scand* Suppl, **101**, 126–38.

Launer, L.J., Andersen, K., Dewey, M.E., Letenneur, L., Ott, A., Amaducci, L.A. *et al.* (1999) Rates and risk factors for dementia and Alzheimer's disease: results from EURODEM pooled analyses. EURODEM Incidence Research Group and Work Groups. European Studies of Dementia. *Neurology*, **52**, 78–84.

Lea, R.A., Dohy, A., Jordan, K., *et al.* (2000) Evidence for allelic association of the dopamine beta-hydroxylase gene (DBH) with susceptibility to typical migraine. *Neurogenetics*, **3**, 35–40.

Lee, P.N. (1994) Smoking and Alzheimer's disease: a review of the epidemiological evidence. *Neuroepidemiology*, **13**, 131–44.

Leidy, N.K., Elixhauser, A., Vickrey, B., *et al.* (1999) Seizure frequency and the health-related quality of life of adults with epilepsy. *Neurology*, **53**, 162–6.

Leonardi, M., Steiner, T.J., Scher, A.T., *et al.* (2005) The global burden of migraine: measuring disability in headache disorders with WHO's Classification of Functioning, Disability and Health (ICF). *J Headache Pain*, **6**, 429–40.

Lhatoo, S.D. and Sander, J.W. (2005) Cause-specific mortality in epilepsy. *Epilepsia*, **46** Suppl 11, 36–9.

LIPPA, C. F., DUDA, J. E., GROSSMAN, M., *et al.* (2007) DLB and PDD boundary issues: diagnosis, treatment, molecular pathology, and biomarkers. *Neurology*, **68**, 812–9.

Lipton, R.B. (1998) Comorbidity in migraine—causes and effects. *Cephalalgia*, **18** Suppl 22, 8–11; discussion 11–4.

Lipton, R.B., B1, M.E., Diamond, M., *et al.* (2007) Migraine prevalence, disease burden, and the need for preventive therapy. *Neurology*, **68**, 343–9.

Lipton, R.B., Stewart, W.F. and Simon, D. (1998) Medical consultation for migraine: results from the American Migraine Study. *Headache*, **38**, 87–96.

Loiseau, J., Picot, M.C. and Loiseau, P. (1999) Short-term mortality after a first epileptic seizure: a population-based study. *Epilepsia*, **40**, 1388–92.

Lopez, O.L., Kuller, L.H., Becker, J.T., *et al.* (2007) Incidence of dementia in mild cognitive impairment in the cardiovascular health study cognition study. *Arch Neurol*, **64**, 416–20.

Lublin, F.D. and Reingold, S.C. (1996) Defining the clinical course of multiple sclerosis: results of an international survey. National Multiple Sclerosis Society (USA) Advisory Committee on Clinical Trials of New Agents in Multiple Sclerosis. *Neurology*, **46**, 907–11.

Lyngberg, A.C., Rasmussen, B.K., Jorgensen, T., *et al.* (2005a) Has the prevalence of migraine and tension-type headache changed over a 12-year period? A Danish population survey. *Eur J Epidemiol*, **20**, 243–9.

Lyngberg, A.C., Rasmussen, B. K., Jorgensen, T., *et al.* (2005b) Prognosis of migraine and tension-type headache: a population-based follow-up study. *Neurology*, **65**, 580–5.

Macclellan, L.R., Giles, W., Cole, J., *et al.* (2007) Probable migraine with visual aura and risk of ischemic stroke: the stroke prevention in young women study. *Stroke*, **38**, 2438–45.

Mackenzie, I.R. and Rademakers, R. (2007) The molecular genetics and neuropathology of frontotemporal lobar degeneration: recent developments. *Neurogenetics*, **8**, 237–48.

Maraganore, D.M., Farrer, M.J., Hardy, J.A., *et al.* (2000) Case–control study of debrisoquine 4-hydroxylase, N-acetyltransferase 2, and apolipoprotein E gene polymorphisms in Parkinson's disease. *Mov Disord*, **15**, 714–9.

Marder, K., Logroscino, G., Alfaro, B., *et al.* (1998) Environmental risk factors for Parkinson's disease in an urban multiethnic community. *Neurology*, **50**, 279–81.

Marder, K., Tang, M.X., Alfaro, B., *et al.* (1999) Risk of Alzheimer's disease in relatives of Parkinson's disease patients with and without dementia. *Neurology*, **52**, 719–24.

Marrie, R.A., Cutter, G., Tyry, T., *et al.* (2005) Changes in the ascertainment of multiple sclerosis. *Neurology*, **65**, 1066–70.

Martyn, C.N. and Hughes, R.A. (1997) Epidemiology of peripheral neuropathy. *J Neurol Neurosurg Psychiatry*, **62**, 310–8.

McDonald, W.I., Compston, A., Edan, G., *et al.* (2001) Recommended diagnostic criteria for multiple sclerosis: guidelines from the International Panel on the diagnosis of multiple sclerosis. *Ann Neurol*, **50**, 121–7.

Mckeith, I.G. (2006) Consensus guidelines for the clinical and pathologic diagnosis of dementia with Lewy bodies (DLB): report of the Consortium on DLB International Workshop. *J Alzheimers Dis*, **9**, 417–23.

Mehta, K.M., Ott, A., Kalmijn, S., *et al.* (1999) Head trauma and risk of dementia and Alzheimer's disease: The Rotterdam Study. *Neurology*, **53**, 1959–62.

Menegon, A., Board, P.G., Blackburn, A.C., *et al.* (1998) Parkinson's disease, pesticides, and glutathione transferase polymorphisms [see comments]. *Lancet*, **352**, 1344–6.

Merikangas, K.R., Fenton, B.T., Cheng, S.H., *et al.* (1997) Association between migraine and stroke in a large-scale epidemiological study of the United States. *Arch Neurol*, **54**, 362–8.

Merikangas, K.R., Whitaker, A.E., Isler, H., *et al.* (1994) The Zurich Study: XXIII. Epidemiology of headache syndromes in the Zurich cohort study of young adults. *Eur Arch Psychiatry Clin Neurosci*, **244**, 145–52.

Mesulam, M., Johnson, N., Krefft, T.A., *et al.* (2007) Progranulin mutations in primary progressive aphasia: the PPA1 and PPA3 families. *Arch Neurol*, **64**, 43–7.

Mikaeloff, Y., Caridade, G., Tardieu, M., *et al.* (2007) Parental smoking at home and the risk of childhood-onset multiple sclerosis in children. *Brain*, **130**, 2589–95.

Minden, K., Niewerth, M., Listing, J., *et al.* (2004) Burden and cost of illness in patients with juvenile idiopathic arthritis. *Ann Rheum Dis*, **63**, 836–42.

Moceri, V.M., Kukull, W.A., Emanuel, I., *et al.* (2000) Early-life risk factors and the development of Alzheimer's disease. *Neurology*, **54**, 415–20.

Mold, J.W., Vesely, S.K., Keyl, B.A., *et al.* (2004) The prevalence, predictors, and consequences of peripheral sensory neuropathy in older patients. *J Am Board Fam Pract*, **17**, 309–18.

Monahan, K. and O'Leary, K.D. (1999) Head injury and battered women: an initial inquiry. *Health Soc Work*, **24**, 269–78.

Morgante, L., Rocca, W.A., Di Rosa, A.E., *et al.* (1992) Prevalence of Parkinson's disease and other types of Parkinsonism: a door-to-door survey in three Sicilian municipalities. The Sicilian Neuro-Epidemiologic Study (SNES) Group. *Neurology*, **42**, 1901–7.

Morimoto, R.I. (2006) Stress, aging, and neurodegenerative disease. *N Engl J Med*, **355**, 2254–5.

Morris, J.C. (2006) Mild cognitive impairment is early-stage Alzheimer disease: time to revise diagnostic criteria. *Arch Neurol*, **63**, 15–6.

Multhaup, G. (2006) Amyloid precursor protein and BACE function as oligomers. *Neurodegener Dis*, **3**, 270–4.

Munger, K.L., Levin, L.I., Hollis, B.W., *et al.* (2006) Serum 25-hydroxyvitamin D levels and risk of multiple sclerosis. *JAMA*, **296**, 2832–8.

Munger, K.L., Peeling, R.W., Hernan, M.A., *et al.* (2003) Infection with Chlamydia pneumoniae and risk of multiple sclerosis. *Epidemiology*, **14**, 141–7.

Murray, M.E., Knopman, D.S. and Dickson, D.W. (2007) Vascular dementia: clinical, neuroradiologic and neuropathologic aspects. *Panminerva Med*, **49**, 197–207.

Nashef, L., Hindocha, N. and Makoff, A. (2007) Risk factors in sudden death in epilepsy (SUDEP): the quest for mechanisms. *Epilepsia*, **48**, 859–71.

Nee, L.E. & Lippa, C.F. (1999) Alzheimer's disease in 22 twin pairs—13-year follow-up: hormonal, infectious and traumatic factors. *Dement Geriatr Cogn Disord*, **10**, 148–51.

Newman, A.B., Fitzpatrick, A.L., Lopez, O., *et al.* (2005) Dementia and Alzheimer's disease incidence in relationship to cardiovascular disease in the Cardiovascular Health Study cohort. *J Am Geriatr Soc*, **53**, 1101–7.

Nicoletti, A., Reggio, A., Bartoloni, A., *et al.* (1998) A neuroepidemiological survey in rural Bolivia: background and methods. *Neuroepidemiology*, **17**, 273–80.

Nicoletti, A., Reggio, A., Bartoloni, A., *et al.* (1999) Prevalence of epilepsy in rural Bolivia: a door-to-door survey. *Neurology*, **53**, 2064–9.

Nielsen, N.M., Westergaard, T., Rostgaard, K., *et al.* (2005) Familial risk of multiple sclerosis: a nationwide cohort study. *Am J Epidemiol*, **162**, 774–8.

Nilsson, L., Farahmand, B.Y., Persson, P.G., *et al.* (1999) Risk factors for sudden unexpected death in epilepsy: a case–control study. *Lancet*, **353**, 888–93.

Nilsson, L., Tomson, T., Farahmand, B. Y., *et al.* (1997) Cause-specific mortality in epilepsy: a cohort study of more than 9,000 patients once hospitalized for epilepsy [see comments]. *Epilepsia*, **38**, 1062–8.

Nordstrom, D.L., Destefano, F., Vierkant, R.A., *et al.* (1998) Incidence of diagnosed carpal tunnel syndrome in a general population. *Epidemiology*, **9**, 342–5.

Noseworthy, J.H., Lucchinetti, C., Rodriguez, M., *et al.* G. (2000) Multiple sclerosis. *N Engl J Med*, **343**, 938–52.

Nourhashemi, F., Gillette-Guyonnet, S., Andrieu, S., *et al.* (2000) Alzheimer disease: protective factors. *Am J Clin Nutr*, **71**, 643S–649S.

Nyholt, D.R., Dawkins, J.L., Brimage, P. J., *et al.* (1998) Evidence for an X-linked genetic component in familial typical migraine. *Hum Mol Genet*, **7**, 459–63.

O'Brien, B., Goeree, R. and Streiner, D. (1994) Prevalence of migraine headache in Canada: a population-based survey. *Int J Epidemiol*, **23**, 1020–6.

Octave, J.N., Essalmani, R., Tasiaux, B., *et al.* (2000) The role of presenilin-1 in the gamma-secretase cleavage of the amyloid precursor protein of Alzheimer's disease. *J Biol Chem*, **275**, 1525–8.

Okie, S. (2005) Traumatic brain injury in the war zone. *N Engl J Med*, **352**, 2043–7.

Olafsson, E. and Hauser, W.A. (1999) Prevalence of epilepsy in rural Iceland: a population-based study. *Epilepsia*, **40**, 1529–34.

Ooi, W.W. and Srinivasan, J. (2004) Leprosy and the peripheral nervous system: basic and clinical aspects. *Muscle Nerve*, **30**, 393–409.

Orchard, T.J., Ce, L.L., Maser, R.E., *et al.* (1996) Why does diabetic autonomic neuropathy predict IDDM mortality? An analysis from the Pittsburgh Epidemiology of Diabetes Complications Study. *Diabetes Res Clin Pract*, **34** Suppl, S165–71.

Orton, S.M., Herrera, B.M., Yee, I.M., *et al.* (2006) Sex ratio of multiple sclerosis in Canada: a longitudinal study. *Lancet Neurol*, **5**, 932–6.

Osuntokun, B.O., Adeuja, A.O., Nottidge, V.A., *et al.* (1992) Prevalence of headache and migrainous headache in Nigerian Africans: a community-based study. *East Afr Med J*, **69**, 196–9.

Palacio, L.G., Jimenez, I., Garcia, H.H., *et al.* (1998) Neurocysticercosis in persons with epilepsy in Medellin, Colombia. The Neuroepidemiological Research Group of Antioquia. *Epilepsia*, **39**, 1334–9.

Parry, O., Mielke, J., Latif, A.S., *et al.* (1997) Peripheral neuropathy in individuals with HIV infection in Zimbabwe. *Acta Neurol Scand*, **96**, 218–22.

Petersen, R.C. (2007) Mild cognitive impairment: current research and clinical implications. *Semin Neurol*, **27**, 22–31.

Petersen, R.C., Smith, G.E., Waring, S.C., *et al.* (1999) Mild cognitive impairment: clinical characterization and outcome [published erratum appears in Arch Neurol 1999 Jun;56(6):760]. *Arch Neurol*, **56**, 303–8.

Petrovitch, H., Ross, G.W., Abbott, R.D., *et al.* (2002) Plantation work and risk of Parkinson disease in a population-based longitudinal study. *Arch Neurol*, **59**, 1787–92.

Pine, D.S., Cohen, P. and Brook, J. (1996) The association between major depression and headache: results of a longitudinal epidemiologic study in youth. *J Child Adolesc Psychopharmacol*, **6**, 153–64.

Polman, C.H., Reingold, S.C., Edan, G., *et al.* (2005) Diagnostic criteria for multiple sclerosis: 2005 revisions to the 'McDonald Criteria'. *Ann Neurol*, **58**, 840–6.

Poser, S. and Kurtzke, J.F. (1991) Epidemiology of MS. *Neurology*, **41**, 157–8.

Power, T., Catroppa, C., Coleman, L., *et al.* (2007) Do lesion site and severity predict deficits in attentional control after preschool traumatic brain injury (TBI)? *Brain Inj*, **21**, 279–92.

Pugliatti, M., Rosati, G., Carton, H., *et al.* (2006) The epidemiology of multiple sclerosis in Europe. *Eur J Neurol*, **13**, 700–22.

Rademakers, R. and Hutton, M. (2007) The genetics of frontotemporal lobar degeneration. *Curr Neurol Neurosci Rep*, **7**, 434–42.

Rasmussen, B.K. (1995) Epidemiology of headache. *Cephalalgia*, **15**, 45–68.

Rayan, G.M. (1999) Carpal tunnel syndrome between two centuries. *J Okla State Med Assoc*, **92**, 493–503.

Rezendes, J.L. (2006) Bicycle helmets: overcoming barriers to use and increasing effectiveness. *J Pediatr Nurs*, **21**, 35–44.

Ritz, B., Ascherio, A., Checkoway, H., *et al.* (2007) Pooled analysis of tobacco use and risk of Parkinson disease. *Arch Neurol*, **64**, 990–7.

Rocca, W.A., Bower, J.H., Ahlskog, J.E., *et al.* (2007) Risk of cognitive impairment or dementia in relatives of patients with Parkinson disease. *Arch Neurol*, **64**, 1458–64.

Rocca, W.A., Cha, R.H., Waring, S.C., *et al.* (1998) Incidence of dementia and Alzheimer's disease: a reanalysis of data from Rochester, Minnesota, 1975–1984. *Am J Epidemiol*, **148**, 51–62.

Rockwood, K., Wentzel, C., Hachinski, V., *et al.* (2000) Prevalence and outcomes of vascular cognitive impairment. Vascular Cognitive Impairment Investigators of the Canadian Study of Health and Aging. *Neurology*, **54**, 447–51.

Roman, G.C. (1994) An epidemic in Cuba of optic neuropathy, sensorineural deafness, peripheral sensory neuropathy and dorsolateral myeloneuropathy. *J Neurol Sci*, **127**, 11–28.

Roman, G.C., Tatemichi, T.K., Erkinjuntti, T., *et al.* (1993) Vascular dementia: diagnostic criteria for research studies. Report of the NINDS-AIREN International Workshop [see comments]. *Neurology*, **43**, 250–60.

Roses, A.D. (1994) Apolipoprotein E is a relevant susceptibility gene that affects the rate of expression of Alzheimer's disease. *Neurobiol Aging*, **15**, S165–7.

Ross, G.W., Abbott, R.D., Petrovitch, H., *et al.* (2000) Association of coffee and caffeine intake with the risk of Parkinson disease. *JAMA*, **283**, 2674–9.

Rothman, K.J. and Greenland, S. (1998) Modern epidemiology, Philadelphia, Pa., Lippincott-Raven.

Rowe, C.C., Ng, S., Ackermann, U., *et al.* (2007) Imaging beta-amyloid burden in aging and dementia. *Neurology*, **68**, 1718–25.

Rowland, L.P. and Merritt, H.H. (1995) *Merritt's textbook of neurology*, Baltimore, Williams & Wilkins.

Russell, M.B., Levi, N. and Kaprio, J. (2007) Genetics of tension-type headache: A population based twin study. *Am J Med Genet B Neuropsychiatr Genet*, **144**, 982–6.

Rutland-Brown, W., Langlois, J.A., Thomas, K.E., *et al.* (2006) Incidence of traumatic brain injury in the United States, 2003. *J Head Trauma Rehabil*, **21**, 544–8.

Sadovnick, A.D., Bulman, D. and Ebers, G. C. (1991) Parent-child concordance in multiple sclerosis. *Ann Neurol*, **29**, 252–5.

Sanchez, A.L., Lindback, J., Schantz, P.M., *et al.* (1999) A population-based, case–control study of *Taenia solium* taeniasis and cysticercosis. *Ann Trop Med Parasitol*, **93**, 247–58.

Scher, A.I., Stewart, W.F., Ricci, J.A., *et al.* (2003) Factors associated with the onset and remission of chronic daily headache in a population-based study. *Pain*, **106**, 81–9.

Schneider, J.A., Arvanitakis, Z., Bang, W., *et al.* (2007) Mixed brain pathologies account for most dementia cases in community-dwelling older persons. *Neurology*, **69**, 2197–204.

Schofield, P.W., Tang, M., Marder, K., *et al.* (1997) Alzheimer's disease after remote head injury: an incidence study. *J Neurol Neurosurg Psychiatry*, **62**, 119–24.

Schumacher, G.A. (1966) Multiple sclerosis. *Arch Neurol*, **14**, 571–3.

Schwartz, B.S., Stewart, W.F. and Lipton, R.B. (1997) Lost workdays and decreased work effectiveness associated with headache in the workplace. *J Occup Environ Med*, **39**, 320–7.

Scordo, M.G., Dahl, M.L., Spina, E., *et al.* (2006) No association between CYP2D6 polymorphism and Alzheimer's disease in an Italian population. *Pharmacol Res*, **53**, 162–5.

Senanayake, N. and Roman, G.C. (1993) Epidemiology of epilepsy in developing countries. *Bull World Health Organ*, **71**, 247–58.

Shackleton, D.P., Westendorp, R.G., Trenite, D.G., *et al.* (1999) Mortality in patients with epilepsy: 40 years of follow up in a Dutch cohort study [see comments]. *J Neurol Neurosurg Psychiatry*, **66**, 636–40.

Shastry, B.S. and Giblin, F.J. (1999) Genes and susceptible loci of Alzheimer's disease. *Brain Res Bull*, **48**, 121–7.

Sherer, M., Struchen, M.A., Yablon, S.A., *et al.* (2008) Comparison of indices of TBI severity: Glasgow coma scale, length of coma, post-traumatic amnesia. *J Neurol Neurosurg Psychiatry*, **79**, 678–85.

Shumaker, S.A., Legault, C., Kuller, L., *et al.* (2004) Conjugated equine estrogens and incidence of probable dementia and mild cognitive impairment in postmenopausal women: Women's Health Initiative Memory Study. *JAMA*, **291**, 2947–58.

Sibley, W.A., Bamford, C.R., Clark, K., *et al.* (1991) A prospective study of physical trauma and multiple sclerosis. *J Neurol Neurosurg Psychiatry*, **54**, 584–9.

Skegg, D.C., Corwin, P.A., Craven, R.S., *et al.* (1987) Occurrence of multiple sclerosis in the north and south of New Zealand. *J Neurol Neurosurg Psychiatry*, **50**, 134–9.

Solomon, D.H., Katz, J.N., Bohn, R., *et al.* (1999) Nonoccupational risk factors for carpal tunnel syndrome. *J Gen Intern Med*, **14**, 310–4.

Sotgiu, S., Arru, G., Soderstrom, M., *et al.* (2006) Multiple sclerosis-associated retrovirus and optic neuritis. *Mult Scler*, **12**, 357–9.

Sperling, M.R., Feldman, H., Kinman, J., *et al.* (1999) Seizure control and mortality in epilepsy. *Ann Neurol*, **46**, 45–50.

St George-Hyslop, P.H. (2000) Molecular genetics of Alzheimer's disease. *Biol Psychiatry*, **47**, 183–99.

Stallings, S.P., Kasdan, M.L., Soergel, T.M., *et al.* (1997) A case–control study of obesity as a risk factor for carpal tunnel syndrome in a population of 600 patients presenting for independent medical examination. *J Hand Surg [Am]*, **22**, 211–5.

Steinlein, O. K. (1999) Gene defects in idiopathic epilepsy. *Rev Neurol (Paris)*, **155**, 450–3.

Stewart, W.F., Bigal, M.E., Kolodner, K., *et al.* (2006) Familial risk of migraine: variation by proband age at onset and headache severity. *Neurology*, **66**, 344–8.

Stewart, W.F., Lipton, R.B. and Liberman, J. (1996a) Variation in migraine prevalence by race. *Neurology*, **47**, 52–9.

STewart, W.F., Simon, D., Shechter, A., *et al.* (1995) Population variation in migraine prevalence: a meta-analysis. *J Clin Epidemiol*, **48**, 269–80.

Stovner, L., Hagen, K., Jensen, R., *et al.* (2007) The global burden of headache: a documentation of headache prevalence and disability worldwide. *Cephalalgia*, **27**, 193–210.

Svendsen, T., Lossius, M. and Nakken, K.O. (2007) Age-specific prevalence of epilepsy in Oppland County, Norway. *Acta Neurol Scand*, **116**, 307–11.

Svenson, L.W., Warren, S., Warren, K.G., *et al.* (2007) Prevalence of multiple sclerosis in First Nations people of Alberta. *Can J Neurol Sci*, **34**, 175–80.

Tagliaferri, F., Compagnone, C., Korsic, M., *et al.* (2006) A systematic review of brain injury epidemiology in Europe. *Acta Neurochir (Wien)*, **148**, 255–68; discussion 268.

Tagliati, M., Grinnell, J., Godbold, J., *et al.* (1999) Peripheral nerve function in HIV infection: clinical, electrophysiologic, and laboratory findings. *Arch Neurol*, **56**, 84–9.

Tesfaye, S., Stevens, L.K., Stephenson, J.M., *et al.* (1996) Prevalence of diabetic peripheral neuropathy and its relation to glycaemic control and potential risk factors: the EURODIAB IDDM Complications Study. *Diabetologia*, **39**, 1377–84.

Thompson, H.J., Mccormick, W.C. and Kagan, S.H. (2006) Traumatic brain injury in older adults: epidemiology, outcomes, and future implications. *J Am Geriatr Soc*, **54**, 1590–5.

Tietjen, G.E. (2000) The relationship of migraine and stroke. *Neuroepidemiology*, **19**, 13–9.

Tolnay, M. and Frank, S. (2007) Pathology and genetics of frontotemporal lobar degeneration: an update. *Clin Neuropathol*, **26**, 143–56.

Tomson, T., Walczak, T., Sillanpaa, M., *et al.* (2005) Sudden unexpected death in epilepsy: a review of incidence and risk factors. *Epilepsia*, **46** Suppl 11, 54–61.

Tonon, C., Guttmann, S., Volpini, M., *et al.* (2002) Prevalence and incidence of cluster headache in the Republic of San Marino. *Neurology*, **58**, 1407–9.

Torelli, P., Beghi, E. and Manzoni, G.C. (2005) Cluster headache prevalence in the Italian general population. *Neurology*, **64**, 469–74.

Trojanowski, J.Q. and Lee, V.M. (2002) Parkinson's disease and related synucleinopathies are a new class of nervous system amyloidoses. *Neurotoxicology*, **23**, 457–60.

Trojanowski, J.Q. and Mattson, M. P. (2003) Overview of protein aggregation in single, double, and triple neurodegenerative brain amyloidoses. *Neuromolecular Med*, **4**, 1–6.

Tsuang, D., Simpson, K., Larson, E.B., *et al.* (2006) Predicting lewy body pathology in a community-based sample with clinical diagnosis of Alzheimer's disease. *J Geriatr Psychiatry Neurol*, **19**, 195–201.

Tyas, S.L., Tate, R.B., Wooldrage, K., *et al.* (2006) Estimating the incidence of dementia: the impact of adjusting for subject attrition using health care utilization data. *Ann Epidemiol*, **16**, 477–84.

Uldall, P., Alving, J., Hansen, L.K., *et al.* (2006) The misdiagnosis of epilepsy in children admitted to a tertiary epilepsy centre with paroxysmal events. *Arch Dis Child*, **91**, 219–21.

Ulrich, V., Gervil, M., Kyvik, K.O., *et al.* (1999) Evidence of a genetic factor in migraine with aura: a population-based Danish twin study. *Ann Neurol*, **45**, 242–6.

Wallin, M.T., Page, W.F. and Kurtzke, J. F. (2004) Multiple sclerosis in US veterans of the Vietnam era and later military service: race, sex, and geography. *Ann Neurol*, **55**, 65–71.

Wang, S.J., Fuh, J.L., Lu, S.R., *et al.* (2001) Quality of life differs among headache diagnoses: analysis of SF-36 survey in 901 headache patients. *Pain*, **89**, 285–92.

Warden, D. (2006) Military TBI during the Iraq and Afghanistan wars. *J Head Trauma Rehabil*, **21**, 398–402.

Werner, C. and Engelhard, K. (2007) Pathophysiology of traumatic brain injury. *Br J Anaesth*, **99**, 4–9.

Whitmer, R.A., Gunderson, E.P., Quesenberry, C.P., JR., *et al.* (2007) Body mass index in midlife and risk of Alzheimer disease and vascular dementia. *Curr Alzheimer Res*, **4**, 103–9.

Winblad, B., Palmer, K., Kivipelto, M., *et al.* (2004) Mild cognitive impairment—beyond controversies, towards a consensus: report of the International Working Group on Mild Cognitive Impairment. *J Intern Med*, **256**, 240–6.

Yuki, N. (2007) Ganglioside mimicry and peripheral nerve disease. *Muscle Nerve*, **35**, 691–711.

Zarrelli, M.M., Beghi, E., Rocca, W.A., *et al.* (1999) Incidence of epileptic syndromes in Rochester, Minnesota: 1980–1984. *Epilepsia*, **40**, 1708–14.

Zhao, J., Fu, Y., Yasvoina, M., Shao, P., *et al.* (2007) Beta-site amyloid precursor protein cleaving enzyme 1 levels become elevated in neurons around amyloid plaques: implications for Alzheimer's disease pathogenesis. *J Neurosci*, **27**, 3639–49.

Ziegler, D.K., Hur, Y.M., Bouchard, T.J., JR., *et al.* (1998) Migraine in twins raised together and apart. *Headache*, **38**, 417–22.

The transmissible spongiform encephalopathies

Richard S.G. Knight and Hester J.T. Ward

Abstract

Prion diseases are a group of animal and human diseases having disparate causes, distributions, and clinical pictures, but are unified by a common neurodegenerative pathology, the common central role of the prion protein, and a shared potential for transmissibility (even in those instances where the primary cause is apparently spontaneous or genetic). This potential transmissibility from animal to man (e.g. variant Creutzfeldt–Jakob disease [vCJD] resulting from bovine spongiform encephalopathy [BSE] dietary contamination) or from human to human (via various means, most recently by blood transfusion) gives these illnesses their specific public health importance.

Introduction

Prion diseases, also known as transmissible spongiform encephalopathies, are a group of animal and human illnesses united by broadly similar pathological features and transmissible potential (Table 9.11.1a). The most common human prion disease is Creutzfeldt–Jakob disease (CJD); this has been divided into four forms on the basis of differing clinicopathological features and cause (Table 9.11.1b). The transmissibility of prion diseases raises important public health concerns, in relation to both animal-to-human and human-to-human disease. To date, the principal occurrences of transmission have been therapy with cadaver-derived human growth hormone (hGH), surgical use of human dura mater grafts, and BSE contamination of human diet. More recently, there has been increasing concern about secondary transmission of vCJD via blood and blood products.

One form of prion disease, kuru, is exclusively an acquired human illness based on person-to-person transmission, albeit by unusual means, namely ritual mourning cannibalism. Kuru is confined to the Fore group in Papua New Guinea and, following the cessation of cannibilistic feasts, a very significant decline in the number of cases, from being the commonest cause of adult female death in the affected area to being a rarity, has been observed (Cervenakova et al. 1998).

The nature of prion diseases

Prion diseases are invariably progressive, ultimately fatal neurological illnesses. The underlying pathological changes in the brain are essentially neurodegenerative, involving neuronal loss, astrocytic hyperplasia, spongiform change, and deposition of an abnormal form of prion protein (the most characteristic feature of these diseases) (DeArmond et al. 2004). Prion protein (PrP) is a normal cellular protein encoded, in humans, by PRNP, the prion protein gene on chromosome 20. The precise function of the normal prion protein (PrP^C) is uncertain. In prion diseases, PrP^C undergoes a post-translational conformational change to an abnormal, disease-related, structure designated PrP^{Sc} (Prusiner 2004a). The pathogenesis of prion diseases is uncertain; the precise relationship between the protein conversion or its tissue deposition and the neuronal damage has not been established. In animals or humans affected by prion diseases, the clinical manifestations are purely neurological; there are no typical systemic responses to infection (such as fever), no detectable antibody responses, and no non-neurological symptoms (even when PrP^{Sc} is found in non-neurological tissues).

When PrP^{Sc} is obtained from prion disease tissue, it has varying molecular features. After treatment with proteases, the protease-resistant fragment has different sizes, and has been termed Type I or Type II on this basis. PrP has two glycosylation sites and thus exists in non-, mono-, and diglycosylated forms. It is now routine practice to classify prion diseases partly according to the PrP^{Sc} type and the ratio of glycoforms found, the most commonly used protein classification being Type I, Type IIA, and Type IIB (Parchi et al. 1996; Head et al. 2004). The exact significance of this protein classification is unclear and it is not entirely straightforward: Different protein types can be found in one brain (Head et al. 2004). However, the classification has utility; for example, Type IIB in humans is unique to vCJD. PRNP, and the equivalent gene in animals, is important for two reasons: Firstly, pathogenic mutations are apparently responsible for genetic forms of prion disease (Kovacs et al. 2002); secondly, polymorphisms in the gene have important potential effects on susceptibility to developing disease, the incubation period, and the resulting clinicopathological phenotype (Parchi et al. 1999).

At codon 129 of PRNP, an individual may code either for methionine (M) or valine (V); therefore, each person can be PRNP-129 MM, PRNP-129 MV, or PRNP-129 VV. The distribution of these different genotypes in normal populations shows some geographic variation (Nurmi et al. 2003). The significance of this is particularly illustrated by the fact that all examined cases of vCJD to date have been of the MM genotype (Clarke & Ghani 2005). In acquired

Table 9.11.1a Prion diseases: the transmissible spongiform encephalopathies

	Disease	Comments
Animal diseases	Scrapie	Natural disease of sheep and goats
	Bovine spongiform encephalopathy (BSE)	Primarily affected cattle Secondary transmission to feline species and exotic ungulates
	Feline spongiform encephalopathy (FSE)	Prion disease caused by BSE transmission to feline species
	Chronic wasting disease (CWD)	Natural disease of cervid species in North America
	Transmissible mink encephalopathy (TME)	Disease of farmed mink
	Atypical scrapie	Recently identified atypical form of scrapie in sheep
	H-type and L-type BSE	Recently described atypical forms of bovine prion disease
Human diseases	Creutzfeldt–Jakob disease (CJD)	The commonest human prion disease. Subclassified into four types (see Table 9.11.1b)
	Gerstmann-Sträussler-Scheinker syndrome (GSSS)	A genetic prion disease
	Fatal familial insomnia (FFI)	A very rare genetic prion disease
	Sporadic fatal insomnia (SFI)	Extremely rare form of prion disease with similar phenotype to FFI, but of sporadic, non-genetic occurrence
	Kuru	A disease confined to a region of Papua New Guinea, spread via cannibalistic mourning rites

Table 9.11.1b The different types of CJD

Type	Comments
Sporadic (sCJD)	Commonest form (but with an annual mortality rate of only 1–2/million). Worldwide distribution; cause unknown. Principally affects the middle-aged and the elderly
Genetic (gCJD)	Resulting from mutations in the *PRNP* gene. Autosomal dominant inheritance
Variant (vCJD)	Due to BSE infection. Most cases in the United Kingdom. Relatively young age group affected compared to sCJD
Iatrogenic (iCJD)	Due to secondary transmission of human prion disease via medical and surgical procedures. Recently, blood transfusions implicated in vCJD transmission (see Table 9.11.2)

direct (giving definitive evidence of transmissibility) but slow and expensive, the incubation period being generally of several months in rodents, for example (Bruce 2003). There are also associated difficulties due to potential differences in susceptibility between humans and, for example, rodents. The second is simpler, quicker, and cheaper from the laboratory standpoint, but indirect (using PrP^{Sc} as a marker of infectivity). Both require appropriate tissue samples, which, in the case of human brain, are not straightforward to obtain in life and may be difficult to obtain after death, because of issues surrounding post-mortems and consent.

Surveillance of CJD

The UK National CJD Surveillance Unit (NCJDSU), Edinburgh, was established by the Department of Health in 1990 following the Southwood Committee Report (www.cjd.ed.ac.uk). The principal aim of the NCJDSU was to identify any changes in CJD in the United Kingdom, in the wake of the BSE epidemic in cattle, that could indicate transmission of BSE to man. Past records of CJD existed from a previous UK MRC-funded study that had run over a 5-year period (1980–84) and had also collected retrospective data from 1970 to 1979 (Will *et al.* 1986; Cousens *et al.* 1990). At the start of the 1990 surveillance period, cases were identified retrospectively for the period 1985–90. In 1996, the NCJDSU reported the emergence of a previously unrecognized form of CJD—vCJD (Will *et al.* 1996). The NCJDSU continues with UK CJD surveillance, identifying all cases of human prion disease, along with associated research particularly to examine risk factors for all UK cases of sCJD and vCJD, to investigate the geographic distribution of CJD, to identify mechanisms of transmission of BSE to humans, to establish short- and long-term trends, to evaluate potential risks of onward transmission, to identify novel forms of human prion diseases, and to evaluate case definitions and diagnostic tests. The UK National Prion Clinic in London has primary responsibility for the identification of UK genetic prion disease. The UK Institute of Child Health in London has primary responsibility for the identification of UK hGH-related CJD.

Many other countries have established CJD surveillance systems and there is active international collaboration that has achieved standardization of methodology, agreed case definitions, and also undertaken many research projects (www.eurocjd.ed.ac.uk)

prion diseases, the codon 129 genotype may affect the incubation period, as has been seen in hGH-related CJD and kuru: Individuals with either MV or VV genotypes may develop vCJD with a longer incubation period than those with the MM genotype (Cervenakova *et al.* 1998; Clarke & Ghani 2005; Huillard d'Aignaux *et al.* 2002a; Brandel *et al.* 2003). In Japan, but not in other countries, another *PRNP* polymorphism (at codon 219) has been shown to have effects on susceptibility and clinicopathological phenotype (Shibuya *et al.* 1998).

Despite their neurodegenerative pathology, prion diseases are transmissible and this gives rise to a number of important public health concerns. In general, transmissibility is associated with PrP^{Sc} and the prevailing view is that PrP^{Sc} is either the infectious agent or its major component (Prusiner 2004b). However, the exact nature of the agent is unknown. This has important implications for research and public health protection with only two methods of detecting infectivity in tissues: Laboratory animal transmission experiments and the identification of PrP^{Sc} in the tissue. The first is

(Pocchiari *et al.* 2004; Ladogana *et al.* 2005). The World Health Organization (WHO) has published guidelines for the diagnosis of prion diseases (World Health Organization 1998, 2002). This international approach allows the accumulation of data on significant numbers of cases in a rare disease and also provides good country comparative data; the initial identification of vCJD was undoubtedly helped by the ability to ascertain that, in 1996, similar cases had not been identified in countries other than the United Kingdom, the country principally affected by BSE.

In most of the European Union countries, cases of prion disease are subject to mandatory reporting rules, but UK surveillance is based on a relatively informal system. One problem of mandatory reporting of prion disease is the case definition for such reporting. There is no simple, non-invasive diagnostic test in life and pre-mortem diagnosis therefore heavily depends on clinical judgement. The internationally agreed, WHO-adopted, clinical diagnostic criteria may not identify clinically atypical cases and also require experience in their application; it is difficult for individual clinicians to obtain this, given the rarity of these diseases. The reporting of definite cases will, of course, identify only those cases with either cerebral biopsy (not a common procedure) or those with autopsy. In the United Kingdom, surveillance is run by local clinicians being asked to refer 'any case suspected of being prion disease' to the NCJDSU. The NCJDSU neurologists then assess the referral, visit the case, interview the family, and review the investigations. In the UK system, about half of the referred living suspect cases are finally classified as prion disease. Pathologists are asked to refer any cases identified by biopsy or at autopsy. Referrals to the NJCDSU also come from death certificates recorded with ICD-10 codes A810 and FO21.

The clinical diagnosis of prion disease is a relatively complex matter, involving a number of neurological differential diagnoses. A number of investigations are required; one cerebrospinal fluid (CSF) test (for 14-3-3 protein) has become an important part of assessment and case classification, especially with respect to sporadic CJD (sCJD) (Green *et al.* 2006). There is a national CSF protein laboratory service located within the NCJDSU. The possibility of obtaining advice or a clinical opinion from neurologists experienced with prion disease, and the provision of CSF laboratory and neuropathological services, encourages referral of cases, including atypical ones. Overlapping, multiple methods of case ascertainment (clinical referral, laboratory test provision, pathology referral, and death certificate review) serve to ensure that surveillance

is as complete as possible. The opportunity for expert, experienced advice, laboratory tests, and neuropathological studies has aided notification of suspect cases in other countries.

Sporadic CJD

Background

Sporadic CJD has a worldwide distribution with an annual mortality rate of around 1–2 per million population per year (Fig. 9.11.1) (Will *et al.* 2004). It is predominantly a disease of mid-to-late life, and with its neurodegenerative pathology, it would be placed alongside other diseases such as Alzheimer's disease, Parkinson's disease, and motor neuron disease, except for its transmissibility (Fig. 9.11.2). The typical clinical profile is of a rapidly progressing encephalopathy: The median duration in most countries is around 4 months (Pocchiari *et al.* 2004; Will *et al.* 2004). Dementia, cerebellar ataxia, and myoclonus are the most characteristic clinical features. The typical pathological findings, including spongiform change and PrP^{Sc} deposition, are confined to the central nervous system. There is, however, some clinicopathological variation, which includes the following: Presentation with a progressive isolated deficit (such as cerebellar ataxia or visual disturbance), atypically young onset, atypically long duration, and different PrP^{Sc} deposition patterns in the brain, including the presence of amyloid plaques in the brain (DeArmond *et al.* 2004; Ladogana *et al.* 2005; Boesenberger *et al.* 2005; Cooper *et al.* 2005; Cooper *et al.* 2006).

Cause

The cause is unknown. The two most favoured theories are spontaneous protein conversion and somatic *PRNP* mutation (Prusiner 2004a). The fact that sCJD is transmissible in the laboratory and can indeed be transmitted from person to person under special circumstances (such as neurosurgery) raises the question as to whether it is, in general, a naturally transmitted disease. There are three ways of exploring this possibility: Investigation of individual cases and their contacts (although this may produce essentially anecdotal evidence), statistical analysis of case clustering, and case–control studies. Despite its rarity, the epidemiology of sCJD has been studied in some detail and case–control studies have been undertaken, involving significant numbers of cases, because of both sustained surveillance over time within individual countries and international collaboration, with data pooling (Harries-Jones *et al.* 1988; Wientjens *et al.* 1996; Van Duijn *et al.* 1998; Collins

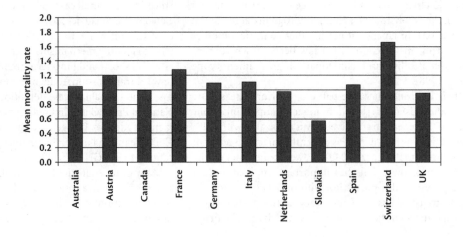

Fig. 9.11.1 Mean annual mortality rates for sCJD in several countries (1993–2006).

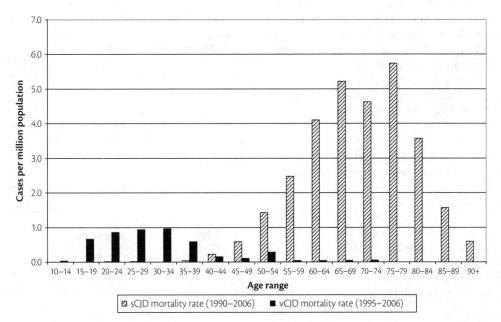

Fig. 9.11.2 Age-specific mortality rates for sCJD cases and variant Creutzfeldt–Jakob disease (vCJD) cases, by 5-year age group (the UK).

et al. 1999; Wilson *et al.* 2000; Zerr *et al.* 2000; Ward *et al.* 2002). Two large case–control studies in Australia and Europe (Collins *et al.* 1999; Ward *et al.* 2002) have shown an increased risk of sCJD associated with any surgery, which in the Australian study increased with increased number of operations. The Australian study found increased risk associated with a range of surgical procedures (carpal tunnel, eye, heart, haemorrhoid, gall bladder, hernia, hysterectomy, varicose vein), and the European study found a small increased risk associated with gynaecological surgery (and a reduced risk associated with tonsillectomy and appendicectomy). 'Other surgery' not categorized a priori into anatomical groups, such as stitches to the skin, was also shown to be associated with increased risk of sCJD in both studies.

Other smaller studies have reported varying findings related to medical risk and sCJD, but have lacked power and/or been subject to bias (Bobowick *et al.* 1973; Kondo & Kuroiwa 1982; Davanipour *et al.* 1985). Examination of clusters, or areas of high incidence of sCJD, has been carried out in various countries; some in fact proved to be due to genetic mutations rather than sCJD infection (in Slovakia, Chile, and among Libyan Jews in Israel) (Kahana *et al.* 1974; Brown *et al.* 1992; Lee *et al.* 1999). However, investigation of smaller clusters has been difficult to interpret (in Australia, England, France, Japan, and the United States) (Matthews 1975; Farmer *et al.* 1978; Will & Matthews 1982; Arakawa *et al.* 1991; Collins *et al.* 2002; Huillard d'Aignaux *et al.* 2002b). One statistical analysis of clustering of sCJD in the United Kingdom reported that cases lived closer together than might be expected by chance and the evidence for this increased the further in the past it was examined. These findings suggest that some sCJD cases may result from exposure to a common external factor years before clinical onset; however, identifying these common factors years after the event is very difficult (Linsell *et al.* 2004).

Although the prion hypothesis allows for the spontaneous conversion of PrP^C to PrP^{Sc}, exposure to an environmental agent, perhaps many years before disease onset, has not been ruled out. As described in the preceding subsection, case–control studies and examination of clusters have not produced convincing evidence of a route or exposure by which public health measures can be implemented to reduce the incidence of sCJD. Of course, it is possible that sCJD is a heterogeneous disease in terms of its cause.

Health risks

Although no definitive evidence that sCJD is a primarily acquired disease exists, it can certainly be secondarily transmitted. Over the years, there have been many instances of transmission, either of sCJD or presumed sCJD, through medical practice: Neurosurgical instruments, depth EEG electrodes, human dura mater grafts, corneal transplantation, and use of human-derived pituitary hormones (Brown *et al.* 2000; 2006) (Table 9.11.2).

Table 9.11.2 Summary of iatrogenic human prion disease

Procedure	Numbers reported[a]	Comments
Human growth hormone treatment	194	
Human dura mater grafts	196	Japan: 123 France: 13 Spain: 10 UK: 7
Neurosurgical instruments	4	
Depth EEG electrodes	2	
Corneal transplants	2	
Human gonadotrophin treatment	4	
Blood transfusion infection of vCJD	4	Three resulted in vCJD; one case of infection but no neurological disease at time of death.

[a] As of April 2007.

vCJD: variant Creutzfeldt–Jakob disease.

In sCJD, infectivity is present in significant amounts in central nervous system (CNS) tissue (including the pituitary gland) and the posterior eye (Peden *et al.* 2004) . Using conventional techniques, PrP^{Sc} is not found in peripheral tissues; particularly sensitive detection methods may reveal PrP^{Sc} deposition in tissues such as spleen and muscle (Glatzel *et al.* 2003a). Abnormal prion protein is not detectable in the dental pulp of sCJD cases (Blanquet-Grossard *et al.* 2000). The WHO recently published guidelines on the infectivity distribution of prion diseases (of both animals and humans) (World Health Organization 2006). The risk of transmission from non-CNS non-ocular tissues is generally very low, although transmission has been reported in experimental settings (Brown *et al.* 1994). Even though transfusion-transmitted vCJD infection has been reported, there have been no reported cases of sCJD transmitted via blood components or plasma products worldwide. As discussed in the preceding subsection, case–control studies of sCJD have not identified blood as a risk factor and have not produced consistent results concerning surgery. These matters are discussed in more detail in the subsections on iatrogenic CJD (iCJD) and public health measures.

Genetic prion diseases

Background

Human genetic prion diseases have been classified into three groups, originally according to clinicopathological characteristics: Genetic CJD, fatal familial insomnia, and Gerstmann–Staussler–Scheinker syndrome. The identification of pathogenic *PRNP* mutations allows for a more rational classification (Kovacs *et al.* 2005). The mode of inheritance is autosomal dominant. Penetrance is reportedly high, but may vary with mutation; in *PRNP* point mutation E200K, penetrance is complete (Spudich *et al.* 1995). A family history is not present in all cases (12–88 per cent); therefore, genetic prion disease cannot be absolutely excluded without *PRNP* sequencing (which can be performed straightforwardly on a blood sample) (Kovacs *et al.* 2005).

Cause

The current belief is that the mutations are directly disease causing. The idea that they represent particular susceptibility factors cannot be absolutely excluded.

Health risks

It is a curious and striking fact that an autosomally inherited gene mutation disease can potentially be transmitted to others who do not have the underlying mutation. Genetic prion disease therefore poses a public health risk one would not expect from its basic genetic cause. It is likely that the tissue distribution of infectivity is similar to that of sCJD (World Health Organization 2006). It is not known whether there is a significant risk of infection from an individual with a *PRNP* mutation in the pre-symptomatic period, but it is wise to assume that such is possibly the case. As is mentioned earlier, not all cases of genetic CJD have a recognized family history. It is assumed that iCJD results from initial sCJD cases; statistically this is probable, but it is possible that some arise from unsuspected genetic cases.

Primary variant CJD

Background

The recognition of BSE in the United Kingdom in 1986 gave rise to concerns that it could be transmitted to humans through diet, and

Table 9.11.3 Worldwide numbers of vCJD cases (as of April 2007)

Country*	Numbers (total)	Comments
United Kingdom	165	162 dietary, three blood transfusions
France	22	
Ireland	4	Two cases considered to have contracted the disease while in the United Kingdom
Italy	1	
United States	3	Two cases considered to have contracted the disease in the United Kingdom, one in Saudi Arabia
Canada	1	Considered to have contracted the disease while in the United Kingdom
Saudi Arabia	1	
Japan	1	Considered to have contracted the disease while in the United Kingdom
The Netherlands	2	
Portugal	1	
Spain	1	

* Cases attributed to country according to normal country of residence at time of illness onset; this may not be the country of exposure to infection (see 'Comments' column).

in 1996, a new form of human prion disease (vCJD) was reported in the United Kingdom (Will *et al.* 1996). There were alarming predictions of thousands or even millions of cases of vCJD but, to date, the epidemic has, fortunately, been much more limited (Clarke & Ghani 2005; Cousens *et al.* 1997).

The earliest recognized case had symptom onset in 1994, and by April 2007, 202 people had been diagnosed with vCJD worldwide, predominantly in the United Kingdom (Table 9.11.3). The basic epidemiology of vCJD is given in Table 9.11.4 (the age distribution among UK cases is also shown in Fig. 9.11.2). It is important to note that, by international agreement, cases of vCJD are attributed to the country where they are normally resident at the time of diagnosis. Especially given the potentially very long incubation period

Table 9.11.4 Basic epidemiology of vCJD in the United Kingdom

Age at onset	Mean: 28 years Median: 26 Range: 12–74
Age at death	Mean: 30 years Median: 28 Range: 14–74
Duration (based on deaths)	Median: 14 months Range: 6–40
Male:Female	92:73
PRNP codon 129*	100 per cent (145 tested)

* All tested cases in other countries have also been *PRNP* codon-129.

of this illness, this is not necessarily the same as the country where they contracted the infection. For example, 3 cases of vCJD have been attributed to the United States, but none of these were thought to have been infected in that country. Judgments as to the likely country of infection have to be based on the residential history of the individual and the estimated risk of BSE infection in that country during the relevant period. After the United Kingdom, France has reported the greatest number of cases, but modelling predicts a limited size to the epidemic, and with a lower total than for the United Kingdom (Alperovitch & Will 2002).

Clinicopathological features and diagnosis

Variant CJD typically presents as an essentially psychiatric disturbance, involving depression, anxiety, social withdrawal, and sometimes, more unusual symptoms such as hallucinations or delusions. The presenting clinical features in the first hundred UK cases have been described in detail by Spencer *et al.* (2002). Symptoms such as chorea, dystonia, and painful sensory disturbances are not uncommon, and with progression, other clearly neurological features appear, including cerebellar ataxia and dementia (Will *et al.* 2004).

The clinical and neuropathological picture is significantly different from that seen in sCJD (DeArmond *et al.* 2004). One particular difference of clinical and public health importance between vCJD and other forms of CJD is that, in vCJD, lymphoreticular tissue (tonsil, appendix, other gut-associated lymphoid tissue, lymph nodes, and spleen) show significant levels of PrPSc deposition and infectivity even during the incubation period (Hilton *et al.* 1998, 2004; Ironside *et al.* 2000). Infectivity in the CNS in vCJD is thought to arise later in the incubation period and reaches much higher infectivity levels than that seen in the lymphoreticular tissues.

Definite diagnosis requires brain tissue and is usually at autopsy, but in some situations, brain biopsy is performed. Clinical diagnosis depends on the exclusion of other possible diagnoses, the presence of characteristic brain MRI findings, and in some cases, tonsil biopsy (Hill *et al.* 1999; Collie *et al.* 2003). Primary vCJD cases, that is, those considered to be due to BSE contamination of foodstuffs, are considered in this subsection. Secondary infection from primary vCJD cases has been so far identified only through blood transfusion (as of August 2008, four reported instances) and is discussed in a separate subsection.

Cause

The causal linkage of vCJD to BSE has three broad bases: vCJD and BSE have the same causative agent, the agent passed from cattle to man, and the passage was via diet (Knight 1999). There are laboratory studies showing that the BSE and vCJD agents have identical biological and molecular properties (although it has to be borne in mind that the agent itself has not been fully characterized) (Bruce *et al.* 1997; Hill *et al.* 1997). All of the epidemiological evidence suggests that the agent passed from cattle to man. BSE-infected material clearly entered human food in significant amounts. There is some support for the dietary cause from a UK case–control study, and possible routes of infection other than diet are not supported by the accumulated epidemiological data (including case–control study) (Ward *et al.* 2006). This causal explanation does not have absolute proof, but it is beyond reasonable doubt.

The main dietary vehicle remains uncertain, but the main exposure was probably via bovine mechanically recovered meat (MRM) and head meat added to pre-prepared foodstuffs, such as burgers, meat pies, and sausages. It is notable that, in the United Kingdom, MRM was prepared from vertebral columns until the end of 1995. There is evidence that such vertebral columns could have contained significant residual spinal cord and also dorsal root ganglia (both materials containing significantly high infectivity) (Will 1998).

An excess of vCJD cases in the north of the United Kingdom, compared with the south, was first described in 2001 (Cousens *et al.* 2001). The excess appears to have declined over time but still remains, with those living in the north of the United Kingdom in 1991 being about one and a half times more likely to have developed vCJD than those residing in the south (rate ratio = 1.46; 95 per cent CIs: 1.07,2.01). The difference remains when the analysis is adjusted for socio-economic status, urban and rural mix, and population density. Although regional variations in diet might explain these observed differences, results of dietary analyses were inconsistent.

Health risks

The relevant health risks can be considered in two parts: The risk of contracting vCJD from BSE infection in diet and the risk of secondary human-to-human transmission, which is discussed in detail in the subsection on secondary vCJD.

Countries have been classified according to BSE risk status by the WHO, according to their particular incidence of BSE in cattle and their potential exposure from imports originating in BSE-affected countries (www.who.int).

From before the first human cases of BSE were recognized in the United Kingdom (in 1986) to approximately mid 1996, the UK population was exposed to BSE in food containing beef and beef products, and therefore was potentially at risk of vCJD (Anderson *et al.* 1996). Although the United Kingdom has had by far the greatest number of cases of BSE in cattle, other countries have been affected as well, with the Republic of Ireland having the next greatest number of cases, France coming third, and Portugal fourth. To some extent, this has been reflected in the number of cases of vCJD to date; however, the risk to a particular country must reflect imports of bovine material from high-risk countries (particularly the United Kingdom) as well as imports of BSE-affected cattle and intrinsic occurrence of BSE. With all diseases, the number of cases identified must depend on the methods of identification. Testing for BSE in cattle was introduced at different times, and in different ways, in different countries. The numbers of reported cases of BSE in cattle depend in part on whether surveillance is passive or active and the population tested; that is, clinically suspect cases, ill animals, animals discovered dead, or healthy animals slaughtered for human consumption. The European Union introduced new testing rules in January 2001, including the need for post-mortem testing of all apparently healthy cattle over 30 months of age at slaughter for human consumption. The figures for BSE in different countries can be obtained through the World Organization for Animal Health (OIE; www.oie.int). The true figures for BSE in many countries in the past remain subject to doubt; it is clear that numbers rose significantly in a number of EU countries after the introduction of the more comprehensive testing policy in 2001. For example, in Germany, only 6 cases of BSE were reported, all in imports, between 1989 and 2000; in 2000, 7 cases were reported, followed by 125 in 2001. In Italy, only 2 cases were reported between 1989 and 2000 (both in imports); in 2001, 48 cases were reported.

Many public health measures have been implemented to prevent transmission of BSE to humans from the 1980s onwards. These can be separated into those that were put in place in order to prevent onward transmission of BSE in cattle and those that were designed to break the chain of transmission from cattle to humans.

Prevention of onward transmission of BSE in cattle

In the United Kingdom, the ban on the use of ruminant protein in feed to ruminants was introduced in 1988, which was extended to pigs and poultry in 1990. In 1994, additional measures were introduced in the United Kingdom to prevent ruminants being fed any form of mammalian protein (with specific exceptions), and in 1996, it became illegal in the United Kingdom to feed any farmed livestock, including fishes and horses, with mammalian meat and bone meal.

Harmonized EU control measures were introduced in 2001, which included the ban on feeding of processed animal proteins to animals which are kept, fattened, or bred for food production. These control measures together with domestic controls have proved successful in significantly reducing the number of BSE cases across EU member states.

Prevention of dietary transmission to humans

Since 1988, under the UK Compulsory Slaughter and Compensation Scheme, all UK cattle suspected of suffering from BSE are slaughtered and sent for diagnosis. All BSE suspects are then destroyed by incineration. In addition, all adult animals presented for slaughter are inspected by veterinary surgeons to make sure that no suspected cases are slaughtered for human consumption.

Controls have existed since 1989 in the United Kingdom that ban certain tissues (specified risk material [SRM]) from cattle, sheep, and goats from entering the human food chain. Since 1989, the European Commission, in close cooperation with its member states, has taken a series of measures to manage the risk of BSE in the European Union. In 2000, harmonized SRM controls were introduced across all EU member states, and in 2001, EU-wide regulations laying down the rules for the prevention, control, and eradication of certain forms of transmissible spongiform encephalopathy (TSE) were introduced. These controls are enforced by domestic legislation.

In 1997 in the United Kingdom, bone-in-beef and beef bones were excluded from the human food chain to protect the public from BSE infectivity, which the UK Spongiform Encephalopathy Advisory Committee (SEAC) had evidence to link to cattle bones. The continuing decline in the BSE epidemic allowed the ban on retail sales to be lifted towards the end of 1999, although it was retained for manufacturing uses of both bone-in-beef and beef bones.

In the United Kingdom in 2005, a system of BSE testing was introduced for slaughtered cattle aged over 30 months (OTM) intended for human consumption. This system replaced the OTM rule that had been in place in the United Kingdom since 1996, which prohibited the sale of beef for human consumption from OTM cattle.

At the height of the BSE epidemic, there was considerable public concern about BSE and the safety of British meat. The UK Government set up an independent committee (SEAC) of leading experts to ensure that it received the best possible scientific advice surrounding TSEs. The UK Food Standards Agency was also established to protect public health and consumers interests in relation to food. In January 1998, the UK 'BSE Inquiry' was set up to 'establish and review the history of the emergence and identification of BSE and

new variant CJD in the United Kingdom, and of the action taken in response to it up to 20 March 1996; to reach conclusions on the adequacy of that response, taking into account the state of knowledge at the time' (www.bseinquiry.gov.uk). Different countries introduced human dietary protection measures at different times. For example, animal CNS material was reportedly still being used in the preparation of certain sausages in Germany in 2000 (Lucker et al. 2000). The present EU testing policy identifies infected animals and thereby prevents their entering human food.

The European Commission produced the TSE Roadmap in 2005 (http://ec.europa.eu/food/food/biosafety/bse/roadmap_en.pdf), which provided an outline of possible future changes to EU measures on BSE in the short, medium, and long term. Since 1995, the Commission has generated 70 primary and implementing acts setting out stringent measures to protect animal and human health at the community level. With indications of a favourable trend in the BSE epidemic, the goal for the coming years is to ensure relaxation of measures while assuring that a high level of food safety is maintained. Relaxation of measures is risk-based and aims to reflect advances in technology and evolving scientific knowledge.

Iatrogenic CJD

Background and cause

Evidence from animal studies and from humans shows that efficiency of transmission of prion diseases depends on the type of prion disease (the agent strain), the species barrier, the route of transmission, the dose of infectivity (relating to the tissue involved and the amount of that tissue), and the susceptibility of the 'host'. The concept of agent strain is a complex and controversial matter. For acquired diseases such as BSE, kuru, and vCJD, it is obviously necessary to consider the nature of the infectious agent; for diseases such as sCJD and gCJD, which are considered not to be acquired, the concept is less clear, although some sort of agent is required for their secondary transmission. Although the currently accepted theory is that the agent is based on PrP^{Sc} itself, the agent has not been finally characterized in any form of prion disease. Different strains of agent do exist, as indicated by persistent, reproducible, different biological behaviours, such as incubation period, neuropathological profile, and biochemical properties of the abnormal prion protein (Bruce 2003; Hill et al. 1997; Somerville et al. 1997; Safar et al. 1998). For example, scrapie infection from one source has a specific incubation period and neuropathological lesion profile distinguishable from those of scrapie from another source (Bruce 2003).

Taking BSE as the cause for vCJD, the BSE agent clearly behaves differently in humans, than the agent from sCJD. The basis of this strain variation is not yet understood. The concept of species barrier in prion disease is also incompletely understood. However, it is a commonly observed experimental feature. The ease of transmission from one species to another varies with species; the incubation period may be initially long, with shortening on serial passage in the new species (Bruce 2003). The route of transmission is very important, and there is no doubt that the most successful means overall is the inoculation of brain tissue directly into recipient brain. However, different diseases and/or agents behave differently and the BSE or vCJD agent appears to be relatively readily transmitted via blood through the intravenous route (Hunter et al. 2002). Further, different tissue distributions of infectivity are associated with different agents and/or diseases; for example, much greater lymphoreticular involvement exists in vCJD than in other human prion diseases. The world summary of iCJD is given in Table 9.11.2.

Two groups account for the majority of the instances: Human dura mater grafts and cadaver-derived human growth hormone treatments. Abnormal prion protein has been detected in the pituitary gland in both sCJD and vCJD (Peden *et al.* 2004). Case-to-case transmission involving brain to brain has happened rarely: Four instances of transmission related to common surgical instruments used in brain surgery and two cases related to normal usage of depth EEG electrodes. There are just two cases linked to corneal transplantation (Brown *et al.* 2006). There is no known risk of transmission of any form of prion disease by normal contact.

As noted, blood components and blood products have not yet been implicated in the secondary transmission of sCJD or gCJD. Recently, blood components have been shown to be a risk for BSE and vCJD. Animal experiments using sheep with BSE have demonstrated that whole blood transfusion is a relatively efficient means of transmission, including blood from preclinical infected animals (Hunter *et al.* 2002). The much greater involvement of lymphoreticular tissue in vCJD compared with other human prion diseases, especially with its preclinical occurrence, raises greater concerns of vCJD transmission via a wide variety of surgical procedures. The specific issue of secondary vCJD is discussed in the following.

Secondary vCJD

Background

The concern that vCJD might be a greater secondary transmission risk than other prion diseases has been justified by the occurrence of blood-transfusion-associated transmissions (Peden *et al.* 2004; Llewelyn *et al.* 2004; Wroe *et al.* 2006; Health Protection Agency 2007). To date, there has been no transmission of vCJD identified through invasive medical procedures, including dentistry, or through receipt of plasma products. The risk of vCJD secondary transmission depends on four factors: Frequency of infected individuals in the general population, presence of significant infectivity in the relevant tissue, route or mode of potential transmission, and susceptibility of the exposed individual. These four factors are considered in detail as follows.

Population prevalence of variant CJD infection

Such cases have, so far, been very limited in number and, in the United Kingdom, are currently declining in number. Naturally, these data need cautious interpretation: There are likely to be later cases in *PRNP*-129 non-MM individuals and there may be other genetic factors that affect incubation period. In addition, increasing numbers of other countries have reported vCJD cases (Table 9.11.3). At present, the chief concern regarding secondary transmission relates to individuals who are preclinically or subclinically infected. Preclinical infection undoubtedly occurs: There are two reported instances of lymphoreticular involvement prior to disease onset in the appendix (up to 2 years before onset), although one appendix specimen was negative 9 years before onset (Hilton *et al.* 1998). It is assumed that all cases of vCJD resulting from BSE dietary contamination have a potentially long period of clinically silent lymphoreticular and blood infectivity. Recently, the idea that truly subclinical vCJD infection of humans may occur has been

considered, with such individuals being a clinically silent source of infection throughout their lifespan. Animal experiments have supported this notion (Bishop *et al.* 2006). Modelling of the present vCJD UK epidemic data also suggests that subclinical infection occurs (Clarke & Ghani 2005).

In addition to the three cases of clinical vCJD transmitted through blood transfusion to date, there has also been one case of vCJD transfusion-transmitted infection without clinical or neuropathological disease reported in the United Kingdom (Peden *et al.* 2004). A patient died from a non-neurological disorder five years after receiving a blood transfusion from a donor who subsequently developed vCJD. Abnormal prion protein was found in the spleen and in a cervical lymph node, but not in the brain or tonsil. The patient was a *PRNP*-129 heterozygote (MV). It is not possible to state whether this represents a truly subclinical infection or someone simply in the preclinical phase, but it proves that vCJD infection is not confined to the *PRNP*-129 methionine homozygous (MM) genotype.

Various methods of determining the prevalence of vCJD infection in the UK population have been carried out or are underway. These include the following:

Retrospective Tonsil and Appendix Study: A study examining routine surgical appendix and tonsil paraffin-embedded blocks from 1995–99 in two centres in the United Kingdom which estimated the total population prevalence of vCJD infection to be 3808 (or 237 per million) in those aged 10–30 years, with wide 95 per cent confidence intervals of 785–11 128 (or 49–692 per million) (Hilton *et al.* 2004). However, this study had recognized limitations (relative small size, only two regions in the United Kingdom, and use of fixed specimens); therefore, the UK National Anonymous Tonsil Archive was established.

UK National Anonymous Tonsil Archive: The aim of this is to establish an unlinked, anonymous archive of routine surgical tonsil specimens, from 100 000 individuals, using what would have otherwise been discarded. A further 3000 tonsil pairs are included from the National Prion Unit, London. Patients are informed of the study preoperatively and given the opportunity to opt out of the study on the routine operation consent form. The UK Health Protection Agency coordinates the study. However, the majority of the tonsillectomies are performed in those under 25 years of age and many of these individuals should have been protected by dietary measures implemented in the 1990s. Therefore, a study that will give more information regarding prevalence in the older population is being established: The UK Post-Mortem Archive.

UK Post-Mortem Archive: This is in the process of being considered in the United Kingdom. It is envisaged that relatives of people referred to the coroner (or equivalent regional official) will be asked to give consent to allow a specimen to be taken from the spleen, in the first instance, and the brain to test for abnormal prion protein. The study would be coordinated by the UK Health Protection Agency and aims to collect over 100 000 specimens, with the majority in the over-65-years age group.

Switzerland has established a cross-sectional, linked anonymous prevalence study in an attempt to determine the population prevalence of vCJD (Glatzel *et al.* 2003b). Tissues used are those obtained from tonsillectomies and autopsies.

Tissue infectivity distribution

In vCJD, the greatest levels of infectivity are found in CNS tissues, but lymphoreticular tissues contain significant levels. Other tissues contain either generally lower levels still or undetectable amounts. The most comprehensive summary of tissue infectivities has been produced by the WHO (2006).

Route of exposure

In general, the evidence, from both animal experiments and human occurrences of secondary transmission, indicates that the direct introduction of infection into the brain is the most efficient transmission route, with the shortest incubation periods. However, other routes are also clearly effective, as indicated by iatrogenic cases resulting from eye surgery and intramuscular injection of human growth hormone. In addition, the intravenous route is a relatively efficient means of infection, as shown in transfusion experiments with BSE-infected sheep and the occurrence of cases of human vCJD following blood transfusion.

Susceptibility of the exposed individual

The only definitively identified susceptibility factor is that of the *PRNP*-129 genotype, as discussed earlier. However, there may be other genetic susceptibility factors.

It is notable that the age of onset of vCJD in the United Kingdom has not changed over the epidemic period. This could suggest that susceptibility to dietary infection is age-related; there is no definitive proof of an age-related susceptibility, and if it exists, its basis is not known (Clarke & Ghani 2005). However, there are known age-related changes in gut-associated lymphoid tissue and these could be relevant. Further, there is no evidence presently to indicate that other modes of infection (e.g. blood transfusion transmission of vCJD) are affected by age at exposure.

An additional important factor in determining the scale of the public health threat from secondary transmission of CJD is to ascertain whether a self-sustaining secondary epidemic is likely. Two studies have modelled data in order to estimate whether blood transfusions could result in a self-sustaining epidemic of vCJD. The first showed that although self-sustaining epidemics were possible (basic reproductive number $R_0 > 1$), they were unlikely when only biologically plausible scenarios, in which the mean incubation period for transfusion-acquired vCJD cases was shorter or similar to that for primary (foodborne), were considered. In addition, public health interventions (leucodepletion and the ban on previously transfused donors; for details, see the next subsection) were likely to be effective (Clarke & Ghani 2005). The second model predicted that vCJD could not become endemic by transfusion alone (Dietz *et al.* 2007). Modelling of the risk of surgical transmission of vCJD demonstrated that self-sustaining epidemics were possible. Key factors determining the scale of such epidemics were the number of times a single instrument was re-used, together with the infectivity of contaminated instruments and the effectiveness of cleaning those instruments (Garske *et al.* 2006).

Public health measures to reduce secondary transmission of CJD

Invasive medical procedures, including surgery and dentistry

In 1998, the UK TSE Working Group of the Advisory Committee in Dangerous Pathogens and the Spongiform Encephalopathy Advisory Committee revised the guidance on the decontamination of instruments and handling of patients known to have CJD, or to be suspect cases of CJD or to be 'at risk' of CJD (www.advisorybodies. doh.gov.uk/acdp/tseguidance/Index.htm). The guidance covers potential exposure in the wider health-care setting, focusing on surgical transmission but including guidance to laboratory staff and mortuary attendants. It is updated online as new advice becomes available.

In addition, prompted by concerns of the theoretical risk of surgical transmission of vCJD in the United Kingdom, the National Decontamination Programme was launched in 1999 to support the NHS (in England) in improving and maintaining standards related to the re-processing of surgical instruments. The key areas of work included development of a national decontamination training scheme, provision of technical advice and guidance, and establishment of a standard output specification (www.dh.gov.uk/en/ Policyandguidance/Organisationpolicy/Estatesandfacilitiesmanage ment/EngineeringEnvironmentAndTechnology/DH_4118225). In 2005, ESAC-Pr (Engineering and Science Advisory Committee, for the decontamination of surgical instruments including prion removal) was formed, which aims to take forward the practical application of relevant research in the area of decontamination in relation to prion removal and deactivation (www.dh.gov.uk/en/Pu blicationsandstatistics/Publications/PublicationsPolicyAndGuidan ce/DH_072443). In the United Kingdom in 2006, the National Institute for Health and Clinical Excellence (NICE) published guidance to further reduce risk of transmission of CJD via surgery, in particular surgery involving high-risk tissues (neurosurgery and posterior ophthalmic procedures) and through neuroendoscopy.

A wholesale move to single-use instruments has not been advocated by NICE or ESAC-Pr. Apart from taking into account their cost, the question of instrument quality is paramount. In England, postoperative haemorrhage following the introduction of single-use instruments for tonsillectomy in 2001 resulted in the reversal of this recommendation shortly afterward. However, in Scotland, where significant complications were not seen, single-use instruments have been recommended for tonsillectomy since 2001, and for dental root canal treatment since 2005. Other countries in the European Union, as well as worldwide, have performed their own risk assessments and implemented various measures accordingly.

Blood, organs, and tissues

As knowledge and potential evidence of the transmission of CJD through blood and plasma product transfusion and organ and tissue transplantation has increased, various public health measures have been implemented in the United Kingdom in an attempt to reduce this likelihood (Table 9.11.5). Countries outside the United Kingdom, including the United States, Canada, New Zealand, Australia, Hong Kong, and several European countries including Germany, Switzerland, Austria, and the Republic of Ireland, have taken the precautionary step of excluding blood donors who have spent more than a defined period in the United Kingdom between 1980 and 1996.

Blood screening tests

There are currently a number of potential tests in development. Most of these are based on the detection of PrP^Sc in blood, as a marker of infectivity. Such tests could have a variety of uses: Diagnostic testing of symptomatic cases, individual presymptomatic diagnosis, population studies to determine the number of

Table 9.11.5 Public health measures implemented in the UK in order to reduce the likelihood of transmission of CJD through blood and plasma product transfusion and organ and tissue transplantation

◆ Withdrawal and recall of any blood components, plasma derivatives, cells, or tissues obtained from any individual who later develops vCJD (December 1997).
◆ Importation of plasma from countries other than the UK for fractionation to manufacture plasma derivatives (fully implemented in October 1999).
◆ Leucodepletion of all blood components (fully implemented in Autumn 1999).
◆ Importation of clinical fresh frozen plasma for patients born after January 1996 (fully implemented in June 2004). Extended to all patients under the age of 16 (July 2005).
◆ Exclusion of whole blood donors who state that they have received a blood component transfusion in the UK since 1st January 1980 (April 2004). Extended to whole blood and apheresis donors who may have received a blood component transfusion in the UK since 1st January 1980 (August 2004) and to any donors who have been treated with UK plasma-derived, intravenous immunoglobulin or have undergone plasma exchange. Extended to those who may have received a blood component transfusion anywhere in the world since 1 January 1980 (November 2005).
◆ Exclusion of live bone donors who have been transfused since 1 January 1980 (July 2005).
◆ Exclusion of blood donors whose blood has been transfused to recipients who later developed vCJD, where blood transfusion cannot be excluded as a source of the vCJD infection and where no infected donor has been identified (July 2005).
◆ Promotion of appropriate use of blood and tissues products and alternatives throughout the National Health Service.

infected individuals, and screening of blood donations for infection. Presently, it is the last of these that is the main driver behind test development. Although the introduction of a screening test for blood has obvious public health advantages (in line with those that have come from screening for HIV, hepatitis C, etc.), there are a number of potential problems, even leaving aside the technical difficulties of detecting a small amount of PrP^{Sc} in the complex matrix of blood that contains normal PrP^{C}. Firstly, the sensitivity of the current potential tests will be defined according to their detection target (as indicated, mostly PrP^{Sc}); this is an indirect measure of infectivity. Secondly, specificity will be difficult to determine; if a positive result is obtained in a normal, healthy individual, it is difficult to know how its significance can be easily and quickly determined. Finally, if the number of infected individuals in the population is relatively small, even a test with high sensitivity and specificity would generate a large number of false-positive results; the management of such individuals would need careful consideration.

CJD Incidents Panel

Many countries throughout the world have assessed the risk to their citizens in relation to the iatrogenic transmission of CJD, especially in view of vCJD. Based on the perceived risk, different actions have been implemented in different countries in an attempt to reduce the risk of onward transmission of CJD.

In 2000, the UK Chief Medical Officers established an expert committee—the CJD Incidents Panel. Its secretariat is provided by the Health Protection Agency on behalf of the Department of Health (http://www.hpa.org.uk/webw/HPAweb&Page&HPAwebA utoListName/Page/1204031511121?p=1204031511121). Incidents involve the potential transmission of CJD between patients through invasive medical procedures, including surgery, blood donations, and organ and tissue donations. Incidents occur when patients diagnosed with (or suspected of having) CJD, or patients identified as 'at risk' of CJD, have undergone invasive medical procedures that may have put other patients at risk.

Patients diagnosed with CJD, or those suspected of having CJD, are referred by the local clinician caring for the patient to the local Consultant in Communicable Disease Control (CCDC) using a standardized format (http://www.cjd.ed.ac.uk/guidance.htm). The CCDC gathers a full invasive medical history with the collaboration of the patient's general practitioner and refers the patient to the CJD Incidents Panel.

Action is decided upon with regards to instruments in surgical incidents and potential 'contacts' who may have been put at risk. This depends on the type of tissue involved (high, medium, or low risk), the type of operation (if surgical), when the incident occurred in relation to the incubation period, and whether 'contacts', who have been put at risk, are traceable via medical records. The CJD Incidents Panel considers individual incidents when there has been no similar incident previously for which a precedent for action has been set. Surgical instruments are quarantined and returned to medical use, destroyed, or given for research purposes.

Designation of groups 'at risk' of CJD

In the United Kingdom, the CJD Incidents Panel advises contacting patients who have been put at additional risk (to that through diet of the background population resident in the United Kingdom between 1980 and 1996) of CJD, of at least 1 per cent through exposure in an incident. Patients are told that they should take certain public health measures to prevent CJD from being spread to other patients. The risk assessment models used to derive this threshold were highly precautionary and based on a number of scientific assumptions and uncertainty. The 1 per cent threshold is seen as a public health tool and not to be used to advise individuals their exact risk of developing CJD.

Table 9.11.6 is a summary of the groups of individuals who are designated 'at risk' of CJD in the United Kingdom, at time of print. In comparison with those who have been informed that they are 'at risk' of CJD through surgery, those 'at risk' of CJD through blood and plasma product incidents are the largest group to date. Plasma product recipients, mainly haemophiliacs treated with Factor VIII,

Table 9.11.6 Groups considered 'at risk' of CJD in the United Kingdom

Surgery related:
◆ Those undergoing high- or medium-risk procedures following a case of CJD.
Transfusion related (variant only):
◆ 'Implicated' red blood cell recipients
◆ 'Implicated' plasma product recipients
◆ Red blood cell donors to cases of vCJD
◆ Other blood component recipients from donors to vCJD cases
At risk of familial forms:
◆ Two or more blood relatives affected by CJD or prion disease, or known genetic mutation in relatives or known genetic mutation in themselves.
Recipients of hormone derived from human pituitary:
◆ Growth hormone and gonadotrophin
Recipients of dura mater grafts:
◆ Those who underwent neurosurgery or operation for tumour or cyst of spine before August 1992

are by far the largest individual group 'at risk' so far. In addition, groups such as those at risk of genetic forms of CJD and recipients of human pituitary-derived growth hormones, have also been designated 'at risk' of CJD. Table 9.11.7 outlines the advice given to those designated 'at risk' of CJD in the United Kingdom.

At present, there are no routine screening tests, for example, on blood, or prophylactic treatments available for those 'at risk' of CJD. If they are developed in the coming years, they will be offered to those at risk if appropriate.

Guidance of the TSE Working Group of the Advisory Committee in Dangerous Pathogens and the Spongiform Encephalopathy Advisory Committee advises as to what precautions should be taken when caring for those 'at risk' of CJD in the health-care setting (www.advisorybodies.doh.gov.uk/acdp/tseguidance/Index.htm).

It is imperative that those designated 'at risk' are followed up for public health and research purposes. In the United Kingdom, the Health Protection Agency is coordinating two different research proposals: The first to look at the psychological and social effects of being put in an 'at risk' of CJD group and the second following up those 'at risk' of CJD over time. Ethical approval has been granted and studies have commenced.

Conclusion

Prion diseases have led to a number of public health concerns and actions, despite their general rarity. Fortunately, the number of

Table 9.11.7 Advice for those designated 'at risk' of CJD in the United Kingdom

◆ Not to donate blood, organs, or tissues
◆ To tell the doctor, dentist, or nurse in charge of their care whenever they are going to have surgery or invasive medical procedures that they are in an 'at-risk' group for CJD
◆ To tell their family in case they require emergency surgery

cases of vCJD due to dietary BSE contamination is likely to be limited, but concerns remain about possible secondary transmission via blood and surgical instruments. The magnitude of this risk depends on the prevalence of preclinical or subclinical BSE or vCJD infection in the United Kingdom and other populations. A number of important public health protective measures are in place. The cause of sCJD remains uncertain. Iatrogenic transmission of sCJD is uncommon, with most cases relating to the use of cadaver-derived human growth hormone and human dura mater grafts, both of which are now avoided. The difficulties of accidental transmission of prion diseases are increased by their long incubation period (when acquired), the uncertain nature of the prion agent, the lack of direct methods of detecting the agent or infectivity, and the unusual resistance of the infection to the usual sterilization methods employed in health services.

Summary

◆ All prion diseases are potentially transmissible, even if the original cause is not an infection.

◆ The prion agent is not fully characterized; there are no simple direct methods of detecting the agent and its infectivity.

◆ Infectivity is resistant to many standard methods of inactivation.

◆ There are no simple, non-invasive, absolute diagnostic tests for human prion diseases, but experienced clinicians can achieve relatively secure clinical diagnosis in the majority of the cases.

◆ Many public health measures are in place in many countries; these should limit the risk of transmission from animal to man and man to man.

References

Alperovitch A., Will R.G. Predicting the size of the vCJD epidemic in France. *Comptes Rendus Biologies* 2002;**325**:33–6.

Anderson R.M., Donnelly C.A., Ferguson N.M. *et al*. Transmission dynamics and epidemiology of BSE in British cattle. *Nature* 1996;**382**:779–88.

Arakawa K., Nagara H., Itoyama Y. *et al*. Clustering of 3 cases of Creutzfeldt-Jakob disease near Fukuoka City, Japan. *Acta Neurologica Scandinavia* 1991;**84**(5):445–7.

Bishop M.T., Hart P., Aitchison L. *et al*. Predicting susceptibility and incubation time of human to human transmission of vCJD. *Lancet Neurology* 2006;**5**:393–8.

Blanquet-Grossard F., Sazdovitch V., Jean A. *et al*. Prion protein is not detectable in dental pulp from patients with Creutzfeldt-Jakob disease. *Journal of Dental Research* 2000;**79**(2):700.

Bobowick A.R., Brody J.A., Matthews M.R. *et al*. Creutzfeldt-Jakob disease: a case-control study. *American Journal of Epidemiology* 1973; **98**:381–94.

Boesenberger C., Schulz-Schaeffer W., Meissner B. *et al*. Clinical course in young patients with sporadic Creutzfeldt-Jakob disease. *Annals of Neurology* 2005;**58**:533–43.

Brandel J-P, Preece M., Brown P. *et al*. Distribution of codon 129 genotype in human growth hormone-treated CJD patients in France and the UK. *Lancet* 2003;**362**:128–30.

Brown P., Brandel J-P, Preece M. *et al*. Iatrogenic Creutzfeldt-Jakob disease: the waning of an era. *Neurology* 2006;**67**:389–93.

Brown P., Galvez S., Goldfarb L.G. *et al*. Familial Creutzfeldt-Jakob disease in Chile is associated with the codon 200 mutation of the PRNP amyloid precursor gene on chromosome 20. *Journal of the Neurological Sciences* 1992;**112**:65–7.

Brown P., Gibbs C.J., Jr., Rodgers-Johnson P. *et al.* Human spongiform encephalopathy: the National Institutes of Health series of 300 cases of experimentally transmitted disease. *Annals of Neurology* 1994;**35**:513–29.

Brown P., Preece M., Brandel J.P. *et al.* Iatrogenic Creutzfeldt-Jakob disease at the millennium. *Neurology* 2000;**55**:1075–81.

Bruce M.E., Will R.G., Ironside J.W. *et al.* Transmissions to mice indicate that 'new variant' CJD is caused by the BSE agent. *Nature* 1997;**389**:498–501.

Bruce M.E. TSE strain variation. *British Medical Bulletin* 2003;**66**:99–108.

Cervenakova L., Goldfarb L.G., Garruto R. *et al.* Phenotype-genotype studies in kuru: implications for new variant Creutzfeldt-Jakob disease (nvCJD). *Proceedings of the National Academy of Sciences USA* 1998;**95**:13239–41.

Clarke P., Ghani A.C. Projections of the future course of the primary vCJD epidemic in the UK: inclusion of subclinical infection and the possibility of wider genetic susceptibility. *Journal of the Royal Society Interface* 2005;**2**:19–31.

Collie D.A., Summers D.M., Sellar R.J. *et al.* Diagnosing variant Creutzfeldt-Jakob disease with the pulvinar sign: MR imaging findings in 86 neuropathologically confirmed cases. *American Journal of Neuroradiology* 2003;**24**:1560–9.

Collins S., Boyd A., Fletcher A. *et al.* Creutzfeldt-Jakob disease cluster in an Australian rural city. *Annals of Neurology* 2002;**52**(1):115–8.

Collins S., Law M.G., Fletcher A. *et al.* Surgical treatment and risk of sporadic Creutzfeldt-Jakob disease: a case-control study. *Lancet* 1999;**353**:693–7.

Cooper S.A., Murray K.L., Heath C.A. *et al.* Isolated visual symptoms at onset in sporadic Creutzfeldt-Jakob disease: the clinical phenotype of the 'Heidenhain variant'. *British Journal of Ophthalmology* 2005;**89**:1341–2.

Cooper S.A., Murray K.L., Heath C.A. *et al.* Sporadic Creutzfeldt-Jakob disease with cerebellar ataxia at onset in the United Kingdom. *JNNP* 2006;**77**:1273–5.

Cousens S., Smith P.G., Ward H. *et al.* Geographical distribution of variant Creutzfeldt-Jakob disease in Great Britain, 1994–2000. *Lancet* 2001;**357**:1002–7.

Cousens S.N., Harries-Jones R., Knight R. *et al.* Geographical distribution of cases of Creutzfeldt-Jakob disease in England and Wales, 1970–84. *Journal of Neurology, Neurosurgery, and Psychiatry* 1990;**53**:459–65.

Cousens S.N., Vynnycky E., Zeidler M. *et al.* Predicting the CJD epidemic in humans. *Nature* 1997;**385**:197–8.

Davanipour Z., Alter M., Sobel E. *et al.* A case-control study of Creutzfeldt-Jakob disease: dietary risk factors. *American Journal of Epidemiology* 1985;**122**:443–51.

DeArmond S.J., Ironside J.W., Bouzamondo-Bernstein E. *et al.* Neuropathology of prion diseases. In: Prusiner SB, editor. *Prion biology and diseases.* New York (NY): Cold Spring Harbour Laboratory Press; 2004. p. 777–856.

Dietz K., Raddatz G., Wallis J. *et al.* Blood transfusion and spread of variant Creutzfeldt-Jakob disease. *Emerging Infectious Diseases* 2007;**13**(1):89–96.

Farmer P.M., Kane W.C., Hollenberg-Sher J. Incidence of Creutzfeldt-Jakob disease in Brooklyn and Staten Island. *New England Journal of Medicine* 1978;**298**:283–4.

Garske T., Ward H.J.T., Clarke P. *et al.* Factors determining the potential for onward transmission of variant Creutzfeldt-Jakob disease via surgical instruments. *Journal of the Royal Society Interface* 2006;**3**:757–66.

Glatzel M., Abela E., Maissen M. *et al.* Extra neural pathologic prion protein in sporadic Creutzfeldt-Jakob disease. *New England Journal of Medicine* 2003a;**349**:1812–20.

Glatzel M., Ott P.M., Linder T. *et al.* Human prion diseases: epidemiology and integrated risk assessment. *Lancet Neurology* 2003b;**2**:757–63.

Green A., Sanchez-Juan P., Ladogana A. *et al.* CSF analysis in patients with sporadic CJD and other transmissible spongiform encephalopathies. *European Journal of Neurology* 2006;**14**:121–4.

Harries-Jones R., Knight R., Will R.G. *et al.* Creutzfeldt-Jakob disease in England and Wales, 1980–1984: a case-control study of potential risk factors. *Journal of Neurology, Neurosurgery, and Psychiatry* 1988;**51**:1113–9.

Head M.W., Bunn T.J.R., Bishop M.T. *et al.* Prion protein heterogeneity in sporadic but not variant Creutzfeldt-Jakob disease: UK cases, 1991–2002. *Annals of Neurology* 2004;**55**:851–9.

Health Protection Agency. Fourth case of transfusion-associated variant-CJD. *Health Protection Report* 2007;**1**(3).

Hill A.F., Butterworth R.J., Joiner S. *et al.* Investigation of variant Creutzfeldt-Jakob disease and other human prion diseases with tonsil biopsy samples. *Lancet* 1999;**353**:183–4.

Hill A.F., Desbruslais M., Joiner S. *et al.* The same prion strain causes vCJD and BSE. *Nature* 1997;**389**:448–50.

Hilton D.A., Fathers E., Edwards P. *et al.* Prion immunoreactivity in appendix before clinical onset of variant Creutzfeldt-Jakob disease. *Lancet* 1998;**352**(9129):703–4.

Hilton D.A., Ghani A.C., Conyers L. *et al.* Prevalence of lymphoreticular prion protein accumulation in UK tissue samples. *Journal of Pathology* 2004;**203**:733–9.

Huillard d'Aignaux J., Cousens S.N., Delasnerie-Laupretre N. *et al.* Analysis of the geographical distribution of sporadic Creutzfeldt-Jakob disease in France between 1992 and 1998. *International Journal of Epidemiology* 2002b;**31**:490–5.

Huillard d'Aignaux J., Cousens S.N., Maccario J. *et al.* The incubation period of kuru. *Epidemiology* 2002a;**13**:402–8.

Hunter N., Foster J., Chong A. *et al.* Transmission of prion diseases by blood transfusion. *Journal of General Virology* 2002;**83**:2897–905.

Ironside J.W., Hilton D.A., Ghani A. *et al.* Retrospective study of prion-protein accumulation in tonsil and appendix tissues. *Lancet* 2000;**355**:1693–4.

Kahana E., Alter M., Braham J. *et al.* Creutzfeldt-Jakob disease: focus among Libyan Jews in Israel. *Science* 1974;**183**:90–1.

Knight R. The relationship between new variant Creutzfeldt-Jakob disease and bovine spongiform encephalopathy. *Vox Sanguinis* 1999;**76**:203–8.

Kondo K., Kuroiwa Y. A case-control study of Creutzfeldt-Jakob disease: association with physical injuries. *Annals of Neurology* 1982;**11**:377–81.

Kovacs G.G., Puopolo M., Ladogana A. *et al.* Genetic prion disease: the EUROCJD experience. *Human Genetics* 2005;**118**:166–74.

Kovacs G.G., Trabattoni G., Hainfellner J.A. *et al.* Mutations of the prion protein gene: phenotypic spectrum. *Journal of Neurology* 2002; **249**:567–1582.

Ladogana A., Puopolo M., Croes E.A. *et al.* Mortality from Creutzfeldt-Jakob disease and related disorders in Europe, Australia, and Canada. *Neurology* 2005;**64**:1586–91.

Lee H-S, Sambuughin N., Cervenakova L. *et al.* Ancestral origins and worldwide distribution of the PRNP 200K mutation causing familial Creutzfeldt-Jakob disease. *American Journal of Human Genetics* 1999;**64**:1063–70.

Linsell L., Cousens S.N., Smith P.G. *et al.* A case-control study of sporadic Creutzfeldt-Jakob disease in the United Kingdom: analysis of clustering. *Neurology* 2004;**63**:2077–83.

Llewelyn C.A., Hewitt P.A., Knight R.S.G. *et al.* Possible transmission of variant Creutzfeldt-Jakob disease by blood transfusion. *Lancet* 2004;**363**:417–21.

Lucker E.H., Eigenbrodt E., Wenisch S. *et al.* Identification of central nervous system tissue in retain meat products. *Journal of Food Protection* 2000;**63**:258–63.

Matthews W.B. Epidemiology of Creutzfeldt-Jakob disease in England and Wales. *Journal of Neurology, Neurosurgery, and Psychiatry* 1975;**38**:210–13.

Nurmi M.H., Bishop M., Strain L. *et al.* The normal population distribution of PRNP codon 129 polymorphism. *Acta Neurologica Scandinavica* 2003;**108**:374–8.

Parchi P., Castellani R., Capellari S. *et al.* Molecular basis of phenotypic variability in sporadic Creutzfeldt-Jakob disease. *Annals of Neurology* 1996;**39**:767–78.

Parchi P., Giese A., Capellari S. *et al.* Classification of sporadic Creutzfeldt-Jakob disease based on molecular and phenotypic analysis of 300 subjects. *Annals of Neurology* 1999;**46**:224–33.

Peden A.H., Head M.W., Ritchie D.L. *et al.* Preclinical vCJD after blood transfusion in a PRNP codon 129 heterozygous patient. *Lancet* 2004;**364**:527–9.

Pocchiari M., Puopolo M., Croes E.A. *et al.* Predictors of survival in sporadic Creutzfeldt-Jakob disease and other human transmissible spongiform encephalopathies. *Brain* 2004;**127**:2348–59.

Prusiner S.B., editor. An introduction to prion biology and diseases. *Prion biology and diseases*. New York (NY): Cold Spring Harbour Laboratory Press; 2004a. pp. 1–87.

Prusiner S.B. Development of the prion concept. In: Prusiner SB, editor. *Prion biology and diseases*. New York (NY): Cold Spring Harbour Laboratory Press; 2004b. pp. 89–141

Safar J., Wille H., Itri V. *et al.* Eight prion strains have PrP^{Sc} molecules with different conformations. *Nature Medicine* 1998;**4**:1157–65.

Shibuya S., Higuchi J., Shin R-W *et al.* Protective prion protein polymorphisms against sporadic Creutzfeldt-Jakob disease. *Lancet* 1998;**351**:419.

Somerville R.A., Chong A., Mulqueen O.U. *et al.* Biochemical typing of scrapie strains. *Nature* 1997;**386**:564.

Spencer M.D., Knight R.S.G., Will R.G. First hundred cases of variant Creutzfeldt-Jakob disease: retrospective case note review of early psychiatric and neurological features. *British Medical Journal* 2002;**324**:1479–82.

Spudich S., Mastrianni J.A., Wrensch M. *et al.* Complete penetrance of Creutzfeldt-Jakob disease in Libyan Jews carrying the E200K mutation in the prion protein gene. *Molecular Medicine* 1995;**1**:607–13.

Van Duijn C.M., Delasnerie-Laupretre N., Masullo C. *et al.* Case-control study of risk factors of Creutzfeldt-Jakob disease in Europe during 1993–95. *Lancet* 1998;**351**:1081–85.

Ward H.J.T., Everington D., Cousens S.N. *et al.* Risk factors for variant Creutzfeldt-Jakob disease: a case-control study. *Annals of Neurology* 2006;**59**:111–20.

Ward H.J.T., Everington D., Croes E.A. *et al.* Sporadic Creutzfeldt-Jakob disease and surgery: a case-control study using community controls. *Neurology* 2002;**59**:543–8.

Wientjens D.P.W.M., Davanipour Z., Hofman A. *et al.* Risk factors for Creutzfeldt-Jakob disease: a reanalysis of case-control studies. *Neurology* 1996;**46**:1287–91.

Will R.G., Alpers M.P., Dormont D. *et al.* Infectious and sporadic prion diseases. In: Prusiner SB, editor. *Prion biology and diseases*. New York (NY): Cold Spring Harbor Laboratory Press; 2004. p. 629–671

Will R.G., Ironside J.W., Zeidler M. *et al.* A new variant of Creutzfeldt-Jakob disease in the UK. *Lancet* 1996;**347**:921–5.

Will R.G., Matthews W.B., Smith P.G. *et al.* A retrospective study of Creutzfeldt-Jakob disease in England and Wales 1970–1979 II: epidemiology. *Journal of Neurology, Neurosurgery, and Psychiatry* 1986;**49**:749–55.

Will R.G., Matthews W.B. Evidence for case-to-case transmission of Creutzfeldt-Jakob disease. *Journal of Neurology, Neurosurgery, and Psychiatry* 1982;**45**:235–8.

Will R.G. New variant Creutzfeldt-Jakob disease. *The Darlington Postgraduate Journal* 1998;**17**(1):35–42.

Wilson K., Code C., Ricketts M.N. Risk of acquiring Creutzfeldt-Jakob disease from blood transfusions: systematic review of case-control studies. *British Medical Journal* 2000;**321**:17–9.

World Health Organization. Guidelines on tissue infectivity distribution in transmissible spongiform encephalopathies. Geneva: World Health Organization; 2006. pp. 1–61.

World Health Organization. Manual for strengthening diagnosis and surveillance of Creutzfeldt-Jakob disease. Geneva: World Health Organization; 1998. pp. 1–75.

World Health Organization. The revision of the surveillance case definition for variant Creutzfeldt-Jakob disease (vCJD). Geneva: World Health Organization; 2002. pp. 1–30.

Wroe S.J., Pal S., Siddique D. *et al.* Clinical presentation and pre-mortem diagnosis of variant Creutzfeldt-Jakob disease associated with blood transfusion: a case report. *Lancet* 2006;**368**:2061–7.

Zerr I., Brandel J.P., Masullo C. *et al.* European surveillance on Creutzfeldt-Jakob disease: a case-control study for medical risk factors. *Journal of Clinical Epidemiology* 2000;**53**:747–54.

Sexually transmitted infections

Mary L. Kamb and John M. Douglas, Jr.

Sexually transmitted infections (STI) are among the world's most common diseases. More than 20 organisms and at least as many syndromes are recognized as being transmissible through vaginal, anal, or oral sex, including human immunodeficiency virus infection (HIV), discussed separately in Chapter 9.13 (Table 9.13.1). Globally, annual incidence of bacterial STI is exceeded only by diarrhoeal diseases, malaria, and lower respiratory infections (World Health Organization 2007). In the United States, two bacterial STI, chlamydia and gonorrhoea, are the first and second most commonly reported of all notifiable diseases (CDC 2006). Even so, the burden of bacterial STI is small when compared to that of viral STI such as human papillomavirus (HPV) and herpes simplex virus-2 (HSV-2), the former leading to persistent long-term infection in many and the latter resulting in lifelong infection in all those infected.

Given the high burden of STI, it is not surprising to find that regardless of a nation's resources, STI symptoms rank among the top five disease categories for which adults seek health-care services (Dallabetta et al. 2007). It is less well-recognized that STI are associated with substantial public health costs because of their profound effects on reproductive health outcomes, causation of a variety of malignancies, and the role they play in enhancing HIV transmission (Over & Piot 1996; World Health Organization 2007). In developing nations, STI are among the most important causes of years of healthy productive life lost overall (Over & Piot 1993, 1996), and for women of reproductive age, STI-associated disability adjusted life years lost is exceeded only by pregnancy-associated maternal morbidity and HIV (World Bank 2003). While overall STI disease burden is most prominent in adolescents and young adults, the most serious adverse health consequences, including adverse pregnancy outcomes and STI-associated cancers, are borne primarily by women and infants. For nations with high STI prevalence, prevention and control of these infections is a critical and cost-effective investment in preventing many of the most important long-term health consequences (World Health Organization 2007).

Since the licensure of the first STI vaccine, against hepatitis B virus (HBV) 25 years ago, a number of important advances have occurred in the field of STI. First, safe and effective vaccines are now available for two STI, including HPV as well as HBV (World Health Organization 2007; Munoz et al. 2003; Szmuness et al. 1980; Villa et al. 2005; CDC 2007; Koutsky et al. 2002; Harper et al. 2004;

Schmiedeskamp & Kockler 2006; CDC 2006). Thus, an opportunity now exists to prevent the two viruses that account for most of the world's STI-related cancer burden (Pisani et al. 1999), although widespread programmatic implementation of HBV vaccine for infants is still limited in many countries and discussions about best ways to roll out HPV vaccines in pre-adolescents are just beginning for HPV vaccines (World Health Organization 2007). Second, since the early 1990s, with the World Health Organization's (WHO) recommendation that low-income countries use locally validated syndromic approaches for STI diagnosis and treatment, the prevalence of bacterial causes of genital ulcer disease and neonatal conjunctivitis have been observed to decline markedly in several low-income settings in Africa (World Health Organization 2007). Third, with the adoption of national screening policies for asymptomatic STI with serious adverse sequelae (e.g. antenatal syphilis screening, gonorrhoea and chlamydia screening for young women, cervical cancer screening) many nations have substantially reduced associated morbidity and mortality (World Health Organization 2007; Berman & Kamb 2007). Fourth, several fairly effective behaviour change approaches have been identified and effectively implemented among high-risk populations in health facilities and community settings (Greenberg et al. 1998; Kamb et al. 1998; Manhart & Holmes 2005; Fenton & Bloom 2007; McFarlane & Bull 2007; Vega & Ghanem 2007), although, again, these have not been widely implemented in most areas. Fifth, improved methods for contacting, counselling, and treating sex partners have been proven to reduce re-infections (Golden et al. 2005; Du et al. 2006; White et al. 2005; Passin et al. 2006; Brewer 2005; Hogben et al. 2007; Trelle et al. 2007). Sixth, better and more acceptable targeted interventions have been developed for highly affected, hard-to-reach populations who—through an improved understanding of STI transmission dynamics—are recognized in certain settings to contribute importantly to spread of infection into the general community (Dallabetta et al. 2007; World Health Organization 2007; Berman & Kamb 2007; Greenberg et al. 1998; Manhart & Holmes 2005; Fenton & Bloom 2007; Sanchez et al. 2003; Levine et al. 1998; Laga et al. 1994; Fleming & Wasserheit 1999; CDC 2001). Finally, aside from the interventions themselves, more efficient and affordable methods have been identified to assess STI health burden, implement STI prevention and control programmes and to evaluate their effects (World Bank 2003; Hassig et al. 1996).

Table 9.12.1 Sexually transmitted pathogens and associated diseases or syndromes

Pathogen	Associated disease or syndrome
Bacteria	
Neisseria gonorrhoeae	Cervicitis, urethritis, proctitis, pharyngitis, Bartholinitis, endometritis, pelvic inflammatory disease (PID), infertility, chronic pelvic pain, orchitis, epididymitis, urethral stricture, prostatitis, perihepatitis, disseminated infection, Reiter's syndrome; enhanced HIV risk; asymptomatic in up to 2/3 (women) and 1/3 (men) of cases. *Maternal:* Ectopic pregnancy, maternal death, preterm rupture of membranes; *Infant:* Neonatal conjunctivitis, corneal scarring, blindness, premature birth, low birth weight
Chlamydia trachomatis	Cervicitis, urethritis, proctitis, pharyngitis, Bartholinitis, endometritis, PID, infertility, chronic pelvic pain, orchitis, epididymitis, urethral stricture, prostatitis, perihepatitis, disseminated infection, Reiter's syndrome; lymphogranuloma venereum (LGV)—anogenital ulcer or inguinal swelling; enhanced HIV risk; asymptomatic in up to 2/3 (women) and 1/3 (men) of cases *Maternal:* Ectopic pregnancy, maternal death, preterm rupture of membranes; *Infant:* Neonatal conjunctivitus, pneumonia, premature birth, low birth weight
Mycoplasma hominis	Postpartum fever, PID
Mycoplasma genitalium	Urethritis, cervicitis; PID, enhanced HIV risk
Ureaplasma urealyticum	Urethritis, chorioamnionitis, premature delivery
Treponema pallidum (syphilis)	Genital ulcer (chancre), local adenopathy, skin rashes, condyloma lata, hepatitis, arthritis, enhanced HIV risk; bone, cardiovascular (e.g. aortic disease) and central nervous system disease (e.g. aseptic meningitis, cerebrovascular accidents, cranial nerve abnormalities, optic atrophy, tabes dorsalis, general paresis) *Maternal:* Spontaneous abortion, stillbirth, preterm delivery, low infant birth weight *Infant:* congenital syphilis
Gardnerella vaginalis (in association with other bacteria)	Bacterial vaginosis, PID, enhanced HIV risk, urethral discharge *Maternal:* Chorioamniotis, prematurity, low birth weight
Haemophilus ducreyi (chancroid)	Genital ulcers, inguinal adenitis, disfiguring lesions, tissue destruction, enhanced HIV risk
Calymmatobacterium granulomatis (granuloma inguinale, Donovanosis)	Nodular swellings and ulcerative lesions of inguinal and anogenital areas
Shigella spp.	Shigellosis in homosexual men
Salmonella spp.	Enteritis, proctocolitis in homosexual men
Campylobacter spp.	Enteritis, proctocolitis in homosexual men
Viruses	
Human immunodeficiency virus, types 1 and 2	HIV-related disease, opportunistic infections, lymphomas, AIDS *Maternal:* Vertical transmission to infants *Infant:* HIV infection
Herpes simplex virus types 1 and 2	Anogenital vesicular lesions and ulcerations, recurrent genital ulcers, cold sores cervicitis, urethritis, pharyngitis, proctitis, chronic pain, arthritis, aseptic meningitis, hepatitis, meningitis, enhanced HIV risk. *Maternal:* Vertical transmission to infants *Infants:* Ulcerations of skin, eye, mucous membranes; encephalitis, disseminated infection with hepatitis, pneumonitis, encephalitis; long-term neurologic abnormalities
Human papilloma virus (more than 30 genital genotypes identified)	Anogenital and oral warts; intraepithelial neoplasia of the cervix, penis, vulva, vagina, anus; carcinoma of the cervix, penis, vulva, vagina, anus; recurrent respiratory papillomatosis, oropharyngeal cancer *Maternal:* Vertical transmission to infant *Infants:* Recurrent respiratory papillomatosis
Hepatitis B virus	Acute hepatitis, liver cirrhosis, end-stage liver disease, hepatocellular cancer *Maternal:* Vertical transmission to infants; *Infants:* Cirrhosis, end stage liver disease, primary liver cancer
Hepatitis A virus	Acute hepatitis A
Hepatitis C virus	Acute hepatitis C, liver cirrhosis, end-stage liver disease, hepatocellular cancer
Cytomegalovirus (CMV)	Heterophil-negative infectious mononucleosis, hepatitis *Infant:* Primary infection of the newborn, hepatitis, sepsis, deafness, mental retardation
Molluscum contagiosum virus	Genital molluscum contagiosum,
Human T-lymphotrophic retrovirus, type 1	Human T-cell leukemia or lymphoma
Human herpesvirus 8 (HHV-8)	Kaposi's sarcoma, primary effusion lymphoma, Castleman's disease

Protozoa	
Trichomonas vaginalis	Vaginitis, cervicitis, urethretis, endometritis, salpingitis, probably enhanced HIV risk
	Maternal: Chorioamniotis, preterm delivery, low birth weight
	Infants: Pneumonitis, fever, vaginal discharge in female infants
Entamoeba histolytica	Amebiasis in men who have sex with men
Giardia lamblia	Giardiasis in men who have sex with men
Fungi	
Candida albicans	Vulvovaginitis, balanitis
Ectoparasites	
Phthirus pubis	Pubic lice infestation
Sarcoptes scabiei	Scabies, Norwegian (disseminated) scabies
	Infants: Norwegian (disseminated) scabies

Global burden of STI

WHO estimates that each year more than 340 million new curable STI (i.e. gonorrhoea, chlamydia, trichomoniasis, and syphilis) occur in reproductive-aged men and women (Fig. 9.12.1) (World Health Organization 2007). This estimate does not include the many millions of new viral STI that occur each year. Genital HPV infection is believed to be the highest incidence STI worldwide, infecting an estimated 50–70 per cent of sexually active persons and accounting for an estimated 5 million new infections each year in the United States alone (Baseman & Koutsky 2005; Weinstock *et al.* 2004). HSV-2 is also extremely common, with reported population prevalences among nations ranging from 20 per cent to 40 per cent

even higher, and is now recognized to be the most common cause of genital ulcer disease worldwide (Paz-Bailey *et al.* 2007). Although not always transmitted sexually, HBV accounts for an estimated 360 million chronic infections globally; and additionally 3 per cent of the world's population is believed to be infected with hepatitis C virus (HCV), including an estimated 170 million people with severe liver disease (Global Burden of Hepatitis C Working Group 2004; Goldstein *et al.* 2005). Additionally, there are approximately 33 million new cases of HIV in adults each year, most of them transmitted sexually (World Health Organization 2007). Viral STI generally cannot be cured and result in either latent infection or active disease that can be transmitted to sex partners. Long-term infection with viral STI may lead to chronic conditions with serious

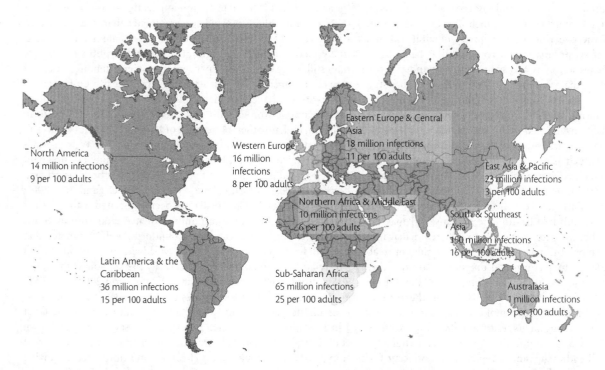

North America
14 million infections
9 per 100 adults

Western Europe
16 million infections
8 per 100 adults

Eastern Europe & Central Asia
18 million infections
11 per 100 adults

East Asia & Pacific
23 million infections
3 per 100 adults

Northern Africa & Middle East
10 million infections
6 per 100 adults

South & Southeast Asia
150 million infections
16 per 100 adults

Latin America & the Caribbean
36 million infections
15 per 100 adults

Sub-Saharan Africa
65 million infections
25 per 100 adults

Australasia
1 million infections
9 per 100 adults

Fig. 9.12.1 Estimated annual numbers and incidence per 100 adults of curable STIs among men and women aged 15–44 years, globally and by region (2001). Each year, an estimated 340 million cases of curable STIs are due to gonorrhoea, chlamydia, syphilis, and trichomoniasis. *Source:* World Health Organization (WHO), An Overview of Selected Curable Sexually Transmitted Diseases, Geneva: WHO, Global Programme on AIDS. 2001.

consequences, such as anogenital cancers associated with HPV and hepatocellular carcinomas and end-stage liver disease associated with HBV and HCV.

Most high- and moderate-income nations that have established national STI control programmes have seen marked declines in bacterial infections, notably gonorrhoea and syphilis (Berman & Kamb 2007). Consequently, 80–90 per cent of the global burden of curable STI currently occurs in developing countries, with incidence and prevalence rates up to 20 times higher than in industrialized nations (World Health Organization 2007; Adler 1996). The highest curable STI prevalence rates occur in sub-Saharan African nations, followed by Latin America and the Caribbean, and South and Southeast Asia (Fig. 9.12.1). For a variety of biologic, behavioural, and socioeconomic reasons, curable STI are most common in young adults and adolescents, particularly those under age 24. Although highest STI prevalence occurs in low-income settings in Africa, the largest overall numbers of curable STI occur in Asian nations with large populations under age 40. Viral STI are remarkably common both in industrialized and in developing countries. National population-based surveys in the United States indicate that 17 per cent of reproductive-aged adults are HSV-2 infected, and that prevalence increases with age (from 1.6 per cent in 14–19-year-olds to 26.3 per cent in 40–49-year-olds), and that prevalence varies considerably by racial/ethnic group (Xu *et al.* 2006). Conversely, because of the synergy between HIV and HSV-2, in which each virus enhances shedding of the other, countries with high HIV prevalence generally see increasingly higher HSV-2 prevalence, resulting in a continuing vicious cycle (Paz-Bailey *et al.* 2007). Some of these situations could change in the future. For example, widespread implementation of primary HPV prevention through newly available vaccines could reduce HPV incidence and prevalence in succeeding generations.

STI are greatly under-recognized and under-treated for several reasons. First, a large proportion of STI, including at least half of bacterial STI and the overwhelming majority of viral STI are asymptomatic or, if symptomatic, not recognized as being STI-related. Second, even when signs and symptoms exist and are recognized, the social stigma associated with these diseases that still exists in virtually every society contributes to their under-detection. Shame around acquiring an STI can lead symptomatic people to seek treatment outside established health care systems, with traditional healers or pharmacists, or to resort to self-treatment through inadequate methods such as douching or over-the-counter remedies. Many people do not seek treatment at all, and signs and symptoms will typically disappear with time, although risk for resultant sequelae persists if STI are not treated. Third, when symptomatic patients present to established health care systems, STI may be missed. Many STI laboratory tests are costly, and therefore may not be ordered, and often practitioners are hesitant to consider or treat an STI without a laboratory-confirmed diagnosis. Additionally, health care providers may be unfamiliar with some STI and their manifestations and may not consider them during the clinical work-up. Finally, the most serious complications associated with STI typically occur after a long latent period and therefore are often not associated with the original infection. In the case of viral STI, the sequelae of AIDS and malignancies typically do not occur for many years or decades after the initial exposure.

If left untreated, STI can cause a vast array of health consequences, ranging from relatively minor discomfort or cosmetic concerns to death (Table 9.12.1). The most important health consequences fall under the general categories of (1) reproductive morbidity and mortality including adverse pregnancy outcomes and infertility; (2) STI-associated cancers; and (3) enhanced transmission and acquisition of HIV. The most common of the serious STI consequences are adverse reproductive outcomes, particularly infertility, generally caused by chlamydia or gonorrhoea. As noted earlier, chlamydia and gonorrhoea are highly prevalent infections, and 10–40 per cent of women with untreated infection may develop pelvic inflammatory disease (PID), up to 25 per cent of which can result in infertility (World Health Organization 2007). These infections also can lead to ectopic pregnancy, which is associated with maternal morbidity and mortality as well as pregnancy loss. Women who have had PID are 6–10 times more likely than women without PID to develop a subsequent ectopic pregnancy, with an estimated 40–50 per cent of all ectopic pregnancies attributed to PID (World Health Organization 2007). Although mortality associated with ectopic pregnancy has declined markedly in industrialized nations (Ebrahim *et al.* 1997), hospital-based studies in some low-income nations have reported from 1 per cent to 3 per cent fatality rates associated with ectopic pregnancy, which is about 10 times higher than fatality rates reported in higher-income nations (Goyaux *et al.* 2003). Limited other data suggest ectopic pregnancy may be the source of as much as 11 per cent of maternal mortality in some developing-world settings (Goyaux *et al.* 2003; Meheus 1992). Chlamydial and gonorrhoeal infections also can lead to the long-term morbidity of chronic pelvic pain in women.

Another large proportion of the reproductive morbidity associated with STI is related to adverse pregnancy outcomes for infants, including foetal loss or stillbirth, premature birth or low birth weight infant, blindness, or neonatal death. Maternal syphilis is the most important cause of adverse pregnancy outcome, accounting for an estimated 750 000 to 1.5 million deaths worldwide each year (Schmid *et al.* 2007), morbidity even greater than that associated with perinatal HIV infection. Although antenatal screening is routinely recommended throughout the world, syphilis prevalence rates still range from 4 to 15 per cent in women attending antenatal care clinics in some African settings (World Health Organization 2007). Studies have documented that 25–40 per cent of all pregnancies among women with untreated early syphilis will result in stillbirth, and a further 14 per cent of these pregnancies will result in neonatal death (World Health Organization 2007; Watson-Jones *et al.* 2007). Universal syphilis screening and treatment of pregnant women would prevent more than 500 000 stillbirths and perinatal deaths each year in Africa alone (World Health Organization 2007; Schmid *et al.* 2007). Chlamydia has been associated with neonatal pneumonia and more commonly with neonatal conjunctivitis which, if left untreated, can lead to blindness. WHO estimated that in 2006, from 1000 to 4000 infants worldwide were blinded from STI-related conjunctivitis, which is easily preventable with topical antimicrobial agents (World Health Organization 2007). Viral STI also can lead to adverse outcomes of pregnancy. HSV-2 can cause neonatal herpes infection which, although unusual (estimated at 1 in 3000 births in the United States), is often severe or fatal (Brown *et al.* 1997) and perinatally transmitted HPV can cause recurrent respiratory papillomatosis, a chronic condition often requiring recurrent surgical procedures. On the other hand, the majority of HBV and HCV infections in infants are asymptomatic, although perinatal HBV infection will often result in chronic infection and subsequent complications (CDC 2006).

The second important category of serious STI-related health consequences are malignancies, including anogenital cancers, hepatocellular cancers, lymphomas (e.g. those associated with HIV), and sarcomas (e.g. Kaposi's sarcoma associated with human herpes virus type 8 [HHV-8]). It is now firmly established that certain HPV subtypes are the causal agents of cervical cancer and likely of other anogenital cancers (e.g. vulvar, vaginal, penile, anal) as well (Zur Hausen 1996; Cogliano et al. 2005). Two carcinogenic HPV subtypes, 16 and 18, are responsible for an estimated 70 per cent of all cervical cancers and likely of 80–90 per cent of anal and penile cancers worldwide (Munoz et al. 2003; Daling et al. 2004, 2005). Cervical cancer is now the most common cancer in women worldwide, after breast cancer, and in developing world settings, it is the leading cause of cancer mortality in women, estimated to account for more than 200 000 deaths per year (World Health Organization 2007). The cellular changes associated with carcinogenic HPV types occur slowly, presenting first with dysplasia and later with localized (in situ) disease before proceeding to invasive cancer, a natural history which allows early detection and treatment through cervical screening programmes (i.e. Pap test or direct cervical visualization). The large disparity in cervical cancer morbidity and mortality between industrialized and developing nations is largely attributed to limited availability of cervical screening and treatment in the latter. In addition, a significant interaction exists between HPV and HIV which can accelerate HPV-related cellular changes and may further contribute to disparities between developed and industrialized settings, at least in high HIV prevalence nations. Routine periodic cervical screening with a Pap test is the standard of care in most high-income nations and in an increasing number of moderate-income nations, with more frequent screening intervals recommended for HIV-infected women. However, in developing-world settings many women have never had a Pap smear (Schmiedeskamp & Kockler 2006).

HBV is a highly prevalent infection in developing-world settings, which is typically related to vertical transmission from mother-to-child. HBV also is commonly transmitted parenterally through tainted blood products, organs, or medical or illicit drug injection equipment. This virus also can be transmitted sexually, and in industrialized nations such as the United States where vertical transmission is unusual, sexual transmission now accounts for a majority of HBV infections, and is especially common among men who have sex with men (MSM). HBV is associated with several serious, long-term complications, including cirrhosis and end-stage liver disease and hepatocellular cancer (primary liver cancer). Hepatocellular cancer is the fifth leading cause of cancer deaths in adults worldwide but ranks third in developing-world settings, accounting for 415 000–500 000 deaths per year, of which 80 per cent occur in Asia and sub-Saharan Africa (Pisani et al. 1999; McGlynn & London 2005). Just over half of hepatocellular carcinomas globally are attributed to chronic HBV infection, with regional estimates varying greatly, ranging from 16 per cent in North America, 47 per cent each in Africa and Southeast Asia, 59 per cent in Eastern Mediterranean countries, and 65 per cent in East Asia (Perz et al. 2006). About 25 per cent of hepatocellular cancers are caused by HCV (which is sexually transmitted in about 20 per cent of cases) (Perz et al. 2006). In addition to malignancies, HBV and HCV also are major contributors to cirrhosis globally (causing 30 per cent and 27 per cent of all cases, respectively) (Perz et al. 2006).

The third important category of adverse STI-associated outcomes is related to HIV transmission and acquisition. Persons co-infected with HIV and certain STI, particularly those causing genital ulcers, have higher levels of HIV shedding than HIV-infected persons without other STI; co-infected individuals are more likely to transmit HIV to an uninfected partner; and successful STD treatment has been documented to reduce viral shedding (Fleming & Wasserheit 1999). Additionally, HIV-uninfected people with certain STI—again particularly genital ulcers—are more susceptible to acquiring new HIV infections from HIV-infected sex partners, probably by disrupting mucosal integrity and by increasing the presence and activation of HIV-susceptible cells in the genital tract (Fleming & Wasserheit 1999). Intervention studies have demonstrated that routine STI clinical services and condom promotion can result in large reductions in HIV incidence or prevention of epidemic increases among high-risk persons such as commercial sex workers (CSW) (Levine et al. 1998; Laga et al. 1994; Plummer et al. 2005). Furthermore, a community randomized trial conducted in Mwanza, Tanzania, in the early 1990s documented that communities receiving an improved programme of management of symptomatic STI had reduced HIV incidence compared with communities with typical STI management programmes—supporting an HIV prevention benefit at the community level (Grosskurth et al. 2000). The lack of a similar effect in subsequent community level intervention trials (i.e. Rakai study of mass treatment; Wawer et al. 1999, and Masaka study of enhanced syndromic management; Korenromp et al. 2005) evaluating various STI control strategies indicates that a community-level HIV benefit is not likely to occur in all circumstances or for all populations but that such benefit may be particularly important in settings of early (non-generalized) epidemics with a high prevalence of bacterial GUD (White et al. 2004). Nonetheless, the individual-level benefit of STI treatment for HIV-infected persons co-infected with curable STI or for HIV susceptible persons with symptomatic STI is compelling. Even in advanced HIV epidemics where STI care has less population-level impact on HIV, it remains an effective intervention at the individual level and may be particularly important in preventing transmission from persons with HIV infection, underlining the importance of offering STI services to those in HIV care. The strong association of genital ulcer disease with HIV transmission, along with the above-noted observation that high HSV-2 prevalence often occurs in countries with high HIV prevalence, raises the question of whether treatment of genital HSV-2 might reduce the likelihood of HSV-2 or HIV shedding (or both) and thus prevent transmission or acquisition of new HIV infections (Paz-Bailey et al. 2007; Weiss 2004). This is of particular interest because some antiviral agents (e.g. acyclovir) that are effective against genital HSV-2 are now off-patent and therefore may be affordably priced even for low-income nations with high HIV prevalence. A recent trial has demonstrated that treatment of HSV-2 infections can reduce HIV shedding in HSV-2/HIV co-infected, asymptomatic persons (Nagot et al. 2007), and a rigorous evaluation involving several larger, multinational randomized controlled trials in various populations is expected to provide additional data about this potential HIV prevention strategy within the next few years.

Conceptual framework for STD prevention

Individual vs. population benefit

STI prevention programmes provide benefits both to individuals and to the larger population. Individual benefits derive from activities that prevent acquisition of infection, ameliorate symptoms, and reduce complications of initial infection, while the general population benefits from efforts that prevent continuing transmission and thus reduce overall prevalence of infection and complications in the population (Aral *et al.* 2005; Douglas & Fenton 2007). Since activities that prevent acquisition of infection (behaviour change, condom use, vaccines) or lead to diagnosis and treatment of curable infections (e.g. screening, clinical care, management) also prevent subsequent transmission, they provide population-level as well as individual-level effects. Alternatively, some interventions may have greater effects on transmission, and thus population benefit, than on personal health. One example is vaccination of males for HPV 16/18, where models indicate that there may be an effect on disease in women but limited benefit for men (Hughes *et al.* 2002). Another example is measures to prevent transmission from persons chronically infected with HSV-2 or HIV (e.g. suppressive antiviral treatment to prevent HSV-2 transmission between sexual partners; maternal antiretroviral treatment to prevent vertical transmission, promotion of condom use; etc.) (White *et al.* 2004). The relative importance of individual versus population benefit can vary by specific subpopulation. For example, substantial STI prevention efforts are focused on subpopulations important in continuing transmission, such as 'core groups' (groups who have high STI prevalence and also high rates of partner change, discussed in depth later). Interventions aimed at core groups have the potential to have greater population-level impact than those targeted at the broader, general population, and thus are often higher priorities for public health programmes (Douglas & Fenton 2007; Aral *et al.* 1996).

Determinants of transmission

An important concept in understanding STI epidemiology in populations and the possible impact of prevention strategies is the STI transmission dynamics model of May and Anderson (1987). The reproductive rate of an STI in a population (R_0), which is the average number of new infections generated by each infected person, is based on three factors: (1) the likelihood of transmission per sexual contact between an infected person and a susceptible partner (B); (2) the average number of new sexual partnerships formed over time between infected and susceptible persons (c); and (3) the average duration of infectiousness (D), where $R_0 = BcD$. Incidence and prevalence of a specific STI within a population will increase when R_0 exceeds 1 and decrease if R_0 falls below 1. Circumstances that reduce any of the three factors will reduce R_0 and population prevalence (Brunham 2005).

A primary focus of STI prevention programmes has been reduction in duration of infectiousness (D) by detecting and treating infected persons. Measures to accomplish this goal include enhancing access to and utilization of health care, improving case finding, and improving completion of treatment after clinical contact. Prevention strategies that reduce transmission efficiency (B) and number of sexual partnerships (c) can affect all STI but are particularly important for those that are not curable by antimicrobial therapy, such as HIV, HSV-2, and HPV. Most approaches to reduce transmission efficiency are behavioural (e.g. efforts to promote male and female condom use; efforts to reduce higher-risk practices such as needle sharing), but a growing number of biomedical approaches shows promise. For example, suppressive antiviral therapy of HSV-2 has been proven to reduce transmission within

discordant sexual partnerships (Corey *et al.* 2005). In addition, male circumcision has been recently shown to reduce transmission of HIV and possibly other STI (Weiss 2007). Most importantly, effective vaccines markedly reduce susceptibility. Vaccination programmes have substantially reduced the incidence of HBV in developed countries (CDC 2006) and may have similar effects in the future on HPV (Goldie *et al.* 2004). Even low-efficacy vaccines or those that reduce viral load without completely preventing infection can have substantial effects at the population level (Anderson & Hanson 2005). Finally, strategies to reduce sexual partnerships between susceptible and infected partners can have the broadest effects, but may be difficult to implement and sustain. For example, although programmes to encourage abstinence by adolescents have been strongly encouraged in the United States, there is growing evidence that such programmes may have limited effectiveness (Santelli *et al.* 2006). Encouraging a reduction in the number of sex partners, particularly among people with frequent sex partner change (e.g. sex workers), may be a more plausible approach, based on experiences in several countries where HIV prevalence has fallen (Shelton *et al.* 2004).

Sexual networks and core groups

In addition to these factors' affecting transmission at the level of individuals and their partners, networks of sexual interaction within populations also influence likelihood of contact between susceptible and infected persons (Aral *et al.* 1996; Adimora & Schoenbach 2005). Sexual networks consist of groups or individuals who are directly or indirectly sexually connected, and the location of an individual in such networks can influence the likelihood of infection as much as or more than personal behaviour by influencing the prevalence of infection in their partners. Larger numbers of sexual linkages in a subpopulation can result in transmission of STI from core groups to the general population, especially if the sexual partnerships are formed concurrently rather than sequentially and involve dissassortative (like-with-unlike) mixing patterns (Aral *et al.* 1996, 2005). Sexual networks can be affected by a variety of contextual factors, such as community norms about sexual behaviour; migration and travel patterns; economic circumstances; and the societal disruptions induced by natural disasters, political conflict, and wars. As noted earlier, a related concept in STI prevention is that of the 'core group', persons with multiple partners at well-connected points in sexual networks who are responsible for continuing STI transmission. From the perspective of STI transmission determinants, they are defined as groups or individuals with sufficient rates of sex partner change to maintain $R_0 > 1$, and their characteristics will vary by their location in the sexual network and by specific STI depending on duration of infection and efficiency of transmission. Targeting core groups with STI prevention efforts such as screening and condom promotion can be more efficient and cost-effective than efforts targeted more broadly (Over & Piot 1996; Douglas & Fenton 2007). Programmes focusing on CSWs, persons living in geographic areas with a high prevalence of reported cases of STD, incarcerated persons, or those with repeat STI infection have used the core group approach (Leichliter *et al.* 2007; Williams & Kahn 2007).

STI prevention programmes

The previous section described why, for communicable diseases such as STI, effective diagnosis and treatment is an important prevention strategy. Prompt and effective treatment of curable STI minimizes their adverse outcomes in the individual patient, but also reduces further spread of STI into the community (making STI exposure less likely). However, clinical case management considered alone has limitations that are illustrated by a tuberculosis management model developed using actual data from rural women in one African nation (Ryan *et al.* 2007; Waaler & Piot 1969). Figure 9.12.2a describes STI prevalence in a community and a series of steps required to ensure effective STI treatment, focusing on the proportion of STI missed (not effectively treated) at each step. The model illustrates that most people with STI, even those with symptoms, are not effectively treated; and even fewer have sex partners effectively treated. These issues can be addressed, however. Figure 9.12.2b shows the potential benefits of (i) well-conducted clinic-based management (i.e. persons coming to health facilities obtain effective STI treatment); (ii) the incremental benefits that might be attained if symptomatic patients who do not come to health facilities could be identified and receive STI services (e.g. through asymptomatic screening, targeted outreach programmes, community-based educational efforts and effective partner management); and (iii) the incremental benefits that primary prevention might bring (e.g. through high coverage of an effective STI vaccine; or widespread community education around STI prevention, whether abstinence, delaying initiation of sex in adolescents, or promotion of safer sex practices such as correct and consistent condom use).

With this concept that STI clinical services cannot, by themselves, control STI in a community, STI prevention programmes are based on several essential components working together. These include STI surveillance, STI prevention interventions, and programme support components.

Surveillance

As for other public health programmes, accurate STI surveillance is critical for assessing the magnitude of the problem, trends over

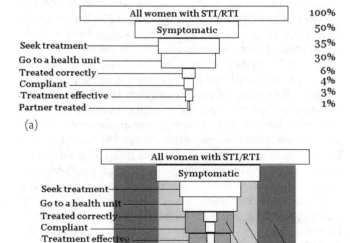

(a)

(b)

Fig. 9.12.2 (a) Piot–Fransen model of STI prevalence and typical STI case management. (b) Potential benefits of additional control strategies in concert with STI case management.

time, emergence of outbreaks or new problems, development of prevention strategies, prioritization of resources, and monitoring public health effects. There are several approaches to surveillance that can provide complementary information (World Health Organization 2007; Douglas & Fenton 2007). First, *case-reporting* provides a measure of new cases of STI or associated syndromes over a specified time interval and is the most common surveillance activity, especially in jurisdictions with functional reporting systems for notifiable infectious diseases. In industrialized countries, gonorrhoea, syphilis, and chlamydia are generally nationally reportable, with reports generated by clinicians, laboratories, or both. In developing countries where national reporting is more difficult, reporting from sentinel clinics can be useful. Second, *prevalence monitoring* can define the prevalence of STI or related syndromes in defined populations undergoing routine assessment (e.g. screening or diagnostic testing for infections, examination for syndromes) and can complement case-reporting in assessing the burden of infection or disease. For example, in the United States, while notifiable cases of chlamydia have continually climbed as screening has increased, prevalence monitoring in STI and family planning clinics has shown little change, indicating that the burden of infection is unlikely to be rising (CDC 2005, 2006). Third, *sentinel surveillance* generally refers to data collection from representative 'sentinel populations' for outcomes not routinely measured, such as antimicrobial resistance or infectious aetiology of various STI-related syndromes, and is often useful for generating broader guidance about appropriate treatment regimens and national lists of essential medications. Fourth, *population-based surveys*, involving collection of data such as prevalence of specific infections from persons considered representative of the general population are difficult to perform but provide the best assessment of population burden. In addition to these approaches for assessing morbidity, periodic surveillance of sexual behaviours or health services can be useful in monitoring the need for or responses to educational and health marketing efforts, and can also provide information on where prevention services are most needed (Douglas & Fenton 2007). Because of the large burden of disease and often limited resources for collection and analysis of STI surveillance data, conducting effective STI surveillance is challenging even in industrialized countries, and there is a critical need to enhance it in developing countries by improving laboratory facilities and surveillance personnel and strengthening reporting mechanisms (World Health Organization 2007).

STI prevention interventions

STI prevention interventions include clinical management, laboratory services, partner management strategies, and health education and behavioural interventions.

Clinical management

STI clinical management (i.e. diagnosis, treatment, and prevention services at a health facility) is generally considered the core intervention for STI prevention efforts. Effective clinical management can provide individual health benefits (e.g. ameliorating symptoms and preventing complications), but it can also provide overall population health benefits. From the perspective of transmission determinants, effective diagnosis and treatment reduce the duration of infection (D) and thus reduce efficiency of further transmission in the community. STI clinical services can be offered in virtually any type of clinical setting, ranging from specialty STI, HIV, and family planning clinics to primary care clinics and antenatal clinic services; additionally, STI screening is increasingly offered in non-clinical outreach settings. Because of the sensitive and often stigmatizing nature of STI, particular attention must be paid to offering services that are nonjudgmental and confidential.

The traditional approach to STI clinical management has been through dedicated specialty clinics classified as STI, genitourinary, or dermato-venereology clinics (Douglas & Fenton 2007). These are typically publicly funded clinics staffed by providers with greater clinical experience and who generally have greater access to comprehensive rapid and conventional diagnostic testing and treatment services than providers in other settings. Especially in wealthier countries, there is often heavy reliance on laboratory testing to establish aetiologic diagnoses that can enhance surveillance and partner services. Such clinics frequently offer a comprehensive range of sexual health services including HIV testing, risk-reduction counselling and condom provision, contraception, referral for other services (e.g. HIV and substance abuse care), Pap testing and immunizations (e.g. HBV vaccine). However, even in countries where such specialty clinic services are available, most STI management is provided in other types of health facilities. In the United States, for example, the majority of all reportable STI now originates from non-STI clinic sites (e.g. primary and secondary syphilis—67 per cent, gonorrhoea—65 per cent, chlamydia—76 per cent) (CDC 2006), with other important sites including family planning, correctional health care, and primary care clinics and specialty providers in both public and private sector settings. In developing countries, STI services are often provided by private providers, traditional healers, or pharmacists, and quality of management may be suboptimal (World Health Organization 2007; Douglas & Fenton 2007). The importance of integrating high quality, comprehensive STI management into a spectrum of other settings including private clinics, is particularly critical in developing countries in order to enhance coverage, access, and ultimately impact (World Health Organization 2007).

In an ideal world, STI clinical management would be guided by use of rapid, point-of-care diagnostic tests (done at the time of the initial clinic visit) that are affordable, easy to use, and highly sensitive and specific. Such rapid STI tests are generally not available, and tests that do exist are often costly and require several days for results. Given the limited availability of reliable, high-quality, or affordable diagnostic tests in most developing countries, WHO has recommended that settings with limited diagnostic infrastructure consider using locally validated syndromic management approaches for care of symptomatic STI and other reproductive tract infections (RTI) (Dallabetta et al. 2007; World Health Organization 2007; Ryan et al. 2007). Syndromic management is based on the identification of a 'syndrome', a constellation of easily elicited symptoms and recognizable clinical signs that are associated with a limited number of defined STI or RTI aetiologies. The approach is practical in that it can be carried out in almost any setting (Dallabetta et al. 2007). It does not require laboratory facilities, and patients are treated at the initial clinical visit, which allows prompt treatment and thus reduces chances for complications to develop or for further STI spread to sex partners. Costs are minimized because laboratory tests are avoided and drug regimens are simplified. The use of standardized algorithms covering all likely conditions reduces treatment failures, eliminating the need for repeated visits or referrals to higher level centres. Standardized regimens also help improve case-reporting for surveillance and, consequently, provide more information for programme management (Dallabetta et al. 2007; Ryan et al. 2007).

The syndromic approach also has important limitations (Dallabetta et al. 2007; World Health Organization 2007). The most critical is that it does not address asymptomatic patients, who account for the majority of curable STI. Asymptomatic women with cervical infections are at risk for serious adverse outcomes including tubal damage and infertility, but they are not covered by this approach. Furthermore, because many genitourinary symptoms are caused by other conditions or situations in the absence of an STI, the syndromic approach can lead to false positive diagnoses and thus to unnecessary drug use, additional costs and potential partner issues. Partner management is a particular issue, as many providers are hesitant to treat sex partners of individuals who are treated without a specific, laboratory-defined STI aetiology, even though re-infection of the patient would be very likely without treatment of a steady sex partner. Additionally, the most common presenting syndrome for women, vaginal discharge syndrome, is usually caused by non-STI related RTIs (e.g. bacterial vaginosis, candidiasis) or by other factors. Vaginitis can be complicated to treat, often requiring multiple visits and repeated presumptive treatment trials, which can be costly and may lead to side effects. Finally, some health care providers, particularly physicians, have been reluctant to adopt syndromic approaches because they have been trained in aetiologic diagnosis-based treatment and often view syndromic management as 'unscientific' (Dallabetta et al. 2007; Ryan et al. 2007).

Programmatic evaluations from a variety of settings indicate that syndromic management approaches are particularly effective for management of genital ulcer syndrome in men and women, urethritis or epididymitis in men, and neonatal conjunctivitis in infants (World Health Organization 2007). Over the past decade, repeated cross-sectional studies in several nations indicate that bacterial causes of genital ulcer syndrome have markedly declined in parts of Africa (World Health Organization 2007). Although this finding may be related to other factors, it suggests that the widespread promotion of syndromic management has had a substantial effect on reducing the prevalence and controlling the bacterial STI most highly associated with HIV transmission and acquisition.

Because the majority of persons with most STI are asymptomatic, screening asymptomatic persons is an important adjunct to providing STI clinical services. However, appropriate screening strategies (e.g. which infection, population, venue, frequency, etc.) must be carefully considered because of implications for resources and infrastructure. Screening programmes are most justifiable when complications are severe; when screening tests are sensitive, specific, and inexpensive; and when treatment options are available. For example, syphilis screening of pregnant women meets these criteria and is widely recommended as part of antenatal care. Within the United States and many other industrialized countries, examples of other STI screening recommendations include annual screening for chlamydia of sexually active women under 25 years of age; screening of pregnant women for syphilis, gonorrhoea, chlamydia, and HIV; annual screening of sexually active MSM for gonorrhoea, chlamydia, syphilis, and HIV; and routine Pap testing (every 1–3 years for women starting at age 21) (CDC 2006; Douglas & Fenton 2007).

Although not traditionally included in STI clinical services, the availability of safe and effective STI vaccines has increased interest in their provision in selected settings. Although HBV vaccine is a routine infant immunization in many countries, settings providing STI care or serving those at high STI risk have been recommended as additional venues for HBV immunization (CDC 2006; Douglas & Fenton 2007). The recent licensure of an HPV vaccine, now recommended in the United States for 11–12-year-old girls routinely and for young women from 13 to 26 years of age as a catch-up vaccine (CDC 2007), creates the possibility of linking a second vaccine to STI services to enhance population coverage. HPV vaccines are projected to be cost-effective even in settings with Pap test screening programmes (Elbasha *et al.* 2007), although they will have the greatest potential impact in developing countries with no organized cervical cancer prevention programmes. Possible ancillary benefit of an STI vaccine widely recommended for young women include the chance to establish vaccine platforms that are relevant to future HIV vaccines, and to destigmatize and normalize STI prevention services.

Laboratory services

Laboratory services are essential for effective surveillance and clinical services. In settings where diagnostic tests are available, they can provide accurate diagnosis of symptomatic persons and exposed sex partners and a means of screening asymptomatic high-risk populations. As noted earlier, for optimal utility, STI laboratory tests should be accurate, rapid, simple, and inexpensive. For curable STI, where administration of a short course of therapy can interrupt transmission as well as resolve symptoms and prevent complications, test sensitivity has traditionally been more important than specificity. However, in recent years, test specificity has been an increasing concern, owing to the growing importance of chronic viral STI (where a diagnosis can have lifelong implications), increased STI screening in asymptomatic populations (where low specificity can reduce positive predictive value and result in an unacceptable level of false positive diagnoses), and greater attention to partner services (where a false positive diagnosis can lead to unnecessary distress or relationship problems) (Cates & Holmes 1998).

In developing countries, insufficient resources and infrastructure limit the capacity of laboratory testing to affect clinical care of individuals. However, in these settings, laboratory services still play a critical role in validating and intermittently re-assessing the appropriateness of algorithms for syndromic case management. For example, as noted above, over the past 10 years, such assessments have pointed to the growing importance of HSV-2 in genital ulcer disease, leading to revised algorithms including empiric antiviral therapy. Laboratory services are also essential for monitoring trends in antimicrobial resistance, particularly for gonorrhoea. Because susceptibility testing for individual patients is impractical, national and regional surveillance systems have been important in detecting emerging gonococcal resistance and altering management guidelines (World Health Organization 2007).

Rapid, point-of-care laboratory tests are especially important for STI prevention for several reasons. In many settings, persons with STI may not return for follow-up visits. In addition, prompt diagnosis expedites the time to treatment and partner services, which can reduce spread of STI in the community. In settings with low rates of follow-up, use of rapid tests can result in more complete treatment of infected persons than can the use of more sensitive but slower conventional tests (Gift *et al.* 1999). Clinics specializing in STI care have emphasized rapid diagnosis in men by use of microscopy for diagnosis of gonorrhoea and urethritis by Gram stain, of trichomoniasis in women by wet mount examination, and of syphilis by darkfield examination. Rapid serologic tests for syphilis (e.g. RPR card tests) have been important in syphilis control, but can be difficult to use properly. Newer generation rapid tests that are simple enough to use in developing country settings offer great promise in screening pregnant women and preventing vertical transmission, and are one of the bases for new global efforts at elimination of congenital syphilis.

Partner management

Partner management has long been integral to STI control programmes, initiated in the first few decades of the twentieth century for syphilis control in many industrialized countries (Brewer 2005; Hogben *et al.* 2007). Its principal goal is notifying sex partners of persons with STI diagnoses of their exposure to enhance early diagnosis and treatment, providing health benefit at both the individual level (to index patients whose risk of re-infection is reduced and to partners, for whom early treatment may avoid complications) and the population level (by preventing continuing transmission). Additional benefits of partner management include fulfilment of an ethical duty to warn persons exposed to serious infections, as well as the opportunity to enhance understanding of sexual and drug-use networks in which STI transmission is occurring.

Two basic approaches are used for partner management services: Provider referral and patient referral (Brewer 2005; Hogben *et al.* 2007). The former involves the use of third parties, usually health care providers or public health workers, to interview the index patient to determine partner names and locating information, with subsequent confidential notification of partners about their exposure and their need for testing and treatment. In contrast, patient referral, which offers a less labour-intensive approach for the many settings with insufficient resources to conduct provider referral, relies upon the index patient to notify their partner(s), preferably assisted by written materials. A hybrid approach known as contract-referral begins with patient referral but is followed by provider referral if contacts have not been notified within a specified time-frame. The primary focus of partner management has been on the curable STI (e.g. syphilis, gonorrhoea, chlamydia, and trichomoniasis), although there is growing interest in partner services for persons with HIV infection, and, in some countries, for other viral STI such as genital HSV and HPV.

The efficacy of partner referral has been summarized in several recent reviews (Passin *et al.* 2006; Brewer 2005; Hogben *et al.* 2007). Provider referral has a similar yield for the curable STI of syphilis, chlamydia, and gonorrhoea, with a range of 0.22–0.25 infected partners identified and treated per index patient. Estimations of the effect of partner services on population transmission are limited, although several reports have described reductions in gonorrhoea incidence following increased partner management efforts (Du *et al.* 2006; Douglas & Fenton 2007; Han *et al.* 1999). Although there have been few direct comparisons, patient referral appears to have a lower yield than provider referral. However, even in industrialized countries, there are insufficient resources to offer provider services to more than a minority of patients. Therefore, novel approaches, such as expedited partner therapy, which relies on the delivery of therapy by patients to partners without a provider examination, are of increasing interest. This approach has been shown to increase partner treatment and to reduce index patient re-infection for both gonorrhoea and chlamydia, and modelling studies indicate that it may allow sufficiently increased population coverage to reduce population prevalence (Golden *et al.* 2005; White *et al.* 2005; Douglas & Fenton 2007). Increased operational research to better understand benefit and acceptability of different approaches, especially in developing countries, is an important STI prevention priority (World Health Organization 2007).

Health education and behavioural interventions

A mainstay of effective STI prevention programmes is the provision of health education and other strategies to promote healthful sexual behaviour. Basic educational messages should include primary prevention strategies such as the benefits of delaying initiation of sexual activity, reducing the number and concurrency of sex partners, and the benefit of the correct and consistent use of condoms in situations where partners are not known to be free of STI. They should also include information about the value of preventive interventions such as testing and immunizations, and the importance of seeking care for possible STI symptoms to facilitate early STI diagnosis and treatment and prevention of transmission to partners (World Health Organization 2007). In addition, for those in whom an STI is diagnosed, information on completing therapy, need for follow-up examinations or testing, notification of sex partners, and STI preventive measures in the future are all important.

Health education can be supplemented by behavioural intervention services that promote healthful sexual behaviour. Such interventions can be conducted at both individual and community levels. Individually focused interventions target behaviour change at the individual level by providing knowledge or strategies to modify attitudes, beliefs, motivation, or skills and such interventions include approaches such as risk-reduction counselling for adolescents, MSM and persons with an STI; outreach and counselling programmes for illicit drug users; and condom promotion and distribution programmes for high-risk individuals such as CSW. Such interventions are most efficiently delivered in settings where high-risk individuals can be easily accessed. Successful examples include risk-reduction counselling delivered in STI clinic settings (Kamb *et al.* 1998) and educational videos promoting safer behaviour in waiting room settings (Warner & Rietmeijer 2006), prevention counselling for persons with HIV infection in HIV care settings (CDC 2003), and street outreach projects targeting high-risk youth and injecting drug users (Greenberg *et al.* 1998). Such interventions may be particularly effective at 'teachable moments', when individuals first learn that they have an STI. In contrast, interventions targeted at the community level address individual risk in the broader context of their social networks and environments and attempt to modify social norms, influence social and sexual networks, and reduce community barriers to healthful sexual behaviour and health-care seeking behaviour (CDC 2001).

Health marketing, also known as social marketing, is an aspect of health communication directed at the community that is of emerging importance both in industrialized and in developing countries. It combines techniques from consumer marketing (e.g. consumer research and marketing) with theoretical models of behaviour change, creating a hybrid form of marketing whose goal is to change awareness, attitudes, beliefs, and behaviours, rather than selling a product (Vega & Ghanem 2007). With the realization that mass media are primary sources of health information for many consumers (Salmon 1989), health marketing campaigns can use a variety of mass media approaches (e.g. printed materials, broadcast media, and the Internet). Although public service announcements (PSAs) have usually been the primary broadcast media approach, these can be effectively complemented by messages conveyed by news reports and entertainment programming, also known as 'edu-tainment'. Recent efforts in the United States to respond to syphilis epidemics in MSM have successfully combined all of these approaches (Vega & Ghanem 2007). The interaction between perceived vulnerability, perceived severity of the health outcome, and efficacy of preventive behaviours is a central issue for development of effective messages. How much such campaigns should emphasize negative consequences has often been controversial, although it appears that appeals to fear can be effective if they are linked to specific protective recommendations and information about how to accomplish the recommendations, while fear appeals without a high-efficacy message can result in denial (Vega & Ghanem 2007; Witte & Allen 2000). STI prevention health marketing should emphasize positive outcomes of prevention (peace of mind, protecting personal and partner health) as well as the normative aspects of the recommended behaviour.

Programme support components

Several programme components are essential to support STI prevention and control interventions. These include leadership and advocacy around STI prevention, STI training for health providers and other public health specialists, monitoring and evaluation of existing programmes to ensure high quality and wide coverage of services, and STI research, including applied programme evaluations or primary research around intervention effectiveness.

Leadership and advocacy

Strong and effective programme leadership is essential for implementing and sustaining effective STI prevention programmes and for effectively integrating the other essential programme components. No matter how effective prevention technologies are, they cannot produce sustainable individual and population benefit without the leadership to develop political will and resources, and to ensure a supportive legal and policy environment for STI prevention and control. The need for effective leadership is especially critical for conditions such as STI because their associated stigma often makes public discussion and community involvement difficult (World Health Organization 2007). Important components of effective leadership include partnerships and collaboration, priority setting and planning, and policy development and implementation.

Given the magnitude of the STI burden, even in countries with dedicated STI prevention programmes and clinics, building effective partnerships and collaborations is increasingly recognized as critical to achieving population coverage and effect (World Health Organization 2007; Douglas & Fenton 2007). Such efforts can include professional organizations, academia, the pharmaceutical industry, the private health care sector, and community-based organizations. Professional organizations can be critical in providing endorsement of prevention activities and training. Regarding community-based organizations, while secular non-governmental organizations have generally been the primary source of partnerships, there has been recent emphasis on collaborations with faith-based organizations, which often have extensive networks including rural locations and which, because of their influence in shaping opinions and attitudes of their members, have great potential for reducing stigmatization (World Health Organization 2007).

To maximize effects and cost-effective use of limited resources, priority setting and planning is an equally important leadership activity. Most countries have developed broad, multisectoral responses to HIV prevention. However, many have not developed similar, comprehensive STI control strategies, and many nations have very limited engagement of private (and sometimes even the public) health sector in STI prevention and control efforts. Some examples of more comprehensive efforts exist, however, such as the national Infertility Prevention Program (CDC 2004) and Syphilis Elimination Plan (CDC 2006) in the United States and the National Strategy for Sexual Health and HIV in the UK (Department of Health 2007). Appropriate surveillance, monitoring, and evaluation are critical for effective priority setting and planning.

Finally, policy development creates an overarching structure for public health programmes and is the key determinant of long-term public health effects. It includes the broad planning efforts described above as well as attention to the legal and regulatory environment, the securing of financial resources, and advocacy for programme priorities. Examples of important legal issues affecting STI prevention include providing confidential (without parental consent) clinical services for young people, ability of non-physician providers to provide services or prescribe drugs, and the permissibility of expedited partner therapy (World Health Organization 2007; CDC 2006). Securing financial resources for STI prevention is a core function with a major effect on population coverage of services since in the private sector the cost of clinical services for low-income users is a major barrier to effective programmes (World Health Organization 2007). Finally, advocacy for and communication of prevention priorities to decision-makers is an increasingly critical policy priority, not only to raise political interest and will but also to mobilize resources. For developing countries, such efforts often involve attempts by multinational organizations such as WHO to work with leaders of possible donor countries.

Training

A well-trained workforce is critical for implementation of all other programme components. As public health and STI prevention have expanded from a largely biomedical focus to include other areas of expertise such as behavioural science, health communications, and informatics, the spectrum of training needs has likewise grown. In addition, with the increasing role of non-categorical STI clinics in providing services, the need to train providers in other sectors—especially primary care and HIV care providers—has increased. The development and dissemination of national guidelines can enhance the quality of care in all sectors (World Health Organization 2007). For example, in the United States, such efforts have included those focused specifically on STI programme operations as well as on more detailed STI management recommendations (CDC 2001, 2006).

Clinical training has historically been provided by health professional schools, but because inclusion of STI training is variable and often suboptimal, retraining of post-graduate staff through on-the-job training, continuing education efforts, and activities by professional organizations (e.g. conferences, journal articles, newsletters, etc.) is of primary importance (World Health Organization 2007). In addition, some countries have provided national training efforts (e.g. the clinical, behavioural, and partner services training provided by the US National Network of STD Prevention Training Centers; (World Health Organization 2007; CDC 2006) sexual health training provided in the UK through the Development Toolkit of the Department of Health). There is increasing interest in the use of the Internet as a low-cost and widely available training medium, particularly in its ability to provide 'just in time' training through rapid access to guidelines for non-specialist providers of STI care (Tietz et al. 2004). Retraining of post-graduates can aid in updating (e.g. on newer tests and therapies) and also introducing new approaches (e.g. on recent vaccines, risk-reduction counselling, expedited partner therapy).

All of these issues are compounded by challenges in workforce capacity both in industrialized and in developing countries which are not specific to STI programmes but which affect them. In the United States, the overall public health workforce is aging, with estimated retirement rates over the next several years of more than 40 per cent and chronic shortages in professional areas such as nursing, epidemiology and laboratory science (ASTHO 2004). In the developing world, there are grave shortages of health care workers in all sectors related to limited resources for education of professionals, but compounded both by 'brain drain', when trained professionals leave to go to wealthier countries experiencing shortages, as well as by donor support for scaling up vertical programmes (e.g. HIV treatment and care), causing a shift in workforce from other health sectors.

Monitoring and evaluation

The purpose of monitoring and evaluation is to ensure high-quality, appropriate services (Hassig et al. 1996). Fundamentally, monitoring and evaluation are tools that allow documentation of the overall value and improvement of an STI prevention and control programme over time. While programme monitoring was once mainly conducted as a periodic activity to assure aspects of programme quality, with funding nowadays increasingly linked to attainment of a programme's targeted goals and objectives, monitoring and evaluation have blossomed into a science in their own right. For best results, monitoring and evaluation should be introduced as part of the design and development of any programme, not only in the implementation phases. A number of useful 'how to' tools have become available to help with this (Salabarria-Pena et al. 2007). When monitoring and evaluation are approached as an expected part of an overall programme, data collection procedures are more likely to be done well and less likely to be considered a burden by members of the staff (Hassig et al. 1996).

Monitoring refers to tracking data that measure the progress of a specific STI prevention or control programme in carrying out the steps that the programme is designed to achieve. The data collected should identify programme strengths and weaknesses, and thus serve to document programme progress, identify resource needs and allocation and make changes needed to improve programmes. Programme monitoring often involves measuring factors such as service delivery, staff performance, adequacy of staffing patterns, client satisfaction, or resource needs and allocation (Hassig et al. 1996). Collecting data on programme operating costs (e.g. staff salaries), commodities, and other resources expended is an important part of programme monitoring, and is also important in the evaluation phase of a programme to measure cost-effectiveness. Examples of indicators monitoring service delivery include the hours of operation of a specific clinical facility, the number of patient encounters that took place during a specified time interval, the numbers of specific STI or disease syndromes diagnosed over a time interval, the numbers of commodities (e.g. condoms, drugs, syringes) dispensed during that interval, average patient waiting time, the number (or type, or training) of staff at the facility, and adequacy of water, lighting and cleanliness.

Ensuring 'good service' is not easy, as adequacy of service is seldom entirely objective. Important first steps for any STI programme are ensuring that expectations are clearly documented in programme procedures manuals, and that staff members receive training on specific programme expectations. Given clear programme expectations, managers have employed a variety of tools to try to measure quality of service delivery. One of these is periodic on-site observation of services by supervisors, using a predetermined checklist of events (e.g. provider treated patient with respect). Ideally, such observation would be followed by constructive feedback to providers while the specifics of a situation were still fresh in the mind. Several peer monitoring techniques have also been employed, such as periodic case conferences where providers are asked to share particularly satisfying or difficult patient interactions, with a chance for colleagues to offer feedback. The use of simulated patients who go through services and report back on how services were delivered has been used by programmes in many nations. Patient satisfaction surveys may also be useful, although they tend to provide fewer data on service quality than other techniques when patients are not aware of the quality of service that they ought to expect. Because providers tend to focus on the services for which they are judged, the focus should be on a small number of indicators that are vitally important to the programme. Ideally, these should be factors that can be easily collected; otherwise data collection may get interfere with service provision (Hassig et al. 1996). Some examples of helpful prevention indicators are the two developed by the WHO Global Programme on AIDS: (1) the proportion of clients presenting for STI diagnosis and treatment who are treated according to national guidelines (PI-6), and (2) the proportion of clients presenting for STI diagnosis and treatment who receive appropriate prevention-related services (PI-7). Both involve a combination of routine data collection and direct observation to assess quality of STI service delivery (World Health Organization 1994; Franco et al. 1997).

Evaluation measures a programme's impact, whether on intermediate-term goals (e.g. reducing chlamydia prevalence in a defined population) or longer-term goals (e.g. preventing chlamydia-related sequelae in a defined population). Evaluation measures may focus on specific disease pathogens, the burden of STI overall, longer-term sequelae, or cost-effectiveness of programmes (e.g. cost per case averted). Sometimes referred to as 'data for decision making', evaluation data are important in determining whether an STI programme is worth continuing, and convincing policy makers about the value of a specific programme. Because programme goals will vary among interested parties, many experts recommend that programme goals and objectives ought to be developed collaboratively by the major stakeholders involved (rather than imposed by outside evaluators); this approach is also likely to increase compliance in data collection (Salabarria-Pena et al. 2007). Some common ways to collect impact data are through evaluation of STI surveillance data (whether case-reports or population-based surveys), STI-related morbidity indicators collected from non-STI service

sites, results of special studies conducted by the STI control programme itself, or by other means (e.g. Demographic and Health Surveys) (Hassig et al. 1996).

Ultimately, the value of findings identified in monitoring and evaluation systems is to modify, strengthen, and improve the programme. This is more likely to take place if simple feedback mechanisms are established to ensure that programme staff members are aware of problems and can make needed changes. Feedback mechanisms may range from simple procedures, such as routine monthly communication from a supervisor or manager to the clinic staff to sophisticated annual reports on all aspects of programme performance (Hassig et al. 1996).

Research

Research helps in identifying more effective ways to conduct current prevention activities and in developing effective approaches to emerging problems. Most of the advances in STI prevention programmes and policy over the past decade were stimulated by research findings in the areas of epidemiology, clinical manifestations, and natural history of infection, diagnostics, therapeutics, and primary prevention approaches such as behavioural strategies, barrier contraceptives, and vaccines. Research is typically not conducted by STI prevention programmes; however, it is increasingly apparent that programme involvement is important, if not essential, for successful research translation. Programme involvement helps ensure that programme-relevant research questions are identified and that appropriate approaches to prevention research are used to evaluate intervention effectiveness, whether at the individual or population level (Aral et al. 2007).

There are many research priorities facing the field of STI prevention. Some are the development of better diagnostic tests (e.g. more accurate, faster, and cheaper); improved therapies, especially for those STI for which antimicrobial resistance is a concern; new vaccines, especially for viral STI; enhanced approaches for partner services; use of new communications technologies for prevention (e.g. Internet, social networking websites); practical use of sexual network analysis to reduce STI transmission; effective strategies for reducing HIV transmission through STI control; and determining the best combinations of interventions to enhance STI control. These efforts will require the involvement of a variety of sectors, including the pharmaceutical industry, academia, government, research networks, and involved communities (Douglas & Fenton 2007).

Special issues for STI prevention

Access to care

Effective STI management requires symptomatic individuals to have access to appropriate quality health services. That is a deceptively simple statement, however, as gaining access to STI care is a remarkably complex transaction in almost all societies. In addition to the general issues surrounding availability, affordability, and acceptability of health services, seeking health care for an STI is a function of attitudes about disease and sex (Dallabetta et al. 2007). In virtually every society, STI are associated with substantial stigmatization and prejudice, and tend to be viewed as 'social diseases' that are dirty, shameful, and somehow deserved. This may be the general norm even in the situation that occurs for many women (and all infants), whose STI exposure may be related to a partner's risk rather their own. Access to STI services requires that services be available; that involves factors such as easy-to-reach locations, convenient hours of operation, and providers trained in effective STI management. Access to effective STI management also requires affordability of the services. In some communities, public clinics may exist which are free of charge, but individuals may be required to pay for drugs prescribed. A recent review found that STI drug treatment (excluding STI management) in low- and middle-income countries cost approximately US$3 for acute, bacterial STI (range US$0.05–35.23); this exceeds the average daily income for low-income nations (Terris-Prestholt et al. 2006). In some settings, individuals must cover all costs of the services, making it less likely that poor or vulnerable populations will have access to the services. Whether or not available STI services are acceptable can also be complicated. Perceived empathy and acceptance by service providers has been observed to have a profoundly positive effect on patients' opinions of services, and perceived judgmental or scolding attitudes have been observed to lead to equally negative opinions of the services, even if they are of otherwise high quality (Dallabetta et al. 2007). Other factors related to acceptability include real and perceived privacy of the setting and confidentiality of services. Adolescents and stigmatized or marginalized groups (e.g. CSW, MSM) are often the least likely to find services in official settings to be acceptable. This situation must be addressed because of the contribution of such groups to STI transmission dynamics in a community.

Antimicrobial resistance

Resistance to previously effective antimicrobial therapies has developed for several STI including gonorrhoea, chancroid, trichomoniasis, syphilis, and HSV-2. Evolving resistance of gonorrhoea to various antimicrobial agents has had the greatest effect, and the emergence of highly resistant strains of gonorrhoea has been deemed by some public health experts to be 'one of the major health care disasters of the twentieth century' (World Health Organization 2007). Gonorrhoea resistance has been increasingly observed throughout the world over the past 30 years. Penicillinase-producing strains were first isolated in South East Asia as early as the 1970s, and subsequently penicillin-resistant gonorrhoea has spread widely throughout the world (WHO 2007). Resistance to other first-line therapies such as spectinomycin and tetracycline emerged in Asia in the 1980s. Fluoroquinolone-resistant gonorrhoea strains were found in several Asian countries in the 1990s, and high levels of fluoroquinolone resistance subsequently spread throughout Asia and other parts of the world (Lawung & Buatiang 2005) including the United States, in which treatment guidelines have recently been revised to no longer recommend the use of fluoroquinolones for treatment against gonorrhoea (CDC 2006; WHO 2007). Globally, WHO no longer recommends a single, first-line treatment for gonorrhoea, and national experts must decide, based on the local resistance data, what drugs to recommend (WHO 2007). That is a problematic situation because many countries cannot afford surveillance and must rely on data from other areas. With loss of fluoroquinolones, at present only a single class of antibiotics—third generation cephalosporins—remains uniformly effective against gonorrhoea. This situation will be seriously compounded if resistance to available cephalosporins develops, and therefore the development of effective alternative treatment regimens is a high STI-control priority. Antimicrobial resistance is also emerging for H. ducreyi, the causative agent of chancroid, although oral antibiotic therapies are still effective against this disease (CDC 2006). Azithromycin resistance in syphilis has been reported in a few settings (Lukehart et al. 2004), although the geographic distribution of resistant strains has not been well established, and T. pallidum remains exquisitely sensitive to penicillin, the first-line recommended therapy against syphilis. Resistance of trichomoniasis to standard treatment with single dose metronidazole occurs occasionally, requiring lengthier drug regimens or alternative treatments (CDC 2006). Additionally, while resistance of HSV-2 to acyclovir and related antiviral regimens is uncommon in immunocompetent patients, it has been observed to occur in up to 5 of HIV-infected patients (Reyes et al. 2003).

Essential drugs

Effective treatment and cure of bacterial STI requires the availability of appropriate drugs, preferably those with minimal side effects, and for which antimicrobial resistance is unlikely to develop. Also, such drugs ideally should not be contraindicated in pregnant or lactating women, and should lend themselves to single-dose, oral administration (World Health Organization 2007). A continual problem for many nations is that the most desirable drugs may not be included on national essential drug formularies, and therefore are generally not available to clients who attend public clinics. Although availability of particular STI drugs is dependant on numerous factors, the most immediate issue for most developing nations is affordability. Local availability also depends on intact and efficient national distribution systems to ensure that STI drugs (as well as other needed commodities such as condoms and syringes) are provided to all levels of the health care system before product expiration dates. Effective treatment requires that health care practitioners provide or prescribe appropriate drugs. Chances of this increase when national or local STI management guidelines are provided and disseminated, when STI training is included in professional school curricula or when refresher training courses are part of licensure or recertification of public and private providers, and when alternative practitioners (such as pharmacists) are included in STI management courses. Correct choice of drugs by providers has been observed to increase when countries adopt national syndromic algorithms, because management then becomes locally validated and standardized (Dallabetta et al. 2007). Some alternative strategies, such as pre-packaged STI drug kits, may also increase the likelihood that effective STI drugs will be provided to clients (Crabbe et al. 1998).

Targeted interventions for high-risk populations

As noted earlier, core groups can contribute significantly to disease burden and to further sustaining or perpetuating STI spread. In many communities, the core groups are CSW or other sex traders (individuals who trade sex for commodities other than money, such as food or drugs), men with highly mobile occupations that take them away from their homes and families (e.g. miners, seafarers, truck drivers) and MSM. Other populations, particularly adolescents, may also be viewed as 'high risk' given their high vulnerability to STI and their adverse consequences, even if the subgroup does not contribute disproportionately to disease transmission in the community. In most settings, the high-risk populations noted here have minimal or reduced access to official health care services either because of stigma, lack of financial resources, lack of time or convenient hours of operation, or because the official services are unacceptable to them. Given the situation of high-frequency transmitters who may have limited access to effective STI management, and often, limited resources, there is growing interest in the use of specialized, highly accessible interventions that are particularly targeted toward core groups or other vulnerable populations (Dallabetta *et al.* 2007; World Health Organization 2007). In the context of STI control, several such targeted interventions have been proven effective in selective community settings (Table 9.12.2). Current research indicates that the utility of any particular intervention is likely highly contextual, and that what works in one community may not work in others. Additionally, effective implementation of even a good, community-specific targeted intervention can be challenging since core groups are often difficult to identify or access, or both (Dallabetta *et al.* 2007). Additionally, the intervention or the persons applying it must not be perceived as stigmatizing or discriminatory toward the targeted group since acceptability of a specific intervention is generally determined by what happens at the first visit.

New opportunities for prevention

New initiatives

In May 2006, WHO announced a new *Global Strategy for Prevention and Control of STI: 2006–2015* and has begun work in supporting development of an Action Plan that could be adapted by nations around the world (World Health Organization 2007). The strategy emphasizes the importance of scaling up STI prevention activities globally and better integrating STI prevention with other prevention programmes. The strategy also highlights specific priority prevention activities for implementation (Table 9.12.3). In addition to scaling up syndromic management for STI in developing settings (which has been a continuing focus since the 1990s), areas that are given particularly high priority in the Global Strategy are the elimination of congenital syphilis as a public health problem; scaling up STI prevention strategies and programmes for HIV-infected persons; increasing STI surveillance within the context of second generation HIV surveillance programmes; and the elimination of bacterial causes of genital ulcer disease.

The Global Strategy's continuing focus on STI diagnosis and treatment illustrates the fundamental importance of high quality STI management in preventing adverse STI-related health outcomes in individuals, and also preventing further disease spread in the community. In contrast, the Global Strategy's priority ranking of congenital syphilis represents a renewed emphasis on the serious, adverse pregnancy outcomes related to syphilis that is timely for several reasons. First, syphilis screening tests and treatment are now readily available, and national policies in most countries support universal syphilis screening for pregnant women. Furthermore, several new opportunities exist, including availability of new rapid diagnostic tests that allow point-of-care screening (and if positive, treatment) at increasingly affordable prices (discussed below); greater attention on improved health care for women and infants as a result of the new Millennium Development Goals (MDGs) of the United Nations; and the global re-interest in advancing and supporting integrated antenatal care services.

The Global Strategy's third priority, an emphasis on STI screening and prevention in HIV-infected persons, is related to an increasing understanding that, even as more and more HIV-infected persons are able to access effective HIV treatments, new cases of HIV continue to occur at an alarming rate. Targeting HIV prevention efforts,

including STI screening and treatment, for persons already in care is recognized as an early (and relatively easy) step in primary HIV prevention, even in countries with limited resources. The Strategy's fourth priority aimed at upgrading STI surveillance illustrates a need for countries to define their STI burden and to understand the population groups and settings where STI are most likely to occur. Many HIV programmes have already developed population-level behavioural and risk surveys, or sentinel surveillance surveys. For many of these, linking STI testing to existing surveillance systems can provide information that is important for both HIV and STI programmes. Control and elimination of bacterial causes of genital ulcer disease is the fifth priority area of the Global Strategy. Although increasingly unusual in many parts of the world, bacterially-caused genital ulcers remain problematic in parts of Africa and the Americas. Of all STI syndromes, genital ulcer disease has been most associated with enhanced HIV acquisition and transmission, with ulcerogenic STI estimated to account for 5–11 per cent of new HIV infections in some settings (Wasserheit 1992). Data from syndromic management validation studies indicate that both syphilis and chancroid have decreased in many settings in Africa and the Caribbean over the past 20 years. Although their decline is likely multifactorial, the promotion by WHO of syndromic management approaches and of regular availability of sufficient and effective antibiotics is playing an important role in this effort.

Rapid diagnostic tests

As noted earlier, rapid diagnostic tests (e.g. point-of-care) facilitate screening and treatment of STI in asymptomatic persons (e.g. chlamydial infections, syphilis infections in pregnant women) in settings where it may be difficult for patients to learn of results and get prompt treatment if test results are positive (e.g. remote, hard-to-reach settings where reference laboratories are limited or have reduced capacity). Rapid tests may also be useful for symptomatic patients where more sensitive and specific diagnostic tests are unaffordable. Although syndromic treatment algorithms are used in many parts of the world for symptomatic patients, the use of appropriate diagnostic tests could greatly increase the specificity of the algorithms and thus reduce unnecessary treatment (e.g. for women with vaginitis). Recognizing the need for simple, affordable diagnostic tests for STI that can be performed during a clinic visit so as to allow immediate treatment, WHO's Sexually Transmitted Disease Diagnostic Initiative (SDI) is dedicated to the development, evaluation and application of rapid diagnostic tests for STI that are appropriate for use in primary health care settings in developing countries (Sexually Transmitted Diseases Diagnostics Initiative 2007). The SDI focus is on tests that meet the 'ASSURED' criteria—*a*ffordable, *s*ensitive, *s*pecific, *u*ser-friendly (simple to perform in only a few steps and with minimal training), *r*apid and robust (to enable treatment at first visit, and not requiring refrigeration), *e*quipment-free (i.e. easy, non-invasive way to collect specimens), and *d*elivered to end users (Sexually Transmitted Diseases Diagnostics Initiative 2007).

To date, the SDI has prioritized evaluation of rapid tests for syphilis, gonorrhoea and chlamydia, as these are the STI most associated with substantial adverse health outcomes in developed settings and for which curative therapy is widely available. Rapid tests for syphilis have been particularly successful, and there are more than a dozen with good performance relative to the reference standard. Also, they are easy to use and often quite affordable (e.g. substantially

Table 9.12.2 Some targeted interventions for high-risk populations that have been found effective in reducing STI in selected community settings

Female sex workers	
Specialized sex worker clinics	STI clinical services, condoms and preventive education and counselling provided by specially trained staff, available at convenient locations and during hours that do not interfere with women's work. Ideally, such clinics can be easily accessed using public transport as many women work in neighbourhoods far from their homes and prefer treatment close to the work site and away from their homes (Dallabetta *et al.* 2007)
Ambulatory clinic vans	Mobile vans that travel from community to community and allow women to come in for routine STI clinical care and other health services. Integrating additional health services helps reduce stigma
Clinics at the work site	CSW establishment owners contract with private practitioners to provide routine on-site STI clinical evaluations and treatment (Dallabetta *et al.* 2007)
Brothel-based 100 per cent condom use programs	Structural intervention whereby brothel managers require clients and women to use condoms with every sexual encounter. Was particularly effective in Thailand
Periodic presumptive therapy	Single empiric mass treatment of sex workers has been found to reduce STI prevalence in some settings, however levels eventually rose again. Periodic empiric mass treatment appears to lower bacterial STI and particularly syphilis (Berman & Kamb 2007)
Men away from home	
Pharmacy-based interventions	Pharmacists trained in syndromic management can provide effective treatment to men with urethritis and GUD who may be unwilling to wait in primary health clinics. Use of prepackaged STI 'treatment kits' that include specific STI drugs, partner referral cards, and condoms has been found to increase rates of effective treatment in some communities and may be particularly useful in pharmacies (Ryan *et al.* 2007)
Clinics at the work-site	Many companies (e.g. shipping companies, mining operations, agricultural estates) provide STI clinical care, condoms and health education to employees. Services seem to be most acceptable if it is perceived that care is not related to employment (e.g. HIV testing may have low uptake if perceived related to employment)
Men who have sex with men	
Specialized clinics or services	Accessible, acceptable clinical services with specialized providers promotes trust and increases likelihood men will come promptly for treatment and refer partners (Peterman *et al.* 2005)
Venue-based interventions	Providing information or clinical services (or referral to services) at bars, bath houses or other venues where MSM are likely to congregate has been effective in some communities. Provision of integrated health services may be more acceptable and less stigmatizing (Blank *et al.* 2005; Ciesielski *et al.* 2005)
Network-based interventions	Internet or local gay press may be ways to provide preventive health information or information about where clinical services can be safely obtained without stigma (McFarlane *et al.* 2005)
Adolescents	
Specialized youth centres	Services catering toward youth and their issues, with specialized counselling. Special care units may be integrated within existing care facilities (e.g. within family planning services, within primary care with special days for youth) or in store-fronts in places easily accessible to youth (World Health Organization 2007)
Internet and mobile telephone interventions	Health education messages or referrals to specialized clinical services may be increasingly used as more adolescents have access to new technologies (Kachur 2007)

less than US$1 in many cases). Many syphilis tests can use whole blood and do not require refrigeration. Thus far, however, all of the licensed rapid syphilis tests have been treponemal tests, recognizing syphilis infection but unable to distinguish between new and prior (treated) infection, which has been the function of the nontreponemal tests (e.g. VDRL, RPR) that are typically used for screening and to quantify disease activity. Use of treponemal tests alone carries the potential for over-treatment, which may be substantial in settings with prior STI control activities, as many of these positive tests will simply indicate prior infection rather than active disease. Therefore, development of a simple, rapid, two-antigen test, including non-treponemal as well as treponemal tests, is an important priority.

Evaluations for rapid gonorrhoea and chlamydia tests are continuing, and some promising candidates are being evaluated now or are to be evaluated in the near future (Lee 2007). The tests developed thus far have had less than ideal sensitivity and specificity, although mathematical models indicate that in certain settings with relatively high STI prevalence even tests with lower than optimal sensitivity and specificity might have a significant effect on disease burden when asymptomatic people who would otherwise not be treated can be reached for screening and treatment (Peeling *et al.* 2006). The SDI notes that recent advances in the understanding about the pathogenesis of STI, and the availability of complete genome sequences for the pathogens causing specific STI syndromes, are likely to support the development of raid tests in upcoming years (Peeling *et al.* 2006).

Table 9.12.3 WHO global strategy for prevention and control of STI 2006–2015: prevention activities for priority implementation in resource-limited settings*

Priority 1 activities	Indicators	National-level targets (to be reached by 2010* or 2015)
1. Scale up STI diagnosis and treatment, using syndromic management where diagnostic resources are limited	◆ Per cent of primary care sites providing comprehensive case management for symptomatic STI ◆ Per cent of STI patients at selected health facilities who are diagnosed, treated and counselled per national guidelines	◆ 90 per cent of primary care sites provide comprehensive STI care ◆ 90 per cent of women and men with STI at health-care facilities are appropriately diagnosed, treated and counselled
2. Control congenital syphilis as a step towards elimination	◆ Per cent of 15–24-year-old pregnant women attending antenatal clinics with a positive serology for syphilis who are treated per national guidelines	◆ 90 per cent of first time 15–24-year-old antenatal care attendees screened for syphilis ◆ 90 per cent of syphilis sero-positive women are treated adequately
3. Scale up STI prevention strategies and programmes for HIV-positive persons	◆ Per cent of HIV-positive patients with STI who receive comprehensive STI care, including advice on condom use and partner notification	◆ Strategies and guidelines for HIV positive persons with STI interventions in place* ◆ 90 per cent of primary point-of-care sites provide effective STI care for HIV infected persons
4. Upgrade STI surveillance within the context of second generation HIV surveillance	◆ Number of STI prevalence studies regularly conducted (at sentinel sites or in sentinel populations) every three to five years ◆ Annual incidence of reported STI (syndromic or etiologic)	◆ At least two rounds of prevalence surveys conducted ◆ Routine STI reporting established and sustained over at least 5 consecutive years
5. Control bacterial genital ulcer disease (GUD)	◆ Per cent of confirmed bacterial GUD cases in patients with genital ulcerative diseases ◆ Per cent of 15–24-year-old pregnant women attending antenatal clinics with a positive serology for syphilis	◆ Zero cases of chancroid identified in GUD patients ◆ Reduction to below 2 per cent of positive syphilis serology among 15–24-year-old antenatal care attendees
Priority 2 activities	**Indicators**	**National-level targets (to be reached by 2010* or 2015)**
6. Implement targeted interventions for high-risk and vulnerable populations	◆ Health needs identified/ national plans developed and implemented for STI/HIV control for key high-risk and vulnerable populations ◆ Per cent of people aged 15-24 years with STI that are detected during diagnostic STI testing	◆ Health needs, policies, legislation and regulations reviewed; plans in place and country-specific targeted interventions implemented* ◆ At least two rounds of prevalence surveys done among groups with high-risk behaviour and among young people
7. Implement age-appropriate comprehensive sexual health education and services	◆ Per cent of schools with at least one teacher who can provide life-skills-based STI/HIV prevention education	◆ Review of policies, development of age-appropriate training and information material for schools completed (by 2007) ◆ Increased number of teachers trained in participatory life-skills-based STI/HIV education
8. Promote partner treatment and prevention of reinfection	◆ Per cent of patients with STI whose partner(s) are referred for treatment	◆ Plans/support materials for partner notification developed; and health-care provider training in place* ◆ Double the proportion of patients who bring in or provide treatment to their partner(s)
9. Roll out of effective vaccines (HBV, HPV and eventually HSV)	◆ Policy and plans for universal vaccination for hepatitis B ◆ Plans and policy reviews and strategies for implementation of HPV and potential HSV-2 vaccines.	◆ Plans in place regarding vaccination for hepatitis B and HPV (by 2008) ◆ Pilot vaccination programmes initiated and scaling up in progress*
10. Universal opt-out HIV voluntary counselling and testing in STI patients	◆ Per cent of STI patients who are routinely counselled and offered confidential HIV testing	◆ HIV testing and counselling available in all settings providing care for STI ◆ Double the proportion of STI patients who receive voluntary counselling and testing for HIV

STI, sexually transmitted infections; HIV, human immunodeficiency virus; GUD, genital ulcer disease; HBV, hepatitis B virus; HPV, human papillomavirus; HSV, herpes simplex virus.
Priority 1: Should be implemented in all nations
Priority 2: Should be implemented if resources exist
* Adapted from World Health Organization. (2007). *Global Strategy for the prevention and Control of Sexually Transmitted Infections 2006–2015*. Geneva, WHO.

Integration of services

Over the past century, the fashions around integrated public health programmes that focus on prevention as well as curative aspects of STD control, versus a more vertical approach that focuses on STI diagnosis and cure, have waxed and waned. With the MDGs clearly addressing women, infants and adolescents, the potential advantages of integrated programmes for some areas of STI control are important considerations. Antenatal service visits and delivery offer the opportunity to integrate a package of preventive services, including maternal syphilis screening and HIV testing (both preferably early in pregnancy), prophylactic treatment for conjunctivitis (at delivery), and neonatal HBV (postnatal period) in appropriate settings where vertical HBV transmission is high (e.g. parts of Asia). In settings where prevention of mother-to-child HIV transmission functions as a separate (often parallel) programme alongside antenatal services, introduction of syphilis testing has the potential both to reduce congenital syphilis infections and to enhance uptake of HIV testing, which can be more stigmatizing than syphilis testing. For reproductive-aged women, family planning services offer an opportunity for STI education and screening that target sexually active women who may be at risk for particular STI. In this setting, consideration must be given to encouraging condoms as a disease-prevention strategy that should be considered in conjunction with (rather than instead of) more effective contraceptive practices such as hormonal contraceptives. For men, on the other hand, opportunities for integrating STI care into other health services have not been particularly effective thus far, as many men do not use traditional public health clinics. Recently, the results of three African clinical trials found a substantial protective effect of adult male circumcision against new HIV infection, and strategies around safe and affordable circumcision may offer an opportunity for integrating STI services for men in those settings (World Health Organization 2007; WHO/UNAIDS Technical Consultation 2007). Many nations with high HIV prevalence are already grappling with best practices of providing circumcision to interested adult males, and public health experts have recognized that additional services around HIV/STI prevention education and counselling, HIV testing, condom promotion and screening for certain STI associated with HIV may be an efficient and cost-effective part of the package.

Conclusion

At the outset of the twenty-first century, STI continue to be a major global health problem, accounting for substantial reproductive, perinatal, and cancer-related morbidity and mortality—in addition to their contributions to HIV transmission. This chapter has outlined a number of successes that have occurred and several upcoming opportunities that exist in the field of STI control both in industrialized countries with established STI control programmes and in developing countries. For example, the use of syndromic case management in developing settings appears to have markedly reduced the burden of curable STI and their sequelae in many nations. Additionally, although viral STI remain highly prevalent in all countries, new tools for their control (e.g. vaccines, suppressive antiviral therapy) offer great promise. However, many challenges remain. In an era of increasingly available and affordable interventions, some very basic STI control programmes (e.g. universal syphilis screening of pregnant women) have not been well-adopted, especially in developing-world settings. New problems are also emerging, such as antimicrobial resistance and social disruption leading to gaps in health care and altered sexual networks, both of which enhance transmission. Because STI are stigmatizing conditions that have their greatest effect in vulnerable or marginalized populations, mobilizing societal and political support for their prevention and control remains challenging in all countries. However, in spite of this challenge, given the societal costs associated with STI and the new approaches available to prevent them, efforts to sustain and scale up effective STI control programmes must remain important global health priorities.

References

Adimora A.A., Schoenbach V.J. (2005). Social context, sexual networks, and racial disparities in rates of sexually transmitted infections. *J Infect Dis* 191 Suppl 1:S115–S122.

Adler M.W. (1996). Sexually transmitted diseases control in developing countries. *Genitourin Med* 72(2):83–88.

Anderson R., Hanson M. (2005). Potential public health impact of imperfect HIV type 1 vaccines. *J Infect Dis* 191 Suppl 1:S85–S96.

Aral S.O., Holmes K.K., Padian N.S. *et al.* (1996). Overview: individual and population approaches to the epidemiology and prevention of sexually transmitted diseases and human immunodeficiency virus infection. *J Infect Dis* 174 Suppl 2:S127–S133.

Aral S.O., Lipshutz J.A., Douglas J.M. (2007). Introduction. In Aral, S.O.; Douglas, J.M.; Lipshutz, J.A. eds., *Behavioral Interventions for Prevention and Control of Sexually Transmitted Diseases*: New York, Springer Science and Business Media, LLC. 60–101.

Aral S.O., Padian N.S., Holmes K.K. (2005). Advances in multilevel approaches to understanding the epidemiology and prevention of sexually transmitted infections and HIV: an overview. *J Infect Dis* 191 Suppl 1:S1–S6.

ASTHO. (2004). State Public Health Employee Shortage Report: A Civil Service Recruitment and Retention Crisis.

Baseman J.G., Koutsky L.A. (2005). The epidemiology of human papillomavirus infections. *J Clin Virol* 32 Suppl 1:S16–S24.

Berman S., Kamb M. (2007). Biomedical Interventions. In Aral, S.O.; Douglas, J.M.; Lipshutz, J.A. eds., *Behavioral Interventions for Prevention and Control of Sexually Transmitted Diseases*: New York, Springer Science and Business Media, LLC. 60–101.

Blank S., Gallagher K., Washburn K. *et al.* (2005). Reaching out to boys at bars: utilizing community partnerships to employ a wellness strategy for syphilis control among men who have sex with men in New York City. *Sex Transm Dis* 32(10 Suppl):S65–S72.

Brewer D.D. (2005). Case-finding effectiveness of partner notification and cluster investigation for sexually transmitted diseases/HIV. *Sex Transm Dis* 32(2):78–83.

Brown Z.A., Selke S., Zeh J. *et al.* (1997). The acquisition of herpes simplex virus during pregnancy. *N Engl J Med* 337(8):509–515.

Brunham R.C. (2005). Parran Award Lecture: insights into the epidemiology of sexually transmitted diseases from Ro = betacD. *Sex Transm Dis* 32(12):722–724.

Cates W. Jr., Holmes K.K. (1998). Public Health and Preventive Medicine. Wallace R, editor. *Sexually Transmitted Diseases*, 14th Edition, 137–155.

CDC. (2001). Community and individual behavior change interventions. Program Operations Guidelines for STD Prevention:1–24.

CDC. (2001). Guidelines for STD Prevention. Program Operations Guidelines for STD Prevention:1–27.

CDC. (2001). Overview. Program Operations Guidelines for STD Prevention:1–26.

CDC. (2003). Incorporating HIV prevention into the medical care of persons living with HIV. MMWR 52(RR-12):1–24.

CDC. (2004). Infertility and Prevention of Sexually Transmitted Diseases. Report to Congress. (Accessed on February 8, 2007, at http://www.cdc.gov/std/infertility/ReportCongressInfertility.pdf).

CDC. (2005). Sexually Transmitted Disease Surveillance. Atlanta, GA. U.S. Department of Health and Services.

CDC. (2006). Expedited partner therapy in the management of sexually transmitted diseases. Atlanta, GA: U S Department of Health and Human Services.

CDC. (2006). Hepatitis B Virus Infection: A comprehensive immunization strategy to eliminate transmission in the United States, Part II immunization of adults. MMWR:1–79.

CDC. (2006). Sexually Transmitted Disease Treatment Guidelines. MMWR 55(RR-11):1–94.

CDC. (2006). The National Plan to Eliminate Syphilis from the United States. Division of STD Prevention.

CDC. (2007). Quadrivalent human papillomavirus vaccine – recommendations of the Advisory Committee on Immunization Practices (ACIP). MMWR:1–24.

CDC. National Network of STD Prevention Training Center (NNPTC) (Accessed January 12, 2006, at http://www.cdc.gov/std/training/courses.htm).

Ciesielski C., Kahn R.H., Taylor M. et al. (2005). Control of syphilis outbreaks in men who have sex with men: the role of screening in nonmedical settings. Sex Transm Dis 32(10 Suppl):S37–S42.

Cogliano V., Baan R., Straif K. et al. (2005). Carcinogenicity of human papillomaviruses. Lancet Oncol 6(4):204.

Corey L., Huang ML., Selke S. et al. (2005). Differentiation of herpes simplex virus types 1 and 2 in clinical samples by a real-time taqman PCR assay. J Med Virol 76(3):350–355.

Crabbe F., Tchupo J.P., Manchester T. et al. (1998). Prepackaged therapy for urethritis: the 'MSTOP' experience in Cameroon. Sex Transm Infect 74(4):249–252.

Daling J.R., Madeleine M.M., Johnson L.G. et al. (2004). Human papillomavirus, smoking, and sexual practices in the etiology of anal cancer. Cancer 101(2):270–280.

Daling J.R., Madeleine M.M., Johnson L.G. et al. (2005). Penile cancer: importance of circumcision, human papillomavirus and smoking in in situ and invasive disease. Int J Cancer 116(4):606–616.

Dallabetta G., Field M., Lage M. et al. (2007). STDs: Global Burden and Challenges for Control. In G. Dallabetta, M. Laga, and Lamptey P. eds. 'Control of Sexually Transmitted Diseases: A handbook for the design and management of programs,' Durham, North Carolina; Family Health International/The AIDS Control and Prevention Project (AIDSCAP). 23–52.

Department of Health. Better prevention, better services, better sexual health - The national strategy for sexual health and HIV. Crown Copyright. July 2001. Accessed January 7, 2007 at http://www.dh.gov.uk/PublicationsAndStatistics/Publications/PublicationsPolicyAndGuidance/PublicationsPolicyAndGuidanceArticle/fs/en?CONTENT_ID=4003133&chk=/iTv%2BN).

Douglas J.M., Fenton K. (2007). STD/HIV Prevention Programs in Developed Countries. In: Sexually Transmitted Disease. Holmes KK. eds, Fourth edition. McGraw-Hill: New York (in press).

Du P., Coles F.B., Gerber T. et al. (2006). Effects of partner notification on reducing gonorrhea incidence rate. Sex Transm Dis:189–194.

Ebrahim S.H., Peterman T.A., Zaidi A.A. et al. (1997). Mortality related to sexually transmitted diseases in US women, 1973 through 1992. Am J Public Health 87(6):938–944.

Elbasha E.H., Dasbach E.J., Insinga R.P. (2007). Model for assessing human papillomavirus vaccination strategies. Emerg Infect Dis 13(1):28–41.

Fenton K., Bloom F. (2007). STD Prevention with Men Who Have Sex with Men in the United States. In: Behavioral Interventions for Prevention and Control of Sexually Transmitted Diseases. Aral S, Douglas J, eds. New York: Springer SBM, LLC.

Fleming D.T., Wasserheit J.N. (1999). From epidemiological synergy to public health policy and practice: the contribution of other sexually transmitted diseases to sexual transmission of HIV infection. Sex Transm Infect 75(1):3–17.

Franco L.M., Daly C.C., Chilongozi D. et al. (1997). Quality of case management of sexually transmitted diseases: comparison of the methods for assessing the performance of providers. Bull World Health Organ 75(6):523–532.

Gift T.L., Pate M.S., Hook E.W., III. et al. (1999). The rapid test paradox: when fewer cases detected lead to more cases treated: a decision analysis of tests for Chlamydia trachomatis. Sex Transm Dis 26(4):232–240.

Global Burden of Hepatitis C Working Group. Accesed on August 17, 2007 at http://jcp.sagepub.com/misc/terms.shtml. (2004). J Clin Phar 44:20–29.

Golden M.R., Whittington W.L., Handsfield H.H. et al. (2005). Effect of expedited treatment of sex partners on recurrent or persistent gonorrhea or chlamydial infection. N Engl J Med 352(7):676–685.

Goldie S.J., Kohli M., Grima D. et al. (2004). Projected clinical benefits and cost-effectiveness of a human papillomavirus 16/18 vaccine. J Natl Cancer Inst 96(8):604–615.

Goldstein S.T., Zhou F., Hadler S.C. et al. (2005). A mathematical model to estimate global hepatitis B disease burden and vaccination impact. Int J Epidemiol 34(6):1329–1339.

Goyaux N., Leke R., Keita N. et al. (2003). Ectopic pregnancy in African developing countries. Acta Obstet Gynecol Scand 82(4):305–312.

Greenberg J.B., MacGowan R., Neumann M. et al. (1998). Linking injection drug users to medical services: role of street outreach referrals. Health Soc Work 23(4):298–309.

Grosskurth H., Gray R., Hayes R. et al. (2000). Control of sexually transmitted diseases for HIV-1 prevention: understanding the implications of the Mwanza and Rakai trials. Lancet 355(9219):1981–1987.

Han Y., Coles F.B., Muse A. et al. (1999). Assessment of a geographically targeted field intervention on gonorrhea incidence in two New York State counties. Sex Transm Dis 26(5):296–302.

Harper D.M., Franco E.L., Wheeler C. et al. (2004). Efficacy of a bivalent L1 virus-like particle vaccine in prevention of infection with human papillomavirus types 16 and 18 in young women: a randomised controlled trial. Lancet 364(9447):1757–1765.

Hassig S., Hoffman I., Hamilton H. (1996). STD Monitoring and Evaluation, In: Control of Sexually Transmitted Diseases; A Handbook for the Design and Management of Programs, eds. Dallabetta, G.; Laga, M.; Lamptey, P.; Family Health International, AIDS Control and Prevention Project. 275–289.

Hogben M., Brewer D.D., Golden M.R. (2007). Partner Notification and Management Interventions. In: Behavioral Interventions for Prevention and Control of Sexually Transmitted Diseases. Aral S., Douglas J., eds. New York: Springer SBM, LLC.

Hughes J.P., Garnett G.P., Koutsky L. (2002). The theoretical population-level impact of a prophylactic human papilloma virus vaccine. Epidemiology 13(6):631–639.

Kamb M.L., Fishbein M., Douglas J.M., Jr. et al. (1998). Efficacy of risk-reduction counseling to prevent human immunodeficiency virus and sexually transmitted diseases: a randomized controlled trial. Project RESPECT Study Group. JAMA 280(13):1161–1167.

Korenromp E.L., White R.G., Orroth K.K. et al. (2005). Determinants of the impact of sexually transmitted infection treatment on prevention of HIV infection: a synthesis of evidence from the Mwanza, Rakai, and Masaka intervention trials. J Infect Dis 191 Suppl 1:S168–S178.

Koutsky L.A., Ault K.A., Wheeler C.M. et al. (2002). A controlled trial of a human papillomavirus type 16 vaccine. N Engl J Med 347(21):1645–1651.

Laga M., Alary M., Nzila N. et al. (1994). Condom promotion, sexually transmitted diseases treatment, and declining incidence of HIV-1 infection in female Zairian sex workers. Lancet 344(8917):246–248.

Lawung R., Buatiang A. et al. (2005). Increasing trend of multiple resistance and genomic mobility of Neisseria gonorrhoeae to penicillin and quinolone. EXCLI Journal 4, 130–140.

Lee H. (2007). A new chlamydia rapid test using non-invasive samples. 17th International Society for STD Research, Seattle, Washington.

Leichliter J., Ellen J., Gunn R. (2007). STD Repeaters: Implications for the Individuals and STD Transmission in a Population In: *Behavioral Interventions for Prevention and Control of Sexually Transmitted Diseases*. Aral S, Douglas J, eds. New York: Springer SBM, LLC.

Levine W.C., Revollo R., Kaune V. et al. (1998). Decline in sexually transmitted disease prevalence in female Bolivian sex workers: impact of an HIV prevention project. *AIDS* 12(14):1899–1906.

Lukehart S.A., Godornes C., Molini B.J. et al. (2004). Macrolide resistance in Treponema pallidum in the United States and Ireland. *N Engl J Med* 351(2):154–158.

Manhart L.E., Holmes K.K. (2005). Randomized controlled trials of individual-level, population-level, and multilevel interventions for preventing sexually transmitted infections: what has worked? *J Infect Dis* 191 Suppl 1:S7–24.

May R.M., Anderson R.M. (1987). Transmission dynamics of HIV infection. *Nature* 326(6109):137–142.

McFarlane M., Bull S.S. (2007). Use of the Interest in STD/HIV Prevention. In: *Behavioral Interventions for Prevention and Control of Sexually Transmitted Diseases*. Aral S, Douglas J, eds. New York: Springer SBM, LLC. 214–231.

McFarlane M., Kachur R., Klausner J.D. et al. (2005). Internet-based health promotion and disease control in the 8 cities: successes, barriers, and future plans. *Sex Transm Dis* 32(10 Suppl):S60–S64.

McGlynn K.A., London W.T. (2005). Epidemiology and natural history of hepatocellular carcinoma. *Best Pract Res Clin Gastroenterol* 19(1): 3–23.

Meheus A. (1992). Women's health: importance of reproductive tract infections, pelvic inflammatory disease and cervical cancer, in A. Germain, K.K. Holmes, P. Piot, and J.N. Wasserheit eds., *Reproductive Tract Infections: Global Impact and Priorities for Women's Reproductive Health*: New York, Plenum Press, p. 61–91.

Munoz N., Bosch F.X., de S.S. et al. (2003). Epidemiologic classification of human papillomavirus types associated with cervical cancer. *N Engl J Med* 348(6):518–527.

Nagot N., Ouedraogo A., Foulongne V. et al. (2007). Reduction of HIV-1 RNA levels with therapy to suppress herpes simplex virus. *N Engl J Med* 356(8):790–799.

Over M., Piot P. (1993). HIV infection and sexually transmitted diseases. In D.T. Jameson, Mosley W.H., Measham A.R., Babadilla J.L., eds. *Disease Control Priorities in Developing Countries*, New York; Oxford University Press. 445–529.

Over M., Piot P. (1996). Human immunodeficiency virus infection and other sexually transmitted diseases in developing countries: public health importance and priorities for resource allocation. *J Infect Dis* 174(Suppl. 2):S162–S175.

Passin W.F., Kim A.S., Hutchinson A.B. et al. (2006). A systematic review of HIV partner counseling and referral services: client and provider attitudes, preferences, practices, and experiences. *Sex Transm Dis* 33(5):320–328.

Paz-Bailey G., Ramaswamy M., Hawkes S.J. et al. (2007). Herpes simplex virus type 2: epidemiology and management options in developing countries. *Sex Transm Infect* 83(1):16–22.

Peeling R.W., Mabey D., Herring A. et al. (2006). Why do we need quality-assured diagnostic tests for sexually transmitted infections? *Nat Rev Microbiol* 4(12):909–921.

Perz J.F., Armstrong G.L., Farrington L.A. et al. (2006). The contributions of hepatitis B virus and hepatitis C virus infections to cirrhosis and primary liver cancer worldwide. *J Hepatol* 45(4):529–538.

Peterman T.A., Collins D.E., Aral S.O. (2005). Responding to the epidemics of syphilis among men who have sex with men: introduction to the special issue. *Sex Transm Dis* 32(10 Suppl):S1–S3.

Pisani P., Parkin D.M., Bray F. et al. (1999). Estimates of the worldwide mortality from 25 cancers in 1990. *Int J Cancer* 83(1):18–29.

Plummer F.A., Countinho R.A., Ngugi E.N. et al. (2005). Sex workers and their clients in the epidemiology and control of sexually transmitted diseases. *Sexually Transmitted Diseases*, Third Edition. [10], 143–150.

Reyes M., Shaik N.S., Graber J.M. et al. (2003). Acyclovir-resistant genital herpes among persons attending sexually transmitted disease and human immunodeficiency virus clinics. *Arch Intern Med* 163(1):76–80.

Ryan C., Kamb M., Holmes K. (2007). STI Care Management. In: *Sexually Transmitted Disease*. Holmes K.K. eds, Fourth edition. McGraw-Hill: New York.

Salabarria-Pena Y., Pat B.S., Walsh C.M. (2007). Practical Use of Program Evaluation among Sexually Transmitted disease (STD) Programs, Atlanta (GA): Centers for Disease Control and Prevention.

Salmon, C.T. (1989)ed., *Information Campaigns: Balancing Social Values and Social Change*, Newbury Park, CA Sage.

Sanchez J., Campos P.E., Courtois B. et al. (2003). Prevention of sexually transmitted diseases (STDs) in female sex workers: prospective evaluation of condom promotion and strengthened STD services. *Sex Transm Dis* 30(4):273–279.

Santelli J., Ott M.A., Lyon M. et al. (2006). Abstinence-only education policies and programs: a position paper of the Society for Adolescent Medicine. *J Adolesc Health* 38(1):83–87.

Schmid G.P., Stoner B.P., Hawkes S. et al. (2007). The need and plan for global elimination of congenital syphilis. *Sex Transm Dis* 34(7 Suppl):S5–10.

Schmiedeskamp M.R., Kockler D.R. (2006). Human papillomavirus vaccines. *Ann Pharmacother* 40(7–8):1344–1352.

Sexually Transmitted Diseases Diagnostics Initiative website accessed on April 11, 2007 at http://www.who.int/std_diagnostics/.

Shelton J.D., Halperin D.T., Nantulya V. et al. (2004). Partner reduction is crucial for balanced 'ABC' approach to HIV prevention. *BMJ* 328(7444):891–893.

Szmuness W., Stevens C.E., Harley E.J. et al. (1980). Hepatitis B vaccine: demonstration of efficacy in a controlled clinical trial in a high-risk population in the United States. *N Engl J Med* 303(15):833–841.

Terris-Prestholt F., Vyas S., Kumaranayake L. et al. (2006). The costs of treating curable sexually transmitted infections in low- and middle-income countries: a systematic review. *Sex Transm Dis* 33(10 Suppl): S153–S166.

Tietz A., Davies S.C., Moran J.S. (2004). Guide to sexually transmitted disease resources on the Internet. *Clin Infect Dis* 38(9):1304–1310.

Trelle S., Shang A., Nartey L. et al. (2007). Improved effectiveness of partner notification for patients with sexually transmitted infections: systematic review. *BMJ* 334(7589):354.

Vega M.Y., Ghanem K.G. (2007). STD Prevention Communication: Using Social Marketing Techniques with an Eye on Behavioral Change. In Aral, S.O.; Douglas, J.M.; Lipshutz, J.A. eds., *Behavioral Interventions for Prevention and Control of Sexually Transmitted Diseases*: New York, Springer Science and Business Media, LLC, pp. 142–169.

Villa L.L., Costa R.L., Petta C.A. et al. (2005). Prophylactic quadrivalent human papillomavirus (types 6, 11, 16, and 18) L1 virus-like particle vaccine in young women: a randomised double-blind placebo-controlled multicentre phase II efficacy trial. *Lancet Oncol* 6(5):271–278.

Waaler H.T., Piot M.A. (1969). The use of an epidemiological model for estimating the effectiveness of tuberculosis control measures. Sensitivity of the effectiveness of tuberculosis control measures to the coverage of the population. *Bull World Health Organ* 41(1):75–93.

Warner L., Rietmeijer C. et al. (2006). A brief waiting room video intervention reduces incident sexually transmitted infections among STD clinic patients. 2006 National STD Prevention Conference, Jacksonville, FL, May 8–11.

Wasserheit J.N. (1992). Epidemiological synergy. Interrelationships between human immunodeficiency virus infection and other sexually transmitted diseases. *Sex Transm Dis* 19(2):61–77.

Watson-Jones D., Weiss H.A., Changalucha J.M. et al. (2007). Adverse birth outcomes in United Republic of Tanzania—impact and prevention of maternal risk factors. *Bull World Health Organ* 85(1):9–18.

Wawer M.J., Sewankambo N.K., Serwadda D. *et al.* (1999). Control of sexually transmitted diseases for AIDS prevention in Uganda: a randomised community trial. Rakai Project Study Group. *Lancet* 353(9152):525–535.

Weinstock H., Berman S., Cates W. Jr. (2004). Sexually transmitted diseases among American youth: incidence and prevalence estimates, 2000. *Perspect Sex Reprod Health* 36(1):6–10.

Weiss H. (2004). Epidemiology of herpes simplex virus type 2 infection in the developing world. *Herpes* 11 Suppl 1:24A-35A.

Weiss H.A. (2007). Male circumcision as a preventive measure against HIV and other sexually transmitted diseases. *Curr Opin Infect Dis* 20(1):66–72.

White P.J., Golden M.R. Thurner K.M.E. *et.al.* (2005). Patient-delivered partner therapy: when and where should it be used? predicting its impact in the USA and U.K. 16th International Society for STD Research, Amsterdam, Netherlands.

White R.G., Orroth K.K., Korenromp E.L. *et al.* (2004). Can population differences explain the contrasting results of the Mwanza, Rakai, and Masaka HIV/sexually transmitted disease intervention trials?: A modeling study. *J Acquir Immune Defic Syndr* 37(4):1500–1513.

WHO Report on Infectious Diseases 2000, Overcoming Antimicrobial Resistance. (Accessed August 18, 2007 at http://www.who.int/infectious-disease-report/2000/.

WHO/UNAIDS Technical Consultation. Male circumcision and HIV prevention: Research implications for policy and programming. Montreaux, 6–8 March, 2007; Conclusions and Recommendations (www.who.int/hiv/mediacentre/MCrecommendations_en.pdf).

Williams S.P., Kahn R.H. (2007). Looking Inside and Affecting the Outside: Corrections-based Interventions for STD Prevention. In: *Behavioral Interventions for Prevention and Control of Sexually Transmitted Diseases.* Aral S, Douglas J, eds. New York: Springer SBM, LLC. 374–396.

Witte K., Allen M. (2000). A Meta-analysis of Fear Appeals: Implications for Effective Public Health Campaigns. *Health Education and Behavior*, 27:591–615.

World Bank (2003). World Bank World Development Report 2004: New York, Oxford University Press.

World Health Organization. (1994). Evaluation of a national programme: a methods package 1. Prevention of HIV infection. Geneva.

World Health Organization. (2007). Global Strategy for the Prevention and Control of Sexually Transmitted Infections 2006–2015. Geneva, World Health Organization.

World Health Organization. Revised Global Burden of Disease 2002 Estimates, Accessed on April 11, 2007 at http://www.who.int/healthinfo/bodgbd2002revised/en/index.html.

Xu F., Sternberg M.R., Kottiri B.J. *et al.* (2006). Trends in herpes simplex virus type 1 and type 2 seroprevalence in the United States. *JAMA* 296(8):964–973.

Zur Hausen H. (1996). Papillomavirus infections--a major cause of human cancers. *Biochim Biophys Acta* 1288(2):F55–F78.

9.13

Acquired immunodeficiency syndrome

Salim S. Abdool Karim,
Quarraisha Abdool Karim, and
Roger Detels

Abstract

In the 25 years since the first reported cases of acquired immunodeficiency syndrome (AIDS), more than 70 million people have been infected with the human immunodeficiency virus (HIV). HIV is a retrovirus that is spread from mother to child, through blood contamination and through sex. Antiretroviral drugs administered to HIV-infected pregnant women and the newborn child, together with exclusive or no breastfeeding, have drastically reduced mother-to-child transmission. Screening of blood supplies, universal safety precautions in medical settings, and needle exchange programmes for intravenous drug users are effective in avoiding bloodborne spread. Reduction in sexual transmission is achievable through sexual abstinence, monogamy, condoms, treatment of concurrent sexually transmitted infections, male circumcision, and HIV counselling and testing.

When spread, HIV specifically infects and replicates in CD4+ cells, leading to the systematic destruction of CD4+ cells over a period of years. The drop in CD4+ T-cell numbers to low levels leads to individuals developing symptoms including weight loss, low-grade fevers, night sweats, frequent fungal infections, and eventually various opportunistic infections and malignancies, which signal the onset of AIDS. Until then, individuals who have been asymptomatic with HIV infection over several years have been infectious, thereby creating the conditions for the efficient spread of this virus. HIV infection is readily diagnosed by assays detecting antibodies, viral components, and the viral genome. More than 25 antiretroviral drugs are known to be effective against HIV. Combinations of these drugs, referred to as highly active antiretroviral therapy, are effective in treating HIV infection.

Globally, it has proven to be a substantial challenge to extend HIV prevention programmes and provide treatment to those who most need it, as a disproportionately large burden of this disease is in poor countries. This pandemic has created many ethical, social, human rights, and political challenges. The estimated 25 million people that have already died from AIDS far exceeds the total killed in all the major wars of the twentieth century. AIDS is the world's most devastating epidemic and the deadliest in the history of humankind.

History of AIDS

First reported cases of AIDS

AIDS was first reported in 1981 by a young physician from the University of California Los Angeles School of Medicine who described the occurrence, without identifiable cause, of *Pneumocystis carinii* pneumonia (PCP) in four gay men in Los Angeles (Gottlieb *et al.* 1981). This new disease was also reported to and published by the US Centers for Disease Control and Prevention (CDC) in June 1981 and marked the beginning of awareness of the epidemic potential of AIDS in the United States. In 1982, the disease was given the name 'acquired immunodeficiency syndrome (AIDS)'. At this time, very little was known about the epidemiology and transmission of AIDS, and initially it was thought that only homosexuals and injecting drug users were affected but reports soon emerged that the disease was also occurring in haemophiliacs and Haitian immigrants in the United States.

A greater understanding of the mode of transmission of AIDS was gained following the reported death, from infections related to AIDS, of a young child who had previously received multiple blood transfusions, causing worldwide concerns about the safety of the blood supply, and the first cases of possible mother-to-child transmission of AIDS. By the time reports emerged that the disease was also transmitted heterosexually, it was apparent that the world was facing a disease of epidemic proportions.

Discovery of HIV as the cause of AIDS

The discovery that HIV caused AIDS was not a simple or direct path and required a substantial collaboration among different groups of scientists and clinicians. Only after the discovery of the human T leukaemia virus types 1 and 2 (HTLV-1 and HTLV-2) in the 1980s, did the scientific community accept that it was possible for retroviruses to infect humans. The marked decline in CD4 cells and possible mode of transmission led scientists to believe that AIDS was possibly caused by a retrovirus. In 1983, a virus was isolated from a patient with lymphadenopathy, which was later named lymphadenopathy-associated virus (LAV). In the same year, two distinct viruses were isolated from an AIDS patient in Haiti, one which cross-reacted with antibodies to HTLV, while the other virus killed target T-cells. It proved to be challenging to make the link between the virus and the clinical disease, AIDS, because the clinical signs of disease develop several years after the infection. However, through persistent isolation of the virus from patients with AIDS, the linkage was made possible (Gallo 2002; Gallo & Montagnier 2003). A series of important papers describing isolates of the new retrovirus, methods for its continuous production, and analyses of its proteins, were published in *Science* and *Lancet* in 1984 and provided the scientific evidence that HIV is the cause of AIDS.

Viral structure and genetic diversity

Viral structure and replication

HIV belongs to the family Retroviridae and the genus *Lentivirus*: Lenti meaning slow due to the long time from infection to disease. HIV, being a retrovirus, encodes the enzyme, reverse-transcriptase, which makes DNA from viral RNA. HIV genetic material, as proviral DNA in the nucleus of infected cells, is able to persist in long-lived reservoirs such as resting T-cells, thwarting efforts to clear HIV from the body.

Viral particles are spherical, about 100 nm in diameter. HIV has two major structural components—the core and the envelope. The core comprises the Gag (group-associated *a*ntigens) proteins, including the matrix protein (p17), which lies just beneath the envelope, and the capsid protein (p24) which encloses the viral RNA. The envelope, a lipid membrane, consists of two 'Env' glycoproteins, gp120 and gp41. These proteins exist as trimers on the viral surface facilitating binding and entry to the host cell. Besides reverse transcriptase, two other enzymes, integrase and protease, collectively known as polymerases, are carried inside the viral particle and are encoded by the 'Pol' gene of HIV. In addition to the major structural proteins, a number of regulatory and accessory proteins are also produced, including: Tat and Rev, which enhance levels of gene expression, and Vif, Vpr, Vpu, and Nef, which function to increase viral production and infectivity. Regulatory and accessory proteins are usually only produced once the virus infects cells and are not present inside the viral particles (Morris & Cilliers 2005).

HIV can attach to any cell that has a CD4+ receptor. Although these receptors are found primarily on the CD4+ lymphocytes, they are also found on a range of mononuclear cells including macrophages, B cells, mature CD8+ cells, and cells in the central nervous system. The process of HIV replication begins when gp120 binds to surface CD4+ and a co-receptor molecule, either CCR5 or CXCR4 (Moore & Doms 2003). Once HIV has successfully attached to the cell, a conformational change occurs allowing gp41 to insert itself into the host cell membrane. The capsid is then intruded into the cytoplasm of the cell where the viral RNA is reverse-transcribed to DNA and transported to the nucleus where, with the aid of the viral enzyme integrase, it is incorporated into human DNA. The transcription process, however, is imperfect, and mutations are common occurrences during replication. The 'errors' in this step are a major reason why HIV is able to escape the immune system and persist (Weiss 2001).

After the viral DNA has been incorporated into the host DNA, it is indistinguishable from the host DNA and is referred to as the 'provirus'. Each time the cell divides, the viral DNA will be passed on to the progeny cells. Proviral DNA can remain quiescent for extended periods of time or become transcriptionally active, particularly in cases where there is inflammation (Simon & Ho 2003).

The virus makes use of the host cell machinery to replicate itself. Messenger RNA directs the production of viral proteins. After cleavage by viral proteases to generate individual proteins, structural proteins aggregate just beneath the plasma membrane surface for inclusion into the new virions. Envelope glycoproteins insert themselves into the cell membrane and mature viral particles are formed when the virus buds through the membrane. Full-length unspliced genomic RNA is transported to the plasma membrane to be incorporated into the viral progeny. As the new HIV is extruded from the host cell, lipid from the cell wall is incorporated onto the virus and forms the envelope of the progeny virus. A single CD4+ cell is capable of producing hundreds of new HIV progeny.

Genetic diversity

There are two HIV types, HIV-1 and HIV-2. HIV-2 is less pathogenic than HIV-1 and largely restricted to West Africa, with limited spread to other countries and is genetically more closely related to SIV than to HIV-1. Numerous HIV-1 subtypes and circulating recombinant forms (CRF) make up the complex mosaic of the global HIV-1 pandemic (McCutchan 2006). Specifically, HIV has been classified into three groups, M, N, and O. The Major Group (Group M) comprises the viruses that are currently dominating the global AIDS epidemic. The Outlier Group (Group O) and the non-M non-O group (Group N) are much less common. Based on their phylogenetic relatedness, the Group M viruses have been further subdivided into nine subtypes or clades; A, B, C, D, F, G, H, J, and K. Two of these, subtypes A and F have been further subdivided into sub-subtypes (referred to as A1, A2 and F1, F2, respectively).

An analysis of 23 874 HIV samples from 70 countries shows that, in terms of viral diversity, subtype C viruses dominate and account for half of all HIV-1 infections worldwide while subtypes A, B, D and G account for 12, 10, 3, and 6 per cent, respectively. Circulating recombinant forms are responsible for 18 per cent of infections worldwide. Subtype C is dominant in Africa and Asia, while subtype B is the commonest subtype in Europe and the Americas (Hemelaar *et al.* 2006).

HIV diversity is generated either through mutations introduced into viral genomes during replication or during the recombination of viral genomes. Mutations are introduced into the viral genome

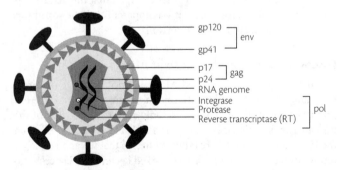

Fig. 9.13.1 Schematic diagram of HIV showing the constituent proteins and enzymes.
Source: Adapted from Morris & Cilliers (2005), with permission from Cambridge University Press.

primarily due to the error-prone nature of the viral replication enzyme, reverse transcriptase. HIV has an average mutation rate of 5×10^{-6} mutations per nucleotide per cycle of virus replication (Smith *et al.* 2005). As a consequence, no two viruses are identical within an infected individual, allowing for rapid adaptation to fluctuating selection pressures such as immune responses and antiretroviral drugs.

Natural history of HIV infection

Following the introduction of HIV into the human body, there is replication in local CD4+ cells before spread to the gut-associated lymphoid tissue, where there is high-level HIV replication leading to virus levels in blood which can exceed ten million viral particles per ml. During viral replication in the gut-associated lymphoid tissue, there is a rapid decline in the numbers of CD4+ T lymphocytes, with the CD4+ cell count dropping by up to 50 per cent within weeks post-infection.

Within a few weeks of the onset of HIV infection, the host immune response curtails viral replication resulting in a decline in the viral load and a slow increase in CD4+ T-cell numbers for a few months before starting its slow progressive decline (Fig. 9.13.2). At the time of the immune response, many infected individuals experience influenza-like symptoms characterized by chills, malaise, and weakness for a few weeks.

Within 6–12 months following the onset of HIV, viral replication reaches a level which is referred to as the 'set point'. The level of the set point correlates with the rate of disease progression. Most individuals remain clinically well (asymptomatic) for an average of 8–9 years although the asymptomatic interval may vary widely. For reasons that are not fully understood, some individuals never develop control over viral replication and progress to AIDS within 1–2 years of infection (rapid progressors) while others have remained disease-free for up to 20 years, often with undetectable viral loads (long-term non-progressors).

Kinetic studies have shown that during the asymptomatic period up to a billion HIV particles and two billion CD4+ T-cells are destroyed and produced each day. Thus, while individuals may be clinically well, the virus continues to replicate, particularly in the lymph nodes, causing a gradual decline in CD4+ T-cell numbers. The drop in CD4+ T-cell numbers to low levels leads to individuals developing AIDS symptoms. With the deterioration of immune function, the viral load increases and, in the absence of treatment, death usually occurs within 6 months to 2 years after an AIDS diagnosis (Burger & Poles 2003). Treatment with Highly Active Antiretroviral Therapy (HAART) significantly extends the time period between AIDS diagnosis and death. There is accumulating evidence that the onset of AIDS may be about 1–2 years shorter following onset of HIV infection, in Africa compared to the developed world (Jaffar *et al.* 2004).

Laboratory assays

The isolation of HIV in 1984 and the establishment of its causal relationship with AIDS led to the development of the first commercially available HIV serological tests by 1985. Subsequently, there has been a rapid evolution in HIV diagnostic technology that has matched the rapidly evolving understanding of the natural history of HIV disease. Currently, a wide range of assays are available for adult and paediatric diagnosis, monitoring disease progression and therapeutic success, as well as for research and surveillance. These assays can be performed on a range of biological tissues such as serum, plasma, saliva, whole blood, urine, seminal fluid, and cervico-vaginal specimens.

Antibody detection

Detection of antibodies using serological tests such as a standard enzyme immunoassay (EIA) is most often used for screening or diagnosis of HIV infection. A major advance has been the availability of rapid HIV antibody tests. The two limitations of these serological tests are, firstly, detection of infection during primary infection when antibody levels are low or absent and secondly, determination of whether a reactive EIA or positive rapid HIV test in newborns is due to infection in the baby or due to passively

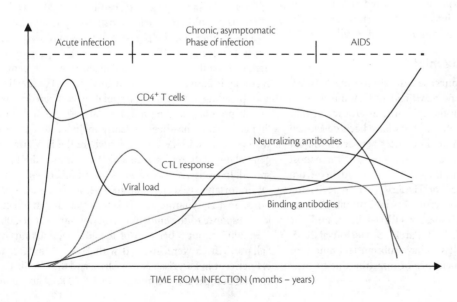

Fig. 9.13.2 Schematic diagram showing the natural history of HIV infection.
Source: Adapted from Morris & Cilliers (2005) with permission from Cambridge University Press.

transferred maternal antibodies. In these instances, the use of polymerase chain reaction technology for detection of viral RNA is helpful.

Antigen detection

Standard EIA tests are available for p24 antigen, which is often the earliest antigen that can be detected in acute HIV infection before the presence of antibodies is detectable. It is therefore used to identify the presence of HIV infection during the window period, the period between onset of HIV infection and the detection of HIV antibodies.

Nucleic acid detection

Plasma viral load is a marker of viral replication and is used to monitor therapeutic success in patients on antiretroviral treatment. A number of commercially available tests provide sensitive quantification as low as 50 copies of HIV RNA per ml (Berger *et al.* 2005). There are also tests for cell-associated HIV which measure branched DNA levels.

CD4+ cell counts

The number of CD4+ T-cells reveals the degree of immunodeficiency and is therefore a key criterion for initiating antiretroviral treatment. At present, flow cytometry analysis is the standard method for quantification of CD4+ cells. Where CD4+ quantification is not readily available, total white cell counts are sometimes used as a proxy marker (Spacek *et al.* 2006).

T-cell immune response detection

Various assays have been developed to assess the presence of a cellular immune response to HIV antigens. The earlier approaches like the Chromium release assay and the tetramer assay have now largely been superseded by the Elispot assay and the Intracellular cytokine stain assay. The latter two assays depend on the release of certain cytokines, such an interferon-gamma, when T-cells from the patient recognize HIV antigens used in the test. These assays are very sensitive and can sometimes be positive in the absence of any other markers of HIV infection—suggesting that the patient has previously encountered and can recognize HIV antigens, perhaps through a previous HIV exposure or aborted HIV infection. The hypotheses of aborted HIV infection and clearance of established HIV infection have not been confirmed empirically.

Assays to identify recent HIV infection

For research and surveillance purposes, differentiating between established/prevalent infection and new/incident HIV infections is critical for monitoring trends in the epidemic or efficacy of new interventions under trial. A number of tests have been developed for this purpose; most are based on differences between antibody responses in early versus established HIV infection. The three most commonly used serologic assays for estimating incidence from prevalent studies are the 'detuned' or STARHS (Serologic Testing Algorithm for Recent HIV Seroconversion) assay, Immunoglobulin G Capture BED-enzyme immunoassay (BED-CEIA), and the Avidity Index (AI) (Dobbs *et al.* 2004, Parekh & McDougal 2005; Janssen *et al.* 1998). All of these assays have substantial limitations and tend to over-estimate the incidence of infection due to their high false-positive rates.

STARHS consists of a less sensitive, first-generation ELISA followed by a later-generation ELISA with increased sensitivity. Recent infection (within the last 129 days, depending on viral sub-type) is indicated if the first-generation ELISA is negative and the second-generation ELISA is positive.

The *BED-CEIA* attempts to identify recent HIV infection by measuring increasing levels of anti-IgG as a proportion of overall IgG. Recent infection (within the last 153 days) is indicated by a ratio of HIV-specific IgG/total IgG less than 0.8.

The *AI* attempts to identify the weak antibody-antigen interaction present early in HIV infection compared to later stages where this interaction is stronger and more difficult to disrupt. Recent infection (within 120 days) is indicated by an Avidity Index less than 80 per cent.

Other assays in development are the Affinity assay, IgG3 isotype assay and anti-HIV p31 assay.

Global epidemiology of HIV

Since the first reported cases of AIDS in 1982, an estimated 70 million HIV infections and about 25 million AIDS-related deaths have occurred globally (UNAIDS 2006). In 2007, UNAIDS estimated that globally there were 33.2 million (upper and lower bound of estimate: 30.6–36.1 million) adults and children living with HIV infection. Furthermore, globally a total of 2.5 million (1.8–4.1 million) new infections occurred and 2.1 million (1.9–2.4 million) people died from AIDS in 2007 (UNAIDS 2007).

Differences in the time of introduction of HIV and rates of HIV transmission in specific countries and populations have resulted in a complex mosaic of epidemics (Abdool Karim *et al.* 2007). In most countries, HIV continues to spread and in countries with limited access to antiretroviral treatment, morbidity and mortality rates are on the rise.

A distinctive feature of the pandemic in the twenty-first century is its increasing burden in women. Women now comprise about 42 per cent of those infected globally, over 70 per cent of whom live in sub-Saharan Africa. Of significance is that a quarter of all new HIV infections occur in young adults under 25 years of age (UNAIDS 2003). Notably, where HIV transmission is predominantly sexual, HIV infection rates are 3–6-fold higher in adolescent girls compared to boys in the same age group (Pettifor *et al.* 2005; UNAIDS 2006).

The HIV epidemic varies substantially from one geographical area to another. For the purpose of epidemiological surveillance at a country level, UNAIDS and WHO have categorized the HIV epidemics broadly as 'low level', 'concentrated', or 'generalized'. The typology is based on the extent to which HIV infection is present and spreading in the general population compared to spread of HIV in sub-populations that are most at risk. An additional scenario 'hyperendemic' has been recently included to describe countries with generalized HIV epidemics where the HIV prevalence in the general population is in excess of 15 per cent and HIV continues to spread. In reality, most countries have a mix of epidemic scenarios. Of importance is keeping up to date on the sources of new infections, as it is dynamic and is key to shaping an effective country level response to the epidemic (Abdool Karim *et al.* 2007).

In 2007, about 5 per cent of the adult population living in sub-Saharan Africa were infected with HIV in contrast to less than 0.4 per cent in East Asia, North Africa and the Middle East, West and Central Europe, and Oceania (UNAIDS 2006). Sub-Saharan Africa is severely affected by HIV and accounts for 67.8 per cent [22.5 million (20.9 million–24.3 million)] of global infections (Fig. 9.13.3) (UNAIDS 2007). It is estimated that 1.7 million (1.4 million–2.4 million) people in this region became newly infected in 2007, while 1.6 million (1.5–2 million) died from AIDS in this period. The majority of infections in sub-Saharan Africa occur through heterosexual contact, where women have about 2–3 times more HIV infection compared to men (Abdool Karim & Abdool Karim 1999).

Southern Africa epitomizes a 'hyper-endemic' scenario and remains at the epicentre of the pandemic (Abdool Karim 2006a). HIV prevalence is >15 per cent in the general adult population fuelled by extensive heterosexual spread, widespread concurrent sexual partnerships, and transmission in discordant stable couples.

Several countries in sub-Saharan Africa have shown a decline in HIV prevalence in recent years, including Kenya, urban areas in Rwanda, Zimbabwe, and urban areas in Burkino Faso (Hallett *et al.* 2006; Kayirangwa *et al.* 2006; UNAIDS 2005, 2006). In contrast, while Uganda has for years been an excellent role-model for successfully impacting the HIV epidemic, more recent data demonstrate an increase in HIV infection in young women (Shafer *et al.* 2006).

HIV prevalence in the Middle East and North Africa is low, and the national HIV prevalence has not exceeded 0.3 per cent, with the exception of Sudan, where national prevalence in 2005 was estimated at 1.6 per cent. A total of 380 000 (270 000–500 000) people were living with HIV in this region in 2007. The main modes of transmission in this region are unprotected sexual contact (including commercial sex and sex between men) and injecting drugs using contaminated equipment. In some countries in North Africa and the Middle East, a significant number of infections still result from contaminated blood products, blood transfusions or lack of infection control measures in healthcare settings although the extent of this has decreased significantly over the last decade.

The HIV epidemics in Latin America and the Caribbean are associated mainly with unsafe sex (both heterosexual and men who have sex with men) and use of contaminated drug injecting equipment, especially among the poor and unemployed. In Latin America, an estimated 1.6 million (1.4–1.9 million) people were living with HIV in 2007. In most Latin American countries, HIV prevalence is highest among men who have sex with men.

In North America, and Western and Central Europe, HIV prevalence has remained below 1 per cent and AIDS mortality has been low because of the widespread availability of antiretroviral therapy. A total of 2.1 million people infected with HIV live in these regions (Fig. 9.13.3), of whom about 1.3 million live in the United States. A total of 77 000 people were newly infected in these regions in 2007 (UNAIDS 2007). Unsafe sexual practices between men and the use of contaminated drug injecting equipment are the most important routes of transmission of HIV in these regions. However, in recent years there has been an increase in heterosexual transmission and more women and members of minority ethnic groups have become infected through unsafe sex.

Epidemic patterns have also been changing in Eastern Europe and Central Asia in recent years, where an increasing number of women are being infected, many of whom acquire HIV infection from their male partners who became infected through injecting drugs using shared, contaminated injecting equipment. The epidemics in this region are continuing to grow. The total number of people living with HIV increased by about 36 per cent from 2003 to 2005 (UNAIDS 2006). UNAIDS estimates that, of the 1.6 million (1.2–2.1 million) people living with HIV in this region, 150 000 (70 000–290 000) were newly infected with the virus in 2007. The Russian Federation and Ukraine account for the majority of infections in this region; most are infected through injecting drugs using contaminated equipment.

In South and Southeast Asia, it is estimated that there were 4 million (3.3 million–5.1 million) people living with HIV at the end of 2007; 340 000 (180 000– 740 000) became newly infected with HIV; and 270 000 (230 000–380 000) died from AIDS during 2007 (UNAIDS 2007). About 69 per cent of all people infected with HIV in this region live in India. However, with a total population of

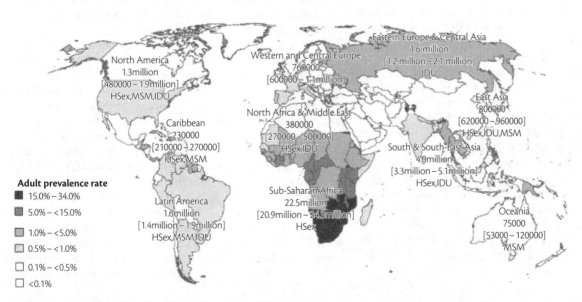

Fig. 9.13.3 Global distribution of people (adults and children) living with HIV in 2005 (33.2 million (30.6–36.1 million)). Major modes of HIV transmission are abbreviated as follows: MSM = men who have sex with men, HSex = heterosexual, and IDU = injection drug use (Adapted from: UNAIDS (UNAIDS 2007)).

over 1 billion people, the adult prevalence in India is still below 1 per cent (NACO 2006). In India, HIV transmission is primarily heterosexual, with female sex workers and their clients being the main drivers of HIV transmission (Mawar *et al.* 2005).

In East Asia (including China, Japan, Mongolia, Republic of Korea, and Democratic People's Republic of Korea) adult prevalence remains low and has not yet reached 0.1 per cent. In most of the rest of the countries in Asia, HIV prevalence remains low; only Cambodia, Thailand, and Myanmar had adult HIV prevalence rates above 1 per cent (1.6 per cent, 1.4 per cent, and 1.3 per cent, respectively) in 2005 (UNAIDS 2006).

Thailand provides an example of the dynamic nature of the evolving epidemic at a country level. The main routes of transmission in the late 1980s and early 1990s were through the use of non-sterile equipment in injecting drug users and through unsafe sexual behaviours. While the 100 per cent condom use policy in brothels made a major impact on preventing sexual spread of HIV to the general population, Thailand's more conservative policy on needle exchange and methadone treatment has enabled HIV to spread rapidly to injecting drug users, who are potentially an important bridge to the general population. In 2005, it was estimated that about 43 per cent of all new infections in Thailand occurred in the low-risk heterosexual population, while 21 per cent of new infections occurred among men who have sex with men (Gouws *et al.* 2006).

Of 75 000 (53 000–120 000) people infected with HIV in Oceania, it is estimated that over 70 per cent are living in Papua New Guinea, where the epidemic started recently, but is growing rapidly. The number of cases of HIV in Papua New Guinea has increased by about 30 per cent per year since 1997 (UNAIDS 2006), reaching an adult prevalence of 2.4 per cent in 2007, with the main mode of transmission being unsafe sex. HIV prevalence in other countries in this region (including Australia, New Zealand, and Fiji) has remained low at about 0.1 per cent (UNAIDS 2006) and is mainly concentrated in men who have sex with men and intravenous drug users.

Transmission of HIV

HIV spreads sexually, vertically from HIV infected mothers to their unborn infants, and through contaminated blood and blood products. It is estimated that sexual transmission (heterosexual and sex between men) accounts for about 84 per cent, injecting drug use for about 7 per cent, mother-to-child transmission for about 6 per cent and unsafe healthcare practices for about 2.5–5 per cent of the global HIV burden in 2006. While the attributable fraction of HIV transmission globally through injecting drug use is relatively small, it accounts for more than 80 per cent of all HIV infections in Eastern Europe and Asia and is an important bridge to the general population.

HIV transmission is sometimes viewed purely from a biomedical perspective of underlying biology and within an epidemiological paradigm of risk groups and risk factors. However, such an approach is inadequate to understand the complexity of HIV transmission. It is important to recognize that social, economic, human rights, and political perspectives are important 'drivers' of HIV transmission that render some groups or populations more vulnerable to HIV acquisition.

Sexual transmission

While the probability of HIV transmission through a single coital act is very low, this risk increases with repeated exposure, co-infection with sexually transmitted infection(s) especially genital ulcers, genital immaturity, receptive anal sex, circumcision status of male sexual partner, higher viral load in the HIV infected person, and the susceptibility of the exposed individual (Vernazza *et al.* 1999). The risk of HIV infection is 3 per 10 000 contacts for the male partner compared to 20 per 10 000 contacts for the female partner in peno-vaginal sex. Hence, on average, women are seven times more likely to become infected. This ratio rises in peno-anal sex, where the risk ratio for the receptive compared to insertive partner exceeds 20:1, highlighting the importance of receptive anal sex as an important factor not only for men but for women as well.

The underlying biological mechanisms of sexual transmission of HIV are poorly understood. Studies have shown that both semen and vaginal secretions have both cell-free virus and T-cells and macrophages which contain HIV. CD4+ positive cells are present both in the male urethra and female vagina—but it remains unclear whether CD4+ cells in the lumen or in the mucosa are involved in the infectious process.

High viral load is associated with more efficient transmission of HIV (Quinn *et al.* 2000). Viral load varies according to the stage of HIV infection, and is elevated during early infection, as well as during advancing HIV disease and progression to AIDS as immunity diminishes. Viral load is also higher during periods where there are other co-infections including herpes simplex virus type 2, malaria, tuberculosis and intestinal parasites. Ulcerative and non-ulcerative sexually transmitted infections contribute to higher HIV transmission and acquisition risk.

The various biological factors that influence the risk of HIV acquisition and transmission occur in a milieu of social, behavioural, and cultural situations which also impact on the spread of HIV. These include poverty, gender-based economic and power differentials, gender-based violence, migrant labour, sex work, and alcohol abuse.

Transmission through blood

Transmission through blood and blood products includes the sharing of needles and syringes during illicit drug use, inadequately screened or unscreened transfusion of blood and blood products, contaminated needles, and/or equipment in healthcare settings or through traditional healing practices.

The risk of HIV transmission via infected donor blood and blood products was recognized early in the HIV epidemic. The implementation of widespread screening of the blood supply has reduced this mode of transmission drastically. However, some national blood screening efforts are impeded by inadequate resources for HIV testing, poor quality assurance of HIV testing procedures, inadequacy of staff training and the quality and choice of laboratory procedures (UNAIDS 2006). A particular challenge for the provision of safe transfusion products is the 'window period', when HIV antibody tests are negative but infectious HIV is present in the blood.

In healthcare settings, HIV can be transmitted between patients and healthcare workers in both directions via blood on sharp instruments, and may also be transmitted between patients through re-use of contaminated instruments. This risk can be reduced through universal precaution practices including use of gloves, standard infection control measures, rigid containers for needles and single use syringes.

The sharing of needles and syringes among injecting drug users is a high-risk practice for HIV transmission. Sterile needle exchange programmes are effective in reducing HIV transmission among injecting drug users. The illicit nature of injection drug use and associated social stigma have compromised efforts to reduce HIV transmission in injecting drug users resulting in continuing high rates of transmission in these populations with bridging transmission to the general population in some instances.

Mother-to-child transmission

HIV is transmitted *in utero* (pre-partum), during the process of childbirth (intra-partum) and post-partum through breastfeeding. In the absence of any intervention, the mother-to-child transmission rate is between 20 per cent and 40 per cent. Most transmission from mother-to-child occurs during childbirth where mother's infected blood in the birth canal infects the baby, resulting in 10–20 per cent of babies becoming infected. About 5 per cent of babies become infected *in utero*. Breastfeeding accounts for 5–20 per cent of babies becoming infected, depending on length and type of breastfeeding. The risk of perinatal HIV transmission is influenced by the severity of HIV disease in the mother (high RNA viral load and low CD4+ count), the route of delivery (Caesarean section versus vaginal delivery), and the type of breastfeeding practices (exclusive breastfeeding or mixed feeding) and duration of breastfeeding. Notable advances have been made in reducing mother-to-child transmission of HIV to very low levels through the use of antiretroviral drugs, obstetric practices including Caesarean delivery, and management of breastfeeding.

As availability of antiretroviral therapy to reduce mother-to-child transmission during childbirth increases, breastfeeding is assuming a proportionately greater role as a source of HIV spread to newborn babies in settings where formula-feeding is not an affordable option.

Breastfeeding, particularly in poor countries, can account for one-third to one-half of all mother-to-child transmissions. This risk is reduced substantially if the mother exclusively breastfeeds her baby since mixed feeding (breastmilk plus formula milk or any other feeds, including water) increases the risk of HIV transmission to the baby. Duration of breastfeeding affects the rate of transmission. A meta-analysis (Coutsoudis *et al.* 2004) of breastfeeding studies from sub-Saharan Africa estimated the cumulative probability of acquiring HIV infection to be 3 per cent at 3 months, 5 per cent at 6 months, 9 per cent at 12 months, and 15 per cent at 18 months.

Obstetric practices, such as vaginal delivery (compared to Caesarean section) and prolonged rupture of membranes (>4 h), increase mother-to-child HIV transmission. Invasive procedures during labour and delivery, such as foetal scalp monitoring, amniocentesis, foetal scalp electrodes, episiotomy, and instrumental delivery, may also increase the risk of transmission. Circulating HIV variants in the mother are selected through immune pressure which is HLA dependent. Where the father has a substantially different HLA profile from the mother, the risk of transmission and/or the viral load in the baby is lower.

HIV prevention strategies

HIV prevention focuses, on the one hand, on reducing the likelihood of and vulnerability to infection in those who are currently uninfected and, on the other hand, on reducing the risk of transmission from those who are currently infected with HIV. The latter is an important new opportunity for enhancing prevention efforts through integration of prevention programmes into the health services which are scaling up AIDS treatment and the prevention of mother-to-child transmission. Knowledge of HIV status is an important gateway for targeted prevention and care efforts. It creates an opportunity to address prevention efforts along a continuum that includes those uninfected who are at high risk of getting infected, those recently infected, those with established infection but asymptomatic and those who have advancing HIV disease and those on antiretroviral treatment. Within this context, groups that are particularly vulnerable can be targeted and their particular needs addressed. Proven interventions are available for preventing HIV through any of its transmission modalities (Table 9.13.1).

Reducing sexual transmission

Globally, the incidence rate of new HIV infections continues to exceed AIDS mortality rates. Reducing sexual transmission, especially heterosexual transmission, of HIV is critical to altering the current epidemic trajectory in many parts of the world. Prevention of sexual transmission can be achieved through reduction in the number of discordant sexual acts and/or reduction of the probability of HIV transmission in discordant sexual acts (Fig. 9.13.4).

There is no risk of HIV infection among those who practice sexual abstinence or lifelong mutual monogamy. Serial monogamy, where there are multiple sequential individual short-lived monogamous partnerships, is associated with an increased risk of HIV, but not to the same extent as the substantial increase in risk of transmission emanating from multiple concurrent sexual partnerships (Morris & Kretzschmar 1997). Reduction in the number of concurrent sexual partnerships and the use of condoms are key components of HIV prevention messages, widely promoted as part of 'ABC' campaigns promoting Abstinence, Be faithful and Condomize.

Male condoms

Condoms are a pivotal part of the fight against HIV/AIDS. They are inexpensive and relatively easy to use and provide protection against acquisition and transmission of HIV, a wide range of other sexually transmitted infections as well as pregnancy. When used correctly and consistently, the latex male condom is highly effective in preventing the sexual transmission of HIV. The strongest evidence for the role of condoms in preventing the transmission of HIV comes from sero-discordant couple studies, which uniformly show that increased condom use is associated with a substantially reduced risk of HIV transmission. However, there are still important questions regarding whether inconsistent condom use (that is, condom use in less than 100 per cent of sexual contacts) is protective. While some studies have suggested that inconsistent condom use may offer more protection than no condom use whatsoever, others have demonstrated that the transmission of HIV among irregular condom users is similar to that of individuals who do not use condoms (Ahmed *et al.* 2001).

To be effective as a prevention option to impact on the growth of the epidemic, access to condoms needs to be drastically scaled up. In 2001, it was reported, that the overall provision of condoms to sub-Saharan Africa was 4.6 per man per year. An estimated 1.9 billion additional condoms would be needed to raise all countries to the average procurement level (about 17 condoms per man per year) of the six African countries that use the most condoms (Shelton & Johnson 2001). It would cost an estimated US$47.5 million a year to fill the 1.9 billion condom gap excluding service delivery costs and production. However, based on data on condoms procured in public sector health facilities across South Africa, the estimated unmet need for condoms is probably closer to 13 billion (Myer *et al.* 2001).

Table 9.13.1 Biomedical technologies for prevention for each mode of HIV transmission

Mode	Technology	Intervention
Blood and blood products	◆ HIV screening for both virus and antibodies	◆ Selection of donors based on lower HIV risk profile ◆ Screening of all blood supplies with best available technology for viral detection during the window period of infection
Occupational exposure in health care settings	◆ Barrier nursing—gloves, goggles, gowns as appropriate ◆ Universal Infection control practices ◆ Proper sharps and other biohazards disposal systems ◆ Post-exposure prophylaxis	◆ Guidelines for universal precautions ◆ Trained health care workers ◆ Availability of post-exposure prophylaxis ◆ Availability of barrier nursing paraphernalia ◆ Availability of disposal systems for sharps and other biohazardous materials
Exposure to infected blood through traditional skin cutting and blood-letting practices	◆ Infection control practices ◆ Barrier nursing	◆ Guidelines for universal precautions ◆ Adequate training of traditional healers ◆ Information to public raising awareness of HIV risk through traditional practices
Injecting drug use	◆ Detoxification centres ◆ Sterile needles and syringes ◆ Maintenance therapy; e.g. buponorphine	◆ Treatment/rehabilitation centres ◆ Free needle exchange programmes
Mother-to-child transmission	◆ Determine mother and/or father's HIV status ◆ Antiretroviral drugs ◆ Alternative baby feeding options ◆ Non-invasive intra-partum procedures ◆ Caesarian section	◆ Implementation of a comprehensive prevention of mother-to-child transmission (PMTCT) programme
Sexual transmission		◆ Abstinence ◆ Delay age of sexual debut ◆ Mutually faithful monogamous relationship between concordant couples ◆ Zero-grazing', i.e. no concurrent multiple partnerships
Consensual sex	◆ Male condoms ◆ Female condoms ◆ HIV testing ◆ Sexually transmitted infection treatment ◆ Male medical circumcision	◆ Implementation of services for condom distribution, HIV education and counselling, HIV testing, sexually transmitted infection treatment, and circumcision services
Non-consensual/coerced sex	◆ Post-exposure prophylaxis ◆ Emergency contraception ◆ Sexually transmitted infection treatment	◆ Availability of health services for post-exposure prophylaxis, sexually transmitted infection treatment and emergency contraception
Experimental prevention tools to reduce sexual transmission (unproven)	◆ Antiretroviral drugs as pre-exposure prophylaxis for HIV uninfected persons ◆ Early antiretroviral therapy for HIV-infected persons ◆ Microbicides ◆ Vaccines	

Notwithstanding the challenges to condom access, a wide range of factors have been implicated as barriers to condom use; the most common being the widespread perception that condoms reduce sexual pleasure and that suggesting the use of condoms represents self-acknowledgement of HIV infection or a lack of trust in the partner. In the context of a marital relationship or stable partnership where pregnancy is desired, or where subordination of women limits their ability to negotiate safer sex practices, attempts to introduce or promote condom use have had limited success.

Several studies have demonstrated that alcohol consumption is associated with inconsistent condom use; this phenomenon is particularly problematic because many individuals meet high-risk sexual

Factors facilitating HIV spread

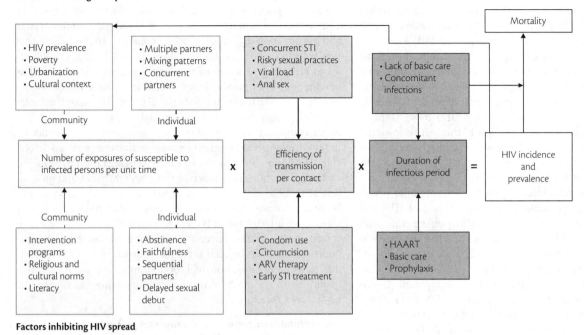

Factors inhibiting HIV spread

Fig. 9.13.4 Interplay between factors influencing sexual transmission of HIV infection.
Source: Department of Health, South Africa (2007).

partners in social settings where alcohol is available. Condoms use is lower in partnerships where an effective form of contraception is being used. This points to the need for interventions that promote dual method use (the simultaneous use of condoms with another form of contraception) among high-risk women. An important predictor of condom use is previous experience using condoms; individuals who have used condoms previously are more likely to use them in the future.

Female condoms

It is generally accepted that the efficacy of the female condom, when used correctly, is at least comparable to that of male condoms. While there are less data on the efficacy of the female condom, it protects essentially the same mucosal surface area as the male condom, and the polyurethane used in the construction of the female condom is stronger and less permeable than the latex used in most male condoms. Furthermore, female condoms do not degrade appreciably after several washings and, if they are cleaned appropriately, can be reused (unlike the male condom) though this practice is not widely recommended.

Sexually transmitted infections

HIV transmission and acquisition during heterosexual intercourse is enhanced in the presence of sexually transmitted infections, particularly ulcerative infections such as syphilis, chancroid, and herpes simplex virus type 2 virus infection. Genital ulceration or inflammation caused by sexually transmitted infections increase the infectiousness of HIV-positive individuals and the susceptibility of HIV negative individuals.

The incidence of curable sexually transmitted infections is highest in sub-Saharan Africa, with 69 million new cases per year in a population of 269 million adults aged 15–49 (WHO 2001). This is an important factor in accelerating the spread of HIV in this region.

In rural South Africa, nearly 9 per cent of adults have syphilis, and almost one in 20 has gonorrhea (Colvin *et al.* 1998). The prevalence of HIV infection in sexually transmitted disease clinic patients has exceeded 70 per cent in Zimbabwe (WHO 2001) and exceeded 50 per cent in Swaziland (UNAIDS 2002). It is estimated that only 14 per cent of those in Africa in need of sexually transmitted disease services are able to access them.

Male circumcision

In 2006/2007, three randomized control trials conducted in Africa consistently demonstrated that medical male circumcision reduces the risk of female to male transmission of HIV by 50–60 per cent (Auvert *et al.* 2005; Bailey *et al.* 2007; Gray *et al.* 2007). There may be an increased risk of HIV infection in men who engage in sex before complete healing of the circumcision wound. It is unclear as to whether male circumcision has any impact on the risk of male to female HIV transmission or on male to male HIV transmission. Mathematical modelling of the introduction of male circumcision suggests that 2–3 million HIV infections could be averted in sub-Saharan Africa. If integrated into a comprehensive package of male sexual and reproductive health services it could mark a critical milestone in increasing male involvement in HIV prevention.

Reducing transmission through blood

Transmission of HIV through exposure to infected blood can occur through transfusion of blood and blood products, through sharing of needles and syringes among injecting drug users and through inadvertent nosocomial transmission (e.g. through needlestick injuries) in healthcare settings.

Injection drug use

Of the estimated 13.2 million injecting drug users worldwide, 78 per cent of them reside in low- and middle-income countries, especially in Eastern Europe, and Central, South, and Southeast Asia. An estimated 10 per cent of the world's HIV infections are attributed to injection drug use, which is the main mode of transmission in certain Asian and European countries. HIV epidemics among injecting drug users are characterized by significant regional inter-country and intra-country variations, and prevalence of HIV infection among injecting drug users has been shown to exceed 50 per cent and in some cases reach even up to 90 per cent of injecting drug users in a very short timeframe (UNAIDS 2004). Ukraine exemplifies how quickly the virus can spread through an injecting population: With the number of diagnosed HIV infections increasing from virtually zero in 1995 to 20 000 a year since 1996; 80 per cent of these new infections are occurring in injecting drug users.

The sharing and reuse of injecting equipment, particularly needles and syringes, is responsible for the transmission of HIV and other bloodborne diseases and is widespread among injecting drug users. Needle sharing is often a consequence of a lack of perceived risk for HIV infection, group norms and rituals, inaccessibility of clean injecting equipment due to scarcity or relative cost of equipment, and/or the inability to carry injecting equipment due to potential negative social or legal consequences (UNAIDS 2004). Although injection drug use is distinct from sexual intercourse as a mode of transmission, the two routes are frequently linked epidemiologically. Injection drug users are often young and sexually active, potentially exposing their sexual partners, children and foetuses to the virus. In addition, injection drug use is common in the commercial sex industry.

Over the past 20 years, research among injecting drug users and the experience from numerous programmes and projects indicate that the HIV epidemics among injecting drug users can be prevented, stabilized and even reversed. Effective programmes typically include; drug dependence treatment, including substitution treatment (e.g. methadone programmes), outreach to injecting drug users to promote safer sex and injecting practices, clean needles and syringes, condoms, voluntary counselling and HIV testing, treatment of sexually transmitted infections, and interventions for special populations-at-risk such as prisoners and sex workers who inject drugs (UNAIDS 2004).

'Needle exchange' or 'syringe exchange' programmes, when part of a comprehensive harm-reduction approach, have been shown to reduce the risk of transmission without contributing to an increase in drug use (Des Jarlais et al. 1996; Vlahov & Junge 1998). Early implementation of needle exchange, community outreach, and access to sterile injection equipment have been critical factors in helping several cities avoid a serious HIV outbreak among injecting drug users (Des Jarlais et al. 1995). An analysis of 81 cities around the world showed that HIV prevalence decreased 5.8 per cent in 29 cities with needle exchange projects compared to a 5.9 per cent increase in HIV prevalence in 52 cities without such programmes (Hurley et al. 1997).

Blood transfusions

The transfusion of HIV-infected blood or blood products is probably responsible for 5–10 per cent of cumulative infections worldwide (UNAIDS 2006), translating to an estimated 160 000 cases of HIV being transmitted every year (WHO 2005a).

In the 1980s and early 1990s, the majority of HIV infections through blood and blood products were in haemophiliacs. In the past 15 years great strides have been made to build up the safety of the blood supply, particularly in low- and middle-income countries. The creation of nationally coordinated blood transfusion services and introduction of a range of policies and procedures, with a particular focus on HIV screening of donated blood to detect antibodies to HIV, the reduction of unnecessary transfusions as well as development of improved donor screening and deferral techniques have helped to virtually eliminate the risk that HIV would be transmitted through donated blood in high-income countries. The ongoing concern is the risk of transmission when blood donors are in the window period where they are infectious but have no detectable HIV antibodies. The use of the newer generation p24 antigen assays, polymerase chain reaction to detect viral RNA and quarantine of first blood donations until subsequent donations prove to be uninfected are some of the strategies used to reduce the risk of transfusing infected blood (Heyns & Swanevelder 2005). Almost all countries have routine screening of blood donations for HIV antibodies (UNAIDS 2006), but some continue to experience problems due to poor organization of blood supply systems, inadequate quality assurance mechanisms, poor staff training and suboptimal laboratory procedures.

Nosocomial transmission and universal precautions

Healthcare workers exposed to blood and body fluids have a low but measurable risk of occupational infection with HIV. In a review of transmission probability estimates, infectivity following a needlestick exposure was estimated to range from 0.00 per cent to 2.38 per cent (weighted mean = 0.23 per cent) (Baggaley et al. 2006). While international guidelines recommend the use of relatively inexpensive auto-disable syringes as the 'equipment of choice' to help prevent HIV transmission in healthcare settings, only 62 per cent of low- and middle-income countries were using such syringes in their national vaccine programmes in 2004 (WHO 2005b). Risk of exposure to blood or other body fluids can be significantly lowered through workers' adherence to 'universal precautions', which involves the routine use of gloves and other protective gear to prevent occupational exposures, safe disposal of sharps, and timely administration of a 4-week prophylactic course of antiretroviral prophylaxis if a worker does get exposed.

Preventing mother-to-child transmission

Over 4 million HIV-infected children under the age of 15 have been born to HIV-infected mothers; in 2005 alone, an estimated 700 000 children became newly infected. With few exceptions, most children acquire their HIV infection from their mothers. Mother-to-child-transmission (MTCT) of HIV occurs in the intrauterine period, during labour and delivery, and postnatally through breastfeeding. Africa bears 70 per cent of the global burden of HIV in all age groups, but has at least 90 per cent of all the HIV-infected children in the world resulting in a reversal of decades of steady progress in child survival.

Substantial progress has been made in preventing MTCT. Before medical interventions became available, approximately one-third of babies of HIV positive mothers became infected with HIV. With a combination of antiretroviral drugs, changes in obstetric practices and alternatives to breastfeeding, MTCT rates below 1 per cent can be attained and MTCT has been virtually eliminated in high-income countries.

The first research breakthrough in MTCT occurred in 1994 when the Paediatric AIDS Clinical Trials Group 076 trial showed that HIV transmission from mother-to-child can be reduced from 25.5 per cent to 8.3 per cent using AZT. This efficacious regimen of AZT from about 12 weeks gestation and through labour and delivery in the infected mother and for a week post-birth to the infant has been widely implemented in industrialized countries. For resource-constrained settings, cheaper interventions using AZT or nevirapine are available. The Thai short course AZT regimen administered to mothers from 36 weeks gestation through the intra-partum period and the HIVNET 012-single dose nevirapine regimen (a dose to the mother at onset of labour and a dose to the infant within 72 h of birth) are preferred in resource-constrained settings. The main advantage of single-dose nevirapine is the ease of administration and low cost; the chief drawback is concern about drug resistance in the mother. Concerns about drug resistant viral strains have led to several trials using combination treatments to reduce transmission during the intra-partum period.

Breastfeeding is not recommended for HIV-positive mothers since this is associated with an increased risk of HIV transmission. However, lack of access to clean running water in resource-constrained settings has precluded the use of formula feeding. While exclusive breast feeding with abrupt weaning is one proven option of reducing breastfeeding risk in these settings, other options are under investigation (Coovadia *et al.* 2007), including studies of whether antiretrovirals given to baby (and mother) during breastfeeding may reduce MTCT.

Despite single-dose nevirapine being a readily implementable effective HIV prevention strategy to reduce MTCT in almost any country, only 9 per cent of pregnant women in low- and middle-income countries were offered services to prevent transmission to their newborns in 2005 (Global HIV Prevention Working Group 2006). A lot more still needs to be done to expand interventions to reduce MTCT.

Voluntary counselling and testing

Knowledge of HIV status is not only a vital entrée to treatment, it is also essential for prevention of MTCT, prevention of transmission through blood transfusions and reducing sexual transmission of HIV infection. Voluntary counselling and testing (VCT) has been shown to be both efficacious in reducing risky sexual behaviours (The VCT efficacy study group 2000) and cost-effective as a prevention intervention. In a large multi-centre study ($n = 4293$), both men and women randomized to receive VCT significantly reduced unprotected intercourse with their primary partners than those receiving only health information (The VCT efficacy study group 2000). In this VCT trial, the centres in Kenya and Tanzania averted an estimated 1104 and 895 HIV infections and this translated into a cost-saving of US$249 and US$346 per HIV infection averted in Kenya and Tanzania, respectively (Sweat *et al.* 2000).

Large numbers of HIV infected people, particularly in low- and middle-income countries, do not know their HIV status and are diagnosed too late (Shisana *et al.* 2005). While the aim is to put all those eligible for antiretroviral therapy (often defined as CD4 <200 cells/ml) on treatment, it is primarily those who are symptomatic and seeking care who are learning their HIV status and accessing care. VCT has traditionally been offered as an out-patient or ambulatory service based at primary care providers or specialized VCT centres. However, stigma, which is a common experience of those infected and affected by HIV, is a major obstacle to HIV testing and acknowledgement of individual risk of infection.

The traditional form of VCT was developed in the pre-ART era in response to human rights and ethical concerns about HIV testing that centred on the need to ensure autonomy and minimize harms for the client (Fylkesnes 1999). At that stage, VCT was mainly for prevention purposes. Unfortunately, this form of VCT has become a major obstacle to care due to the lack of capacity of health services to provide this time-consuming approach to VCT.

In an attempt to overcome this limitation, a number of different models to promote HIV testing have started to emerge, each designed to meet different goals, including:

a. Individual pre- and post-test counselling, which is the classic model that is client initiated and is typical of most free-standing VCT sites

b. Group information opt-in individual pre- and post-test counselling, which is widely used in high-prevalence settings

c. Group information opt-out individual testing with individual post-test counselling for sero-positives, which is widely used during routine medical screening, e.g. antenatal clinics

d. Group information opt-in couple/family pre-test counselling with individual post-test counselling

e. No specific pre-test information and testing is an opt-out option with individual post-test counselling, e.g. antenatal and sexually transmitted disease clinics

Routine opt-out testing, with a right to decline, was pioneered in Botswana in 2004. A population-based study on attitudes, practices, and human rights concerns showed that of 1268 adults interviewed, 81–93 per cent were in favour of opt-out HIV testing as it enhanced access to treatment. Barriers to testing included fear of learning one's status (49 per cent), lack of perceived HIV risk (43 per cent), and fear of having to change sexual practices with a positive HIV test (33 per cent) (Weiser *et al.* 2006). In the United States, routine opt-out testing in healthcare settings has been recommended since 2006.

While alternate models of VCT have engendered some concern about coercion of clients to participate in HIV testing, most of these concerns are readily remedied. Some have argued for a move away from the 'HIV exceptionalism' approach to a 'HIV normalization' approach wherein HIV is treated as any other infectious disease. In this context VCT is essential for both HIV prevention and early diagnosis for timely access to treatment (De Cock & Johnson 1998).

Community interventions for HIV prevention

Community intervention strategies can be categorized according to three approaches: Mass media (e.g. television, radio, newspapers/magazines, posters); community mobilization, through which the community becomes a participant in the design of the intervention; and interpersonal communication involving direct, face-to-face approaches such as counselling.

A common theoretical model used in developing behavioural interventions (Bertrand *et al.* 2006) requires the direct impact of the intervention to increase knowledge, change attitudes, and enhance self-efficacy, leading to a reduction in risk behaviours, greater utilization of health services and, ultimately, a reduction in HIV prevalence. An overall approach to the way interventions are designed and implemented suggests that for an intervention to be successful, it needs to be based on behavioural theory, designed to change specific risk behaviours, delivered by health professionals, delivered in an intensive manner, delivered to individuals, delivered as part of routine health services; and should incorporate skill-building (Crepaz et al. 2006).

The mass media approach targets the general population, regardless of level of HIV risk. Thus, the message that is delivered through the mass media must carefully consider the impact of the content and approach of their messages. In the early 1980s in the United States, mass media messages tended to emphasize the severity of the disease and the fatal outcome. The unexpected outcome of that approach was to induce fear and cause many people to shun individuals in high-risk groups and persons with AIDS, resulting in stigmatization. Stigmatization is now one of the major barriers to effective control of the epidemic, and has compromised efforts to promote HIV testing.

A systematic review (Bertrand et al. 2006) of interventions using the mass media in low- and middle-countries found that only two of the desired outcomes were achieved in 50 per cent or more of the trials: Knowledge of HIV transmission and reduction of high-risk activities (multiple partners, visiting sex workers, etc.). Few of the mass media intervention studies resulted in an increase in reported use of condoms.

A review (Eke et al. 2006) of community-based programmes, suggested that success was dependent on the interventions being tailored to respond to the unique contexts in which risk behaviours occur (e.g. in Thailand and Cambodia, a high proportion of sexual risk behaviour occurs in brothels, which then become a logical target for intervention), addressing contextual variables and practices such as sociocultural norms (e.g. acceptance that extra-marital sex is to be expected), and the provision of adequate resources with which to implement the intervention.

A successful example of a community mobilization strategy (Wu et al. 2002), aimed at new drug users in southern Yunnan Province in China, produced a two-thirds reduction in HIV incidence within one year. Another successful example of an intervention targeting a specific community is the Sonagachi Project, which organized commercial sex workers in Kolkata, India, to promote safer sex, better working conditions, better health-seeking behaviours, and better access to healthcare (Jana et al. 2004).

Community intervention strategies, like the successful examples above, can prevent HIV infection, but they must be carefully designed, and should mobilize the target population to participate in the intervention design and implementation.

Post-exposure prophylaxis

HIV infection is thought to initially established within the dendritic cells of the skin and mucosa before spreading through lymphatic vessels and developing into a systemic infection. Thus, there is a 'window of opportunity' following exposure for the use of antiretroviral therapy to prevent systemic infection.

There are several groups who could benefit from post-exposure prophylaxis (PEP). These include health workers, laboratory personnel, and individuals with likely exposure to HIV through sexual contact (including rape) or breast milk. The success of PEP in preventing established infection depends on a number of factors, including route and dose of exposure, efficacy of drug(s) used, interval between exposure and initiation of drug(s), and level of adherence to the drug. The dose of exposure depends primarily on the route of infection and the stage of infection of the source. Thus, receptive anal intercourse and deep accidental needle sticks carry the highest risk of exposure and the greatest challenge for effective PEP. People who are in the acute or terminal stages of HIV disease will also have the highest levels of HIV, and thus present the highest risk to those exposed to them.

It is unlikely that placebo-controlled double-blinded clinical trials of PEP will ever be conducted for logistical and ethical reasons. A case–control study of PEP following occupational exposures (Cardo et al. 1997) showed 81 per cent protection against HIV infection. A study of PEP following sexual exposure, primarily through anal intercourse, also showed a protective effect (Roland et al. 2005).

An important issue in implementing PEP is whether it will lead to behavioural disinhibition, i.e. individuals believing, because of PEP, they can safely engage in high-risk activities. Thus, counselling on the need for reduction of risk exposures should be an integral part of any PEP programme.

The US Centers for Disease Control and Prevention has issued guidelines for management of occupational, sexual, and other exposures to HIV (Panlilio et al. 2005). The current consensus is that combination antiretroviral therapy should be initiated as soon as possible after exposure, and continued for at least 4 weeks.

Scaling up prevention interventions

Despite substantial increases in knowledge of what works in preventing HIV infection, and resources for their implementation, the virus continues to spread. The inability to curb the epidemic in many settings is due to the inability to implement proven HIV prevention strategies at the necessary scale and magnitude to those who need it most, and not recognizing the link between HIV prevention and broader development needs especially in resource-constrained settings.

In 2006, the gap between HIV prevention needs and provision of prevention programmes was substantial. A significant constraint to prevention efforts has been the inability to integrate HIV prevention: (i) within a comprehensive AIDS strategy, including prevention integrated with AIDS treatment; (ii) within other national development programmes; (iii) into poverty reduction strategies; iv) into education programmes; (v) into health services, especially sexual and reproductive health services; (vi) into programmes aimed at reducing gender inequalities; and (vii) into initiatives to enhance economic and political opportunities for women and girls.

Prevention efforts have generally targeted whole communities or those who are HIV negative. There is a steady shift in prevention efforts from a narrow focus on HIV uninfected persons to a more effective continuum of prevention that includes those who are uninfected, recently infected, infected but asymptomatic as well as those with advancing HIV disease and on antiretroviral therapy.

To improve the impact of known effective HIV prevention interventions, implementation needs to be done to scale, targeting the key populations in the epidemic with integrated approaches that recognize that prevention planning and implementation needs to take the context into account.

New HIV prevention technologies under investigation

Several trials of new HIV prevention technologies are currently underway. Antiretroviral prophylaxis, microbicides, and vaccines are being tested and may have great potential in the future.

Pre-exposure prophylaxis

Certain groups are repeatedly exposed to possible infection by HIV. These include health workers, laboratory personnel, sex workers, injection drug users, and both homosexual and heterosexual individuals who have multiple partners and are unwilling to take precautions (as well as their spouses and/or regular partners). The concept of pre-exposure prophylaxis is not new, but has now gained considerable popularity as a possible strategy for reducing the risk of infection among high-risk groups.

However, there are many issues inherent in long-term prophylaxis with any drug. These include the need for inexpensive drugs, the potential for serious toxic side effects, development of viral resistance to the drug with repeated use, the potential impact on behavioural disinhibition (i.e. increasing risky behaviour and decreasing condom use), the possible need for multiple drug combinations, and assuring an acceptable cost:benefit ratio.

Several studies of the antiretroviral drug, tenofovir, were initiated to assess its effectiveness as pre-exposure prophylaxis (Liu *et al.* 2006). Results from one pre-exposure trial conducted in Ghana, Cameroon, and Nigeria (Peterson *et al.* 2007) showed no increased risk of drug-associated toxicity from oral tenofovir, and did not observe any increase in high-risk behaviour.

Whether pre-exposure prophylaxis becomes a widely implemented, acceptable prevention strategy will depend on the results of these trials evaluating efficacy/effectiveness, toxicity and behavioural disinhibition. If pre-exposure prophylaxis is shown to be safe and effective, implementation programmes of this potential prevention strategy will need to emphasize the concomitant use of other prevention strategies such as condoms.

Microbicides

Topical microbicides, products designed to prevent the sexual transmission of HIV and other sexually transmitted pathogens, are one of the most promising prevention tools currently under development that women can use to protect themselves from HIV (Stone 2002). Potentially, they can be applied vaginally to prevent both male-to-female and female-to-male transmission.

Currently in the research pipeline are over 60 substances that are being studied as possible microbicides. Some 50 of these substances are in pre-clinical development, and 11 have entered various stages of human clinical testing.

Microbicides in human trials have one of four mechanisms of action:

a. Surfactants, e.g. nonoxynol-9 and C31G (Savvy), which act by disrupting cell membranes

b. Vaginal defence enhancers, which boost the body's natural defences against infection by maintaining the naturally acidic environment of the vagina by increasing lactobacilli or by rapidly acidifying alkaline ejaculate, e.g. BufferGel

c. Attachment and fusion inhibitors, which bind to pathogens or to receptors on healthy human cells thereby preventing attachment, e.g. Carraguard, PRO2000, and Cellulose Sulphate

d. Replication inhibitors, or antiretroviral agents, which act locally in the reproductive tract mucosa at various steps in the HIV replication cycle and therefore have a narrow spectrum of activity, e.g. Tenofovir gel, Dapivirine, and UC781

Early studies of the spermicide, nonxynol-9, showed this product, which acts by disrupting cell membranes, to be harmful as it caused lesions in the genital tract and increased the risk of HIV infection. Subsequent studies of Savvy, another product in the same class, were halted due to low HIV incidence rates in the trial sites. Trials of Cellulose Sulphate, were stopped in 2007 due to safety concerns. Gel formulations of inhibitors of the chemokine receptor, CCR5 have shown promise in animal models and are currently being developed for early human studies.

There are significant challenges in conducting microbicide effectiveness trials, including the ethical need to promote condoms thereby undermining the ability to show the effect of the microbicide, low HIV incidence rates in some trial populations, poor adherence to study products and high rates of pregnancy as study products are discontinued during pregnancy.

Vaccines

A safe, protective and inexpensive vaccine would be the most efficient, effective, and possibly the only way to control the HIV pandemic. Despite intensive research, development of such a candidate vaccine remains elusive. Safety concerns prohibit the use of whole killed HIV or live attenuated virus as immunogens (Sheppard 2005). Many different approaches using recombinant technologies have been pursued over the past two decades. Initially, efforts were focused on generating neutralizing antibodies using recombinant monomeric envelope gp120 (AIDSVAX) as immunogen. This vaccine did not induce neutralizing antibodies and the phase III trials failed to show protection against HIV acquisition. Antibody-mediated HIV neutralization is complicated by the high genetic diversity of the variable Env regions, epitopes masked by a carbohydrate shield (glycosylation) and conformational rearrangements (Garber *et al.* 2004).

Since CD8+ T-cell responses have been shown to control viral replication *in vivo*, recent vaccine development has focused on eliciting cellular immune responses. Unfortunately, safety and immunogenicity studies of adenovirus vector-based T-cell vaccine have failed to show a protective effect and may be associated with an increased risk of HIV infection.

Vaccine development is severely hampered by the lack of any immune correlate which has been shown to prevent viral infection or clear initial viral infection. The human immune system generally fails to spontaneously clear HIV infection and so there is no natural immune process for the vaccine candidates to mimic. It is, however, believed that approaches aimed at eliciting both humoral and cell mediated immunity are most promising to prevent or at least control retroviral infection (Ho & Huang 2002).

Most of the efforts to produce a vaccine have concentrated on looking at components of the virus that may stimulate protective immunity and substrates that may enhance the immune response. While natural immunity has not been observed in HIV/AIDS, several researchers (Clerici *et al.* 1992; Detels *et al.* 1994; Detels *et al.* 1996) have identified groups of men who have sex with men and female sex workers who have been repeatedly exposed to HIV and have not become infected. Some of these individuals were shown to lack the CCR-5 receptor on CD4+ cells to which the HIV attaches (Dean *et al.* 1996). However, these individuals comprise only a subset of 'resistant' individuals. If the factors that allow these individuals to resist infection can be identified, it might be possible to confer the 'resistance factor' on individuals lacking it, thus artificially providing them some measure of protection against HIV infection. This approach would represent an alternative approach to the traditional strategies of vaccine development and might overcome the apparent lack of natural immunity to HIV.

The spectrum of clinical manifestations of AIDS

Opportunistic infections, which seldom cause serious disease in immunocompetent people, are common in HIV-infected individuals. Indeed, most of the morbidity and mortality associated with HIV infection is almost always as a consequence of opportunistic diseases or malignancies that occur when immunity is impaired, usually corresponding with a CD4+ count below 200 cells/ml. Infections caused by more virulent pathogens, such as *Mycobacterium tuberculosis* or *Streptococcus pneumoniae*, often occur with lesser degrees of immune suppression. Over 100 opportunistic infections by viruses, bacteria, fungi, and protozoa have been associated with AIDS. The spectrum of clinical manifestations includes:

Dermatological manifestations

Cutaneous abnormalities are common and some of the conditions are unique and virtually pathognomonic for HIV disease, e.g. Kaposi's sarcoma.

Neurological manifestations

Apart from dementia, HIV-infected patients are at risk for a wide range of neurologic diseases. Global cerebral disease can present with altered mental status or generalized seizures, whereas focal disease often produces hemiparesis, hemisensory loss, visual field cuts, or disturbances in language use. Fungal, viral, and mycobacterial meningoencephalitis are the most common causes of global cerebral dysfunction, and progressive multifocal leukoencephalopathy (PML), primary CNS lymphoma, and toxoplasmosis account for the majority of focal presentations.

Pulmonary manifestations

HIV-associated pulmonary conditions include both opportunistic infections and neoplasms. The opportunistic infections include bacterial, mycobacterial, fungal, viral, and parasitic pathogens. Some of the more common respiratory infections associated with HIV patients include: Pneumonia, tuberculosis, and pulmonary Kaposi's sarcoma.

Endocrine manifestations

A number of endocrine abnormalities develop in patients with HIV infection; some due to infiltration of endocrine glands by tumour or infection.

HIV wasting

This condition was first recognized as an AIDS-defining illness by the US Centers for Disease Control and Prevention in 1987. The 'wasting syndrome' is defined as a weight loss of at least 10 per cent in the presence of diarrhoea or chronic weakness and documented fever for at least 30 days that is not attributable to a concurrent condition other than HIV infection itself.

Haematologic manifestations

Clinically significant haematologic abnormalities are common in persons with HIV infection. Impaired haematopoiesis, immune-mediated cytopaenias, and altered coagulation mechanisms have all been described in HIV-infected individuals.

Renal manifestations

Renal disorders during HIV infection range from fluid and electrolyte imbalances commonly seen in hospitalized HIV-infected patients, to HIV-associated nephropathy, which can progress rapidly to end-stage renal disease.

Gastrointestinal manifestations

Common gastrointestinal disorders include diarrhoea, dysphagia and odynophagia, nausea, vomiting, weight loss, abdominal pain, anorectal disease, jaundice and hepatomegaly, gastrointestinal bleeding, interactions of HIV and hepatotropic viruses, and gastrointestinal tumours (Kaposi's sarcoma and non-Hodgkin's lymphoma).

Ophthalmic manifestations of HIV

Numerous ophthalmic manifestations of HIV infection may involve the eye including tumours of the periocular tissues, a variety of external infections, HIV-associated retinopathy, and a number of opportunistic infections of the retina and choroid.

Otolaryngologic manifestations

HIV disease is associated with a variety of problems in the head and neck region; as many as 70 per cent of HIV-infected patients eventually develop such conditions.

Oral manifestations

Oral manifestations of HIV disease are common and include oral lesions and novel presentations of previously known opportunistic diseases. Some are caused by fungal infections, e.g. candidiasis; while others are due to viral infections, e.g. herpes simplex, herpes zoster, human papillomavirus, cytomegalovirus, hairy leukoplakia, and Epstein–Barr virus. Other oral complications include periodontal disease, neoplastic lesions, and lymphomas.

Rheumatologic and musculoskeletal manifestations

Musculoskeletal syndromes that occur in HIV-infected patients include manifestations of drug toxicity, reactive arthritis, Reiter's syndrome, infectious arthritis, and myositis.

Tuberculosis and HIV

In resource-constrained settings, the most common presenting illness of AIDS is tuberculosis (TB). TB is a global public health problem that has been exacerbated by the HIV epidemic. In 2003 an estimated 8.8 million new cases of TB were diagnosed and 1.7 million people died from the disease. The most severely affected region has been sub-Saharan Africa, where TB notifications have, on average, trebled since the mid-1980s, and death rates on treatment have reached 20 per cent compared with the 5 per cent that can be achieved by good TB-control programmes without HIV (WHO 2005c).

AIDS has changed the profile of TB patients globally; from a disease of the malnourished, elderly and men to a disease of young people, predominantly women. Extra-pulmonary TB is common in

AIDS patients; together with other reasons for smear-negative TB, this has created a major diagnostic problem. The result is large numbers of patients being treated for TB without microbiological confirmation of infection. The rapid growth of the HIV epidemic has resulted in a rapidly growing TB epidemic. Rising TB incidence rates in those who are HIV infected has had a spillover effect of rising TB incidence rates even among those who do not have HIV infection.

In much of sub-Saharan Africa, the strain of growing TB and HIV epidemics has led to the emergence of extensively drug resistance TB. Global increases in multidrug-resistant (MDR-TB) and extensively drug-resistant (XDR-TB), are threatening both TB and HIV treatment programmes worldwide. The former is defined as resistance to both isoniazid and rifampin, whereas the newly defined XDR-TB consists of MDR and resistance to a fluroquinolone and at least one injectable second-line TB drug (kanamycin, amikacin, or capreomycin). Together, they raise concerns of a global epidemic of untreatable TB and pose a huge threat to TB control. In high-prevalence TB and HIV areas of the developing world, the current DOTS (Directly Observed Treatment, Short Course) strategy is proving ineffective because available resources are being outstripped by the large number of patients in need of treatment. As a consequence TB treatment and outcomes are sub-optimal and MDR and XDR TB are on the rise.

Treatment

Antiretroviral therapy (ART)

The ART era started in 1987 with the approval of AZT (also known as zidovudine), a thymidine nucleoside analogue that interrupts the transcription of viral RNA to viral DNA by blocking the action of the reverse transcriptase enzymes. During the late 1980s additional nucleoside reverse transcriptase inhibitors (NRTIs) were developed. As more antiretroviral drugs of different classes became available, triple combination therapy was shown to have greater and more durable benefits than either mono- or dual therapy. The big treatment breakthrough occurred in 1996 with the introduction of protease inhibitors (PIs) that are capable of blocking the assembly of the progeny HIV within the CD4+ cell, marking the beginning of the era of highly active antiretroviral therapy (HAART). A third class of antiretrovirals, the non-nucleoside reverse transcriptase inhibitors (NNRTIs) was developed soon after the first PIs became available.

Combinations of drugs from these three classes of antiretrovirals are widely used as the 'standard of care' (Wood 2005). The currently recommended regimens for adults that demonstrate the most potent virologic and immunologic efficacy are those composed of two NRTIs together with either a NNRTI or a PI (DHHS Panel on Antiretroviral Guidelines for Adults and Adolescents 2006b). Although HAART is not a cure, it has dramatically improved rates of mortality and morbidity, improved quality of life, revitalized communities and transformed perceptions of AIDS from a plague to a manageable, chronic illness.

Several international HIV treatment guidelines exist to guide clinicians in the management of HIV-infected individuals and are based on a combination of evidence from randomized clinical trials, observational cohorts and expert opinion.

Since the advent of HAART in 1996, most guidelines have evolved to keep up with new evidence. For example, the United States Department of Health and Human Services (US DHHS) guidelines initially advocated a more aggressive therapy but have subsequently moved towards a more conservative approach. The 2006 DHHS guidelines (DHHS Panel on Antiretroviral Guidelines for Adults and Adolescents 2006b) recommend initiation of treatment in all asymptomatic patients with <200 CD4+ cells/ml and allowing clinical judgement to be exercised at earlier stages of disease.

The WHO recommendations for expanded access in low- and middle-income countries (WHO 2004) take into account the lack of medical and laboratory infrastructure in many countries that have a high AIDS burden. The WHO guidelines emphasize treatment of patients with significant symptomatic disease and those with CD4+ cell count < 200 cells/ml. A substitute for the CD4+ cell count criterion in resource-constrained settings where a CD4+ cell count is not available is a total lymphocyte count <1200 cell/ml. All of the guidelines emphasize initiation of ART for symptomatic patients with HIV-related symptoms (WHO stages 3 & 4), while the decision to initiate treatment of asymptomatic patients is more complex and is based on the patient's readiness to adhere to long-term therapy, together with an assessment of the level of existing immunodeficiency, the risk of disease progression and the risks and costs of therapy. In resource-constrained settings, the threshold for entry into an ART programmatic will also need to take cognizance of the resultant numbers to be treated, available financial and medical infrastructure and the resources necessary to identify treatment beneficiaries.

The dynamics of HIV in paediatric patients is distinct from that of adults. Most children infected with HIV have contracted the disease through vertical transmission from their mothers. The mean survival of vertically HIV infected children ranges from 75–90 months and only a fraction of the HIV-infected children survive to around 10 years of age without ART. In countries where it has been successfully introduced, ART has substantially changed the face of HIV infection in children, with many HIV-infected infants and children now surviving to adolescence and adulthood. Guidelines for treatment of HIV-infected children are also continually evolving. The decision to start therapy and what drugs to choose for children is complex (DHHS Panel on Antiretroviral Guidelines for Adults and Adolescents 2006a). While HIV-infected children suffering from impaired growth and development may benefit from earlier initiation of HAART, the criteria for treatment initiation is based on CD4+ percentage, viral load and clinical condition.

Prophylaxis and treatment of co-morbidities

The best way to prevent opportunistic infections is to prevent exposure to the infectious agent. However, this is not possible for all opportunistic infections because several are thought to be caused by a reactivation of latent infection, e.g. tuberculosis, herpes simplex virus, cytomegalovirus, and toxoplasmosis.

Improvement in immune function following the initiation of HAART can significantly lessen the morbidity of opportunistic infections. Furthermore, the incidence of a number of opportunistic infections and associated mortality can also be reduced through the use of prophylactic agents like cotrimoxazole.

Specifically targeted interventions like preventive therapy for tuberculosis in high-risk patients, chemoprophylaxis for malaria for HIV infected pregnant women in malaria endemic areas, and vaccinations against pneumococcal infections and influenza in HIV infected adults can be used to lessen the morbidity and mortality from opportunistic infections. Although not generally regarded as an opportunistic infection, vaccinations against hepatitis B should be considered in selected patients who are shown to be non-immune because of the effect that HIV has on the natural history of hepatitis B (Maartens 2005).

Challenges in ART provision

Since 2000, the collective efforts of activists, researchers, service providers, pharmaceutical companies, policy makers, and international agencies have generated real momentum in scaling up AIDS treatment and prevention across the globe, particularly in low- and middle-income countries. Coverage of ART in the developing world has more than doubled—increasing from 400 000 in 2003 to approximately 1 million by June 2005 (WHO 2006). While still short of the WHO goal of '3 by 5', the momentum in expanding treatment access is a remarkable achievement despite the initial challenges in implementing AIDS treatment programmes, especially in Africa where the burden is largest. The scale of ART provision was guided by what WHO refers to as the 'Public health approach to AIDS treatment'. This involved standardizing first and second line ART regimens, creating algorithms for determining who was eligible for ART, and how to manage patients on ART. This standardization enabled healthcare workers who are not physicians to become involved in AIDS care. Indeed, in much of Africa, nurse practitioners or intermediate-level clinicians are the main providers of ART. However, many challenges with respect to the scale up and sustained provision of treatment remain. These include constraints in scaling up VCT, stigma and discrimination, challenges in achieving high levels of treatment adherence, and side effects and toxicity such as hyperlipidaemia, insulin resistance, frank diabetes mellitus, acute life-threatening lactic acidosis, asymptomatic lactic acidaemia, chronic myopathy, peripheral neuropathy, and gastrointestinal intolerance.

While these challenges are being resolved, new challenges are emerging in scaling up the treatment and sustaining the ART provision in resource-constrained settings. While the various practical and political challenges in ART provision have changed since 2000, three over-arching challenges—under-developed, overburdened healthcare services, the persistence of stigma, and the failure to integrate prevention into care–continue to hamper the effort to maximize the benefits of ART implementation (Abdool Karim 2006b).

Impact of AIDS

Impact of AIDS on mortality

Globally, AIDS has joined the leading causes of premature death among both women and men 15–59 years of age (Piot 2006). In the worst affected countries like South Africa, AIDS is the single largest contributor to premature loss of life and accounts for about half of the disability adjusted life years lost. In Africa, one important feature of AIDS related mortality is its age and gender frequency distribution. While the overall AIDS related mortality rates are highest in the 20–40-year age group, women experience higher AIDS mortality rates at younger ages in Africa.

The introduction of ART has helped slow the rising mortality due to AIDS. In high-income countries the introduction of HAART

led to significant declines in AIDS mortality rates (Palella *et al.* 1998; Detels *et al.* 1998) (See http://www.cdc.gov/hiv/topics/surveillance/resources/slides/trends/index.htm). Unfortunately, this trend has not yet become evident in most poor countries, where mortality rates due to AIDS continue to climb. However, as ART becomes more widely available in poor countries, it is hoped that mortality will start to fall.

Impact of AIDS on society

The social impact of AIDS is more pronounced in generalized epidemics and in settings where heterosexual transmission is dominant. For example, the AIDS epidemic in sub-Saharan Africa has had widespread impact on many sectors of society, impacting beyond the individual, to the family structure and society at large. High death rates in the socially and economically most active sectors of society are impacting dramatically on economic activity, financial wellbeing and social progress. Indeed, AIDS has become the biggest threat to the continent's development for the current generation of young adults as well as the next generation. UNAIDS estimates that AIDS is reducing the per capita growth rate by 0.5–1.2 per cent annually in sub-Saharan Africa. Life expectancy has halved in some countries and millions of adults are dying in their economically productive years, thereby impacting on the economic dependency ratio. Many families are losing their income earners and the families of those who die have to find money to pay for their funerals.

As the epidemic progresses, social cohesion in already fragile communities is being further eroded. An increasing number of households are either grandmother or child-headed. Children who are orphaned struggle to survive without parental care and frequently cease attending school because they cannot afford school fees and uniforms or have to look after younger siblings (Johnson 2001). A decline in school enrolment is one of the most visible effects of the HIV/AIDS epidemic on education in Africa.

Private industry and companies of all types face higher costs of training, insurance, benefits, absenteeism and illness. A number of skilled personnel in important areas of public management and core social services are being lost to AIDS. Essential services are being depleted and scarce resources are put under greater strain. As the epidemic matures, the health sector suffers the additional pressures of caring for those with AIDS. Not only has health utilization increased, but other illnesses that deserve attention (such as diabetes, malaria, hypertension, etc.) are being crowded out by the increasing morbidity that AIDS brings.

The worst of the epidemic impact has yet to come. In the absence of massively expanded prevention, treatment and care efforts, the AIDS death toll on the continent of Africa is expected to continue rising before peaking around the end of this decade.

Ethical and human rights issues

Human rights challenges in AIDS treatment provision

The continued spread of HIV globally and the immense and growing burden of AIDS places a moral, scientific and ethical imperative on individuals and societies to mobilize political will and resources to respond to the pandemic. This imperative extends to the urgent need to conduct research to find new ways of preventing and treating AIDS. The immediacy of the challenge and need for solutions has redefined the way medical practitioners, governments, and health service providers, amongst others, respond to an infectious disease and the way in which researchers conduct research and clinical trials.

During the early days of the epidemic, AIDS was identified with already socially and/or legally marginalized or stigmatized groups, such as men who have sex with men, injecting drug users, racial minorities, and sex workers. The uncertainty of the cause of the new disease and how it is spread created conflict between human rights activists and public health practitioners. Classical infectious diseases approaches of 'isolate and contain', as practised in the sanitoria of Cuba, the closure of bath-houses in San Francisco, and restrictions on entry of HIV infected persons to the United States were at odds with the ongoing campaigns in the gay community to secure their rights. As knowledge of natural history of infection grew, levels of social stigma and discrimination did not diminish but an uneasy balance was struck between respect of the right of the infected person and public good. A phrase coined by Bayer (Bayer & Fairchild 2006), 'HIV exceptionalism', captures the outcome of this balance between the rights of those infected with broader rights of society to be protected from an incurable infectious disease.

In the pre-HAART era, the manifestation of protection of the rights of the individual infected person was most apparent in HIV testing policies. All HIV testing had to be voluntary, client-initiated, and done in the context of pre- and post-test counselling by a trained person. In contrast to management of other health conditions where the clinician made decisions about what diagnostic tests are undertaken, HIV set new standards of patient autonomy to make this decision in an informed manner. Furthermore, disclosure was the prerogative of the infected person. Several precedent-setting judgements in the courts of law reinforced this right in several countries (Jonsen 1990; Kirp 1989; Kirp & Bayer 1992). Prohibitions on pre-employment HIV testing in the workplace are another of the human rights achievements in response to workplace-based discriminatory policies against those with AIDS.

Research showing the substantial benefit of AZT in reducing mother-to-child transmission of HIV re-opened some of the early HIV testing debates in industrialized countries, focusing now on whether HIV testing should be compulsory for all pregnant women in light of potential benefit to the unborn baby. These debates were echoed in poor countries as single-dose nevirapine became available for prevention of mother-to-child transmission of HIV. Despite the high HIV prevalence in pre-natal settings, many women choose not to test because of real or perceived fear of testing positive, fear emanating from the social consequences of having HIV infection. The status of women in these settings, as well as fear of violence and discrimination, impact a number of decisions infected mothers make—whether to have an HIV test, take their intra-partum dose of medication, ensure their babies receive nevirapine, or breastfeed their babies.

The introduction of HAART in industrialized countries in the late 1990s highlighted the economic disparities between north and south. Global activism, spurred on by social movements of people living with AIDS, community groups, professional organizations and advocacy groups, resulted in major reductions in drug prices. Importantly, it also led to the establishment of International Assistance Funds to help countries provide these life-saving drugs; the Global Fund against AIDS, Tuberculosis and Malaria and the US President's Emergency Plan for AIDS Relief (PEPfAR).

These initiatives have set important precedents for how the global community responds to public health crises. Other long-standing public health challenges are benefiting, such as maternal and child health, reproductive health services, tuberculosis and malaria. Importantly, these funds are supporting efforts to increase access to ART, expand training of healthcare workers, strengthen healthcare services, and build new facilities including laboratory infrastructure and drug distribution systems in resource-constrained settings. While these efforts cannot undo the historical inequities between north and south, they demonstrate the importance of global commitment and joint action.

Ethical challenges in AIDS research

The disparities between north and south in the context of HIV prevention trials have led to substantial debate on research ethics. In the mid-1990s, a prominent medical journal questioned the ethics of conducting placebo-controlled trials for the prevention of MTCT in Africa and Thailand. The argument was that PACTG 076 regimen of AZT, which has been shown to be effective in reducing MTCT in the United States, should be the control intervention in all subsequent MTCT trials. The counter-arguments were that the PATCG 076 regimen of AZT was not implementable in resource-constrained settings and hence the need to assess the efficacy of short implementable courses of antiretrovirals against the existing standard of care in the countries hosting the trials. The centrepiece of these debates is whether placebo-controlled trials were justifiable when an intervention exists regardless of whether the intervention was not affordable or feasible in the host country, as was the case with the AZT regimen emanating from the PACTG 076 trial. A certain level of paternalism dominated these debates—issues of exploitation, duties of sponsors, and questions about the voluntariness of the informed consent process in poor and low-literate populations. This debate led to the revision of several international ethical guidelines to clarify when placebo controlled trials are ethically justifiable.

New standards in HIV prevention and treatment research have emerged that pay particular attention to community engagement and participation through formalized structures such as Community Advisory Boards; assessments of comprehension of the informed consent process prior to enrolling volunteers into trials; upfront provision for post-trial access and provision of ancillary care. In contrast to non-HIV research, additional responsibilities are placed on HIV researchers to provide therapies unrelated to the study interventions, e.g. provision of HAART for HIV vaccine trial participants who become infected. In some instances, the pendulum has swung too far across and researchers have become over-protectionist and risk averse in the conduct of HIV prevention research in these settings.

Conclusion

The last 25 years has seen the emergence of a completely new pathogen and its devastating consequences. The magnitude of the global HIV epidemic also spurred the scientific community to develop several interventions that are proven to prevent HIV infection and over 25 new drugs that are effective in treating AIDS. For each of the three main modes of HIV transmission, there are effective strategies to prevent HIV infection using existing technologies (like circumcision and male condoms) or new technologies like antiretrovirals to prevent MTCT, female condoms, and new HIV tests to protect the blood supply. The challenge has been to implement these interventions to scale given the historical under-development of public health systems in the countries worst affected by AIDS.

While medical research has made enormous strides in the prevention of MTCT and bloodborne spread, changing sexual behaviour to reduce HIV risk has proved more challenging. However, there are notable exceptions. Thailand reversed its HIV epidemic through its 100 per cent condom programme in brothels, and Uganda has been able to alter the course of its epidemic through political will for programmes that reduced high-risk behaviours. Vaccines have been key to infectious disease control and, in some instances, eradication. Developing an HIV vaccine has proven to be elusive, due mainly to the absence of identifiable natural immunity against HIV infection in humans. The enormity of this vaccine development challenge led to the creation of the AIDS vaccine enterprise, which is a global collaboration amongst scientists to work towards the common goal of a safe and effective AIDS vaccine.

AIDS has redefined the way in which doctors relate to their patients, the way in which research is conducted and the way in which activism has forced redress in global inequities to life-saving medical care. The experiences of the AIDS epidemic over almost three decades has illustrated that AIDS is more than a medical problem; it is also a social and development problem with profound consequences on the very fabric of society. It is impacting on security, social cohesion, and economic growth, and is even reversing some of the health gains of the last century.

References

Abdool Karim Q. and Abdool Karim S.S. (1999). Epidemiology of HIV infection in South Africa. *AIDS*, **13**, S4-S7.

Abdool Karim S.S. (2006a). The African Experience. In Mayer K. and Pizer H.F., ed. *The AIDS Pandemic: Impact on science and society*, pp. 351–73. Elsevier Academic Press, San Diego, California.

Abdool Karim S.S. (2006b). Durban 2000 to Toronto 2006: The evolving challenges in implementing AIDS treatment in Africa. *AIDS*, **20**, N7–N9.

Abdool Karim S.S., Abdool Karim Q., Gouws E. *et al.* (2007). Global Epidemiology of HIV. *Infectious Disease Clinics of North America*, **21**, 1–18.

Ahmed S.T., Lutalo T., Wawer M. *et al.* (2001). HIV incidence and sexually transmitted disease prevalence associated with condom use: a population study in Rakai, Uganda. *AIDS*, **15**, 2171–9.

Auvert B., Taljaard, D., Lagarde E. *et al.* (2005). Randomized, controlled intervention trial of male circumcision for reduction of HIV infection risk: the ANRS 1265 Trial. *PLoS Med*, **2**, e298.

Baggaley R.F., Boily M.C., White R.G. *et al.* (2006). Risk of HIV-1 transmission for parenteral exposure and blood transfusion: a systematic review and meta-analysis. *AIDS*, **20**, 805–12.

Bailey R.C., Moses S., Parker C.B. *et al.* (2007). Male circumcision for HIV prevention in young men in Kisumu, Kenya: a randomised controlled trial. *Lancet*, **369**, 643–56.

Bayer R. and Fairchild A.L. (2006). Changing the Paradigm for HIV Testing—The End of Exceptionalism. *N Engl J Med*, **355**, 647–9.

Berger A., Scherzed L., Sturmer M. *et al.* (2005). Comparative evaluation of the Cobas Amplicor HIV-1 Monitor Ultrasensitive Test, the new Cobas AmpliPrep/Cobas Amplicor HIV-1 Monitor Ultrasensitive Test and the Versant HIV RNA 3.0 assays for quantitation of HIV-1 RNA in plasma samples. *J Clin Virol*, **33**, 43–51.

Bertrand J.T., O'Reilly K., Denison J. *et al.* (2006). Systematic review of the effectiveness of mass communication programs to change HIV/AIDS-related behaviors in developing countries. *Health Educ Res*, **21**, 567–97.

Burger S. and Poles M.A. (2003). Natural history and pathogenesis of human immunodeficiency virus infection. *Semin Liver Dis*, **23**, 115–24.

Cardo D.M., Culver D.H., Ciesielski C.A. *et al.* (1997). A case-control study of HIV seroconversion in health care workers after percutaneous exposure. Centers for Disease Control and Prevention Needlestick Surveillance Group. *N Engl J Med*, **337**, 1485–90.

Clerici M., Giorgi J.V., Chou C.C. *et al.* (1992). Cell-mediated immune response to human immunodeficiency virus (HIV) type 1 in seronegative homosexual men with recent sexual exposure to HIV-1. *J Infect Dis*, **165**, 1012–9.

Colvin M., Abdool Karim S.S., Connolly C. *et al.* (1998). HIV infection and asymptomatic sexually transmitted infections in a rural South African community. *Int J STD & AIDS*, **9**, 548–50.

Coovadia H.M., Rollins N.C., Bland R.M. *et al.* (2007). Mother-to-child transmission of HIV-1 infection during exclusive breastfeeding in the first 6 months of life: an intervention cohort study. *Lancet*, **369**, 1107–16.

Coutsoudis A., Dabis F., Fawzi W. *et al.* (2004). Late postnatal transmission of HIV-1 in breast-fed children: an individual patient data meta-analysis. *J Infect Dis*, **189**, 2154–66.

Crepaz N., Lyles C.M., Wolitski R.J. *et al.* (2006). Do prevention interventions reduce HIV risk behaviours among people living with HIV? A meta-analytic review of controlled trials. *AIDS*, **20**, 143–57.

De Cock K.M. and Johnson A.M. (1998). From exceptionalism to normalisation: a reappraisal of attitudes and practice around HIV testing. *BMJ*, **316**(7127), 290–3.

Dean M., Carrington M., Winkler C. *et al.* (1996). Genetic restriction of HIV-1 infection and progression to AIDS by a deletion allele of the CKR5 structural gene. Hemophilia Growth and Development Study, Multicenter AIDS Cohort Study, Multicenter Hemophilia Cohort Study, San Francisco City Cohort, ALIVE Study. *Science*, **273**, 1856–62.

Department of Health. (2007). HIV and AIDs and STI Strategic Plan for South Africa, 2007-2011. Department of Health, Pretoria. Available online at http://www.doh.gov.za/docs/misc/stratplan-f.html Accessed 30 January 2008.

Des Jarlais D.C., Hagan H., Friedman S.R. *et al.* (1995). Maintaining low HIV seroprevalence in populations of injecting drug users. *JAMA*, **274**, 1226–31.

Des Jarlais D.C., Marmor M., Paone D. *et al.* (1996). HIV incidence among injecting drug users in New York City syringe-exchange programmes. *Lancet*, **348**(9033), 987–91.

Detels R., Liu Z., Carrington M. *et al.* (1994). Resistance to HIV-1 infection. Multicenter AIDS Cohort Study. *Journal of Acquired Immune Deficiency Syndrome*, **7**, 1263–9.

Detels R., Mann D., Carrington M. *et al.* (1996). Persistently seronegative men from whom HIV-1 has been isolated are genetically and immunologically distinct. *Immunol Lett*, **51**, 29–33.

Detels R., Munoz A., McFarlane G. *et al.* (1998). Effectiveness of potent antiretroviral therapy on time to AIDS and death in men with known HIV infection duration. Multicenter AIDS Cohort Study Investigators. *JAMA*, **280**, 1497–503.

DHHS Panel on Antiretroviral Guidelines for Adults and Adolescents (2006). *Guidelines for the Use of Antiretroviral Agents in HIV-1-Infected Adults and Adolescents*. Available online at http://aidsinfo.nih.gov/ Accessed (8 March 2007), Office of AIDS Research Advisory Council (OARAC), National Institutes of Health.

DHHS Panel on Antiretroviral Guidelines for Adults and Adolescents (2006). *Guidelines for the Use of Antiretroviral Agents in Pediatric HIV Infection*. Available online at http://aidsinfo.nih.gov/ Accessed (8 March 2007), Office of AIDS Research Advisory Council (OARAC), National Institutes of Health.

Dobbs T., Kennedy S., Pau C.P. *et al.* (2004). Performance characteristics of the immunoglobulin G-capture BED-enzyme immunoassay, an assay to detect recent human immunodeficiency virus type 1 seroconversion. *J Clin Microbiol*, **42**, 2623–8.

Eke A.N., Mezoff J.S., Duncan T. *et al.* (2006). Reputationally strong HIV prevention programs: lessons from the front line. *AIDS Educ Prev*, **18**, 163–75.

Fylkesnes K., Haworth, A., Rosenvard, C. *et al.* (1999) HIV counseling and testing: overemphasizing high acceptance rates threat to confidentiality and the right not to know. *AIDS*, **13**:2469–74

Gallo R.C. (2002). Historical essay. The early years of HIV/AIDS. *Science*, **298**,1728–30.

Gallo R.C. and Montagnier L. (2003). The discovery of HIV as the cause of AIDS. *N Engl J Med*, **349**, 2283–5.

Garber D.A., Silvestri G. and Feinberg M.B. (2004). Prospects for an AIDS vaccine: three big questions, no easy answers. *Lancet Infect Dis*, **4**, 397–413.

Global HIV Prevention Working Group (2006). New approaches to HIV prevention—accelerating research and ensuring future access. Available from www.gatesfoundation.org and www.kff.org Accessed 18 January 2008.

Gottlieb M.S., Schroff R., Schanker H.M. *et al.* (1981). Pneumocystis carinii pneumonia and mucosal candidiasis in previously healthy homosexual men: evidence of a new acquired cellular immunodeficiency. *N Engl J Med*, **305**, 1425–31.

Gouws E., White P.J. Stover J. *et al.* (2006). Short term estimates of adult HIV incidence by mode of transmission: Kenya and Thailand as examples. *Sex Transm Infect*, **82**(Suppl 3), iii51–55.

Gray R.H., Kigozi G., Serwadda D. *et al.* (2007). Male circumcision for HIV prevention in men in Rakai, Uganda: a randomised trial. *Lancet*, **369**, 657–66.

Hallett T.B., Aberle-Grasse J., Bello G. *et al.* (2006). Declines in HIV prevalence can be associated with changing sexual behaviour in Uganda, urban Kenya, Zimbabwe, and urban Haiti. *Sex Transm Infect*, **82**(Suppl 1), i1–8.

Hemelaar J., Gouws E., Ghys P.D. *et al.* (2006). Global and regional distribution of HIV-1 genetic subtypes and recombinants in 2004. *AIDS*, **20**, W13–23.

Heyns A. and Swanevelder J.P. (2005). Safe Blood Services. In Abdool Karim SS and Abdool Karim Q, ed. *HIV/AIDS in South Africa*. pp. 203–16. Cambridge University Press, Cape Town.

Ho D.D. and Huang Y. (2002). The HIV-1 vaccine race. *Cell*, **110**, 135–8.

Hurley S.F., Jolley D.J. and Kaldor J.M. (1997). Effectiveness of needle-exchange programmes for prevention of HIV infection. *Lancet*, **349**, 1797–800.

Jaffar S., Grant A.D., Whitworth J., Smith P.G. and Whittle H. (2004). The natural history of HIV-1 and HIV-2 infections in adults in Africa: a literature review. *Bull World Health Organ*, **82**, 462–9.

Jana S., Basu I., Rotheram-Borus M.J. *et al.* (2004). The Sonagachi Project: a sustainable community intervention program. *AIDS Educ Prev*, **16**, 405–14.

Janssen R.S., Satten G.A., Stramer S.L. *et al.* (1998). New testing strategy to detect early HIV-1 infection for use in incidence estimates and for clinical and prevention purposes. *JAMA*, **280**, 42–8.

Johnson L. and Dorrington R. (2001). The Impact of AIDS on orphanhood in South Africa: A Quantitative Analysis: Monograph No.4. University of Cape Town: Centre for Actuarial Research.

Jonsen A.R. (1990). The Duty to Treat Patients with AIDS and HIV Infection. In Gostin LO ed. *AIDS and the Health care System*, pp. 155–68, 270–1. Yale University Press, New Haven.

Kayirangwa E., Hanson J., Munyakazi L. *et al.* (2006). Current trends in Rwanda's HIV/AIDS epidemic. *Sex Transm Infect*, **82**(Suppl 1), 127–31.

Kirp D.L. (1989). *Learning by Heart: AIDS and Schoolchildren in America's Communities*. Rutgers University Press, New Brunswick, New Jersey.

Kirp D.L. and Bayer R. (1992). *AIDS in the Industrialized Democracies. American Civil Liberties Union Epidemic of Fear: A Survey of AIDS Discrimination in the 1980s and Policy Recommendations for the 1990s (ACLU AIDS Project,1990) for other economically advanced democracies.* Rutgers University Press, New Brunswick New Jersey.

Liu A.Y., Grant R.M. and Buchbinder S.P. (2006). Preexposure prophylaxis for HIV: unproven promise and potential pitfalls. *JAMA*, **296**, 863–5.

Maartens G. (2005). Prevention of opportunistic infections in adults. In Abdool Karim SS and Abdool Karim Q (eds.) *HIV/AIDS in South Africa*, pp. 454–462 Cambridge University Press, Cape Town.

Mawar N., Saha S., Pandit A. *et al.* (2005). The third phase of HIV pandemic: social consequences of HIV/AIDS stigma & discrimination & future needs. *Indian J Med Res*, **122**, 471–84.

McCutchan F.E. (2006). Global epidemiology of HIV. *J Med Virol*, **78** (Suppl 1), S7-S12.

Moore J.P. and Doms R.W. (2003). The entry of entry inhibitors: a fusion of science and medicine. *Proc Natl Acad Sci USA*, **100**, 10598–602.

Morris L. and Cilliers T. (2005). Chapter 5: Viral structure, replication, tropism, pathogenesis and natural history. In Abdool Karim SS and Abdool Karim Q. *HIV/AIDS in South Africa*. pp 79–88. Cambridge University Press, Cape Town.

Morris M. and Kretzschmar M. (1997). Concurrent partnerships and the spread of HIV. *AIDS*, **11**, 641–8.

Myer L., Mathews C., Little F. (2001). Condom gap in Africa is wider than study suggests. *BMJ*, **323**, 937.

NACO (2006). HIV/AIDS epidemiological Surveillance & Estimation report for the year 2005. Delhi, National AIDS Control Organization, Ministry of Health & Family welfare, Government of India (Available at www. nacoonline.org Last accessed 22 January 2008).

Needle R.H., Coyle S.L., Normand J. *et al.* (1998). HIV prevention with drug-using populations - current status and future prospects: introduction and overview. *Public Health Reports*, **113**(Supp 1), 4–18.

Palella F.J., Delaney K.M., Moorman A.C. *et al.* (1998). Declining morbidity and mortality among patients with advanced human immunodeficiency virus infection. *N Engl J Med*, **338**, 853–60.

Panlilio A.L., Cardo D.M., Grohskopf L.A. *et al.* (2005). Updated U.S. Public Health Service guidelines for the management of occupational exposures to HIV and recommendations for postexposure prophylaxis. *MMWR Recomm Rep*, **54**(RR-9), 1–17.

Parekh B.S. and McDougal J.S. (2005). Application of laboratory methods for estimation of HIV-1 incidence. *Indian Journal for Medical Research*, **121**, 510–518.

Peterson L., Taylor D., Roddy R. *et al.* (2007). Tenofovir disoproxil fumarate for prevention of HIV infection in women: a phase 2, double-blind, randomized, placebo-controlled trial. *PLoS Clin Trials* **2**, e27.

Pettifor A.E., Rees H.V., Kleinschmidt I. *et al.* (2005). Young people's sexual health in South Africa: HIV prevalence and sexual behaviors from a nationally representative household survey. *AIDS*, **19**, 1525–34.

Piot P. (2006). AIDS: from crisis management to sustained strategic response. *Lancet*, **368**, 526–30.

Quinn T.C., Wawer M.J., Sewankambo N. *et al.* (2000). Viral load and heterosexual transmission of human immunodeficiency virus type 1. *N Engl J Med*, **342**, 921–9.

Roland M.E., Neilands T.B., Krone M.R. *et al.* (2005). Seroconversion following nonoccupational postexposure prophylaxis against HIV. *Clin Infect Dis*, **41**, 1507–13.

Shafer L.A., Biraro S., Kamali A. *et al.* (2006). *HIV prevalence and incidence are no longer falling in Uganda—a case for renewed prevention efforts: evidence from a rural population cohort 1989–2005, and from ANC surveillance [Abstract: THLB0108]*. XVI International AIDS Conference, Toronto, Canada.

Shelton J.D. and Johnson B. (2001). Condom gap in Africa: evidence from donor agencies and key informants. *BMJ*, **323**, 139.

Sheppard H.W. (2005). Inactivated- or killed-virus HIV/AIDS vaccines. *Curr Drug Targets Infect Disord*, **5**, 131–41.

Shisana O., Rehle T., Simbayi L.C. *et al.* (2005). South African National HIV prevalence, HIV incidence, behaviour and communication survey. Cape Town, Human Sciences Research Council Press.

Simon V. and Ho D.D. (2003). HIV-1 dynamics in vivo: implications for therapy. *Nat Rev Microbiol*, **1**, 181–90.

Smith R.A., Loeb L.A. and Preston B.D. (2005). Lethal mutagenesis of HIV. *Virus Res*, **107**, 215–28.

Spacek L.A., Shihab H.M., Lutwama F. *et al.* (2006). Evaluation of a low-cost method, the Guava Easy CD4 assay, to enumerate CD4-positive lymphocyte counts in HIV-infected patients in the United States and Uganda. *J Acquir Immune Defic Syndr*, **41**, 607–10.

Stone A. (2002). Microbicides: a new approach to preventing HIV and other sexually transmitted infections. *Nature Reviews*, **1**, 977–85.

Sweat M., Gregorich S., Sangiwa G., Furlonge C., Balmer D., Kamenga C. *et al.* (2000). Cost-effectiveness of voluntary HIV-1 counselling and testing in reducing sexual transmission of HIV-1 IN Kenya and Tanzania. *Lancet*, **356**, 113–21.

The Voluntary HIV-1 counseling and testing efficacy study group (2000). Efficacy of voluntary HIV-1 counseling and testing in individuals and couples in Kenya, Tanzania, and Trinidad: a randomised trial. *Lancet*, **356**, 103–12.

UNAIDS (2002). *Report on the global HIV/AIDS*. Geneva, Switzerland, UNAIDS.

UNAIDS (2003). *AIDS epidemic update December 2003*. Geneva, UNAIDS and WHO.

UNAIDS (2004). Chapter 1: The World Drug Problem: a status report. In UNAIDS *World Drug Report includes latest trends, analysis and statistics*, pp. 47–51. United Nations Office on Drugs and Crime (UNODC), Geneva, Switzerland.

UNAIDS (2005). *Evidence for HIV decline in Zimbabwe: a comprehensive review of the epidemiological data*. Joint United Nations Programme on HIV/AIDS. Geneva, Switzerland.

UNAIDS (2006). *2006 Report of the global AIDS epidemic*. Joint United Nations Programme on HIV/AIDS (Available at www.unaids.org). Geneva, Switzerland.

UNAIDS (2007). *2007 AIDS Epidemic Update*. http://data.unaids.org/pub/ EpiSlides/2007/2007 EpiUpdate_en.pdf (Accessed 27 November 2007). Joint United Nations Programme on HIV/AIDS. Geneva, Switzerland.

Vernazza P.L., Eron J.J., Fiscus S.A. *et al.* (1999). Sexual transmission of HIV: infectiousness and prevention. *AIDS*, **13**, 155–66.

Vlahov D. and Junge B. (1998). The role of needle exchange programs in HIV prevention. *Public Health Rep*, **113**(Suppl 1), 75–80.

Weiser S.D., Heisler M., Leiter K. *et al.* (2006). Routine HIV Testing in Botswana: A Population-Based Study on Attitudes, Practices, and Human Rights Concerns. *PLoS Med*, **3**, e261.

Weiss R.A. (2001). Gulliver's travels in HIVland. *Nature*, **410**, 963–7.

World Health Organization (WHO) (2001). Global Prevalence and incidence of selected curable sexually transmitted infections. Overview and estimates, World Health Organisation, Geneva, Switzerland.

WHO (2006). Progress on Global Access to HIV Antiretroviral Therapy: A report on 3 by 5 and Beyond. Geneva, World Health Organisation and United Nations Programme on HIV/AIDS.

WHO (2004). Scaling up antiretroviral therapy in resource-limited settings: Treatment guidelines for a public health approach. A revision. World Health Organisation, Geneva, Switzerland.

WHO (2005). The safety of immunization practices improves over last five years, but challenges remain. World health Organisation, Geneva, Switzerland.

WHO (2005). World alliance for patient safety: Global patient safety challenge, World Health Organisation, Geneva, Switzerland.

WHO (2005). Global tuberculosis control: surveillance, planning, financing. Geneva, Switzerland, World Health Organisation, Geneva, Switzerland.

Wu Z., Detels R., Zhang J., Li V. *et al.* (2002). Community-based trial to prevent drug use among youths in Yunnan, China. *Am J Public Health*, **92**, 1952–7.

Tuberculosis

Dermot Maher, Marcos Espinal, and Mario Raviglione

Abstract

We begin the chapter by describing the natural history of *Mycobacterium tuberculosis* infection. This underpins our understanding of tuberculosis epidemiology and the principles of tuberculosis control, for which the main stratagems are then briefly discussed. We continue with an historical account of the global tuberculosis epidemic as the necessary background to a description of the current burden of tuberculosis and recent trends. A brief account of tuberculosis control in the era of anti-tuberculosis chemotherapy serves as the backdrop to the development and implementation of the World Health Organization (WHO) strategy for tuberculosis control known as DOTS (a brand name derived from Directly Observed Treatment, Short-Course) and its adaptations. The next section reviews the basic principles in tuberculosis care which underpin the public health approach to tuberculosis control. We provide an assessment of the progress made towards the international targets for tuberculosis control for 2005, and then outline recent events in the evolving international response to the challenge of tuberculosis, including the development of the Stop TB Strategy and the Global Plan to implement it. We conclude with an assessment of the prospects for tuberculosis control in the future, looking forward to 2015 (the target year for the United Nations' Millennium Development Goals) and then beyond to 2050 (the target year for the elimination of tuberculosis as a global public health problem).

Introduction

Tuberculosis still represents a threat and a challenge to humanity today as it has done throughout history. There were an estimated 1.6 million tuberculosis deaths and 8.8 million new tuberculosis cases worldwide in 2005 (WHO 2007a), of which about 1 million cases (11 per cent) occur in children aged less than 15 years. Low- and middle-income countries suffer the brunt of the tuberculosis epidemic. Overall, it is estimated that 95 per cent of the world's tuberculosis cases and 98 per cent of the tuberculosis deaths occur in the developing world (Raviglione *et al.* 1995). Tuberculosis was the third leading cause of death (after HIV/AIDS and ischaemic heart disease) in adults aged 15–59 years in low- and middle-income countries in 2001 (Lopez *et al.* 2006).

The paradox is that tuberculosis continues to pose a great threat at a time when we are potentially well equipped to respond to the challenge. The explanation to the paradox lies in collective neglect. We have not yet dedicated enough effort and resources firstly, in technological innovation to replace the current generally old technologies for tuberculosis prevention and control; and secondly, in public health practice to ensure worldwide equitable access to the benefits of our understanding of the disease and of the means to control it.

The natural history of tuberculosis

In the practice of public health regarding tuberculosis prevention and control, the natural history of *M. tuberculosis* infection and tuberculosis disease underpins our understanding of tuberculosis epidemiology and the principles of tuberculosis control. A description of the contagious nature of pulmonary tuberculosis dates back to the tenth-century book *Qanun fi'l-Tibb* (The Canon of Medicine) by Avicenna (also known as Ibn Sina) (http://www.ummah.net/history/scholars/ibn_sina). Koch confirmed Avicenna's description 900 years later, by identifying the tubercle bacillus and its causative role in tuberculosis. Bacelli observed in 1882 that the tubercle bacillus is a necessary, but not a sufficient, cause of tuberculosis: '*Il bacillo non é ancora tutta la tuberculosi*' (The bacillus is not yet all there is to tuberculosis.) (quoted by Bloom 1994). Tuberculosis can only occur following infection with *M. tuberculosis*, but occurs in a small minority of those infected. The risk of *M. tuberculosis* infection is largely exogenous in nature, determined by the characteristics of the source case, environment and duration of exposure. In contrast, the risk of tuberculosis following *M. tuberculosis* infection is largely endogenous, determined mainly by the individual's immune status. Although tubercle bacilli may vary in virulence, the influence of the genetic diversity of the infecting organisms on the course of infection is not very well understood. The natural history of tuberculosis comprises the sequence of events following exposure to an infectious case: Transmission of *M. tuberculosis* infection, the process of becoming infected, the development of tuberculosis as one of the consequences of infection, and the completion of the disease cycle by transmission of *M. tuberculosis* by new or recurrent infectious cases.

Exposure to infection with *M. tuberculosis* and transmission of infection

The transmission of *M. tuberculosis* is almost exclusively airborne. The patient with pulmonary tuberculosis who is coughing (or talking, sneezing, spitting, or singing) produces droplets that may contain tubercle bacilli (Loudon & Roberts 1966). As the droplets expelled into the air evaporate, some form droplet nuclei (i.e. infectious particles of respiratory secretions usually less than 5 µm in diameter containing one or a few tubercle bacilli). A single cough can produce 3000 droplet nuclei which can remain suspended in the air for several hours. Whereas larger particles either fall to the ground or, if inhaled, are trapped either in the nose or in the mucociliary system of the tracheobronchial tree, droplet nuclei are so small that they avoid the defences of the bronchi and penetrate into the terminal alveoli of the lungs where infection begins. The particles containing tubercle bacilli on the clothing, bed-covers, or belongings of a tuberculosis patient cannot be dispersed in aerosols, so do not play a significant part in transmission of infection.

Those people with respiratory tract tuberculosis who produce the most tubercle bacilli are the most infectious. The number of tubercle bacilli found in sputum specimens reflects infectiousness (Frieden 2004). The most potent sources of infection are patients with sputum smear-positive pulmonary tuberculosis. This was demonstrated by the higher risk of tuberculosis found among contacts of sputum smear-positive than among contacts of smear-negative index cases in special studies and in classical contact tracing (Liippo et al. 1993). More recently, the use of molecular fingerprinting techniques has shown that the relative transmission rate from sputum smear-negative compared with sputum smear-positive source cases was 0.22 (Behr et al. 1999). Patients with extrapulmonary tuberculosis do not generally constitute a source of infection.

Risk of infection

Risk of infection depends on the extent of an individual's exposure to droplet nuclei and on susceptibility to infection.

Exposure to droplet nuclei

The two factors that determine an individual's risk of exposure are the concentration of droplet nuclei in contaminated air and the length of time spent breathing that air. The extent of an individual's exposure to droplet nuclei is determined by the proximity and duration of contact with an infectious source case.

The concentration of droplet nuclei depends on the number of infectious droplets expelled and the volume of air into which they are expelled. Risk of exposure is therefore much greater indoors than outdoors. Ventilation dramatically dilutes the concentration of droplet nuclei, and so is the most important environmental measure to decrease risk of infection among exposed persons. The simplest and least expensive way of ventilating a room or hospital ward is to maximize natural ventilation through open windows (WHO 1999a). Transmission generally occurs indoors since the concentration of droplet nuclei in contaminated air falls very quickly outdoors, and direct sunlight kills tubercle bacilli in 5 minutes.

A susceptible individual's risk of infection is therefore high with close, prolonged, indoor exposure to a person with sputum smear-positive pulmonary tuberculosis (generally considered 'close contact'). A contact tracing study in the Netherlands that cast the contact tracing 'net' very widely showed that the closer the contact of a susceptible individual to an infectious source case, the greater the chance of infection (Veen 1992). The number of cases of infection in a particular exposure group (defined by closeness to the source case) is the product of the risk and the number of people in the group.

Thus, more cases of infection occur in a large group of distant, low-risk contacts than in a small group of close, high-risk contacts—an example of the Rose axiom (Rose 1985). Conventional contact tracing generally identifies the close, high-risk contacts and therefore identifies a minority of the contacts infected by a source case. The extent of an individual's exposure to infection determines not only risk of infection but also affects the risk of disease, since those with greater intensity of exposure are at greater risk of developing disease (Houk et al. 1968).

Susceptibility to infection

It has been difficult to separate the influence of the genetic and exogenous (socioeconomic and environmental) factors that determine susceptibility to infection. The role of genetic factors in determining susceptibility was suggested by a study in the United States of nursing home residents with apparently the same risk of exposure which found a higher risk of infection among black than white residents (Stead et al. 1990). Susceptibility to infection is affected by the ability of macrophages to phagocytose and destroy the bacilli that reach the terminal alveoli and begin the process of implantation and infection (Schluger & Rom 1998). Since several genes are involved in this process, the study of human genomics has the potential to increase our understanding of differences between individuals and populations in their susceptibility to infection (Davies & Grange 2001).

Some exogenous factors may cause increased susceptibility to infection by impairing the local immune response in the respiratory tract, e.g. silicosis and inhalation of smoke from cooking fires and industrial pollution, or by damaging the respiratory endothelium and mucociliary stairway, e.g. cigarette smoking (Aubry et al. 2000). In practice it has been difficult to separate the possible influence of these exogenous factors on susceptibility to infection versus progression of infection to disease. HIV may increase susceptibility to infection with *M. tuberculosis*. The evidence for this mainly depends on comparisons in hospital outbreaks of the outcome of exposure to source cases of tuberculosis, with higher rates of development of tuberculosis in HIV-positive than HIV-negative patients exposed. Assuming that the secondary cases have primary tuberculosis, the higher rates of tuberculosis in HIV-positive people reflect higher rates of *M. tuberculosis* infection and therefore increased susceptibility to infection with *M. tuberculosis*.

Primary infection and its outcomes

Primary infection occurs in persons without previous exposure to tubercle bacilli. When droplet nuclei are inhaled into the lungs, those small enough to avoid the mucociliary defences of the bronchi are ingested by alveolar macrophages. Bacilli virulent enough to withstand the proteolytic enzymes in the macrophage phagolysosomes multiply and initiate infection. About 2–4 weeks after infection, cell-mediated immunity results in the formation of granulomas, which usually constrain the spread of the bacilli. The initial focus of infection in the lungs (the Ghon focus) together with the related hilar lymphadenopathy comprise the primary complex, which develops without symptoms. The development of the immune response (delayed hypersensitivity and cellular immunity) about 4–6 weeks after the primary infection is indicated by a positive tuberculin skin test and occasionally by clinical hypersensitivity reactions.

The balance between host immunity and bacillary multiplication determines the outcome of infection. The immune response in most cases stops bacillary multiplication, but in a few cases is insufficient to prevent bacillary multiplication, and progression from infection to disease occurs within a few months. Young children are at increased risk of primary tuberculosis since the immune system may not be mature enough to contain the initial infection. Primary tuberculosis results from local bacillary multiplication and spread in the lung or spread in the blood from the primary complex throughout the body, with seeding of bacilli in various tissues and organs. In some cases dormant bacilli may persist and cause disease on later reactivation. The possible outcomes of primary infection with *M. tuberculosis* are therefore: (1) latent infection (with a positive tuberculin skin test and no clinical disease)—the usual outcome in 90 per cent of cases or more; (2) hypersensitivity reactions; (3) pulmonary and pleural complications; and (4) disseminated disease.

Progression of *M. tuberculosis* infection to disease

Once infected with *M. tuberculosis,* a person remains infected for many years, probably for life. The vast majority (90 per cent) of people without HIV infection who are infected with *M. tuberculosis* do not develop tuberculosis (Sutherland 1976). In contrast to the risk of *M. tuberculosis* infection that is largely determined by exogenous factors, the risk of tuberculosis following *M. tuberculosis* infection is largely endogenous, determined by the individual's immune status. Why some people with latent *M. tuberculosis* infection develop tuberculosis and others do not is still an unanswered question.

The 5–10 per cent of people infected with *M. tuberculosis* who develop tuberculosis in their lifetime do so mostly within 5 years of infection (Comstock & Cauthen 1993). The chance of developing disease is greatest shortly after initial infection and then steadily lessens over time. Various conditions or emotional stresses may trigger progression of infection to disease. The most important trigger is weakening of immune resistance, especially by HIV infection, but also by immunosuppressive therapies. The medical conditions that increase risk of progression to disease include diabetes mellitus, malnutrition, substance abuse, silicosis, malignancies, malabsorption, and chronic renal failure (Rieder 1999).

Impact of HIV co-infection on progression of *M. tuberculosis* infection

HIV increases the risk of progression to active tuberculosis both in people with recently acquired (DiPerri *et al.* 1989) and with latent (Selwyn *et al.* 1989) *M. tuberculosis* infection (for which HIV is the most powerful known risk factor for reactivation). This risk increases with increasing immunosuppression (Antonucci *et al.* 1995). As HIV infection progresses, CD4+ T-lymphocytes steadily decline in number and function, with a concomitant decreased ability to restrict tubercle bacilli to a few infected macrophages.

The impact of HIV on the outcome of primary infection is an increased risk and speed of progression to primary tuberculosis through local and disseminated bacillary spread. The tuberculin skin reaction is also suppressed. HIV increases not only the risk but also the speed of progression of latent *M. tuberculosis* infection to disease. Overall, compared to an individual who is not infected with HIV, an individual with untreated HIV infection has a 10 times increased risk of developing tuberculosis (Selwyn *et al.* 1989).

First episode (primary or post-primary) or recurrent tuberculosis

First episode of tuberculosis

A first episode of tuberculosis may be primary, i.e. occurring through progression of primary infection, or post-primary, i.e. occurring after a latent period of months or years after primary infection.

Primary tuberculosis

Primary tuberculosis mainly occurs in childhood since this is when most *M. tuberculosis* infections occur. Since HIV dramatically increases the risk of rapid progression of *M. tuberculosis* infection to disease, adults with HIV infection who become infected with *M. tuberculosis* often develop primary tuberculosis. The incidence of primary tuberculosis is therefore increased in countries with high HIV prevalence. The manifestations of primary tuberculosis mainly result from pulmonary and pleural complications and dissemination of primary infection.

Post-primary tuberculosis

Post-primary tuberculosis may occur either by reactivation of the dormant tubercle bacilli that have persisted in tissues for months or years after primary infection or by re-infection. The patient's immune response results in a characteristically localized pathological lesion, often with extensive tissue destruction and cavitation. Post-primary tuberculosis usually affects the lungs but can involve any part of the body. Patients with post-primary pulmonary tuberculosis often have extensive lung destruction with cavitation and positive sputum smear on microscopy, and are the main transmitters of infection in the community. People with latent *M. tuberculosis* infection who become infected with HIV are at increased risk of progression of infection to disease. The clinical picture depends on the degree of immunodeficiency, with disease dissemination more likely as immunodeficiency progresses.

Recurrent tuberculosis

A recurrent episode of tuberculosis is one that occurs after a previous episode has been considered cured, and may be due to relapse (reactivation of the same strain causing the original disease) or reinfection (indicating the lack of effectiveness of acquired immunity) (Lambert 2003). HIV increases the rate of recurrent tuberculosis (Korenromp *et al.* 2003), with increased likelihood of reinfection in settings of intense *M. tuberculosis* transmission.

Natural history of untreated tuberculosis (in the absence of HIV infection)

Studying the natural history of untreated tuberculosis would nowadays be unethical. However, in South India during the 1960s a study of untreated patients with sputum smear-positive pulmonary tuberculosis in a rural population found that five out of ten died within 5 years, three self-cured, and two remained ill with chronic, infectious tuberculosis (National Tuberculosis Institute, Bangalore 1974). As a rule of thumb in tuberculosis epidemiology (Styblo 1991), this finding is embodied in practically every conceptual model—qualitative or quantitative—of the way tuberculosis affects populations (Dye 2006a).

The disease cycle

In the absence of HIV infection, up to 10 per cent of people infected with *M. tuberculosis* will develop active tuberculosis (whether from progression of recent infection or from reactivation), of whom about one half will be infectious (usually with sputum smear-positive pulmonary disease) (Sutherland 1976). Thus, only one in 20 people infected with *M. tuberculosis* develops infectious tuberculosis, and each infectious case in turn needs to infect about 20 people in order to generate one further infectious case. This is the situation of stable tuberculosis incidence (i.e. the case reproduction number is one). Key determinants of the case reproduction number are the number of people infected by an infectious case, and the proportion of people infected with *M. tuberculosis* who develop active tuberculosis. Any factors that increase the number of people infected by an infectious case (e.g. lack of or inadequate anti-tuberculosis treatment) or that increase the proportion of people infected with *M. tuberculosis* who develop active tuberculosis will push the case reproduction number above one, with consequent increasing tuberculosis incidence.

Stratagems for tuberculosis control

The primary stratagem of tuberculosis control is to reduce the average number of people infected by each infectious case so that the case reproduction number is less than one. This can be achieved by prompt diagnosis and effective treatment, which lie at the heart of the approaches to tuberculosis control developed in the era of anti-tuberculosis chemotherapy (see 'The development of the approach to tuberculosis control in the chemotherapy era'). Other stratagems target individuals at risk of developing tuberculosis and are aimed at decreasing risk of primary infection with *M. tuberculosis*, risk of progression of *M. tuberculosis* infection to a first episode of disease, or risk of a recurrent episode of disease (whether due to relapse or reinfection).

Prompt diagnosis and effective treatment

The correct application of anti-tuberculosis drugs can cure over 90 per cent of new smear-positive tuberculosis patients who have neither tuberculosis resistance to first-line drugs nor HIV infection. Before the spread of HIV, countries that met the two international targets of at least 70 per cent case detection (among incident cases of sputum smear-positive pulmonary tuberculosis) and at least 85 per cent treatment success of those detected could expect to see a decline in tuberculosis incidence rates of 5–10 per cent per year or more (Dye *et al.* 1998). This expected epidemiological impact has been demonstrated in, for example, Peru (Suarez *et al.* 2001), and has been supported by observed reductions in prevalence, for example in the areas of China that have implemented the DOTS strategy (China Tuberculosis Control Collaboration 2004).

BCG immunization

A tuberculosis vaccine could potentially interrupt the disease cycle by decreasing risk of infection with *M. tuberculosis* or risk of progression of *M. tuberculosis* infection to disease. BCG provides protection against tuberculosis by decreasing risk of progression of *M. tuberculosis* infection to disease. Since BCG has a protective efficacy of 70–80 per cent against disseminated and severe forms of tuberculosis (e.g. meningeal and miliary tuberculosis) in children, WHO in 1996 recommended BCG vaccination for all neonates in countries with high tuberculosis incidence. Most of the infants vaccinated with BCG worldwide are therefore protected to a large extent against disseminated and severe tuberculosis for the first few years of their lives (WHO 1995). Although a meta-analysis of the published literature on efficacy of BCG in the prevention of tuberculosis found that, on average, BCG reduced the risk of tuberculosis by 50 per cent (Colditz *et al.* 1994), protective efficacy varies considerably in different populations (Fine & Rodrigues 1990). Most people who are vaccinated as children in countries with high tuberculosis incidence will not be protected against pulmonary tuberculosis as adults because the vaccine is unlikely to protect for longer than 15 years and, in many populations, often has low efficacy against adult pulmonary disease. BCG is therefore not expected to have any significant global impact in reducing *M. tuberculosis* transmission and tuberculosis incidence.

Preventive treatment

Preventive treatment can be aimed at decreasing risk of primary infection with *M. tuberculosis*, risk of progression of *M. tuberculosis* infection to a first episode of disease, or risk of a recurrent episode of disease (whether due to relapse or reinfection). The most common example of preventive treatment aimed at decreasing risk of primary infection with *M. tuberculosis* is the administration of isoniazid to an infant born to a mother with sputum smear-positive pulmonary tuberculosis and therefore at high risk of becoming infected. Most individuals who receive preventive treatment are those who are infected with *M. tuberculosis* and at high risk of developing tuberculosis, i.e. they receive treatment for latent *M. tuberculosis* infection. Isoniazid preventive treatment (IPT) for 6 months is recommended for such high-risk individuals, including children who are household contacts of an infectious case of tuberculosis and who, after screening, are found not to have active tuberculosis themselves (WHO 2006a) and people infected with HIV, since up to 15 per cent of tuberculin-positive, HIV-positive adults will develop tuberculosis each year (WHO 1999b). Preventive treatment is also of benefit in decreasing the risk of tuberculosis recurrence after successful treatment of a first tuberculosis episode in people who are HIV-infected (Fitzgerald *et al.* 2000).

Although cheap, IPT is at present used mostly for the protection of individuals, rather than to prevent transmission. This is because children rarely develop infectious tuberculosis, and because of the difficulties in large-scale administration of IPT to healthy adults. Since at least 6 months' daily consumption of isoniazid is difficult for health services and patients alike, many people who could benefit from treatment drop out before completion. The proportion of HIV-infected people who do complete a course of IPT is typically small (Aisu *et al.* 1994). For IPT to be effective in preventing a large number of tuberculosis cases, ways need to be found to maximize the detection of people infected with *M. tuberculosis* and at high risk of tuberculosis, and minimize the IPT dropout rate. For tuberculosis associated with HIV, maximizing the detection of people infected with *M. tuberculosis* depends on expanded provision of voluntary counselling services for HIV-positive patients (Hawken & Muhindi 1999).

Physical measures to decrease transmission

Removal of tuberculosis patients from their homes and their isolation in sanatoria may well have played a role in decreasing the transmission of *M. tuberculosis* in the pre-chemotherapy era. In the early years of chemotherapy, the usual policy for administration of treatment was through hospitalization. This changed following a study in Chennai, India, which showed that ambulatory anti-tuberculosis chemotherapy was effective and not associated with an increased risk of tuberculosis among the household contacts of infectious index cases (Kamat et al. 1966). This is because chemotherapy rapidly results in tuberculosis patients becoming no longer infectious, so the vast majority of household contacts who were infected by the index cases became infected before the diagnosis of tuberculosis was made and treatment started.

Physical measures are very important to prevent nosocomial transmission. In providing care for patients with or suspected of having tuberculosis, clinicians and persons responsible for healthcare facilities should take measures that reduce the potential for transmission of M. tuberculosis to healthcare workers and to other patients. Implementation of local, national, or international guidelines for infection control is particularly important in areas or specific populations with a high prevalence of HIV infection (WHO 1999a).

The history of the global tuberculosis epidemic

M. tuberculosis is a very successful pathogen, infecting about one-third of the world's population (Dye et al. 1999). Understanding the history of M. tuberculosis and of the global tuberculosis epidemic can provide the key to explaining this success, and how to tilt the balance of the pathogen–host interaction in favour of the human host.

Tuberculosis and our ancestors' ancestors

The success of M. tuberculosis as a human pathogen reflects the extremely long and close relationship it has enjoyed with humanity. M. tuberculosis has an extremely low level of genetic variation. Until recently it was thought that this meant that the entire population of members of the M. tuberculosis complex (MTBC) resulted from clonal expansion following an evolutionary bottleneck around 35 000 years ago. However, genetic analysis of human tubercle bacilli discovered in East Africa indicate that they represent a much broader progenitor species as old as three million years from which the MTBC clonal group evolved (Gutierrez et al. 2005). This suggests that our remote early hominid ancestors may have suffered from tuberculosis. It is possible that, similarly to humans, tubercle bacilli emerged in Africa and then underwent early diversification, followed by recent expansion of a successful clone to the rest of the world, possibly coinciding with the waves of human migration out of Africa. Louis Leakey's aphorism 'The past is the key to the future' is as true for our understanding of the history of M. tuberculosis as it is for Homo sapiens (two species that have emerged together from East Africa). The co-evolution of MTBC with humanity over the past three million years has profound implications for our understanding of the natural selection effect of tuberculosis on human populations and of how the remarkable ability of tubercle bacilli to persist for decades in host tissues has evolved.

The origins of today's tuberculosis epidemic

Bates and Stead (1993) have provided an excellent review of the slow worldwide progress of the tuberculosis epidemic. We have no direct evidence of the nature of the interaction between MTBC and our early hominid ancestors, but this interaction has left its indelible mark on human populations through the development of natural resistance over many generations of continued selective pressure. Direct evidence of human disease caused by MTBC is provided by paleopathology, with tuberculous spondylitis having been recognized in Egyptian mummies as early as 3700 BC (Zimmerman 1977).

In the prehistoric era, before people began to settle in villages, there was little potential for the person-to-person spread of MTBC. Settlements of 25 000 or more tipped the balance between M. tuberculosis and the human host, favouring the pathogen. In populations exposed to M. tuberculosis over hundreds and thousands of years, natural selection has favoured the retention of protective genes. The nature of the tuberculosis epidemic in a particular population thus depends on the degree of natural resistance, the effect of any exogenous influences on immunity, and the degree to which environmental conditions favour transmission.

The development of crowded cities in the middle ages in Europe heralded the importance of the tubercle bacillus as an important cause of disease. In the 1600s, the tuberculosis epidemic increased rapidly, spreading throughout western Europe over the next 200 years as the high population densities and low living standards in the enlarging cities facilitated the airborne transmission of M. tuberculosis. Europe was probably the epicentre of the subsequent global epidemic, with spread to North America, Asia, and Africa by European migrants and colonizers. Historical records point to the rarity of tuberculosis in indigenous populations living generally in conditions of low population density before the arrival of Europeans. For example, Livingstone found little or no tuberculosis on his extensive travels in Africa between his arrival in 1840 and his death in 1873. While the tuberculosis epidemic peaked in Europe at the time of the industrial revolution in the late 1700s and early 1800s and has since steadily declined, this was only the beginning of the new tuberculosis epidemics in most parts of the world, where epidemic spread was promoted by a combination of low natural resistance and dramatic social changes with increasingly the crowded living conditions associated with urbanization.

In summary, the pattern of tuberculosis in a population depends to a large extent on the maturity of the epidemic. At the beginning of the twenty-first century, the tuberculosis epidemic in populations of European origin is mature and characterized by low morbidity and mortality, with most cases arising among older people by reactivation of latent infection often acquired several decades previously. However, the epidemic in most other populations is generally much less mature and characterized by high morbidity and mortality mainly among young adults and children, usually due to recent infection or reinfection (Dye 2006b). The HIV epidemic has exacerbated this situation in many countries in sub-Saharan Africa, causing 'a perfect storm' of tuberculosis (see 'HIV-related tuberculosis').

Tuberculosis case notification trends during the twentieth century

Little is known about the tuberculosis burden and its trend throughout most of the twentieth century in low- and middle-income countries, since they generally started developing reliable systems for case notification towards the end of the century. However, it is likely that the tuberculosis epidemic was generally uncontrolled, since there was little political commitment and funding for tuberculosis control, little improvement in socioeconomic conditions, little if any social support for tuberculosis patients, and few facilities for the care and isolation of tuberculosis patients.

Information on trends in tuberculosis case notifications during the course of the twentieth century is available mainly from industrialized countries. Case notifications steadily declined throughout most of the twentieth century, beginning before the introduction of anti-tuberculosis chemotherapy (Styblo 1991). This was largely because of socioeconomic improvements and possibly also because of the isolation of infectious cases in sanatoria. Tuberculosis caused by *M. bovis* (transmitted from cattle through ingestion of infected milk) was controlled by veterinary measures to ensure cattle herds remained free from bovine tuberculosis and by milk pasteurization. The effective application of chemotherapy in the latter half of the twentieth century further accelerated the decline, which reached up to 10–13 per cent annually.

From the mid-1980s onwards, however, several industrialized countries saw a failure of the expected continued decline, and others saw the trend reversed, with case notifications increasing for the first time in many years. For example, in the United States, after 30 years of previous steady decline, tuberculosis incidence increased regularly between 1985 and 1992 (Cantwell *et al.* 1992). Factors responsible for the continuing problem of tuberculosis in industrialized countries have included increased poverty among marginalized groups in inner city areas, immigration from countries with high tuberculosis prevalence, the impact of HIV, and the failure to maintain the necessary public health infrastructure under the mistaken belief that tuberculosis was a problem of the past.

Tuberculosis case notification rates are still high in the countries of the former Soviet Union (WHO 2007a), in many of which the previous continued decline in case notifications stopped or reversed from the early 1990s onwards. For example, annual notification rates doubled in Russia from 1990 to 2002, with an increased proportion of cases in young adults (WHO 2007a). Dramatic social changes following the end of the Soviet Union engendered a combination of factors responsible for the reversal of the previous trend, probably through increased susceptibility to infection and increased breakdown to disease after infection. These factors include increased poverty and poor living conditions (resulting in malnutrition, crowding, and stress) and in some cases civil conflicts and wars, deteriorating health services, and lack of drugs, resulting in decreased rates of cure of tuberculosis patients and continued transmission in the community. The high prevalence of drug-resistance contributed to the tuberculosis crisis in many countries of the former Soviet Union. The spread of HIV in some countries, particularly the Russian Federation and Ukraine, has the potential, if unchecked, to fuel the tuberculosis epidemic further. In the past few years, the increasing case notification rates in the countries of the former Soviet Union have been checked, probably as a result of improvement both in socioeconomic conditions and public health infrastructure.

The current status of the global burden of tuberculosis and recent trends

Quantifying the size of the burden of tuberculosis is important since it draws attention to the scale of the problem, thereby helping to mobilize resources for tuberculosis control. Changes in indicators of the size of the burden indicate the extent of progress in tuberculosis control. The burden in terms of cases and deaths may be quantified using reported tuberculosis case notifications and deaths or through a process of estimation.

Tuberculosis case notifications and reported deaths

Since national tuberculosis notification data are important for monitoring the global tuberculosis situation they are routinely reported by WHO (WHO 2007a). At the country level, a system of recording and reporting tuberculosis cases and their treatment outcomes (including death) is an intrinsic part of the DOTS strategy, i.e. the policy package for tuberculosis control comprising five elements (see 'The development of the approach to tuberculosis control in the chemotherapy era') (WHO 1994). Therefore as the number of countries implementing the DOTS strategy has increased, routine national tuberculosis programme (NTP) data on tuberculosis cases and deaths have become more widely available (WHO 2007a).

Tuberculosis case notifications

Notification data reflect health service coverage and the efficiency of case-finding and reporting activities of NTPs. Thus, in low- and middle-income countries where tuberculosis incidence is generally high, access to health services may be limited, and NTP performance may be suboptimal, notification data often represent only a fraction of the true incident cases. In industrialized countries, however, where tuberculosis incidence is generally low, health service coverage is generally universal, and NTPs are effective, notifications of cases often closely approximate the true incidence of tuberculosis. In any country, under stable programme conditions, case notifications may provide useful data on the trend of incidence and a means for obtaining rates by age, sex, and risk group.

Despite the limitations of tuberculosis case notifications, WHO has since 1997 published worldwide data provided by its member states. Every year, WHO requests information from NTPs or relevant public health authorities in 212 countries/areas via a standard data collection form. In each country aggregated national data is compiled from the standard data reported by districts (Maher & Raviglione 2004). A total of 199 countries/areas reported 5 million episodes of tuberculosis (new patients and relapses) under the DOTS strategy in 2005 (WHO 2007a).

Three WHO regions dominate the worldwide distribution of cases notified under the DOTS strategy: The Southeast Asian Region (36 per cent of cases), the Western Pacific Region (25 per cent of cases) and the African Region (24 per cent of cases). The three other WHO regions have much smaller proportions of the cases notified worldwide: The Eastern Mediterranean Region (6 per cent), the European Region (5 per cent), and the Region of the Americas (4 per cent).

Reported tuberculosis deaths

Data on tuberculosis deaths are reported through national vital registration systems and through the routine NTP recording and reporting system. Few low- and middle-income countries have comprehensive vital registration systems for the accurate reporting of deaths. Routine NTP data on tuberculosis deaths are becoming more widely available in low- and middle-income countries. NTPs report these tuberculosis cohort deaths (the number and proportion of tuberculosis patients dying during treatment) without specifying cause, because the cause of death can rarely be determined in countries where income is low and the prevalence of tuberculosis is high (WHO 2003). Inaccurate routine NTP reporting of cohort deaths and incomplete NTP coverage of all incident cases in many countries limit the extent to which tuberculosis cohort deaths reflect tuberculosis mortality.

Death, as a treatment outcome not associated with ongoing tuberculosis transmission, is not relevant to the public health objective of cutting the cycle of disease transmission. However, death is an extremely adverse outcome for tuberculosis patients and their families. Since the reduction of tuberculosis deaths is one of the aims of tuberculosis control, death is an important indicator in NTP monitoring. Global health targets agreed as part of the Millennium Development Goals include the reduction of tuberculosis deaths (Dye *et al.* 2006). Tuberculosis deaths as an indicator of the impact of tuberculosis control measures are therefore important in the epidemiological surveillance of progress towards these targets (Maher *et al.* 2005a). These considerations are particularly important in countries with high HIV prevalence, with substantially increased reported cases and deaths (Mukadi *et al.* 2001). Tuberculosis deaths are also closely linked to HIV prevalence. Routine NTP data on tuberculosis cohort deaths are important in programme monitoring, and improvements in recording and reporting of deaths would help to overcome limitations in their accuracy. As routine NTP data on tuberculosis cohort deaths are insufficient as an indicator in epidemiological surveillance regarding the impact of NTPs on tuberculosis mortality, measuring progress towards targets for reduced tuberculosis deaths depends on improved national vital registration systems for a more accurate determination of tuberculosis mortality (Maher *et al.* 2005a).

Estimated tuberculosis incidence and deaths

Because of the limitations of tuberculosis notifications and the difficulties in directly measuring the numbers of cases and deaths, it is necessary to estimate the size of the tuberculosis disease burden. WHO estimates of tuberculosis incidence and deaths are based on a variety of inputs, including surveys of prevalence of *M. tuberculosis* infection and disease, vital registration data, and independent assessments of quality of surveillance systems (Dye *et al.* 1999; Corbett *et al.* 2003; WHO 2007a).

In 2005, there were an estimated 8.8 million new cases of tuberculosis worldwide (WHO 2007a). A total of 1.6 million people died of tuberculosis, including 199 000 people co-infected with HIV. Table 9.14.1 summarizes tuberculosis incidence and mortality estimates in 2005 by WHO regions (WHO 2007a). After more than a

decade of increase, the global annual incidence rate (136 per 100 000 population in 2005) appears to have stabilized and may be now declining. In four WHO regions (the Americas, Southeast Asia, Eastern Mediterranean and Western Pacific), the annual incidence rate has been stable or falling slowly over the past decade. In the other two regions (Africa and Europe) the rate had been increasing for more than a decade but appears to have reached a peak (WHO 2007a).

The importance of the tuberculosis problem for individual countries is expressed as the annual incidence (absolute number of cases occurring yearly) and as the incidence rate (cases per 100 000 population). WHO provides the estimated annual tuberculosis incidence and incidence rate by country, with also a ranking of countries by annual incidence to draw attention to the 22 countries that account for roughly 80 per cent of the global tuberculosis burden (WHO 2007a). Figure 9.14.1 shows estimated tuberculosis incidence rates by country in 2005 (WHO 2007a).

Tuberculosis incidence rates are generally much lower in industrialized than in low- and middle-income countries. Among the 15 countries with the highest estimated tuberculosis incidence rates, 13 are in sub-Saharan Africa (Swaziland, Djibouti, Namibia, Lesotho, Botswana, Kenya, Zimbabwe, Zambia, South Africa, Sierra Leone, Mozambique, Malawi, and Cote d'Ivoire)—the other two are Timor Leste and Cambodia—and in most of these countries HIV prevalence among tuberculosis patients is high (WHO 2007a).

HIV-related tuberculosis

HIV fuels the tuberculosis epidemic where the population infected with *M. tuberculosis* overlaps with the population infected with HIV. Sub-Saharan Africa carries the greatest share of HIV-related tuberculosis since about one-third of the population is infected with *M. tuberculosis* (Dye *et al.* 1999) and the region carries two-thirds of the global burden of HIV (UNAIDS and WHO 2006). By the end of 2000, of the 11 million people worldwide co-infected with *M. tuberculosis* and HIV, about 8 million (70 per cent) were in sub-Saharan Africa (WHO 2002b). The spread of HIV has driven the incidence of tuberculosis in sub-Saharan Africa upwards: In countries with high HIV prevalence, the annual increase in tuberculosis incidence from 1990 to 2004 ran parallel to the change in HIV prevalence in the general population (WHO 2007a). The annual tuberculosis

Table 9.14.1 Tuberculosis incidence and mortality estimates in 2005 by WHO regions (WHO 2007a)

WHO Region	Population 1000s	Incidence (all forms)[a]		Mortality (all forms)		HIV prevalence in incident TB cases in adults (15–49 years)
		Number 1000s	Per 100 000 population per year	Number 1000s	Per 100 000 population per year	
AFR	738 083	2529	343	544	74	28
AMR	890 757	352	39	49	5.5	7.9
EMR	541 704	565	104	112	21	2.1
EUR	882 395	445	50	66	7.4	4.6
SEAR	1 656 529	2993	181	512	31	3.9
WPR	1 752 283	1927	110	295	17	1.0
Global	6 461 751	8811	136	1577	24	11

Abbreviations: AFR, African; AMR, Americas; EMR, Eastern Mediterranean; EUR, European; SEAR, Southeast Asia; WPR, Western Pacific.
[a] All estimates include tuberculosis in people with HIV.

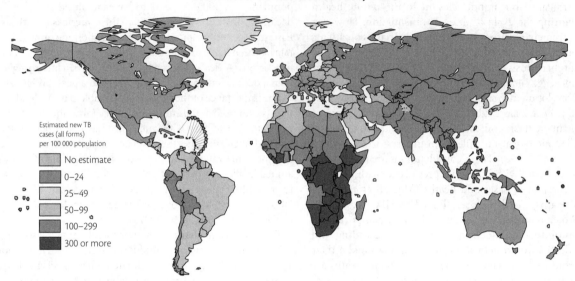

Estimated TB incidence rate, 2005

Estimated new TB
cases (all forms)
per 100 000 population

- No estimate
- 0–24
- 25–49
- 50–99
- 100–299
- 300 or more

Fig. 9.14.1 Estimated tuberculosis incidence rates by country in 2005
Source: WHO (2007a).

incidence rate (343 per 100 000 in 2005) may now be stabilizing in sub-Saharan Africa as HIV prevalence has reached a plateau.

Globally, in 2005, an estimated 11 per cent of adults aged 15–49 years with newly diagnosed tuberculosis were infected with HIV, with great variation among regions—from 28 per cent in the African region to 1 per cent in the Western Pacific region (Table 9.14.1). Figure 9.14.2 maps the distribution of HIV among tuberculosis patients. The prevalence of HIV among patients with tuberculosis has so far remained below 1 per cent in several of the large countries with very high tuberculosis burden, including Bangladesh, China, Indonesia, and Pakistan, in contrast with the particularly high rates in countries of eastern and southern Africa (which have high HIV prevalence in the general population). HIV infection is now the most important single predictor of tuberculosis incidence in Africa (Corbett *et al.* 2003). Of the 22 high-burden countries that constitute 80 per cent of the global burden of tuberculosis, nine are in Africa (WHO 2007a).

Because HIV infection rates in sub-Saharan Africa are generally higher in women than men, more tuberculosis cases are being reported among women, especially those aged 15–24 years. Although tuberculosis case notifications typically show a predominance among men, in several African countries with high rates of HIV infection, the majority of notified tuberculosis cases are now women (WHO 2007a).

Multidrug-resistant (MDR) tuberculosis

Drug resistance and eventually MDR (i.e. resistance to at least isoniazid and rifampicin) are expected to occur wherever there is inadequate application of antituberculosis chemotherapy (Crofton *et al.* 1997). An assessment of the number and distribution of drug-resistant tuberculosis cases is important for planning tuberculosis control because the treatment of resistant cases is more costly, toxic

and complex when second-line drugs are used, with more frequent failures and deaths. The distinction between resistance among new cases (previously known as primary resistance) and resistance among previously treated cases (previously known as acquired resistance) is important because of their different implications for NTPs.

Assessment of the extent of the problem of MDR tuberculosis

Assessment of the extent of the problem of MDR tuberculosis is based on routine surveillance data, survey data, and estimates.

Routine surveillance data

Industrialized countries provide good routine surveillance data on MDR tuberculosis since their diagnostic services generally include routine culture and drug susceptibility testing (DST). However, routine surveillance data from low- and middle-income countries, where most MDR tuberculosis cases arise, are limited since they provide culture and DST only for a small group of tuberculosis cases selected on a clinical basis usually among patients who fail treatment. The long-term vision for control of MDR tuberculosis includes routine drug resistance surveillance and treatment of MDR tuberculosis as standard components of all NTPs.

Survey data

Until this vision is realized by a massive scale-up of culture and DST services, survey data will be crucial in assessing the extent and trends of the problem of MDR tuberculosis. The Global Drug Resistance Surveillance Project coordinated by WHO and the International Union Against Tuberculosis and Lung Disease (IUATLD) has now generated three rounds of survey data (1997, 2000, and 2004) on drug resistance among new and previously treated cases (Pablos-Mendez *et al.* 1998; Espinal *et al.* 2001; Aziz *et al.* 2006).

Estimated HIV prevalence in new TB cases, 2005

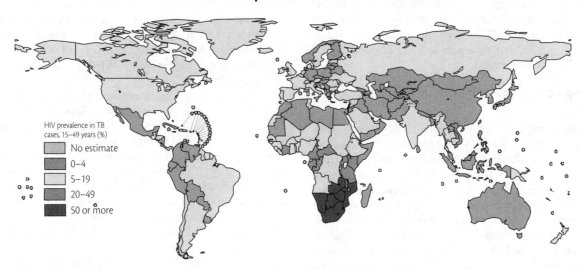

Fig. 9.14.2 Estimated HIV prevalence in new tuberculosis cases, 2005
Source: WHO (2007a)

The decrease in any resistance in Cuba and Hong Kong could well be the result of stable and well-performing tuberculosis control programmes (Aziz *et al.* 2006). At present, trend data are limited from most low-income countries, and no trend data are available from African countries, with the exception of Botswana, which reported an increasing prevalence of MDR tuberculosis (Aziz *et al.* 2006). More representative geographic coverage of global drug resistance surveillance, with further data from longitudinal studies, will enable more accurate and comprehensive monitoring of global trends in the spread of MDR tuberculosis. Increases in prevalence of resistance can be caused by poor or worsening tuberculosis control, immigration of patients from areas of higher resistance, outbreaks of drug-resistant disease, and variations in surveillance methodologies. Although drug-resistant tuberculosis is present in all settings surveyed, the prevalence of MDR is high only in certain settings, e.g. countries of the former Soviet Union and some provinces of China. Because good tuberculosis control practices are generally associated with lower or decreasing levels of resistance, the findings of the WHO/IUATLD Global Project emphasize the vital importance of strengthening tuberculosis control worldwide, by expanding and improving the quality of implementation of the DOTS strategy to prevent the emergence of further drug resistance. National programmes need to manage MDR tuberculosis cases, regardless of prevalence, through application of the DOTS-Plus strategy (see 'Adaptation of the DOTS strategy in response to TB/HIV and MDR-TB').

Estimated incidence

WHO has used the most recent survey data to analyse the predictors of multidrug-resistance and generate global, regional, and national incidence estimates of multidrug-resistance among new and re-treatment tuberculosis cases in 2004 (Zignol *et al.* 2006). About 4 per cent of all the new tuberculosis cases that arise globally

each year are estimated to be MDR (Zignol *et al.* 2006), although the frequency among previously treated cases is higher. With an estimated global incidence of over 400 000 MDR tuberculosis cases in 2004, most patients are not correctly diagnosed or treated, since facilities to diagnose and treat MDR tuberculosis are not yet widely available (WHO 2007a).

Extensively drug-resistant (XDR) tuberculosis

The worldwide emergence of *M. tuberculosis* strains resistant to second-line drugs reflects improper treatment of MDR tuberculosis. Although the scale of the XDR tuberculosis problem globally is not yet known, extensive drug resistance was identified during 2000–2004 in MDR tuberculosis isolates reported worldwide (Centers for Disease Control and Prevention 2006). The initial definition of XDR (MDR with further resistance to three or more of the six classes of second-line drugs), has been replaced by a new definition (WHO 2006c). The report in 2006 of cases of XDR tuberculosis in South Africa with HIV infection and extremely high mortality highlighted the problem of HIV-associated XDR tuberculosis (Gandhi *et al.* 2006). The worldwide emergence of XDR tuberculosis highlights the need to ensure high-quality management of MDR tuberculosis patients within strengthened basic tuberculosis control programmes (Raviglione & Smith 2007).

The development of the approach to tuberculosis control in the chemotherapy era

The following account draws on the excellent review of tuberculosis control in the chemotherapy era by Holme (1997). In the pre-chemotherapy era, the aim of tuberculosis treatment was to strengthen host resistance (through special diets and rest in bed in a sanatorium) and to rest the diseased part of the lung (by various techniques of collapse therapy). Sanatorium treatment was expensive and associated with a 5-year case fatality of at least 50 per cent (Styblo 1991). Before the 1950s, of the many tuberculosis patients worldwide, only a select few among those living in industrialized countries had access to treatment.

The development of anti-tuberculosis treatment regimens

The development in the late 1940s and early 1950s of specific anti-tuberculosis chemotherapy heralded a revolution in tuberculosis control. Control of the disease became possible based on interruption of its transmission through the rapid identification and cure of infectious cases (see 'The disease cycle'). With proper treatment, a person with infectious tuberculosis very quickly becomes non-infectious—probably most often in less than two weeks (Rouillon et al. 1976)—and so can no longer spread disease to others. Waksman discovered streptomycin, the first specific anti-tuberculosis drug, in 1944. Streptomycin became available in 1946 and its efficacy was demonstrated in a pioneering randomized controlled clinical trial in 1948 run by the British Medical Research Council (MRC) Tuberculosis Research Unit established under Philip D'Arcy Hart. The trial was the first high-profile demonstration of the therapeutic benefit of a drug using the principles of the randomized controlled trial developed by Austin Bradford Hill to eliminate bias.

This trial not only secured the scientific basis of chemotherapy as a revolution in tuberculosis control, but also pioneered the controlled trial as the gold standard in medicine for the evaluation of therapeutic interventions. However, the initial promise of streptomycin often proved a disappointment as the problems of resistance and toxicity soon became apparent. A subsequent MRC trial of streptomycin and PAS showed for the first time that combination chemotherapy decreased the emergence of drug resistance and provided the basis for anti-tuberculosis chemotherapy for the next 20 years.

Following the advent of isoniazid in 1952, Sir John Crofton led the team that developed the 'Edinburgh approach'. This was based on the administration of triple combination chemotherapy (streptomycin, PAS and isoniazid) with intensive support to ensure adherence throughout the 18 months of treatment and scrupulous monitoring of each patient's progress through bacteriological analysis (Ross et al. 1958). By 1954, this combination of the first three anti-tuberculosis drugs discovered had been conclusively demonstrated to cure virtually all tuberculosis patients, however severe their disease (in the absence of drug resistance). The very high cure rates under this approach coupled with intensive case-finding had a swift public health impact, with tuberculosis case notification rates falling by half between 1954 and 1957 (Crofton 1960).

The Styblo model of tuberculosis control

The principles of tuberculosis control based on case-finding and effective treatment were rapidly and successfully applied in industrialized countries but not the low- and middle-income countries. The widespread benefits of the anti-tuberculosis chemotherapy revolution had to wait until Karel Styblo's pioneering development in the 1970s of a model of tuberculosis control applicable in resource-poor countries. This model was based on the sound epidemiological principles of case-finding among symptomatic patients and the application of chemotherapy and was delivered using the existing district-based government health infrastructure. The model encompassed the comprehensive organizational and managerial approach to tuberculosis control that had previously been lacking (WHO 1999c), despite it being clearly spelled out in the recommendations of the Report of the WHO Expert Committee on Tuberculosis (WHO 1974).

The use of standard long-course treatment (1 year of isoniazid and thiacetazone, with streptomycin in addition in the initial phase of treatment) in the first few years of pioneering this approach did not achieve high rates of treatment success. It was therefore abandoned in favour of short-course chemotherapy, with rifampicin during the initial 2 months' phase. The model made use of the available government district hospitals, relying on hospitalization to ensure adherence to treatment during the initial phase of treatment. This was controversial since ambulatory treatment was quickly becoming the norm at the time (see 'Stratagems for tuberculosis control').

The Tanzania National Tuberculosis Programme (NTP) was the first of the IUATLD model programmes with successful nationwide coverage. From the 1980s, many NTPs, especially in sub-Saharan Africa, relied on hospitalization for supervised administration of treatment during the initial phase. Between 1978 and 1991, the IUATLD supported NTPs in nine resource-poor countries with high tuberculosis incidence in implementing the recommended policy package for tuberculosis control.

The DOTS strategy

1991 marked the end of the pilot phase of implementing the Styblo model—the basis of WHO's new strategy for global tuberculosis control (Kochi 1991)—and the beginning of scale-up through a global alliance of partners (Maher & Nunn 1998; Raviglione & Pio 2002). Following WHO's declaration of tuberculosis as a global emergency in 1993, from 1994 to 1995 onwards WHO promoted the DOTS strategy which was formulated as a five-point policy package (WHO 1994), subsequently further refined (WHO 2002a) and then later incorporated in the Stop TB Strategy (see Box 9.14.1).

In the new era of renewed interest in tuberculosis control in the 1990s, the principles and policies that proved practical and effective in implementing the new strategy were those established by the WHO Expert Committees on Tuberculosis during the doldrums of global tuberculosis control in the 1960s and 1970s. For example, the four principles formulated for NTPs by the WHO Expert Committee that met in 1973 remain valid—the NTP should be: (1) integrated into general health services, within the Ministry of Health; (2) nationwide; (3) permanent because of the nature and chronicity of the disease; and (4) adapted to the needs of the people, with tuberculosis services being as close to the community as possible to facilitate diagnosis, treatment and follow-up (WHO 1974).

In 1991, the World Health Assembly established two targets for global tuberculosis control by the year 2000: To detect 70 per cent of cases and to cure 85 per cent of sputum smear-positive patients with pulmonary tuberculosis under treatment (WHO 1991). The choice of these levels of performance reflected the need to have a significant epidemiological impact through reaching targets that field experience had demonstrated were feasible in countries with high incidence rates of tuberculosis. Despite considerable progress in scaling up the DOTS strategy, towards the end of the 1990s it

Box 9.14.1 Components of the WHO Stop TB strategy and implementation approaches

1. Pursue high-quality DOTS expansion and enhancement

- Political commitment with increased and sustained financing
- Case detection through quality-assured bacteriology
- Standardized treatment with supervision and patient support
- An effective drug supply and management system
- Monitoring and evaluation system, and impact measurement

2. Address HIV-related tuberculosis, MDR tuberculosis, and other challenges

- Implement collaborative TB/HIV activities
- Prevent and control MDR tuberculosis
- Address prisoners, refugees, and other high-risk groups, and special situations

3. Contribute to health system strengthening

- Actively participate in efforts to improve system-wide policy, human resources, financing, management, service delivery, and information systems
- Share innovations that strengthen systems, including the Practical Approach to Lung Health
- Adapt innovations from other fields

4. Engage all care providers

- Public–public and public–private mix approaches
- International standards for TB care

5. Empower people with TB, and communities

- Advocacy, communication, and social mobilization
- Community participation in tuberculosis care
- Patients' Charter for Tuberculosis Care

6. Enable and promote research

- Programme-based operational research
- Research to develop new diagnostics, drugs, and vaccines

Source: Raviglione & Uplekar (2006).

became apparent that the year 2000 targets would not be met. The World Health Assembly in 2000 therefore postponed the date to achieve those targets to 2005, with the final report of progress against the targets being made in 2007 (see 'Progress towards the international targets for tuberculosis control by 2005').

Adaptation of the DOTS strategy in response to TB/HIV and MDR-TB

The particular threats to successful implementation of the DOTS strategy posed by the HIV epidemic and the emergence of anti-tuberculosis drug-resistance necessitated adaptations to the strategy.

Strategy of expanded scope to counter HIV-associated tuberculosis

HIV has dramatically fuelled tuberculosis in populations with high HIV prevalence (Corbett et al. 2003). The implications of HIV for tuberculosis control (Maher et al. 2005b) necessitated the development of a WHO strategy of expanded scope to counter the HIV-driven tuberculosis epidemic. The strategy comprises measures aimed directly against tuberculosis—full implementation of the DOTS strategy with intensified case-finding (Corbett et al. 2007) and preventive treatment (WHO 1999b)—and measures against HIV, including prevention of HIV transmission and provision of antiretroviral drugs (WHO 2002b).

Strategy for managing drug-resistant tuberculosis

Recognition of the extent of the global problem of drug-resistant tuberculosis (Pablos-Mendez et al. 1998) led to the adaptation of the DOTS strategy as 'DOTS-Plus' to counter MDR tuberculosis (Espinal et al. 1999). The inadequate response of patients with drug-resistant tuberculosis to standard short-course chemotherapy based on first-line anti-tuberculosis drugs indicated the need for treatment regimens including second-line drugs (Espinal et al. 2000). The DOTS strategy is the starting point for managing drug-resistant tuberculosis, which also involves quality-assured drug-susceptibility testing and the use of second-line drugs in recommended treatment regimens (WHO 2006b). The feasibility and cost-effectiveness of standardized second-line drug treatment for patients with drug-resistant tuberculosis within programme conditions has been demonstrated in Peru (Suarez et al. 2002) and the Philippines (Tupasi et al. 2006).

The establishment by a group of partners of the Green Light Committee hosted by WHO enabled the negotiation of lower prices with the drug industry, the use of a mechanism for pooled procurement, and the coordination of technical assistance to ensure the quality of programmatic management of patients with MDR tuberculosis (Gupta et al. 2001). Epidemiological modelling suggests that MDR-tuberculosis will remain a locally severe problem rather than become a global one, provided that cases are managed in line with recommended guidelines (WHO 2006b) and that MDR-tuberculosis strains are actually less fit than drug-susceptible ones (Dye & Espinal 2001).

Basic principles in tuberculosis care

Prompt diagnosis and effective treatment of tuberculosis are at the heart of the DOTS strategy, since they are not only the key elements in the public health response to tuberculosis and the cornerstone of tuberculosis control, but also essential for good patient care (Maher 1999; Tuberculosis Coalition for Technical Assistance 2006). All healthcare providers who undertake evaluation and treatment of tuberculosis patients are not only delivering care to an individual, but also assuming an important public health function.

These basic principles of care for persons with, or suspected of having, tuberculosis are the same worldwide: (1) a diagnosis should be established promptly and accurately; (2) standardized treatment regimens of proven efficacy should be used with appropriate treatment support and assessment; (3) the response to treatment should be monitored; and (4) the essential public health responsibilities must be carried out (Tuberculosis Coalition for Technical Assistance 2006). *Toman's Tuberculosis* provides a comprehensive account of the evidence base underpinning current recommendations for case detection, treatment, and monitoring (Frieden 2004). The basic principles in tuberculosis care are fully consistent with the approach to tuberculosis control formulated as the DOTS strategy.

Establish prompt and accurate diagnosis

In populations with high tuberculosis incidence identification of acid-fast bacilli in samples from a suspected site of disease provides immediate diagnosis with a high degree of specificity and is the practical gold standard. Since culture confirmation of *M. tuberculosis* usually takes up to 8 weeks, it does not provide useful diagnostic information at the time a clinician needs to make the diagnosis. Notwithstanding the delay in results, proving a diagnosis of tuberculosis by culture is useful in confirming an immediate diagnosis made by sputum smear microscopy and establishing drug susceptibility, in diagnosing sputum smear-negative pulmonary tuberculosis and other cases of diagnostic doubt (especially in populations with high HIV prevalence), and in managing suspected drug-resistant tuberculosis. The reliability of sputum smear microscopy and culture for *M. tuberculosis* depends on an effective national system of laboratory quality assurance.

Use effective standardized drug treatment

Effective treatment regimens

WHO provides guidelines on patient categorization and management for all tuberculosis patients—pulmonary (sputum smear-positive and smear-negative) and extrapulmonary, adults and children, with and without HIV (WHO 2003). These guidelines emphasize use of effective standardized, short-course regimens, and of fixed-dose drug combinations (FDCs) to facilitate adherence to treatment and to reduce the risk of the development of drug resistance. Separate WHO guidelines are also available for management of patients with drug-resistant tuberculosis (WHO 2006b).

Comprehensive approach to promoting adherence

A high standard of care is essential to restore the health of individuals with tuberculosis, to prevent the disease in their families and others with whom they come into contact, and to protect the health of communities (Hopewell *et al.* 2006). Substandard care results in poor patient outcomes (treatment failure, relapse, death, and drug resistance) and poor public health outcomes (continued infectiousness with transmission of *M. tuberculosis* to family and other community members, and generation and propagation of drug resistance). Ensuring that treatment leads to the best possible patient and public health outcomes depends on the extent to which patients complete the prescribed treatment regimen, i.e. on adherence to treatment. All providers (public and private) who undertake to treat a patient with tuberculosis have two specific responsibilities regarding tuberculosis treatment, as a matter not only of individual health but also of public health: (1) they must prescribe a recommended standard treatment regimen; and (2) they must promote and assess adherence to ensure that treatment is completed.

The importance of providing intensive support to tuberculosis patients to promote adherence to treatment was recognized in the 1950s when combination anti-tuberculosis chemotherapy was pioneered (Fox 1958). NTPs have the responsibility to ensure a comprehensive approach to promoting adherence, aimed at service providers

and patients. Recommended measures aimed at promoting adherence include placing the patient at the centre of tuberculosis control activities, ensuring confidentiality and consideration of patients' needs, organizing tuberculosis services so that the patient has treatment as close to home as possible, addressing factors that may make patients interrupt or stop treatment by identifying potential problems in advance, considering incentives, keeping accurate address records and taking defaulter actions (WHO 2003). There is increasing recognition of the role in promoting adherence of a treatment partner or supporter who is acceptable to the patient and is trained and supervised by health services, and of patient and peer support groups. Support for patients must be context-specific and patient-sensitive, with particular attention paid to groups with particular needs, including prisoners and intravenous drug users.

Assessment of adherence

Assessment of adherence is crucial to determine the success of measures to promote adherence and ensure completion of treatment. Direct observation of treatment provides a practical means of assessing, rather than of promoting, adherence (Bayer & Wilkinson 1995). Direct observation of treatment by a trained health worker or community member responsible for promoting adherence may be undertaken at a health facility, in the workplace, in the community or at home (Maher 2003). Recognition of non-adherence enables immediate action to be taken to identify the reason and take corrective action. Direct observation of treatment has generally been found to be a more practical way of assessing treatment adherence than pill-counting or urinary isoniazid metabolite testing.

Promote individual civil liberties and public health

Approaches to tuberculosis control should promote the protection of both individual civil liberties and of public health. Although authorities in high-income, low tuberculosis incidence countries have sometimes adopted authoritarian and coercive measures to ensure treatment adherence (Coker 2000), such measures have been found unnecessary in some low tuberculosis incidence settings (Levy & Alperstein 1999) and are almost unheard of in low-income, high-tuberculosis-incidence countries. The government and health service responsibility is to ensure health provider adherence to treatment recommendations and to provide the resources and organizational requirements for the range of support measures necessary for tuberculosis patients to be able to adhere to treatment, without recourse to coercion (Coker 1999).

Safeguard patients' rights and promote responsibilities

The Patients' Charter for Tuberculosis Care sets out patients' rights and responsibilities, including 'the responsibility to follow the prescribed and agreed treatment plan . . . to protect the patient's health, and that of others' (World Care Council 2006). An agreement (known as concordance) between a tuberculosis patient and healthcare provider reinforces their mutual contribution and responsibility to achieve successful treatment (Maher *et al.* 2003). Concordance is therefore a key step at the start of the dynamic process of supporting a patient throughout treatment. An enhanced concept of concordance embraces the initial agreement between patient and healthcare provider and also measures for ongoing support for patients to enable them to complete treatment and obtain the successful treatment outcome desirable for the individual and for public health.

Just as good care for individuals with tuberculosis is in the best interest of the community, the community has an interest in promoting good care of individuals. Community contributions to tuberculosis care and control are increasingly important in raising public awareness of the disease, providing treatment support, encouraging adherence, reducing the stigma associated with tuberculosis, and demanding that healthcare providers in the community adhere to a high standard of tuberculosis care (Hadley & Maher 2000).

Ensure access to treatment

Many people face physical, financial, social and cultural—as well as health system—barriers to accessing tuberculosis treatment services. Improving access to treatment involves taking locally appropriate measures to identify and address these barriers. The poorest and most vulnerable population groups deserve particular attention. Appropriate actions may include expanding treatment services in the poorest rural and urban settings and involving providers close to where patients live, e.g. through engaging community contribution to tuberculosis care (Maher 2003). Other appropriate actions may include ensuring that services are free or heavily subsidized, offering psychological and legal support, addressing gender issues, improving staff attitudes and undertaking advocacy and communication activities.

Monitor the response to treatment

Patient monitoring is necessary to evaluate response to treatment and to identify adverse drug reactions. Sputum smear microscopy is the most practical method to judge the response of pulmonary tuberculosis to treatment. Ideally, where quality-assured laboratories are available, sputum cultures, as well as smears, should be performed for monitoring. Having a positive sputum smear at completion of five months of treatment defines treatment failure, indicating the need for determination of drug susceptibility and initiation of a re-treatment regimen (WHO et al. 2001). Radiographic and clinical assessments, although used commonly, have been shown to be unreliable for evaluating response to treatment (Santha 2004). However, in patients with extrapulmonary tuberculosis and in children, clinical evaluations may be the only available means of assessing response to treatment.

Carry out essential public health responsibilities

Healthcare providers who undertake evaluation and treatment of patients with tuberculosis assume an important public health function. Delivering care to an individual entails a high level of responsibility to the community, as well as to the individual patient. The essential public health responsibilities of health providers include contact tracing and reporting of cases to the statutory health authority, as well as case-finding and treatment.

Contact tracing

All providers of care for patients with tuberculosis should ensure that persons (especially children under 5 years of age and persons with HIV infection) who are in close contact with patients who have infectious tuberculosis are evaluated and managed in line with international recommendations (WHO 2006d). Children under 5 years of age and persons with HIV infection who have been in contact with an infectious case should be evaluated for both latent *M. tuberculosis* infection and for active disease (WHO 2006a).

Reporting

Reporting tuberculosis cases to the local tuberculosis control programme is an essential public health function, and in many countries is legally mandated. Ideally, the reporting system design, supported by a legal framework (WHO 2001), should be capable of receiving and integrating data from several sources, including laboratories and healthcare institutions, as well as individual practitioners. An effective reporting system enables a determination of overall NTP effectiveness, of resource needs, and of the true distribution and dynamics of the disease within the population as a whole, not just the population served by the government NTP. In most countries, tuberculosis is a reportable disease. A system of recording and reporting information on tuberculosis cases and their treatment outcomes is one of the key elements of the DOTS strategy in ensuring accountability of health providers and programmes: The system serves not only to monitor progress and treatment outcomes of individual patients but also to evaluate the overall performance of the tuberculosis control programmes, at the local, national, and global levels, and to indicate programmatic weaknesses (Maher & Raviglione 2004).

Progress towards the international targets for tuberculosis control by 2005

Progress in implementing the DOTS strategy has mainly been assessed in relation to the targets for global tuberculosis control by 2005 of detecting 70 per cent of new patients with sputum smear-positive pulmonary tuberculosis and curing 85 per cent of those detected (WHO 1991). WHO provided the final report of progress against these targets in 2007. The DOTS strategy was being applied in 187 countries in 2005; 89 per cent of the world's population lived in areas where the DOTS strategy had been implemented by public health services. 26.5 million patients were notified under the DOTS strategy by programmes between 1995 and 2005, and 10.8 million new smear-positive cases were registered for treatment under the DOTS strategy by programmes between 1994 and 2004.

Since practice varies considerably between countries in documenting negative sputum smears on completion of treatment, for practical purposes the treatment success rate (cure + treatment completion) is considered as a proxy for cure rate (WHO 2007a). The latest global estimates of progress against the targets for 2005 indicate that, among patients with sputum smear-positive pulmonary tuberculosis diagnosed and treated under the DOTS strategy, the case-detection rate was 60 per cent (for the cohort of patients diagnosed in 2005) and the treatment success rate was 84 per cent (for the cohort of patients treated in 2004) (Table 9.14.2).

All WHO regions have made progress, with the Western Pacific Region having achieved and surpassed the targets, but with considerable variation among different countries. In all countries, the expected epidemiological impact on incidence, prevalence and mortality depends on NTPs performing well in ensuring the highest possible case-detection and treatment-success rates. Maximizing the expected epidemiological impact on the tuberculosis burden depends, for countries that have not reached the targets by 2005, on reaching them as soon as possible, and, for countries that have reached the targets for 2005, on sustaining and surpassing this achievement.

Table 9.14.2 Progress towards the tuberculosis control targets for 2005 (WHO 2007b)

WHO Region	Progress towards targets for 2005				
	Case detection rate (in 2005) (%)	Number of countries achieving 70% detection target	Treatment success rate (in 2004) (%)	Number of countries achieving 85% treatment-success target	Number of countries achieving both targets
African	50	9	74	7	1
Americas	65	18	80	7	4
Southeast Asia	64	5	87	7	3
European	35	13	74	11	5
Eastern Mediterranean	44	7	83	7	5
Western Pacific	76	15	91	18	8
Global	60	67	84	57	26

Italics indicate rates that exceed the targets.

Achievement of global rates of 60 per cent for case detection and 84 per cent for treatment success by 2005 represents tremendous progress in tuberculosis control since the respective targets of 70 per cent and 85 per cent were established in 1991. At that time no system existed for measuring the global burden of tuberculosis and the worldwide effort to implement the DOTS strategy was in its early stage. With the establishment of the global monitoring and surveillance system in the mid-1990s, the rates were determined for the first time: 11 per cent for case detection in 1995 and 77 per cent for treatment success in 1994. Not only has the case-detection rate risen substantially over the past decade but it has doubled over the past five years, from 30 per cent in 2001. The treatment-success rate has increased at the same time as an approximate tenfold increase in cases detected.

The evolving international response to the challenge of tuberculosis

Roles of international partners

The Stop TB Partnership

When the first *ad hoc* committee on the tuberculosis epidemic met in London in 1998 and reviewed the barriers to faster progress, one of the key recommendations was to form a global alliance to harness the efforts of, and obtain synergy from, the increasing number and range of stakeholders in global tuberculosis control. A global alliance of partners met in Amsterdam in 2000 as the Global Tuberculosis Initiative, which in 2001 became the Stop TB Partnership (http://www.stoptb.org). The Stop TB Partnership represents a global movement to accelerate social and political action to stop the spread of tuberculosis. It consists of a network of over 500 international organizations, countries, donors (public and private sector), governmental and non-governmental organizations, foundations, corporate sector representatives, and individuals, all united by the common goal of tuberculosis elimination by 2050. The Partnership's mission is to ensure that every tuberculosis patient has access to effective diagnosis, treatment and cure; to stop transmission of tuberculosis; to reduce the inequitable social and economic toll of tuberculosis; and to develop and implement new preventive, diagnostic and therapeutic tools and strategies to Stop TB. One of

the ways by which the Partnership improves access to effective treatment for tuberculosis is through the Partnership's Global Drug Facility which was established in 2001 and by the end of 2006 had made available 10 million tuberculosis treatments (Stop TB Partnership 2007).

Role of the WHO

WHO plays a key role in tuberculosis control as the lead United Nations agency for health and as the institution that houses the Stop TB Partnership secretariat. The objectives of WHO's Stop TB Department are: (1) to develop global policies, strategies and standards for tuberculosis control; (2) to support the tuberculosis control efforts of WHO member states; (3) to measure progress towards global targets for tuberculosis control, and assess NTP performance, financing and impact; (4) to facilitate partnerships, advocacy and communications, in pursuit of achieving global targets for tuberculosis control; and (5) to promote research (http://www.who.int/tb/en).

The Stop TB Strategy

In 2003, WHO and the Stop TB Partnership convened the second *ad hoc* Committee on the tuberculosis epidemic to find ways of speeding up progress in global tuberculosis control. The committee's recommendations reflected recognition that progress in tuberculosis control can contribute to improved health and poverty reduction, and depends on strengthening not only the specifics of traditional tuberculosis control programme activities but also general health systems. The key recommendations to Stop TB partners were to: (1) consolidate, sustain, and advance achievements; (2) enhance political commitment (and its translation into policy and action); (3) address the health workforce crisis; (4) strengthen health systems, particularly primary care delivery; (5) accelerate the response to the TB/HIV emergency; (6) mobilize communities and the corporate sector; (7) invest in research and development to shape the future (Stop TB Partnership and WHO 2004).

These recommendations informed the formulation of WHO's new Stop TB Strategy, which was endorsed by the Stop TB Partnership and launched in March 2006 (WHO 2006d). The Strategy (Box 9.14.1) is aimed at achieving the Stop TB Partnership's targets for 2015, which are linked to the United Nations Millennium Development

Goals (MDGs) (Raviglione & Uplekar 2006). The goal relevant to tuberculosis (Goal 6, Target 8) is 'to have halted and begun to reverse incidence by 2015'. In addition to interpreting Target 8 as an incidence rate that should be falling by 2015, the Stop TB Partnership has endorsed international targets linked to Target 8, to decrease tuberculosis prevalence and deaths by half by 2015 (in comparison with a 1990 baseline) (Dye *et al.* 2006b).

In 2007, the Stop TB Partnership and WHO established the Stop TB Research Movement as an alliance of stakeholders to enable and promote tuberculosis research across the spectrum of basic science, research and development of new tools, and applied research (http://www.stoptb/researchmovement.org).

The Global Plan to Stop TB, 2006–2015

How all Stop TB partners will implement the Stop TB Strategy is set out in the Partnership's Global Plan to Stop TB, 2006–2015, launched in 2006 at the World Economic Forum in Davos, Switzerland (Stop TB Partnership and WHO 2006). Developed through a process of extensive consultation, the Plan sets out the steps in research and development for new tools (diagnostics, drugs, and vaccines) and the implementation of currently available interventions to help achieve the global targets for 2015. These activities include scaling up interventions against MDR tuberculosis and against HIV-related tuberculosis. Regarding research and development for new diagnostics, drugs and vaccines, Box 9.14.2 shows the expected outcomes under the Plan. Regarding the expected outcomes of implementation of currently available interventions, from 2006 to 2015, 50 million people will be treated for tuberculosis under the Stop TB Strategy. The total of 50 million people treated includes 800 000 patients with MDR-tuberculosis, and 3 million patients with both tuberculosis and HIV infection who will be enrolled on antiretroviral therapy. This would result in 14 million lives saved compared to a situation without implementation of the DOTS strategy.

The Plan sets out the resources needed for actions, underpinned by sound epidemiological analysis with robust budget justifications. The Plan's total cost (US$56 billion) over 10 years includes US$47 billion for implementation of currently available interventions and US$9 billion for research and development. The estimated funding gap is US$31 billion, since an estimated US$25 billion is

likely to be available based on projections of current domestic and external funding trends.

Conclusion—prospects for tuberculosis control in the future

Tuberculosis control in the near future depends on the extent to which the human and financial resources are made available for successful implementation worldwide of the Global Plan to Stop TB, 2006–2015. Since health systems are crucial for the effective implementation of any disease-specific package, the Stop TB Strategy embraces those health system components that are relevant to tuberculosis control. Developments in sectors beyond health will also certainly affect the future of tuberculosis control in the medium term looking towards the international targets for 2015 and particularly in the long term looking towards the goal of tuberculosis elimination by 2050. The broad determinants of health include poverty, urbanization, housing, nutrition and education, which are often shaped by socioeconomic forces that are part of globalization. These 'upstream' determinants are directly relevant to tuberculosis control, including through conditions that are normally beyond the reach of those directly involved in tuberculosis control, yet within the health system capacity to influence them, e.g. tobacco use, diabetes, malnutrition, indoor pollution, and, of course, HIV infection. Those interested in tuberculosis control share a common cause with those interested in concerted health sector advocacy for the relevant sectors of society to address the socioeconomic determinants of a wide range of illnesses (www.who.int/social_determinants/en).

Prospects for faster progress in tuberculosis control depend on the development of new and improved tools that are equally effective in people with or without HIV-infection: New sensitive and specific diagnostic tests for tuberculosis and for latent *M. tuberculosis* infection that are cost-effective and robust enough for use at the peripheral level of the health system, along with the means of predicting risk of future progression to active disease to enable targeted preventive therapy; new drugs that would allow a marked reduction of the duration of treatment to 1–2 months or less, be effective against MDR tuberculosis, be compatible with antiretroviral therapy and also effective against latent *M. tuberculosis* infection; and new vaccines to prevent tuberculosis in children and adults (Brosch & Vincent 2007). Projections show that continued implementation of the planned interventions under the Global Plan at the level of scale-up reached in 2015 will not result in the Partnership's goal of tuberculosis elimination by 2050 (see Fig. 9.14.3). At the average rate of decline in tuberculosis incidence of 5–6 per cent per year expected globally between 2010 and 2015 under the Global Plan, the incidence rate in 2050 will still be about 100 times larger than the elimination target of 1 per million. A revolutionary new technology for tuberculosis control will be needed for any realistic prospect of achieving this goal.

Increased investment in the development of these new tools must be accompanied by increased investment in the basic research that underpins progress. For example, the sequencing of the *M. tuberculosis* genome holds out the prospect of a dramatic impact on drug discovery research (Cole *et al.* 1998). The development of such new tools, and the full implementation of the interventions currently available to control tuberculosis, represent the two-pronged approach needed to tilt the balance in the long relationship between humanity and *M. tuberculosis* in irreversible favour of the human host.

Box 9.14.2 Expected outcomes of planned research and development for new tools

Drugs
The first new TB drug for 40 years will be introduced in 2010, with a new short TB regimen (1–2 months) shortly after 2015.
Diagnostics
By 2010, diagnostic tests at the point of care will allow rapid, sensitive and inexpensive detection of active TB. By 2012, a diagnostic toolbox will accurately identify people with latent TB infection and those at high risk of progression to disease.
Vaccines
By 2015, a new, safe, effective, and affordable vaccine will be available with potential for a significant impact on TB control in later years.

Source: Stop TB Partnership and WHO (2006).

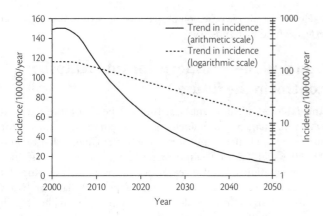

Fig. 9.14.3 Projected tuberculosis incidence 2000–2050 plotted against a linear scale and a logarithmic scale
Courtesy of: Christopher Dye, WHO, Geneva

Key points

♦ *M. tuberculosis* has been a constant companion of humanity, probably going back 3 million years to the time of our remote early hominid ancestors.

♦ After more than a decade of increase, the global annual tuberculosis incidence rate appears to have stabilized by 2005 and since then may be declining.

♦ The balance between *M. tuberculosis* and the human host may now be tipping in favour of humanity.

♦ Turning around the global tuberculosis epidemic requires sustained commitment to investing in full implementation of the Stop TB Strategy, to ensure universal access to the benefits of the current means of prevention and treatment.

♦ Any realistic prospect of achieving the goal of tuberculosis elimination by 2050 depends on the development and widespread introduction of revolutionary new technology for tuberculosis control.

References

Aisu T., Raviglione M.C., van Praag E. *et al.* (1994). Preventive chemotherapy for HIV-associated tuberculosis in Uganda: an operational assessment at a voluntary counseling and testing centre. *AIDS*, **9**, 267–73.

Antonucci G., Girardi E., Raviglione M. *et al.* (1995). Risk factors for tuberculosis among HIV-infected persons. *Journal of the American Medical Association*, **274**, 1345–9.

Aubry M.C., Wright J.L., Myers J.L. (2000). The pathology of smoking-related lung diseases. *Clinical Chest Medicine*, **21**, 11–35.

Aziz M.A., Wright A., Laszlo A. *et al.* (2006) Epidemiology of antituberculosis drug resistance (the Global Project on Anti-tuberculosis Drug Resistance): an updated analysis. *Lancet*, **368**, 2142–54.

Bates J.H. and Stead W.W. (1993).The history of tuberculosis as a global epidemic. *Tuberculosis*, **77**, 1205–16.

Bayer R. and Wilkinson D. (1995). Directly observed therapy for tuberculosis: history of an idea. *Lancet*, **345**, 1545–8.

Behr M.A., Warren S.A., Salamon H. *et al.* (1999). Transmission of *Mycobacterium tuberculosis* from patients smear-negative for acid-fast bacilli. *Lancet*, **353**, 444–9.

Bloom B.R. (1994). Quotation by Bacelli G. in *Tuberculosis. Pathogenesis, Protection and Control*. (Barry R. Bloom, editor). ASM Press, Washington, DC.

Brosch R. and Vincent V. (2007). Cutting edge science and the future of tuberculosis control. *Bulletin of the World Health Organization*, **85**, 410–12.

Cantwell M.F., Snider Jr. D.E., Cauthen G.M. *et al.* (1994). Epidemiology of tuberculosis in the United States, 1985 through 1992. *Journal of the American Medical Association*, **272**, 535–9.

Centers for Disease Control and Prevention (2006). Emergence of *Mycobacterium tuberculosis* with extensive resistance to second-line drugs—worldwide, 2000–2004. *Morbidity and Mortality Weekly Review*, **55**, 301–5.

China Tuberculosis Control Collaboration (2004). The effect of tuberculosis control in China. *Lancet*, **364**, 417–22.

Coker R. (1999). Public health, civil liberties, and tuberculosis. *British Medical Journal*, **318**, 1434–5.

Coker R.J. (2000) *From chaos to coercion: detention and the control of tuberculosis*. St Martin's Press, New York.

Colditz G.A., Brewer T.F., Berkey C.S. *et al.* (1994). Efficacy of BCG vaccine in the prevention of tuberculosis. Meta-analysis of the published literature. *Journal of the American Medical Association*, **271**, 698–702.

Cole S.T., Brosch R., Parkhill J. *et al.* (1998) Deciphering the biology of *Mycobacterium tuberculosis* from the complete genome sequence. *Nature*, **393**, 537–44.

Comstock G.W. and Cauthen G.M. (1993). In Reichman L.B., Hershfield E.S., eds. *Tuberculosis. A Comprehensive International Approach*. Vol. 66 pp. 23–48. Marcel Dekker Inc., New York.

Corbett E.L., Watt C.J., Walker N. *et al.* (2003). The growing burden of tuberculosis: global trends and interactions with the HIV epidemic. *Archives of Internal Medicine*,**163**, 1009–21.

Corbett E.L., Bandason T., Cheung Y.B. *et al.* (2007). Epidemiology of tuberculosis in a high HIV prevalence population provided with enhanced diagnosis of symptomatic disease. *PLoS Medicine*, **4** (**1**) e22, 1–9.

Crofton J. (1960). Tuberculosis undefeated. *British Medical Journal*, **2**, 679–87.

Crofton J., Chaulet P. and Maher D. (1997). *Guidelines for the management of drug-resistant tuberculosis*. WHO/TB/1996.210. WHO, Geneva.

Davies P. and Grange J. (2001). The genetics of host resistance and susceptibility to tuberculosis. *Annals of the New York Academy of Sciences*, **953**, 151–6.

DiPerri G., Cruciani M., Danzi M.H. *et al.* (1989). Nosocomial epidemic of active tuberculosis in HIV infected patients. *Lancet*, **2**, 1502–4.

Dye C., Garnett G.P., Sleeman K. *et al.* (1998). Prospects for worldwide tuberculosis control under the WHO DOTS strategy. Directly Observed Short-Course Therapy. *Lancet* **352**, 1886–91.

Dye C., Scheele S., Dolin P. *et al.*, for the WHO Global Surveillance and Monitoring Project (1999). Global burden of tuberculosis: estimated incidence, prevalence and mortality by country. *Journal of the American Medical Association*, **282**, 677–86.

Dye C., Espinal M.A. Will tuberculosis become resistant to all antibiotics? (2001). *Proceedings of the Royal Society, London*, B **268**, 45–52.

Dye C., Maher D., Weil D. *et al.* (2006). Targets for global tuberculosis control. *International Journal of Tuberculosis and Lung Disease*, **10**, 460–2.

Dye C. (2006a). India's leading role in tuberculosis epidemiology and control (Editorial). *Indian Journal of Medical Research*, 123, 481–4.

Dye C. (2006b). Global epidemiology of tuberculosis. *Lancet*, **367**, 938–40.

Espinal M.A., Dye C., Raviglione M. *et al.* (1999). Rational "DOTS Plus" for the control of MDR-TB. *International Journal of Tuberculosis and Lung Disease*, 3, 561–3.

Espinal M.A., Kim S.J., Suarez P.G. *et al.* (2000). Standard short-course chemotherapy for drug-resistant tuberculosis. Treatment outcomes in 6 countries. *Journal of the American Medical Association*, **283**, 2537–45.

Espinal M.A., Laszlo A., Simonsen L. *et al.* (2001). Global trends in resistance to antituberculosis drugs. *New England Journal of Medicine*, **344**, 1294–303.

Fine P. and Rodrigues L.C. (1990). Modern vaccines. Mycobacterial diseases. *Lancet*, **335**, 1016–20.

Fitzgerald D.W., Desvarieux M., Severe P. *et al.* (2000). Effect of post-treatment isoniazid on prevention of recurrent tuberculosis in HIV-1-infected individuals: a randomized trial. *Lancet*, **356**, 1470–4.

Fox W. (1958). The problem of self-administration of drugs; with particular reference to pulmonary tuberculosis. *Tubercle*, **39**, 269–74.

Frieden T.R., ed. (2004). *Toman's tuberculosis: case detection, treatment, and monitoring* (2nd ed). WHO, Geneva.

Gandhi N.R., Moll A., Sturm W. *et al.* (2006). Extensively drug-resistant tuberculosis as a cause of death among patients co-infected with tuberculosis and HIV in a rural area in South Africa. *Lancet*, **368**, 1575–80.

Gupta R., Kim J.Y., Espinal M.A. *et al.* (2001). Responding to market failures in tuberculosis control. *Science*, **293**, 1049–51.

Gutierrez M.C., Brisse S., Brosch R. *et al.* (2005). *PLoS Pathogens*, **1 (1)** e5, 1–7.

Hadley M. and Maher D. (2000). Community involvement in tuberculosis control: lessons from other health care programmes. *International Journal of Tuberculosis and Lung Disease*, **4**, 401–8.

Hawken M. and Muhindi D.W. (1999). Tuberculosis preventive therapy in HIV-infected persons: feasibility issues in developing countries. *International Journal of Tuberculosis and Lung Disease*, **3**, 646–50.

Holme C.I. (1997). Trial by TB. *Proceedings of the Royal College of Physicians of Edinburgh*, **27 (1)** Suppl 4.

Hopewell P., Pai M., Maher D. *et al.* (2006). International standards for tuberculosis care. *Lancet Infectious Diseases*, **6**, 710–25.

Houk V.N., Rent D.C., Baker J.H. *et al.* (1968). The Byrd study, an analysis of a micro-outbreak of tuberculosis in a closed environment. *Archives of Environmental Health*, **16**, 26.

Kamat S.R., Dawson J.J.Y., Devadatta S. *et al.* (1966). A controlled study of the influence of segregation of tuberculosis patients for one year on the attack rate of tuberculosis in a 5-year period in close family contacts in South India. *Bulletin of the World Health Organization*, **34**, 517–32.

Kochi A. (1991). The global tuberculosis situation and the new control strategy of the World Health Organization. *Tubercle*, **72**, 1–6.

Korenromp E.L., Scano F., Williams B.G. *et al.* (2003). Effects of human immunodeficiency virus infection on recurrence of tuberculosis after rifampin-based treatment: an analytical review. *Clinical Infectious Diseases*, **37**, 101–112.

Lambert M-L, Hasker E., Van Deun A. *et al.* (2003). Recurrence in tuberculosis: relapse or reinfection? *Lancet Infectious Diseases*, **3**, 282–7.

Levy M. and Alperstein G. (1999). Patients with tuberculosis can be managed effectively in the community. *British Medical Journal*, **319**, 455 (letter).

Liippo K.K., Kulmala K. and Tala E.O.J. (1993). Results of tuberculosis contact tracing by smear grading of index cases. *American Review of Respiratory Diseases*, **148**, 235–6.

Lopez A.D., Mathews C.D., Ezzati M. *et al.* (2006). *Global burden of disease and risk factors*. Oxford University Press, New York, and World Bank, Washington, DC.

Loudon R.G. and Roberts R.M. (1966). Droplet expulsion from the respiratory tract. *American Review of Respiratory Diseases*, **95**, 435–42.

Maher D. and Nunn P. (1998). Commentary: making tuberculosis treatment available for all. *Bulletin of the World Health Organization*, **76**, 125–6.

Maher D. (1999). Smear-positive pulmonary tuberculosis: good clinical management is good public health. *Africa Health*, **21**, 6–9.

Maher D., Uplekar M., Blanc L. *et al.* (2003). Editorial. Treatment of tuberculosis. Concordance is a key step. *British Medical Journal*, **327**, 822–3.

Maher D. (2003). The role of the community in the control of tuberculosis. *Tuberculosis*, **83**, 177–182.

Maher D. and Raviglione M.C. (2004). Why is a recording and reporting system needed, and what system is recommended? In: Frieden TR, ed. *Toman's tuberculosis. Case detection, treatment and monitoring*, 2nd edition. WHO, Geneva.

Maher D., Watt C.J., Williams B.G. *et al.* (2005a). Tuberculosis deaths in countries with high HIV prevalence: what is their use as an indicator in tuberculosis programme monitoring and epidemiological surveillance? *International Journal of Tuberculosis and Lung Disease*, **9**, 123–7.

Maher D., Harries A. and Getahun H. (2005b). Tuberculosis and HIV interaction in sub-Saharan Africa: impact on patients and programmes; implications for policies. *Tropical Medicine and International Health*, **10 (8)**, 734–42.

Mukadi Y.D., Maher D. and Harries A. (2001). Tuberculosis case fatality rates in high HIV prevalence populations in sub-Saharan Africa. *AIDS*, **15**, 143–52.

National Tuberculosis Institute, Bangalore (1974). Tuberculosis in a rural population of South India: a five-year epidemiological study. *Bulletin of the World Health Organization*, **51**, 473–88.

Pablos-Mendez A., Raviglione M.C., Laszlo A. *et al.* (1998) Global surveillance for antituberculosis-drug resistance, 1994-1997. *New England Journal of Medicine*, **338**, 1641–9.

Raviglione M.C., Snider D. and Kochi A. (1995). Global epidemiology of tuberculosis: morbidity and mortality of a worldwide epidemic. *Journal of the American Medical Association*, **273**, 220–6.

Raviglione M.C. and Luelmo F. (1996). *Update on the global epidemiology of tuberculosis*. Current Issues in Public Health, **2**, 192–7.

Raviglione M.C. and Pio A. (2002). Evolution of WHO policies for tuberculosis control, 1948-2001. *Lancet*, **359**, 775–80.

Raviglione M. and Uplekar M. (2006). The new Stop TB Strategy of WHO. *Lancet*, **367**, 952.

Raviglione M.C. and Smith I.M. (2007). XDR tuberculosis - implications for global public health. *New England Journal of Medicine*, **356**, 656–9.

Rieder H.L. (1999). *Epidemiologic basis of tuberculosis control* (1st edn). International Union Against Tuberculosis and Lung Disease, Paris.

Rose G. (1985). Sick individuals and sick populations. *International Journal of Epidemiology*, **14**, 32–8.

Ross J.D., Grant I.W.B., Horne N.W. *et al.* (1958). Hospital treatment of pulmonary tuberculosis. *British Medical Journal*, **1**, 237–42.

Rouillon A., Perdrizet S. and Parrot R. (1976). Transmission of tubercle bacilli: the effects of chemotherapy. *Tubercle*, **57**, 275–99.

Santha T. (2004). How can the progress of treatment be monitored? In: Frieden TR, ed. *Toman's tuberculosis. Case detection, treatment and monitoring*, 2nd edition. WHO, Geneva. 250–2.

Schluger N.W. and Rom W.N. (1998). The host immune response to tuberculosis. *American Journal of Respiratory and Critical Care Medicine*, **157**, 679–91.

Selwyn P.A., Hartel D., Lewis V.A. *et al.* (1989). A prospective study of the risk of tuberculosis among intravenous drug users with human immunodeficiency virus infection. *New England Journal of Medicine*, **320**, 545–50.

Stead W.W., Senner J.W., Reddick W.T. *et al.* (1990). Racial differences in susceptibility to infection by *M. tuberculosis. New England Journal of Medicine*, **322**, 422–7.

Stop TB Partnership and WHO (World Health Organization) (2004). Report on the meeting of the second ad hoc Committee on the TB epidemic, Montreux, Switzerland: 18–19 September 2003. Recommendations to Stop TB partners. WHO/HTM/STB/2004.28. WHO, Geneva.

Stop TB Partnership and WHO (2006). Global Plan to Stop TB 2006-2015. Actions for life - towards a world free of tuberculosis. WHO/HTM/STB/2006.35. WHO, Geneva.

Stop TB Partnership (2007). Global Drug Facility achievements report. (WHO/HTM/STB/2007.40). WHO, Geneva.

Styblo K. (1991). *Epidemiology of tuberculosis*. (2nd ed). Royal Netherlands Tuberculosis Association, The Hague.

Suarez P.G., Watt C.J., Alarcon E. *et al.* (2001). The dynamics of tuberculosis in response to 10 years of intensive control effort in Peru. *Journal of Infectious Diseases*, **184**, 473–8.

Suarez P.G., Floyd K., Portocarrero E. *et al.* (2002). Feasibility and cost-effectiveness of standardised second-line drug treatment for chronic tuberculosis patients: a national cohort study in Peru. *Lancet*, **359**, 1980–1989.

Sutherland I. (1976). Recent studies in the epidemiology of tuberculosis, based on the risk of being infected with tubercle bacilli. *Advances in Tuberculosis Research*, **19**, 1–63.

Tuberculosis Coalition for Technical Assistance (2006). *International standards for tuberculosis care*. Tuberculosis Coalition for Technical Assistance, The Hague.

Tupasi T.E., Gupta R., Quelapio M.I.D. *et al.* (2006). Feasibility and cost-effectiveness of treating multidrug-resistant tuberculosis: a cohort study in the Philippines. *PLoS Medicine*, **3**, e352, 1–10.

UNAIDS (Joint United Nations Programme on HIV/AIDS) and WHO (World Health Organization) (2006). AIDS epidemic update, December 2006. UNAIDS and WHO, Geneva.

Veen J. (1992). Microepidemics of tuberculosis: the stone-in-the-pond principle. *Tubercle and Lung Disease*, **73**, 73–6.

World Care Council (2006). *Patients' charter for tuberculosis care*. World Care Council, Geneva.

WHO Expert Committee on Tuberculosis. (1974). 9th Report. World Health Organization Technical Report Series No. 552. WHO, Geneva.

WHO (1991). Forty-fourth World Health Assembly. Resolutions and decisions. Resolution WHA 44.8. WHA44/1991/REC/1. WHO, Geneva.

WHO (1994). *Framework for effective tuberculosis control*. WHO/TB/94.179. WHO, Geneva.

WHO (1995). Global Tuberculosis Programme and Global Programme on Vaccines. Statement on BCG Revaccination for the Prevention of Tuberculosis. *Weekly Epidemiological Record*, **70**, 229–36.

WHO (1999a). *Guidelines for the prevention of tuberculosis in health care facilities in resource-limited settings*. WHO, Geneva.

WHO (1999b). Preventive Therapy against Tuberculosis in People Living with HIV. *Weekly Epidemiological Record*, **74**, 385–98.

WHO (1999c). *What is DOTS? A guide to understanding the WHO-recommended tuberculosis control strategy known as DOTS*. WHO/CDS/CPC/TB/99.270. WHO, Geneva.

WHO (2001). *Good practice in legislation and regulations for TB control: an indicator of political will*. WHO/CDS/TB/2001.290. WHO, Geneva.

WHO/IUATLD/KNCV (2001). Revised international definitions in tuberculosis control. *International Journal of Tuberculosis and Lung Disease*, **5 (3)**, 213–5.

WHO (2002a). *An expanded DOTS framework for TB control*. WHO/CDS/TB/2002.297. WHO, Geneva.

WHO (2002b). *Strategic framework to decrease the burden of TB/HIV*. WHO/CDS/TB/2002.296 WHO/HIV_AIDS/2002.2.WHO, Geneva.

WHO (2003). *Treatment of tuberculosis: guidelines for national programmes* (3rd ed). WHO/CDS/TB/2003.313. WHO, Geneva.

WHO (2006a). *Guidance for national tuberculosis programmes on the management of tuberculosis in children*. WHO, Geneva.

WHO (2006b). *Guidelines for the programmatic management of drug-resistant tuberculosis*. WHO/HTM/TB/2006.361. WHO, Geneva.

WHO (2006c). Addressing the threat of tuberculosis caused by extensively drug-resistant *Mycobacterium tuberculosis*. *Weekly Epidemiological Record*, **81**, 385–396.

WHO (2006d). *The Stop TB Strategy*. WHO/HTM/TB/2006.368. WHO, Geneva.

WHO (2007a). *Global tuberculosis control: surveillance, planning, financing. WHO Report 2007*. WHO/HTM/TB/2007.376. WHO, Geneva.

WHO (2007b). Progress towards the 2005 international targets for tuberculosis control. *Weekly Epidemiological Record*, 82, 178-180

Zignol M., Hosseini M.S., Wright A. *et al.* (2006). Global incidence of multidrug-resistant tuberculosis. *Journal of Infectious Diseases*, **194**, 479–85.

Zimmerman M.R. (1977). The mummies of the tomb of Nebevenef: paleopathology and archeology. *Journal of the American Research Center, Egypt*, **14**, 33.

Malaria

Richard H. Morrow and William J. Moss

Abstract

Although malaria remains a major public health hazard in many low- and middle-income countries, the overwhelming problems with malaria are in the high-transmission areas of Africa where everyone receives infectious bites every day. One consequence of this high transmission is that clinical malaria in children differs from other parts of the world; it strikes abruptly and kills in 18–72 h. A second consequence is that standard vector control methods effective elsewhere have less impact on reducing malaria disease.

The main malaria control methods have been vector control and antimalarial drug treatment. The most important vector control method has been residual insecticide spraying in households that kill vectors when, after a blood meal, they rest on a sprayed wall. The use of dichlorodiphenyltrichloroethane (DDT) in this fashion was dramatically successful in many parts of the world. But then, problems with insecticide resistance and ecological damage (from use in agriculture) led to widespread breakdowns of these control efforts. In most of Africa, vector control by residual insecticides has never been an option because of transmission rates many times more than elsewhere in the world. Until recently, the only control method in Africa has been antimalarial treatment of symptomatic individuals.

The use of chloroquine for treatment of malaria was highly successful for decades with low cost and negligible adverse reactions. However, with the emergence and spread of drug-resistant *Plasmodium falciparum* malaria throughout the world, combination therapy with artmesinin is now universally recommended despite its cost.

Malaria is the most intense stimulator of the human immune system known; all immunologic defence systems are activated with massive production of antibodies, cellular immune responses, and cytokine cascades. Although malaria parasites have evolved complex mechanisms of evasion, the overwhelming evidence is that humans do develop protective immune responses. Effective vaccines should be possible and have been expected for decades, but to date none has been sufficiently effective. With recent progress, however, more than 40 candidate vaccines are currently undergoing clinical trials.

New malaria control approaches are becoming much more widely used: Insecticide-treated bed nets; intermittent preventive therapy for infants, sick children, and pregnant women; and immediate treatment at home can effectively reduce child mortality even in high-transmission areas.

History of malaria

Malaria is an ancient disease. Nearly 5000 years ago, the Chinese *Nei Ching* (The Canon of Medicine) described patients with malaria, and ancient Sumerian, Egyptian, Vedic, and Brahmanic texts dating nearly as far back did so as well (Kakkilaya 2006). Since the sixth century BCE, the Greeks and then the Romans understood the relation of fever to swamps and low-lying water and built their cities on hills. Indeed, the name 'malaria' is derived from medieval Italian meaning 'bad air', reflecting the association with foul-smelling, stagnant swamp water (Bruce-Chwatt 1988).

The discoveries that a protozoan parasite of infected red blood cells cause malaria and that mosquitoes transmit it from human to human were crucial scientific advances made towards the end of the nineteenth century. Although Charles Laveran, a French army doctor working in Algeria, first described the parasite in 1880, he was awarded the Nobel Prize only in 1907. In the interim, Ronald Ross was awarded the Nobel Prize in Medicine in 1902 for his work on malaria and its transmission cycle. Chemotherapy preceded a basic understanding of malaria epidemiology by hundreds of years. Extracts from the wormwood plant, *Artemisia annua*, were used for centuries in China. Cinchona bark was used to treat fevers in Peru and Ecuador prior to the arrival of Europeans (Desowitz 1991). Quinine, extracted from cinchona bark in the early nineteenth century, became the first effective antimalarial drug in the Western world.

Advances in controlling mosquito breeding through drainage and environmental control were key to building the Panama Canal and have continued as major methods for malaria control. During World War II, two major biochemical and pharmaceutical advances in unrelated fields revolutionized malaria control and its treatment: DDT as an insecticide was found to be highly effective against anopheline vectors and chloroquine for the treatment of malaria replaced quinine as the principle antimalarial drug. With these new tools, plans for the reduction and control of malaria were envisioned, but beyond that the exciting prospect of total eradication of this horrendous disease began to be discussed. Residual spraying of DDT on the walls of households was the principal weapon to be employed and, in nearly all early trials, was remarkably effective in killing those mosquitoes which had just enjoyed a blood meal from a sleeping household resident.

Following World War II, the newly formed World Health Organization (WHO) formulated a plan for worldwide malaria eradication at the 8th World Health Assembly in 1955. It was estimated that eradication using DDT residual spraying could be accomplished at a cost of less than 25 cents per person per year; the total cost for the first 5 years would be half a billion US dollars (IDAB 1956). Plans were put into action in many areas of the world, and truly dramatic success was achieved in some regions. By 1958, the most inspirational, ambitious, complex, and costly health campaign ever undertaken was well underway (WHO 1967). Early campaign efforts in many countries in Europe, Asia, and Latin America were enormously successful. Indeed, in Malta the anopheline vector was completely eliminated (Russell *et al.* 1963). However, as time passed, there was little effect in many continental tropical countries of Asia and South America. In Africa, where malaria was by far of greatest importance, virtually nothing was even attempted. Unfortunately, with the great emphasis on logistics and organizational activities, there was a comparable de-emphasis on scientific research. For 20 years, virtually no innovative research on malaria was undertaken.

By the mid-1960s, it was clear that eradication would fail. The complex logistical and operational needs were too much for the weak infrastructures in most tropical countries; moreover, basic biological developments emerged, including anopheline resistance to insecticides and parasite resistance to antimalarials (WHO 1969; Krishna 1997). The malaria eradication campaign came to be viewed as a major failure; in fact, large numbers of lives were saved and major economic activities were spurred.

Today, major advances have taken place in the molecular biology of the malaria parasite; parasite and vector genomics and proteomics; the immunology of malaria infection and vaccine development; vector control methods and a variety of other innovative strategies for malaria control. Yet, despite these advances, a resurgence of severe malaria and an increased number of deaths, particularly in Africa, have taken place. Perhaps the term 'resurgence' is not entirely apt in Africa since malaria was never under any sort of control there. Only quite recently is malaria being viewed as a genuine priority in Africa. Roll Back Malaria (RBM) was launched in 1998 by the World Health Organization, UNICEF, UNDP, and the World Bank to provide a coordinated international approach to fighting malaria. The Roll Back Malaria Partnership is a global initiative—made up of more than 90 partners—whose goal is to halve the burden of malaria by 2010. The first 5 years were devoted to coordinating efforts of the many stakeholders, working toward an in-depth understanding of the ecology, biology, and epidemiology of malaria, particularly in Africa, developing comprehensive and cohesive planning, and raising funds and political support.

Public health importance

The impact of malaria in human populations varies greatly in different parts of the world. Figure 9.15.1 shows a map of the malaria distribution according to the level of endemicity (see geographical areas according to intensity of transmission). Although *Plasmodium vivax* malaria is a major cause of morbidity in parts of China, Southeast Asia, and Latin America, the overwhelming problems of malaria as a life-threatening disease are in those countries with *P. falciparum* malaria, especially in Africa. Much of this chapter will focus on issues related to tropical Africa, where malaria is of greatest importance and where approaches to control have had the least success.

The public health significance of a disease depends upon its incidence and resulting disability and mortality. Incidence is defined as the number of new episodes of disease in a specified population per time period. In many areas where malaria is hypo- or mesoendemic, the incidence of malaria has meaning and can be expressed as the number of new episodes per thousand persons per year. In holoendemic areas, however, with an entomological inoculation rate (EIR) ranging from dozens to hundreds of infectious bites per person per year, everyone is infected all the time and is

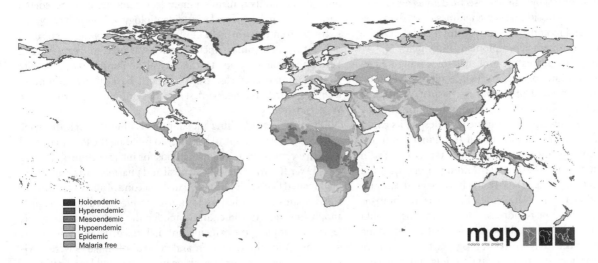

Fig. 9.15.1 The Lysenko map of global malaria endemicity.
Endemicity as used by Lysenko is defined by the parasite rate in the 2–10 year cohort (hypoendemic < 0.1; mesoendemic 0.1–0.5; hyperendemic 0.51–0.75; holoendemic >0.75 (using the parasite rate in the 1-year-old age group). The black line represents the 2002 limit of malaria risk. Note that the 'epidemic' class is of historical interest only and consists of hypoendemic areas restricted to temperate regions.
Source: Hay, S.I. *et al.* The global distribution and population at risk of malaria: past, present, and future. *Lancet Infect Dis*, 2004. **4**: 327–36.

re-infected every few days. The very idea of incidence, or indeed prevalence (the proportion of the population infected at a given time), has little meaning. The health status of an individual in these situations results from a balance between the parasite and host immunity. Elimination of parasites from the host occurs only when the person is treated with an effective antimalarial. Reinfection and, thus, 'a new incident' case occurs as soon as the level of the antimalarial drug drops below the effective therapeutic level and recently injected sporozoites develop into blood stage parasites.

The figure that from one to two million children die of malaria every year has remained the quoted estimate since first put forth by the WHO in the early 1950s (Oaks et al. 1991). In the 2004 World Health Report (data from 2002), a total of 1 272 000 malaria deaths were estimated globally, of which 1 136 000 were in Africa. In addition, malaria accounted for 46 486 000 disability-adjusted life years (DALYs) lost globally, of which 40 855 000 were in Africa. Whatever the estimate, the reality in Africa is that malaria is a major cause of mortality in infants and children and of disability in adults. An indirect indicator of the historical importance of malaria mortality is the frequency of sickle-cell trait (AS) in tropical Africa (ranging from 16 to 29 per cent AS haemoglobin in adults). To account for this frequency, the case fatality rate in West Africa attributed to malaria must have been in the order of 15–20 per cent of all children born with AA haemoglobin (Morrow 1984).

Malaria parasites

Malaria parasites and their life cycle

Four species of protozoan parasites of the genus *Plasmodium* infect humans: *P. falciparum*, *P. vivax*, *P. ovale*, and *P. malariae* (Table 9.15.1). Although *P. vivax* is the most widespread form of malaria infection in the world, *P. falciparum* causes the most severe disease and is responsible, by far, for most deaths and serious morbidity associated with malaria.

The parasite undergoes multiple transformations within the mosquito and human host; at least a dozen separate steps have been identified. The complex life cycle of the malaria parasite is given in Fig. 9.15.2. As an infected female anopheline mosquito takes a blood meal (first arrow), the parasite as the sporozoite form is transmitted to humans. Sporozoites enter the venous blood system from the subcutaneous tissues through the capillary bed, and within minutes those that avoid the defending reticuloendothelial (RE) system and innate immune system invade liver cells. Over the next 5–15 days, each sporozoite nucleus replicates thousands of times to develop into a hepatic (tissue) schizont within the liver cells.

When released from the swollen liver cells into the bloodstream, each schizont splits into tens of thousands of daughter parasites called merozoites. Merozoites attach to specific erythrocyte surface receptors (Duffy blood group antigen for *P. vivax* (Miller *et al.* 1976), glycophorins for *P. falciparum*) and penetrate into the erythrocyte. Each intra-erythrocytic merozoite differentiates into a trophozoite that ingests human haemoglobin, enlarges and divides into 6–24 intra-erythrocytic merozoites forming a schizont (lower right of Fig. 9.15.2). The red cell swells and bursts, releasing the next batch of approximately 20 merozoites, which then attach and penetrate new erythrocytes to begin this cycle again. Along with the liberation of merozoites, the resultant haemolysis and release of 'pyrogens' from infected red cells and the host's response to these toxins correspond with clinical paroxysms of fever and chills. When synchronous, the simultaneous release from many red cells account for the periodicity of these symptoms in some patients. This second stage of asexual division takes about 48 h for *P. falciparum*, *P. vivax,* and *P. ovale*, or 72 h for *P. malariae* (Russell *et al.* 1963). A single *P. falciparum* sporozoite potentially can lead to 10 billion new parasites through these recurrent cycles. After a number of cycles within red cells, some merozoites differentiate into sexual forms called gametocytes, specifically female macrogametocytes and male microgametocytes, which are ingested by an anopheline during its next blood meal.

Sporogonic development

Once in the mosquito, the red cells are digested, freeing the gametocytes, which then begin sexual reproduction leading to sporogonic development. The male and female gametes fuse, providing for genetic recombination, to form a zygote. Over the next 12–14 h, the zygote elongates and forms an ookinete, which in turn penetrates the wall of the mosquito's stomach and becomes an oocyst (lower left of Fig. 9.15.2). During the next several days, the oocyst enlarges, forming more than 10 000 sporozoites, and ruptures into the coelomic cavity. The sporozoites migrate to the salivary glands, ready to be injected back into the human host to complete their life cycle. Once infected with malaria, a female anopheline remains infected for life and can transmit sporozoites with each blood meal (Russell *et al.* 1963; Garnham 1966).

This extrinsic cycle, or sporogonic phase, of parasite development generally takes from 7 to 12 days, depending upon the species of the parasite and the ambient temperature. Under optimal conditions with the temperature at 30°C, *P. falciparum* requires only 9 days; but at 20°C it takes 23 days—a difference of 14 days for a temperature differential of 10°C. Though anopheline females can survive up to

Table 9.15.1 Malaria parasites of humans

Species	Intra-RBC schizont period	Type of RBC	Relapse (hypnozoite)	Global distribution
P. vivax	48 hours	Reticulocytes	Yes	Everywhere except Africa
P. ovale	48 hours	Reticulocytes	Yes	Africa
P. malariae	72 hours	Older RBCs	No	Everywhere
P. falciparum	48 hours (±)	All	No	Tropical regions

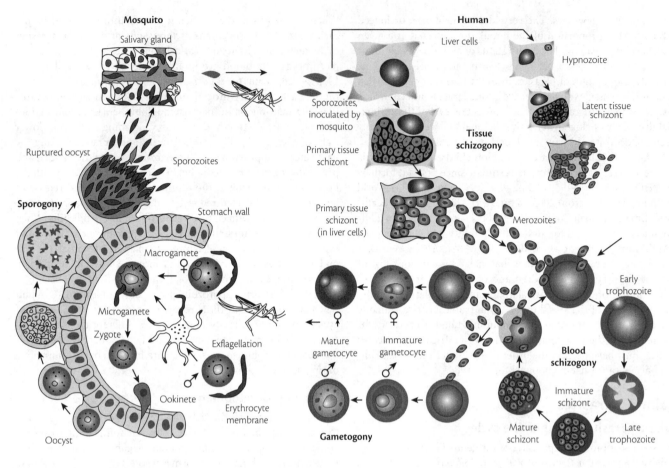

Fig. 9.15.2 Life cycle of malaria parasite.

30 days, the average life span for most is less than 21 days. Thus, the ambient temperature is critical to successful transmission.

During sporogonic development, each female–male pair of gametocytes can potentially produce over 10 000 sporozoites for inoculation. Since dozens to thousands of gametocytes can be ingested with one blood meal, the potential exists for millions of sporozoites to be injected with one bite. Perhaps related to damage to the mosquito from such heavy loads or insufficient nutrients and metabolites available to support these levels of parasitaemia, such high inocula counts are not observed. Limited studies of naturally infected mosquitoes have found sporozoite loads (the number of sporozoites in the salivary glands) from 10 to over 100 000 (Beier *et al*. 1991). *In vitro* studies using experimentally infected mosquitoes have shown most infected mosquitoes transmit fewer than 25 sporozoites per bite, but about 5 per cent can transmit hundreds (Beier 1998).

Biological differences among malaria species

There are important species-specific differences in this generic life cycle (Table 9.15.1). With *P. vivax* and *P. ovale*, some sporozoites entering hepatic cells do not immediately proceed to tissue schizogony, but become hypnozoites (Krotoski *et al*. 1982) (upper right of Fig. 9.15.2) and lie dormant for months to years. Later, these hypnozoites can differentiate into hepatic schizonts, leading to the cycle of erythrocytic schizogony and consequent relapse of symptoms.

This biologic capability accounts for the relapses characteristic of *P. vivax* and *P. ovale* and the need for specific drug treatment targeted to the hypnozoite stage (primaquine). There is no diagnostic test available to determine the presence of hepatic hypnozoites. *P. falciparum* and *P. malariae* do not produce hypnozoites and do not relapse following effective treatment, but untreated or inadequately treated infections may lead to persistent low-grade parasitaemia and sometimes to recrudescent clinical disease. Relapse refers to renewed infection from survival of the parasite in hepatic cells as hypnozoites; recrudescence refers to renewed infection from surviving erythrocytic forms.

The different species of human malaria parasites have affinities for particular types of erythrocytes. *P. vivax* and *P. ovale* parasites only invade the young reticulocytes; density of peripheral parasitaemia in these infections rarely exceeds 3 per cent. *P. malariae* is limited to older red cells. However, *P. falciparum* infects erythrocytes of all ages, and for this reason is able to produce high-density parasitaemias with serious morbidity and high mortality (Russell *et al*. 1963; Garnham 1966). There are also important differences in gametocyte production among species. After infection with *P. vivax*, infective gametocytes appear in the peripheral blood almost as soon as the asexual blood-stage forms. Gametocytes are usually present when vivax malaria is first diagnosed and before antimalarial treatment has been started. In contrast, following infection with *P. falciparum*, gametocytes appear only after several intra-erythrocytic cycles, first appearing at least 10 days after infection. Early treatment of *P. falciparum* with an effective drug will kill blood stage schizonts, preventing gametocytes from developing and blocking transmission. However, gametocytes that do develop will be derived from malaria parasites that survived drug treatment and may carry drug resistance genes. The difference in timing of gametocyte emergence may be a major factor accounting for the much higher rate of drug resistance in *P. falciparum* as compared to *P. vivax* (Mendis *et al.* 2001).

Aspects of the molecular biology of the malaria parasite

Understanding the molecular biology of malaria parasites has been greatly advanced by the publication of the genome sequence of *P. falciparum* in 2002 (Gardner *et al.* 2002). Genome sequencing of *P. vivax* is expected to be published soon. Functional and comparative genomics and proteomics of the malaria parasite, during different stages of its life cycle, will lead to improved understanding of plasmodium biology and pathogenesis, and hopefully to the identification of new drug and vaccine targets.

The genome of *P. falciparum* consists of 14 chromosomes, containing over 5000 predicted genes. Several aspects of the molecular biology of *P. falciparum* are relevant to the epidemiology and control of malaria. A large proportion of identified genes are involved in immune evasion and host–parasite interactions. *P. falciparum* contains three families of highly variable genes; the most important is the *var* gene family, comprising 59 genes encoding for the *P. falciparum* erythrocyte membrane protein 1 (PfEMP1). Transcriptional switching between different *var* genes allows the parasite to evade immune responses directed against PfEMP1. These genes may also be modified by the exchange of material between chromosome ends, where these genes are located. PfEMP1 is located on the surface of infected red blood cells and mediates adherence to endothelial cells. One *var* gene encodes a protein that mediates adherence to chondroitin sulphate A in the placenta and is responsible for the severe disease observed in pregnant women. This gene family encodes for an important virulence factor responsible for the sequestration of infected red blood cells in various organs of the infected human (Rowe *et al.* 2002).

Identification of potential antigens for vaccine development may result from careful study of the *P. falciparum* genome, particularly the identification of conserved sequences expressed on cell surfaces during different stages of parasite development (Hoffman *et al.* 2002). However, as the scientists responsible for the genome sequencing of *P. falciparum* wrote, 'genome sequences alone provide little relief to those suffering from malaria', and much work needs to be done to convert this knowledge into effective control strategies (Gardner *et al.* 2002). Although the malaria genome project focused on a single clone of *P. falciparum*, great genetic diversity is found among parasites from different geographical regions. Improved understanding of the genetic differences among strains will provide insights into transmission patterns, virulence, and drug resistance.

Anopheline mosquito vectors

Of the approximately 400 *Anopheles* species, about 70 are capable of transmitting malaria to humans, but no more than 40 are considered important vectors. Only females transmit malaria and require protein derived from vertebrate blood to produce eggs. There is great variation among anopheline species in host feeding preference, in biting and resting behaviour, and in selection of larval habitat for laying eggs. Some anophelines feed on a variety of vertebrates (zoophilic), whereas others are particular and take blood meals only from one host, for example, humans (anthropophilic). Some feed only indoors (endophagic), whereas others may occasionally or exclusively feed outdoors (exophagic). Whether they rest indoors (endophilic) or outdoors (exophilic) after feeding is critical in understanding transmission and effective approaches to control, specifically indoor residual insecticide spraying. Nearly all anophelines prefer clean water for laying eggs, but some have very specific preferences, e.g. *Anopheles stephensi* breed in tin cans or other confined water spaces, whereas *Anopheles gambiae*, the most important vector in Africa, prefers small, open sunlit pools. Knowledge of these variations is critical for effective vector control.

The mosquito goes through four stages of growth during its life cycle, from egg to larva to pupa and to adult. Shortly after emerging as an adult and before the first blood meal, anopheline females mate. They usually mate only once and store the sperm, laying a total of 200–1000 eggs in 3–12 batches over their lifetime (Russell *et al.* 1963). A fresh blood meal is required for development of each egg batch. After hatching, an anopheline larva feeds at the water's surface and develops over 5–15 days before pupation. Within 2–3 days an adult mosquito emerges from the pupal case. The entire cycle requires a total of 7–20 days, depending upon the anopheline species and the environmental conditions. Under favourable conditions of high humidity and moderate temperatures, female anophelines can survive up to 30 days, time enough for the parasite to develop into sporozoites in the salivary glands for injection with the next blood meal. Thereafter, the mosquito transmits malaria with each human blood meal, taken every 2–3 days for the remainder of its life. Therefore, the longevity of the anopheline mosquito is critically important in determining the efficiency of transmission.

Mosquitoes are able to seek out their host in response to a combination of chemical and physical stimuli, including carbon dioxide, body odours, warmth, and movement. Most anophelines feed at night, but some species may feed in the late afternoon or early morning. During feeding, the mosquito injects salivary fluid containing enzymes that diffuse through the surrounding tissue and increase blood flow, facilitating both the blood meal and transfer of sporozoites to the capillary bed. Anophelines generally feed on people sleeping indoors. Some species, however, bite outdoors, especially those that are forest dwellers, such as *Anopheles dirus*. After feeding, the engorged female seeks a resting place on a nearby wall or in a secluded spot outdoors. Some species change behaviour in the presence of DDT or other insecticides, becoming irritated and fly outside to seek refuge. Engorged mosquitoes usually rest for 24–36 h to digest the blood meal before they search for an oviposition site.

Simultaneous with the publication of the genome sequence of *P. falciparum*, a first draft of the genome sequence of *An. gambiae* was published in 2002 (Holt 2002). Identification of polymorphisms within the *An. gambiae* genome will aid in the detection of insecticide resistance genes (e.g. detoxifying enzymes), genetic factors responsible for transmission efficiency of malaria parasites, and gene flow within mosquito populations. Genetic studies should also lead to a better understanding of the determinants of anopheline behaviours, including mechanisms by which the mosquito identifies human hosts, as well as metabolic targets for insecticide development.

Vectorial capacity and entomological inoculation rate

Understanding the dynamics of transmission is fundamental to understanding how best to reduce transmission through vector control measures. The entomological inoculation rate (EIR) and vectorial capacity (VC) are two basic indices of malaria transmission. These measures are closely related, but it is important to know how they are derived and how they are used. Both are applied to a defined ecological area and both vary greatly in place and time (MacDonald 1957; Molineaux & Gramiccia 1980). The EIR is usually expressed as the average number of infected bites that each person receives per year in a specified population. An EIR of 50 indicates that each person receives on average 50 infective bites in a year—about one each week. It is calculated by multiplying the human landing rate (HLR) by the sporozoite rate (SR). The HLR, previously termed the human biting rate, is obtained by capturing all mosquitoes that land on a person, the 'bait', during a night and is expressed as the number of mosquitoes landing (bites) per person per night. The SR is determined by microscopic examination of dissected salivary glands to detect sporozoites in these captured mosquitoes, expressed as the ratio of infected anophelines to the total collected. The EIR provides a direct measure of malaria transmission and the risk of human exposure to the bites of infected mosquitoes. In contrast to the EIR, the VC measures the rate of *potentially* infective contact, i.e. the potential for malaria transmission, and is based solely on key vector parameters in a particular area (Molineaux & Gramiccia 1980).

It is important to understand the nonlinear relation among these variables (Dye *et al.* 1996). In Fig. 9.15.3, the prevalence of parasitaemia in children age two to nine is charted against the average annual EIR. Note that at low levels of EIR, small increases result in a rapid rise in the prevalence of parasitaemia; thereafter, a long plateau is reached, where large changes in the EIR do not change the level of parasitaemia. This is the situation in most of tropical Africa. In these areas, reduction of several 100- or even a 1000-fold in the EIR will not change the prevalence of malaria (although it may change the frequency and nature of severe malaria). Effective vector control has been possible only in areas with EIRs well under 100; therefore, malaria control for holoendemic areas, as in much of tropical Africa, must involve a 'peaceful' coexistence rather than elimination of malaria.

Geographical areas according to intensity of transmission

Traditionally, geographical patterns of transmission have been classified into four broad categories according to the intensity of transmission and based upon the percentage of children aged two to nine with enlarged spleens and malaria parasites (Molineaux 1988). These are:

1. *Holoendemic:* Areas of intense transmission with continual high EIRs (50–2000+) where virtually everyone is infected with malaria parasites all the time. Classification as above: Splenomegaly and parasitaemia rates of over 75 per cent.

2. *Hyperendemic:* Regions with regular, often seasonal, transmission but where the immunity in some of the population does not confer protection at all times (EIR 10–50). Classification as above: Splenomegaly and parasitaemia from 50 to 75 per cent.

3. *Mesoendemic:* Areas that have malaria transmission fairly regularly but at much lower levels (EIR less than 10 and variable). The danger in these areas is occasional epidemics involving those with little immunity and resulting in fairly high morbidity and mortality. Classification as above: Splenomegaly and parasitaemia from 10 to 50 per cent.

4. *Hypoendemic:* Areas with limited malaria transmission and where the population will have little or no immunity (EIR usually not measurable). These areas can sometimes have severe malaria epidemics involving all age groups. Classification as above: Splenomegaly and parasitaemia less than 10 per cent.

Pathogenesis of malaria

Infection and disease

The distinction between infection and disease is particularly important in malaria. Infection with the malaria parasite does not necessarily result in disease, especially in highly endemic areas with high levels of partial immunity. In these regions, children may have

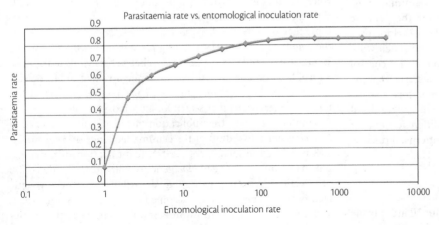

Fig. 9.15.3 Prevalence of parasitaemia in human population and average annual entomological inoculation rate (EIR). See text.

parasitaemia prevalence rates of 50 per cent or more and yet few will have symptoms. Disease is the result of the combination of parasite multiplication and the host reaction to the parasite. The classic description of periodic shaking chills, severe fever and drenching sweats every two or three days can be seen in non-immune adults infected with *P. vivax* (every other day) or *P. malariae* (every third day). The symptoms in these cases result from the host response to synchronous lysis and release of pyrogens from infected red cells. However, with falciparum malaria, clinical manifestations range from asymptomatic parasitaemia to severe overwhelming disease and rapid death. Children may present with drowsiness, coma, convulsions or simply listlessness and fever with nonspecific symptoms. Abdominal cramping, cough, headaches, muscle pains, and varying levels of mental disorientation are common. Severe and complicated malaria due to falciparum malaria is a medical emergency.

Host response

Malaria, on a population basis, is the most intense stimulator of the human immune system known. Many immunologic defence systems are activated in response to malaria infections, including the RE system with enhanced phagocytosis in the spleen, lymph nodes, and liver to remove infected RBCs, an intense production of antibodies and a range of cellular immune responses and cytokine cascades. Some of these responses are protective and others contribute to pathology (and often to both). For example, pro-inflammatory cytokines, severe metabolic acidosis, as well as the classical sequestration of infected RBCs that cause cerebral anoxia may all contribute to the pathogenesis of cerebral malaria; at the same time, the pro-inflammatory response and acidosis evidently account for why some patients survive without neurological complications (Miller *et al.* 2002).

The host response to malaria can go wrong in several ways. For example, the pathogenesis of 'big spleen disease' (tropical splenomegaly) is caused by an excessive and inappropriate host response to malaria. Tropical splenomegaly is fairly common among relatively non-immune populations who, because they move to a malarious area or experience a change in climate, are exposed to more intense transmission. The disease starts in childhood, progressing through adolescence to young adulthood with severe anaemia, high levels of IgM and antimalarial antibodies, a decrease in platelets and a huge spleen. Malaria parasites rarely are detectable. If untreated, tropical splenomegaly is often fatal, usually from a secondary infection, but if treated with long-term antimalarials, the condition regresses.

Malaria parasites have evolved complex mechanisms to evade host immune responses and establish persistent or repeated infections. Understanding the basis of effective immune responses that prevent infection or reduce disease severity is important for vaccine development. Protective immunity following repeated natural infections takes years to develop. However, no immunodominant response has been identified, and an effective immune response likely is the sum of cellular and humoral responses to multiple parasite antigens. Antibodies to the circumsporozoite protein can protect from sporozoite challenge and prevent the binding of sporozoites to liver cells. Cellular immune responses, specifically interferon-γ secreting T cells, are important in killing infected liver cells. Antibodies play a role in killing parasitized red blood cells, though cell-mediated immunity contributes to blood-stage protection as well. The great antigenic variability of *P. falciparum*, as described above, is in large part responsible for the ability of the parasite to evade effective host immune responses.

Differences in disease related to malaria species

The reasons disease resulting from infection with *P. falciparum* can be so severe is due to the rapid development of a heavy parasite load and its capacity to evade effective host defences. Unlike other malaria species, *P. falciparum* invades all forms of RBCs, and more than one parasite can invade the same RBC. A total human body parasite count can be 10^{12}, a 1000-fold greater than any other human malaria species.

P. vivax has the widest geographic distribution of the malaria species that infect humans, although it is absent in West Africa because it requires the Duffy receptor for RBC attachment. The Duffy receptor is not found in West African populations. Different genetic strains give rise to hypnozites with differing relapse times. *P. vivax*, which infects only reticulocytes, has a coordinated 48-h schizont phase leading to classic tertian fever. *P. ovale*, similar to *P. vivax* in that it infects only reticulocytes, also forms hypnozoites. It has a 48-h schizont period but does not require the Duffy receptor. Mainly seen in Africa, *P. ovale* is not a common infection and is often misdiagnosed as *P. vivax*. It can have very long relapse time of up to 5 years. *P. malariae*, the cause of classic quartan fever with a 72-h schizont period, is relatively infrequent but has widespread geographic distribution including all areas where other human malaria species are found. *P. malariae* can only invade older red cells and is thus not a cause of high-density infection. In East Africa, it has been associated with the nephrotic syndrome.

Human genetic factors

As humans, mosquitoes, and malaria parasites have evolved together, many human genetic characteristics that provide partial protection against malaria have emerged. These genetic polymorphisms mostly involve the red blood cell, and include structural variants in the β globin chain of haemoglobin such as sickle-cell trait (haemoglobin S) and haemoglobins C (West Africa) and E (Southeast Asia); altered α and β globin chain production leading to the α and β thalassaemias (Mediterranean anaemia); erythrocyte enzyme deficiencies including glucose-6-phosphate dehydrogenase (G6PD); red cell cytoskeletal abnormalities such as ovalocytosis; and changes in the red cell membrane such as the absence of the Duffy blood group factor (West Africa) (Miller *et al.* 1994). The mechanism that provides protection seems clear for sickle-cell trait—when red cells are invaded, they sickle and are preferentially removed by the RE system thus reducing parasite density levels (Luzatto *et al.* 1970)—but mechanisms have not been fully elucidated for other genetic polymorphisms.

Many polymorphisms exact a heavy burden on the homozygous individual, e.g. haemoglobin SS or sickle cell disease. To account for the frequency of sickle-cell trait (AS) in tropical Africa (16–29 per cent in adults), the historical case fatality ratio due to malaria in children with the AA haemoglobin genotype must have been 10–20 per cent (Morrow 1984).

Undernutrition and micronutrient deficiencies

Malaria is prevalent in regions where childhood malnutrition is common, and nutritional deficiencies interact with malaria infection in complex ways. Early observational studies (Gilles 1957) suggested that undernourished children suffered lower morbidity and mortality than adequately nourished children. These early reports often involved selected groups or were conducted during famine, and re-feeding severely malnourished children may worsen apparent disease severity. However, more recent studies have not confirmed this association with undernutrition *per se*. Pooled analyses of two cohort studies that examined the relationship between underweight and the severity of malaria found that malnourished children were more likely to die from malaria than adequately nourished children (Caulfield *et al.* 2004).

Iron deficiency is the most common micronutrient deficiency, and is associated with defects in immune responses and a number of poor health outcomes. However, early observations suggested that infants with iron deficiency had less severe malaria than children without iron deficiency, and that providing iron supplementation may increase disease severity (Gilles 1957). These observations were confirmed in a meta-analysis of iron supplementation given to children in malarious areas. Pooled analyses indicated a small but significant increase in parasitaemia, and a small but not significant increase in splenomegaly and clinical attack rates, in those given iron (Shankar & Stolfus 1998). However, severe anaemia was reduced by 50 per cent and there was no increase in severe malaria. The authors concluded that the value of iron supplementation outweighed the minor intensification of malaria parasitaemia.

Vitamin A is essential for the proper functioning of the immune system in response to malaria. In contrast to the effects of iron, a trial of vitamin A supplementation in preschool children in Papua New Guinea found that vitamin A reduces clinical episodes of malaria, splenic enlargement and parasite density, particularly in children one to 3 years of age. Extrapolating from this single trial, the fraction of malaria morbidity attributable to vitamin A deficiency was estimated to be 20 per cent worldwide (Caulfield *et al.* 2004). Zinc is another micronutrient that is essential for both cellular and humoral immunity. In randomized trials in Papua New Guinea and The Gambia, zinc supplementation reduced malaria morbidity and mortality (Shankar *et al.* 2000). The fraction of malaria morbidity attributable to zinc deficiency was estimated to be 20 per cent worldwide, similar to that for vitamin A (Caulfield *et al.* 2004).

The diversity of disease due to *Plasmodium falciparum*

Disease due to *P. falciparum* is a major cause of death in children wherever there is a high intensity of infection. Results from community-based intervention studies (Alonso *et al.* 1991) indicate that malaria accounts for nearly half the mortality of children younger than 5 years in high-transmission areas. In hospitals throughout tropical Africa, a large proportion of under-5 admissions and deaths are due to malaria. However, these are a small proportion of malaria cases and deaths in the community. In rural tropical Africa, more than 80 per cent of under-5 deaths occur at home. The pattern of disease as seen in hospitals is determined by access and health seeking behaviour as well as by the nature of the disease and, thus, may not provide a good guide to the pattern of disease in the community.

In high-transmission areas in Africa, severe disease in children does not progress from mild or moderate illness; it strikes abruptly without warning. Mothers are frequently unable to get their infants and young children to a health centre in time to provide treatment before the child dies, even when facilities with trained health workers are readily available. If they do manage to reach a hospital, many die within 24 h of admission despite treatment efforts (Marsh *et al.* 1995; Molyneux *et al.* 1989). Rapid progression to severe disease is not characteristic in areas with less intense transmission. In Southeast Asia, malaria typically progresses gradually in severity over several days in both children and in adults. Early effective treatment before the onset of the severe phase is the key to reducing mortality in these circumstances, an option difficult to achieve with the fulminant African form. Although these gradually progressive types are also seen in Africa, they are less common in intense transmission areas than the rapid severe forms in children.

The three major clinical manifestations of severe malaria are cerebral malaria, pulmonary oedema, and severe anaemia. The classical histopathological picture of cerebral malaria is intense sequestration of infected cells in the cerebral microvasculature (McPherson *et al.* 1985), clinically associated with case-fatality ratios of 10–50 per cent. Cerebral malaria is heterogeneous and includes four overlapping syndromes fulfilling the WHO definition of cerebral malaria with different pathogenic mechanisms: (1) prolonged post-ictal state, characterized as deep sleep, headache, confusion, and muscle soreness; (2) covert status epilepticus, characterized by continual seizures; (3) severe metabolic derangement (particularly with hypoglycaemia and metabolic acidosis); and (4) children with a primary neurological syndrome. Commonly more than one of these situations co-exists. A child may be acidotic, have hypoglycaemia and be in status epilepticus. Recognition and proper management of all three, in addition to treatment of the malaria, is critical (Marsh & Snow 1997).

Pulmonary oedema, often seen with acute respiratory distress syndrome (ARDS), is included in the WHO criteria for severe malaria and has long been recognized as a serious, frequently fatal complication of malaria in non-immune adults (Warrell *et al.* 1990). Respiratory distress *per se* did not appear in the original WHO criteria, but it is a valuable defining characteristic because with minimum training the clinical signs can be applied with good inter-observer consistency. The clinical signs of hyperventilation, driven by efforts to reduce CO_2, are highly sensitive and specific for the diagnosis of respiratory distress (English *et al.* 1996).

The third major clinical manifestation of severe malaria is severe anaemia, which also has a complex pathogenesis and varies considerably geographically, partly due to the extent of interaction with malnutrition and iron deficiency. It tends to be the predominant form in areas of the most intense transmission and is common in the youngest age groups.

Epidemiological features of severe malaria

Though it now seems useful to consider three main severe malaria syndromes as discussed above, most descriptions of severe malaria in African children have focused on differentiating those with severe anaemia from those with cerebral and neurological involvement (Greenwood *et al.* 1991; Molyneux *et al.* 1989). Clear epidemiological differences parallel these distinctive clinical forms of severe malaria. Intensity of transmission varies widely among geographical areas in Africa; with higher intensity, the proportion of those with severe malaria as compared to non-severe shifts to younger age groups. Because of earlier development of immunity among children who survive, the proportion with asymptomatic malaria among those with malaria infection is shifted to younger ages. In areas with the most intense transmission, severe malaria and death is restricted largely to children younger than 5 years, and most clinical disease is seen in the younger age groups (Molineaux 1996).

In holoendemic areas in Africa, about the same proportion of under-5 children will have severe malaria, but within any endemic area, the type of severe morbidity varies with age. Severe anaemia predominates in younger children (median age, 15–24 months), whereas coma is more common in older children (median age, 36–48 months). Among holoendemic areas with different levels of transmission intensity, there may be a marked difference in the relative importance of different clinical syndromes. An additional factor that apparently affects the nature of severe malaria in a population is the constancy of transmission. An area of intense perennial transmission has a higher incidence of severe anaemia, whereas an area with intense seasonal transmission has a higher rate of cerebral malaria (Marsh *et al.* 1996).

Malaria in pregnancy

Women infected with malaria while pregnant are at much greater risk of serious consequences than women who are not pregnant (or than men). Host defence mechanisms are much dampened during and for several weeks post pregnancy with reductions in both cell-mediated and humoral responses (Brabin 1991). In all areas endemic for malaria, pregnant women are more likely to be bitten by malaria vectors. This increased risk of bites is related to the higher metabolic rate during pregnancy which increases body temperature and CO_2 release, both of which are attractants for mosquitoes. Pregnant women are also more likely to develop severe, complicated malaria and die than non-pregnant women. Adverse outcomes of their pregnancies are also higher, related to active malarial infection of the placenta (Nosten *et al.* 2004).

The maternal mortality ratio (MMR) for pregnant women infected with malaria ranges from 100 to over 1000 per 100 000 and relative risks for maternal mortality for women with malaria as compared to those without range from two to tenfold. The MMR is as high in low-transmission areas as it is in high transmission, but the nature of the complications and those at greatest risk are different. In low-transmission areas, pregnant women across the spectrum of parity die from severe, complicated malaria, particularly with cerebral symptoms, hypoglycaemia and acute respiratory distress syndrome. MMRs of up to 1000 per 100 000 live births are reported during malaria epidemics in low-transmission areas. In areas of high transmission, the risk of severe disease and death is mainly among women in their first pregnancy (over 1000 per 100 000 MMR) even though they had acquired a high level of immunity prior to their pregnancy; mortality is mainly related to severe anaemia (Steketee *et al.* 2001).

Pregnant women with malaria have a higher rate of low-weight birth infants and of stillbirths than those without malaria. The proportion of low-birth-weight (LBW) infants is elevated in both low- and high-transmission areas, but the reasons for the low weight may be different. Pre-term delivery is common in low-transmission areas especially in association with acute febrile episodes due to malaria in the third trimester, whereas in high-transmission areas there is fetal growth retardation associated with chronic placental inflammatory damage throughout pregnancy.

Malaria and HIV infection

Especially in Africa, the MMR has actually increased in the last decade in concert with the emergence of drug-resistant *P. falciparum* and the HIV epidemic. HIV infection impairs the ability of pregnant women to control parasitaemia and shifts the usual gravidity-specific pattern of malaria burden from the primigravidae to all pregnant women (ter Kuile *et al.* 2004). Where severe anaemia from malaria requires blood transfusion, the dangers of HIV and hepatitis B virus transmission are added risks to the consequences of malaria.

Early investigations concluded that there were no significant interactions between HIV and malaria co-infection, with the exception of malaria in HIV-infected pregnant women. Subsequently, HIV-infected Ugandan adults were observed to have twice as many episodes of symptomatic parasitaemia than HIV-uninfected adults, and the parasite density and clinical signs and symptoms were correlated with the degree of immunosuppression (Whitworth *et al.* 2000). In Malawi, plasma HIV-1 RNA levels in adults were almost twice as high during periods of malaria parasitaemia (Kublin *et al.* 2005) but resolved within a few weeks after antimalarial treatment, suggesting malaria may enhance HIV disease progression and aid HIV transmission. Few studies have investigated malaria in HIV-infected children, the age group at greatest risk of morbidity and mortality due to malaria. These studies suggest malaria may be more severe and less responsive to therapy in HIV-infected children and that malaria may adversely affect HIV disease progression.

Human activities and the epidemiology of malaria

Human activities, particularly at the population level, but also at the individual behavioural level, strongly influence the epidemiological pattern of malaria and the efforts to control it. Agricultural development, population movement and urbanization are important determinants of the pattern of malaria transmission. Malaria has long been linked to farming practices. In sub-Saharan Africa, the clearing of forest for crop production has increased breeding of *An. gambiae*, the most efficient vector of human malaria, which prefers sunlit open pools of standing water to the full shade of tropical forest. The formation of small towns, dams and irrigation schemes arising in concert with agricultural development in much of Africa has concentrated populations of humans and vectors in relatively confined areas near water supplies. Additionally, agricultural use of pesticides has been a major factor in the development and spread of insecticide-resistant vectors. Thus, the very efforts to promote economic development and improve human conditions have increased the intensity of malaria transmission.

Population movements throughout Africa have contributed toward an increased intensity of malaria transmission. Traditionally, in many parts of Africa seasonal migration has been a part of life with people moving from their village settlements to rural farms during the early months of the wet season when cultivation, planting and weeding are carried out. Often intensity of transmission is much higher in these areas than in their settled home villages where water supplies are controlled. In a similar way, many pastoral Africans are exposed to higher transmission as they move their livestock between highlands and lowland pastures with the seasons. Other reasons for population movement are related to population expansion, with movement into previously unoccupied and more marginally productive areas. The living and working conditions in these areas often result in greater exposure to malaria vectors. Africa has been especially afflicted with drought, famine, war and political upheavals resulting in mass population displacement and refugee movements, all of which are frequently associated with increased malaria transmission. These groups frequently are poorly served by government health and malaria control programmes, and have less access to antimalarials and other aspects of health care. Disasters and conflicts, so prominent in Africa for decades, greatly contribute to the transmission of malaria and hinder malaria control efforts.

Approximately one-third of malaria deaths in sub-Saharan Africa occur in countries affected by complex emergencies. Factors facilitating malaria mortality in complex emergencies include migration of non-immune people to hyperendemic areas, overcrowding, interruption of vector control programmes and inadequate access to health care (Connolly et al. 2004). Multiple interventions, including provision of shelter, vector control, case management and surveillance, are required for malaria control in complex emergencies. Insecticide-treated plastic sheeting used for shelter may be an effective means of vector control in complex emergencies.

In contrast to the types of population movement described above, the major secular migrations to urban areas throughout Africa generally have little influence on malaria transmission. Although malaria in Africa is principally a rural rather than an urban disease, some anopheline species have come to be well adapted to city life. For example, An. arabiensis has become a transmitter of malaria in many cities of Nigeria (Oaks et al. 1991). Generally, this vector is restricted to semi-urban slum areas rather than the highly concentrated population areas in urban centres.

Although malaria can infect and cause severe disease in anyone, it is principally a disease of the poor and uninformed. Loss of healthy life due to malaria is much higher in poor rural areas of Africa than in the better-developed urban areas. Some notion of the difference in impact on different social groups can be seen in the studies by Oduntan (1974) in Nigeria, who found that the sickle-trait rate amongst elite school children in Ibadan was under 20 per cent whereas in rural children of the same age not attending school, the AS rate was 26.3 per cent. To account for this marked differential, the mortality rate due to malaria among those with AA haemoglobin in the poor must be many times greater than that in the elite who would have had better nutrition and access to health services. If one assumes that at birth the distributions of AA, AS, and SS genotypes were the same, and that none of the elite with AA died by school age, then 30 per cent of those with AA in the non-elite would have died from malaria. However, with the strong tendency for social classes to intermarry, it is likely that the genotype distributions would not have been the same and that at least some of this marked differential could be attributed to lower malaria mortality and less benefit from AS in the last generation or two among the elite. The interplay between environmental factors (malaria) and genetics (haemoglobin genotypes) ensures that sickle-trait rate will continue to be reduced among the better off in whom the balanced polymorphism from selective protection for sickle-trait no longer holds. The dramatic differential in mortality from malaria by social class provides clear evidence that malaria control efforts should contribute to improved equity of health status.

Individual and community behaviour are important factors influencing the population effects discussed above and are crucial in determining the success of malaria control. In Africa, there is great diversity in cultures and community structures. Understanding and acting in accord with the prevailing belief systems are essential; otherwise these beliefs may serve as barriers to adoption of effective interventions. Health-seeking behaviour, key for obtaining timely treatment, depends upon understanding the need for treatment; thus people's perceptions of malaria and its causes are very important.

Even in communities that have an appreciation of the importance of malaria and the need to obtain appropriate treatment, the symptoms of cerebral malaria may be misunderstood because it produces convulsions and confusion. People frequently do not recognize these as signs for urgent treatment for malaria; indeed such symptoms often are attributed to belief of supernatural causes, not something that modern medicine can affect, and the advice of traditional healers is often sought (Winch et al. 1996; Tarimo et al. 2000).

Travel to endemic regions for many reasons continues to escalate; tourism, business matters, military movements, migration to escape from natural or man-made disasters—all expose non-immune populations to malaria and account for an increasing source of malaria cases and potential for the spread of drug resistant malaria strains particularly with the diversity of advice about antimalarials given to travellers. In fact, the CDC (Centers for Disease Control and Prevention, http://www2.ncid.cdc.gov/travel/yb/utils/ybGet.asp?section=dis&obj=index.htm) provides excellent, detailed, and up-to-date information about all malaria risk areas, approaches to personal protection, a checklist for travellers to malarious areas, drugs to take and their adverse reactions with special notes about drug resistant malaria, about relapses following P. vivax and P. ovale infection, and important details concerning children and pregnant women.

Diagnosis of malaria

A definitive diagnosis of malaria is made by demonstration of parasites in red blood cells. The standard technique is microscopic examination of a Giemsa stained thick and thin smear of blood on glass microscope slides. This technique will likely remain the gold standard. The thick smear is the more sensitive method for the detection of parasites. With thin films, skilled technicians can determine not only the species of malaria, but also can obtain reliable estimates of the number of parasites (parasite density). The ability to detect parasites depends on the number of fields examined and the experience of the technician viewing the slide.

Although this approach continues as standard, there are numerous problems of practical implementation and of interpretation. At the practical level, work is tedious and demanding, and rigorous maintenance of equipment and staining materials is critical. Quality control and good morale among the technicians are essential. The problems of interpretation of blood smears are twofold. First, peripheral smears may be falsely negative before red blood cells are infected and later during schizogony when infected red blood cells are sequestered in the capillary beds. Second, the peripheral smear may be 'falsely' positive in the sense that the presence of parasites in a febrile patient in an endemic area does not necessarily mean that the symptoms are due to malaria. Most children in holoendemic areas have malaria parasites all the time. In this situation there is no satisfactory approach to diagnosing clinical disease: Patients are presumptively treated based on clinical symptoms alone and any child with fever is given antimalarials (Nicoll 2000). Such an approach may be necessary to provide early treatment to young children with severe malaria, but it also can result in serious over use of antimalarials with the high cost, increased risk of adverse reactions, and in missed diagnosis of other serious causes of fever such as bacterial pneumonia and meningitis.

Many efforts have been expended to develop rapid methods of diagnosis that do not involve the demanding discipline and technical skills of microscopic examination of blood smears. A variety of immunochromatographic assays have been developed that detect different malaria antigens, including histidine-rich protein 2 (HRP2) and lactate deydrogenase (LDH) (Murray *et al.* 2003). These rapid diagnostic tests have been designed for use as dipsticks, and are easy to use in health centres without equipment and with minimal training. Trials of a dipstick assay based upon antigen capture of HRP2 antigen (ParaSight-F test) showed high sensitivity and specificity with moderate parasite densities, but reduced sensitivity at lower parasite densities (Moody 2002). The need for simple, inexpensive and rapid diagnostic tests for malaria is of increasing importance as countries in Africa shift from low-cost antimalarials (chloroquine, sulphadoxine/pyrimethamine) to more expensive combination regimens (artemisinin-based combination therapy) in the face of widespread drug resistance.

Although not appropriate for the diagnosis of malaria in endemic areas, the use of polymerase chain reaction (PCR)-based assays can provide high sensitivity in persons with low-level parasitaemia. These molecular diagnostic tools can distinguish infections with multiple *Plasmodia* species and can provide quantitative measures using real-time PCR that may prove useful in following responses to treatment (de Monbrison *et al.* 2003). PCR-based genotyping is valuable in the analysis of malaria parasites in drug efficacy trials by distinguishing recrudescences from new re-infections. Molecular epidemiology also assists in analysing parasite populations during and after vaccine trials and changes in parasite populations resulting from vector control or environmental alterations.

Treatment of malaria

Antimalarial drugs

The history of drug treatment of malaria goes back hundreds of years: Cinchona bark used by Peruvian healers for generations and extracts of wormwood used in China for centuries. Quinine is the active ingredient in cinchona bark and continues as an important therapeutic agent for drug-resistant falciparum malaria (Bruce-Chwatt 1988; Russell *et al.* 1963). A family of highly effective antimalarials, the artemisinins, was derived from wormwood and is coming into widespread use in combination with other antimalarials for drug-resistant malaria. During the World War II, several compounds were found to be highly effective against malaria, including chloroquine, primaquine and sulphadoxine-pyrimethamine.

Chloroquine is rapidly absorbed after oral administration and is active against the asexual stages of all human species except for strains of *P. falciparum* that have become resistant. Chloroquine interferes with the degradation of haeme in the parasite, allowing the accumulation of toxic metabolic products that kill the parasite within the red blood cell. It is well tolerated even when taken for long periods, and is safe for young children and pregnant women. The only important adverse reaction of chloroquine taken in doses recommended for antimalaria treatment or prophylaxis is intense pruritis reported uniquely but frequently by black Africans. However, long-term, high-dosage chloroquine treatment as used for rheumatology patients can lead to irreversible visual loss from chloroquine-induced retinopathy (Taylor & White 2004). Because of its effectiveness, low cost, and low toxicity, chloroquine was the drug-of-choice to treat malaria for decades following World War II. Only after parasite resistance to chloroquine was demonstrated were serious efforts focused on developing alternative antimalarials.

Primaquine is the only drug effective against both sporozoites and the hepatic forms, and can be used to prevent infection in the liver (referred to as a 'causal' prophylaxis) and to eliminate the hypnozoite stages of *P. vivax* and *P. ovale* that lead to relapse (anti-relapse treatment) (Wernsdorfer 1994). It is also effective in eliminating gametocytes, and could play a role in reducing transmission and preventing the spread of drug-resistant strains. Primaquine causes hemolysis in persons with glucose-6-phosphate dehydrogenase (G6PD) deficiency, common in those of African and Mediterranean descent.

Sulphadoxine-pyrimethamine (Fansidar, SP), originally developed for its efficacy against chloroquine-resistant *P. falciparum*, has been widely used for treatment to replace chloroquine in areas of drug-resistance. Both sulphadoxine and pyrimethamine inhibit enzymes in the folic acid synthesis pathway. Because it is single-dose therapy and inexpensive, SP has been widely used in Africa to treat malaria, was the preferred antimalarial for pregnant women and can be used for intermittent prophylactic treatment of young children. Adverse reactions, including Stevens-Johnson syndrome, have been reported when SP is used for prophylaxis. Now combination regimens with artemisinins as discussed below are recommended.

Mefloquine, a synthetic compound structurally related to quinine and quinidine, was developed for its activity against chloroquine-resistant *P. falciparum* in the late 1960s. Mefloquine has an unusually long half-life, is used for chemoprophylaxis and for treatment in combination with artesunate in Thailand. However, resistance to mefloquine has emerged in southeast Asia, and frequent reports of adverse mental and emotional disturbances have led to reduction in its use.

Artemisinin and related compounds (e.g. artesunate, arthemether), the active agent of the Chinese herbal medicine, are metabolized to the active form, dihydroartemisinin, and act by inhibiting the calcium pumping enzyme *P. falciparum* ATP6. These drugs quickly clear blood stage parasites and gametocytes and provide a rapid clinical response reducing the risk of severe malaria. Importantly, resistance to artemisinins has not been observed yet. The major disadvantages are high cost and, related to high demand, serious problems of availability. A minor disadvantage as compared with SP is the need for a 3-day regimen.

The most significant change in the treatment of malaria has not been the introduction of novel antimalarials but the use of older drugs in combination. Because of rapid and widespread emergence of resistant parasites in Southeast Asia, combination therapy, particularly of artesunate and mefloquine, has been used there for many years. With the spread of drug resistance through out the world, combination therapy is now universally recommended. Many combinations of antimalarials without artemisinin have been used, but the most widely recommended combinations include an artemisinin, referred to as artemisinin-based combination therapy (ACT). Examples include artemether/lumefantrine, artesunate/amodiaquine, and artesunate/mefloquine.

Antimalarial drug resistance

The emergence and spread of drug resistant malaria, particularly of chloroquine and sulphadoxine-pyrimethamine resistant *P. falciparum*, is of major public health importance and likely responsible for the doubling of child mortality attributable to malaria in parts of Africa (White 2004). These once highly effective, affordable, and safe drugs are no longer useful in many malaria endemic regions, forcing countries to switch to more expensive artemisinin-based combination therapies. Resistance to more recently introduced antimalarials, such as mefloquine and atovaquone, developed quickly, and many experts believe it is only a matter of time before resistance develops to artemisinins. The emergence of drug resistance to the artemisinins may be delayed because of their short half-life and ability to reduce gametocyte carriage. Antimalarial drug resistance is largely a problem with *P. falciparum* infection, although chloroquine-resistant *P. vivax* is prevalent in Papua New Guinea and Irian Jaya. Clinically-relevant drug resistance in *P. malariae* and *P. ovale* has not been documented (Wongsrichanalai *et al.* 2002).

Many factors contribute to the emergence and spread of antimalarial drug resistance, including pharmacologic properties of the drug, host immunity, parasite genetics, and transmission characteristics. For example, use of antimalarials with a prolonged half-life (such as sulphadoxine-pyrimethamine), poor compliance or inappropriate use can expose parasites to sub-therapeutic drug levels, thus increasing the risk of emergence of drug-resistant parasites. An effective host immune response can clear drug-resistant parasites that escape being killed, making the transmission of drug resistance more likely in immunologically naïve hosts (Wongsrichanalai *et al.* 2002).

Antimalarial drug resistance can be assessed in several ways, including evaluation of therapeutic responses *in vivo*, measurement of parasite growth *ex vivo*, and identification of genetic mutations associated with resistance. However, there is great need for a rapid, simple and inexpensive field test to detect antimalarial drug resistance.

The traditional method of *in vivo* resistance testing was developed by the WHO (Wernsdorfer 1994). Infected patients are given an antimalarial drug according to an established regime, and parasite counts are performed at the start of therapy, at 24 h, at 7 days, and at 28 days after the start of treatment. If parasites are not detectable at the end of 7 days (and still not detectable at 28 days), the malaria parasites are considered sensitive to the drug. If there is clearance of parasites at 7 days, but recrudescence 8 or more days after the start of treatment, the parasites are stage RI resistant. If there is reduction in parasitaemia but not complete clearance at 7 days, the parasites are considered stage RII resistant. If there is no evidence of response, the parasites are considered to be fully resistant, RIII.

In the absence of molecular epidemiologic tools distinguishing recrudescence from re-infection (new inoculation) by parasite counts is not possible. To overcome this limitation in regions of intense transmission, WHO introduced a modified protocol based on clinical response rather than parasitaemia. The results are categorized as an adequate clinical response (sensitive), a late treatment failure (partial resistance), or an early treatment failure (fully resistant). A limitation in interpreting *in vivo* testing is that persons with immunity will clinically improve even if the parasites are moderately resistant to the drug.

In vitro testing of *P. falciparum* drug resistance relies on short-term culture of malaria parasites. Blood from a parasitaemic individual is prepared for culture and incubated with increasing concentrations of an antimalarial drug. Several assay endpoints have been developed to measure parasite growth in the presence of different drug concentrations, including schizont maturation, radioisotope incorporation, and detection of the parasite enzyme LDH or HRP2 (Noedl *et al.* 2003). The advantages of *in vitro* resistance testing are that these assays are independent of individual variation in drug levels and immune responses.

Genetic polymorphisms are associated with drug resistance and are best characterized for chloroquine and sulphadoxine-pyrimethamine resistance. Chloroquine resistance is associated with mutations in the *pfcrt* gene that codes for a membrane transporter protein that allows the parasite to excrete chloroquine so that intracellular concentrations do not reach toxic levels. One particular mutation, the substitution of threonine for lysine in codon 76 (T76), is highly associated with chloroquine resistance. More is known about the mutations that decrease the binding affinity of *P. falciparum* enzymes to sulphadoxine-pyrimethamine. At least five different point mutations in the gene encoding the enzyme dihydropteroate synthetase (*dhps*) confer resistance to sulphadoxine. Resistance to pyrimethimine is due to specific point mutations in the gene encoding dihydrofolate reductase (*dhfr*). Accumulation of three or four mutations confers high-level resistance to pyrimethamine. Mutations in the *pfmdr1* gene are associated with resistance to mefloquine, chloroquine, and other antimalarials (Reed *et al.* 2000).

Although not feasible for case management, identification of these polymorphisms in clinical isolates is a useful but expensive tool for monitoring drug resistance in populations. However, the identification of specific mutations does not always correlate with *in vivo* drug resistance. For example, the presence of the Th76 mutation in the *pfcrt* gene predicted only a third of treatment failures, although the absence of this mutation was highly predictive of chloroquine susceptibility (Djimde *et al.* 2001).

Epidemiology of drug resistance in malaria

Chloroquine resistance in *P. falciparum* was first reported in the late 1950s in South America in areas between Venezuela and Colombia, and in Southeast Asia along the borders between Thailand and Cambodia and between Thailand and Burma (Maberti 1960; Harinasuta *et al.* 1962). Although it was nearly 20 years later that resistance was first demonstrated in Africa, chloroquine-resistant malaria is now widespread in Africa. Only in Central America and the Caribbean has chloroquine resistance not yet been documented.

P. falciparum was first noted to be resistant to sulphadoxine-pyrimethamine along the Thai–Cambodian border in the mid-1960s. In Africa, resistance to sulphadoxine-pyrimethamine was first noted in the late 1980s, with high-level resistance and treatment failures most common in east Africa. Mefloquine resistance also was first observed near the Thai–Cambodian border, in the late 1980s.

The origins and mechanisms of spread of drug resistant strains of *P. falciparum* are of great public health importance. Chloroquine resistance is conferred by a complex set of genetic mutations, making multiple independent origins unlikely. Resistance to chloroquine appears to have originated only four times, and to have spread from Asia to Africa (Wootton *et al.* 2002). Because of the less complex nature of resistance to sulphadoxine-pyrimethamine, and the ease in which resistance mutations can be induced in the laboratory, resistance to sulphadoxine-pyrimethamine was thought to have multiple, independent origins. However, genotyping of microsatellite markers flanking the *dhfr* gene suggests that high-level resistance to sulphadoxine-pyrimethamine (i.e. triple or quadruple mutant *dhfr* alleles) originated in Southeast Asia and subsequently spread to Africa (Roper *et al.* 2004).

Of considerable debate is whether drug resistance evolves faster in areas of high or low malaria transmission (Hastings 2003; Mharakurwa 2004). This question has important public health implications, as interventions to reduce transmission could impact rates of drug resistance. Lower transmission was hypothesized to increase rates of drug resistance by enhancing parasite inbreeding, thus lowering the rate of genetic recombination and increasing the probability that drug resistance mutations would spread in the parasite population. Inbreeding is more frequent when transmission rates are lower as infection with multiple different strains is less likely. The frequent emergence of resistance along the Thai–Cambodian border supports the hypothesis that lower transmission facilitates the emergence of drug resistance. However, the true situation is more complex than this simple analysis suggests (Hastings 2003). Reduced transmission in Zimbabwe through residual insecticide spraying of households was associated with suppressed levels of drug resistance, suggesting that malaria control measures that reduce transmission will not increase drug resistance.

Vaccines against malaria

Prospects for a successful vaccine against malaria have been considered bright for several decades; unfortunately, they have remained prospects and to date no vaccine has been sufficiently effective to warrant widespread use. However, progress has been made. Vaccine development has largely focused on *P. falciparum*, although efforts have been made to develop vaccines against *P. vivax*. The overwhelming evidence that humans develop protective immune responses against *P. falciparum* when repeatedly exposed to infection indicates that development of an effective vaccine should be possible. By the age of 6 years, most children in holoendemic regions have acquired substantial immunity. These children are protected from severe and fatal malaria, even though they may have parasitaemia and occasional bouts of fever. The population will have paid a high price for this protection, however, since under-5 mortality from malaria is very high. Early studies by Ian McGregor *et al.* (1963) demonstrated that serum from immune adults in the Gambia could be used to treat young children with malaria in East Africa. In the early 1970s, David Clyde and others demonstrated that injection of sporozoites derived from irradiated *P. falciparum*-infected mosquitoes provided protective immunity against challenge (Clyde *et al.* 1975). However, the immunologic basis of protection induced by natural infection or irradiated sporozoites is not completely understood.

In addition to the empirical evidence for an effective acquired immune response, important advances have taken place in sequencing the genomes of *P. falciparum*, the *An. gambiae* vector and the human host, with hopes that genomics and proteomics will spur novel vaccine development. In addition, progress has been made in understanding the immunology and pathogenesis of malaria, and advances have been made in vaccinology. Sub-unit vaccines composed of synthetic peptides or recombinant proteins, newer vaccine strategies (e.g. prime-boost and the targeting of dendritic cells), and novel adjuvants and protein conjugates, give hope that the formidable impediments to malaria vaccine development will be overcome.

Several high-risk groups would greatly benefit from a malaria vaccine that decreases morbidity and mortality, including young children and primagravida women in endemic areas. In addition, immunologically naïve travellers to malaria endemic regions would benefit from a vaccine that prevents infection. These different risk groups necessitate different types of vaccine. The different stages of the malaria parasite outlined in Fig. 9.15.2 provide potential targets for immunization. Vaccine development has focused largely upon three parasite stages: (1) pre-erythrocytic sporozoite and hepatic forms to prevent infection; (2) asexual erythrocytic forms to reduce morbidity and mortality; and (3) sexual forms within the mosquito to prevent transmission. By the end of 2006, over 100 malaria vaccine candidates were in various stages of development, with many in clinical trials in humans. Table 9.15.2 outlines malaria vaccine strategies according to the strategy for protection, the stage in the malaria life cycle with presumed time period of exposure, and the target antigens with examples of vaccine candidates.

Much effort has gone into development of sporozoite vaccines because immunity was induced by immunization with irradiated sporozoites (Clyde *et al.* 1975), even though there is little evidence of effective natural immunity to sporozoites. A single sporozoite that evades the immune response could potentially generate thousands of merozoites capable of infecting red blood cells. Efforts to develop a pre-erythrocytic vaccine have focused largely on targeting the circumsporozoite (CS) protein, a major component of the sporozoite surface. One of the more promising CS vaccines, RTS,S/AS02A, consists of recombinantly expressed *P. falciparum* CS peptides fused to a portion of the hepatitis B virus surface antigen and administered with an adjuvant (AS02A). In a much publicized clinical trial, both the first clinical episode of malaria and episodes of severe malaria were reduced in Mozambican children for 6 months following vaccination (Alonso *et al.* 2004). However, protective efficacy for the first clinical episode of malaria was only 30 per cent and antibody titres decayed rapidly. In addition to this subunit vaccine,

Table 9.15.2 Malaria vaccine strategies

Vaccine strategy	Stage in malaria life cycle	Vaccine targets (examples)
Prevent infection by killing sporozoites	Sporozoite Intra-vascular (3–5 minutes)	Sporozoite antigens (CSP)
or	⇓	
Prevent infection by killing liver stage parasites	Liver stage Intra-hepatocytic (1–2 weeks)	Liver stage antigens (LSA1)
	⇓	
Prevent disease by targeting infected red blood cells	Asexual blood stage Intra-erythrocytic (2+ day cycle)	Merozoite antigens (MSP-1, AMA-1) Schizont antigens (PEMP-1)
	⇓	
Prevent transmission by targeting gametocytes	Sexual blood stage	Gametocyte antigens (Pfs 45/48)
or	⇓	
Prevent transmission by targeting sexual stages within the mosquito	Anopheles mosquito Intra-mosquito mostly (10–14 days)	Sexual stage antigens (Pfs 25/28)

CSP = circumsporozoite protein
LSA = liver stage antigen
MSP = merozoite surface protein
AMA = apical merozoite antigen
Pfs = antigen on *Plasmodium falciparum* sexual stages
PfEMP = *Plasmodium falciparum* erythrocyte membrane protein

other vaccine constructs targeting the pre-erythrocytic stages include using viral vectors or plasmid DNA to express recombinant CS, thrombospondin-related adhesion protein (TRAP) or liver-stage antigen (LSA). Other approaches include the pursuit of a radiation-attenuated sporozoite vaccine and vaccines based on genetically modified sporozoites (Mueller et al. 2005). Vaccines against asexual blood stages of P. falciparum would seem a promising approach, as passive transfer of immunity has been shown with anti-merozoite immunoglobulin (McGregor et al. 1963). However, as described above, the P. falciparum genome contains a number of highly polymorphic gene families, most importantly the var genes encoding the surface protein PfEMP1 that allows successive waves of parasites to express new variant surface antigens. Antibodies directed against these variable surface proteins are unlikely to remain effective for long; however, protective immunity apparently can be established against a limited number of conserved surface antigens (Gratepanche et al. 2003). Children surviving repeated malaria eventually mobilize a sufficiently diverse set of antibodies to protect against severe disease. In holoendemic Africa, where the entomological inoculation rate may be hundreds a year, protective immunity takes place over several years, representing thousands of inoculated parasites. The hope is to develop a vaccine that can induce similar levels of immunity by age 6 months rather than 6 years. Most current vaccine candidates against blood-stage parasites are directed toward merozoite surface proteins (e.g. MSP-1) or apical membrane antigens (e.g. AMA).

Finally, substantial work has been done on vaccines directed against gametocytes that block parasite development within the mosquito, termed 'transmission blocking' vaccines. These vaccines represent an interesting approach in that the vaccine does not protect the vaccinated individual but would reduce transmission from those who are infected, analogous to the use of residual insecticides in households. Preclinical studies have demonstrated that antibodies against sexual stage antigens expressed by P. vivax and P. falciparum can prevent the development of infectious sporozoites in the mosquito salivary gland. Actual interruption of malaria transmission in communities, however, would require sustained high levels of vaccine coverage.

Approaches to control

The malaria transmission cycle illustrated in Fig. 9.15.2 displays many opportunities for stopping or slowing transmission of malaria parasites between vectors and human hosts. Additionally many opportunities exist for altering the course of disease in humans as discussed in the section on Pathogenesis. In this section we review a wide range of malaria control methods. Selection of the most cost-effective set of methods is highly place and time dependent. Detailed knowledge of the ecological and epidemiological circumstances, and of the human economic, cultural, and social situation, is as vital for determining how best to intervene as are the specifics of the vector, parasite, and intervention tool itself.

Vector control methods

The array of vector control methods is based on attacking the mosquito in various stages of its life cycle: Control of breeding sites to reduce vector density by drainage and waterway engineering and application of specific larvacides and biological agents; the use of mosquito netting, screens, and repellents for personal protection

from bites; aerosol distribution of insecticides to reduce adult mosquito densities; killing adult mosquitoes after they have taken a blood meal by use of residual insecticides within households; and the development of insecticide-impregnated bed nets and curtains that kill or reduce those adults seeking a blood meal.

Breeding site and larva control

After the discovery of the role of mosquito vectors, efforts were directed towards elimination or reduction of vector breeding sites by swamp drainage and environmental control, including water source diversion, water management with flushing and sluicing, covering of wells, clearing vegetation, and reforestation. DDT, other insecticides, and larvacides added further breeding site control methods, particularly in urban settings. In addition to these engineering and insecticide approaches, biological control of breeding sites include larva predators such as larvivorous fish and anti-larval toxins produced by bacteria such as B. thuringensis, can be selectively used. Reduction of breeding sites continue to play a major role in malaria control strategies.

Adult vector control

The use of DDT for household residual spraying had great impact on malaria control in many areas of the world, and its initial successes served as the rationale for the eradication efforts in the 1950s and 1960s. The conceptual foundation for eradication through use of residual insecticides was based upon anopheline resting behaviour after a blood meal. The success of this approach depends upon the biting and resting behaviour of the mosquito and upon the willingness of the human population to have their households sprayed. The effect is upon the mosquito that has already bitten an infected human in the household and rests nearby after engorgement. No protection is provided to those in the treated household itself. Instead, the protection is to those in other households whom these mosquitoes would have bitten for their next blood meal. The dilemma is that to reduce transmission, almost all households in the neighbourhood must be sprayed. The higher the intensity of transmission the more difficult it is to achieve a sufficient level of coverage. Success with residual household spraying was achieved in large areas of Europe, Asia and Latin America, but in areas with EIRs of dozens or more per year as in much of tropical Africa, control by residual spraying alone is not possible.

Where residual spaying with DDT was successful, however, other obstacles to its use arose: Anopheline resistance to DDT became widespread and DDT was widely restricted from use because of its deleterious ecological effects. The root problem was its widespread use in agriculture that led to anopheline resistance. Although other insecticides were substituted for malaria control, they were generally difficult to formulate for residual spraying and were much more expensive and toxic to humans and other mammals. Actually, residual spraying of DDT for malaria control requires minute amounts that are absorbed by the wall material and fully contained indoors. Because of this, anti-malaria use of DDT is not a factor in the development of anopheline resistance or in the devastation of bird populations by DDT thinning of eggshells. But the ecological effects from agricultural use led to major restrictions and, in many countries, complete banning of DDT for any use. As production dropped, the cost of DDT increased. Sadly, these restrictions and their economic consequences adversely affected antimalarial residual spraying programmes, curtailing an effective public health tool. Nevertheless, the use of household residual insecticides, even DDT in some countries, continues as an important vector control measure in many countries.

Insecticide-treated bednets

In the last 10 years, increasing experience with insecticide-treated bed nets (ITNs) demonstrated that their use leads to reductions in transmission, clinical disease, and overall childhood mortality (Binka *et al.* 1996; Nevill *et al.* 1996). Although not all studies demonstrated positive benefits (D'Alessandro *et al.* 1997) and there were major concerns about adequate coverage and sustainability, further work in western Kenya confirmed the value of ITNs in reducing all-cause post-neonatal mortality, maternal mortality, stillbirths and prematurity, and all-cause hospital admissions in a cost-effective manner (Nahlen *et al.* 2003). The three key determinants of effectiveness were coverage (proportion of households with ITNs), adherence (the proportion of individuals properly deploying ITNs each night), and net treatment care (the proportion of nets properly treated with insecticide). These three determinants can serve as the foundation for implementation of national ITN programmes (Hawley *et al.* 2003).

Treatment strategies

Passive case finding and treatment

In tropical Africa, anti-malaria programmes have focused on the use of antimalarial drugs in passive case finding and treatment of those who present to clinics or pharmacies with symptoms of malaria (Buck 1986). Health workers in Africa are taught about the major symptoms of malaria and the need to treat it promptly with an appropriate antimalarial drug and treatment of malaria in childhood is accorded a prominent place in the Integrated Management of Childhood Illnesses (IMCI).

Unfortunately, severe malaria kills children so rapidly in most of Africa that often mothers cannot get their children to facility-based treatment in time. An effective case-treatment strategy for reducing under-5 mortality must include community mobilization and education for families, particularly for the mother or caretaker, to understand the urgency to obtain treatment of their sick child. The range of IMCI activities now extend beyond the health facility to include critical family and community aspects, but so far there has been little impact in reducing under-5 mortality from malaria.

Home treatment

A relatively untried strategy for timely provision of antimalarial drugs is to teach mothers to recognize symptoms of malaria in their children and to treat immediately at home. If mothers are taught to recognize and promptly treat their children and have an appropriate antimalarial supply immediately at hand, many children could be saved in high-transmission areas who are dying under current health care conditions. This approach was tested in a randomized trial in Tigray, Ethiopia. Village-based mother coordinators (MCs) received training and supervision to teach neighbouring mothers to recognize symptoms of malaria in their children and to promptly administer the antimalarial. Overall, under-5 mortality was reduced by 40 per cent at very low cost (Kidane & Morrow 2000). Training private drug vendors about appropriate drugs and dosages for malaria treatment may be a useful supplement, but the primary need is to empower mothers to treat their children at home.

Prophylaxis

Prophylaxis with antimalarials has been the standard procedure for travellers and short-term residents of endemic areas. It has also been an effective approach for selected 'captive' populations, such as plantation workers or miners. From the public health viewpoint, prophylaxis has also been shown to be highly beneficial in pregnancy, both for the pregnant woman and for the fetus, especially for first and second pregnancies (McGregor 1984). This strategy now has been replaced by intermittent preventive (full) treatment (IPT) that involves administration of a full treatment course each month during antenatal care.

The role of prophylaxis for infants and young children is still not clear. In pilot studies in The Gambia, prophylaxis was more effective than use of nearby primary health care facilities for treatment of children (Alonso *et al.* 1993). There have been two major concerns about antimalarial prophylaxis: It might suppress development of an immune response and it might favour development of drug resistance, but there is little firm evidence for either. Even in tightly run prophylaxis programmes, little retardation in development of immunological defences has been observed. In many respects, household treatment of possible malaria symptoms as discussed above would be equivalent, would not inhibit host defence mechanisms, would require less antimalarial distribution and would provide for a natural stopping age for use of antimalarials.

Intermittent preventive treatment

An alternative strategy to prevent malaria in young children is the use of intermittent preventive treatment (IPT). This strategy differs from chemoprophylaxis in that infants and children receive periodic full treatment doses of antimalarials rather than prophylactic regimens. IPT can be offered at the time of routine childhood immunization, a strategy referred to as intermittent preventive treatment in infants (IPTi). Large trials of IPTi have demonstrated high levels of effectiveness against clinical malaria and severe anaemia (Schellenberg *et al.* 2001; Massaga *et al.* 2003). The logic would suggest that IPT be given to every child under age five when seen for any other reason including all IMCI visits. There is no evidence that IPT interferes with immune responses to childhood vaccines (Rosen & Breman 2004).

Strategies for vaccine use

Even after development of one or several vaccines, the most appropriate vaccine and its use will depend on the epidemiological situation (see Table 9.15.2). A pre-erythrocytic stage vaccine is designed to prevent infection. A potential danger, however, is that if any sporozoite bypasses host defences and invades a liver cell, a full-blown malaria episode could follow. An anti-sporozoite vaccine is likely to have a limited duration of protection and to have limited, if any, natural boosting. Thus, it could be useful for visitors to endemic areas, but would not be as effective for those living in endemic areas. An asexual stage vaccine, however, would mimic natural immunity, and could be targeted to children and pregnant women in holoendemic areas. Natural infection could provide a booster effect. In such a situation, it could be counterproductive to reduce transmission since the transmission would be the method for vaccine boosting.

The use of vaccines directed against the sexual, gamete forms (the 'transmission blocking' vaccine) is more problematic. It might be useful as an additional control component in areas of relatively unstable malaria where other control measures are in place, and might be a particularly useful supplement to reduce the spread of drug-resistant parasites. Its only use would be where malaria control efforts were focused on reduction or elimination of transmission; it would be counter-productive where the booster effect of natural infection is needed as with an asexual, blood form vaccine used to reduce the severity of disease rather than to reduce transmission.

The future

Doing better with what we have

The first order of business for any country facing malaria is to improve the current antimalaria programme. This requires strengthened planning based on detailed epidemiological data combined with improved management and operational research capacity of the health system, particularly that of primary health care and its support systems at the local community and district levels. It also will require basic human development improvements including strengthened infrastructural and institutional support for enhanced employment opportunities, strengthened women's groups, better access to microcredit, augmented community and family education, and better communication and transport systems. These general development improvements are needed because the strategies as elaborated above to achieve effective malaria control require understanding and concerted action at the household and community level. The fundamental institutional and profound structural reconstruction required to achieve these basic changes are only recently being enacted in a handful of African countries. The sector-wide approach programmes (SWAPs), in which all donors contribute to a common 'basket' for which host country decision makers are responsible, should assist in these changes when undertaken by countries with a sufficient technical and political competence to effectively use and account for the funding. Globally, the need for improved equity to generate the capacity for all countries and locales to make decisions for themselves not only must be recognized, but the wealthy nations must be convinced that it is in their long-term interest.

Operational research to support better planning and management, largely country- and even locale-specific, is needed with special attention to quality management and support supervision to enhance health worker performance. In particular, if the antimalaria strategies discussed above are to be effective, more work must be devoted to the following: (1) IPT added to EPI, IMCI, and antenatal care; (2) approaches to training of trainers for distribution and use of antimalarial drugs by mothers in the household to treat their children; (3) community-based programmes for distribution, use and continuing re-treatment of insecticide treated bed nets; (4) increased monitoring for drug resistance; (5) support for communities to work through their own approaches to take community actions to control malaria including reduction of vector habitats especially in areas with marginal or highly variable transmission; and (6) continued improvement in immunization coverage particularly to the under-served populations in anticipation of an effective antimalarial vaccine.

New resources for development and research at last

Despite the large number of control methods reviewed above, there is evident need for new and improved interventions and support tools.

Research on nearly all aspects of control measures languished until quite recently. Finally, in 1996, the World Bank publication, *Investing in Health Research and Development* (Ad Hoc Committee on Health Research 1996) gave some sense of priority for global health research. With the initiation of Roll Back Malaria in 1998, there was a renewal of interest in malaria research. With the Multilateral Initiative on Malaria, the Malaria Vaccine Initiative, the Global Fund against AIDS, Malaria and TB, the [US] President's Malaria Initiative, and further support from the Gates Foundation, there is now a much stronger international effort focused on malaria control and related research.

Research and development priorities include:

- Development of asexual stage vaccines, especially now that health infrastructures in many African countries are sufficiently developed to deliver childhood vaccines to a large part of their population
- Continued efforts to develop new antimalarial drugs
- Continued work to understand the molecular biology of the parasite, especially the metabolic pathways contributing to virulence that might be amenable to rational drug development
- Continued development of mathematical modelling done in direct concert with field investigations may facilitate a deeper understanding of the critical quantitative relationships involved in transmission control
- Improved entomological field methods for better understanding of micro-epidemiological variation and for local anopheline control efforts
- Better understanding of the mechanisms underlying drug resistance and factors contributing to its spread will likely require a combined understanding of genetics, entomology, and epidemiology
- Simple, inexpensive, rapid, and robust diagnostic tests that would provide for quantification of parasite density and indicate drug resistance
- Re-engineering anophelines so they do not adequately support the parasite through completion of the sporogonic cycle

References

Ad Hoc Committee on Health Research Relating to Future Intervention Options. *Investing in Health Research and Development*. World Health Organization, Geneva. 1996 (Document TDR/Gen96.1).

Alonso P.L., Lindsay S.W., Armstrong J.R.M. *et al.* (1991) The effect of insecticide-treated bed nets on mortality of Gambian children. *Lancet*, **337**, 1499–1502.

Alonso P.L., Lindsay S.W., Armstrong Schellenberg J.R. *et al.* (1993) A malaria control trial using insecticide-treated bed nets and targeted chemoprophylaxis in a rural area of The Gambia, West Africa. 6. The impact of the interventions on mortality and morbidity from malaria. *Transactions of the Royal Society of Tropical Medicine and Hygiene*, **87**, 37–44.

Alonso P.L., Sacarlal J., Aponte J.J. *et al.* (2004) Efficacy of the RTS,S/AS02A vaccine against *Plasmodium falciparum* infection and disease in young African children: randomised controlled trial. *Lancet*, **364**, 1411–1420.

Beier J.C. (1998) Malaria parasite development in mosquitoes. *Annual Review of Entomology*, **43**, 519–43.

Beier J.C., Onyango K., Ramadhan M. *et al.* (1991) Quantitation of malaria sporozoites in the salivary glands of wild Afrotropical Anopheles. *Medical and Veterinary Entomology*, **5**, 63–70.

Binka F., Kubaje A., Adjuik, M. *et al.* (1996) Impact of permethrin impregnated bednets on child mortality in Kassena-Nankana District, Ghana: A Randomized Controlled Trial. *Tropical Medicine & International Health*, 1, 147–54.

Brabin B.J. (1991) The risks and severity of malaria in pregnant women. *TDR/Applied Field Research in Malaria Reports, No. 1*. Geneva, World Health Organization.

Bruce-Chwatt L.J. (1988). History of malaria from prehistory to eradication. In Wernsdorfer W.H., McGregor I., eds. *Malaria: Principles and Practice of Malariology*. pp. 1–69. Churchill Livingstone, Edinburgh.

Buck A.A., ed. (1986) Proceeding of the Conference on Malaria in Africa: Practical Considerations on Malaria Vaccines and Clinical Trials, American Institute of Biological Sciences, Washington.

Caulfield L.E., Richard S.A. and Black R.E. (2004) Undernutrition as an underlying cause of malaria morbidity and mortality in children less than five years old. *American Journal of Tropical Medicine and Hygiene*, 71(Suppl 2), 55–63.

Clyde D.F., McCarthy V.C., Miller R.M. *et al.* (1975) Immunization of man against falciparum and vivax malaria by use of attenuated sporozoites. *American Journal of Tropical Medicine and Hygiene*, 24, 397–401.

Connolly M.A., Gayer M., Ryan M.J. *et al.*(2004) Communicable diseases in complex emergencies: impact and challenges. *Lancet*, 364, 1974–83.

Creasey A., Fenton G., Walker A. *et al.*(1990) Genetic diversity of *Plasmodium falciparum* shows geographic variation. *American Journal of Tropical Medicine and Hygiene*, 42, 403.

D'Alessandro U., Olaleye B., Langerock P. *et al.* (1997) The Gambian National Impregnated Bed Net Programme: evaluation of effectiveness by means of case-control studies. *Transactions of the Royal Society of Tropical Medicine and Hygiene*, 91, 638–42.

De Monbrison F., Angei C., Staal A. *et al.*(2003) Simultaneous identification of the four human Plasmodium species and quantification of Plasmodium DNA load in human blood by real-time polymerase chain reaction. *Transactions of the Royal Society of Tropical Medicine and Hygiene*, 97, 387–390.

Desowitz R.S. (1991). *The Malaria Capers: More Tales of Parasites and People*. W.W. Norton, New York.

Djimde A., Doumbo O.K., Cortese J.F. *et al.* (2001) A molecular marker for chloroquine-resistant falciparum malaria. *New England Journal of Medicine*, 344, 299–302.

Dye C., Lines J.D. and Curtis C.F. (1996) A test of the malaria strain theory. *Parisitology Today*, 12, 88–9.

English M., Waruiru C., Amukoye E. *et al.* (1996) Deep breathing reflects acidosis and is associated with poor prognosis in children with severe malaria and respiratory distress. *Journal of Tropical Medicine and Hygiene*, 55, 521–4.

Gardner M.J., Hall N., Fung E. *et al.* (2002). Genome sequence of the human malaria parasite *Plasmodium falciparum*. *Nature* 419, 498–511.

Garnham P.C.C. (1966) *Malaria Parasites and Other Hemosporidia*. Blackwell Scientific Publications, Oxford.

Gilles H.M. (1957) The development of malarial infection in breast-fed Gambian infants. *Annals of Tropical Medicine and Parasitology*, 51, 58–72.

Gratepanche S., Gamain B., Smith J.D. *et al.* (2003) Induction of crossreactive antibodies against the *Plasmodium falciparum* variant protein. *Proceedings of the National Academy of Sciences*, 100, 13007–12.

Greenwood B., Marsh K. and Snow R. (1991) Why do some African children develop severe malaria. *Parasitology Today*, 7, 277–81.

Harinasuta T., Migasen S. and Boonag D. (1962) UNESCO 1st Regional Symposium on Scientific Knowledge of Tropical Parasites. University of Singapore.

Hastings I.M. (2003) Malaria control and the evolution of drug resistance: an intriguing link. *Trends in Parasitology*, 2, 70–3.

Hawley W.A., Ter Kuile F.O., Steketee R.S. *et al.* (2003) Implications of the western kenya permethrin-treated bed net study for policy, program implementation, and future research. *American Journal of Tropical Medicine and Hygiene*, 68(Suppl 4), 168–73.

Holt R.A., Subramanian G.M., Halpern A. *et al.* (2002). The genome sequence of the malaria mosquito *Anopheles gambiae*. *Science*, 298, 129–49.

International Development Advisory Board (1956). Malaria Eradication: Report and Recommendations of the International Development Advisory Board, International Development Advisory Board.

Ito J., Ghosh A., Moreira L.A. *et al.* (2002) Transgenic anopheline mosquites imparied in transmission of a malaria parasite. *Nature*, 417, 452–5.

Kakkilaya B.S. (2006). Malaria in Ancient Literature. Dr. B.S. Kakkilaya's Malaria Web Site. www.malariasite.com/malaria/history literature.htm

Kidane G. and Morrow R.H. (2000) Teaching mothers to provide home treatment of malaria in Tigray, Ethiopia: a randomized trial. *Lancet*, 356, 550–5.

Krishna S. (1997) Malaria. *British Medical Journal*, 315, 730–2.

Krotoski W.A. Collins W.E. Bray R.S. *et al.* (1982) Demonstration of hypnozoites in sporozoite-transmitted *Plasmodium vivax* infection. *American Journal of Tropical Medicine and Hygiene*, 31, 1291–3.

Kublin J.G., Patnaik P., Jere C.S. *et al.* (2005) Effect of *Plasmodium falciparum* malaria on concentration of HIV-1-RNA in the blood of adults in rural Malawi: a prospective cohort study. *Lancet*, 365, 233–40.

Luzatto L., Nwachuku-Jarret E.S. and Reddy S. (1970) Increased sickling of parasitised erythrocytes as mechanism of resistance against malaria in the sickle-cell trait. *Lancet*, 1, 319–21.

Maberti S. (1960) Desarollo de resistencia a la pirimetamima. Presentacion de 15 casos estudiados en Trujillo. *Med. Trop. Paras. Med.*, 3, 239–59.

MacDonald G. (1957) *The Epidemiology and Control of Malaria*. Oxford University Press, Inc., London.

Marsh K., English M., Crawley J. *et al.* (1996) The pathogenesis of severe malaria in African children. *Annals of Tropical Medicine and Parasitology*, 90, 396–402.

Marsh K., Forster D., Waruiru C. *et al.* (1995) Indicators of life-threatening malaria in African children. *New England Journal of Medicine*, 322, 1399–404.

Marsh K. and Snow R.W. (1997) Host–parasite interaction and morbidity in malaria endemic areas. *Philosophical Transactions of the Royal Society of London B: Biological Sciences*, 352, 1385–94.

Massaga J.J., Kitua A.Y., Lemnge M.M. *et al.* (2003) Effect of intermittent treatment with amodiaquine on anaemia and malarial fevers in infants in Tanzania: a randomised placebo-controlled trial. *Lancet*, 361, 1853–60.

McGregor I.A. (1984) Epidemiology, malaria and pregnancy. *American Journal of Tropical Medicine and Hygiene*, 33, 517–25.

McGregor I.A., Carington S.P. and Cohen S. (1963) Treatment of East African *P. falciparum* malaria with West African human gammaglobulin. *Transactions of the Royal Society of Tropical Medicine and Hygiene*, 57, 170-5.

McPherson G.G., Warrell M.J., White N.J. *et al.* (1985) Human cerebral malaria: a quantitative ultrastructural analysis of parasitized erythrocyte sequestration. *American Journal of Pathology*, 119, 385–401.

Mendis N. Sina B.J. Marchesini P. *et al.* (2001) The neglected burden of *Plasmodium vivax* malaria. *American Journal of Tropical Medicine and Hygiene*, 64, S97–S106.

Mharakurwa S. (2004) *Plasmodium falciparum* transmission rate and selection for drug resistance: a vexed association or a key to successful control? *International Journal for Parasitology*, 34, 1483–7.

Miller L.H. (1994) Impact of Malaria on genetic polymorphism and genetic diseases in Africans and African-Americans. *Proceedings of the National Academy of Sciences*, 91, 2415–9.

Miller L.H., Baruch D.I., Marsh K. *et al.* (2002) The pathogenic basis of malaria. *Nature*, 415, 673–9.

Miller L.H., Mason S.J., Clyde D.F. *et al* (1976) The resistance factor to *Plasmodium vivax* in blacks: The Duffy Blood-group genotype, Fy-Fy. *New England Journal of Medicine*, 295, 302.

Molineaux L. (1988) The epidemiology of human malaria as an explanation of its distribution including some implications for its control. In Wernsdorfer WH Mcgregor I (Eds.) *Malaria: Principles and Practices of Malariology*, Churchill Livingstone, Edinburgh.

Molineaux L. (1996) *Plasmodium falciparum* malaria: some epidemiological implications of parasite and host diversity. *Annals of Tropical Medicine and Parasitology*, **90**, 379–93.

Molineaux L. and Gramiccia G. (1980). The Garki Project: Research on the Epidemiology and Control of Malaria in the Sudan Savanna of West Africa. World Health Organization, Geneva.

Molyneux M.E., Taylor T.E., Wirima J.J. *et al.* (1989) Clinical features and prognostic indicators in pediatric cerebral malaria: a study of 131 comatose malarian children. *Quarterly Journal of Medicine*, **71**, 441–59.

Moody A. (2002) Rapid diagnostic tests for malaria parasites. *Clinical Microbiology Reviews*, **15**, 66–78.

Morrow R.H. (1984) The application of a quantitative approach to the assessment of the relative importance of vector and soil transmitted diseases in Ghana. *Social Science and Medicine*, **19**, 1039–49.

Mueller A.K., Labaied M., Kappe S.H. *et al.* (2005) Genetically modified Plasmodium parasites as a protective experimental malaria vaccine. *Nature*, **433**, 164–7.

Murray C.K., Bell D., Gasser R.A. *et al.*(2003) Rapid diagnostic testing for malaria. *Tropical Medicine & International Health*, **8**, 875–83.

Nahlen B.L., Clark J.P. and Alnwick D. (2003) Insecticide-treated bed nets. *American Journal of Tropical Medicine and Hygiene*, **68** (Suppl 4), 1–2.

Nevill C., Some E., Mung'ala V. *et al.* (1996) Insecticide-treated bednets reduce mortality and severe morbidity from malaria among children on the Kenyan coast. *Tropical Medicine and International Health*, **1**, 139–46.

Nicoll A. Integrated management of childhood illness in resource-poor countries: an initiative from the World Health Organization. *Transactions of the Royal Society of Tropical Medicine and Hygiene*, 2000, **94**(1):9–11.

Noedl H., Wongsrichanalai C. and Wernsdorfer W.H. (2003) Malaria drug-sensitivity testing: new assays, new perspectives. *Trends in Parasitology*, **19**, 175–81.

Nosten F., Rogerson S.J., Beeson J.G. *et al.* (2004) Malaria in pregnancy and the endemicity spectrum: what can we learn? *Trends in Parasitology*, **20**, 425–32.

Oaks S.C., Jr., Mitchell V.S., Pearson G.W. *et al.* (1991) *Malaria: Obstacles and Opportunities*. National Academy Press, Washington, D.C.

Reed M.B., Saliba K.J., Caruana S.R. *et al.* (2000) Pgh1 modulates sensitivity and resistance to multiple antimalarials in *Plasmodium falciparum*. *Nature*, **403**, 906–9.

Roper C., Pearce R., Nair S. *et al.* (2004) Intercontinental spread of pyrimethamine-resistant malaria. *Science*, **305**, 1124.

Rosen J.B. and Breman J.G. (2004) Malaria intermittent preventive treatment in infants, chemoprophylaxis, and childhood vaccinations. *Lancet*, **363**, 1386–8.

Rowe J.A., Kyes S.A., Rogerson S.J. *et al.* (2002) Identification of a conserved *Plasmodium falciparum var* gene implicated in malaria in pregnancy. *The Journal of Infectious Diseases*, **185**, 1207–11.

Russell P.F., West L.S., Maxwell R.D. *et al.* (1963). *Practical Malariology*. Second Ed, Oxford University Press, London.

Schellenberg D., Menendez C., Kahigwa E. *et al.* (2001) Intermittent treatment for malaria and anaemia control at time of routine vaccinations in Tanzanian infants: a randomised, placebo-controlled trial. *Lancet*, 1471–7.

Shankar A.H., Genton B., Baisor M. *et al.* (2000) The influence of zinc supplementation on morbidity due to *Plasmodium falciparum*: a randomized trial in preschool children in Papua New Guinea. *American Journal of Tropical Medicine and Hygiene*, **62**, 663–9.

Shankar A.H. and Stoltzfus R.J. (1998) A meta-analysis of controlled trials of iron supplementation to infants and children in malarious areas.

Steketee R.W., Nahlen B.L., Parise M.E. *et al.* (2001) The burden of malaria in pregnancy in malaria-endemic areas. *American Journal of Tropical Medicine and Hygiene*, **64**, 28–35.

Tarimo D.S., Lwihula G.K., Minjas J.N.A. *et al.* (2000) Mothers' perception and knowledge on childhood malaria in holoendemic Kibaha district, Tanzania: implications for malaria control and the IMCI strategy. *Tropical Medicine & International Health*, **5**, 179–84.

Taylor W.R.J. and White N.J. (2004) Antimalarial drug toxicity: A review. *Drug Safety*, **27**, 25–61.

Ter Kuile F.O., Parise M.E., Verhoeff F.H. *et al.* (2004) The burden of co-infection with human immunodeficiency virus type 1 and malaria in pregnant women in sub-saharan Africa. *American Journal of Tropical Medicine and Hygiene*, **71**(2 Suppl), 41–54.

Warrell D.A., Molyneux M.E. and Beales P.F. (1990) Severe and complicated malaria. *Transactions of the Royal Society of Tropical Medicine and Hygiene*, **84**, 1–65.

Wernsdorfer W.H. (1994) Epidemiology and drug resistance in malaria. *Acta Tropica*, **56**, 143–56.

White, N.J. (2004) Antimalarial drug resistance. *Journal Clinical Investigation*, **113**, 1084–92.

Whitworth J., Morgan D., Quigley M. *et al.* (2000) Effect of HIV-1 and increasing immunosuppression on malaria parasitaemia and clinical episodes in adults in rural Uganda: a cohort study. *Lancet*, **356**, 1051–6.

Winch P.J., Makemba A.M., Kamazima S.R. *et al.* (1996) Local terminology for febrile illnesses in Bagamoyo district, Tanzania and ite impact on the design of a community-bsed malaria control programme. *Social Science and Medicine*, **42**, 1057–67.

Wongsrichanalai C., Wernsdorfer W.H. and Meshnick S.R. (2002) Epidemiology of drug-resistant malaria. *The Lancet Infectious Diseases*, **2**, 209–18.

Wootton J.C., Feng X., Ferdig M.T. *et al.* (2002) Genetic diversity and chloroquine selective sweeps in *Plasmodium falciparum*. *Nature*, **418**, 320–3.

World Health Organization Expert Committee on Malaria (1967). WHO Technical Report Series No. 357, Geneva.

World Health Organization (1969). *Re-examination of the Global Strategy of Malaria Eradication*. WHO Official Records No. 176.

World Health Organization (2004). *World Health Report*. Geneva, Switzerland.

Chronic hepatitis and other liver disease

Pierre van Damme, Koen Van Herck, Peter Michielsen, Sven Francque, and Daniel Shouval

Abstract

Approximately one of every 40 deaths worldwide can be attributed to liver cirrhosis and primary liver cancer (hepatocellular carcinoma, HCC). In this chapter, we will focus on the epidemiology and public health impact of the main aetiologies of chronic liver disease, i.e. viral hepatitis B and C, and alcoholic as well as non-alcoholic fatty liver diseases. Hepatitis B virus (HBV) and hepatitis C virus (HCV) infections are major risk factors in the development of HCC either by inducing cirrhosis or by direct oncogenic effects. Hepatitis B is a significant health issue across the world, mainly in Asia and Africa but also in the industrialized countries. However, unlike hepatitis C and HIV, it has not captured sufficient attention from policymakers, advocacy groups or the general public. Globally, 57 per cent of cirrhosis cases and 78 per cent of HCC have been attributed to either HBV or HCV. As hepatitis B and C share modes of transmission their combined occurrence is not uncommon, particularly in areas where both viruses are endemic, and in individuals at high risk of parenteral infection (e.g. drug users).

It has long been known that alcohol consumption is responsible for increased illness and death. The spectrum of liver pathology caused by alcohol consumption goes from steatosis, over cirrhosis to hepatocellular carcinoma. Thirty-two per cent of all cases of cirrhosis worldwide are estimated to be attributable to alcohol. Worldwide, alcoholic liver disease may increase in the next several decades. Recent data indicate that alcohol consumption is increasing in low- and middle-income countries. In addition, rates of excessive alcohol intake appear to be rising in women.

Non-alcoholic fatty liver disease and non-alcoholic steatohepatitis are chronic liver diseases associated with the metabolic syndrome. This tends to take epidemic proportions in the Western population, and to constitute a major health problem in the near future.

Despite the availability and widespread use of vaccines against hepatitis B, it will still take many years before its chronic consequences will be effectively controlled on a global scale. In the meantime, hepatitis C prevention and control will form a major challenge to those involved in public health, especially since the development of vaccines against hepatitis C still has not resulted in a success. On top of the chronic liver diseases caused by viral hepatitis, increasing alcohol consumption and the rising epidemiology of non-alcoholic chronic liver diseases will increasingly require our attention in the future.

Hepatitis B

Aetiological agent

HBV is a double-stranded, enveloped virus of the *Hepadnaviridae* family. The *Hepadna* virus family has the smallest genome of all replication competent animal DNA viruses. The single most important member of the family is HBV. Eight genotypes of HBV have been identified, termed A–H. The hepatitis B virion consists of a surface and a core, which contains a DNA polymerase and the e antigen. The DNA structure is double-stranded and circular with four major genes: The S (surface), the C (core), the P (polymerase) and the X (transcriptional transactivating). The S gene consists of three regions—S, pre-S1, and pre-S2—that encode the envelope protein (HBsAg). HBsAg is a lipoprotein of the viral envelope that circulates in the blood as spherical and tubular particles. The C gene is divided into two regions, the pre-core and the core, and codes for two different proteins, the core antigen (HBcAg) and the e antigen (HBeAg).

The course of hepatitis B virus infection is controlled by cellular and humoral immune responses. It can be tracked through serological detection of these virus particles or the antibodies raised by the immune system to target the virus. The presence of hepatitis B surface and/or hepatitis B core antibodies (anti-HBs and anti-HBc) in the absence of HBsAg is generally taken to indicate resolution of infection and provides evidence of previous HBV infection. Persistence of HBV infection is diagnosed by the detection of HBsAg in the blood for at least 6 months or through detection of HBV-DNA even in the absence of detectable HBsAg in patients with occult HBV infection. HBeAg is an alternatively processed protein of the pre-core gene that is only synthesized under conditions of high viral replication. Since a few years HBV-DNA is used as an indicator for viral replication expressed as IU/ml or copies/ml. There is a clear association between serum HBV-DNA levels (viral load) and prognosis: The cumulative incidence of cirrhosis or hepatocellular carcinoma being 4.5 and 1.3 per cent, respectively, in persons with DNA levels less than 300 copies/ml (corresponding to 50 IU/ml), while it is 36.2 and 14.9 per cent, respectively, in persons with DNA levels of more than or equal to 10^6 copies/ml (corresponding to $>2 \times 10^5$ IU/ml). This is the rationale for treating patients with high levels of HBV DNA (Tan & Lok 2007; Lok & McMahon 2007).

Epidemiology

Globally, hepatitis B is one of the most common infectious diseases. Estimates indicate that at least 2 billion people have been infected with HBV, with over 378 million people being chronic carriers (6 per cent of the world population). On the basis of sero-epidemiological surveys, the World Health Organization (WHO) has classified countries into three levels of endemicity according to the prevalence of chronic HBsAg carriage (Fig. 9.16.1): High (8 per cent or greater), intermediate (2–8 per cent), and low (less than 2 per cent) (WHO 2004a).

HBV is transmitted by either percutaneous or mucous membrane contact with infected blood or other body fluid. The virus is found in highest concentrations in blood and serous exudates (till 10^9 virions/ml). The primary routes of transmission are perinatal, early childhood exposure (often called horizontal transmission), sexual contact, and percutaneous exposure to blood or infectious body fluids (i.e. injections, needle stick, blood transfusion).

Most perinatal infections occur among infants of pregnant women with chronic HBV infection. The likelihood of an infant developing chronic HBV infection is 70–90 per cent for those born to HBeAg-positive mothers (corresponding to high titres of HBV DNA) and less than 15 per cent for those born to HBeAg-negative mothers. Most early childhood infections occur in households of

persons with chronic HBV infection. The most probable mechanism involves unapparent percutaneous or permucosal contact with infectious body fluids (e.g. bites, breaks in the skin, dermatologic lesions, skin ulcers). Sexual transmission has been estimated to account for 50 per cent of new infections among adults in industrialized countries. The most common risk factors include multiple sex partners and history of a sexually transmitted infection. Finally, unsafe injections and other unsafe percutaneous procedures are a major source of bloodborne pathogen transmission (HBV, HCV, HIV) in many countries: The risk of HBV infection from needle stick exposure to HBsAg-positive blood is ~30 per cent. Worldwide unsafe injection practices account for ~8–16 million HBV infections each year.

In areas of high endemicity, the lifetime risk of HBV infection is more than 60 per cent, and most infections occur during the perinatal period (transmission from mother to child) or during early childhood. In areas of intermediate endemicity, the lifetime risk of HBV infection varies between 20 and 60 per cent, and infections occur in all age groups through the four modes of transmission, but primarily in infants and children. In areas of low endemicity, infection occurs primarily in adult life by sexual or parenteral transmission (e.g. through drug use). Although the acute infection is more clinically expressed in adults, infections in infants and pre-school age children are at greatest risk of becoming chronic, thereby increasing the risk of cirrhosis and primary HCC later in life. The precise mechanism by which carrier rates are influenced by age of infection is unknown but probably relates to the effect of age on the immune system's ability to clear and eliminate the infection.

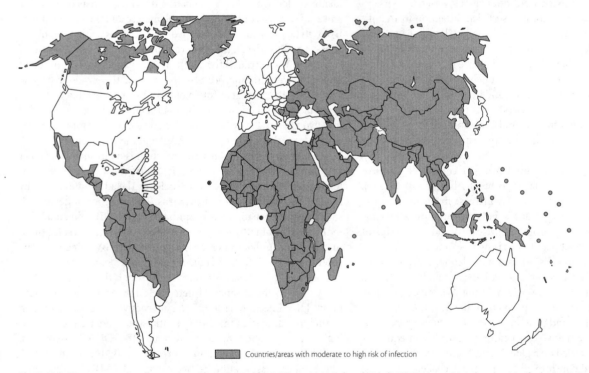

Countries/areas with moderate to high risk of infection

Fig. 9.16.1 Map representing all countries with moderate (2–8% HBsAg positivity) and high (≥8% HBsAg positivity) endemicity for hepatitis B. *Source*: http://www.who.int/ith/maps/hepatitisB2007.jpg.

Approximately 75 per cent of the world's chronic hepatitis B carriers live in Asian countries. China ranks highest, with ~100 million hepatitis B carriers, and India the second highest, with a carrier pool of ~35 million (Tandon & Tandon 1997). Importantly, chronic carriers of HBV are not only at risk of developing the long-term progression of the infection but also represent a significant source of infection to others.

A model was recently developed to estimate HBV-related morbidity and mortality at country, regional, and global levels (http://aim.path.org/en/vaccines/hepb/assessBurden/model/index.html). This model calculates the age-specific risk of acquiring HBV infection, acute HBV (illness and fulminant disease), and progression to chronic HBV infection (Goldstein et al. 2005). HBV-related deaths among chronically infected persons were determined from HBV-related cirrhosis and HCC mortality curves, adjusted for background mortality. For the year 2000, the model estimated 620 000 persons died worldwide from HBV-related causes: 580 000 (94 per cent) from chronic infection-related cirrhosis and HCC and 40 000 (6 per cent) from acute HBV infection. Infections acquired during the perinatal period, in early childhood (<5 years old), and 5 years of age and older accounted for 21 per cent, 48 per cent, and 31 per cent of deaths, respectively.

Besides the age at which the infection is acquired, some of the variation in outcome of HBV infection may be related to the genetic heterogeneity of the virus. Eight genotypes (A–H) have been described, genotype A being most common in the United States and Northern Europe, B and C in Asia, and D in Mediterranean countries and the Middle East. Chronic infection with genotype B appears to have a better prognosis than genotype C. Pre-core mutant infection is also most common in genotypes B, C, and D, which explains why pre-core mutant infection is more common in Asia and Southern Europe.

Clinical manifestations

Acute hepatitis B has a long incubation period (90 days on average) during which the individual is infectious. Individual responses to the infection vary greatly. One-third of the individuals have sub-clinical infection; one-third experience a mild 'flu-like' illness without jaundice; and the remaining one-third develop jaundice with dark urine, extreme fatigue, anorexia, and abdominal pain. Jaundice usually peaks within one to 2 weeks and then gradually subsides. About 90 per cent of adults recover completely, although this may require 6 months or more with persistent tiredness and intolerance to alcohol which can last for a year or more. A small proportion (1 per cent) of adults develops fulminant hepatitis, an exceptionally severe form of the disease which is almost always fatal unless liver transplantation is performed (Sherlock 1993). About 5–10 per cent of acutely infected adults and 50–90 per cent of newborns will become chronically infected and remain infectious.

The natural history of chronic HBV infection can vary dramatically between individuals. Risk factors which affect progression to chronic hepatitis, cirrhosis, and HCC include male gender, viral load, elevated ALT, genotype, and degree of fibrosis on liver biopsy. Some patients with persistent HBV infection will develop the condition commonly referred to as a chronic carrier state. These patients, who are still potentially infectious, have no symptoms and no abnormalities on laboratory testing. Nonetheless, some of these patients will have evidence of hepatitis on liver biopsy. Some individuals with chronic HBV infection will have clinically insignificant or minimal liver disease and never develop complications. Others will have clinically apparent chronic hepatitis. Chronic infection with HBV can be either 'replicative' or 'non-replicative'. The 'replicative' phase or immune tolerance phase, characterized by positive HBeAg and high viral load, is often present in newborns and children of HBsAg-positive mothers. In 'non-replicative' infection, the rate of viral replication in the liver is low, serum HBV DNA concentration is generally low, and HBeAg is not detected. In these inactive HBsAg carriers, reactivation can occur either spontaneously or by immune suppression. In replicative infection, the patient usually has a relatively high serum concentration of viral DNA (viral load) and detectable HBeAg. Patients with chronic HBV and replicative infection, defined by the presence of detectable HBeAg and high viral load, have a generally worse prognosis and a greater chance of developing cirrhosis and/or HCC than those without HBeAg (Chen 2006). In rare strains of HBV with mutations in the pre-core gene, replicative infection can occur in the absence of detectable serum HBeAg (Worman 1999).

Treatment

The main goal of therapy for chronic HBV infection is to significantly suppress replication of HBV, thus preventing liver disease progression to cirrhosis and its complications, and reducing secondary spread of the infectious disease. Treatment of chronic HBV infections has some limited success. Anti-viral therapy will only rarely lead to complete resolution of persistent HBV infection. Furthermore, residual HBV DNA in the form of intra-nuclear cccDNA may still be present in patients who lost HBsAg and seroconverted to anti-HBs, a situation which leads to occult HBV infection. In patients who are HBeAg-positive, the goal of treatment is HBeAg seroconversion with sustained suppression of HBV DNA and rarely HBsAg seroconversion. In those who are HBeAg-negative, the goal of treatment is sustained suppression of HBV DNA and liver injury as measured by ALT levels as well as HBsAg seroconversion (which is achieved only on rare occasions).

Recommendation for therapy is dictated by the level of HBV DNA and liver enzymes. Several therapies are licensed: Nucleo(t)side analogues and interferon-based therapy. Depending on the defined outcome, approximately one-third of patients respond to a 1-year course of α-interferon therapy. Currently, interferon-based therapy appears to be superior to nucleo(t)side analogues, due to the relatively higher rate of anti-HBe seroconversion, the limited duration of treatment as compared to nucleos(t)ide analogues, the potential, albeit rare, HBsAg loss after 1 year therapy, the lower overall cost and the absence of resistance (Hoofnagle 2007). Treatment with nucleos(t)ide analogues is very effective in suppressing viral load but the endpoint of treatment is undetermined and long-term treatment is required, which remains costly and unavailable to the majority of those affected. Combination therapy (interferon-based and nucleo(t)side) does not lead to a better viral response.

Public health impact

HBV infection is a serious global health problem. Of the approximately 2 billion people who have been infected worldwide, more than 350 million are chronic carriers of HBV. Approximately 15–40 per cent of infected patients will develop cirrhosis, liver failure or hepatocellular carcinoma. HBV infection accounts for an estimated 600 000 deaths each year, mainly due to the consequences of chronic hepatitis, such as cirrhosis and liver cancer (Lavanchy 2004; Goldstein *et al.* 2005; Perz *et al.* 2006a). Because these complications mainly occur in adults who quite often were infected with HBV as children, most of the benefits of vaccination initiated ~20 years ago have yet to be realized. Table 9.16.1 summarizes the global prevalence and mortality of HBV versus the observed prevalence and mortality of hepatitis C virus (HCV) and human immunodeficiency virus/acquired immunodeficiency syndrome (HIV/AIDS).

Prevention

All major health authorities agree that the most effective approach to reducing the burden of HBV is primary prevention of infection through universal vaccination and control of disease transmission. Interrupting the chain of infection requires knowledge of the mode of disease transmission and modification of behaviour through individual education to practice safe sex and good personal hygiene. Screening of all donated blood and maintenance of strict aseptic technique with invasive health treatments has reduced the likelihood of contracting HBV.

Safe and effective HBV vaccines have been available since the 1980s, and immunization with HBV vaccine remains the most effective means of preventing HBV disease and its consequences worldwide. Although the vaccine will not cure chronic hepatitis, it is 95 per cent effective in preventing chronic infections from developing, and is the first vaccine against a major human cancer.

After the development of plasma-derived vaccines (in 1982), which continue to be used mostly in the low- and middle-income countries, recombinant DNA technology has allowed the expression of HBsAg in other organisms (Szmuness *et al.* 1981). As a result, different manufacturers have successfully developed recombinant DNA vaccines against HBV (commercialized in 1986).

Moreover, apart from monovalent vaccines against hepatitis B, a broad range of combination vaccines that include an HBV component exists, especially for vaccination during infancy and early childhood. Most of these simultaneously immunize against tetanus, diphtheria, and pertussis (with either a whole-cell or an acellular component); they may also include antigens for vaccination against polio and/or *H. influenzae* b. For each of these combination vaccines, it has been shown that the respective components remain sufficiently immunogenic, and that the combination vaccine is safe.

More recently, the so-called third-generation hepatitis B vaccines—based on the S-, preS1-, and preS2-antigens, or using new adjuvants—have been and are being developed. These vaccines specifically aim to enhance the immune response in immunocompromised persons and nonresponders (Shouval *et al.* 1994; Rendi-Wagner *et al.* 2006).

Immunization against hepatitis B requires the intramuscular administration of three doses of vaccine given at 0, 1, and 6 months.

More rapid protection (i.e. for healthcare workers exposed to HBV or the susceptible sexual partner of a patient with acute hepatitis B) can be achieved through the adoption of an accelerated schedule using three doses of vaccine administered at 0, 1, and 2 months followed by a booster dose given at 12 months. The extensive use of both plasma-derived and recombinant HBV vaccines since their becoming available has confirmed their safety and excellent tolerability (Niu 1996). Side effects are generally mild, transient, and confined to the site of injection (erythema, swelling, induration). Systemic reactions (fatigue, slight fever, headache, nausea, abdominal pain) are uncommon. However, in recent years, the safety of hepatitis B vaccine has been questioned, particularly in some countries. In 1998, several case reports from France raised concern that hepatitis B vaccination may lead to new cases or relapse of multiple sclerosis (MS) or other demyelinating diseases, including Guillain–Barré syndrome; however, no causal relation has been established (Duclos 2003). Hepatitis B vaccination is not contraindicated in pregnant or lactating women. The only absolute contraindications are known hypersensitivity to any component of the vaccine or a history of anaphylaxis to a previous dose.

Seroprotection against HBV infection is defined as having an anti-HBs level ≥ 10 IU/l after complete immunization (Szmuness *et al.* 1981; CDC 1987). Reviews on the use of HBV vaccine in neonates and infants report seroprotective levels of anti-HBs antibodies at one month after the last vaccine dose for all schedules in 98–100 per cent of vaccines (Safary & André 1999; Venters *et al.* 2004). Another review that included studies conducted mainly in newborns reported seroprotection rates ranging from 92.6 to 100 per cent one month after the 0, 1, 6 months schedule and from 97 to 98 per cent 1 month after an accelerated 0, 1, 2 month or 0, 1, 3 month schedule (Keating & Noble 2003). Indeed, while HBV vaccines generally induce an adequate immune response in over 95 per cent of fully vaccinated healthy persons, a huge interpersonal variability has been demonstrated in the immune response in healthy subjects. As such, fast/high, intermediate, slow/poor and even non-responders can be discriminated based on the magnitude and the kinetics of the immune response to HBV vaccination (Dienstag *et al.* 1984). The antibody response to hepatitis B vaccine has been shown to depend on the type, dosage and schedule of vaccination used, as well as on the age, the gender, genetic factors, co-morbidity and the status of the immune system of the vaccinee (Hollinger 1989; Hadler & Margolis 1992). Immunodeficient patients, such as those undergoing hemodialysis or immunosuppressant therapy, require higher doses of vaccine and more injections (at months 0, 1, 2 and 6) to achieve an adequate and sustained immune response.

Follow-up studies have shown that vaccine-induced antibody persists over periods of at least 10–15 years and that duration of

Table 9.16.1 Global disease burden for hepatitis B, hepatitis C, and HIV/AIDS, 2004

	Hepatitis C		Hepatitis B		HIV/AIDS	
	Per cent	Numbers	Per cent	Numbers	Per cent	Numbers
Global prevalence	3	170 million	35	1.2 billion	0.5	36.1 million
Chronic infection	2.3	129 million	6	350 million	0.5	36.1 million
Number of deaths per year		476 000		< 1 million		2.8 million

Source: Lavanchy (2005).

anti-HBs positivity is related to the antibody peak level achieved after primary vaccination (Jilg *et al.* 1984, 1988). Follow-up of successfully vaccinated people has shown that the antibody concentrations usually decline over time, but clinically significant breakthrough infections are rare. Those who have lost antibody over time after a successful vaccination usually show a rapid anamnestic response when boosted with an additional dose of vaccine given several years after the primary course of vaccination or when exposed to the HBV. This means that the immunological memory for HBsAg can outlast the anti-HBs antibody detection, providing long-term protection against acute disease and the development of the HBsAg carrier state (West & Calandra 1996; Banatvala & Van Damme 2003). Hence, for immunocompetent children and adults the routine administration of booster doses of vaccine does not appear necessary to sustain long-term protection (European Consensus Group 2000). Such conclusions are based on data collected during the first 10–20 years of vaccination in countries of both high and low endemicity (Kao & Chen 2005; Zanetti *et al.* 2006).

Since the availability of hepatitis B vaccines in industrialized countries, strategies for HBV control have stressed immunization of high-risk groups (e.g. homosexual men, healthcare workers, patients in sexually transmitted infection clinics, sex workers, drug users, people with multiple sex partners, household contacts with chronically infected persons, some categories of patients) and the screening of pregnant women. As observed and reported in many countries, and though it is certainly desirable to immunize these persons, it is unlikely that such a programme limited to high-risk groups will control HBV infection in the community.

In 1991, the World Health Organization (WHO) called for all children to receive the HBV vaccine. Substantial progress has been made in implementing this WHO recommendation: By the end of 2006, 168 countries had implemented or were planning to implement a universal HBV immunization programme for newborns, infants and/or adolescents. Of these, 119 (62 per cent) countries reported HBV infant vaccination coverage over 80 per cent after the third dose; these countries are mainly situated in Europe, North and South America, Northern Africa, and Australia (WHO 2006).

High coverage with the primary vaccine series among infants has the greatest overall impact on the prevalence of chronic HBV infection in children (WHO 2004a). According to model-based predictions, universal HBV infant immunization (without administration of a birth dose of vaccine to prevent perinatal HBV infection), would prevent up to 75 per cent of global deaths from HBV-related causes, depending on the vaccination coverage for the complete series. Adding the birth dose would increase the proportion of deaths prevented up to 84 per cent (Goldstein *et al.* 2005).

In countries with high or intermediate disease endemicity, the most effective strategy is to incorporate the vaccine into the routine infant immunization schedule or to start immunization at birth (<24 h). Countries with lower prevalence may consider immunization of children or adolescents as an addition or an alternative to infant immunization (WHO 2004a, 2006).

Indeed, the effectiveness of hepatitis B newborn and infant immunization programmes has already been demonstrated in a variety of countries and settings (André & Zuckerman 1994; Lee 1997; WHO 2001). The results of effective implementation of universal hepatitis B programmes have become apparent in terms of reduction not only in the incidence of acute hepatitis B infections, but also in the carrier rate in immunized cohorts and in hepatitis-B-related

mortality—two ways to measure the impact of a hepatitis B vaccination programme (Coursaget *et al.* 1994).

In Taiwan, the HBsAg prevalence in children under 15 years of age decreased from 9.8 per cent in 1984 to 0.7 per cent in 1999 (Chan *et al.* 2004). The average annual incidence of HCC among children aged 6–14 years was 0.7/100 000 for the period 1981–1986, and declined to 0.36/100 000 in 1990–1994 (Chang *et al.* 1997). In the Gambia, childhood HBsAg prevalence decreased from 10 per cent to 0.6 per cent since the introduction of the universal infant immunization programme (Whittle *et al.* 1995; Viviani *et al.* 1999). In Malaysia, HBsAg seroprevalence in children aged 7–12 years went down from 1.6 per cent in 1997 to 0.3 per cent in 2003 since the implementation of a universal infant programme in 1990 (Ng 2005). Recent data in Hawaii show a 97 per cent reduction in the prevalence of HBsAg since the start of the infant hepatitis B vaccination programme in 1991. The incidence of new acute hepatitis B infections in children and adults was reduced from 4.5/100 000 in 1990 to 0 in the period 2002–2004 (Perz *et al.* 2006b). In Bristol Bay, Alaska, 3.2 per cent of children were HBsAg positive before universal hepatitis B immunization; 10 years later, no child under 10 years of age was HBsAg positive (Wainwright *et al.* 1997). Finally, surveillance data from Italy, where a universal programme was started in 1991 in infants as well as in adolescents, have shown a clear overall decline in the incidence of acute hepatitis B cases from 11/100 000 in 1987 to 3/100 000 in 2000 (Romano *et al.* 2004).

Hepatitis C

Aetiological agent

HCV is classified in the family *Flavivridae*. Like other flaviviruses, HCV is an enveloped RNA virus with an inner nucleoprotein core. Its envelope contains two glycoproteins, E1 and E2, which form heterodimers (to form a functional subunit) at the surface of the virion. Efforts to isolate the virus by standard immunologic and virologic techniques were unsuccessful and HCV was finally identified by direct cloning and sequencing of its genome. Although the virus was identified 15 years ago, its pathogenesis and replication are still not fully understood. An important feature of HCV is that the viral genomes display extensive genetic heterogeneity at the local as well as the global level. Even within a host, the HCV genome population circulates as a 'quasi-species' of closely related sequences. Worldwide, a high degree of genetic variation exists, resulting in at least six major genotypes and more than 100 distantly related subtypes (Forns & Bukh 1999). It has been reported that virus pathogenicity and sensitivity to current standards of treatment appear to vary with different subtypes (genotypes 2 and 3, responding better than genotype 1). These characteristics of HCV, much like HIV, make it a moving target for vaccine design.

Epidemiology

HCV is a major cause of acute hepatitis and chronic liver disease, including cirrhosis and HCC. Globally, an estimated 170 million persons are chronically infected with HCV and 3–4 million persons are newly infected each year (Alter 2007). The worldwide prevalence of HCV ranges from 1 per cent in high-income countries to around 10 per cent in low- and middle-income countries (Fig. 9.16.2). Table 9.16.1 summarizes the global prevalence and mortality of HCV versus the observed prevalence and mortality of HBV and HIV/AIDS.

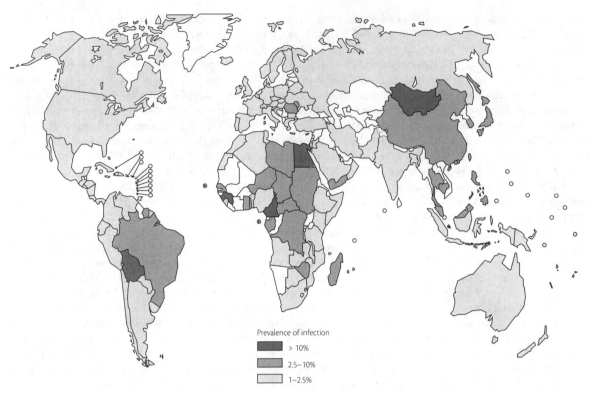

Fig. 9.16.2 Map representing countries with low (1–2.5%), moderate (2.5–10%), and high (>10%) hepatitis C virus prevalence.
Source: http://www.who.int/ith/maps/hepatitisc2007.jpg.

The reported seroprevalence in the Nile delta ranges from 19 per cent in the 10–19-year-old age group to ~60 per cent in the 30-year-old age group, and is associated with a high prevalence of liver cirrhosis in Egypt. The higher prevalence in the Nile delta is reported to be linked to parenteral anti-schistosomiasis therapy, which was carried out with inadequately sterilized injection material (Frank *et al.* 2000). Current estimates in the United States are that 3.9 million Americans are chronically infected with HCV, with prevalence rates as high as 8–10 per cent in African Americans. Haemodialysis patients, haemophiliacs, drug addicts, and people transfused with blood before 1990 are particularly affected by the disease. Despite infection control precautions, healthcare providers remain at risk for acquiring bloodborne viral infections due to accidental exposure. Therapeutic injections are reported as accounting for 2 million new HCV infections each year. Many of these injections are performed in less than ideal conditions, often with reuse of needles or multi-dose vials and mainly, but not exclusively, in low- and middle-income countries. The residual risk of transmitting HCV through blood transfusion is very low in industrialized countries but safety of blood supply remains a major source of public concern in low- and middle-income countries.

In Europe, up to 60–70 per cent of intravenous drug users living in urban areas are seropositive for HCV antibodies. The rate of infection depends on the length of drug use, with 25 per cent of infections occurring during the first year of addiction, 50 per cent after 5 years and up to 90 per cent for more than 5 years of intravenous drug use.

Transmission

The global epidemic of HCV infection emerged in the second half of the twentieth century and has been attributed, at least in part, to the increasing use of parenteral therapies and blood transfusion during that period. In high-income countries, the rapid improvement of healthcare conditions and the introduction of anti-HCV screening for blood donors have led to a sharp decrease in the incidence of iatrogenic HCV (Prati 2006). Injectable drug use remains the main route of transmission, accounting for nearly 90 per cent of new HCV infections. Mother-to-child transmission has been widely documented. The risk of perinatal infection ranges from 3 per cent to 10 per cent in different populations. Transmission is believed to occur *in utero*, as a consequence of a high viral load in the mother (in particular, from mothers who are HIV-co-infected) (Kato *et al.* 1994). Sexual transmission is thought to be relatively infrequent; however, an epidemiological review of current literature shows that, in many cases, no recognizable transmission factor or route is identified (Memon & Memon 2002).

It appears that HCV is inefficiently transmitted sexually; however, the large reservoir of HCV carriers provides multiple opportunities for exposure to potentially infected partners. Individuals with multiple sexual partners, prostitutes and their clients, patients with common sexually transmitted infections, and partners of HCV and HIV co-infected persons are at the highest risk of acquiring HCV sexually.

Clinical manifestations

The incubation period for hepatitis C before the onset of clinical symptoms ranges from six to seven weeks on average. In acute infections, the most common symptoms are fatigue and jaundice; however, the majority of cases (between 60 and 70 per cent), even those who develop chronic infection, are asymptomatic for years. Fulminant hepatitis C forms are rarely observed. While most patients with acute HCV infection have mild symptoms or no symptoms, 50–85 per cent of those infected develop chronic disease.

Chronic disease is difficult to recognize because symptoms are mild and infection passes silently and insidiously from the acute to the chronic phase. In fact, the vast majority of those affected are symptom free for at least 20 years. Serological diagnosis of acute HCV infection is based upon the detection of HCV RNA. Persistence of HCV infection is diagnosed by the presence of HCV RNA in the blood for at least 6 months.

The mechanisms of HCV persistence are currently unknown, although it is known that HCV chronicity develops despite humoral and cellular responses to HCV proteins. Factors associated with development of chronic disease appear to include older age at the time of infection, male gender, and an immunosuppressed state such as HIV infection (Lauer *et al.* 2001).

Treatment

The primary goals for treatment of HCV infection are to reduce morbidity and mortality through complete clearance of HCV and normalisation of liver enzymes, reducing disease progression, improving quality of life and reducing the reservoir of chronic carriers, thereby controlling further transmission. Treatment is recommended for patients with an increased risk of developing cirrhosis; most of these patients (but not all) have persistently elevated liver enzymes and high levels of HCV RNA (>60 IU/ml). Effective sustained virological response has been obtained in about 50 per cent of HCV patients with genotype 1 and 80 per cent of patients with genotype 2 and 3 who had received combined pegylated interferon-based treatment with ribavirin for 48 weeks (Chevalier & Pawlotsky 2007; Tan & Lok 2007). As with HBV treatment, therapy for chronic HCV is often too costly for most patients in low- and middle-income countries to afford.

Public health impact

HCV has been compared to a 'viral time bomb'. The WHO estimates that about 170 million people, some 3 per cent of the world's population, are infected with HCV, 130 million of whom are chronic HCV carriers at risk of developing liver cirrhosis and/or HCC. It is estimated that 3–4 million persons are newly infected each year and that 20 per cent of those infected with HCV progress to cirrhosis within the first 10 years after infection (Gerberding & Henderson 1992; Alter 2007). Furthermore, chronic HCV disease is the primary cause of liver transplantation in industrialized countries.

Prevention

There is no vaccine against HCV. Research is in progress, but the high mutability of the HCV genome complicates vaccine development. Although 20 per cent of patients with acute HCV infection clear the virus spontaneously, lack of knowledge of any protective immune response following HCV infection impedes vaccine research. Although some studies have shown the presence of virus-neutralizing antibodies, it is not fully clear whether and how the immune system is able to eliminate the virus. Thus, from a global perspective, the greatest impact on HCV disease burden will likely be achieved by focusing efforts on reducing the risk of HCV transmission from nosocomial exposures (e.g. screening of blood, rigorous implementation of infection control, reducing unsafe injection practices) and high-risk behaviours (e.g. injection drug use).

Adherence to fundamental infection control principles, including safe injection practices and appropriate aseptic techniques, is essential to prevent transmission of bloodborne viruses in healthcare settings. Educational programmes aimed at the prevention of drug use and, for those already addicted, aimed at the prevention of shared needles and other equipment can decrease this source of infection. Some countries have established syringe exchange programmes that provide easy access to sterile syringes, accompanied by counselling and health education and instructions on the safe disposal of used syringes.

Alcoholic liver disease

Alcoholic beverages have been used in human societies since the beginning of recorded history. It has long been known that alcohol consumption is responsible for increased illness and death. Alcohol has been shown to be related to more than 60 different medical conditions (Room *et al.* 2005). Worldwide, alcohol causes 1.8 million deaths (3.2 per cent of total) and 58.3 million (4 per cent of total) of Disability Adjusted Life Years (World Health Organization 2004b). The burden is not equally distributed among the countries. The highest disease load attributable to alcohol is found in the heavy-drinking former socialist countries of Eastern Europe and in Latin America (Fig. 9.16.3). For most diseases there is a dose–response relation to volume of alcohol consumption, with the risk of the disease increasing with higher volume. Thirty-two per cent of all cases of cirrhosis worldwide are estimated to be attributable to alcohol (Room *et al.* 2005).

Alcoholic liver disease, resulting from the chronic and excessive consumption of alcoholic beverages, represents a considerable burden for the practising clinician, constituting the commonest reason for admitting patients with liver disease to hospital. Alcoholic liver disease is currently the second leading indication for liver transplantation in Europe and the United States after chronic hepatitis C, representing 17–33 per cent of transplants (European Liver Transplant Registry 2007) (Fig. 9.16.4).

The costs to society from alcohol abuse cannot be overemphasized. In 1998, overall costs in the United States amounted to US$186.6 billion, out of which healthcare costs accounted for US$26.5 billion, and hospital-related costs US$600 million to US$1.8 billion (Harwood 2000). In the United Kingdom, alcohol costs the country approximately £20 billion per year (Pincock 2003). Despite this burden, surprisingly little consensus exists on disease pathogenesis and on the factors that determine susceptibility.

Worldwide patterns of alcoholic intake and burden of disease in general and alcoholic liver disease in particular

Patterns of alcohol intake are constantly evolving as well as prevalence and incidence of alcoholic liver disease. The average volume of drinking was highest in established market economies in Western Europe and North America, and in the former Socialist economies in Eastern Europe, and lowest in the Eastern Mediterranean region and parts of Southeast Asia including India (Rehm 2003).

Overall, 4 per cent of the global burden of disease is attributable to alcohol. This is as much as the burden of disease from tobacco (4.1 per cent) (Room *et al.* 2005). Internationally, the highest disease load attributable to alcohol is found in the heavy-drinking former socialist countries in Eastern Europe, where 12.1 per cent of disease burden is related to alcohol. North America, Western Europe, Japan, and Australasia have a 6.8 per cent disease burden (Room *et al.* 2005). In most low- and middle-income countries,

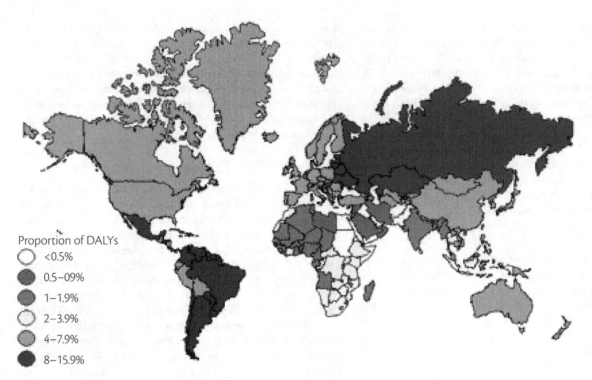

Fig. 9.16.3 Distribution of burden of disease attributable to alcohol in the world, expressed as disability adjusted life years (DALYs) (World Health Organization 2004b: http://www.who.int/topics/alcohol_drinking).

alcohol consumption is still relatively low, with a 1.3 per cent of the burden of disease in the Islamic Middle East and Indian subcontinent, and 2 per cent in the poorest countries of Africa and America (Room *et al.* 2005).

Given the relationship between alcohol consumption and cirrhosis, it would be expected that there is a lag period between changes in per capita alcohol consumption and cirrhosis-related mortality. Data regarding this lag effect have been conflicting. In fact, a long latency time is not observed, and the usual lag period is only one year or less (Kerr *et al.* 2000).

In Europe, 20–30 per cent of the population is estimated to consume excessive amounts of alcohol (Corrao *et al.* 1997). There was an increase in alcohol consumption until the late 1970s, followed by a period of stabilization. Along with this, there has been a pattern of stabilization to decline in cirrhosis mortality since the 1970s (Corrao *et al.* 1997; Ramstedt 2001).

In the United States, per capita consumption of all alcoholic beverages increased between 1962 and the early 1980s, and then decreased until 1998. Since then, there has a slight but persistent increase (Roizen *et al.* 1999). The cirrhosis mortality rate in the United States declined sharply in the early and mid-1970s in spite of the increase of overall per capita consumption till the early 1980s. The factors responsible for the discordance between US alcohol consumption and mortality rates have included better alcoholic liver disease treatments, increased 'Alcoholics Anonymous' memberships, and improved nutrition.

Despite a reduction of alcohol consumption in Europe in the 1970s, mortality rates for alcoholic liver disease decreased only in Western and Southern Europe, but did not change in Eastern and Northern Europe (Corrao *et al.* 1997). Studies in Australia (Saunders & Latt 1993) and Canada (Halliday *et al.* 1991) showed that cirrhosis-related mortality rates declined at almost the same time as the decrease per capita alcohol consumption. A similar pattern of almost simultaneous decrease in cirrhosis mortality and per capita alcohol consumption occurred in Europe during World Wars I and II, as well as in the United States during the Prohibition from 1919 to 1932 (Corrao *et al.* 1997; Saunders & Latt 1993).

In Japan alcohol consumption and all-type cirrhosis mortality increased for the past 50 years (Hasumura & Takeuchi 1991). The proportion of alcohol-induced liver disease increased to 5.1 per cent in 1968 to 10.7 per cent in 1977 and 14.1 per cent of cases in 1986. On the other hand, the Eastern Mediterranean Region—mostly countries with majority Muslim populations—displays a steady low alcohol consumption over a period of almost 40 years (World Health Organization 2004b).

In other parts of the world, including the most populous parts of the world, the trends have been alarming, showing increasing alcohol consumption, especially in the form of spirits, along with a tendency toward unhealthy patterns of alcohol intake (Campollo *et al.* 2001). This is the case in the Southeast Asian Region and the Western Pacific Region, driven by economic growth and aggressive marketing (Fig. 9.16.5) (World Health Organization 2004b; Pearson 2004). Without intervention, experts predict a future wave of alcohol-related problems in these countries. Korea has undergone dramatic socioeconomic transformation in the last 35 years. The per capita alcohol consumption rose from 1 l in 1970 to 7 l per year in 1980. There is also heavier consumption of distilled beverages. The proportion of patients in Korea with alcohol as aetiology of

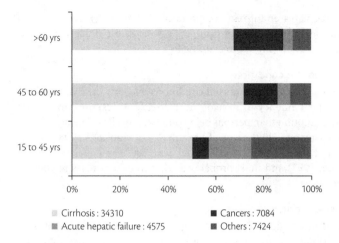

Fig. 9.16.4 Primary indications of liver transplantation in adult recipients (January 1988 to June 2006).
(*Source*: European Liver Transplant Registry, http://www.eltr.org/publi/IMG/gif/DIA8-2.gif).

liver disease increased from 1.5 per cent in 1980 to 24 per cent in 1993 (Park *et al.* 1998).

Morphology and natural history of alcoholic liver disease

Fatty liver (steatosis)

The first and most predictable hepatic change attributable to alcohol is the development of large droplet (macrovesicular) steatosis. This disorder usually resolves within two weeks if alcohol consumption is discontinued (Diehl 1997). In the past, it was assumed that alcoholic fatty liver was a benign process. However, it is now assumed that 5–15 per cent of patients will develop cirrhosis during a 10-year follow-up period (Sorensen *et al.* 1984).

Alcoholic steatohepatitis

The spectrum of alcoholic steatohepatitis includes fatty infiltration of hepatocytes associated with hepatocellular injury including: Ballooning degeneration, Mallory bodies inflammation with neutrophils and/or lymphocytes, and fibrosis with a perivenular, perisinusoidal, and pericellular disposition. These changes are present in 10–35 per cent of all alcoholics. It is not a benign process. Some patients will develop fatal decompensation. In addition, the risk of developing cirrhosis is increased. It is estimated that the probability of developing cirrhosis is ~10–20 per cent per year and ~70 per cent of patients with alcoholic hepatitis will eventually develop cirrhosis (Diehl 1997).

Cirrhosis

Worldwide, cirrhosis kills nearly 150 000 people each year (Corrao *et al.* 1997). Alcoholic cirrhosis accounts for ~38–50 per cent of all cirrhosis-related deaths (Stinson *et al.* 2001; Bellentani *et al.* 1997). The long-term prognosis of alcoholic cirrhosis improves with abstinence. The 5-year survival in compensated cirrhosis patients who continue to drink is <70 per cent, but can be as high as 90 per cent if they abstain from further alcohol intake. In patients with decompensated cirrhosis, the 5-year survival drops to <30 per cent in individuals who continue to drink, but is 60 per cent in those who stay abstinent (Diehl 1997; Alexander *et al.* 1971).

Hepatocellular carcinoma

Alcohol can be considered both as a primary cause of HCC and as a co-factor for the development of HCC. Most of the studies on incidence of HCC in alcoholic cirrhosis date from before the identification of the hepatitis C virus. As hepatitis C is relatively frequent in alcoholics, most of the reported HCC incidence rates in earlier studies are likely to be overestimated. Although the exact incidence rate of HCC in alcoholic cirrhosis is unknown, it is estimated to be over 1.5 per cent, making it worthwhile to offer patients surveillance (Bruix & Sherman 2005).

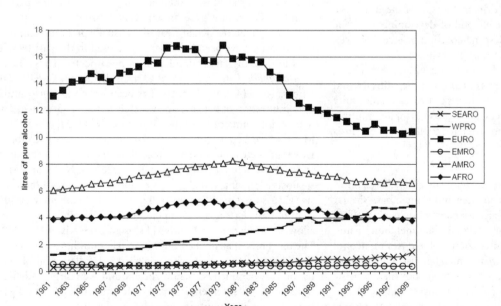

Fig. 9.16.5 Population-weighted means of the recorded adult per capita alcohol consumption in the WHO Regions 1961–1999 (World Health Organization 2004b: http://www.who.int/topics/alcohol_drinking)

Factors influencing the risk of alcoholic liver disease

Alcohol consumption can lead to steatohepatitis and cirrhosis. Most authors agree that persons who drink heavily (50–60 g of ethanol daily) represent a population at increased risk of developing liver disease (Becker et al. 2002). However, the absolute risk of acquiring alcoholic hepatitis or cirrhosis is relatively low (6.9 per cent in the two above-mentioned studies). This suggests that genetic factors and/or environment play a role in disease risk. Many studies that address the risk factors refer to their effect on 'alcoholic liver disease' in general rather than any specific aspect of alcoholic liver disease such as steatohepatitis.

Amount of alcohol

There is a general agreement that excessive alcohol consumption is associated with an increased risk of cirrhosis. However, the exact dose or a specific dose–response relationship for cirrhosis has not been agreed on. Measuring alcohol use in an individual or country has limitations. Most studies rely on interviews with patients and their families to estimate the amount, frequency and duration of alcohol consumption. Patients may not accurately report the quantity of alcohol they consume. The definition of a 'standard drink' varies from country to country: 8 g ethanol in the United Kingdom, 14 g in the United States, 19.75 g in Japan (Pearson 2004). The easiest would be to consider a standard drink containing 10 g of ethanol.

Evidence suggests that there is an increased risk for alcoholic liver disease with the ingestion of >60–80 g/day of alcohol in men and >20 g/day in women (Day 2000). 'Safe' limits of alcohol consumption for the liver are up to two drinks per day for women, and up to four drinks per day for men, with at least three alcohol-free days per week (Michielsen & Sprengers 2003).

Drinking behaviour

Researchers from Denmark showed in a large survey of 30 630 persons that beer or spirits are more likely to promote liver disease than wine (Becker et al. 2002). At present, it is uncertain whether wine per se is responsible for this reduced risk of liver disease compared to the other alcoholic beverages, or whether it represents a surrogate for other healthy behaviours such as increased consumption of fruits/vegetables (Everhart et al. 2003).

According to a Chinese study, drinking outside of mealtimes is a habit that might increase the likelihood of developing alcoholic liver disease (Lu et al. 2004). Researchers from France, however, found no such evidence (Pelletier et al. 2001).

Binge-drinking, an exaggerated form of non-mealtime drinking, has been reported to increase the risk of alcoholic hepatitis fivefold (Barrio et al. 2005), and to increase the risk of all-cause mortality in men and women (Tolstrup et al. 2004). Also drinking multiple types of drinks has been shown to be related to the risk of cirrhosis and non-cirrhotic liver disease (Naveau et al. 1997).

Gender

It is well recognized that women are more susceptible to alcohol-induced health disorders than men. Men and women have similar sized livers and when the rate of alcohol metabolism is normalized to liver mass, men and women have similar metabolic rates. However, blood alcohol levels after comparable doses of alcohol will usually be higher in women than in men because of their lower body volume and the higher percentage of their body mass consisting of fat. Evidence from animal models has suggested that oestrogen increases the gut permeability to endotoxin and accordingly upregulates endotoxin receptors of Kupffer cells leading to an increased production of tumour necrosis factor alpha in response to endotoxin (Enomoto et al. 1999).

Co-morbid conditions

Individuals with co-morbid conditions affecting the liver exhibit a greater tendency to develop liver disease in response to alcohol consumption than persons being otherwise healthy. This was clearly demonstrated in the case of hepatitis C (Corrao et al. 1998), hereditary haemochromatosis (Fletcher et al. 2002) and obesity (Naveau et al. 1997) and most probably applies to other causes of chronic hepatitis.

Genetic polymorphisms

Epidemiologic evidence is strong for the existence of heritable susceptibility to alcoholic liver disease. This appears related to several gene polymorphisms, some of which impact alcohol metabolism and others that influence hepatic immune responses.

Non-alcoholic fatty liver disease (NAFLD) and non-alcoholic steatohepatitis (NASH)

Definitions

Steatosis is defined as the accumulation of fat in the liver parenchymal cells or hepatocytes. A distinction is made between macrovesicular and microvesicular steatosis. Macrovesicular steatosis implies the presence of large fat vacuoles, containing predominantly triglycerides, and occupying a large part of the cell cytoplasm, displacing the nucleus towards the cell border. The hepatocytes may be enlarged by the presence of these fat vacuoles. Macrovesicular steatosis is graded according to the percentage of hepatocytes containing fat vacuoles: <5 per cent is minimal or no steatosis; >5 and ≤30 is mild steatosis; >30 and ≤60 is moderate; and >60 per cent is considered to be severe macrovesicular steatosis (D'Allessandro et al. 1991). In microvesicular steatosis, bipolar lipids are forming micelles, which are spread over the cytoplasm, and which do not displace the nucleus. The cells usually have normal dimensions. Grading is less complex: >45 per cent is considered to be severe microvesicular steatosis (Sheiner et al. 1995). In many patients, both types of steatosis are present, called mixed type steatosis. In those cases, macrovesicular steatosis is usually predominant.

Two terms have been interchangeably used in the past two decades to describe fat accumulation in hepatocytes. These include Non-alcoholic Fatty Liver (NAFL) and Non-alcoholic Fatty Liver Disease (NAFLD). While NAFL has been linked to constitutional fatty infiltration of hepatocytes, which is not necessarily associated with an inflammatory response or fibrosis, NAFLD has been linked to an active hepatic injury pattern, inflammation and fibrosis. However, there is no consensus regarding the use of these two terms and the distinction between them. Regardless, in NAFL or NAFLD, steatosis is present, and alcohol is excluded as a cause of the steatosis (Harrison et al. 2004). As >20 g of alcohol daily may be sufficient to induce steatosis, the maximum daily alcohol consumption allowed for the definition of NAFLD is 20 g (Harrison et al. 2004). The diagnosis of alcohol consumption relies on thorough anamnesis and hetero-anamnesis, with a detailed 7-day diary of alcohol use. Laboratory parameters are non-specific and even carboxy-deficient transferrin measurement is not very accurate in excluding significant alcohol consumption. In addition, the differential diagnosis cannot be made histologically, as the histological features of alcoholic and non-alcoholic liver disease seem to be identical. The diagnosis of the aspect of 'non-alcoholic' therefore constitutes a first problem in the interpretation of any data on the prevalence and natural history of NAFLD.

Non-alcoholic steatohepatitis (NASH) is a subgroup of NAFLD, in which liver steatosis is accompanied by signs of liver cell damage (especially ballooning of hepatocytes) and/or inflammation. In these patients, fibrous tissue may be generated, and patients can evolve to cirrhosis and its complications, including HCC. Although still debated, it is generally believed that pure steatosis does not lead to fibrogenesis and that only the NASH patients may present progressive liver disease (Angulo 2002).

Although not reflected by the name, NAFLD also implies the exclusion of other chronic liver diseases, including chronic viral hepatitis, toxic hepatitis (due to industrial toxins or solvents or to pharmacological agents), autoimmune liver disease, haemochromatosis, Wilson's disease, and some rare metabolic disorders. Hepatitis C, especially genotype 3, and Wilson's disease are two classical examples of liver diseases accompanied by steatosis, but they are not NAFLD. As will be discussed further, steatosis is no longer regarded as an innocent bystander, therefore the term NAFLD is preferred over NAFL.

Diagnosis

As already mentioned, a first problem is the diagnosis of the aspect 'non-alcoholic'. Laboratory tests, including elevation of AST (aspartate transaminase) more than ALT (alanine transaminase), elevation of γGT (gamma-glutamyl transpeptidase) or CDT (carboxy-deficient transferrin) measurement may be helpful, but are inaccurate. Thorough anamnesis and hetero-anamnesis is the cornerstone of the diagnosis, which therefore may always remain questionable.

A second problem is the diagnosis of steatosis and steatohepatitis. Abdominal ultrasound has a sensitivity of 70–75 per cent and a specificity of 60–70 per cent in diagnosing moderate to severe steatosis (Bellentani et al. 2000). CT scan and MRI are equally specific (100 per cent) and sensitive (75 per cent) in making the same distinction (Rinella et al. 2001). These non-invasive tools are thus not very sensitive, not able to accurately grade the steatosis, and not able to diagnose the presence of inflammation or fibrosis, and hence do not distinguish between NAFLD and NASH. Magnetic Resonance Spectroscopy can accurately quantify the fat content of a liver sample, but the need for specific software and practical considerations limits its use to specific research centres. Scores based on laboratory parameters are not validated for the diagnosis of steatosis (Miele et al. 2007). The gold standard for the diagnosis is still liver biopsy. The invasive character of that procedure, however, limits its use on a larger scale.

The diagnosis of steatohepatitis is even more complicated. Laboratory tests, especially the elevation of aminotransferase levels, are inaccurate, although frequently regarded as a sign of liver cell damage and hence inflammation, as patients with elevated liver tests may have pure steatosis without inflammation on liver biopsy, and 50 per cent of the patients with biopsy-proven steatohepatitis have normal transaminases (Prati et al. 2002). The cut-off values for normal aminotransferase levels have recently been questioned, and lowering the upper limit of normal to ≤30 U/l in males and ≤19 U/l in females increases the sensitivity for the diagnosis of NASH from 42 per cent to 80 per cent, but specificity decreases

from 80 per cent to 42 per cent (Kunde et al. 2005). Scoring systems based on laboratory parameters are unvalidated to date. Imaging cannot distinguish steatosis from steatohepatitis. Again liver biopsy is the gold standard. This also holds true for the diagnosis of fibrosis. Laboratory parameters are not useful, except for a stage of cirrhosis, where more specific laboratory features can be present. Scoring systems based on laboratory parameters can distinguish between no or mild fibrosis versus advanced fibrosis and cirrhosis in hepatitis C (Rosenberg et al. 2004), but have not been validated in NASH. Imaging is not useful for the staging of fibrosis, and is only of value if signs of cirrhosis indicate advanced liver disease. Elastography, an ultrasound-based technique measuring liver stiffness (Ganne-Carrie et al. 2006), has been validated in hepatitis C, but not in NASH, and, like the laboratory scoring systems, only roughly distinguishes between no or mild versus severe fibrosis and cirrhosis. Also for fibrosis, liver histology is still the gold, or at least the best, standard (Miele et al. 2007).

Prevalence of steatosis, NAFLD, and NASH

As already mentioned, the difficulty in diagnosing of non-alcoholic steatosis, and the lack of accuracy of the tools for the diagnosis of steatosis, constitute two major problems in the acquisition of precise epidemiological data. Sample selection constitutes a third problem, as some categories of patients are more at risk. This will be discussed in the next section.

In screening studies with ultrasound, prevalence varies between 16 per cent and 23 per cent (Bellentani et al. 2000). In an autopsy series of traffic accidents, steatosis was histologically diagnosed in 24 per cent of cases. The prevalence was clearly age-related: In those aged <20 years the prevalence was 1 per cent, while in those >60 years the prevalence rose to 39 per cent (Hilden et al. 1997). In a series of cadaveric donor livers, 17.5 per cent were steatotic (Crowley et al. 2000). If specific lipid stainings are used, prevalence up to 50 per cent can be noted (Urena et al. 1998). Based on these figures, and making the distinction with alcoholic steatosis, the prevalence of non-alcoholic steatosis is estimated at 15–20 per cent in the general adult population (Angulo 2002). Exact data on the prevalence of NASH in the general population are scarce. In an autopsy series, a prevalence of 6.3 per cent was reported. The prevalence is usually estimated at 2 per cent, but this highly depends on sample selection. As a number of risk factors can be identified (see below), prevalence rates may vary geographically (Neuschwander-Tetri et al. 2003).

NAFLD and NASH and the metabolic syndrome

The metabolic syndrome, associating visceral overweight, dyslipidaemia, hyperinsulinaemia or diabetes mellitus, and arterial hypertension, as defined by the Third Report of the National Cholesterol Education Expert Panel on Detection, Evaluation, and Treatment of High Blood Cholesterol in Adults (Adult Treatment Panel-ATP III) (Expert Panel 2001), seems to be closely related with NAFLD and NASH. Some authors consider NAFLD and NASH as the hepatic manifestation of the metabolic syndrome. Many epidemiological data are at least in favour of a close relationship between the two entities.

In patients with NAFLD, the metabolic syndrome, according to the criteria of the ATP III, is fully present in 30 per cent of males and 60 per cent of females. Visceral adiposity is present in 40 per cent and 65 per cent of males and females, respectively, and diabetes in

10 per cent and 30 per cent, respectively. These prevalence rates are significantly higher than in the control population. The metabolic syndrome is significantly more prevalent in patients with NASH compared to patients with simple steatosis (38 per cent vs. 14 per cent, $p = 0.004$) (Marchesini et al. 2003).

In patients with obesity, steatosis is present in 60–95 per cent, according to the selection of patients and the way of diagnosis (e.g. ultrasound or histology in a series of patients undergoing bariatric surgery). The body mass index is an independent predictive factor for the accumulation of fat in the liver (Marchesini et al. 2003). Liver steatosis is more specifically associated with visceral obesity. Increasing obesity is also associated with an increased risk of NASH. Patients with NASH have visceral obesity in 48 per cent of cases versus 31 per cent of patients with pure steatosis ($p = 0.005$) (Marchesini et al. 2003). In morbid obese patients undergoing bariatric surgery, the prevalence of NASH is 15–25 per cent (compared to 2 per cent in the general population) (Kunde et al. 2005). In obesity, the relative risk of morbidity and mortality related to terminal liver failure is 4 (Ioannou et al. 2003), and the known increased risk for malignancy is largely related to the increased risk for developing HCC.

In patients with type 2 diabetes, cirrhosis and its complications are the second cause of disease-specific mortality (de Marco et al. 1999). NAFLD, as diagnosed by liver ultrasound, is present in 69.5 per cent, in an age-dependent manner (65.4 per cent in patients aged 40–59 years and 74.6 per cent in those aged ≥ 60 years) (Angulo 2002). Diabetes mellitus is a major risk factor for NASH: 15 per cent of patients with diabetes have simple steatosis, but 56 per cent have NASH. Among patients with NAFLD and diabetes, 23.9 per cent develop cirrhosis and 19 per cent experience liver-related death in 19 per cent, compared to 10.6 per cent and 2 per cent in NAFLD patients without diabetes, respectively (Abrams et al. 2004).

The close association between NAFLD/NASH and the metabolic syndrome and its components explains the variance in prevalence data according to the patient selection. The prevalence of NAFLD/NASH is therefore high in the Western population, and will increase, parallel with the increasing prevalence of the components of the metabolic syndrome. The prevalence of obesity is 31 per cent in the adult US population and is projected to be 45 per cent in 2025 (Mokdad et al. 2003). In Belgium, 15 per cent of the adult population is obese (Moreau et al. 2004). In Africa and Asia, the prevalence of overweight is <10 per cent (Kosti et al. 2006). The increase of the prevalence of overweight in children and adolescents is of particular concern. The prevalence of diabetes is also increasing, and is currently estimated at 5–6 per cent worldwide (Adeghate et al. 2006). In the United States, 22 per cent of the adult population fulfils the criteria of the metabolic syndrome (Lin et al. 2007).

The natural history of NAFLD/NASH

Data on the natural history of NAFLD and NASH have the same three problems as outlined for the prevalence data. In patients with NASH, 45 per cent will exhibit fibrosis progression and 19 per cent will ultimately develop cirrhosis (Fassio et al. 2004). In patients with NAFLD, lifetime progression to cirrhosis is estimated at 2–5 per cent (Dam-Larsen et al. 2004; Ekstedt et al. 2006).

It is not clear whether only NASH patients will progress, or if pure steatosis may also lead to progressive fibrosis and ultimately cirrhosis. A recent long-term follow-up study (mean follow-up of 13.7 years) showed no increase in mortality in patients with elevated liver enzymes and pure steatosis on an initial biopsy. Patients with biopsy-proven NASH, on the other hand, had a higher risk of dying from cardiovascular disease (15.5 per cent vs. 7.5 per cent, $p = 0.04$) and from liver-related causes (2.8 per cent vs. 0.2 per cent, $p = 0.04$). Disease progression was, however, noted: 41 per cent had fibrosis progression and 5.4 per cent of patients developed cirrhosis, and this did not depend on features of inflammation on the initial biopsy (Ekstedt et al. 2006).

In patients with cryptogenic cirrhosis, >60 per cent have features that might have been associated with NASH and in these patients cirrhosis is believed to be an end stage of NASH (Ekstedt et al. 2006). Actually cryptogenic cirrhosis accounts for 8 per cent of the indications for liver transplantation in Europe (European Liver Transplant Registry). NASH may recur after liver transplantation, further enforcing the concept of NASH as an aetiology of cryptogenic cirrhosis (Maheshwari et al. 2006).

HCC has been reported in patients with NASH-associated cirrhosis. Data on prevalence and risk, however, are scarce. In the Ekstedt series (Ekstedt et al. 2006), 2.3 per cent developed HCC or 43 per cent of those with documented cirrhosis. It is thus not clear whether the risk is comparable to the 10 per cent cumulative risk usually reported in cirrhosis of any aetiology, but it might be higher (Smedile et al. 2005). HCC has not been reported without cirrhosis or extensive fibrosis.

Risk factors reported to be associated with an increased risk of fibrosis are: Age (>40 or >50 years of age), the presence of diabetes, BMI > 25 or > 28 or > 30, hypertriglyceridaemia, elevated transaminases >2 times the upper limit of normal, and AST/ALT >1 (Angulo et al. 1999; Adams et al. 2005). As already mentioned, patients with NAFLD and diabetes have a higher probability of cirrhosis and liver-related death, compared to NAFLD patients without diabetes (Abrams et al. 2004). In the Ekstedt series (Ekstedt et al. 2006), the 41 per cent progression of fibrosis was associated with higher levels of ALT, a higher weight gain during follow-up, more severe insulin resistance and more pronounced fatty infiltration. As stated previously, patients with NASH more frequently meet the criteria of the metabolic syndrome and are more likely to have visceral obesity compared to patients with simple steatosis. As it is believed that NASH is a subgroup of NAFLD at risk for progressive fibrosis, the metabolic syndrome and its components clearly constitute a risk factor for fibrosis and cirrhosis, which will be a major burden of disease in view of the epidemic of obesity and diabetes and their related conditions.

HCC may also be the ultimate result of NAFLD-related cirrhosis, as stated earlier. A significant proportion of HCC (7–30 per cent) develops in patients with cryptogenic cirrhosis, suggesting that the risk of developing a HCC is higher than from other aetiologies of cirrhosis. Diabetes also seems to be a major risk factor for developing HCC (Bugianesi 2005).

Overall conclusion

In spite of the availability of safe and effective vaccines and their proven effectiveness in reducing the chronic consequences of HBV infections, the current burden of disease associated with hepatitis B remains substantial. To finally achieve the WHO goal of HBV elimination, continuous efforts will be required to keep prevention of hepatitis B on the agenda of public health officers worldwide, and to continue to improve treatment options for those already suffering chronic hepatitis B.

Even if the present burden of disease caused by hepatitis C is somewhat less impressive, the lack of an effective vaccine despite major efforts in its development, and the limited success of treatment pose a substantial future threat to public health.

Alcoholic liver disease remains a major cause of morbidity and mortality worldwide. There is concern that, worldwide, alcoholic liver disease may increase in the next several decades. Recent data indicate that alcohol consumption is increasing in low- and middle-income countries. In addition, rates of excessive alcohol intake appear to be rising in women. Although alcohol-related cirrhosis mortality rates decreased in many countries during the past 30 years, rates are no longer declining in several countries and are actually increasing in low- and middle-income countries.

Although data on the prevalence and natural history of NAFLD/NASH are scarce and suffer from multiple methodological problems, it is clear that, because of its association with the metabolic syndrome and its components, which tend to take epidemic proportions in the Western population, NAFLD and NASH will constitute a major health problem in the near future.

Key points

◆ Liver cirrhosis and primary liver cancer are important public health problems worldwide.

◆ Viral hepatitis B and C, and alcoholic as well as non-alcoholic fatty liver disease, represent the major causes for these chronic liver diseases.

◆ Despite the availability and widespread use of effective hepatitis B vaccines, efforts will be required to keep the immunization programmes on the political and donor agenda.

◆ As the development of a hepatitis C vaccine has not yet resulted in success, prevention and control measures will form a major challenge to all those involved in public health.

◆ In low- and middle-income countries experts predict a future wave of alcohol-related liver diseases.

◆ Fatty liver disease and steatohepatitis, chronic liver diseases associated with the metabolic syndrome, tend to take epidemic proportions in the near future in Western populations.

References

Abrams G.A., Kunde S.S., Lazenby A.J. et al. (2004). Portal fibrosis and hepatic steatosis in morbidly obese subjects: a spectrum of non-alcoholic fatty liver disease. *Hepatology*, **40**, 475–83.

Adams L.A., Lymp J.F., St Sauver J. et al. (2005). The natural history of nonalcoholic fatty liver disease: a population-based cohort study. *Gastroenterology*, **129**, 113–21.

Adeghate E., Schatter P., and Dunn E. (2006). An update on the etiology and epidemiology of diabetes mellitus. *Ann N Y Acad Sci*, **1084**, 1–29.

Alexander J.F., Lischner M.W., Galambos J.T. (1971). Natural history of alcoholic hepatitis. II. The long-term prognosis. *The American Journal of Gastroenterology*, **56**, 515–25.

Alter M.J. (2007). Epidemiology of hepatitis C virus infection. *World Journal of Gastroenterology*, **13**, 2436–41.

André F.E. and Zuckerman A.J. (1994). Review: protective efficacy of hepatitis B vaccines in neonates. *J Med Virol*, **44**, 144–51.

Angulo P., Keach J.C., Batts K.P. et al. (1999). Independent predictors of liver fibrosis in patients with steatohepatitis. *Hepatology*, **30**, 1356–62.

Angulo P. (2002). Nonalcoholic fatty liver disease. *N Engl J Med*, **346**, 1221–31.

Banatvala J.E., Van Damme P. (2003). Hepatitis B vaccine—do we need boosters? *J Hepatol* **10**, 1–6.

Barrio E., Tome S., Rodriguez I. et al. (2005). Liver disease in heavy drinkers with and without alcohol withdrawal syndrome. *Alcoholism, Clinical and Experimental Research*, **28**, 131–6.

Becker U., Gronbaek M., Johansen D. et al. (2002). Lower risk for alcohol-induced cirrhosis in wine drinkers. *Hepatology*, **35**, 868–75.

Bellentani S., Saccoccio G., Masutti F. et al. (2000). Prevalence of and risk factors for hepatic steatosis in northern Italy. *Ann Intern Med*, **132**, 112–17.

Bruix J. and Sherman M. (2005). AASLD Practice Guideline. Management of hepatocellular carcinoma. *Hepatology*, **42**, 1208–36.

Bugianesi E. (2005). Review article: steatosis, the metabolic syndrome and cancer. *Aliment Pharmacol Ther*, **22**(Suppl 2): 40–3.

Campollo O., Martinez M.D., Valencia J.J. et al. (2001). Drinking patterns and beverage preferences of liver cirrhosis patients in Mexico. *Substance Use & Misuse*, **36**, 387–98.

Centers for Disease Control and Prevention (1987). Recommendations of the Immunization Practices Advisory Committee. Update on hepatitis B prevention. *Morbid Mortal Wkly Rep*, **36**, 353–60.

Chan C.Y., Lee S.D., Lo K.J. (2004). Legend of hepatitis B vaccination: the Taiwanese experience. *J Gastroenterol Hepatol*, **19**, 121–6.

Chang M.H., Chen C.J., Lai M.S., et al. (1997). Universal hepatitis B vaccination in Taiwan and the incidence of hepatocellular carcinoma in children. Taiwan Childhood Hepatoma Study Group. *N Engl J Med*, **336**, 1855–9.

Chen C.J., Yang H.I., Su J. et al. (2006). Risk of HCC across a biological gradient of serum HBV-DNA levels. *JAMA*, **295**, 65–73.

Chevalier S. and Pawlotsky J.M. (2007). Hepatitis C virus: virology, diagnosis and management of antiviral therapy. *World J Gastroenterol*, **7**, 2461–6. Review.

Corrao G. and Arico S. (1998). Independent and combined action of hepatitis C virus infection and alcohol consumption on the risk of symptomatic liver cirrhosis. *Hepatology*, **27**, 914–9.

Corrao G., Ferrari P., Zambon A. et al. (1997). Are the recent trends in liver cirrhosis mortality affected by the changes in alcohol consumption? Analysis of the latency period in European countries. *Journal of Studies on Alcohol*, **57**, 486–94.

Coursaget P., Leboulleux D., Soumare M. et al. (1994). Twelve-year follow-up study of hepatitis B immunisation of Senegalese infants. *J Hepatol*, **21**, 250–4.

Crowley H., Lewis D., Gordon F. et al. (2000). Steatosis in donor and transplant liver biopsies. *Human Pathology*, **31**, 1209–13.

D'Allessandro A., Kalayoglu M., Sollinger H. et al. (1991). The predictive value of donor liver biopsies for the development of primary non-function after orthotopic liver transplantation. *Transplantation*, **51**, 157–63.

Dam-Larsen S., Franzmann M., Andersen I.B. et al. (2004). Long term prognosis of fatty liver: risk of chronic liver disease and death. *Gut*, **53**, 750–55.

Day C.P. (2000). Who gets alcoholic liver disease: nature or nurture? *Journal of the Royal College of Physicians of London*, **34**, 557–62.

de Marco R., Locatelli F., Zoppini G. et al. (1999). Cause-specific mortality in type 2 diabetes. The Verona Diabetes Study. *Diabetes Care*, **22**, 756–61.

Diehl A.M. (1997). Alcoholic liver disease: natural history. *Liver Transplantation and Surgery*, **3**, 206–11.

Dienstag J.L., Werner B.G., Polk B.F. et al. (1984). Hepatitis B vaccine in health care personnel: safety, immunogenicity, and indicators of efficacy. *Ann Intern Med*, **82**, 8168–72.

Duclos P. (2003). Safety of immunization and adverse events following vaccination against hepatitis B. *J Hepatol*, **39**, S83–S88.

Ekstedt M., Franzen L.E., Mathiesen U.L. et al. (2006). Long-term follow-up of patients with NAFLD and elevated liver enzymes. *Hepatology*, **44**, 865–73.

El Serag H.B. (2005). Epidemiology of hepatocellular carcinoma. *Clin Liver Dis*, **5**, 87–107.

Enomoto N., Yamashina S., Schemmer P. *et al.* (1999). Estriolsensitizes rat Kupffer cells via gut-derived endotoxin. *American Journal of Physiology*, **277**, G671–7.

European Consensus Group on Hepatitis B immunity (2000). Are booster immunisations needed for lifelong hepatitis B immunity? *Lancet*, **355**, 561–65.

European Liver Transplant Registry (2007). Available at: http://www.eltr.org/publi/IMG/gif/DIA8-2.gif Accessed 15 September 2007.

Everhart J.E. (2003). In vino veritas? *Journal of Hepatology*, **38**, 411–9.

Expert Panel on Detection, Evaluation and Treatment of High Blood Cholesterol in Adults (2001). Executive Summary of The Third Report of The National Cholesterol Education Program (NCEP) Expert Panel on Detection, Evaluation and Treatment of High Blood Cholesterol in Adults (Adult Treatment Panel III). *JAMA*, **285**, 2486–97.

Fletcher L.M., Dixon J.L., Purdie D.M. *et al.* (2002). Excess alcohol greatly increases the prevalence of cirrhosis in hereditary hemochromatosis. *Gastroenterology*, **122**, 281–9.

Forns X. and Bukh J. (1999). The molecular biology of hepatitis C virus. Genotypes and quasispecies. *Clin Liver Dis*, **3**, 693–716.

Frank C., Mohamed M.K., Strickland G.T. *et al.* (2000). The role of parenteral antischistosomal therapy in the spread of hepatitis C virus in Egypt. *Lancet*, **355**, 887–91.

Ganne-Carrie N., Ziol M., de Ledighen V. *et al.* (2006). Accuracy of liver stiffness measurements for the diagnosis of cirrhosis in patients with chronic liver diseases. *Hepatology*, **44**, 1511–17.

Gerberding J.L. and Henderson D.K. (1992). Management of occupational exposures to bloodborne pathogens: hepatitis B virus, hepatitis C virus, and human immunodeficiency virus. *Clin Infect Dis*, **14**, 1179–85.

Goldstein S.T., Zhou F., Hadler S.C. *et al.* (2005). A mathematical model to estimate global hepatitis B disease burden and vaccination impact. *Int J Epidemiol*, **34**, 1329-39. Available at: http://aim.path.org/en/vaccines/hepb/assessBurden/model/index.html Accessed on 18 December 2007.

Hadler S.C. and Margolis H.S. (1992). Hepatitis B immunization: vaccine types, efficacy, and indications for immunization. In: Remington J.S., Swartz M.N., eds. Current Topics In Infectious Diseases (vol. 12), pp. 282–308. Boston, Blackwell Scientific Publications.

Halliday M.L., Coates R.A. and Rankin J.G. (1991). Changing trends of cirrhosis mortality in Ontario, Canada, 1911–1986. *International Journal of Epidemiology*, **20**, 199–208.

Harrison S.A. and Neuschwander-Tetri B.A. (2004). Nonalcoholic fatty liver disease and non-alcoholic steatohepatitis. *Clinics in Liver Disease*, **8**, 861–79.

Harwood H. (2000). Updating estimates of the economic costs of alcohol abuse in the United States: estimates, update, methods and data. *National Institute on Alcohol Abuse and Alcoholism, Bethesda, MD*.

Hasumura Y. and Takeuchi J. (1991). Alcoholic liver disease in Japanese patients: a comparison with Caucasians. *Journal of Gastroenterology and Hepatology*, **6**, 520–7.

Hilden M., Christoffersen P., Juhl E. *et al.* (1997). Liver histology in a "normal" population-examination of 503 consecutive fatal traffic casualties. *Scand J Gastroenterol*, **12**, 593–98.

Hollinger F.B. (1989). Factors influencing the immune response to hepatitis B vaccine, booster dose guidelines and vaccine protocol recommendations. *Am J Med*, **87**(suppl3A), 36–40.

Hoofnagle J.H., Doo E., Liang T.J. *et al.* (2007). Management of hepatitis B: summary of a clinical research workshop. *Hepatology*, **45**, 1056–75. Review.

Ioannou G.N., Weiss N.S., Kowdley K.V. *et al.* (2003). Is obesity a risk factor for cirrhosis-related death or hospitalization? A population-based cohort study. *Gastroenterology*, **125**, 1053–59.

Jilg W., Schmidt M., Zachoval R. *et al.* (1984). Hepatitis B vaccination: how long does protection last? *Lancet*, **2**, 458.

Jilg W., Schmidt M. and Deinhardt F. (1988). Persistence of specific antibodies after hepatitis B vaccination. *J Hepatol*, **6**, 201–7.

Kato N., Ootsuyama Y., Nakazawa T. *et al.* (1994). Genetic drift in hypervariable region I of the viral genome in persistent hepatitis C virus infection. *J Virol*, **68**, 4776–84.

Kao J-H and Chen D.S. (2005). Hepatitis B vaccination: to boost or not to boost? *Lancet*, **366**, 1337–38.

Keating G.M. and Noble S. (2003). Recombinant hepatitis B vaccine (Engerix-B): a review of its immunogenicity and protective efficacy against hepatitis B. *Drugs*, **2003**, 63:1021–51.

Kerr W.C., Fillmore K.M. and Marvy P. (2000). Beverage-specific alcohol consumption and cirrhosis mortality in a group of English-speaking beer-drinking countries. *Addiction*, **95**, 339–46.

Kosti R.I. and Panagiotakos D.B. (2006). The epidemic of obesity in children and adolescents in the world. *Cent Eur J Public Health*, **14**, 151–9.

Kunde S.S., Lazenby A.J., Clements R.H. *et al.* (2005). Spectrum of NAFLD and diagnostic implications of the proposed new normal range for serum ALT in obese women. *Hepatology*, **42**, 650–6.

Lauer G.M. and Walker B.D. (2001). Hepatitis C virus infection. *N Engl J Med*, **345**, 41–52.

Lavanchy D. (2004). Hepatitis B virus epidemiology, disease burden, treatment, and current and emerging prevention and control measures. *J Viral Hep*, **11**, 97–107.

Lavanchy D. (2005). Worldwide epidemiology of HBV infection, disease burden, and vaccine prevention. *J Clin Virol*, **34 (Suppl 1)**, S1–3.

Lee W.M. (1997). Hepatitis B virus infection. *N Engl J Med*, **337**, 1733–45.

Lin S.X. and Pi-Sunyer E.X. (2007). Prevalence of the metabolic syndrome among US middle-aged and older adults with and without diabetes: a preliminary analysis of the NHANES 1999-2002 data. *Ethn Dis*, **17**, 35–9.

Lok A.S. and McMahon J. (2007) Chronic hepatitis B: AASLD Practice Guidelines. *Hepatology*, **45**, 507–39.

Lu X.L., Luo J.Y., Tao M. *et al.* (2004). Risk factors for alcoholic liver disease in China. *World Journal of Gastroenterology*, **10**, 2423–6.

Maheshwari A. and Thuluvath P.J. (2006). Cryptogenic cirrhosis and NAFLD: are they related? *Am J Gastroenterol*, **101**, 664–8.

Marchesini G., Bugianesi E., Forlani G. *et al.* (2003). Nonalcoholic fatty liver, steatohepatitis, and the metabolic syndrome. *Hepatology*, **37**, 917–23.

Memon M.I. and Memon M.A. (2002). Hepatitis C: an epidemiological review. *J Viral Hepat*, **9**, 84–100.

Michielsen P.P. and Sprengers D. (2003). Who gets alcoholic liver disease: nature or nurture? (summary of the discussion). *Acta Gastroenterologica Belgica*, **66**, 292–3.

Michielsen P.P., Francque S.M. and van Dongen J.L. (2005). Viral hepatitis and hepatocellular carcinoma. *World J Surg Oncol*, **20**, 3: 27.

Miele L., Forgione A., Gasbarrini G. *et al.* (2007). Noninvasive assessment of liver fibrosis in non-alcoholic fatty liver disease (NAFLD) and non-alcoholic steatohepatitis (NASH). *Transl Res*, **149**, 114–25.

Mokdad A.H., Ford E.S., Bowman B.A. *et al.* (2003). Prevalence of obesity, diabetes and obesity-related health risk factors. *JAMA*, **289**, 76–9.

Moreau M., Valente F., Mak R. *et al.* (2004). Obesity, body fat distribution and incidence of sick leave in the Belgian workforce: the Belstress study. *Int J Obes Relat Metab Disord*, **28**, 574–82.

Naveau S., Giraud V., Borotto E. *et al.* (1997). Excess weight risk factor for alcoholic liver disease. *Hepatology*, **25**, 108–11.

Neuschwander-Tetri B.A. and Caldwell S.H. (2003). Nonalcoholic fatty liver disease: summary of an AASLD Single Topic Conference. *Hepatology*, **37**, 1202–19.

Ng K.P., Saw T.L., Baki A. *et al.* (2005). Impact of expanded programme on immunization against hepatitis B infection in school children in Malaysia. *Med Microbiol Immunol*, **194**, 163–8.

Niu M.T. (1996). Review of 12 million doses shows hepatitis B vaccine safe. *Vaccine Weekly*, **4**, 13–5.

Park S.C., Oh S.I. and Lee M.S. (1998). Korean status of alcoholics and alcohol-related health problems. *Alcoholism, Clinical and Experimental Research*, 22, 170S–172S.

Pearson H. (2004). Public health: The demon drink. *Nature*, 428, 598–600.

Pelletier S., Vaucher E., Aider R. *et al.* (2002). Wine consumption is not associated with a decreased risk of alcoholic cirrhosis in heavy drinkers. *Alcohol and Alcoholism*, 37, 618–22.

Perz J.F., Armstrong G.L., Farrington L.A. *et al.* (2006a). The contributions of hepatitis B virus and hepatitis C virus infections to cirrhosis and primary liver cancer worldwide. *J of Hepatol*, 45, 529–38.

Perz J.F., Elm JL J.R., Fiore A.E. *et al.* (2006b). Near elimination of hepatitis B infections among Hawaii elementary school children universal infant hepatitis B vaccination. *Pediatrics*, 118, 1403–8.

Pincock S. (2003). Binge drinking on the rise in UK and elsewhere. Government report shows increases in alcohol consumption, cirrhosis, and premature deaths. *Lancet*, 362, 1126–7.

Prati D., Taioli E., Zanella A. *et al.* (2002). Updated definitions of healthy ranges for serum alanine aminotransferase levels. *Ann Intern Med*, 137, 1–10.

Prati D. (2006). Transmission of hepatitis C virus by blood transfusions and other medical procedures: a global review. *J Hepatol*, 45, 607–16.

Ramstedt M. (2001). Per capita alcohol consumption and liver cirrhosis mortality in 14 European countries. *Addiction*, 96 (Suppl 1), S19–33.

Raza S.A., Clifford G.M., Franceschi S. (2007). Worldwide variation in the relative importance of hepatitis B and hepatitis C viruses in hepatocellular carcinoma: a systematic review. *British Journal of Cancer*, 96, 1127–34.

Rehm J., Rehn N., Room R. *et al.* (2003). The global distribution of average volume of alcohol consumption and patterns of drinking. *European Addiction Research*, 9, 147–56.

Rendi-Wagner P., Shouval D., Genton B. *et al.* (2006). Comparative immunogenicity of a PreS/S hepatitis B vaccine in non- and low responders to conventional vaccine. *Vaccine*, 24, 2781–2789.

Rinella M., Alonso E., Rao S. *et al.* (2001). Body mass index as a predictor of hepatic steatosis in living liver donors. *Liver Transplant*, 7, 409–13.

Roizen R., Kerr W.C., Fillmore K.M. (1999). Cirrhosis mortality and per capita consumption of distilled spirits, United States, 1949-1994: trend analysis. *The Western Journal of Medicine*, 171, 83–7.

Romano L., Mele A., Pariani E. *et al.* (2004). Update in the universal vaccination against hepatitis B in Italy: 12 years after its implementation. *Eur J Public Health*, 14(Suppl), S19.

Room R., Babor T. and Rehm J. (2005). Alcohol and public health. *Lancet*, 365, 519–30.

Rosenberg W.M.C., Voelker M., Thiel R. *et al.* on behalf of the European Liver Fibrosis Group (2004). Serum markers detect the presence of liver fibrosis: a cohort study. *Gastroenterology*, 127, 1704–13.

Safary A. and André F. (1999). Over a decade of experience with the yeast recombinant hepatitis B vaccine. *Vaccine*, 18, 57.

Saunders J.B. and Latt N. (1993). Epidemiology of alcoholic liver disease. *Ballières Clinics in Gastroenterology*, 7, 555–79.

Sheiner P., Emre S., Cubukcu O. *et al.* (1995). Use of donor livers with moderate-to-severe macrovesicular fat. *Hepatology*, 22, 205A.

Sherlock S. (1993). Clinical features of hepatitis. In Zuckerman A.J., Thomas H.S., eds. *Viral Hepatitis*, pp. 1–11. Churchill Livingstone, London.

Shouval D., Ilan Y., Adler R. *et al.* (1994). Improved immunogenicity in mice of a mammalian cell-derived recombinant hepatitis B vaccine containing pre-S_1 and pre-S_2 antigens as compared with conventional yeast-derived vaccines. *Vaccine*, 12, 1453–1459.

Smedile A. and Bugianesi E. (2005). Steatosis and hepatocellular carcinoma risk. *Eur Rev Med Pharmacol Sci*, 9, 291–293.

Sorensen T.I., Orholm M., Bentsen K.D. *et al.* (1984). Prospective evaluation of alcohol abuse and alcoholic liver injury in men as predictors of development of cirrhosis. *Lancet*, 2, 241–44.

Stinson F.S., Grant B.F. and Dufour M.C. (2001). The critical dimensions of ethnicity in liver cirrhosis mortality statistics. *Alcoholism, Clinical and Experimental Research*, 25, 1181–7.

Szmuness W., Stevens C.E., Zang E.A. *et al.* (1981). A controlled clinical trial of the efficacy of the hepatitis B vaccine (Hepatavax B): a final report. *Hepatology* 5, 377–85.

Tan J. and Lok A. (2007). Update on viral hepatitis: 2006. *Gastroenterology*, 23, 263–267.

Tandon B.N. and Tandon A. (1997). Epidemiological trends of viral hepatitis in Asia. In Rizzetto M., Purcell R.H., Gerin J.L., Verme G., eds. *Viral Hepatitis and Liver Disease*, pp. 559–561. Edizioni Minerva Medica, Turin.

Tolstrup J.S., Jensen M.K., Tjonneland A. *et al.* (2004). Drinking pattern and mortality in middle-aged men and women. *Addiction*, 99, 323–30.

Urena M., Ruiz-Delgado F., Moreno Gonzalez E. *et al.* (1998). Hepatic steatosis in liver transplant donors: common feature of donor population? *World J Surg*, 22, 837–44.

Venters C., Graham W. and Cassidy W. (2004). Recombivax-HB: perspectives past, present and future. *Expert Rev Vaccines*, 3, 119–29.

Viviani S., Jack A., Hall A.J. *et al.* (1999). Hepatitis B vaccination in infancy in the Gambia: protection against carriage at 9 years of age. *Vaccine*, 17, 2946–50.

Wainwright R., Bulkow L.R., Parkinson A.J. *et al.* (1997). Protection provided by hepatitis B vaccine in a Yupik Eskimo Population: results of a 10 year study. *J Infect Dis*, 175, 674–7.

West D.J. and Calandra G.B. (1996). Vaccine induced immunologic memory for hepatitis B surface antigen: implications for policy on booster vaccination. *Vaccine*, 14, 1019–27.

Whittle H.C., Maine N., Pilkington J. *et al.* (1995). Long-term efficacy of continuing hepatitis B vaccination in infancy in two Gambian villages. *Lancet*, 345, 1089–92.

World Health Onganization (2001). Expanded Programme on Immunization. Introduction of hepatitis B vaccination into childhood immunization services: management guidelines, including information for health workers and parents (WHO/V&B/01.31). Geneva, World Health Organization, 2001. Available at http://www.who.int/vaccines-documents/DocsPDF01/www613.pdf (accessed 12 December 2006).

World Health Organization (2004a). Hepatitis B vaccines (WHO position paper). *Weekly Epidemiol Rec*, 79, 255–63.

World Health Organization (2004b). Global Status Report on Alcohol 2004. Available at http://www.who.int/topics/alcohol_drinking Accessed 20 December 2007

World Health Organization (2006). Vaccines and Biologicals. WHO vaccine preventable disease monitoring system. Global summary 2006 (data up to 2005). Available at http://www.who.int/vaccines-documents/GlobalSummary.pdf Accessed on 15 September 2007.

Worman H.J. (1999). Acute versus chronic disease. In: The Liver Disorders Sourcebook, pp. 12–15. Lowell House, Chicago, Illinois.

Zanetti A.R., Mariano A., Romanò L. *et al.* (2005). Long-term immunogenicity of hepatitis B vaccination and policy for booster: an Italian multicentre study. *Lancet* 366, 1379–84.

Emerging and re-emerging infections

David L. Heymann

Introduction

The microbial world is complex, dynamic and constantly evolving. Infectious agents reproduce rapidly, mutate frequently, cross the species barrier between animal hosts and humans, and adapt with relative ease to their new environments. Because of these traits, infectious agents are able to alter their epidemiology, their virulence, and their susceptibility to anti-infective drugs.

When disease is caused by a microbe that is newly identified and not known previously to infect humans, it is commonly called an emerging infectious disease, or simply an emerging infection. When disease is caused by an infectious agent previously known to infect humans that has re-entered human populations or changed in epidemiology or susceptibility to anti-infective drugs, it is called a re-emerging infection. A report published by the United States Institute of Medicine in 1992 first called attention to emerging and re-emerging infectious diseases as evidence that the fight against infectious diseases was far from won, despite great advances in the development of antimicrobials and vaccines (Lederberg *et al.* 1992).

All forms of infectious agents—bacteria, viruses, parasites, and prions—are able to emerge or re-emerge in human populations, and it is estimated that 70 per cent or more of all emerging infections have a source in animals. When a new infectious agent enters human populations there are several potential outcomes. In some instances, infected humans become ill, while in others, infections are asymptomatic. Once humans are infected, human-to-human transmission may or may not occur. If it occurs, it may be limited to one, two, or more generations, or it may be sustained indefinitely. Among those infectious agents that cause disease, some maintain their virulence, while others attenuate over time. Changes in the epidemiological characteristics of infectious agents may occur gradually, or they may occur abruptly as the result of a sudden genetic change during reproduction and/or replication.

Epidemiology of emerging and re-emerging infections

Rabies and variant Creutzfeldt–Jakob disease are clear examples of human infections that cause illness but cannot transmit from human to human unless there is an iatrogenic cause of transmission through non-sterile medical procedures, blood transfusion, or organ transplant. In several instances, corneal transplantation from a person who died undiagnosed with rabies-infection has caused rabies in transplant recipients. The recent identification of several humans with vCJD associated with blood transfusion demonstrates its potential to spread iatrogenically within the human population.

Human monkeypox provides a clear example of an infectious agent that can infect humans but not sustain transmissibility. Thought to have a rodent reservoir in the sub-Saharan rain forest, the monkeypox virus infects humans who come in contact with an infected animal. Transmission is sustained through one or two generations and then ceases. In the first generation of cases, the case fatality rate can approach 10 per cent, but with passage through human populations the virulence and case fatality of human monkeypox decreases as its transmissibility declines.

The human immunodeficiency virus (HIV) is an example of an infectious agent that has been able to infect humans, maintain virulence and sustain transmission. A long incubation period for HIV has ensured sustained transmission resulting in endemnicity worldwide, causing an estimated 2 million deaths in 2007 alone. It is hypothesized that HIV entered human populations from a non-human primate sometime in the early twentieth century. It escaped detection in the late 1970s when human-to-human transmission was being amplified on the African continent, in island nations of the Caribbean, and in North America. By the time it was first identified in the early 1980s, it had spread widely throughout the world.

The short incubation period in persons infected with the Ebola virus, and the high case fatality rates are less compatible with long-term human-to-human transmission. Ebola endemnicity in humans has not developed, though frequent re-emergence and localized outbreaks with human-to-human transmission continue to be documented. The potential for attenuation of the Ebola virus with passage is unknown, though in its present form it is unlikely that it will be able to become endemic in human populations because of its short incubation period and rapid progression to death in the majority of those infected.

The RNA virus that causes seasonal influenza is highly unstable genetically and mutates frequently during replication, requiring annual antigenic modifications in seasonal influenza vaccines to ensure protection. Avian influenza viruses are likewise unstable and at times infect humans and cause sickness and death. Occasionally, avian influenza viruses cause human influenza pandemics. The trigger virus for the influenza pandemic of 1918 is thought to have been an avian influenza virus. One hypotheses of its origin is that over time it circulated among birds and possibly some mammals, and through adaptive mutation, the virus gradually assumed a form that could infect humans and easily transmit.

Two other influenza pandemics of the twentieth century, in 1957 and 1968, are thought to have been caused by more abrupt genetic reassortment during the intracellular replication process in an animal dually infected with a human and an avian influenza virus. Risk factors for emergence of influenza viruses in humans are thought to be highest in areas such as South China and Southeast Asia where there are large populations of aquatic birds (the hosts of many different types of avian influenza viruses) and where humans live in close proximity to animals that may be infected by these aquatic birds.

Currently, H5N1, an avian influenza virus that was first identified as the cause of human illness in 1997, continues to cause occasional severe infections in humans but remains a zoonotic human infection and does not transmit easily from human to human. Most scientists agree that this virus, like many other avian influenza viruses, has the potential to mutate and gain the epidemiological characteristics that would permit it to spread easily from human to human and cause a pandemic.

Susceptibility of infectious agents to anti-infective drugs

Bacteria, viruses, and parasites can develop resistance to anti-infective drugs through spontaneous mutation and natural selection, or through the exchange of genetic material between strains and species. They then transmit from human to human, replacing more susceptible organisms with resistant strains. Soon after development of the first antibiotics, warning signs of microbial resilience began to appear. By the end of the 1940s, resistance of hospital strains of *Staphylococcus aureus* to penicillin emerged in the United Kingdom with resistance levels as high as 14 per cent, and by the end of the 1990s, levels had risen to of 95 per cent or greater (Fig. 9.17.1).

In addition to acquiring genes encoding resistance to all penicillins—including methicillin and other narrow-spectrum β-lactamase-resistant antibiotics—*S. aureus* has developed resistance to methicillin. Methicillin-resistant *S. aureus* (MRSA) first identified in the United Kingdom in 1961, is now widespread in hospitals throughout the world.

By 1976, chloroquine-resistant *Plasmodium falciparum* malaria was highly prevalent in Southeast Asia and 10 years later was found worldwide, as was high-level resistance to two second-line drugs, sulphadoxine-pyrimethamine and mefloquine. Today combination therapy with two antimalarial drugs with different targets is required to ensure effective treatment, as is surveillance to measure the continuing evolution of antimalarial drug resistance.

The bacterial and viral infections that contribute most to human disease are also those in which antimicrobial resistance is rapidly emerging: Diarrhoeal diseases such as dysentery; respiratory tract infections, including pneumococcal pneumonia and tuberculosis; sexually transmitted infections such as gonorrhoea and HIV; and infectious agents that have now accumulated resistance genes to virtually all currently available anti-infective drugs such as MRSA and extremely resistant tuberculosis (XDR-TB).

Geographic distribution of emerging and re-emerging infections

Emerging infections have the potential to occur in every country and on every continent (Fig. 9.17.2). Though the term emerging infections was newly introduced in the early 1990s, the previous 30 years had seen panoply of newly identified infections in humans on every continent. The year 1976 was especially illustrative of this phenomenon with the identification of the swine flu virus (H1N1), thought to be a direct descendant of the virus that caused the pandemic of 1918, at a military base in the Fort Dix (United States); the identification of *Legionella pneumophila* as the cause of an outbreak of severe respiratory illness among a group of veterans staying at a hotel in downtown Philadelphia (United States), initially feared to be a human outbreak of swine influenza (H1N1); and the identification of the Ebola virus as the cause of simultaneous outbreaks of haemorrhagic fever in Sudan and the Democratic Republic of Congo (then called Zaire).

Nine years earlier, in 1967, the Marburg virus had been identified in an outbreak in Germany that caused 25 primary infections and seven deaths among laboratory workers who were infected by handling monkeys from Uganda, and six secondary cases in health workers who took care of primary cases, with subsequent spread to family members. A member of the same filovirus family as Ebola, the Marburg virus has caused sporadic small outbreaks in Africa during the 1970s and 1980s, and larger outbreaks in 1998 in the Democratic Republic of Congo and 2005 in Angola. Since the Marburg virus was first identified in 1967 there have been over 40 other newly identified infectious agents in humans, an average of one per year.

Health workers and emerging/re-emerging infections

As clearly recorded during the Marburg outbreak of 1967, laboratory and health workers are at especially high risk of emerging and re-emerging infections. Outbreaks of Marburg, Ebola, and recently of severe acute respiratory syndrome (SARS), provide clear examples of the potential for health workers to become infected, and in some instances to sustain and amplify transmission in hospitals, and through their patients and family members, to the community. In the 1995 outbreak of Ebola haemorrhagic fever in Kikwit (Democratic Republic of Congo), almost one third of those infected were health workers, and in the 2003 SARS outbreak in Singapore, 10 health workers were thought to have been infected while treating an infected health worker colleague who is also thought to have infected her husband, three other patients and seven visitors to the hospital. Laboratory workers are also at risk of infection: The last human case of smallpox was caused by a laboratory accident in the United Kingdom, and the last-known human cases of SARS occurred in laboratory accidents in Singapore and China.

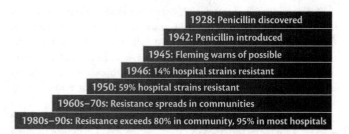

Fig. 9.17.1 Evolution of penicillin resistance in *Staphylococcus aureus*.

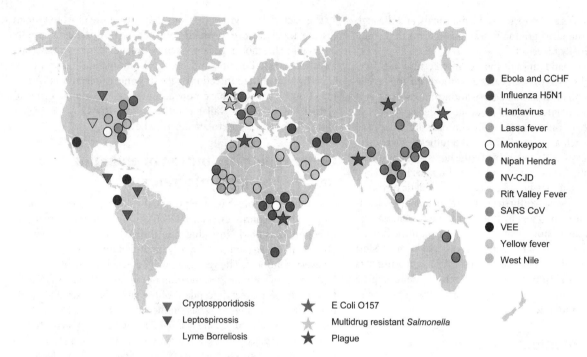

Fig. 9.17.2 Selected emerging and re-emerging infectious diseases: 1996–2004.

Economic impact of emerging and re-emerging infections

Outbreaks caused by emerging and re-emerging infections are costly (Fig. 9.17.3). They consume health-care resources and divert them from endemic disease problems, result in productivity loss, and decrease trade and tourism revenue. At times they economically devastate entire sectors. This has occurred after major outbreaks of emerging or re-emerging infections during the past 20 years, with economic losses ranging from an estimated US$39 million after the reemergence of cholera in Tanzania in 1998, to approximately US$39 billion after the emergence of bovine spongiform encephalopathy in the United Kingdom during the period 1990–1998.

SARS was likewise responsible for sizeable economic losses and insecurity in financial markets across Asia and worldwide. With fewer than 9000 cases, the outbreak was estimated by the Asian Development Bank to have cost Asian countries an estimated US$20 billion in gross domestic product (GDP) terms for 2003, and up to US$60 billion of gross expenditure and business losses.

The main drivers of the economic impact of outbreaks caused by emerging and re-emerging infections are travel, tourism, trade and consumer confidence. Fear of transmission causes international tourists to choose alternative holiday locations, and local population to avoid any perceived source of infection such as restaurants and other public leisure venues—sectors of the economy that are significant contributors to the GDP of many countries.

Factors influencing emergence and re-emergence

Many external factors provide opportunities for enhanced emergence or re-emergence of infectious diseases. They range from weakened public health infrastructure and failure of safety procedures/ regulations to increases in population; anthropogenic activities or natural variances in climate; civil disturbance/human displacement; and human behaviour that varies from occupation and misperceptions about the use of anti-infective drugs to the safety of public health interventions and the desire to deliberately cause terror and harm.

Weakened public health infrastructure

Weakening of public health infrastructure resulted in part from decreased investment in public health during the second half of the twentieth century. *Aedes aegypti* has now become well established in many large cities worldwide following the deterioration of mosquito control campaigns during the 1970s. The resurgence of the *Aedes* species has been confounded by the adoption of modern consumer habits in urban areas where discarded household appliances, tyres, plastic food containers, and jars create abundant artificial mosquito breeding sites.

Along with the increase in *Aedes* species there has been an increased risk of outbreaks of dengue. Prior to 1970, nine countries, mainly in Latin America, reported outbreaks of dengue. Thirteen years later, during 1983, 13 countries in Latin America and Asia reported dengue outbreaks, and by 1998, 1.2 million cases were reported from 56 countries.

During 2001, 69 countries reported outbreaks of dengue, and it is now endemic in more than 100 countries in Africa, the Americas, the Eastern Mediterranean, Southeast Asia, and the Western Pacific. During 2003 there were approximately 1.4 million cases and 6600 deaths reported to WHO. Major dengue outbreaks have occurred in Brazil, Indonesia, Thailand, Viet Nam, Bangladesh, and India.

In 2005, the Chikungunya virus, likewise transmitted by *Aedes aegypti*, emerged and spread throughout several southern Pacific islands. A total of 3100 human infections were reported by a sentinel network on La Réunion within the first 6 months of the outbreak,

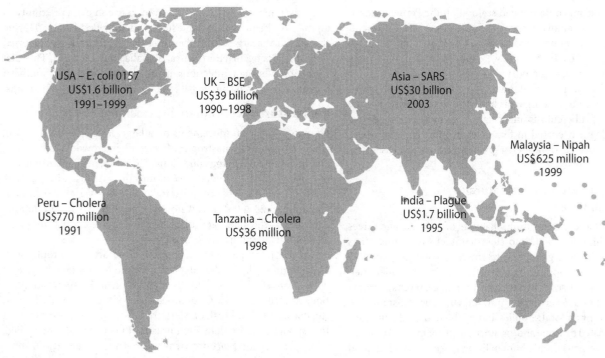

a Excludes economic impact of human sickness and death.

Fig. 9.17.3 Direct economic impact of selected infectious disease outbreaks, 1990–2003a.

leading to an estimate of over 204 000 human infections by March 2006. In 2007, the Chikungunya virus spread north to Europe, where it caused an outbreak in northern Italy.

Lapses in childhood immunization coverage due to weakened childhood immunization programmes in Russia in the early 1990s resulted in the re-emergence of diphtheria, with major epidemics in the early 1990s. Reported cases of diphtheria in the Russian Federation increased from just over 1200 in 1990 to 3897 in 1992 to over 5000 in 1993. Likewise, lapses in yellow fever vaccination programmes in sub-Saharan Africa since the 1950s have left large susceptible populations in both rural and urban areas of sub-Saharan Africa, with sporadic urban outbreaks in cities in Côte d'Ivoire (2001), Senegal and Guinea (2002), and Burkina Faso (2004).

Most epidemiologists recognize that it was in part because of weak surveillance systems in developing countries that HIV rapidly spread during the late 1970s, and was not detected until it was first identified when it began to transmit in the United States.

Failure of safety procedures/regulations

Sub-standard universal precautions and hospital regulations during the 1980s led to breaches in sterile injection practices and nosocomial infections of HIV in the former USSR and Romania, together infecting over 250 children, accompanied by high levels of hepatitis B in both patients and health workers. Likewise sub-standard universal precautions led to nosocomial outbreaks of Ebola haemorrhagic Fever in the Democratic republic of Congo in 1976 and 1995, where syringes and/or failed barrier nursing amplified the transmission to patients, health workers, and the community. Lapses in universal precautions led to nosocomial transmission of SARS in hospitals in China and Hong Kong, Singapore, Vietnam, and Canada, where outbreaks then spread from hospitals to communities.

Changes in the process of rendering the carcasses of ruminant animals for the preparation of bone meal fed to other ruminant animals are thought to have been the cause of the outbreak of borine spongiform encephalopathy (BSE) in cattle that also led, in May 1995, to the death of a 19-year male in the United Kingdom, the first human death from what is now known to be variant Creutzfeldt–Jakob Disease (vCJD) or human Bovine Spongiform Encephalopathy (hBSE). The BSE and hBSE outbreaks demonstrate the health consequences of regulations for rendering that had changed over a 10-year period prior to 1995, inadvertently permitting rendered parts of cattle infected with the BSE-causing prion to contaminate bone meal made from rendered carcasses and used for livestock feed. The most likely source of human infection is thought to be through the consumption of contaminated meat. The BSE outbreak led to the recognition of the need for stronger government intervention along the entire 'feed to food' continuum to ensure the safety of foodstuffs for human consumption.

Population increase

The world's population more than doubled in the second half of the twentieth century, accelerating most rapidly in the developing countries of the tropics and sub-tropics. Rural–urban migration has resulted in inadequacy of water and sanitation systems, crowded living conditions and other basic infrastructure associated with population growth. In 1950, there were two urban areas in the world with populations greater than 7 million; by 1990, this number had risen to 23, and by 2005 to 30.

Population increases in Latin America resulted in breakdowns in sanitation and water systems in large coastal cities. In 1991, when cholera re-emerged in Peru after having been quiescent for approximately 100 years, it rapidly spread throughout Latin America. Thought to have originated from contaminated seafood on the Peruvian coast, the disease spread rapidly across the South American continent, causing nearly 400 000 reported cases and over 4000 deaths in 16 countries that year. By 1995, there were more than 1 million cases and just over 10 000 deaths reported in the Americas.

Urbanization, and the subsequent crowding with sub-standard and living conditions in slum areas has likewise contributed to the re-emergence of tuberculosis and plague. The most recent serious outbreak of plague occurred in five states in India in 1994, where almost 700 suspected bubonic or pneumonic plague cases and 56 deaths were reported.

Anthropogenic activities or natural variance in climate

Deforestation that disrupts natural habitats of animals, and forces animals, searching for food, into closer contact with humans has been linked to the emergence and re-emergence of Lassa Fever in West Africa, and sine nom virus in North America. First identified in 1969 when two nurses died with a haemorrhagic fever syndrome in Nigeria, the Lassa Fever virus is now known to be transmitted to humans from human food supplies and/or the household environment contaminated by urine and/or other excreta of infected rodents. In many instances, rats invade human living spaces in search of food because rainforests, a natural habitat, have been destroyed and can no longer support their needs. Sin nombre virus is a hantavirus, first identified in an outbreak in the southwestern part of the United States in 1993. It is now known to spread from infected rodents to humans through aerosolized excreta found in dust of homes that have been invaded by rodents as they scavenge for food.

In Latin America, Chagas disease re-emerged as an important human disease after mismanagement of deforested land caused triatomine populations to move from their wild natural hosts to involve humans and domestic animals in the transmission cycle, eventually transforming the disease into an urban infection that can be transmitted by blood transfusion. Other emerging infections influenced by changing habitats of animals include Lyme borreliosis in Europe and North America, transmitted to humans who come into contact with ticks that normally feed on rodents and deer, the reservoir of *Borrelia burgdorfi* in nature.

The narrow band of desert in sub-Saharan Arica, in which epidemic *Neisseria meningitides* infections traditionally occur, has enlarged as drought spread south so that Uganda and Tanzania experience epidemic meningitis. Climate extremes, whether involving excessive rainfall or drought, can likewise displace animal species and bring them into closer contact with human settlements, or increase vector breeding sites. A 1998 outbreak of Japanese encephalitis in Papua New Guinea has been linked to extensive drought, which led to increased breeding sites for the *culex* mosquito as rivers dried into stagnant pools. Mosquitoes then transmitted the Japanese encephalitis virus from infected pigs and or wild birds to humans. The Japanese encephalitis virus is now widespread in Southern Asia from India and Thailand to Malaysia, and as far north as Korea and Japan.

Above-normal rainfall associated with the occurrence of the warm phase of the El Niño Southern Oscillation phenomenon is thought to have caused extensive flooding in East Africa from December 1997 to March 1998, increasing the number of pooled-water breeding sites of *aedes* mosquitoes. Mosquitoes then facilitated the transfer of the Rift Valley Fever virus from infected cattle, sheep, and/or goats to humans who had been forced to live in close proximity to animals on islands of dry land surrounded by flood water. During this period, the largest Rift Valley fever (RVF) outbreak ever reported in East Africa occurred in Kenya, Somalia, and Tanzania. The total number of human infections in northern Kenya and southern Somalia alone was estimated at 89 000 with an estimated 478 deaths.

Civil disturbance/human displacement

Human population movements on a large-scale as a result of war, conflict, or natural catastrophe often result in crowded, unhygienic, and impoverished living conditions. This in turn heightens the risk of emergence and re-emergence of infectious diseases. In the aftermath of civil disturbance in Rwanda in 1994, over 48 000 cases of cholera and 23 800 deaths were reported within 1 month among Rwandans who had been displaced to refugee camps in Goma, Democratic Republic of Congo.

A collateral impact of war, conflict, or natural catastrophe such as earthquakes is the destruction or weakening of health systems with diminished capacity to detect, prevent, and respond to infectious disease outbreaks. One consequence of the 27-year civil war in Angola was the outbreak of Marburg haemmorhagic fever in 2004 that spread to more than 200 humans, 90 per cent of whom died. Emergence of the Marburg virus was detected late and transmission was amplified in overcrowded and understaffed health facilities where lack of investment during the war had resulted in sub-standard infection control.

Another large outbreak of Marburg virus infection was identified in late 1998 in the Democratic Republic of Congo, also a conflict-ravaged country. This emergence resulted in sporadic cases with small chains of transmission over a 2-year period in a remote area where civil war had interrupted supply lines and communication to health facilities in the region.

Human behaviour

Occupation

Throughout history, human occupations have been associated with infectious diseases. Anthrax, for example, has been called wool-sorters disease because of transmission of anthrax spores from infected animals to humans who sheer sheep and other wool-producing animals. It has also been associated with butchers who come into contact with infected animals at the time of slaughter or during preparation of meat for markets. Anthrax spores infect humans either intra-dermally, causing cutaneous anthrax, or by inhalation, causing pulmonary or inhalation anthrax.

Though intensive research has failed to confirm the origins of Ebola fever outbreaks, infection is thought to occur as humans encounter animal sources, possibly infected bats and/or non human primates, somewhere in the transmission cycle. An outbreak of Ebola haemorrhagic fever in humans in 1995 was linked to a woodsman, who worked deep within the tropical rainforest making charcoal, and who is somehow thought to have become infected with the Ebola virus that he then carried back to his home village and family members. A Swiss researcher infected with the Ebola virus while searching for the cause of a major die-out of chimpanzees in a forest reserve in West Africa is thought to have become infected while conducting chimpanzee autopsies in search of the cause of death.

In 2003, a veterinarian in the Netherlands became infected with the influenza A (H7N7) virus during an investigation of influenza outbreaks in poultry and later died in acute respiratory failure. A total of 89 humans, including the veterinarian, were confirmed to have H7N7 influenza virus infection associated with this poultry outbreak and no further deaths occurred. The majority of human infections are thought to have occurred as a result of direct contact with infected poultry; but there were three possible instances of transmission of infection from poultry workers to family members.

Mistrust and misinformation

During 2003, unsubstantiated rumours circulated in northern Nigeria that the oral polio vaccine (OPV) was unsafe and could cause infertility by vaccination of young children. Mistrust and misinformation that followed led to the government-ordered suspension of polio immunization in two northern states and substantial reductions in polio immunization coverage in those states, and a large number of others. The result was a polio outbreak across northern Nigeria that then spread to previously polio-free areas in sub-Saharan Africa. Over 70 per cent of all children worldwide who were paralyzed by polio during the following year, 2004, were living in Nigeria—or in other parts of sub-Saharan Africa that had been reinfected by polio virus genetically linked to viruses that had a Nigerian origin.

Misinformation about the safety of vaccines against pertussis, measles, and hepatitis B has likewise led to decreases in vaccine uptake among children, and in some instances industrialized country outbreaks of pertussis and measles.

Anti-infective drug prescription and use

Behaviours such as over- or under-prescribing of antibiotics by health workers, and excessive demand for antibiotics by the general population, have had a remarkable impact on the selection and survival of resistant microbes, rapidly increasing levels of microbial resistance.

The selection and spread of resistant infectious agents is paradoxically facilitated by either over or under-prescribing of drugs, and/or poor compliance to their use and unregulated sale that makes them available to any who have the ability to purchase them. In Thailand, among 307 hospitalized patients in the late 1990s, 36 per cent who were treated with anti-infective drugs did not have an infectious disease. Over-prescribing of anti-infective drugs occurs in most other countries as well. In Canada, it has been estimated of the more than 26 million people treated with anti-infective drugs, up to 50 per cent were treated inappropriately. Findings from community surveys of *Escherichia coli* in the stool samples of healthy children in China, Venezuela, and the United States suggest that although multiresistant strains were present in each country, they were more widespread in Venezuela and China, countries where less control is maintained over antibiotic prescribing and sales.

Animal husbandry and agriculture use large amounts of anti-infective drugs, sometimes indiscriminately, resulting in the selection of resistant bacterial strains. Antibiotics are used as growth-promoting agents in animal feed in some countries, and for spraying of fruit trees, rice paddies, and flowers to avoid bacterial blights. Some of the infectious agents that infect animals freely circulate between animals and humans, providing opportunities for swapping or exchanging resistant genes, increasing the speed with which anti-infective resistance evolves in both agriculture and human populations.

From January 2005 to March 2006, 44 of 53 patients with multidrug resistance to tuberculosis (MDR-TB) were further diagnosed with extreme drug resistant tuberculosis (XDR-TB). All were found to be HIV-positive as well. Widespread infection with HIV provides fertile ground for the transmission of all forms of TB, including XDR-TB, facilitated by inappropriate prescribing behaviour of health workers and poor adherence to treatment regimes by patients.

Deliberate use to cause terror and harm

The potential of organisms used as weapons of biological warfare or bioterrorism was graphically illustrated in 1979 in an accident involving anthrax in Sverdlovsk, 1400 km east of Moscow, in the then Soviet Union. Attributed at first by government officials to the consumption of contaminated meat, it was later shown to have been caused by the unintentional release of anthrax spores from a Soviet military microbiology facility. It is estimated that up to 358 humans were infected and that between 45 and 199 died.

In the United States in late September 2001, the deliberate dissemination of potentially lethal anthrax spores in four known letters sent through the United States Postal Service caused massive disruption of postal services in the United States and many other countries around the world. The anthrax letters—dated 11 September 2001, and postmarked 7 days later—caused huge public alarm and prompted a massive public health response. A total of 22 persons are thought to have been infected by anthrax spores sent through the postal system; 11 developed cutaneous anthrax and the remaining 11 developed inhalation anthrax, of whom five died. Twenty of the 22 patients were exposed to work sites that were found to be contaminated with anthrax spores. Nine of them had worked in mail processing facilities through which the anthrax letters had passed.

Other bacteria, viruses, mycotic agents, and biological toxins are also considered to have the potential for deliberate use to cause harm to humans. Great concern has been expressed by many countries about the potential health consequences that could be caused by the deliberate introduction of infectious agents such as the variola virus into a human population where smallpox vaccination is no longer practised, or the plague bacillus that could potentially cause an outbreak of pneumonic plague.

Public health security: Globalization and emerging/re-emerging infectious disease agents

Emerging and re-emerging infections enter a world of increased human mobility and interdependence that facilitates the transfer of infectious agents from country to country, and from continent to continent. Infectious agents efficiently travel in humans, insects, food and animals, and can spread around the globe and emerge in new geographic areas with ease and speed. Some are transported by the flights of migratory birds. Others, such as disease-carrying mosquitoes, travel in the passenger cabin or luggage hold of jets, to cause tropical infections in temperate countries when they bite airport workers or those who live nearby. They thus threaten public health security—our collective vulnerability to acute infectious disease outbreaks (Heymann 2003).

In 2000, among 312 athletes participating in an international triathlon held in Malaysia, 33 became infected with leptospirosis and returned to their home countries during the incubation period. While leptospirosis lacks human transmissibility and therefore did not set up local foci or transmission, another event in 2003—the outbreak of SARS, clearly demonstrates the full potential of emerging infectious agents for international spread. From a medical doctor who was infected by patients that he was treating in the Guangdong Province of China, and then unknowingly carried the newly emerged infectious agent to a Hong Kong hotel, SARS spread in individual chains of transmission form infected hotel guests to 8422 persons reported infected in North and South America, the Middle East, Europe, and Asia with a case-fatality rate of approximately 11 per cent.

During the years 1969–2003, 18 instances of airport malaria were reported to WHO—malaria infections in workers at airports or in persons who live nearby who had not travelled to malaria-endemic countries. Their infection originated from malaria-infected *anopheles* mosquitoes that had travelled from countries with endemic malaria and took a blood meal from airport workers or other persons upon landing, clearly demonstrating that insects, like humans, can transport infectious agents around the world to emerge in places where they are not endemic.

Livestock, animal products, and food can also carry infectious agents that emerge or re-emerge in non-endemic countries. Rift Valley Fever emerged in humans in Yemen and Saudi Arabia in 2000, 2 years after a major outbreak of Rift Valley Fever in East Africa. Infection has since become endemic in livestock in the Arabian Peninsula, and is thought to have been imported from East Africa in livestock traded across the Red Sea. In 1996, imported raspberries contaminated with *Cyclospora* caused an outbreak in the United States. It is hypothesized that the raspberries imported from Guatemala were contaminated when surface water was used to spray them with fungicide before harvest.

Concern about the international spread of emerging and re-emerging infections and the need for strong public health security are not new. By the fourteenth century, governments recognized the capacity for international disease transmission and legislated preventive measures, as reflected in the establishment of quarantine in the city state of Venice. Arriving ships were not permitted to dock for 40 days, in order to attempt to keep plague from entering by sea.

Many European leaders of the mid-nineteenth century, worried by the cholera pandemic of the time; threats of plague; and the weakness of quarantine measures, began to recognize that controlling the spread of infectious diseases from one nation to another required cooperation between those nations. International conventions were organized and draft covenants signed, almost all of which related to some type of quarantine regulations.

From 1851 to 1897, 10 international sanitary conferences were held among a group of 12 European countries, focusing exclusively on the containment of epidemics in their territories. The inaugural 1851 conference in Paris lasted 6 months and was followed in 1892 by the first International Sanitary Convention that dealt with cholera. Five years later, at the 10th International Sanitary Conference, a similar convention that focused on plague was signed.

New policies then emerged in the late nineteenth century, such as the obligatory telegraphic notification of first cases of cholera and plague, a model that a small group of South American nations followed when they signed the first set of international public health agreements in the Americas during the 1880s. In addition to cholera and plague, often carried by immigrants arriving from Europe, the agreements in the Americas covered yellow fever that was endemic in much of the American region at that time, and that from time to time caused major urban epidemics.

During the following decade, 12 countries attended the First International Sanitary Convention of the American Republics in Washington, DC, leading to the creation of the Pan American Sanitary Bureau (now called the Pan American Health Organization) in 1902. Its counterpart in Europe was the Office International d'Hygiène Publique (OIHP), established in 1907, and based in Paris.

In 1951, 3 years after its founding, WHO adopted a revised version of the International Sanitary Regulations (1892) that remained focused on the control of cholera, plague and yellow fever and rooted firmly in the preceding agreements of nineteenth and twentieth centuries.

The international health regulations

In 1969 the Member States of the World Health Organization agreed to new set of regulations—the International Health Regulations (IHR)—aimed at better ensuring public health security with minimal interruption in travel and trade. In addition to requiring reporting of four infectious diseases—cholera, plague, yellow fever, and smallpox—the IHR (1969) were aimed at stopping the spread of disease by pre-established control measures at international borders. They included requirements such as yellow fever and smallpox vaccination for passengers arriving from countries where yellow fever or smallpox outbreaks had been reported, and thus provided a legal framework for global surveillance and response, with the potential to decrease the world's vulnerability to four infectious diseases that were know to cross international borders.

By 1996, it had become clear, however, that the IHR (1969) were not able to ensure public health security as had been envisioned—countries reported the occurrence of cholera, plague and yellow fever late or not at all because of fear of stigmatization and economic repercussions (smallpox had been removed from the list when it was certified eradicated in 1980). At the same time it was realized that the IHR (1969) did not meet the challenges caused by emerging and re-emerging infectious diseases and the rapid global transit of these infections, sometimes still in the incubation period, by humans, insects, animals, and goods. From 1996 until 2005, the Member States of WHO therefore undertook a process to examine and revise the IHR (1969).

The result—the IHR (2005)—provide a more up-to-date legal framework requiring reporting of any public health emergency of international concern (PHEIC), and the use of real-time evidence to recommend measures to stop their international spread. A PHEIC is defined as an extraordinary event that could spread internationally or might require a coordinated international response (World Health Organization).

Under the IHR (2005) an event is evaluated for its potential to become a PHEIC by the country in which it is occurring, using a decision tree instrument developed for this purpose (Fig. 9.17.4). If the criteria for a PHEIC are met, an official notification must be provided to WHO. Notification is also required for even a single occurrence of a disease that would always threaten global public health security—smallpox, poliomyelitis caused by a wild-type poliovirus, human influenza caused by a new virus subtype, and SARS. In addition, there is a second list that includes diseases of documented—but not inevitable—international impact. An event involving a disease on this second list, which includes cholera, pneumonic plague, yellow fever, Ebola, and the other haemorrhagic fevers, still requires the use of the decision tree instrument to determine if it is a PHEIC. Thus, two

ANNEX 2
DECISION INSTRUMENT FOR THE ASSESSMENT AND NOTIFICATION OF EVENTS THAT MAY CONSTITUTE A PUBLIC HEALTH EMERGENCY OF INTERNATIONAL CONCERN

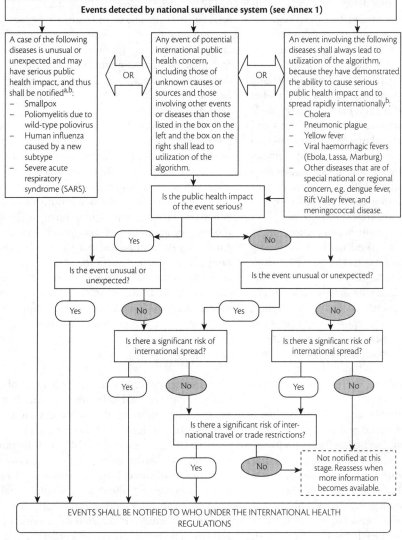

Fig. 9.17.4 Decision tree for assessment of a potential public health event of international concern.

[a] As per WHO case definitions.
[b] The disease list shall be used only for the purpose of these Regulations.

safeguards create a baseline of public health security by requiring countries to respond, in designated ways, to well-known threats.

In contrast to previous regulations, the IHR (2005) introduced a set of core capacity requirements for surveillance and response. All countries must meet these requirements during the first 5 years of implementation of the IHR (2005) in order to detect, assess, notify, report, and contain the events covered by the regulations so that their potential for international spread and negative economic impact are minimized. The IHR (2005) likewise require collective action by all WHO Member States in the event that an emerging or re-emerging infectious disease threatens to spread internationally, and the free-sharing of information pertaining to this threat. They thus provide a safety net against the international spread of emerging or re-emerging infections, requiring collaboration between all states to ensure the timely availability of surveillance information and technical resources that better guarantee international public health security.

Other international frameworks have also been developed to contain and curtail the international spread of emerging infections. Among them are the WHO global strategy for containment of antimicrobial resistance (World Health Organization 2001). Though not legally binding, this framework calls on countries to work across the human health, animal health, and agricultural sectors to ensure more rational use of anti-infective drugs in order to limit the factors that accelerate the selection and proliferation of anti-infective-drug-resistant microbes.

National and international surveillance and response

For emerging and re-emerging infections that are able to transmit from person to person, the window of opportunity for effective intervention often closes quickly. The most important defence against their international spread is highly sensitive national surveillance systems, public health laboratories that can rapidly detect outbreaks caused by emerging and re-emerging infections, and mechanisms that permit timely containment. These are the core capacities required by the IHR (2005). The same systems that detect and contain naturally occurring outbreaks also permit detection and initial response to deliberately caused outbreaks of infectious disease, although the scale of a deliberately caused outbreak could be large, similar to an outbreak caused by an event such as an influenza pandemic.

The collaborative action required by IHR (2005) when emerging or re-emerging infections threaten to spread internationally likewise provides a framework for global surveillance and response that is a departure from previous international conventions and regulations. The IHR (2005) explicitly acknowledge that non-state sources of information about outbreaks often pre-empt official notification, especially in situations when countries may be reluctant to reveal an event in their territories. Within the framework of the IHR (2005), WHO is therefore authorized to take into account information sources other than official notifications.

Collaboration among countries for public health security in the face of emerging and re-emerging infections has been occurring since 1997 when the Global Outbreak Alert and Response Network (GOARN) was first envisaged. This collaboration now sits firmly within the framework of the HIR (2005). By design, GOARN is a network of networks that interlinks electronically, and in real time, over 140 existing laboratory and disease reporting and response networks. Together, these networks possess much of the data, technical expertise, and skills needed to keep the international community constantly alert and ready to respond to emerging diseases within countries and internationally if and when they spread across national borders.

GOARN was formalized in April 2000 and is supported by a customized artificial intelligence engine for real-time gathering of disease information, the Global Public Health Intelligence Network (GPHIN) maintained by Health Canada. This computer application heightens vigilance by continuously and systematically crawling web sites, news wires, local online newspapers, public health email services, and electronic discussion groups in six different languages in order to identify reports of outbreaks (Grein *et al.* 2000).

Other sources of information linked together in GOARN include government and university centres, ministries of health, academic institutions, other UN agencies, networks of overseas military laboratories, and nongovernmental organizations having a strong presence in epidemic-prone countries such as Medecins sans Frontières and the International Federation of Red Cross and Red Crescent Societies. Information from all these sources is assessed and verified on a daily basis by WHO and its partners in GOARN, and validated information is made public on the WHO web site.

If an outbreak of emerging or re-emerging infectious disease occurs in a country that requires international assistance to help in containment activities, as agreed upon in confidential pro-active consultation with the affected country and with experts in the network, electronic communications are used to describe the technical expertise required and to then provide prompt assistance and support. To this end, global databases of professionals with expertise in specific diseases or epidemiological techniques are maintained, together with nongovernmental organizations present in countries and in a position to reach remote areas. Such mechanisms, which are further supported by the WHO network of Collaborating Centres (national laboratories and institutes throughout the world serving as international reference centres), help the world make the maximum use of expertise and resources.

From July 1998 to August 2001, GOARN verified 578 outbreaks in 132 countries, indicating the system's broad geographical coverage (Fig. 9.17.5). The most frequently reported outbreaks were of cholera, meningitis, haemorrhagic fever, anthrax, and viral encephalitis. During this same period, the network launched effective international cooperative containment activities in many developing countries such as Afghanistan, Bangladesh, Burkina Faso, Côte d'Ivoire, Egypt, Ethiopia, Kosovo, Sierra Leone, Sudan, Uganda, and Yemen.

GOARN reached its full potential during the SARS outbreak in 2003. It was not only instrumental in detecting the outbreak, but also in coordinating an international response for the first time using real-time evidence to make recommendation for epidemic containment and control, ways of working that were later incorporated in the IHR (2005). Since the SARS outbreak, operational protocols which set out standardized procedures for the alert and verification process, communications, coordination of an epidemic response, emergency evacuation, research, monitoring, ownership of data and samples, and relations with the media have been finalized and are available on the World Wide Web (WHO). By setting out a chain of command, and bringing order to the containment response, such protocols ensure collective action as required by the IHR (2005) and help ensure public health security.

The future

The vision embraced by the IHR (2005) is of a world on the alert and ready to respond collectively to the threat of emerging and re-emerging infections that represent an acute threat to public health security (Heymann & Rodier 2001).

To achieve this vision, the IHR (2005) requires an unbroken line of defence within countries and globally, using the most up-to-date technologies of surveillance and response. If a country had to concern itself only with the domestic public health issues caused by emerging and re-emerging infections, ensuring core capacities domestically would suffice. In today's world of international travel and trade, no politically drawn borders can absolutely prevent the spread of disease, and all countries have an obligation to develop and maintain these core capacities. They also have an obligation to be part of an interconnected system engaged in risk management activities that collectively reduce international vulnerability to threats to public health security.

Adherence to the IHR (2005) requires adherence to new norms and standards for reporting and responding to emerging and re-emerging infections despite the economic consequences that may result. Their full achievement will provide the highest level of public health security possible. National core capacities as described in the IHR (2005) must be put in place within the national public health system that can detect, investigate, communicate, and contain events that threaten public health security as soon as they appear. An interconnected system must be operating at the national and international levels, engaged in specific threat and risk assessment and management activities that minimize collective vulnerability to public health events.

These two goals are interdependent and must be sustained. They involve measures that the international community must continually invest in, strive to achieve, and assess for progress. In today's mobile,

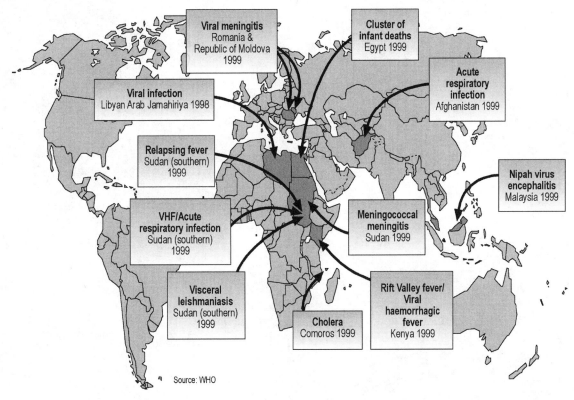

Fig. 9.17.5 Sample of international epidemic response missions during the first 12 months, Global Outbreak Alert and Response Network, 1998–1999.

interdependent, and interconnected world, threats arising from emerging and epidemic-prone diseases affect all countries. Such threats reinforce the need for shared responsibility and collective action in the face of universal vulnerability, in sectors that go well beyond health.

References

Grein T., Kamara K.B.O., Rodier G. *et al.* (2000) Rumours of disease in the global village: outbreak verification. *Emerging Infectious Diseases*, **6**, 97–102.

Heymann D.L. (2003) The evolving infectious disease threat: implications for national and global security. *Harvard University/Commission on Human Security for Global Health, Journal of Human Development*, **4**, 191–207.

Heymann D.L. and Rodier G. (2001) Hot spots in a wired world: Who surveillance of emerging and re-emerging infectiou diseases. *Lancet*, **1**, 345–53.

Lederberg J., Shope R.E., Oaks S.C. Jr., eds. *Emerging infections: microbial threats to health in the United States*, Washington DC: National Academy Press, 1992.

World Health Organization. International Health Regulations (2005), Geneva. Available at: http://www.who.int/gb/ebwha/pdf_files/WHA58/WHA58_3-en.pdf

World Health Organization. (2001) *WHO Global Strategy for Containment of Antimicrobial Resistance*. Geneva. Available at: http://www.who.int/drugresistance/WHO%20Global%20Strategy%20-%20Executive%20Summary%20-%20English%20version.pdf

SECTION 10

Prevention and control of public health hazards

Tobacco

Samira Asma, Douglas W. Bettcher,[1]
Jonathan Samet, Krishna M. Palipudi, Gary Giovino,
Stella Bialous, Katherine DeLand,[1] June Leung,
Daniel Ferrante,[1] Gemma Vestal,[1]
Gonghuan Yang, and Derek Yach

Abstract

Tobacco use is the single-most preventable cause of death and is unique in terms of its current and projected future impacts on global mortality. If current trends of tobacco use continue, the number of people killed by tobacco will reach 8.3 million annually by the year 2030. Tobacco is also the only legal consumer product that can harm everyone exposed to it, and it kills up to half of those who use it as intended. Despite the crises, there is also an opportunity. The current national and global momentum to promote smoke-free societies offers opportunity to apply proven strategies. The World Health Organization (WHO) Framework Convention on Tobacco Control, a multilateral legal framework, presents a blueprint for countries to reduce both supply and demand for tobacco. In addition, the WHO MPOWER package offers recommendations for countries to implement the most proven strategies. This chapter examines the history of tobacco use and dependence, and the current and projected pattern of the tobacco epidemic, reviews the structure, conduct, and strategies of the tobacco industry, and proposes proven tobacco control strategies, which may have relevance throughout the world.

Introduction

Today, tobacco use is the single-most preventable cause of death and is unique in terms of its current and projected future impacts on global mortality. If current trends of tobacco use continue, the number of people killed by tobacco will reach 8.3 million annually by the year 2030 (Mathers & Loncar 2006). Tobacco is also the only legal consumer product that harms every user, killing up to half of those who use it as intended. Tobacco use is widespread due to insufficient public awareness about its dangers, aggressive marketing and promotion of the products, and lack of strong, countering public health policies.

Nonetheless, there are substantial opportunities to slow the epidemic. After decades of implementing, evaluating, and fine-tuning tobacco control programmes, there is now a substantial evidence base identifying and supporting those policies that can be expected to have the greatest positive effect. Promisingly, this evidence base has not been neglected; in the face of the unprecedented toll caused by tobacco use and the worrying projections for the future, the global health community has taken strong steps toward reducing and eventually eliminating the morbidity and mortality caused by the tobacco epidemic; most notably, in the negotiation and implementation of the WHO Framework Convention on Tobacco Control (WHO FCTC).

The WHO FCTC is a multilateral evidence-based treaty, providing the legal framework for countries to reduce both supply and demand for tobacco. With over 160 Parties, the WHO FCTC is one of the most universal treaties in UN history. Over the next several years, its substantial impact should be felt in Parties and, insofar as tobacco is a transnational concern, also in non-Party jurisdictions. Building on this momentum, WHO launched an implementation strategy for the WHO FCTC as part of the WHO Report on the Global Tobacco Epidemic, 2008. The MPOWER technical assistance package contains a set of six proven strategies, each of which reflects one or more provisions of the WHO FCTC.

In addition to these two major global initiatives, the very way in which the tobacco debate is perceived has shifted with the multiple disclosures of internal industry documents revealing the tactics of the tobacco industry. Thus armed, the tobacco control community has expanded inroads for vigilant monitoring of the industry as it seeks to maintain and expand its markets, particularly in less-developed countries and among women.

The purpose of this chapter is to explore the opportunities to limit the epidemic by (a) examining the history of tobacco use and its dependence, and the current and projected pattern of the tobacco epidemic, (b) reviewing the structure, conduct, and strategies of the tobacco industry, and (c) encouraging the use of already proven tobacco control strategies, which have relevance throughout the world.

The tobacco epidemic

In this section, we review the history of tobacco use and dependence, the epidemiological model, and the characteristics of the

[1] The author is a staff member of the World Health Organization. The author alone is responsible for the views expressed in this publication and they do not necessarily represent the decisions or the stated policy of the World Health Organization.

tobacco epidemic. The characteristics of the epidemic include production of tobacco, patterns of tobacco use, smoking cessation and nicotine dependence, exposure to second-hand smoke (SHS), and the pattern and burden of tobacco-related diseases.

The history of tobacco use and dependence

The tobacco plant (*Nicotiana tabacum*) originates from South America, where tobacco was used for ceremonial and shamanistic purposes long before Columbus arrived; however, it was not consumed regularly. By the arrival of Columbus in 1492, tobacco was being chewed, smoked, or snuffed in many areas of both North and South America. In the 1700s and the early 1800s, large quantities of tobacco were being snuffed by the aristocracy of Europe and chewed by the American settlers. By the middle of the 1800s, the technology for making cigarettes in large quantities with a machine and the flue-curing of tobacco had been developed, and the chewing of tobacco was beginning to be considered unhygienic. The converging development of several technologies between the late-nineteenth and early-twentieth centuries made the modern cigarette possible. New tobacco blends and curing processes were developed, which produced a tobacco product that, when burned, could be inhaled. Machinery for manufacturing cigarettes cheaply was perfected, the safety match was invented, and advertising and promotion techniques promoted the products of the tobacco industry. By the start of the twentieth century, the mass production of cigarettes had begun and smoking among men in industrial countries began to rise dramatically. Cigarette smoking became increasingly accepted among women in industrial countries, starting about the time of World War II. At this time, smoking also began to rise in men in developing countries. Today, tobacco is cultivated commercially in more than 100 countries. The major producers are China, Brazil, India, the United States, Angola, Indonesia, Turkey, Greece, Italy, and Pakistan. Tobacco is consumed in all countries of the world (FAO 2006).

The epidemiological model

The epidemiological triad of agent, host, vector, and environment long used for infectious diseases also facilitates the understanding of factors that influence patterns, determinants, and consequences of tobacco use (Orleans & Slade 1993). An agent is traditionally defined as a factor whose presence is essential for the occurrence of disease (Last 1995). In this model, the myriad components of tobacco and tobacco smoke-cause disease. Tobacco and tobacco smoke contain over 3500 chemicals, including hundreds that are toxic or carcinogenic (USDHHS 1989, 2006; Hecht 1999). Tobacco also contains nicotine, an addictive compound that serves to maintain people's use of the agent even when they want to quit (USDHHS 1988; Giovino *et al.* 1995; FDA 1996). The bioavailability of nicotine can be increased by raising the pH of the product (FDA 1996; Fant *et al.* 1999). Many tobacco products (e.g. so-called 'low tar' cigarettes) may appear to be less dangerous than others on the basis of 'tar' and 'nicotine' ratings derived from a smoking machine. However, such products are rated by a machine testing system that does not represent smokers' intake of the toxic components of the cigarette, the way that smokers compensate for reduced nicotine yield, and their availability may undermine smokers' motivations to quit (USDHSS 1996; Kozlowski *et al.* 1998a,b).

The host in this model is the person who uses the product, i.e. one who smokes tobacco (through a cigarette, cigar, pipe, or other smoking device), chews or dips oral tobacco, or inhales snuff. Host factors

found to be determinants of smoking include demographic characteristics, knowledge, attitudes, and behaviours, tobacco use by friends and family members, and genetic susceptibility to addiction and disease (USDHHS 2006). One significant challenge to tobacco control lies in understanding why some people who experiment with smoking easily discontinue, whereas others progress to become regular dependent users. Host factors can influence why some dependent smokers quit and others continue, and why some lifelong smokers develop smoking-attributable diseases while others do not.

Because SHS, also known as environmental tobacco smoke (ETS),[2] which is the combination of sidestream smoke and exhaled mainstream smoke inhaled by non-smokers causes disease in many exposed persons who do not consume tobacco products (SCOTH 1998; Samet & Wang 2000; California Environmental Protection Agency 2005; USDHHS 2006), the complete disease model also includes involuntary smokers as incidental hosts (DiFranza & Lew 1995; USDHHS 2006). The vector serves to transport the agent to susceptible individuals (Last 1995). Just as we understand, e.g. the role of the rat in the spread of the plague or the mosquito in the spread of malaria, we need to understand that tobacco has a vector—tobacco products' manufacturers. Thus, in the development of nicotine addiction and tobacco-attributable disease, tobacco products' manufacturers produce the agent and distribute it in ways that make the product appealing to both users and non-users. The industry uses packaging, advertising, and promotion to reach and influence as many people as possible to use their products. The price of the product (the lower the price, the more will be sold) and the ease with which it can be obtained (from vending machines, over-the-counter displays, and sales by street vendors) are also key distribution factors. In the case of tobacco, the vector also serves to undermine public health attempts to limit use by denying for decades the health consequences of use, and resisting many health-promoting programmes and policies (Hilts 1996; Kluger 1996; Jamieson 1998) in order to maintain the product affordable, to maintain the ability to market the product and to maintain the social acceptability of tobacco use. This vector actively markets products that tacitly claim to be less hazardous and engages in sophisticated public relations campaigns to promote itself as a responsible corporation, and while in some cases admitting the harmful effects of tobacco use (while continuing to deny the health impact of SHS), continues to deny any responsibility over the individual harm caused to smokers and the social harms caused by marketing (Hirschhorn 2004; Lee & Bialous 2006; McDaniel *et al.* 2006, 2008). Additionally, for decades, the vector has manipulated the product in ways that have made it more addictive and potentially more harmful. For example, by the manipulation of pH, manufacturers have enhanced the bioavailability of nicotine to the smoker (Ferris Wayne *et al.* 2006; Hammond *et al.* 2006).

---

[2] Several alternative terms are commonly used to describe the smoke emitted from the burning end of a cigarette or from other tobacco products usually in combination with the smoke exhaled by the smoker. The term 'second-hand smoke' is the preferred term used in the guidelines adopted by the Conference of the Parties for implementation of the WHO Framework Convention on Tobacco Control (WHO 2007a), and thus will be used in this chapter thereafter. Other terms such as 'passive smoking' or 'involuntary exposure to tobacco smoke' are best avoided as the tobacco industry may use these terms to support a position that 'voluntary exposure' is acceptable.

The environment includes diverse cultural, historical, economic, and political factors. In many countries, tobacco growing and tobacco product manufacturing have been, for decades, respected and lucrative businesses that wielded tremendous economic and political influence (World Bank 1999). When the health effects became known, and more recently when the industry's malfeasant activities became apparent, attitudes towards the industry changed precipitously. Nevertheless, the powerful effects of pro-tobacco forces have influenced many political decisions (Francey & Chapman 2000; Saloogee & Dagli 2000; Muggli *et al.* 2001; Neuman *et al.* 2002; McDaniel *et al.* 2008). In addition, the industry often attempts to gain cultural and political favour by sponsoring cultural events and promoting smoking prevention campaigns (Dewhirst & Hunter 2002; Barbeau *et al.* 2004; Anderson *et al.* 2006; Brandt 2007).

Economic and cultural influences in regions where tobacco is grown and/or where tobacco products are produced often result in reduced support for tobacco control activities, in comparison with areas that not affected by tobacco industry activities. Environmental factors also include efforts by the tobacco control community, whether governmental or non-governmental, to counter pro-tobacco influences.

This epidemiological model has proved useful for both research and intervention. Past and ongoing research addresses each of the components of this model, as well as the interactions among its elements. Most research has focused on host factors, although more recent attention has also turned to policy factors. With the widespread dissemination of industry documents, our understanding of the vector has increased and led to legal and regulatory strategies to better control it.

Interventions address different levels in a continuum that extends from the individual smoker to the national and international levels. Some attempt to influence host factors, e.g. by educating people about the dangers of tobacco use, how to quit, and ways to resist pro-tobacco influences from the peers and the media. Recent activities attempt to influence the environment, e.g. by promoting policy changes and mass media interventions. The industry

is changing the agent, e.g. by developing nicotine-delivery products that heat (as opposed to burn) tobacco. Regulatory efforts strive to control both the agent and the activities of the vector; a global initiative has been launched with the advent of the World Health Organization's Framework Convention on Tobacco Control (WHO FCTC).

Characteristics of the tobacco epidemic

In this section, we provide an overview of the characteristics of the global tobacco epidemic, which will include tobacco production and its patterns of use. It will also describe smoking cessation and nicotine dependence, and discuss the exposure to SHS. Finally, we will conclude by reviewing the literature on the patterns and burden of tobacco-related diseases.

Tobacco production

In this section, we classify and describe the various tobacco products available, tobacco growing, and the world market in manufactured tobacco products.

Types of tobacco products

There are two main forms of tobacco in common use: Smoking tobacco and smokeless tobacco. Smoking tobacco includes manufactured cigarettes (filter and unfiltered) and 'roll-your-own' cigarettes. *Kretek* (clove-flavoured cigarettes), from Indonesia, are sticks made from a local variety of sun-cured tobacco known as *brus* and wrapped in cigarette paper. These are indigenous to Indonesia, but are also available in the United States (WHO 2006). *Bidis* (small hand-rolled cigarettes consisting of sun-dried tobacco wrapped in a *tendu* leaf) are smoked throughout Southeast Asia, particularly in India (Stratton *et al.* 2001). They are also becoming increasingly popular among teenagers in the United States (Malson & Pickworth 2002). Cigars are made of air-cured and fermented tobacco with a tobacco leaf wrapper, and come in many shapes and sizes, from cigarette-sized to 10-g double coronas. Pipes are used predominantly in Europe, America, and Southeast Asia; e.g. clay pipes known as *sulpa*, *chilum*, and *hookli* are common in Asia. *Chutta* is an Indian home-made cigar. Reverse smoking of *chutta* (with burning

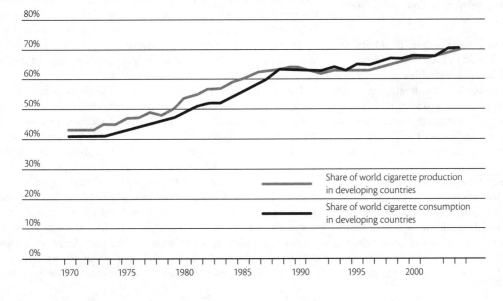

Share of cigarette production and consumption in developing countries

Fig. 10.1.1 Shifting epidemic (the tobacco industry reaches new markets in developing countries).
Source: Based on data from Food and Agriculture Organization FAOSTAT, United Nation Commodity Trade Statistic Database, United Nation Common Database, United States Department of Agriculture Economic Research Service, World Health Organization Statistics Information System, and ERC Group Plc's World Cigarettes Report (2005).

end inside the mouth) is prevalent among women in the rural communities of Andhra Pradesh (Van der Eb *et al.* 1993). Water pipes, also known as *hookah, gaza, narghile*, hubble-bubble, and *shisha*, are in common use in Eastern Mediterranean region, parts of Asia and North Africa.

Smokeless tobacco products, consisting of tobacco leaf and a wide variety of flavouring and other ingredients, are used either orally or nasally. Smokeless tobacco includes chewing tobacco and snuff (dry and moist varieties), used in South Asia, Western Europe and North America and parts of Africa. Chewing tobacco is produced by shredding tobacco leaf. The leaf can be consumed loosely, or by pressing into bricks (plugs), or by drying and forming twist. Snuff, which may be sniffed or placed in the mouth, has a much finer consistency than chewing tobacco and is made from powdered or finely cut tobacco leaves. Moist snuff taken orally has been used for many years in Sweden, where it is known as snus, and in the United States. Smokeless tobacco is being actively marketed as a popular form of tobacco among children and adolescents in the United States and Scandinavia (Tomar 2007). About 40 per cent of total tobacco consumption in India is in the form of smokeless or chewing tobacco (Reddy & Gupta 2004; WHO 2008).

Tobacco growing

Tobacco is grown in more than 115 countries on almost 4 million hectares of land, a third of which is in China (FAO 2006). In 1970, 4.7 million tons of tobacco were produced worldwide, by 1997 leaf production had peaked to almost 9 million tons and by 2006 had fallen to 6.7 million tons (FAO 2006). China is the world's leading producer of tobacco, with production increasing from 0.81 million tons in 1970 (17 per cent of total world output) to 2.75 million tons in 2006 (41 per cent of total world output). In 2006, the other nine leading producers were Brazil, India, the United States, Angola, Indonesia, Turkey, Greece, Italy, and Pakistan.

The pattern of production has shifted significantly in recent decades. Whereas exports from the United States have fallen slightly, those from Brazil, China and Zimbabwe have increased significantly (FAO 2006). According to the Food and Agricultural Organization (FAO) projections, developing countries will account for 87 per cent of world tobacco by 2010. FAO estimates revealed that China is projected to remain the largest producer of tobacco in the world. Brazil (0.91 million metric tons) and India (0.55 million metric tons) are also among top tobacco-producing nations (FAO 2006).

Manufactured tobacco products

Although tobacco is mainly grown in developing countries, the world market is dominated by a handful of American, European, and Japanese companies, which have a controlling presence not only in all Western countries but throughout the developing world. China is an exception, with its own tobacco products mainly used in the domestic market. About 5.5 trillion cigarettes were manufactured worldwide in 2004; four countries (China, the United States, Russia, and Japan) accounted for over half of global production (USDA 2004).

During the late 1990s, two major trends emerged which were significant for the future of the tobacco industry. First, the multinationals merged into a few major conglomerates. Second, state monopolies were increasingly privatized and merged with multinationals. For example, as seen in the companies' own websites, in the past decade, United Kingdom-based British American Tobacco acquired Cigarrera La Moderna in Mexico, merged with Rothmans in Canada, gained control of Peru's Tabacalera Nacional, Italy's ETI, and Serbia's Duvanska Industrija Vranje. It also combined the business of United States-based Brown and Williamson with RJ Reynolds Tobacco Company to form Reynolds American, where BAT has a 42 per cent share. Japan Tobacco International was established in 1999 as a separate division of Japan Tobacco group after the acquisition of RJ Reynolds International division, and recently, of United Kingdom-based Gallaher. Altadis, created from the merge of France's Seita with Spain's Tabacalera has recently acquired Morocco's Regie de Tabacs and United Kingdom's Imperial. Philip Morris International (PMI), similarly, has in the past decade acquired interests in tobacco companies in Greece, Serbia, Colombia, Pakistan and acquired Sampoerna Tobacco in Indonesia and in 2006 announced an agreement with the China National Tobacco Company for the licensed production of Marlboro in China. In March 2008, the parent corporation, Altria, finalized the spin-off of PMI, which becomes a separate tobacco company.

In some countries, state-owned tobacco companies continue to dominate within their own market; the most notable of these is the China National Tobacco Company, which is the largest tobacco company in the world in terms of number of cigarettes sold (WHO 2008). Increasingly, however, the multinationals are moving into countries formerly controlled by state monopolies and introducing aggressive marketing programmes (Szilagyi & Chapman 2003; Lawrence & Collin 2004; Gilmore *et al.* 2005, 2007; Lee K *et al.* 2008). For example, in the 1980s, the American tobacco companies relied upon the United States government, and the threat of trade sanctions, to open the cigarette markets in Japan, Taiwan, South Korea, and Thailand (Chaloupka & Corbett 1998). The shift in focus of the multinationals also comes at a time when they are under increasing attack in their home bases as new disclosures become public, detailing how the tobacco industry built and maintained its markets through decades of improper conduct. These disclosures, in addition to shedding important historical light on the tobacco industry, also provide sobering and relevant insight as the tobacco industry expands to conquer new markets.

Patterns of tobacco use

The continuum of tobacco use in a smoker's lifetime has been described in terms of five stages in one model: Pre-contemplation, contemplation, preparation, action, and maintenance (Prochaska *et al.* 1997). These dynamic processes are major contributors to a given population's patterns of tobacco use. (Differential mortality and immigration also contribute to a country's patterns of use, but to a lesser extent.)

The tobacco epidemic has been conceptualized as having four stages as it evolves within a country (Lopez *et al.* 1994). In the first stage, the prevalence of smoking among males is comparatively high, while among females, it is low (about 15 per cent), which is largely because of sociocultural factors that discourage smoking among women. Death and disease due to smoking are not yet evident. In the second stage, the prevalence of smoking among men rises rapidly, reaching a peak between 50 and 80 per cent. The proportion of ex-smokers is relatively low. Smoking prevalence among women typically lags behind that of males by 10–20 years, but increases rapidly. In the third stage, the prevalence of smoking among males begins to decline, falling to about 40 per cent by the end of this stage, which may last for several decades. The prevalence

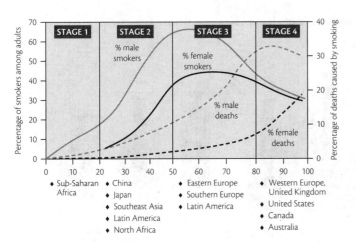

Fig. 10.1.2 Four-stage tobacco epidemic.
Source: Lopez *et al.* (1994).

tends to be lower among middle-aged and older men, many of whom have become ex-smokers. Most importantly, the end of the third stage is characterized by an initial decline in smoking among females. There is also likely to be a marked age gradient in prevalence among women, with about 40–50 per cent of all young women being regular smokers but with relatively few smokers (about 10 per cent) among women above 55–60 years of age. Another characteristic of this period is the rapid increase in smoking-attributable mortality, which rises from about 10 per cent of all deaths in males to about 25–30 per cent within three decades. In middle age (35–69 years), the proportionate mortality of males due to tobacco is even higher (about one in three deaths). The tobacco-related death rate among women is still comparatively low (about 5 per cent of all deaths) but rising. In the fourth stage, smoking prevalence for both sexes continues to decline more or less in parallel, but only slowly, 20–40 years after reaching its peak.

Although the prevalence of smoking has decreased and quitting rates have increased in some developed countries in recent decades, the overall global pattern of tobacco consumption is of major public health concern. Approximately 70 per cent of the world's smokers live in low- and middle-income countries. Nearly two-thirds of the world's smokers live in 10 countries, namely China, India, Indonesia, Russian Federation, the United States, Japan, Brazil, Bangladesh, Germany, and Turkey (WHO 2008).

The current smoking rate for the world's population is 25.3 per cent: 41.2 per cent among males and 9.3 per cent among females. In developed countries, the prevalence of smoking for males and females is 39.8 and 21.7 per cent, respectively. In developing countries, the gender difference in smoking prevalence is larger, with 41.6 per cent of males and 5.7 per cent of females smoking (unpublished data from WHO Tobacco Free Initiative).[3]

Trends in the consumption of tobacco

Trends in cigarette consumption rates have varied worldwide and also across WHO regions (WHO 2004, 2008). Overall, the world has seen an average annual increase of approximately 1 per cent in adult per capita consumption over the last two decades. The most rapid declines have been in countries such as Canada and the United Kingdom, where average annual decreases of 1.8 and 1.6 per cent, respectively, have been recorded since the early 1970s. These have not been matched by equivalent declines in prevalence.

In contrast, over the same time period, there have been dramatic average annual increases in per capita consumption in China (8 per cent), Indonesia (6.8 per cent), Syria (5.5 per cent), and Bangladesh (4.7 per cent). These high rates of increase are occurring from a low starting base, but China and Syria have already reached the per capita consumption levels of the United Kingdom; and in both countries, the rates of smoking among women remain low. There is a growing concern about the efforts of the tobacco industry to increase smoking rates among women in developing countries (WHO 1997a, 2008).

In many countries, people begin smoking at young ages, with the median age of initiation usually being under 15 years. The prevalence of smoking in youth continues to increase in both developed and developing countries, even where the overall prevalence of tobacco use is declining (WHO 1997b, 2008). Between 2000 and 2007, data for Global Youth Tobacco Survey (GYTS) were obtained

---

[3] The global and income aggregates represent adjusted prevalence estimates. Crude estimates received from WHO Member States are adjusted to obtain nationally representative prevalence estimates for current smokers of tobacco for the same year and age groups. These estimates are not age-standardised (i.e. do not remove the effects of the underlying age structures across countries) and should be used with caution when making comparisons of smoking prevalence across regions/income groups. For this reason, these estimates differ to those published in WHS (2008).

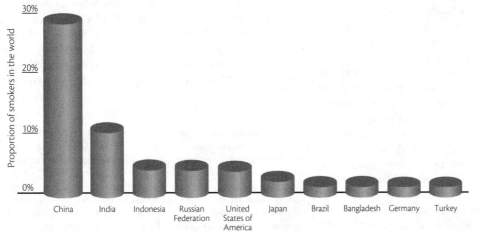

Fig. 10.1.3 Nearly two-thirds of the world's smokers live in 10 countries. *Sources*: WHO (2008a).

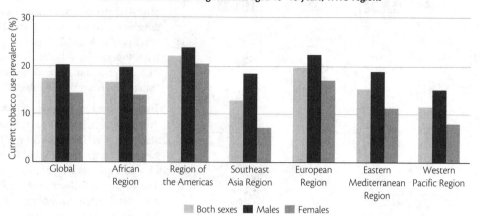

Fig. 10.1.4 Risk factor transition: High prevalence of tobacco use, youth worldwide.
Source: Worren *et al.* (2008a).

over 140 WHO Member States, six territories (American Samoa, British Virgin Islands, Guam, Monserrat, Puerto Rico, and the US Virgin Island), two geographic regions (Gaza Strip and West Bank), one United Nations administered province (Kosovo), one special administrative region (Macau) and one Commonwealth region (northern Mariana Islands). Among the students (aged 13–15 years) who were surveyed, it was revealed that overall 9 per cent of students currently smoke cigarettes. The rates were the highest in the European Region (19.2 per cent) and lowest in the Eastern Mediterranean Region (4.9 per cent). One in 10 (10.1 per cent) students currently used tobacco products other than cigarettes (e.g. pipes, water pipes, smokeless tobacco, and bidis), with the highest prevalence in the East Mediterranean Region (12 per cent) and lowest in the Western Pacific Region (6.6 per cent). Among students who had never smoked cigarettes, 19.1 per cent indicated they were susceptible to initiate smoking during the next year. The rate was highest in the European Union (29.8 per cent) and lowest in the Western Pacific Region (13.4 per cent). Cigarette smoking rates were significantly higher than other tobacco-use rates in the Americas, European Region, and Western Pacific Region; while other tobacco use was significantly more prevalent than cigarette smoking in the East Mediterranean Region and South East Asia Region. There was no difference between cigarette and other tobacco-use rates in the African Region or across all sites. Susceptibility rates were significantly higher than current cigarette smoking rates overall and in every region, except the Western Pacific Region, where no difference was reported (Warren *et al.* 2006; CDC 2008b).

Data from the 2005 United States Youth Risk Behavior Survey indicate that the prevalence of current cigarette smoking among American high-school students increased from 27.5 per cent in 1991 to 36.4 per cent in 1997, declined to 21.9 per cent in 2003, and remained stable (23 per cent) from 2003 to 2007 (CDC 2008a). The GYTS showed that the level of cigarette smoking between boys and girls is similar in many sites; the prevalence of cigarette smoking and use of other tobacco products is similar; and susceptibility to initiate smoking among never smokers is similar among boys and girls and is higher than cigarette smoking in the majority of sites.

In China, the current cigarette smoking prevalence in 2002 was 31.4 per cent, while in 1996, the prevalence of any tobacco smoking was 35.3 per cent. Although both surveys are not comparable, smoking prevalence did not appear to have decreased significantly, and the number of smokers in fact increased by 30 million between 1996 and 2002 (Yang *et al.* 2002). In the Kurdistan region of Iraq, among students aged 13–15, approximately 1 in every 10 ever-smokers of both sexes initiated smoking before 10 years of age. The initiation rates are slightly higher for girls than for boys (CDC 2006).

Many studies have shown that sociodemographic, environmental, behavioural, and personal factors are associated with the onset of tobacco use. Environmental factors include availability and advertising of cigarettes, the perception that tobacco use is the norm, peer and sibling attitudes, and lack of parental support during adolescence (Reid *et al.* 1995). Ease of acquiring cigarettes is another environmental factor that can have an impact on smoking among adolescents. Parental attitudes towards smoking, in particular towards their own children's smoking, has been shown to be related to adolescent smoking. Also important are school performance and psychosocial factors, including low academic achievement, rebelliousness, low self-esteem, alienation from school, and lack of skills to resist offers of cigarettes (Tyas & Pederson 1998). These findings are mainly from Western countries (Conrad *et al.* 1992; Tyas & Pederson 1998); although several studies from developing countries such as China have shown similar results (Wang *et al.* 1994b; Zhu *et al.* 1996). Additionally, data indicate that daily tobacco smoking is most prevalent among the lowest-income households in developing economies—that is, among the poorest of the poor (WHO 2007h).

Tobacco use by women

Tobacco use is one of the major causes of premature disease and death, and is an emerging global public health problem especially among girls and women. According to WHO, currently more than 200 million women smoke cigarettes worldwide, and this figure excludes those using other forms of tobacco (Unpublished data from WHO Tobacco Free Initiative).[4] It is estimated that between 80 000 and 100 000 young people start smoking everyday, and

---

[4] The global and income aggregates represent adjusted prevalence estimates. Crude estimates received from WHO Member States are adjusted to obtain nationally representative prevalence estimates for current smokers of tobacco for the same year and age groups. These estimates are not age-standardised (i.e. do not remove the effects of the underlying age structures across countries) and should be used with caution when making comparisons of smoking prevalence across regions/income groups. For this reason, these estimates differ to those published in WHS 2008.

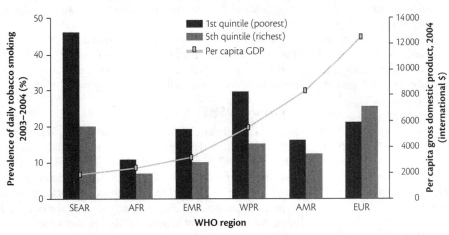

Daily tobacco smoking among adults aged 18 years and older, by income quintile and WHO region

Legend:
- 1st quintile (poorest)
- 5th quintile (richest)
- Per capita GDP

SEAR, Southeast Asia; AFR African; EMR, Eastern Mediterranean; WPR, Western Pacific; AMR, Americas; EUR, European

Fig. 10.1.5 Tobacco use and poverty: High prevalence among the world's poorest.
Source: WHO (2007h).

many of these are girls. An estimated 9.3 per cent of women smoke globally; about 21.7 per cent of women smoke in developed countries, while 5.7 per cent of women smoke in developing countries (estimates for adult population ≥15 years old for 2005, unpublished data from WHO Tobacco Free Initiative[4]). Again, these statistics do not include forms of tobacco use other than cigarettes. For example, in India, 30.8 per cent of men and only 2.8 per cent of women currently smoke (WHO 2008). On the other hand, the prevalence of other forms of tobacco use, i.e. chewing tobacco, is about 9.9 per cent (IIPS and Macro International 2007). Historically, smoking has been more common among men than among women in the majority of countries. In countries for which reliable data are available for assessing trends in smoking (primarily industrialized countries), peak prevalence among women occurred some years after it did so for men (Garfinkel 1997). While there are minor gender differences in smoking rates in some industrialized countries (such as the United States, New Zealand, and Australia), disparities between male and female current smoking rates in Asia are striking, specifically in Japan (43.3 per cent of men and 12 per cent of women), Korea (52.8 per cent of men and 5.8 per cent of women), and China (57.4 per cent of men and 2.6 per cent of women) (WHO 2008).

At the same time, smoking rates are rising among young women in many countries in Asia and the Pacific regions, where smoking is sometimes perceived as a symbol of women's liberation from traditional gender roles. There is an even greater cause for alarm here as statistics on cigarette consumption do not reflect the widespread use of smokeless tobacco among women in South Asia. For example, in Kerala, India, 22 per cent of rural women chew tobacco in a betel leaf. In the Bihar region and parts of Punjab and Haryana, women also smoke *bidis* and *hookahs*, while rural Indian women in the state of Goa rub and plug burnt powdered tobacco inside their mouths (Aghi *et al.* 2001). A major setback in public health would result if more women in developing countries began to smoke, similar to the trend observed in developed countries, and continued to use other forms of tobacco.

A contributing factor to this rising epidemic of tobacco use among women is the proliferation of seductive tobacco advertising worldwide, which may lead women and girls to believe that smoking

is socially desirable. Typically, women's brands in developing countries feature false images of slimness, sophistication, emancipation, and modernity. To sell such images, tobacco companies are producing a range of brands aimed at women and feminized cigarettes which are long, extra slim, low-tar, light-coloured, or menthol.

The Kobe Declaration adopted in 1999 by women and youth leaders, scientists and policy-makers 'demanded a global ban on direct and indirect advertising, promotion and sponsorship by the tobacco industry across all media and in all forms of entertainment; and demanded public funding for counter-advertising that disconnects women's liberation and tobacco use and that reaches women and girls in all cultural contexts' (WHO 1999a, 2000a). WHO also recommends that gender issues be incorporated into the planning and implementation of tobacco control measures, in order to address the specific needs of women and men more effectively (WHO 2007g).

Tobacco use by indigenous people

Tobacco use is an important factor that impacts negatively on the health of indigenous peoples who have the highest rates of tobacco use in the world. It is not unusual for the rates of smoking of indigenous peoples to be twice that of the general population of the country in which they live. A survey among the Inuit of Greenland found that currently 82 per cent of Inuit men and 78 per cent of Inuit women are smokers. Furthermore, in the area of Disko Bay, approximately 65 per cent of pregnant women are smokers (AMAP 1998). Therefore, it is not surprising that the incidence and mortality of tobacco-related cancers are very high among the Inuit of Greenland (AMAP 1998). Similar patterns of smoking and smoking-related disease are evident among other groups of indigenous peoples, including the Maori of New Zealand, the First Nations and Inuit peoples of Canada, and the Aborigines and Torres Strait Islanders of Australia (Durie 1998). By 2006/2007, the rate of smoking among the Maori of New Zealand (42.2 per cent of Maori aged 15 years and over) was twice the rate of non-Maori New Zealanders. After adjusting for age, Maori women were more than twice as likely to be current smokers than women in the total population (Ministry of Health, New Zealand 2008). In 1997, 62 per cent of

First Nations and Labrador Inuit of Canada adults (aged 15 years and over) were smokers. The ratio for indigenous and non-indigenous peoples of the Northwest Territories of Canada in 1996 was similar (S. Gauthier, unpublished report, 1999). The Aborigines and Torres Strait Islanders of Australia have twice the rate of smoking of the non-indigenous Australian population (54 per cent of indigenous men and 46 per cent of indigenous women, compared with 28 and 22 per cent of non-indigenous men and women, respectively) (Australian Bureau of Statistics 2002).

Given the high level of tobacco use by many indigenous peoples around the world, it is essential that their distinctive needs are addressed in national and global public health efforts to control the tobacco epidemic. Tobacco control among indigenous peoples is not adequately addressed within the framework of minority groups or vulnerable populations; more specific approaches are needed to address their distinctive tobacco control needs.

Smoking cessation and nicotine dependence

Smoking cessation decreases health risks, even at older ages (USDHHS 2004). However, many smokers try to quit but fail. Nicotine dependence is the major reason for relapse after quitting. Nicotine, an alkaloid, is a constituent of all tobacco products and a drug that leads to addiction (USDHHS 1988). Nicotine administration can lead to tolerance and physiological dependence. Tolerance is indicated by the diminished response to repeated doses of nicotine. Nicotine-induced physiological dependence and withdrawal are specific to the administration or removal of nicotine itself. Cessation from tobacco following chronic use results in withdrawal symptoms, including a craving for nicotine, impaired ability to concentrate, disrupted cognitive performance, mood changes, and impaired brain function (Hatsukami et al. 1985).

Cessation of smoking is a dynamic process with a cyclical nature. Over the course of time, many people alternate between smoking and non-smoking. Smoking cessation is not a discrete process but rather a complex process involving several stages. As mentioned previously, the trans-theoretical model, which uses stages of change to integrate processes and principles of change on people's behaviour, conceives behavioural change as a process involving five stages: Pre-contemplation, contemplation, preparation, action, and maintenance (Prochaska et al. 1997). Pre-contemplation is defined as a stage in which current smokers have no intention to give up smoking within the next 6 months. During contemplation, current smokers intend to give up smoking within the next 6 months. Current smokers in the preparation stage are seriously preparing to give up smoking within the next 30 days and take some steps in this direction, such as reading relevant materials. The action stage is defined as the first 6 months after smokers stop smoking. Lastly, maintenance continues from 6 months after stopping smoking until the person is a confirmed non-smoker without relapse.

There may be different stage profiles of smoking cessation across different countries and population groups. Understanding the various stage profiles might help public health officials to target messages and projects more appropriately. Tobacco control efforts or other forms of support aimed at smokers who are less ready to quit may promote their intention to quit. For example, results from a 2006 survey of 1750 smokers, aged 16–59, from five different European countries showed that the majority of smokers (73.5 per cent) wanted to stop smoking, and between 62.6 and 77.7 per cent of smokers can be categorized in the pre-contemplation stage.

The study demonstrated that in countries with a high level of tobacco control, the proportion of people in the pre-contemplation stage is lower than in countries with low tobacco control activity (Thyrian et al. 2008).

The stage profile of cessation is different in developing countries. The 1996 National Prevalence Survey in China reported that about 72 per cent of smokers never intended to give up smoking and only about 16 per cent intended to do so (Yang et al. 2001).

Exposure to SHS

Non-smokers inhale SHS, the combination of sidestream smoke that is released as the cigarette burns and the mainstream smoke exhaled by active smokers (USDHHS 2006). SHS is a complex mixture of particles and gases that changes in character as it ages subsequent to its formation. Indicators of exposure to the SHS range from surrogate indicators, such as marriage to a smoker, to direct measurements of exposure and of biomarkers.

Detailed reviews of exposure assessment for SHS are provided in several recent reports from the United States: The 2005 report of the California Environmental Protection Agency and the 2006 report of the US Surgeon General (California Environmental Protection Agency 2005; USDHHS 2006). Questionnaires have proved effective for epidemiological research as have biomarkers; the extent of misclassification associated with questionnaires has been characterized in a number of populations, using biomarkers or other 'gold standards'.

In some countries, in which male smoking prevalence exceeds female smoking prevalence, one useful index at the national level is the husband's smoking status as an estimate of SHS exposure for wives. This index is potentially incomplete because it does not capture smoking by other family members or exposure outside of the home (Wang et al. 1994). Indirect measures used for research and surveillance include self-reported exposure and description of the source of SHS in relevant microenvironments, most often the home and workplace, obtained by using standardized questionnaires.

Nicotine and its metabolite cotinine have long been used as measures of tobacco smoke intake, whether from active smoking or inhaling SHS. The concentrations of serum and urinary cotinine in non-smokers increase significantly with the reported number of cigarettes smoked by their spouses; cotinine can be used to identify second-hand smokers and is sensitive to the extent of tobacco smoke exposure (California Environmental Protection Agency 2005; USDHHS 2006). However, cotinine with a half-life of about 20 h in nonsmokers provides a measurement of exposure within the last few days and does not reflect the long-term exposure to second-hand smoking.

Second-hand smoking exposure of a non-smoker is influenced by the number of smokers in the indoor environment, the intensity of their smoking, the duration of exposure, the volume of the indoor environment, and its ventilation characteristics (USDHHS 2006). The doses of SHS components reaching the respiratory tract further depend on one's breathing pattern and activity level. Homes, workplaces, and public places can all be loci of exposure to SHS, particularly the home for women and children in many societies (Wipfli et al. 2008). The prevalence of SHS exposure remains high, particularly in countries where the prevalence of smoking is high among men and low among women. For example, in a 2002 survey in China, 53 per cent of non-smokers reported that they were exposed to SHS (Yang et al. 2002). The prevalence rate of SHS exposure in females (54.6 per cent) was higher than that in males (49.1 per cent). The highest exposure to SHS (up to 60 per cent) was in middle-aged women. The majority of second-hand smokers were exposed every day, with 82 per cent reporting exposure at home, 35 per cent reporting exposure in their work environments, and 67 per cent being exposed in public places (Yang personal communication).

Studies document substantial exposures of younger children to SHS as well. Children's exposure to SHS is involuntary, arising from smoking, mainly by adults, in the places where they live, work, and play. WHO estimates that about 700 million, or almost half, of the world's children breathe air polluted by tobacco smoke, particularly at home (WHO 1999b). The GYTS data show that approximately 4 in 10 students (42.5 per cent) were exposed to smoke in their home, approximately half (55.1 per cent) of all students were exposed to SHS in public places during the week preceding the survey and more than three-fourths (78.3 per cent) of students in all WHO regions thought smoking should be banned in all public places (CDC 2008). In Hong Kong, China, from data on 8327 newborns in April and May 1997, 41.2 per cent were exposed to SHS at home, mainly from smoking by the father (Leung et al. 2004). For older children, the proportion of SHS exposure at home ranges from 42.1 to 47 per cent, and SHS exposure outside their homes from 35.2 to 67.3 per cent (WHO 2008). In a recent 31-country study, Wipfli and colleagues (2008) measured air nicotine in homes with and without smokers as well as nicotine concentration in the hair of women and children living in the homes. Having a smoking parent was associated with a doubling of the hair nicotine concentration. Air concentrations were substantially higher if smokers lived in the home. Importantly, in only a few percentage of homes was a policy in force with regard to smoking in the home.

Patterns and burden of tobacco-related diseases

Toxicology of tobacco smoke

Tobacco smoke is generated by the burning of a complex organic material, tobacco, together with various additives and paper at a high temperature, reaching several thousand degrees Celsius in the tip during puffing. The resulting smoke, comprising numerous gases and particles, contains many toxic components that can cause injury through inflammation and irritation, asphyxiation, carcinogenesis, and other mechanisms. Active smokers inhale mainstream smoke, i.e. the smoke that is drawn directly through the end of the cigarette. Passive smokers inhale SHS, as noted earlier. Concentrations of SHS are far below the levels of mainstream smoke inhaled by the active smoker, but there are qualitative similarities between SHS and mainstream smoke, as SHS comes predominantly from mainstream smoke (USDHHS 2006).

Both active and second-hand smokers absorb tobacco smoke components through the lung's airways and alveoli, and many of these components, such as the gas carbon monoxide, enter into the circulation and are distributed throughout the body. There is also uptake of some components, such as benzo[a]pyrene, directly into the cells that line the upper airways and the lung's airways. Some of the carcinogens undergo metabolic transformation into their active forms. The genitourinary system is exposed to toxins in tobacco smoke through the excretion of these compounds in the urine. The gastrointestinal tract is exposed through direct deposition of smoke in the upper airways and the clearance of smoke-containing mucus from the trachea through the glottis into the oesophagus. Not surprisingly, tobacco smoking has proved to be a cause of disease in almost all organs of the body in addition to diminishing health generally (USDHHS 2004).

There is a vast bank of scientific literature on the mechanisms by which tobacco smoking causes disease, disability, and death (USDHHS 1989, 2004; WHO 2004d). This literature includes characterization of many of the toxic components in smoke, which include well-known toxins such as hydrogen cyanide, carbon monoxide, and nitrogen oxides. The toxicity of smoke has been studied by exposing animals to tobacco smoke, in cellular and other laboratory toxicity assays, and by assessing smokers for evidence of injury by tobacco smoke using biomarkers such as tissue changes and levels of damaging enzymes and cytokines. The data from these studies amply document the powerful toxicity of tobacco smoke. For example, young smokers in their twenties already show evidence of permanent damage to the small airways of the lung (Niewoehner et al. 1974; PDAY Research Group 1990), and lavage of the lungs of smokers shows increased numbers of inflammatory cells and higher levels of markers of injury compared with non-smokers (USDHHS 1990). The new tools of molecular and cellular biology have provided evidence of tobacco-induced changes at the molecular level as well. For example, an activated tobacco-smoke carcinogen has been shown as binding to the same codon in the p53 gene where mutations are found in smokers with lung cancer (Denissenko et al. 1996). A variety of genetic changes are also found in epithelial cells in smokers' lungs (Wistuba et al. 1997).

WHO and the International Union Against Tuberculosis and Lung Disease have recently confirmed an association between active smoking and tuberculosis mortality through a qualitative systematic review (WHO 2007f), which examined five studies investigating the role of active smoking and tuberculosis mortality. All the studies showed strong effects of smoking on tuberculosis mortality, with the risk ratio ranging from 1.02 to 6.62. This effect appears to be independent of the effects of alcohol use, socioeconomic status, and a large number of other potential confounders.

The most useful epidemiological studies for assessing the health risks of tobacco were the cohort studies initiated in the 1950s, 1960s, and 1970s, together with the follow-up mortality analyses pertaining to this period (Lopez 1999). All are limited to the study of mortality, and give quantitatively similar results for the relative risks of smoking for various diseases (and all causes of death), despite the fact that the cohorts were recruited from countries as diverse as the United States, Sweden, Japan, Canada, and the United Kingdom. These findings have complemented the results of numerous case–control studies, some including thousands of cases (USDHHS 1989, 1997, 2001, 2006).

In the United States, the United Kingdom, and Canada, where men had been smoking in large numbers for decades before these studies were carried out, smoking was typically associated with 70–80 per cent excess mortality from all causes (Peto et al. 1996). The relative risks varied substantially by disease, and were largest for cancers of the lung and upper aerodigestive tract (mouth, pharynx, larynx and oesophagus), and lowest for vascular diseases that have complex multicausal aetiologies. Typically, lung cancer death rates were 10–12 times higher in smokers than in non-smokers, with the notable exception of Japanese men and American women for whom the excess risks were three to four times that of non-smokers. Similarly, the all-cause mortality ratios (relative risks) were substantially lower in these two studies, reflecting the fact that tobacco use in the two populations had been much lower than in other cohorts.

Relative risks of lung cancer for American women smokers versus lifelong non-smokers increased from 2.7 in 1959–1965 to 11.9 in 1982–1986, reflecting the dominant role of duration of exposure in determining lung cancer hazards (USDHHS 1989, 2006).

Two large cohort studies have produced evidence on health hazards from smoking, which have emphasized the increasing hazards of smoking with longer duration of use. These two studies are the 50-year follow-up of the 1951 British doctors cohort (Doll et al. 2004) and the second American Cancer Society Cancer Prevention Study (CPS-II) cohort of over 1.2 million adults monitored since 1982, for which comparisons can be made with CPS-I, initiated 20 years earlier (Thun et al. 1997).

The alarming size of the hazards observable in populations that have been smoking for many decades is now apparent. In the first 20 years of follow-up of the British doctors cohort (1951–1971), smokers had, on an average, about a 1.5–2-fold higher death rate at each age, similar to the excess reported in other studies around that time (Doll et al. 1994, 2004). With a longer duration of smoking, the death rates of smokers increased substantially, so that during the second period of follow-up (1971–1991), the death rate of middle-aged smokers was three times higher than that of non-smokers (Doll et al. 1994, 2004). A similar excess mortality ratio was found in the CPS-II cohort based on follow-up in the latter half of the 1980s. These relative risks suggest that, on an average, a smoker who begins smoking in young adult life and continues to smoke has at least a 50 per cent chance of eventually being killed by tobacco in either middle or old age (Peto et al. 1994).

The evidence from these two studies of the disease-specific risks associated with smoking is similar (Lopez 1999). Current smokers have about a 20-fold higher death rate from lung cancer than never-smokers, among whom lung cancer death rates have remained low and constant. There is epidemiological evidence to suggest that this is also the case in other populations. For example, based on the two American Cancer Society studies with follow-up to 1959–1965 and 1982–1986, respectively, lung cancer death rates among lifelong non-smokers were remarkably constant at 15.4 and 14.7 per 100 000 (age-standardized) for men, and 9.6 and 12 for women; the rates for current smokers were 187.1 and 341.3 for men, and 26.1 and 154.6 for women (Thun et al. 1997). A more recent study on the CPS-II cohort showed that relative risks of colorectal cancer mortality ranged from 1.32 in male to 1.41 in female smokers when compared with never smokers (Chao et al. 2000). Smokers also incur a 10–20-fold excess mortality from chronic obstructive lung disease (primarily chronic bronchitis and emphysema), and a risk of death from major vascular diseases that is about twice that of non-smokers.

The excess mortality of smokers from vascular disease is particularly noteworthy. Vascular disease death rates are typically much higher than those for cancer or other causes associated with smoking. Therefore, cardiovascular diseases (especially ischaemic heart disease and stroke) contribute more to smoking-attributable deaths at a population level than other causes, including lung cancer for which the relative risk is much higher, although this pattern will change as cardiovascular disease mortality declines. Finally, it is worth noting that the all-age excess mortality ratio of about two from cardiovascular diseases masks a very significant age gradient in relative risks. At younger ages (<50 years), smokers have a 5–6-times higher death rate than non-smokers, with the relative excess declining with age. These data suggest that if a smoker dies from vascular disease before the age of about 50 years, there is a 70–80 per cent chance that death was caused by smoking, and that vascular disease is the chief mechanism through which smoking causes a threefold excess mortality rate in middle age (Parish et al. 1995). However, cigarette smoking is only one of several causative factors of cardiovascular disease. This is especially true for ischaemic heart disease, where smoking interacts synergistically with other factors such as hypercholesterolemia and hypertension to increase risk of heart disease substantially. Evidence suggests that the independent risk attributable to smoking is comparable with that of other major risk factors (USDHHS 2004). The interaction with dietary parameters probably explains the historically lower proportions of ischaemic heart disease attributable to smoking in populations such as China where low-fat diets have predominated (Liu et al. 1998).

Smoking by women adversely affects reproduction. Smoking during pregnancy reduces birth weight by approximately 200 g on an average (USDHHS 1990); and the degree of reduction is dose-related. With successful cessation by the third trimester, much of the weight reduction can be avoided. Smoking also increases rates of spontaneous abortion, placenta praevia and perinatal mortality, and smoking during pregnancy is now considered to be a cause of sudden infant death syndrome. There is more limited evidence suggesting that smoking may increase childhood cancer incidence and congenital defects (Charlton 1996; SCOTH 1998).

Cigarettes have changed substantially over the last 50 years (USDHHS 1997). Filtered cigarettes now dominate the market, and tar and nicotine yields, as assessed by smoking machines, have declined substantially. Although tar and nicotine deliveries to smokers have little relationship to machine-measured levels (USDHHS 1997), early epidemiological evidence comparing switchers to filtered cigarettes with continued use of non-filtered cigarettes showed some reduction in lung cancer risk. Subsequent epidemiological evidence on cancer risk in relation to yield of tar has shown little indication of reduced risk for lung cancer; in fact, comparisons of risks of lung cancer in smokers over time show an increase in relative risk, compared with never smokers (USDHHS 2001, 2004). A reduction has not been observed for cardiovascular disease in association with lower yield, as measured by a machine (USDHHS 2001, 2004). Although rising relative risks of smoking have been documented across recent decades when the lower-delivery products came into widespread usage (Doll et al. 1994), this is due to a longer duration of exposure and not to a change in the hazard.

Evidence on health risks of SHS

Evidence on the health risks of SHS comes from epidemiological studies which have directly assessed the associations of SHS exposure with disease outcomes and also from knowledge of the components of SHS and their toxicities. Judgements as to the causality of association between SHS exposure and health outcomes are based not only on this epidemiological evidence, but also on the extensive evidence derived from epidemiological and toxicological investigation of active smoking. The evidence is clear: Exposure to SHS causes illness and death. As US Surgeon General Richard Carmona commented in releasing his 2006 report on SHS, the scientific community has reached consensus on this point (USDHHS 2006).

In the United States, it is estimated to cause as many as 50 000 premature deaths each year, making it the third leading preventable cause of death (California Environmental Protection Agency 2005).

Additionally, studies using biomarkers of exposure and dose, including the nicotine metabolite cotinine and white cell adducts, document the absorption of SHS components by exposed non-smokers, adding to the plausibility of the observed associations of SHS with adverse effects.

Second-hand smoke exposure of the infant and child has adverse effects on respiratory health, including increased risk for more severe lower respiratory infections, middle-ear disease, chronic respiratory symptoms, and asthma, as well as a reduction in the rate of lung function growth during childhood. Maternal smoking during gestation and subsequent SHS exposure increase risk for sudden infant death syndrome (California Environmental Protection Agency 2005; USDHHS 2006). There is more limited evidence suggesting that SHS exposure of the mother reduces birth weight (Zhang & Ratcliffe 1993) and that child development and behaviour are adversely affected by parental smoking (Eskenazi & Castorina 1999; WHO 1999b). There is no strong evidence at present that SHS exposure increases childhood cancer risk (WHO 2004d; USDHHS 2006).

In adults, SHS exposure has been causally associated with lung cancer and may also increase the risk of ischaemic heart disease. In 1986, the conclusion was reached by a number of agencies that SHS caused lung cancer, including the United States Surgeon General (USDHHS 1986), and the US National Research Council (NRC 1986). The International Agency for Research on Cancer (IARC) also concluded that SHS must give rise to some risk of cancer. Arguments that the association of SHS exposure with lung cancer risk in never-smokers could reflect confounding or information bias were considered and set aside in these and subsequent reports. Since 1986, other expert groups have also found SHS to be a cause of lung cancer in non-smokers (EPA 1992; Australian National Health and Medical Research Council 1997; California Environmental Protection Agency 1997, 2005; SCOTH 1998; WHO 2004d; USDHHS 2006).

The risk has been quantified in several meta-analyses, beginning with the 1986 US National Research Council report (NRC 1986). The risk associated with marriage to a smoker has been around 20–30 per cent; a meta-analysis by IARC (WHO 2004d) of 46 studies and 6257 cases yielded a point estimate of 24 per cent (95% CI: 14–34 per cent). Several other recent meta-analyses further quantify the association between SHS and lung cancer. Stayner et al. performed a meta-analysis of 22 studies published through 2003 on workplace SHS exposure and lung cancer, in which the pooled relative risk was found to be 1.24 (95% CI: 1.18–1.29). Among highly exposed workers, the relative risk was 2.01 (95% CI: 1.33–2.60) (Stayner et al. 2007). Taylor et al. performed a meta-analysis to calculate a pooled estimate of relative risk of lung cancer associated with exposure to SHS in never-smoking women exposed to smoking spouses. Using 55 studies (7 cohort, 25 population-based case–control, and 23 non-population-based case–control studies) published through 2006, the authors found a pooled relative risk for lung cancer of 1.27 (95% CI: 1.17–1.37) (Taylor et al. 2007).

Coronary heart disease has also been causally associated with SHS exposure on the basis of observational and experimental evidence (Barnoya & Glantz 2005; California Environmental Protection Agency 2005; USDHHS 2006). Exposure to SHS has been shown to unfavourably affect blood clotting parameters and endothelial cell function. The meta-analysis prepared for the 2006 US Surgeon General's Report estimated the pooled excess risk for coronary heart disease from SHS exposure from marriage to a smoker as 27 per cent (95% CI: 19–36 per cent) (USDHHS 2006). There is also evidence linking SHS to other adverse effects in adults, including stroke (Bonita et al. 1999), exacerbation of asthma, reduced lung function and respiratory symptoms (USDHHS 2006).

Summarizing the health risks of SHS, the 2006 US Surgeon General Report examined the topics of toxicology of SHS, assessment and prevalence of exposure to SHS, reproductive and developmental health effects, respiratory effects of exposure to SHS in children and adults, cancer among adults, cardiovascular diseases, and the control of SHS exposure (USDHHS 2006). This report included six overall conclusions which are provided below.

'The scientific evidence with regard to the involuntary exposure of nonsmokers to tobacco smoke, supports the following major conclusions:

♦ Second-hand smoke causes premature death and disease in children and in adults who do not smoke.

♦ Children exposed to SHS are at an increased risk for sudden infant death syndrome, acute respiratory infections, ear problems, and more severe asthma. Smoking by parents causes respiratory symptoms and slows lung growth in their children.

♦ Exposure of adults to SHS has immediate adverse effects on the cardiovascular system and causes coronary heart disease and lung cancer.

♦ The scientific evidence indicates that there is no risk-free level of exposure to SHS.

♦ Many millions of Americans, both children and adults, are still exposed to SHS in their homes and workplaces despite substantial progress in tobacco control.

♦ Eliminating smoking in indoor spaces fully protects non-smokers from exposure to SHS. Separating smokers from non-smokers, cleaning the air, and ventilating buildings cannot eliminate exposures of non-smokers to SHS'.

Burden of tobacco-related diseases

In 1953, Levin proposed an epidemiological statistic, now referred to as the population attributable risk, for estimating the burden of disease caused by a particular factor in a population (Levin 1953). He was motivated to do so by the emerging information on the association of lung cancer with smoking and the consequent need to understand the related burden of disease. His basic approach has now been widely applied. The global and regional projections of mortality and burden of disease by cause had been published by Murray and Lopez in 1997, and were based on data from 1990. In 2006, Mathers and Loncar updated the projection using more recent data (Mathers & Loncar 2006). They applied the same method applied in the original Global Burden of Disease Study. In relation to tobacco-related deaths, the smoking impact ratios (SIR) were used as an indirect indicator of accumulated smoking risk based on excess lung cancer mortality. Smoking impact ratio measures the absolute excess lung cancer mortality due to smoking in the study population, relative to the excess lung cancer mortality in lifelong smokers of the reference population. Estimated tobacco attributable deaths were 5.4 million in 2005, 6.4 million in 2015 and 8.3 million in 2030. Tobacco attributable deaths are expected to decline in developed countries (9 per cent decrease between

2002 and 2030), but double in low- and middle-income countries (from 3.4 to 6.8 million). By 2015, smoking is expected to cause 50 per cent more deaths than HIV/AIDS, and will be responsible for 10 per cent of all deaths.

Certain countries have contributed to a significant proportion of the world's burden of disease and deaths attributed to tobacco. In China, tobacco killed 1 million smokers by 2000, and by 2020, 2 million will die if the number of smokers continues to grow at present rate (Gan *et al.* 2007). In India, in a national-and population-based case–control study that included 1.1 million households, prevalence of smoking was compared in 74 000 deceased subjects with 78 000 living unmatched subjects. The authors estimated that smoking was associated with higher risk of death in women (risk ratio 2) and in men (risk ratio 1.7). Smoking was associated with a reduction in life expectancy of 8 years in women and 6 years in men. By 2010, if the actual smoking prevalence remains unchanged, almost 1 million deaths will be attributed to tobacco, with 70 per cent of them occurring in middle-aged people (Jha *et al.* 2008).

The tobacco industry

A distinguishing feature of the tobacco epidemic has been the role of major corporations—some of the largest in the world—in promoting tobacco use and, as a consequence, death and disease. This presents a unique challenge for the public health community. The adversary is not only disease or natural forces. It also includes powerful corporations whose actions are antithetical to public health as discussed earlier in the chapter.

As the 21st century begins, the transnational tobacco companies are increasing their presence in global markets. While total consumption of cigarettes is falling in several high-income countries, consumption in low- and middle-income countries is increasing (WHO 2008).

Given the growing influence of the multinationals, an understanding of their history, conduct, and behaviour is essential to help guide strategies for tobacco control. In the mid- to late-1990s, the public health community gained an unprecedented view of the tobacco industry through the release of millions of pages of previously secret internal tobacco company documents (Bero 2003). These documents were obtained primarily through court proceedings in lawsuits against tobacco companies in the United States.

The global corporate actors

While tobacco in diverse forms has been used since antiquity, the modern cigarette did not become a popular phenomenon until the twentieth century, with the invention of the mechanical cigarette rolling machine. With a dramatically increased production capacity, the modern tobacco industry was born (Detels *et al.* 2002). Currently, much of the world's cigarette market is dominated by a few transnational tobacco companies, as articulated earlier in this chapter.

Decades of deceit

Starting in the mid-to-late 1990s, millions of pages of previously secret internal documents from mostly United States-based tobacco companies or companies doing business in the United States, were publicly released in the country secondary to a series of court cases against tobacco companies (WHO 2000b, 2004; Hirschhorn 2005).

Analyses of these documents paint a damning picture of an industry which for decades suppressed scientific research and information on the health hazards and addictiveness of smoking, manipulated the amount and/or form of nicotine to exploit the addictive potential of tobacco, and targeted marketing campaigns at youth (Detels *et al.* 2002; Bero 2003). Recently, other sources of information about the tobacco companies' behaviour are also being used in the development of reports to guide policy-making in tobacco control (Hiilamo & Hirschhorn 2006).[5] One of the most comprehensive analyses of the tobacco companies' deceptive practices can be found in the final report of the United States Department of Justice case against the tobacco companies operating within the country (US Department of Justice 2004, 2006); while dozens of papers and reports have been published looking at the information contained in the tobacco companies' internal documents.[6]

The above documents make clear that many transnational tobacco companies, often in collaboration with each other, have engaged in a decades-long campaign to publicly deny the harmful effects of tobacco use and the addictive powers of nicotine, while these companies' internal research confirmed what was being said by academics and public health professionals. At the same time, these tobacco companies had developed technology in the production of cigarettes to enhance their addictive powers and had manipulated the cigarette development process so as to attract a larger number of consumers across different groups, such as women and ethnic minorities (Wayne & Connolly 2002; Cook *et al.* 2003; Ferris Wayne *et al.* 2006; Hammond *et al.* 2006; Lewis & Wackowski 2006; Milberger *et al.* 2006). The companies have also engaged in joint programmes to deny the harmful effects of SHS exposure, which is yet to be clearly accepted by tobacco companies, and developed sophisticated public relations and political campaigns to stop or deter public policies promoting smoking bans in public places (Ong & Glantz 2000; Drope & Chapman 2001; Samet & Burke 2001; Dearlove *et al.* 2002; Assunta *et al.* 2004). It is also clear how tobacco companies have used funding to subvert the scientific process, igniting the debate of the role of tobacco companies' funding in science and research and calls for such funding to be banned (Malone & Bero 2003; Parascandola 2003; Bero 2005; Chapman 2005; Thomson & Signal 2005; Hirschhorn *et al.* 2006).

In many instances, the tobacco companies indirectly exert their influence on tobacco control policy-making through the funding or creation of front groups and alliances, in order to avoid any negative publicity that might be associated with a tobacco company (Chapman 2003; Smith & Malone 2006; Apollonio & Bero 2007). Additionally, the internal documents show how the tobacco companies work in the political sphere at the local, national, and international levels to stop effective tobacco control policies from moving forward, including strategies to monitor and influence the development of the WHO FCTC and tobacco control advocacy efforts (Francey & Champman 2000; Jamrozik 2000; Saloojee & Dagli 2000; Bialous & Yach 2001; Carter 2002; Gilmore & McKee

---

5   These documents can be found online at: http://legacy.library.ucsf.edu/ and http://bat.library.ucsf.edu/.

6   A list of these publications can be found online at: http://www.library.ucsf.edu/tobacco/docsbiblio.html#mar.

2004; MacKenzie *et al.* 2007; Tong & Glantz 2004; McDaniel *et al.* 2006, 2008; Gilmore *et al.* 2007). Awareness of these strategies could better prepare policy-makers and public health officials to counter the industry efforts of derailing tobacco control (Ling & Glantz 2002; Thomson & Wilson 2005; Chapman 2006).

In the area of advertising and promotion, the tobacco companies have developed target marketing campaigns, including sponsorship of cultural and sports events, have worked to circumvent marketing restrictions when attempts to prevent or modify marketing restrictions had failed and have developed new products to continue to appeal to young people (Dewhirst & Hunter 2002; Pollay & Dewhirst 2002; Neuman *et al.* 2002; Wakefield *et al.* 2002; Assunta & Chapman 2004; Barbeau *et al.* 2004; Smith & Malone 2004; Anderson *et al.* 2005; Carpenter *et al.* 2005; LeGresley *et al.* 2006; MacKenzie *et al.* 2007). There is also an evidence of the tobacco companies' involvement, or at least, awareness of contraband of its products in several regions of the world (Joosens & Raw 2002; WHO 2003a; Collin *et al.* 2004; Lee & Collin 2006).

More recently, several transnational tobacco companies have engaged in efforts to present themselves as socially responsible corporations, when analysis of the industry documents demonstrate that these efforts are no more than public relations campaigns in response to increasing litigation against the industry, as well as increasing public perception of the tobacco companies as untrustworthy (Hirschhorn 2004; McDaniel & Malone 2005; Palazzo & Richter 2005; Szczypka *et al.* 2007).

As the multinational tobacco companies shift their attention to emerging markets, an understanding of the structure and behaviour of the tobacco industry becomes imperative as public health professionals attempt to fashion strategies to deal with a growing epidemic. These strategies cannot be formed and implemented in a vacuum. The tobacco industry is the vector, and only by knowing its history and conduct, monitoring its current behaviour, and regulating and restricting the environment in which the industry operates, can public health strategies be effective.

Tobacco control

The preventive potential for tobacco control to reverse the given forecast of a global tobacco epidemic is still high in many countries. We now have an improved understanding of the complexity of the tobacco epidemic, which will assist us to improve and activate interventions. The main focus of any strategy should be to prevent initiation of tobacco use, to promote quitting among the young and adults and to eliminate non-smokers' exposure to tobacco smoke. Cost-effective strategies are available and have already been proven to make a positive impact in many countries. To build on those successes, a comprehensive tobacco control strategy can provide a road map for national and global action. In this section, we explore the key components of a comprehensive tobacco control strategy that is applicable locally, regionally, and globally. A multifaceted strategy is needed to assure success of global tobacco control. The components of such a strategy will broadly include education and information, legislative measures, economic measures, cessation efforts, crop substitution and diversification, advocacy, litigation, and administration and management. Appropriate monitoring, evaluation, and surveillance are essential to assess the effectiveness of specific interventions. Strong political commitment on both national and global levels is essential for sustaining success.

The following sections will first provide the background and status of the WHO FCTC, followed by an outline of the MPOWER package as essential components of a comprehensive, WHO FCTC-based tobacco control strategy. Additionally, these sections will highlight other important measures such as product regulation, youth access, crop substitution and diversification, and litigation. Finally, the role of management and administration in establishing a sustained strategy will also be discussed.

The WHO framework convention on tobacco control

In May 1999, the WHO Member States unanimously paved the way for negotiations to begin on the WHO FCTC, a multilateral treaty addressing the tobacco epidemic, and possible related protocol agreements. Under Article 19 of its Constitution, WHO has the legal authority to serve as a platform for the development of binding treaties on health-relevant issues, which includes potentially all aspects of tobacco control, national and transnational. Major tobacco growers and exporters, as well as several countries in the developing and developed world that face the brunt of the tobacco industry's marketing and promotion, strongly supported the need for an international treaty to address the tobacco control epidemic.

The framework convention protocol approach has been used to address a wide range of international concerns, including environmental, arms control, and human rights issues. The term 'framework convention' does not have a particular technical meaning in international law. It is used to describe a variety of legal agreements which establish a general system of governance for an issue area, such as global tobacco control. Framework conventions, unlike more comprehensive forms of treaties, do not attempt to resolve all significant issues in a single document. Rather, they divide the negotiation of separate issues into separate agreements. States first adopt a framework convention, which creates an institutional forum in which states can co-operate and negotiate for the conclusion of separate implementing protocols containing detailed obligations or added institutional commitments. The framework convention/protocol approach is a dynamic and incremental process of global law-making that allows the political will of states, as signatories to international legal agreements, to be titrated gradually into legally binding commitments. The WHO FCTC is open for ratification, acceptance, approval, formal confirmation and accession indefinitely for States and eligible regional economic integration organizations wishing to become parties to it (WHO 2008). As of 1 February 2009, there were a total of 168 signatories and 162 Parties (WHO 2008).

The WHO FCTC entered into force on 27 February 2005, and WHO convened the first session of the COP, the treaty's governing body, in Geneva from 6 to 17 February 2006, in accordance with the Convention's Article 23 *Conference of the Parties*. During that first session, the Parties agreed on a number of procedural and substantive matters, formalized as decisions. They adopted Rules of Procedure to guide their interactions and a budget, funded exclusively by voluntary assessed contributions from Parties, and Financial Rules and Regulations to provide the necessary monetary structure for the work of the Convention. Additionally, the Conference established the Convention Secretariat in decision FCTC/COP1(10), which was confirmed and adopted by reference by the Health Assembly in May 2006. The Convention Secretariat is part of the WHO structure, reporting to the COP on technical and treaty matters and to the WHO Director General on administrative and certain technical matters. The Convention Secretariat is mandated to work closely and synergistically with TFI to provide the necessary support to implement the WHO FCTC.

At its first session, the COP also established two kinds of intersessional groups to move the work of the treaty forward. Working groups, composed of interested Parties and invited experts from civil society were formed to develop guidelines for the implementation of Article 8 *Protection from exposure to tobacco smoke* and Articles 9 and 10 *Regulations of the contents of tobacco products* and *Regulation of tobacco product disclosures*, respectively. Expert groups, comprising of four experts from each of the six WHO regions and invited experts from civil society, were established to draft templates for protocols on advertising, promotion and sponsorship of tobacco products and the illicit trade in tobacco products. The reports of the Working Groups and the Expert Groups were submitted to the Parties for their consideration at the second session of the COP, held in Bangkok, 30 June–6 July 2007.

At its second session, the Conference made important strides forward in the efforts to control tobacco use globally. Among the decisions taken in Bangkok, the Parties adopted guidelines for the implementation of Article 8 *Protection from exposure to tobacco smoke* that include strong language regarding the need for areas to be entirely smoke free. The work of the Articles 9 and 10 Working Group was continued and three new guideline development working groups were created, one each for Articles 5.3 *General Obligations*, Article 11 *Packaging and labelling of tobacco products*, Article 12 *Education, communication, training and public awareness* and Article 13 *Tobacco advertising, promotion and sponsorship*. At its third session, held in Durban, 17-22 November 2008, the Conference adopted guidelines for implementation of Articles 5.3, 11, and 13 and established two new working groups to develop

guidelines, one each for Article 12 *Education, communication, training and public awareness* and Article 14 *Demand reduction measures concerning tobacco dependence and cessation*. Additionally, the Parties decided to enter into negotiation of a protocol on illicit trade in tobacco products. As such, the Conference established an intergovernmental negotiating body (INB), a subsidiary body of the Conference, mandated to negotiate the text of the protocol, using the template developed by the expert group as the basis for initiating its work. The INB has met twice in Geneva, the first time from 11 to 16 February 2008 and the second time from 20 to 25 October 2008. A Chairperson's text was submitted to the INB for its consideration at its second session; a revised Chairperson's text will be submitted for consideration at the third session, scheduled to take place from 28 June to 5 July 2009, in Geneva.

As noted in the chapter on International Public Health Instruments, the WHO FCTC provides an effective instrument for counteracting the globalization of the tobacco pandemic by serving as a platform for multilateral commitment, co-operation, and action to address the rise and spread of tobacco consumption. The globalization of the tobacco epidemic restricts the capacity of countries to control tobacco unilaterally within their sovereign borders (Bettcher & Yach 1998). All transnational tobacco control issues, including trade, smuggling, advertising and sponsorship, prices and taxes, control of toxic substances, and tobacco package design and labelling, require multilateral cooperation and effective action at the global level. It is clear that national and transnational dimensions of tobacco control must be addressed in tandem; in the absence of effective international co-operation even the most comprehensive national control programmes can be unravelled (Bettcher *et al.* 2000).

The adoption and entry into force of the WHO FCTC was the start of a unique new chapter in global public health. WHO's ongoing

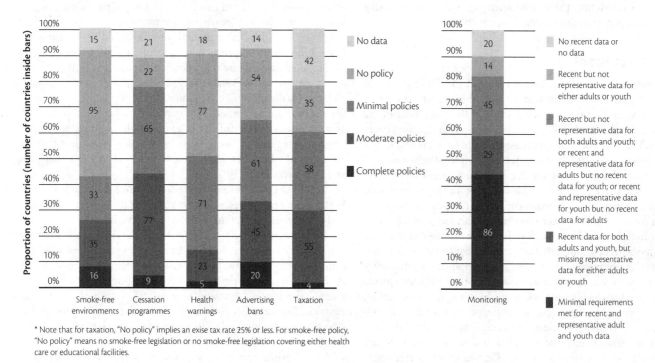

* Note that for taxation, "No policy" implies an exise tax rate 25% or less. For smoke-free policy, "No policy" means no smoke-free legislation or no smoke-free legislation covering either health care or educational facilities.

Fig. 10.1.6 The state of tobacco control policies in the world.
Source: WHO (2008a).

commitment to the WHO FCTC and global tobacco control implementation has been supported by its selection as a partner in the Bloomberg Initiative to Reduce Tobacco Use. The WHO FCTC and the MPOWER implementation strategy combine an overwhelming scientific evidence base with an evolving global social movement. This work links science and international relations at the global level as a vehicle for addressing a totally preventable man-made epidemic.

MPOWER

The WHO FCTC provides the foundation and context for effective global tobacco control policy intervention. As WHO's technical assistance package for the WHO FCTC, WHO released the MPOWER package of six cost-effective mechanisms proven to reduce tobacco use, each of which reflects at least one provision of the WHO FCTC (WHO 2008). Each of the elements of MPOWER reflects one or more provisions of the WHO FCTC. The six proven strategies of MPOWER are:

♦ Monitor tobacco use and prevention policies (Articles 20 and 21 of the WHO FCTC)

♦ Protect people from tobacco smoke (Article 8 of the WHO FCTC)

♦ Offer help to quit tobacco use (Article 14 of the WHO FCTC)

♦ Warn about the dangers of tobacco (Articles 11 and 12 of the WHO FCTC)

♦ Enforce bans on tobacco advertising, promotion and sponsorship (Article 13 of the WHO FCTC)

♦ Raise taxes on tobacco (Article 6 of the WHO FCTC)

Although there has been progress in recent years, no government is fully implementing all of these key interventions.

This translates to only a small portion—not more than 5 per cent in any circumstance—of the world's population being covered by comprehensive tobacco control policies (WHO 2008a).

Monitoring, surveillance and evaluation

Countries need accurate measures of tobacco use to effectively plan, implement, and evaluate tobacco control strategies. An effective national or international monitoring system must track several indicators, which include prevalence of tobacco use; impact of policy interventions; and tobacco industry marketing, promotion, and lobbying (WHO 2008). Comprehensive monitoring informs leaders of governments and civil society about the extent of the tobacco epidemic in their countries, helps them allocate tobacco control resources accordingly and shows them how effective the existing policies are.

Surveillance refers to the systematic and ongoing process of collection, collation, and analysis of data at national, regional, and global levels, as well as the timely dissemination of this information. Surveillance of tobacco use can guide policy decisions, research initiatives, and the development and evaluation of intervention programmes (Giovino 2000; WHO 2008). An ideal surveillance system would monitor variables contained in the traditional epidemiological model of agent, host, vector, and environment (Orleans & Slade 1993). Surveillance of agent factors (i.e. various tobacco products) may include monitoring of toxic constituents, pH, and additives. Most surveillance work monitors host factors (i.e. smoker/user or potential smoker/user) and the measures may include: Patterns of initiation, susceptibility of tobacco use, indicators of dependence, quitting patterns and methods, receipt of advice to quit from physicians and dentists, mental health indicators, use of behaviours, sources of tobacco, prices paid for cigarettes, usual brand, receptivity to marketing, awareness of tobacco control programmes and opinions about tobacco control policies. Surveillance of vector (i.e. tobacco product manufacturers) includes chronicling tobacco industry public relations, lobbying, and marketing activities. Environmental surveillance (economic, cultural, political, and historical) includes national tobacco control legislation and programmes, exposure to health messages; and tobacco promotions, prices, and placements (Giovino 2000).

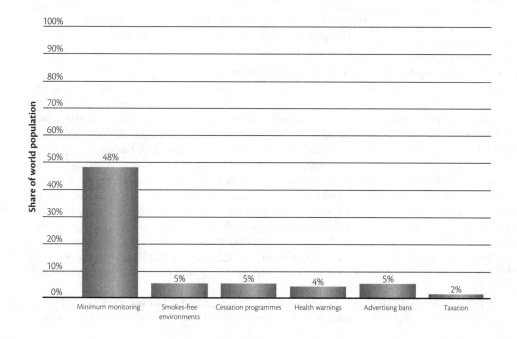

Fig. 10.1.7 Share of the world population covered by tobacco control policies.
Source: WHO (2008a).

For instance, the WHO Global Tobacco Surveillance System (GTSS) includes the collection of standard and comparable data through four surveys: Global Youth Tobacco Survey (GYTS), Global School Personal Survey (GSPS), Global Health Professions Students Survey (GHPSS) and Global Adult Tobacco Survey (GATS). The purpose of the GTSS is to enhance the capacity of countries to design, implement, and evaluate their national comprehensive tobacco action plan (GTSS Collaborative Group 2005). The GYTS focuses on youth aged 13–15 and collects information in schools. The GSPS surveys teachers and administrators from the same schools who participate in the GYTS. The GHPSS focuses on third-year students pursuing degrees in dentistry, medicine, nursing, and pharmacology. The GATS, a household survey, monitors tobacco use among adults aged 15 and above. The surveys cover a wide range of topics related to tobacco, including tobacco use prevalence (smoking and other tobacco products); exposure to SHS; cessation; risk perceptions; knowledge and attitudes; exposure to media; price and taxation on tobacco products; and sociodemographic characteristics.

Surveillance is also a crucial part of evaluation research. In order to ensure that the utility of both surveillance and evaluation research are maximized, programme evaluations should be built upon and complement tobacco-related surveillance systems. However, it is also important that specific evaluation surveys and data collection systems are implemented to evaluate individual programme activities. Ensuring that surveillance and evaluation are used in concert will serve to link programmes at national, regional, and global levels to facilitate progress towards intermediate and primary outcome objectives in tobacco control. It must also be highlighted that findings from the surveillance system must be effectively disseminated and used, especially in the policy-making process.

Protect people from tobacco smoke

Smoke-free environments are becoming increasingly popular, and such policies are important because they protect non-smokers from exposure to tobacco smoke, reduce smoker's consumption of cigarettes and induce some smokers to quit (Brownson et al. 1997; Chapman et al. 1999). Many countries are enacting comprehensive smoke-free legislation in all enclosed public spaces and workplaces (such as healthcare facilities, government offices, schools and universities, restaurants and bars, day-care centres, and transport facilities).

Studies conducted in the United States of America and Australia have attributed between 13 and 22 per cent of the declines in the tobacco consumption in these countries in recent years to the impact of smoke-free environments (Chapman et al. 1999). Smoke-free policies also alter tobacco use behaviour in young adults. Chaloupka and Wechsler (1997) found that relatively strong restrictions on smoking in public places discourage college students from smoking; while Evans et al. (1999) discovered that workplace smoking bans reduce smoking prevalence by 4–6 per cent and average daily consumption among smokers by 10 per cent. Smoke-free policies in workplaces in several industrialized countries have reduced total tobacco consumption among workers by an average of 29 per cent (Fichtenberg & Glantz 2002). Smoke-free legislation proposed in Ireland in 2006, which included pubs, showed no negative impact on business or profits (Howell 2005; Fong et al. 2006).

Uruguay was the first country in the Americas in 2006 to become 100 per cent smoke-free by enacting a ban on smoking in all public spaces and workplaces, including bars, restaurants and casinos. About half of all Americans and 90 per cent of Canadians live in areas where public spaces and workplaces are smoke-free (PAHO 2007). It is clear that there is growing support from countries to enact comprehensive smoke-free legislation. In this regard, WHO recommends a step by step approach to creating and enforcing smoke-free environments (WHO 2004a).

Offer help to quit tobacco use

Integrating tobacco cessation within primary healthcare systems and available healthcare services can be effective. Programmes that assist young and adult smokers to stop smoking can produce quicker public health benefits through incorporating cessation services in primary care, offering quit lines, providing affordable pharmacological treatment options and government support. Smokers who quit before the age of 50 halve their risk of dying in the next 15 years (USDHHS 1990). In addition, the cost savings from reduced tobacco use resulting from the implementation of moderately priced and effective smoking cessation interventions would more than pay for these interventions within 3–4 years (Wagner et al. 1995).

Evidence shows that advice from healthcare practitioners can increase cessation rates (Fiore et al. 2000). Quit lines linked to counselling and treatment are also effective, and if well-designed and managed, can be accessible widely.

On the other hand, pharmacological therapy such as nicotine replacement therapies (NRT) are generally expensive, considered to be less cost-effective than physicians' advice and quit lines and more difficult to obtain in many countries. However, NRT have been demonstrated to double or triple quit rates (Tobacco Advisory Group 2000; Silagy et al. 2004), and could increase demand for and effectiveness of cessation efforts (Fiore et al. 2000). Over-the-counter forms of NRT include nicotine patches, gum, nasal spray, inhaled nicotine and sublingual nicotine. Prescription drugs such as Bupropion and Varenicline have also proven to be effective. Access to low-cost pharmacological therapy is helpful to tobacco users who want to quit.

It is important for governments to provide support for tobacco users to quit in the context of robust public policies. Furthermore, treatment for tobacco dependence should be adapted to local conditions and cultures, and tailored to individual preferences and needs (WHO 2008).

Warn about the dangers of tobacco

Evidence about the addictive nature of nicotine, and other harmful effects of tobacco use, needs to be widely disseminated. Most of the consumers are unaware of the risks of tobacco use and merely regard it as a bad habit (Hammond et al. 2006b). The public learn about this information mainly through published scientific and epidemiological research (or simplified summaries of studies), the media and public health campaigns. These avenues must all be utilized in order to successfully convey the dangers of tobacco use. It is necessary to change the image of tobacco so that people begin to associate tobacco with extreme addictiveness and dangerous health consequences, and to see it as socially negative and undesirable. This aim can be achieved by implementing anti-tobacco counter-advertising campaigns and pack warnings on all tobacco products.

Anti-tobacco counter-advertising campaigns that use graphic images of the harms of tobacco are particularly effective in promoting users to quit (Siahpush *et al.* 2006). They should also be professionally designed and produced, relevant to the context of the country and strategically placed in all forms of media. By publicizing the full extent of tobacco's dangers, these campaigns have the potential to prevent use, promote quitting and expose the tobacco industry tactics, while promoting a tobacco-free society. The downside to counter-advertising is that effective campaigns can be expensive. The United States Centers for Disease Control and Prevention recommend that governments spend about 15–20 per cent of total tobacco control programme costs on counter-advertising campaigns (USDHHS 2007). In addition to paid advertising, 'earned media' in the form of television and radio coverage, news stories in print, broadcast and online media and letters to the editor and opinion articles can be a highly effective and inexpensive way to communicate the harms of tobacco, increase attention on tobacco control initiatives and counter tobacco industry misinformation.

Warnings on the packaging of tobacco products also play a pivotal role in conveying the health risks of tobacco to its users. Health warnings increase smokers' awareness of their risk (Hammond *et al.* 2006b), and their ultimate goal is to cause cessation. Evidence shows that the effectiveness of these warnings increases with their prominence—larger warnings with pictures have more impact compared to smaller, text-only health warnings. WHO also recommends that packaging of tobacco products should not contain deceptive terms such as 'low tar', 'light', or 'mild'—all of which create the false impression that a particular product is less harmful than others, but do not actually signify any reduction in health risk (WHO 2006).

Enforce bans on tobacco advertising, promotion and sponsorship

Tobacco marketing is a strong impediment to tobacco control efforts. It has the potential to 'normalize' tobacco, encourage potential users, mislead the consumer with false information and strengthen industry influence over the media. Tobacco advertising and promotion activities stimulate adult consumption and increase the risk of youth initiation (USDHHS 1994). Children buy the most heavily advertised brands (USDHHS 1994) and are three times more susceptible to advertising than are adults (Pollay *et al.* 1996).

The success of the Marlboro cigarettes advertising campaign highlights the obstacles in altering consumer behaviour (Elliot 1995). By projecting the image of a free-spirited, masculine cowboy, the Marlboro Man falsely associates smoking with independence, enjoyment, relaxation, and 'being cool'. Deceptive marketing strategies such as this make it difficult for the public to understand the hazards of smoking. In light of these ubiquitous and sustained pro-tobacco use messages, counter-marketing efforts of comparable intensity are needed to alter the environmental context of tobacco use.

Since 1972, the most high-income countries have introduced stronger restrictions on advertising and promotion of tobacco products across more media and on various forms of sponsorship. A study of 22 high-income countries based on data from 1970 to 1992 concluded that comprehensive bans on cigarette advertising and promotion can reduce smoking, while more limited partial bans have little or no effect. The study concluded that if the most comprehensive restrictions were in place, tobacco consumption would fall by more than 6 per cent in high-income countries (World Bank 1999). Another study of 100 countries compared consumption trends over time in those with relatively complete bans on advertising and promotion and those with no such bans. In the countries with nearly complete bans, the downward trend in consumption was much steeper (World Bank 1999).

There are reasons to believe that young people are more receptive to advertising than are adults (Pierce *et al.* 1991; McCann 1992); hence a comprehensive advertising ban may prevent potential users, mostly young people, from trying tobacco and consequently becoming long-term users. There is also growing evidence that the tobacco industry is directing increasing shares of its advertising and promotion activity towards markets where there is judged to be growth or potential for growth, including some youth markets and specific minority groups among whom tobacco use has been uncommon until recently (USDHHS 1998).

It must be emphasized that advertising, promotion, and sponsorship bans should be complete and apply to all marketing and promotional categories in order to be effective (WHO 2004a). Partial bans enable the tobacco industry to retain their marketing power, particularly towards young people who are potential users and adults who want to quit. If only certain marketing channels are blocked, e.g. television and radio, the tobacco industry will shift its budgets to other avenues such as magazines, newspapers, billboards, and the Internet. If only these traditional advertising channels are blocked, the industry can then replace advertising with sponsorship of events that are particularly attractive to young people. There is also a growing need for international bans as more tobacco companies are advertising and selling their products through the Internet. Comprehensive marketing bans must be regularly amended so as to keep up with the innovations in industry tactics and media technology (WHO 2008).

Raise taxes on tobacco

Evidence from several countries shows that increases in price on tobacco products are highly cost-effective in reducing demand. Higher taxes induce some smokers to quit and prevent others from starting. They also reduce the number of ex-smokers who return to cigarettes and reduce consumption among continuing smokers. On an average, a price rise of 10 per cent on a pack of cigarettes would be expected to reduce demand for cigarettes by about 4 per cent in high-income countries and by about 8 per cent in low- and middle-income countries (World Bank 1999). Evidence also shows that a 70 per cent increase in the price of tobacco could prevent up to a quarter of all smoking-related deaths worldwide (Jha *et al.* 2006). Children and adolescents are more responsive to price rises than older adults, and so this intervention would have a significant impact on them. Currently, four-fifths of high-income countries tax tobacco at more than 50 per cent of retail price while less than a quarter of low and middle income countries tax tobacco at 50 per cent or more of the retail price (WHO report 2008).

Several myths exist in the economics of tobacco control. First, it is often believed that smokers always bear the costs of their consumption choices. The reality is that smokers do impose certain costs on non-smokers. These costs include health damage, nuisance, and irritation from exposure to SHS. In addition, smokers can impose financial costs on others (e.g. treatment of diseases caused by exposure to second-hand smoke and bearing a portion of smokers' excess healthcare costs). In high-income countries, smokers' healthcare costs on an average exceed those of non-smokers in any given year (Warner 2000). Second, it is often argued that tobacco control will result in permanent job losses for an economy.

In actuality, tobacco control policies will lead to only a slow decline in global tobacco use so that the transition will be phased over several decades. Furthermore, money not spent on tobacco will be spent on other goods, generating alternative employment. Third, many believe that governments will lose revenues if they increase cigarette taxes, because people will buy fewer cigarettes. The reality is at complete variance with this claim. The evidence is clear: Calculations show that even substantial cigarette tax increases will still reduce consumption and increase tax revenues. This is in part because the proportionate reduction in demand does not match the proportionate size of the tax increase. Historically, raising tobacco taxes has led to increases in cigarette tax revenues. Fourth, it is often claimed that cigarette taxes have a disproportionate impact on the poor. Although less-wealthy individuals tend to smoke more, it does not necessarily follow that the poor pay a greater share of their income in tobacco taxes. This reasoning ignores the effect that tax increases have on the prevalence and initiation of tobacco use, and also ignores the benefits of cessation; it ignores the evidence that shows that the young and the poor are more responsive to price increases. It is also instrumental to note that the main concern of policy-makers should be the distributional impact of the entire tax and expenditure system, and not particular taxes in isolation. Finally, contrary to claims by the tobacco industry, tax increases do not necessarily promote smuggling. Other factors contribute to smuggling such as corruption, weak policies to tackle smuggling, and porous borders, among others. An interesting example is Spain, which for years had lower tobacco taxes and more smuggling than most other European countries. When the Spanish government raised tobacco taxes and stepped up law enforcement in the 1990s, tobacco revenues increased by 25 per cent while smuggling took a dramatic decline (WHO 2003b).

In summary, it is important to note that higher tax increases government revenues and effectively decreases consumption, in particular among the young and the poor. Smuggling, on the other hand, can only effectively be tackled through strict customs policies and law enforcement. Given the importance of controlling smuggling, the Parties to the WHO FCTC are currently negotiating a legally binding protocol on illicit trade that will counter smuggling and counterfeiting. This protocol should markedly increase international cooperation on this critical issue.

Other measures

Product regulation

As WHO seeks to minimize the impacts of tobacco on morbidity and mortality, it must create and endorse public health policies that rest on firm scientific foundation. In the area of tobacco product regulation, which is defined by WHO as the governmental oversight and enforcement of how tobacco products are manufactured (ingredients and emissions), distributed, packaged, and labelled in order to promote public health protection, the regulation of tobacco products is encompassed within a set of provisions contained in Articles 9, 10, and 11 of the Framework Convention that are targeted at the regulation of the manufacture and distribution of tobacco products. The scientific basis for the principles guiding the implementation of Articles 9 and 10 establishes the rationale for the principles guiding the implementation of Article 11. For this reason, and in order to achieve the synergistic effect of these provisions, all three articles should be treated as a single set of interrelated and mutually reinforcing regulations.

To assist countries in improving their capacity to regulate tobacco products, WHO has created an expert Study Group, working groups, and a global network of tobacco testing and measuring laboratories in order to increase capacity to inform policymakers as they make decisions at the international, regional, and national level. The work of these groups addresses the effects of nicotine, tobacco contents and emissions, smokeless tobacco, harm reduction products, and other tobacco product regulation issues, in accordance with Article 9, which provides for the adoption of guidelines on the testing and measuring of contents and emissions of tobacco products, and for the regulation of such contents and emissions, and Article 10, which sets forth requirements for product disclosures (WHO 2005).

Research and scientific evidence informed the negotiation of Articles 9, 10, and 11 of the WHO FCTC (WHO 2006), which govern tobacco product regulation. To help establish the content of Articles 9–11, WHO created an *ad hoc* Scientific Advisory Committee on Tobacco Product Regulation (SACTob), which held its first meeting in October 2000 (WHO 2004c). SACTob provided sound scientific information on tobacco product regulation, which eventually 'served as the basis for negotiations and subsequent consensus reached on the language of these three articles of the Convention' (WHO 2007e). In November 2003, recognizing the continuing critical importance of tobacco product regulation, the WHO Director-General changed the status of the SACTob from an *ad hoc* committee to a formal study group, the WHO Study Group on Tobacco Product Regulation (TobReg). TobReg is composed of experts on product regulation, tobacco-dependence treatment, and the laboratory analysis of tobacco ingredients and emissions. Its work is based on cutting edge research on tobacco product issues and recommends research and testing in order to fill in the regulatory gaps of tobacco control (WHO 2007b).

As mentioned earlier, to implement Articles 9, 10, and 11, government regulatory authorities require some degree of laboratory capacity and global uniformity to guide and validate tobacco product testing (WHO 2004b). Responding to this need, and to a TobReg recommendation, WHO Tobacco Free Initiative created the WHO Tobacco Laboratory Network (TobLabNet). TobLabNet is a global network of government, academic, and independent laboratories that furthers the objectives of Article 9 by addressing tobacco product testing and research on product contents and emissions on a global level. TobLabNet is unique in its scientific treatment of tobacco and in its consideration of the fact that 'temporal and geographical variations are important sources of product variability that should be included in any examination of the differences within and across products' (WHO 2005). Thus, TobLabNet strengthens national and regional capacity for the research and verification testing of the contents and emissions of tobacco products. Once capacity is established, TobLabNet will be a main source of laboratory support, methods development and validation, and scientific information for tobacco testing and research, allowing national governments to meet the requirements prescribed by the WHO FCTC (WHO 2007d).

The WHO Tobacco Free Initiative currently serves as the Secretariat and coordinating body for both TobReg and TobLabNet (WHO 2007d). In recognition of the valuable work of TobReg and TobLabNet and to avoid redundancy, the Conference of the Parties (COP) to the WHO FCTC at its first session in February 2006 (WHO 2007c) decided to set up a working group of Parties to develop guidelines for the implementation of Articles 9 and 10 of the WHO FCTC, referring to the work of TobReg and TobLabNet. The working group provided a progress report to the COP at its second session in July 2006 and another progress report at its third session in November 2008. The progress report provides an outline for future work that will take several years to accomplish. Therefore, the efforts by the working group are ongoing and TobReg and TobLabNet continue to provide expert and technical advice as needed (WHO 2007b). For example, and further to the work on the guidelines development for product regulation, TobLabNet is currently preparing to perform international validation of test methods for three contents (nicotine, ammonia, and humectants) and emissions (tobacco-specific nitrosamines, benzo[a]pyrene, aldehydes, and volatile organic compounds).

WHO looks forward to a day when tobacco, a product that kills half of its consumers when used as intended by manufacturers, is forced to operate under a heavily regulated environment such that regulatory agencies will have the information and resources to collaborate with other regulatory agencies (such as, trend data and product characteristic and design features linked to exposure and harm biomarkers) and to act to prevent further harm to the public. Some current WHO recommendations related to product regulation are as follows:

- Ban the use of misleading terms such as 'light', 'mild', and other words or imagery (including certain brand names), which have the aim or effect of implying a reduced health risk attributable to low tar or nicotine measurements on tobacco products and in advertising/promotional material.

- Remove tar and nicotine measures derived from International Organization for Standardization methods from packages. Warning labels should emphasize the addictiveness of tobacco products.

- Require tobacco manufacturers to disclose the contents, purpose, and effects of constituents in all their products at regular intervals.

- Develop and implement a comprehensive long-term communication programme to accompany all the above actions that stresses that there is no safe cigarette and that nicotine addiction is a major public health concern.

- In order to reduce the addictiveness of tobacco products, research is urgently needed to evaluate the benefits and/or hazards of reducing nicotine and other possible addictive constituents in tobacco products over time. Particular attention should be given in research to determining whether a threshold exists for addictiveness.

- Determine whether countries should forbid addition of all new additives and explicitly address the possibility of reducing the use of additives that make tobacco products more attractive and/or taste better.

These recommendations are likely to be implemented in some form over the next few decades by many countries and represent a significant new focus of tobacco control efforts.

Youth access laws

As recognized in Article 16 of the WHO FCTC, youth access laws limit the supply of tobacco products to youths who are too young to comprehend the risks of consuming tobacco products. Youth access laws are designed to limit the availability of tobacco to minors from commercial sources (stores, pharmacies, vending machines, samples from distributors). The rationale for governments enacting youth access restrictions rests primarily on the fact that minors should be protected from the inherent dangers of tobacco as they do not know how to access or accurately appreciate the risks of becoming addicted to nicotine (USDHHS 1994). Jurisdiction attempts to prohibit the sale of cigarettes to minors by establishing minimum age-at-sale laws, banning self-service displays, limiting vending machines to adult-only locations or banning them completely, banning the sale of loose cigarettes, and outlawing the distribution of free samples to minors. Additionally, some jurisdictions require retail vendors to be licensed to sell tobacco products, and some laws include revocation of the license if retailers repeatedly violate minimum age-at-sale laws. In general, youth restrictions are difficult to enforce, because youths often obtain cigarettes from their older peers and sometimes from their parents. There have been several unsuccessful attempts to impose restrictions on the sale of cigarettes to teenagers in many developed countries. In many developing countries where tobacco consumption is rising, the infrastructure and resources needed to implement and enforce such restrictions are not available.

The literature provides mixed evidence on the effectiveness of youth access laws in reducing youth smoking prevalence. Retailer compliance with laws prohibiting sales to minors can be increased through active enforcement (DiFranza & Brown 1992; Cummings et al. 1998; Forster & Wolfson 1998), educational interventions (Altman et al. 1991; Feighery et al. 1991; Gemson et al. 1998), and community involvement (Forster et al. 1998). Forster and Wolfson (1998) summarize workable policies to restrict youth access to tobacco. Strong youth access intervention programmes should enforce one or all of the following means of restricting supply:

- Complete restrictions on distribution, such as bans on free samples and coupons

- Regulation of the means of sale through bans or locks on vending machines, placement of tobacco products behind service counters to limit self-service, and prohibitions on the single/loose cigarettes

- Regulation of the seller through tobacco products licensing requirements, which includes possible revocation and the passage of minimum age-at-sale laws whose violation results in stiff penalties and fines

Even successful efforts to reduce sales in stores can be undermined in two ways. First, young people can often locate the small percentage of stores that continue to sell to minors. Additionally, young people often can find an older (or older appearing) friend or acquaintance who will purchase tobacco for them.

Crop substitution and diversification

Historically, tobacco is a highly attractive crop to the farmers, providing a higher net income yield per unit of land than most cash crops and substantially more than food crops. In the best tobacco-growing areas of Zimbabwe, tobacco is approximately 6.5 times more profitable than the next best alternative crop. Farmers also find tobacco an attractive crop for more practical reasons because the global price of tobacco is relatively stable, the tobacco industry provides in-kind supports and loans to the farmers, tobacco is less perishable than many other crops, and the industry assists with delivery or collection (World Bank 1999).

There have been a number of experimental schemes to substitute other crops for tobacco. For example, in developing countries, a number of alternative crops have been identified, which include cassava in Brazil, sugarcane in Kenya, and chillies, soya beans, cotton, and mustard in India (Reddy & Gupta 2004). However, there is no hard evidence, except in Canada, that these schemes succeed, where a tobacco diversification plan provided incentives to stop growing tobacco and develop alternatives to assist the orderly downsizing the tobacco industry (PAHO 1992).

An important development in this area has been the establishment of the study group on economically sustainable alternatives to tobacco growing by the COP at its first session in February 2006. The aims of the study group include summarizing the uptake of existing economically viable alternatives for tobacco-related workers, growers and, as the case may be, individual sellers; recommending to the COP mechanisms to assess the impact over time of the tobacco companies practices; reporting on initiatives that are being taken at national level in accordance with Article 17; and recommending cost-effective diversification initiatives. The study group met for the first time in February 2007 in Brasilia, Brazil. Background documentation prepared for the meeting intended to summarize existing literature and research on the issues related to tobacco growing and crop substitution. One of the key conclusions of the meeting was that there was insufficient research on health, environmental and socioeconomic impacts of tobacco growing and that there was a need for deeper analysis of financial factors of crop substitution, particularly targeting at the case of small farmers. The second meeting of the study group was convened in June 2008 in Mexico and aimed particularly to expand the scope of work by updating experiences from the first study group meeting (current progress of case studies, focusing on challenges and lessons learned), and introducing additional relevant cases. Another objective is to review cross-national analysis in selected topics: Drawing common aspects, understanding different contexts, and identifying best practices.

Litigation

The WHO FCTC acknowledges that litigation can be an effective public health intervention in the area of tobacco control. This has been demonstrated most dramatically by recent events in the United States. In the mid- and late-1990s, there was a new wave of litigation against the tobacco industry in the United States. There were a variety of forms of litigation, including lawsuits filed by individual smokers, class action lawsuits by large groups of smokers, and lawsuits filed by victims of SHS. To date, the most successful litigation against the tobacco industry in the United States has been a series of actions brought by the Attorneys General of individual states.

The lawsuits brought by the Attorneys General focused on the conduct of the tobacco industry, not merely the product *per se*. Among other things, these lawsuits sought to recover the enormous sums of money that the states spent in healthcare costs for persons with smoking-related disease. These lawsuits alleged that the tobacco industry had misrepresented and concealed the health risks and addictiveness of smoking, manipulated the form and/or amount of nicotine in cigarettes to ensure their addictive potential, conspired to suppress health research, and targeted youth in their advertising

and marketing campaigns. Thus, the legal bases for these lawsuits generally focused on consumer protection and antitrust statutes (JAMA 1995).

The Attorneys General lawsuits were all successfully resolved by settlement with the tobacco industry in 1997 and 1998. The settlement agreements resulted in the payment of billions of dollars to the states. While the ultimate disposition of this money is not entirely resolved, and in some cases is the subject of fierce political battles, some of the funds have been dedicated to tobacco control efforts, infusing the tobacco control community with unprecedented levels of funding. In addition, beyond the monetary terms, the settlements provided for a variety of injunctive relief, including the prohibition of marketing to children, the banning of certain types of advertising and promotion (i.e. billboards and movie placements), and the dissolution of two of the tobacco industry's longtime trade groups, the Tobacco Institute and the Council for Tobacco Research. The Attorneys General litigation and settlements also resulted in the release of millions of pages of previously secret documents from the files of the tobacco industry. These documents paint a damning picture of the tobacco industry's conduct for decades, and contain a wealth of information that can help guide public health activities for years to come.

The US Department of Justice filed a landmark lawsuit under the civil racketeering (RICO) law on 22 September 1999, to hold Philip Morris International legally accountable for decades of illegal and harmful practices. The trial in the case lasted from 21 September 2004 to 9 June 2005. It was recommended that the tobacco company be required to pay US$130 billion to fund cessation and prevention programmes, however in the end no financial remedies were given. The company was found guilty of decades of deception and fraud and was banned from making future deceptive statements, eliminating misleading descriptor words such as 'light' and 'mild', improving health warnings, and making all internal documents open to the government and public.

Class action lawsuits have also been successful. In Florida, a group of flight attendants filed a lawsuit on behalf of non-smoking flight attendants exposed to SHS. The case was settled in October 1997 in exchange for a US$300 million fund to research the diagnosis and treatment of diseases caused by SHS.

The litigation was successful in the United States in large part because new successful alliances forged between attorneys and the public health community. The American Medical Association, in an unusual step, recommended in 1995 that 'all avenues of individual and collective redress should be pursued through the legal system' (JAMA 1995). Prominent public health professionals provided invaluable assistance in the litigation by serving as expert witnesses.

Litigation against the tobacco industry is now being pursued in a number of countries, including Canada, France, India, Israel, Ireland, Germany, Australia, Poland, South Korea, Nigeria, and the Marshall Islands. In many countries, this type of litigation is unusual, and it is still too early to anticipate how the various actions will play out. The risks and challenges of litigation against the tobacco industry (which fiercely opposes lawsuits with virtually unlimited resources) are very large. In the United States, e.g. litigation against the tobacco industry began in 1954, and for more than 40 years (until the breakthroughs in the 1990s), the tobacco industry won every single case. Thus, the prospect of litigation needs to be carefully evaluated before any decisions to proceed are undertaken. However, the potential rewards in terms of public health objectives can be enormous. In some jurisdictions, where there are promising theories of liability and sufficient resources, litigation may be one way to achieve tobacco control objectives in a forum—the courts—which may not be subject to the same political influences as legislative bodies.

Administration and management

An effective global tobacco control requires a well-designed and efficient management structure to facilitate co-ordination of programme components at the country, regional, and global levels. Experience from other successful public health programmes such as smallpox, tuberculosis, and poliomyelitis has demonstrated the importance of an organized administrative and management systems. Because a comprehensive programme involves multiple partners, programme management and co-ordination is a challenging task. Furthermore, co-ordinating efforts require adequate resources, training and communication systems. Administration and management activities include (a) recruiting and training qualified, technical, programme, and administrative staff, (b) coordinating implementation across programme areas and assessing programme performance, (c) creating an effective communication system, and (d) developing a sound fiscal management and reporting systems.

Acknowledgements

The authors would like to acknowledge the following people for their contributions towards the chapter: A.D. Lopez, Derek Yach, Anne-Marie Perucic, Ayda Yurekli, Dongbo Fu, and Daniel Ferrante.

References

Aghi, M., Asma, S., Yeong, C.C., Vaithinathan, R. (2001). Initiation and maintenance of tobacco use among girls and women. In J.M. Samet and S.Y. Yoon, eds. *Women and the tobacco epidemic: Challenges for the 21st century*. WHO, Geneva.

Altman, D.G., Rasenick-Douss, L., Foster, V., Tye, J.B. (1991). Sustained effects of an educational program to reduce sales of cigarettes to minors. *American Journal of Public Health*, 81, 891–3.

AMAP (Arctic Monitoring and Assessment Programme) (1998). *AMAP assessment report: Arctic pollution issues*. AMAP, Oslo.

Anderson, S.J., Glantz, S.A., Ling, P.M. (2005). Emotions for sale: Cigarette advertising and women's psychosocial needs. *Tobacco Control*, 14, 127–35.

Anderson, S.J., Dewhirst, T., Ling, P.M. (2006). Every document and picture tells a story: Using internal corporate document reviews, semiotics, and content analysis to assess tobacco advertising. *Tobacco Control*, 15(3), 254–61.

Apollonio, D.E., Bero, L.A. (2007). The creation of industry front groups: The tobacco industry and "Get Government off our Back". *American Journal of Public Health*, 97(3), 419–27.

Assunta, M., Chapman, S. (2004). 'The world's most hostile environment': How the tobacco industry circumvented Singapore's advertising ban. *Tobacco Control*, 13(2), ii51–7.

Assunta, M., Fields, N., Knight, J., Chapman, S. (2004). Care and feeding: The Asian environmental tobacco smoke (ETS) consultants programme. *Tobacco Control*, 13(2), ii4–12.

Australian Bureau of Statistics (2002). *National aboriginal and torres strait islander social survey*, p. 13. ABS, Canberra.

Australian National Health and Medical Research Council (1997). *The health effects of passive smoking. A scientific information paper*. Australian Government Publishing Service, Canberra.

Barbeau, E., Leavy-Sperounis, A., Balbach, E. (2004). Smoking, social class, and gender: What can public health learn from the tobacco industry about disparities in smoking? *Tobacco Control*, 13, 110–20.

Barnoya, J., Glantz, S.A. (2005). Cardiovascular effects of secondhand smoke: Nearly as large as smoking. *Circulation*, 111, 2684–98.

Bero, L.A. (2003). Implications of the tobacco industry documents for public health and policy. *Annual Review of Public Health* 24, 267–88.

Bero, L.A. (2005). Tobacco industry manipulation of research. *Public Health Reports*, 120, 200–8.

Bettcher, D., Yach, D. (1998). The globalization of public health II: The convergence of self-interest and altruism. *American Journal of Public Health*, 88, 839.

Bettcher, D., Yach, D., Guindon, G.E. (2000). Global trade and health: Key linkages and future challenges. *Bulletin of the World Health Organization*, 78, 521–34.

Bialous, S., Yach, D. (2001). Whose standard is it anyway? How the tobacco industry determines the International Organization for Standardization (ISO) standards for tobacco and tobacco products. *Tobacco Control*, 10, 96–104.

Bonita, R., Duncan, J., Truelsen, T., Jackson, R.T., Beaglehole, R. (1999). Passive smoking as well as active smoking increases the risk of acute stroke. *Tobacco Control*, 8, 156–60.

Brandt, A.M. (2007). *The cigarette century: The rise, fall and deadly persistence of the product that defined America*. Basic Books, New York.

Brownson, R.C., Eriksen, M.P., Davis, R.M., Warner, K.E. (1997). Environmental tobacco smoke: Health effects and policies to reduce exposure. *Annual Review of Public Health*, 18, 163–85.

California Environmental Protection Agency (1997). *Health effects of exposure to environmental tobacco smoke: Fnal report*. California Environmental Protection Agency, Office of Environmental Health Hazard Assessment, Sacramento, CA.

California Environmental Protection Agency (2005). *Proposed identification of environmental tobacco smoke as a toxic air contaminant*. California Environmental Protection Agency, Office of Environmental Health Hazard Assessment, Sacramento, CA.

Carpenter, C.M., Wayne, G.F., Pauly, J.L., Koh, H.K., Connolly, G.N. (2005). New cigarette brands with flavours that appeal to youth: Tobacco marketing strategies. *Health Affairs*, 24, 1601–10.

Carter, S.M. (2002). Mongoven, Biscoe & Duchin: Destroying tobacco control activism from the inside. *Tobacco Control*, 11, 112–8.

CDC (Centers for Disease Control and Prevention) (2008a). Youth Risk Behavior Surveillance United States 2005. Surveillance Summaries, *Morbidity and Mortality Weekly Report* 2008, 57 (No. 25).

CDC (Centers for Disease Control and Prevention) (2008b). Global youth tobacco surveillance, 2000–2007. Surveillance summaries. *Morbidity and Mortality Weekly Report 2008*, 55 (No. SS-1).

Chaloupka, F.J., Wechsler, H. (1997). Price, tobacco control policies and smoking among young adults. *Journal of Health Economics*, 16, 359–73.

Chaloupka, F.J., Corbett, M. (1998). Trade policy and tobacco: Towards an optimal policy mix. In I. Abedian, ed. *The economics of tobacco control*, pp. 129–45. Applied Fiscal Research Center, University of Cape Town. Cape Town, South Africa.

Chao, A., Thun, M.J., Jacobs, E.J., Henley, S.J., Rodriguez, C., Calle, E.E. (2000). Cigarette smoking and colorectal cancer mortality in the Cancer Prevention Study II. *Journal of the National Cancer Institute*, 92(23), 1888–96.

Chapman, S., Borland, R., Scotto, M., Brownson, R.C., Dominetto, A., Woodward, S. (1999). Impact of smoke-free workplaces on declining cigarette consumption in Australia and United States. *American Journal of Public Health*, 89, 1018–23.

Chapman, S. (2003). 'We are anxious to remain anonymous': The use of third party scientific and medical consultants by the Australian tobacco industry, 1969 to 1979. *Tobacco Control*, 12(3), 31–7.

Chapman, S. (2005). Research from tobacco industry affiliated authors: Need for particular vigilance. *Tobacco Control*, 14, 217–9.

Chapman, S. (2006). Regulating the global vector for lung cancer. *Lancet*, **367**, 706–8.

Charlton, A. (1996). Children and smoking: The family circle. *British Medical Bulletin*, **52**, 90–107.

Collin, J., LeGresley, E., MacKenzie, R., Lawrence, S., Lee, K. (2004). Complicity in contraband: British American Tobacco and cigarette smuggling in Asia. *Tobacco Control*, **13**(2), ii104–11.

Conrad, K.M., Flay, B.R., Hill, D. (1992). Why children start smoking cigarettes: Predictors of onset. *British Journal of Addiction*, **87**, 1711–24.

Cook, B., Wayne, G., Keithly, L., Connolly, G. (2003). One size does not fit all: How the tobacco industry has altered cigarette design to target consumer groups with specific psychological and psychosocial needs. *Addiction*, **98**, 1047–61.

Cummings, K.M., Hyland, A., Saunders-Martin, T., Perla, J., Coppola, P.R., Pechacek, T.F. (1998). Evaluation of an enforcement program to reduce tobacco sales to minors. *American Journal of Public Health*, **88**, 932–6.

Dearlove, J., Bialous, S., Glantz, S.A. (2002). Tobacco industry manipulation of the hospitality industry to maintain smoking in public places. *Tobacco Control*, **11**, 94–104.

Denissenko, M.F., Pao, A., Tang, M., Pfeifer, G.P. (1996). Preferential formation of benzo[*a*]pyrene adducts at lung cancer mutational hotspots in P53. *Science*, **274**, 430–2.

Detels, R., McEwen, J., Beaglehole, R., Tanaka, H., eds (2002). *Oxford textbook of public health, 4th ed.* Oxford University Press, New York.

Dewhirst, T., Hunter, A. (2002). Tobacco sponsorship of Formula One and CART auto racing: Tobacco brand exposure and enhanced symbolic imagery through co-sponsors' third party advertising. *Tobacco Control*, **11**, 146–50.

DiFranza, J.R., Brown, L.J. (1992). The Tobacco Institute's 'It's the Law' campaign. Has it halted illegal sales of tobacco to children? *American Journal of Public Health*, **82**, 1271–3.

DiFranza, J.R., Lew, R.A. (1995). Effect of maternal cigarette on pregnancy complications and sudden death infant syndrome. *Journal of Family Practice*, **40**, 385–94.

Doll, R., Peto, R., Wheatley, K., Gray, R., Sutherland, I. (1994). Mortality in relation to smoking: 40 years observations on male British doctors. *British Medical Journal*, **309**, 901–11.

Doll, R., Peto, R., Boreham, J., Sutherland, I. (2004). Mortality in relation to smoking: 50 years' observations on male British doctors. *British Medical Journal*, **328**, 1519.

Drope, J., Chapman, S. (2001). Tobacco industry efforts at discrediting scientific knowledge of environmental tobacco smoke: A review of internal industry documents. *Journal of Epidemiology and Community Health*, **55**, 588–94.

Durie, M.H. (1998). *Whaiora–Maori health development.* Oxford University Press, Auckland.

Elliot, S. (1995). Uncle Sam is no match for the Marlboro Man. *The New York Times*, 27 August, C1.

EPA (Environmental Protection Agency) (1992). *Respiratory health effects of passive smoking: Lung cancer and other disorders.* EPA/600/006F. US Government Printing Office, Washington, DC.

Eskenazi, B., Castorina, R. (1999). Association of prenatal maternal or postnatal child environmental tobacco smoke exposure and neurodevelopmental and behavioral problems in children. *Environmental Health Perspectives*, **107**, 991–1000.

Evans, W.N., Farrelly, M.C., Montogomery, E. (1999). Do workplace smoking bans reduce smoking? *American Economic Review*, **89**, 728–47.

Fant, R.V., Henningfield, J.E., Nelson, R.A., Pickworth, W.B. (1999). Pharmacokinetics and pharmacodynamics of moist snuff in humans. *Tobacco Control*, **8**, 387–92.

FAO (Food and Agricultural Organization) (2006). *FAOSTAT database.* [Online]. Available at: http://faostat.fao.org/site/567/DesktopDefault.aspx?PageID=567.

FDA (Food and Drug Administration) (1996). Regulations restricting the sale and distribution of cigarettes and smokeless tobacco to children and adolescents: final rule. *Federal Register*, **61**, 44395–618.

Feighery, E., Altman, D.G., Shaffer, G. (1991). The effects of combining education and enforcement to reduce tobacco sales to minors. *Journal of the American Medical Association*, **266**, 3168–71.

Ferris Wayne, G., Connolly, G.N., Henningfield, J.E. (2006). Brand differences of free-base nicotine delivery in cigarette smoke: The view of the tobacco industry documents. *Tobacco Control*, **15**(3), 189–98.

Fichtenberg, C.M., Glantz, S.A. (2002). Effect of smoke-fee workplaces on smoking behaviour: Systematic review. *British Medical Journal*, **325**(7357), 188.

Fiore, M.C., Hyland, A., Borland, R. *et al.* (2000). Treating tobacco use and dependence: A public health service clinical guidelines. US Department of Health and Human Services, Rockville, MD, press briefing.

Fong, G.T., Bailey, W.C., Cohen, S.J. *et al.* (2006). Reductions in tobacco smoke pollution and increase in support for smoke-free public places following the implementation of comprehensive smoke-free workplace legislation in the Republic of Ireland: Findings from the International Tobacco Control (ITC) Ireland, UK Survey. *Tobacco Control*, **15** (Suppl. 3), iii51–8.

Forster, J.L., Wolfson, M. (1998). Youth access to tobacco: Policies and politics. *Annual Review of Public Health*, **19**, 203–35.

Forster, J.L., Murray, D.M., Wolfson, M., Blaine, T.M., Wagenaar, A.C., Hennrikus, D.J. (1998). The effects of community policies to reduce youth access to tobacco. *American Journal of Public Health*, **88**, 1193–8.

Francey, N., Chapman, S. (2000). Operation Berkshire: The international tobacco companies' conspiracy. *British Medical Journal*, **321**, 371–4.

Gan, Q., Smith, K.R., Hammond, S.K., Hu, T.W. (2007). Disease burden of adult lung cancer and ischaemic heart disease from passive tobacco smoking in China. *Tobacco Control*, **16**, 417–22.

Garfinkel, L. (1997). Trends in cigarette smoking in the United States. *Preventive Medicine*, **26**, 447–50.

Gemson, D.H., Moats, H.L., Watkins, B.X., Ganz, M.L., Robinson, S., Healton, E. (1998). Laying down the law: Reducing illegal tobacco sales to minors in central Harlem. *American Journal of Public Health*, **88**, 936–9.

Gilmore, A.B., McKee, M. (2004). Moving east: How the transnational tobacco companies gained entry to the emerging markets of the former Soviet Union. Part I: Establishing cigarette imports. *Tobacco Control*, **13**, 43–100.

Gilmore, A., Radu-Loghin, C., Zatushevski, I., McKee, M. (2005). Pushing up smoking incidence: Plans for a privatised tobacco industry in Moldova. *Lancet*, **365**, 1354–9.

Gilmore, A., Collin, J., Townsend, J. (2007). Transnational tobacco company influence on taxation policy during privatization: The case of BAT in Uzbekistan. *American Journal of Public Health*, **97**, 2001–9.

Giovino, G.A., Henningfield, J., Tomar, S.L., Escobedo, L.E., Slade, J. (1995). Epidemiology of tobacco use and dependence. *Epidemiologic Reviews*, **17**, 48–65.

Giovino, G.A. (2000). World's best practice in tobacco control. Surveillance of patterns and consequences of tobacco use: USA. *Tobacco Control*, **9**, 232.

GTSS (Global Tobacco Surveillance System Collaborating Group) (2005). Global Tobacco Surveillance System: Purpose, production, and potential. *Journal of School Health*, **75**, 15–24.

Hatsukami, D., Hughes, J.R., Pickens, R. (1985). Characterization of tobacco withdrawal: Physiological and subjective effects. In J. Grabowski and S.M. Hall, eds. *Pharmacological adjuncts in smoking cessation*, pp. 56–67. DHHS Publication (ADM) 85–1333. US Department of Health and Human Services, Public Health Service, Alcohol and Drug Abuse and Mental Health Administration, Washington, DC.

Hammond, D., Collishaw, N., Callard, C. (2006a). Tobacco industry research on smoking behaviour and product design. *Lancet*, **367**, 781–7.

Hammond, D., Fong, G.T., McNeill, A., Borland, R., Cummings, K.M. (2006b). Effectiveness of cigarette warning labels from informing smokers about the risk of smoking: Findings from the international Tobacco Control (ITC) Four Country Survey. *Tobacco Control*, **15** (Suppl. 3), iii19–25.

Hecht, S.S. (1999). Tobacco smoke carcinogens and lung cancer. *Journal of the National Cancer Institute*, **91**, 1194–210.

Hiilamo, H., Hirschhorn, N. (2006). Tobacco industry documents from outside sources: New perspectives on industry strategies on local levels. *Central European Journal of Public Health*, **14**(4), 175–9.

Hilts, P.J. (1996). *Smoke screen. The truth behind the tobacco industry cover-up.* Addison-Wesley, New York.

Hirschhorn, N. (2004). Corporate social responsibility and the tobacco industry: Hope or hype? *Tobacco Control*, **13**(4), 447–53.

Hirschhorn, N. (2005). *The tobacco industry documents. What they are, what they tell us, and how to search them. A practical manual. 2nd ed.* [Online]. Available at: http://www.who.int/tobacco/communications/TI_manual_content.pdf

Hirschhorn, N., Bialous, S., Shatenstein, S. (2006). The Philip Morris external research program: Results from the first round of projects. *Tobacco Control*, **15**(3), 267–9.

Howell, R. (2005). Smoke-free bars in Ireland: A runaway success. *Tobacco Control*, **14**(2), 73–4.

International Institute for Population Sciences (IIPS) and Macro International (2007). *National Family Health Survey (NFHS-3), 2005–2006: India: Volume, I.* IIPS, Mumbai.

JAMA (1995). The Brown and Williamson documents. Where do we go from here? *Journal of the American Medical Association*, **274**, 256–7.

Jamieson, K.H. (1998). '*Tax and spend' vs. 'little kids': Advocacy and accuracy in the tobacco settlement ads of 1997–1998.* Annenberg Public Policy Center, University of Pennsylvania, Philadelphia, PA.

Jamrozik, K. (2000). Barbarians inside the gate: How the tobacco industry penetrated the World Health Organization: Report of the Committee of Experts on Tobacco Industry Documents. Tobacco company strategies to undermine tobacco control activities at the World Health Organization. Geneva: World Health Organization, 2000, pp. 247. *International Journal of Epidemiology*, **30**, 633–4.

Jha, P., Chaloupka, F., Moore, J. *et al.* (2006). Tobacco Addiction. In D.T. Jamison, J.G. Breman, A.R. Measham. *et al.*, eds. *Disease control priorities in developing countries, 2nd ed*, pp. 869–85. Oxford University Press, New York and World Bank, Washington, DC.

Jha, P., Jacob, B., Gajalakshmi, V. *et al.* (2008). A nationally representative case–control study of smoking and death in India. *New England Journal of Medicine*, **13**, **358**(11), 1137–47.

Joosens, L., Raw, M. (2002). *Turning off the tap: An update on cigarette smuggling in the UK and Sweden, with recommendations to control smuggling.* [Online]. Cancer Research UK and National Institute of Public Health, Sweden. Available at: http://old.ash.org.uk/luk/lukdocs/turningoffthetap.pdf

Kluger, R. (1996). *Ashes to ashes. America's hundred-year cigarette war, the public health, and the unabashed triumph of Philip Morris.* Alfred, A. Knopf, New York.

Kozlowski, L.T., Pillitteri, J.L., Ahern, F.M. (1998a). Advertising fails to inform smokers of official tar yields of cigarettes. *Journal of Applied Biobehavioral Research*, **3**, 55–64.

Kozlowski, L.T., Goldberg, M.E., Yost, B.A., White, E.L., Sweeney, C.T., Pillitteri, J.L. (1998b). Smokers' perceptions of light and ultra-light cigarettes may keep them smoking. *American Journal of Preventive Medicine*, **15**, 9–16.

Last, J.M., ed. (1995). *A dictionary of epidemiology, 3rd ed.* Oxford University Press, New York.

Lawrence, S., Collin, J. (2004). Competing with kreteks: Transnational tobacco companies, globalisation and Indonesia. *Tobacco Control*, **13**(2), ii96–103.

Lee, K., Bialous, S.A. (2006). Corporate social responsibility: Serious cause for concern. *Tobacco Control*, **15**(6), 419.

Lee, K., Collin, J. (2006). "Key to the Future": British American Tobacco and cigarette smuggling in China. *PLoS Med*, **3**(7), e228.

Lee, K., Kinh, H., MacKenzie, R., Gilmore, A., Minh, N., Collin, J. (2008). Gaining access to Vietnam's cigarette market: British American Tobacco's strategy to enter 'a huge market which will become enormous.' *Global Public Health*, **3**(1), 1–25.

LeGresley, E., Muggli, M.E., Hurt, R.D. (2006). Movie moguls: British American Tobacco's covert strategy to promote cigarettes in Eastern Europe. *The European Journal of Public Health*, **16**(5), 505–8.

Leung, G.M., Ho, L.M., Lam, T.H. (2004). Secondhand smoke exposure, smoking hygiene, and hospitalization in the first 18 months of life. *Archives of Paediatric and Adolescent Medicine*, **158**(7), 687–93.

Levin, M.L. (1953). The occurrence of lung cancer in man. *Acta Union International Contra Cancer*, **9**, 531–41.

Lewis, M.J., Wackowski, D. (2006). Dealing with an innovative industry: A look at flavoured cigarettes promoted by mainstream brands. *American Journal of Public Health*, **96**(2), 244–51.

Ling, P.M., Glantz, S. (2002). Using tobacco-industry marketing research to design more effective tobacco-control campaigns. *Journal of the American Medical Association*, **287**, 2983–9.

Liu, B.Q., Peto, R., Chen, Z.M. *et al.* (1998). Emerging tobacco hazards in China: Retrospective proportional mortality study of one million deaths. *British Medical Journal*, **317**, 1411–22.

Lopez, A.D. (1999). Measuring the health hazards of tobacco. *Bulletin of the World Health Organization*, **77**, 82–3.

Lopez, A.D., Collishaw, N.E., Piha, T. (1994). A descriptive model of the cigarette epidemic in developed countries. *Tobacco Control*, **3**, 242–7.

MacKenzie, R., Collin, J., Sriwongcharoen. K. (2007). Thailand – lighting up a dark market: British American Tobacco, sports sponsorship and the circumvention of legislation. *Journal of Epidemiology and Community Health*, **61**(1), 28–33.

MacKenzie R, Collin J, Sriwongcharoen K, Muggli ME. 'If we can just "stall" new unfriendly legislations, the scoreboard is already in our favour': transnational tobacco companies and ingredients disclosure in Thailand. *Tobacco Control*. 2004 Dec;**13** Suppl 2:79–87.

Mathers, C., Loncar, D. (2006). Projections of Global Mortality and burden of Disease from 2002 to 2030. *PLoS Medicine*, **3**(11:e442), 2011–30.

Malone, R.E., Bero, L.A. (2003). Chasing the dollar: Why scientists should decline tobacco industry funding. *Journal of Epidemiology and Community Health*, **57**, 546–8.

Malson, J.L., Pickworth, W.B. (2002). Bidis – Hand-rolled, Indian cigarettes: Effects on physiological, biochemical and subjective measures. *Pharmacology Biochemistry and Behaviour*, **72**, 443–7.

McCann, J. (1992). Tobacco logo recognition. *Journal of Family Practice*, **34**, 681–4.

McDaniel, P.A., Malone, R.E. (2005). Understanding Philip Morris's pursuit of US government regulation of tobacco. *Tobacco Control*, **14**, 193–200.

McDaniel, P.A., Smith, E.A., Malone, R.E. (2006). Philip Morris's Project Sunrise: Weakening tobacco control by working with it. *Tobacco Control*, **15**(3), 215–23.

McDaniel, P.A., Intinarelli, G., Malone, R.E. (2008). Tobacco industry issues management organizations: Creating a global corporate network to undermine public health. *Global Health*, **4**, 2.

Milberger, S., Davis, R., Douglas, C. *et al.* (2006). Tobacco manufacturers' defense against plaintiffs' claims of cancer causation: Throwing mud at the wall and hoping some of it will stick. *Tobacco Control*, **15**(4), iv17–26.

Ministry of Health, New Zealand (2001). *Inhaling inequality – tobacco's contribution to health inequality in New Zealand.* Available at: http://www.moh.govt.nz/moh.nsf/0/eb38a31c067f8776cc256af0000f6f1e/$FILE/InhalingInequality.pdf

Ministry of Health, New Zealand (2008) Tobacco Use In: A portrait of health - Key results of the 2006/07 New Zealand Health Survey. Available at: http://www.moh.govt.nz/moh.nsf/pagesmh/7440/$File/second-hand-smoke-and-tobacco-use-nz-health-survey-jun08.pdf

Muggli, M., Forster, J., Hurt, R., Repace, J. (2001). The smoke you don't see: Uncovering tobacco industry strategies aimed against environmental tobacco smoke. *American Journal of Public Health*, **91**, 1419–23.

Murray, C.J.L., Lopez, A.D. (1997a). Global mortality, disability, and the contribution of risk factors: Global burden of disease study. *Lancet*, **349**, 1436–42.

Murray, C.J.L., Lopez, A.D. (1997b). Alternative projections of mortality and disability by cause, 1990–2020: Global burden of disease study. *Lancet*, **349**, 1498–504.

National Research Council (NRC) (1986). *Environmental tobacco smoke: Measuring exposures and assessing health effects*. National Academy Press, Washington, DC.

Neuman, M., Bitton, A., Glantz, S. (2002). Tobacco industry strategies for influencing European Community tobacco advertising legislation. *Lancet*, **359**, 1323–30.

Niewoehner, D.E., Kleinerman, J., Rice, D.B. (1974). Pathologic changes in the peripheral airways of young cigarette smokers. *New England Journal of Medicine*, **291**, 755–8.

Ong, E., Glantz, S. (2000). Tobacco industry efforts subverting the International Agency for Research on Cancer's second-hand smoke study. *Lancet*, **355**, 1253–9.

Orleans, C.T., Slade, J. (1993). Preface. In C.T. Orleans and J. Slade, eds. *Nicotine addiction. Principles and management*. Oxford University Press, New York.

PAHO (Pan American Health Organization) (1992). *Tobacco or Health: Status in the Americas*. Scientific Publication Number 536. PAHO, Washington, DC.

PAHO (Pan American Health Organization) (2007). *Smoke free inside*. PAHO, Washington, DC.

Palazzo, G., Richter, U. (2005). CSR business as usual? The case of the tobacco industry. *Journal of Business Ethics*, **61**, 387–401.

Parascandola, M. (2003). Hazardous effects of tobacco industry funding. *Journal of Epidemiology and Community Health*, **57**, 548–9.

Parish, S., Collins, R., Peto, R. *et al.* (1995). Cigarette smoking, tar yields, and non-fatal myocardial infarction: 14 000 cases and 32 000 controls in the United Kingdom. *British Medical Journal*, **311**, 471–7.

PDAY Research Group (1990). Relationship of atherosclerosis in young men to serum lipoprotein cholesterol concentrations and smoking. A preliminary report from the Pathological Determinants in Youth (PDAY) Research Group. *Journal of the American Medical Association*, **263**, 3018–24.

Peto, R., Lopez, A.D., Boreham, J., Thun, M., Heath, C. (1994). *Mortality from smoking in developed countries, 1950–2000*. Oxford University Press, Oxford.

Peto, R., Lopez, A.D., Boreham, J., Thun, M., Heath, C., Doll, R. (1996). Mortality from smoking worldwide. *British Medical Bulletin*, **52**, 12–21.

Pierce, J.P., Gilpin, E., Burns, D.M. *et al.* (1991) Does tobacco advertising target young people to start smoking? Evidence from California. *Journal of the American Medical Association*, **266**(22):3154–8.

Pollay, R.W., Siddarth, S., Siegel, M. *et al.* (1996). The last straw? Cigarette advertising and realized market shares among youths and adults, 1979–1993. *Journal of Marketing for Professions*, **60**, 1–16.

Pollay, R.W., Dewhirst, T. (2002). The dark side of marketing seemingly "light" cigarettes: Successful images and failed fact. *Tobacco Control*, **11**(1), i18–31.

Prochaska, J.O., Redding, C.A., Evers, K.E. (1997). The trans-theoretical model and stages of change. In K. Glantz, F.M. Lewis and B.K. Rimer, eds. *Health behaviour and health education, theory, research, and practice*. Jossey-Bass, San Francisco, CA.

Reddy, S.K., Gupta, P.C., eds. (2004). *Report on Tobacco Control in India*. Ministry of Health and Family Welfare, Government of India, New Delhi.

Reid, D.J., McNeill, A., Glynn, T.J. (1995). Reducing the prevalence of smoking in youth in Western countries: An international review. *Tobacco Control*, **4**, 266–77.

Saloojee, Y., Dagli, E. (2000). Tobacco industry tactics for resisting public policy on health. *Bulletin of the World Health Organization*, **78**, 911–2.

Samet, J.M., Wang, S.S. (2000). Environmental tobacco smoke. In M Lippmann, ed. *Environmental toxicants: Human exposures and their health effect. 2nd ed.* Wiley, New York.

Samet, J.M., Burke, T.A. (2001). Turning science into junk; the tobacco industry and passive smoking. *American Journal of Public Health*, **91**, 1742–4.

SCOTH (Scientific Committee on Tobacco and Health) (1998). *Report of the Scientific Committee on Tobacco and Health*. HMSO, London.

Siahpush, M., McNeill, A., Hammond, D., Fong, G.T. (2006). Socioeconomic and country variations in knowledge of health risks of tobacco smoking and toxic constituents of smoke: Results from the 2002 International Tobacco Control (ITC) Four Country Survey. *Tobacco Control*, **15**(3), iii65–70.

Silagy, C., Lancaster, T., Stead, L., Mant, D., Fower, G. (2004). Nicotine Replacement therapy for smoking cessation. *Cochrane Database Systematic Review*, **3**, C000146.

Smith, E.A., Malone, R.E. (2004). "Creative Solutions": Selling cigarettes in a smoke-free world. *Tobacco Control*, **13**, 57–63.

Smith, E.A., Malone, R.E. (2006). 'We will speak as the smoker': The tobacco industry's smokers' rights groups. *European Journal of Public Health*, **17**(3), 306–13.

Stayner, L., Bena, J., Sasco, A.J. *et al.* (2007). Lung cancer risk and workplace exposure to environmental tobacco smoke. *Americal Journal of Public Health*, **97**(3), 545–51.

Stratton, K., Shetty, P., Wallace, R., Bondurant, S., eds. (2001). Products for tobacco exposure reduction. In *Clearing the smoke. Assessing the science base for tobacco harm reduction*, pp. 78–98. National Academy Press, Washington, DC.

Szczypka, G., Wakefield, M., Emery, S., Terry-McElrath, Y., Flay, B., Chaloupka, F. (2007). Working to make an image: An analysis of three Philip Morris corporate image media campaigns. *Tobacco Control*, **16**(5), 344–50.

Szilagyi, T., Chapman, S. (2003). Hungry for Hungary: Examples of tobacco industry's expansionism. *Central Europe Journal of Public Health*, **11**, 38–43.

Taylor, R., Najafi, F., Dobson, A. (2007). Meta-analysis of studies of passive smoking and lung cancer: Effects of study type and continent. *International Journal of Epidemiology*, **36**(5), 1048–59.

Thomson, G., Signal, L. (2005). Associations between universities and the tobacco industry: What institutional policies limit these associations? *Social Policy Journal of New Zealand*, **26**, 186–204.

Thomson, G., Wilson, N. (2005). Directly eroding tobacco industry power as a tobacco control strategy. *New Zealand Medical Journal*, **118**, U1683.

Thun, M.J., Day-Lally, C., Myers, D.G. *et al.* (1997). Trends in tobacco smoking and mortality from cigarette use in Cancer Prevention Studies I (1959–1965) and II (1982–1988). In *Changes in cigarette-related disease risks and their implication for prevention and control, smoking and tobacco control monograph 8*, pp. 305–82. US Department of Health and Human Services, Public Health Service, National Institutes of Health, Bethesda, MD.

Thyrian, J.R., Panagiotakos, D.B., Polychronopoulos, E., West, R., Zatonski, W., John, U. (2008). The relationship between smokers' motivation to quit and intensity of tobacco control at the population level: A comparison of five European countries. *BMC Public Health*, **8**, 2.

Tomar, S.L. (2007). Epidemiologic perspectives on smokeless tobacco marketing and population harm. *American Journal of Preventive Medicine*, **33**(6), S387–97.

Tong, E.K., Glantz, S.A. (2004). ARTIST (Asian Regional Tobacco Industry Scientist Team): Philip Morris' attempt to exert a scientific and regulatory agenda on Asia. *Tobacco Control*, **13**(2), ii118–24.

Tyas, S.L., Pederson, L.L. (1998). Psychosocial factors related to adolescent smoking: A critical review of the literature. *Tobacco Control*, **7**, 409–20.

Tobacco Advisory Group of the Royal College of Physicians (2000). *Nicotine addiction in Britain; a report of the Tobacco Advisory Group of the Royal College of Physicians*. Royal College of Physicians of London, London.

USDA (US Department of Agriculture) (2004). *Global cigarette production, distribution and supply 2000–2004*. [Online]. Available at: http://www.fas.usda.gov/tobacco/circular/2004/092004/CIGARETTE2004.PDF

USDHHS (US Department of Health and Human Services) (1986). *The health consequences of involuntary smoking: A report of the Surgeon General*. DHHS Publication 87–8398. US Department of Health and Human Services, Centers for Disease Control, Center for Health Promotion and Education, Office on Smoking and Health, Rockville, MD.

USDHHS (US Department of Health and Human Services) (1988). *The health consequences of smoking: Nicotine addiction. A report of the Surgeon General*. DHHS Publication 88–8406. US Department of Health and Human Services, Public Health Service, Centers for Disease Control, Center for Health Promotion and Education, Office on Smoking and Health, Rockville, MD.

USDHHS (US Department of Health and Human Services) (1989). *Reducing the health consequences of smoking: 25 years of progress. A report of the Surgeon General*. DHHS Publication 89–8411. US Department of Health and Human Services, Public Health Service, Centers for Disease Control, Center for Chronic Disease Prevention and Health Promotion, Office on Smoking and Health, Rockville, MD.

USDHHS (US Department of Health and Human Services) (1990). *The health benefits of smoking cessation. A report of the Surgeon General*. DHHS Publication 90-8416. US Department of Health and Human Services, Public Health Service, National Centre for Chronic Disease Prevention and Health Promotion (Centers for Disease Control and Prevention), Office on Smoking and Health, Rockville, MD.

USDHHS (US Department of Health and Human Services) (1994). *Preventing tobacco use among young people. A report of the Surgeon General*. DHHS Publication 017-001-00491-0. US Department of Health and Human Services, Centers for Disease Control and Prevention, National Center for Chronic Disease Prevention and Health Promotion, Office on Smoking and Health, Atlanta, GA.

USDHHS (US Department of Health and Human Services) (1996). The FTC cigarette test method for determining tar, nicotine, and carbon monoxide yields of US cigarettes. Report of the National Cancer Institute Expert Committee. NIH Publication 96-4028. US Department of Health and Human Services, Public Health Service, National Institutes of Health, National Cancer Institute, Bethesda, MD.

USDHHS (US Department of Health and Human Services) (1997). *Smoking and tobacco control monograph 8: Changes in cigarette-related disease risks and their implication for prevention and control*. NIH Publication 97-1213, US Department of Health and Human Services, Public Health Service, National Institutes of Health, Bethesda, MD.

USDHHS (US Department of Health and Human Services) (1998). *Tobacco use among US racial/ethnic minority groups—African Americans, American Indians and Alaska Natives, Asian Americans and Pacific Islanders, and Hispanic. A report of the Surgeon General*. US Department of Health and Human Services, Centers for Disease Control and Prevention, National Center for Chronic Disease Prevention and Health Promotion, Office on Smoking and Health, Atlanta, GA.

USDHHS (US Department of Health and Human Services) (2001). *Smoking and tobacco control monograph 13: Risks associated with smoking cigarettes with low tar machine-measured yields of tar and nicotine*. National Cancer Institute, National Institutes of Health, Rockville, MD.

USDHHS (US Department of Health and Human Services) (2004). *The Health Consequences of Smoking: A report of the Surgeon General*. US Department of Health and Human Services, Centers for Disease Control and Prevention, National Center for Chronic Disease Prevention and Health Promotion, Office on Smoking and Health. Washington, DC.

USDHHS (US Department of Health and Human Services) (2006). *The Health Consequences of Involuntary Exposure to Tobacco Smoke: A report of the Surgeon General*. NIH Publication 97-1241, US Department of Health and Human Services, Public Health Service, National Institutes of Health, Bethesda, MD.

USDHHS (US Department of Health and Human Services) (2007). *CDC recommended annual per capita funding levels for state programs*. US Department of Health and Human Services, Centers for Disease Control and Prevention, Atlanta, GA.

United States Department of Justice (2004). United States of America, plaintiff v. Philip Morris *et al*. defendants. United States' Final Proposed Findings of Fact. United States District Court for the District of Columbia, Civil Action No. 99-CV-02496 (GK). Available at: http://www.usdoj.gov/civil/cases/tobacco2

United States Department of Justice (2006). United States of America, plaintiff v. Philip Morris. *et al*. defendants. Final Opinion. United States District Court for the District of Columbia, Civil Action No. 99-CV-02496 (GK). Available at: http://www.library.ucsf.edu/tobacco/litigation/uspm.html

Van der Eb, M.M., Leyten, E.M., Gavarasana, S., Vandenbroucke, J.P., Kahn, P.M., Cleton, F.J. (1993). Reverse smoking as a risk factor for palatal cancer: A cross sectional study in rural Andhra Pradesh, India. *International Journal of Cancer*, **54**, 754–8.

Wagner, E.H., Curry, S.J., Grothaus, L., Saunders, K.W., McBride, C.M. (1995). The impact of smoking and quitting on health care use. *Archives of Internal Medicine*, **155**, 1789–95.

Wakefield, M., Morley, C., Horan, J., Cummings, K. (2002). The cigarette pack as image: New evidence from tobacco industry documents. *Tobacco Control*, **11**(1), i73–80.

Wang, F.L., Love, E.J., Liu, N., Dai, X.D. (1994a). Childhood and adolescent passive smoking and the risk of female lung cancer. *International Journal of Epidemiology*, **23**, 223–30.

Wang, S.Q., Yu, J.J., Zhu, B.P., Liu, M., He, G.Q. (1994b). Cigarette smoking and its risk factors among senior high school students in Beijing, China, 1988. *Tobacco Control*, **3**, 107–14.

Warner, K.E. (2000). The economics of tobacco: Myths and realities. *Tobacco Control*, **9**, 78–89.

Warren, C.W., Jones, N.R., Eriksen, M.P., Asma, S., Global Tobacco Surveillance System (GTSS) collaborative group (2006). Patterns of global tobacco use in young people and implications for future chronic disease burden in adults. *Lancet*, **367**(9512), 749–53.

Wayne, G., Connolly, G. (2002). How cigarette design can affect youth initiation into smoking: Camel cigarettes 1983–1993. *Tobacco Control*, **11**(1), i32–9.

WHO (World Health Organization) (1997a). *Tobacco or health: A global status report*. WHO, Geneva.

WHO (World Health Organization) (1997b). *Smoking, drinking and drug taking in the European region*. WHO Regional Office for Europe, Copenhagen.

WHO (World Health Organization) (1999a). *World health report 1999*. WHO, Geneva.

WHO (World Health Organization) (1999b). *Tobacco free initiative consultation report, international consultation on environmental tobacco smoke (ETS) and child health*. WHO/TFI/99.10, WHO, Geneva.

WHO (World Health Organization) (2000a). *Kobe Declaration*. Tobacco Free Initiative Report. WHO, Geneva.

WHO (World Health Organization) (2000b). *Tobacco company strategies to undermine Tobacco Control activities at the World Health Organization*. Report of the Committee of Experts on Tobacco Industry Documents. WHO, Geneva.

WHO (World Health Organization) (2003a). *The cigarette "transit road" to the Islamic Republic of Iran and Iraq. Illicit tobacco trade in the Middle East*. WHO Regional Office for the Eastern Mediterranean, Cairo.

WHO (World Health Organization) (2003b). *Report on smuggling control in Spain*. WHO, Geneva. Available at: http://www.who.int/tobacco/training/success_stories/en/best_practices_spain_smuggling_control.pdf

WHO (World Health Organization) (2004a). Tobacco Free Initiative. *Building blocks for tobacco control: A handbook*. WHO, Geneva.

WHO (World Health Organization) (2004b). *Recommendation 6: Guiding principles for the development of tobacco product research and proposed protocols for the initiation of tobacco product testing*. [Online]. WHO Study Group on Tobacco Product Regulation. Available at: http://repositories.cdlib.org/context/tc/article/1172/type/pdf/viewcontent/

WHO (World Health Organization) (2004c). *Scientific advisory committee on tobacco product regulation*. [Online]. Tobacco Free Initiative. Available at: http://www.who.int/tobacco/sactob/en/ [Accessed on 3 November 2007].

WHO (World Health Organization) (2004d). *IARC monographs on the evaluation of carcinogenic risks to humans: Tobacco smoke and involuntary smoking, Vol.83*, pp. 53–119. International Agency for Research on Cancer, WHO, France.

WHO (World Health Organization) (2005). *The first meeting of the WHO Tobacco Laboratory Network (TobLabNet) on 28 & 29 April 2005 in the Hague, the Netherlands*. [Online]. Tobacco Free Initiative. Available at: http://www.who.int/tobacco/global_interaction/tobreg/laboratory/en/ [Accessed on 23 April 2008].

WHO (World Health Organization) (2006). *Tobacco: Deadly in any form or disguise*. WHO, Geneva.

WHO (World Health Organization) (2007a). *Elaboration of guidelines for implementation of the Convention (decision FCTC/COP1(15)) – Article 8: Protection from exposure to tobacco smoke*. [Online]. The Second Session of Conference of the parties to the WHO Framework Convention on Tobacco Control. Available at: http://www.who.int/gb/fctc/PDF/cop2/FCTC_COP2_7-en.pdf

WHO (World Health Organization) (2007b). *Elaboration of guidelines for implementation of the Convention (decision FCTC/COP1(15)) – Article 9: Product regulation*. [Online]. The Second Session of Conference of the parties to the WHO Framework Convention on Tobacco Control. Available at: http://www.who.int/gb/fctc/PDF/cop2/FCTC_COP2_8-en.pdf

WHO (World Health Organization) (2007c). *The first session of the Conference of the Parties to the WHO Framework Convention on Tobacco Control*. [Online]. Tobacco Free Initiative. Available at: http://www.who.int/tobacco/fctc/cop/en/index.html [Accessed on 3 November 2007].

WHO (World Health Organization) (2007d). *WHO Tobacco Laboratory Network (TobLabNet)*. [Online]. Tobacco Free Initiative. Available at: http://www.who.int/tobacco/global_interaction/toblabnet/history/en/index.html [Accessed on 3 November 2007].

WHO (World Health Organization) (2007e). *The scientific basis of tobacco product regulation*. WHO Technical Report Series 945. WHO, Geneva.

WHO (World Health Organization) (2007f). *A WHO/The Union monograph on TB and tobacco control: Joining efforts to control two related global epidemics*. WHO, Geneva. Available at: http://whqlibdoc.who.int/publications/2007/9789241596220_eng.pdf

WHO (World Health Organization) (2007g). Gender and tobacco control: A policy brief. WHO, Geneva. Available at: http://www.who.int/tobacco/resources/publications/general/policy_brief.pdf.

WHO (World Health Organization) (2007h). World health statistics 2007. WHO, France; 15.

WHO (World Health Organization) (2008a). *WHO Report on the Global Tobacco Epidemic, 2008: The MPOWER package*. WHO, Geneva.

WHO (World Health Organization) (2008b). World health statistics 2008. WHO, Geneva; 66–75.

Wipfli, H., Avila-Tang, E., Navas-Acien, A. *et al.* (2008). Secondhand smoke exposure among women and children: Evidence from 31 countries. *American Journal of Public Health*, **98**(4), 672–9.

Wistuba, I.I., Lam, S., Behrens, C. *et al.* (1997). Molecular damage in the bronchial epithelium of current and former smokers. *Journal of the National Cancer Institute*, **89**, 1366–73.

World Bank (1999). *Curbing the epidemic: Governments and the economics of tobacco control*. World Bank, Washington, DC.

Yang, G., Ma, J., Chen, A. *et al.* (2001). Smoking cesation in China: Findings from the 1996 national prevalence survey. *Tobacco Control*, **10**(2), 170–4.

Yang, G.H., Ma, J.M., Liu, N., Zhou, L.N. (2005). Smoking and passive smoking in Chinese, 2002. [Article in Chinese]. *Zhonghua Liu Xing Bing Xue Za Zhi*, **26**(2), 77–83.

Zhang, J., Ratcliffe, J.M. (1993). Paternal smoking and birthweight in Shanghai. *American Journal of Public Health*, **83**, 207–10.

Zhu, B.P., Liu, M., Shelton, D., Liu, S., Giovino, G.A. (1996). Cigarette smoking and its risk factors among elementary school students in Beijing. *American Journal of Public Health*, **86**, 368–75.

Drug abuse

Don C. Des Jarlais and Robert L. Hubbard

Abstract

Abuse and dependence on alcohol and other drugs is a particularly complex and very important public health problem. Drug dependence disorders involve biomedical, pharmacological, psychological, and social factors. Drug abuse often involves multiple pharmacological agents used within a complex social environment in which some substances are legal and others illegal. The consequences of drug abuse are many and varied. Over the last 40 years, there have been major advances in prevention and treatment of drug abuse, but given present worldwide trends, the problems associated with psychoactive drug use are likely to continue increasing. Human immunodeficiency virus (HIV), the virus that causes acquired immunodeficiency syndrome (AIDS) has emerged as the most dramatic adverse consequence of drug use. HIV is not transmitted through drug use *per se*, but through the sharing of equipment to inject drugs and through unsafe sexual activities that are often facilitated by drug use. Sharing of injection equipment can lead to extremely rapid transmission of HIV, with half or more of a local drug user population becoming infected over a period of a few years. Conversely, programmes such as community outreach and syringe exchange can be highly effective in reducing injection-related HIV transmission. It is possible to prevent epidemics of HIV among injecting drug users. The main problems have been not implementing programmes to prevent HIV among injecting drug users at all, but waiting until after an epidemic has already occurred to implement programmes, or implementing programmes on an inadequate scale. The HIV/AIDS crisis has spurred development of the 'harm reduction' perspective towards the problems of psychoactive drug use. This perspective is based in a human rights approach to drug users—drug users should be treated with dignity and respect—and a pragmatic, public health perspective on drug related problems. It is not likely that the problems associated with drug use can be eliminated, so public health policy should focus on the many different ways in which those problems can be minimized.

Abuse and dependence on alcohol and other drugs is a particularly complex public health problem. The complexity of alcohol and other drug abuse is a function of its diverse nature. Dependence disorders involve biomedical, pharmacological, psychological, and social factors. Substance abuse often involves multiple pharmacological agents used within a complex social environment in which some

substances are legal and others illegal. Furthermore, the distinctions among use, abuse, and dependence are often blurred. The consequences of substance abuse are many and varied. Some are acute and put an individual at immediate risk, such as driving while intoxicated. Use of addictive substances by biologically vulnerable individuals may result in long-term consequences such as criminal behaviour and loss of employment. Sharing of injection equipment by intravenous drug users immediately increases their risk of exposure to HIV and, once exposed, their life-styles compromise health and may lead to accelerated development of AIDS. Thus, simple definitions, explanations, or solutions for substance abuse are inadequate, inefficient, and potentially counterproductive. The evolution of research on the individuals using drugs, prevention, and treatment was summarized in a 2006 conference reflecting on 40 years of substance abuse research (Sloboda 2008). This chapter indicates some of the broad concepts necessary to understand substance abuse and dependence disorders, their consequences, and potential solutions.

The focus in the first section of the chapter is dependence on drugs other than alcohol, which is discussed in another chapter. While recognizing that problems of alcohol and drug abuse occur worldwide and across diverse cultures (Babor 1986), this discussion is limited by both space and data to the United States. In the United States, the problem is most profound. The history and current conditions in the United States illustrate many of the issues that exist or can be expected to emerge in many countries in the future. The abuse of alcohol (Aaron & Musto 1981) and other drugs (Brecher *et al.* 1972) has persisted for centuries. Since 1900, attention to alcohol and other drug abuse has waxed and waned in the United States (Jaffe 1979). Some of the foremost reasons for renewed attention on alcohol and drug abuse in the 1980s and the 1990s are the increasing costs for treatment for dependence, the violent crime associated with cocaine distribution, and the role of intravenous drug use in the transmission of HIV. Intravenous drug use is now the second most common risk behaviour associated with AIDS. It is also the major contributing factor to paediatric and heterosexual AIDS cases in the United States (Turner *et al.* 1989). In the last 5 years, rates are rapidly escalating among minorities and underserved populations in rural communities outside traditional epicentres (Reif *et al.* 2006).

This first section describes the definition, epidemiology, aetiology, and consequences of alcohol and drug abuse. The major efforts made in the United States to prevent and treat alcohol and other drug abuse are reviewed and their effectiveness documented. The chapter concludes with a discussion of the critical role of intravenous drug use in the HIV/AIDS epidemic. The last section incorporates a broader worldwide view. Within each section, a broad array of perspectives on these problems are presented. These perspectives range from the biomedical search for genetic markers to legal attempts to control alcohol and other drug use. A full discussion of all perspectives is beyond the scope of one particular presentation. Because of the orientation of the authors, this presentation necessarily has a social/psychological orientation. This is not to suggest that the other approaches are not important to consider, only that the authors of this chapter are most qualified to deal with the research literature in their own discipline.

Definition of dependence on drugs

Various approaches have been used to characterize the use, abuse, and dependence on drugs. Numerous personal interviews and self-report inventories have been developed to obtain a comprehensive history of use as well as assessments of current use patterns, dependence, and drug- and alcohol-related problems (Skinner & Horn 1984; Babor et al. 1988). No single measure has yet been accepted as fully characterizing use, abuse, or dependence. From an epidemiological perspective, frequency of use, and total number of times used in a lifetime are often the principal measures. Abuse refers to usage levels that have short-term acute personal or social consequences. Psychiatric diagnosis of dependence requires evidence of consequences over an extended period of time. The clinical definition of dependence, which is now undergoing careful review, has evolved over the past decade to include psychological as well as physiological components.

Assessment of alcohol dependence and problems has received more attention than diagnosis of drug abuse problems or dependence. Research on alcohol dependence has fostered interest in the measurement of drug dependence syndromes, using similar diagnostic criteria (Edwards et al. 1981). Many of the assessments that were used to measure alcohol abuse have been modified for drug abuse research. A factor analytical study (Skinner & Horn 1984) identified a general cluster resembling the alcohol dependence syndrome postulated by Edwards et al. (1976). The salient markers of this factor include loss of behavioural control over drinking, withdrawal symptoms, and obsessive-compulsive drinking style. Early validation research (Skinner & Horn 1984) indicates that the drug dependence symptoms correlate in predictable ways with clinic attendance, physical symptoms, and psychosocial problems.

Perhaps the most ambitious and theoretically sound approach to assessing dependence has been taken by Rounsaville et al. (1986) on the structured clinical interview for the revised edition of the Diagnostic and Statistical Manual of Mental Disorders (DSM-III-R). The structured clinical interview is designed to determine diagnoses and symptoms of substance use disorder according to the American Psychiatric Association's revised Diagnostic and Statistical Manual of Mental Disorders (Spitzer & Williams 1987). The structured clinical interview provides a more comprehensive assessment of alcohol and drug dependence symptoms than the substance use disorders section of the Diagnostic Interview Schedule, and provides diagnoses that can be applied to both the third edition and the third revised edition of the Diagnostic and Statistical Manual of Mental Disorders.

The criteria have been substantially revised (Rounsaville et al. 1986) and are designed to reflect aspects of the dependence syndrome (Edwards et al. 1981). Symptoms include: (1) more use than intended; (2) inability to reduce use; (3) amount of time seeking substance; (4) physical effects of use; (5) use replaces other activities; (6) continued use in spite of problems; (7) tolerance; (8) withdrawal symptoms; or (9) use to avoid withdrawal symptoms. Dependence severity is assessed by considering the number of symptoms reported and the extent of impairment, and the indication of level of dependence (mild, moderate, severe, partial remission, full remission) rather than simply the presence or absence of dependence or abuse. Abuse is defined as sporadic non-dependent patterns of use in spite of problems or physical hazards. Rounsaville (2002) reviewed the two emergent systems, International Classification of Diseases 10 (WHO 1992) and Diagnostic and Statistical Manual of Disease IV (APA 2000), and identified needs for consistency across the two systems, a consistency that may be achieved more easily for dependence.

Initial attempts to define alcohol and drug dependence have been confounded by increased multiple use of various drugs during the 1970s and 1980s (Clayton 1985; Hubbard et al. 1986) and the rise of cocaine use during the 1980s. A very complex typology is needed to capture the full extent of alcohol and other drug use. In fact, many individuals who use alcohol heavily also report the use of marijuana and, increasingly, the use of cocaine. Among those using marijuana, almost all will have used alcohol. At another extreme, most intravenous heroin users have used alcohol, cocaine, and marijuana (Hubbard et al. 1986). To address this problem, Spitzer and Williams (1987) introduce a general category of polydrug dependence to include dependence on three or more specific psychoactive substances or dependence on psychoactive substances in general. These emerging approaches to definition within and across the complex array of usage patterns offer the promise of a more comprehensive understanding of abuse and dependence (Cacciola & Woody 2005).

Epidemiology

Since the 1960s in the United States, national attention has been focused on the rapidly expanding problem of drug abuse. In particular, the concern was the involvement of adolescents with alcohol and other drugs. To trace these high levels of use, three series of national probability sample surveys have been conducted in the United States. Each year since 1974, a national sample of high school senior students has completed self-administered questionnaires on alcohol and drug use (Johnston et al. 1989). In the years 1972, 1974, 1975, 1979, 1982, 1985, and 1988, and annually since 1991, personal interviews on drug use have been conducted with a national sample of American household residents, stratified by ages 12–17, 18–25, and 26 years or older (National Institute on Drug Abuse 1989). These surveys have documented relative stability in alcohol use, but a rapid escalation from 1972 to 1979 in lifetime and current use of other drugs, particularly marijuana and cocaine. After 1979, the use of marijuana and, since 1985, cocaine, dropped rapidly (Table 10.2.1). For youth, the rates of marijuana use then began to increase in the mid-1990s, but since 2000, a gradual decline has been noted (Johnston et al. 2005).

Table 10.2.1 Trends in prevalence of self-reported use of marijuana, cocaine, and alcohol in the National Household Survey on Drug Abuse in the United States, 1974–2005

Year of survey	1974	1979	1985	1991	1995	2000	2005
Lifetime prevalence for youths aged 12–17							
Marijuana	23%	26.7%	20.1%	11.1%	16.2%	18.3%	17.4%
Cocaine	3.6%	5.5%	4.7%	2.4%	2%	2.4%	2.3%
Alcohol	54%	70.8%	56.1%	46.9%	40.6%	41.7%	40.6%
Past year prevalence for young adults aged 18–25							
Marijuana	34.2%	44.2%	34%	22.9%	21.8%	23.7%	28%
Cocaine	8.1%	17%	13.6%	6.7%	4.3%	4.4%	6.9%
Alcohol	77.1%	84.6%	84.2%	80.7%	76.5%	74.5%	77.9%
Past year prevalence for older adults aged 26–34							
Marijuana	3.8%	20.5%	20.2%	11.6%	11.8%	5%	6.9%
Cocaine	–	5.7%	10.5%	4.4%	3.1%	1%	1.5%
Alcohol	62.7%	81.7%	81.9%	79.1%	77%	63.7%	69%

The spectrum of problems associated with drug use persists, and now includes the crucial role of intravenous heroin and cocaine use in the transmission of HIV infection. The large-scale household or school-based surveys do not provide useful information on the relatively rare and hidden populations of intravenous drug users. Estimates of the size and usage patterns of this population are derived largely from studies of convenience samples, statistical models, and informed guesses.

Youth and young adults

While alcohol and other drug abuse occur at all income levels and in virtually all age groups, the high levels of abuse among youths and young adults causes the most concern. In the United States, approximately 70 per cent of all youth have at least experimented with illegal drugs by the time they leave high school (Johnston *et al.* 1999), and one in three senior students report current heavy drinking (five or more drinks in a row in the past 2 weeks). A survey of 7500 youth aged 11–14 years has shown that initiation of alcohol and drug abuse rises exponentially through the years of early adolescence (Hubbard *et al.* 1988). By the age of 14, two of five adolescents have at one time consumed two or more drinks or reported trying drugs for non-medical reasons. The patterns of use have also varied greatly since the first national surveys were conducted in 1972.

The trends in the use of drugs by youth showed a levelling off from the mid-1970s to the early 1980s, a rapid decline in the late 1980s, an increase in the mid-1990s, and fairly consistent rates through 2005 (Table 10.2.1). Percentages of youth who had ever tried marijuana, 26.7 per cent in 1979, had fallen to 20.1 per cent in 1985 and to 9.9 per cent in 1993, before beginning an annual increase to 17 per cent in 1998, where the figure has remained. Cocaine use rose rapidly from 1.5 per cent in 1972 to 5.5 per cent in 1979 to 6.1 per cent in 1982, but fell to 2.4 per cent in 1991 and to 1.1 per cent by 1993, then climbed to 2.2 per cent by 1998, where it has remained through 2005. Although the percentages of youths aged 12–17 years

who used drugs in 2005 are lower than the 1979 figures, rates have fluctuated, but now appear to have been relatively stable from 2000 through 2005 (Substance Abuse and Mental Health Services Administration 1999, 2007).

The levels and trends for youth in the household surveys have paralleled those for high-school senior students, which show a downward trend in the use of marijuana and other illicit drugs from 1979 to 1993, with rates increasing through 1998 (Johnston *et al.* 1999). Beginning in 2000, a gradual trend in decreasing rates has been observed (Johnston *et al.* 2006). Cocaine use was an exception to this rapid downward trend, having stabilized through 1986 at the levels attained in the late 1970s. Rates decreased from 1986 through 1993 before beginning to climb again through 1998. By 1986, about one of every six high-school senior students reported trying cocaine, and one in 20 reported use in the 30 days prior to the survey. By 1998, about one of every 10 high-school senior students reported trying cocaine, and only one in 40 reported use in the last 30 days. Between 1983 and 1986, the proportion of seniors reporting daily cocaine use in the month before the survey and the proportion who had been unable to stop using in the prior year had both doubled. Between 1986 and 1998, the proportion of seniors reporting daily cocaine use in the month before the survey had fallen to the 1983 level. The proportion who had smoked crack cocaine, a more dangerous and effective route of administration, had also doubled from 1983 to 1986, but rapidly declined from 5.7 per cent (1986 level) to 1.5 per cent by 1991. In 1986, only half of the senior students thought there was much risk associated with occasional cocaine use. The 1988 survey, however, shows a marked decline in cocaine use coupled with a heightened perception of risk. One in eight report lifetime use, and one in 30 reported use in the past 30 days. About 7 in 10 high-school senior students viewed occasional cocaine use as harmful. By 1993, rates of lifetime use of cocaine had decreased to 6 per cent, and less than 2 per cent of high school senior students used cocaine in the 30 days prior to the survey. The 1993 data also reported an increased number of drugs used and less negative attitudes towards drugs. By 2005, only 8 per cent of high school seniors reported ever using cocaine, and in 2007, only 3 per cent of 8th graders reported ever using cocaine.

Although use among young adults also declined during the 1980s, many continue to use various types of drugs. The National Household Survey on Drug Abuse conducted in 1979 showed that 44.2 per cent of persons aged 18–25 years had used marijuana in the year before the survey (Table 10.2.1). There was a general downward trend until the mid-1990s (21.8 per cent in 1995), with an increase to 24.1 per cent in 1998. Cocaine use decreased from a high of 17 per cent in 1979 to 4.3 per cent in 1995, before rising slightly to 4.7 per cent in 1998. Self-reports of any illicit drug in the year before the survey fell from a high of 45.5 per cent in 1979 to around 25 per cent through 1998. Lifetime cocaine use prevalence for 19–28-year-olds was 32 per cent in 1986, but had dropped steadily to 12.3 per cent by 1998 (Johnston *et al.* 1999). The 2005 data from the national household survey shows a troubling increase in the rate of use in the past year to 28 per cent for marijuana and 6.9 per cent for cocaine, trends that parallel the trend for alcohol use (Substance Abuse and Mental Health Administration 2007).

Adults

Levels of drug use for adults (aged 26–34 years old) have not fluctuated as dramatically as those for youth and young adults. About 9 in 10 of older adults reported some experience with alcohol. Lifetime rates of marijuana (45 per cent in 1979, to 54.9 per cent in 1993, to 47.9 per cent in 1998) and cocaine use (13.4 per cent in 1979 to 25.4 per cent in 1993 to 17.1 per cent in 1998) have shown the same trends as youth and young adults. Use of all drugs in the past year remained relatively low (around 10 per cent for marijuana and under 5 per cent for cocaine) throughout the years of the household survey (Table 10.2.1).

More detailed and reliable data on dependence are available from a consortium of community epidemiological studies conducted from 1980 to 1982. In three American cities, lifetime rates between 11.5 and 15.7 per cent for alcohol abuse/dependence disorders and between 5.5 and 5.8 per cent for drug abuse/dependence were found for the adult residents interviewed in households (Robins *et al.* 1984). Current 6-month prevalence rates for men ranged between 8.2 and 10.4 per cent for alcohol dependence and 2.5 and 3.0 per cent for drug dependence (Myers *et al.* 1984). Rates for females were between 4.5 and 5.7 per cent for alcohol abuse/dependence and 1.8 and 2.2 per cent for drug abuse/dependence. Both of these data sets indicate that a substantial proportion of individuals in the United States have self-recognized problems with alcohol and drugs, and many meet the third edition criteria for dependence of the Diagnostic and Statistical Manual of Mental Disorders. Observations from community-based observers in 22 geographically dispersed communities have tracked trends from various data sources (e.g. emergency rooms, law enforcement, treatment) since the 1970s (Community Epidemiology Work Group 2007). They have reported geographically disparate rates of use of methamphetamine and prescription opioids, which cannot be easily accessed through household or school-based survey methodology.

Intravenous drug users

Estimating the number of intravenous drug users is an imprecise art. The problem of estimation is further hampered by differing definitions of past and current behaviour that qualifies an individual as an intravenous drug user. Spencer (1989) reviewed the variety of indirect estimates (derived from statistical models of indicators such as emergency room and medical examiner reports), direct estimates (based on surveys of convenience samples, back extrapolation, and capture-recapture estimates) or informed guesses. Considering all sources, Turner *et al.* (1989) conclude that a reasonable guess of the number of intravenous drug users in the United States is between 500 000 and 2 million. In the latest NSDUH, a likely underestimate, 3.8 million Americans, were projected to have used heroin, and 338 000 were projected to have used in the past month (SAMHSA 2007).

Consequences

Drug abuse costs were US$47 billion in 1980 (Harwood *et al.* 1984). The major contributors to these costs are lost productivity and treatment costs. Lost productivity attributed to drug abuse was estimated to be US$26 billion. Treatment services related to drug abuse were just over US$1 billion. This represents direct health services provided to victims, including long- and short-term hospitalization, services from physicians, and other sources. The overall costs also include the economic costs of crime, and violent crime due to drug abuse, premature mortality resulting from drug overdoses, liver disease, suicide, homicide, motor vehicle crashes, and other causes. Drug abuse costs US$2 billion for accidental overdoses. Drug addiction cost society approximately US$9 billion because of the addicts' pursuit of non-productive and criminal careers, another US$6 billion for criminal justice expenses, and US$1.5 billion for incarceration. These costs alone place drug abuse as one of the main contributors to the social cost of health-related problems in the United States. The costs were estimated to rise about 5 per cent a year, reaching US$181 billion in 2002 (Office of National Drug Control Policy 2004).

With the emergence of the AIDS epidemic in the 1980s, every drug abuser who contracts AIDS adds another US$80 000 in medical care costs to the equation (Scitovsky & Rice 1987). As described below, intravenous drug users play an important role in the AIDS epidemic, as they are second only to male homosexuals in the ranking of high-risk groups for AIDS in the United States (Turner *et al.* 1989). Intravenous drug use is also a major factor in cases involving children, heterosexuals, blacks, and Hispanics (Day *et al.* 1988; Des Jarlais & Friedman 1988). Regardless of sexual orientation, past or present intravenous drug users represent over one-quarter of reported AIDS cases in the United States, and the proportion continues to increase. Tests for HIV have shown that 10–58 per cent of sampled intravenous drug users are seropositive (Robert-Guroff *et al.* 1986; Chaisson *et al.* 1987; Des Jarlais *et al.* 1989). This increased risk of infection resulted in estimates of costs of US$2.5 to US$3.5 billion in the mid-1990s, with potentially greater costs due to the increased number of HIV/AIDS patients being treated (Office of National Drug Control Policy 2004).

Aetiology

The goal of efforts to deal with alcohol and drug abuse involves identifying those at risk and intervening to prevent or treat the problem. Information on risk factors to help target prevention, treatment, and rehabilitation efforts is largely limited to youth and young adults. Research is moving closer to uncovering basic biological and psychosocial mechanisms in alcohol and other drug use, but it does not appear likely that any simple explanation will be found. Being the child of a substance abuser has been found to be a consistent predictor of abuse. Both genetic and family environmental factors have been cited as influential agents (Kandel *et al.* 1978; Schuckit 1980; Cloninger *et al.* 1981; Goodwin 1985; Petrakis 1985).

Delinquent behaviour, including alcohol and drug abuse, often occur together (Jessor *et al.* 1980; Robins 1980). Many of the studies conclude that involvement in delinquent behaviour precedes drug use (Bachman *et al.* 1978; Elliott *et al.* 1985; Kandel *et al.* 1986), and that both behaviours have the same aetiological sources (Elliott *et al.* 1985; Hawkins *et al.* 1985). Early delinquent behaviour, usually before the age of 10, has also been linked to earlier initiation (Kandel *et al.* 1986) and frequent drug use (Kandel *et al.* 1978; Johnston *et al.* 1978; Kellam & Brown 1982; Rachal *et al.* 1982; Robins & Przybeck 1985; Kaplan *et al.* 1986). Other social factors such as low socio-economic status of parents, social isolation, and poor living conditions have also been found to be related to chronic delinquency and drug use (Farrington 1985; Hawkins *et al.* 1987). Studies have also identified an association of alcohol and drug abuse with depression, low self-esteem, and psychological distress (Kandel *et al.* 1978; Kaplan *et al.* 1982; Aneshensel & Huba 1983).

One of the areas that has received relatively little attention in aetiological research is the examination of factors leading to cessation. Kandel and Raveis (1989) found that health and social factors discouraging use among young adults were predictive of cessation and a more extensive degree of previous involvement in drug use was predictive of continuation. Interpretation of these correlates of the likelihood of stopping use will require a more comprehensive understanding of use, abuse, and dependence (Meyer 1989), including the relative role of pharmacological, social, and physiological factors combined with the level and nature of involvement.

Another area where data is lacking is the dynamics of the initiation into intravenous drug use. Des Jarlais *et al.* (1986) suggest that initiation is often an unanticipated behaviour. Turner *et al.* (1989) conclude that some of the same factors contributing to initiation of other types of illicit use (such as peer groups) also predict initiation of intravenous use and continuation of usage. The uncertainty surrounding initiation, particularly in the face of the AIDS epidemic, dictates the need for more extensive and intensive research on initiation, development, maintenance, and cessation of intravenous drug use. More recent research has focused on the cessation rather that initiation of substance use. Laudet (2007) identified recovery as a multifaceted concept. The Betty Ford Institute Consensus Panel (2007) defined recovery as 'a voluntarily maintained lifestyle characterized by sobriety, personal health and citizenship'.

Prevention

Identifying youth at risk for alcohol/drug initiation and continued use is a potentially efficient and effective means for targeting prevention efforts. In the United States, however, youth in general are at risk for drug initiation (Hubbard *et al.* 1988). Surveys of high school students have shown that non-medical drug use begins in the early teens, peaks in early adulthood, and declines sharply thereafter (Kandel 1980). Initiation to marijuana is almost completed by the age of 20, and to psychedelic drugs by the age of 21 (Kandel & Logan 1984). More than half of inhalant, phencyclidine, and barbiturate users initiate use before tenth grade (15–16 years old). Prior to the crack epidemic, most cocaine users initiated use in the last 2 years of high school (Johnston *et al.* 1984).

Drug use prevention programmes should ideally first reach youth prior to adolescence, then reinforce the message throughout adolescence. Research findings suggest that prevention efforts oriented towards delaying the age of onset of initiation may prevent the initiation of other perhaps more dangerous drugs (Kandel 1982), a greater frequency of use (Rachal *et al.* 1982), and the involvement in other delinquent acts (Brunswick & Boyle 1979).

Prevention strategies seek to prevent substance abuse by informing, educating, and training individuals so that they have the necessary information, skills, and confidence to choose not to abuse alcohol or other drugs. Environmental approaches seek to restrict the opportunity for exposure to alcohol and other drugs. Prevention programmes and organizations offering prevention services often adopt one or more strategies (Tobler 1986):

1. Information activities are designed to provide accurate and timely information about alcohol and other drugs and their effects on the individual, family, and community.

2. Education activities use a structured process to assist individuals in learning and improving basic life skills (decision-making, problem-solving, community, and peer/social resistance skills).

3. Alternatives programmes provide challenging positive growth experiences in which individuals can develop the self-discipline, confidence, personal awareness, self-reliance, and independence they need to become socially mature individuals by offering positive alternatives to alcohol and other drug-using behaviours.

4. Intervention services identify individuals with early substance abuse problems, help them assess their problems and take action to resolve them, and provide emotional support and practical guidance during the early stages of recovery.

5. Environmental controls include efforts to make alcohol and other drugs less accessible by raising drinking ages, increasing enforcement, or otherwise reducing access to alcohol and other drugs.

Most of the drug education programmes are based on a knowledge/attitude, value/decision-making, or social competency theoretical approach (Moskowitz 1983). The knowledge/attitude approach has been used most widely, although empirical support for the assumed causal links between knowledge of the consequences of drug use, attitudes concerning use, and use behaviour is limited (Hanson 1980; Kinder *et al.* 1980; Goodstadt 1981). The effectiveness of the value/decision-making approach (Huba *et al.* 1980; Goodstadt 1981), which assumes that logical weighing of the costs and benefits of drug use takes place, is also not well supported. Studies measuring the effects of the teaching of social skills on drug use prevention among adolescents show promising results. Pentz (1983) concluded that teaching skills such as assertiveness, initiating/maintaining conversation, non-verbal expression, expressing feelings/empathy, decision-making, expressing an opinion or request, self-control, praise, and responding to criticism reduces drug use and related behaviours among adolescents. Similarly, Botvin (1983), after instituting a prevention programme teaching life skills to adolescents, found a 50 per cent reduction in new cigarette smoking 1 year after the programme.

Prevention efforts have been implemented and developed primarily in three social realms—the school, the family, and the community.

Educational programmes presented in schools are the most frequently employed approach to drug abuse prevention. Evaluative studies (Schaps *et al.* 1984) and reviews (Goodstadt 1980; Schaps *et al.* 1981), however, provide little support for the effectiveness of school-based programmes. Goodstadt (1980), in a review of several drug education programmes, observed that most had mixed results; i.e. they produced negative results on some attitudinal and behavioural dimensions and positive results on others. He concluded that although education programmes do not appear to be as harmful or counterproductive as some detractors claim, their results are not as strongly positive as one would like. While these educational programmes have reported some positive results, both the programmes and the evaluations of them have been criticized because of an inadequate theoretical base. They assume, albeit implicitly, that attitudes are strongly related to behaviours, and that a single exposure will have enduring effects throughout the adolescent years. Attitudes are usually not good predictors of behaviour (Fishbein & Ajzen 1975), and most programmes do not consider the complex development stages of adolescence (Greenspan 1985).

Many theories have addressed the importance of involving parents in any type of intervention. Bry (1983) notes the significance of modelling and the necessity for communication skills to teach young people how to say 'no' when dealing with the pressures of substance abuse behaviours and other negative behaviours. McAlister (1983) points specifically to the significance of prevention programmes that address low self-esteem, poor skills for coping with stress, and alienation from school and family. He addresses the significance of self-image being more related to family relationships than to school relationships. These theories give credence to involving parents with their children in a family approach to prevention.

Descriptions of community action programmes in alcohol (Hewitt & Blane 1984) and drug abuse (Flay & Sobel 1983) have generally focused on media campaigns. Project STAR (Students Taught Awareness and Resistance), a community-based drug and alcohol abuse prevention programme in Kansas City, MO, however, is a comprehensive approach that works through a liaison between the programme implementers and researchers (Pentz *et al.* 1986). Programme components are implemented, and progress is observed and tested for any effect on drug use. The component is then refined according to the evaluation results before the initiation of the next programme component. Data from the delayed implementation of this multicommunity trial (Pentz *et al.* 1989) indicate the potential effectiveness of comprehensive intervention. The interventions included a combination of mass media, school-based programmes, parental involvement, and community support. Prevalence of alcohol, tobacco, and marijuana was lower in the sites where the intervention had been implemented compared to control sites where the intervention had been delayed, 17 versus 24 per cent for cigarettes, 11 versus 16 per cent for alcohol, and 7 versus 10 per cent for marijuana. The rate of increase in usage was also lower in the sites where the intervention had been implemented.

Based on the success of public information campaigns to reduce smoking and the results of prevention research, a media effort to reduce drug use among youth was launched throughout the United States in 1998 (Westat 2003). While exposure to (70–80 per cent) and recall of (58–76 per cent) of the messages were high for both youth and parents, the effects were weak or absent. Parents did seem to be more likely to talk to youth about drugs and engaged in more activities. Although believing monitoring was important, those exposed to messages did not increase their monitoring behaviour. There was 'little evidence of direct favourable campaign effects on youths' beliefs, intentions or behaviour'. Delayed effect analyses have been planned, but are not yet available.

Treatment

Treatment in one form or another for both alcohol and drug abuse have been available since the turn of the century. It is, however, only in the late 1960s and early 1970s that both alcohol and drug abuse treatment have become major parts of the public health system in the United States. The administration of the public treatment system in America shifted from the federal government to states under the Omnibus Reconciliation Act of 1981. Treatment systems rapidly evolved to meet the demands of cost containment in the 1990s. In the next millennium, the evolution of treatment programmes and the system that supports them has continued. There is a major transformation to fee for service and evidence-based practice (Lewin Group 2005; Roman *et al.* 2006).

Approaches

The alcohol treatment system emerged from an effort in the late 1960s to establish community-based alcohol treatment centres throughout many parts of the United States. Combined with this public approach was the availability of proprietary inpatient programmes based on the Minnesota model treatment protocol (Laundergan 1982; Cook 1988). These short-term inpatient regimens help guide alcohol abusers through the first phases of the 12 steps of the Alcoholics Anonymous recovery programme.

The rapid escalation of heroin addiction in communities in the late 1960s, coupled with the high rates of addiction among returning Vietnam veterans, led to the establishment of a national system of drug abuse treatment programmes to deal with the increasing rates of addiction and associated crime (Jaffe 1979). Since these early years, there have been far-reaching changes in the drug abuse treatment system. The three major modalities or types of treatment developed and currently being administered under public funding in the United States are outpatient methadone clinics, therapeutic communities, and outpatient drug-free programmes. Outpatient methadone programmes treat opioid abusers, most of whom use heroin intravenously. After stabilization with medically prescribed doses of methadone, clients receive a variety of counselling and other services to help them resume productive lives. Therapeutic communities use group counselling with all types of drug abusers over long stays in a 24-h community environment. Outpatient drug-free programmes tend to be oriented towards non-opioid users, emphasizing counselling, often in community mental health centre settings. Among the three modalities, there are great variations in programme size, structure, therapeutic approach, services, and funding. Treatment for drug abuse, particularly cocaine, began to be provided in chemical dependency programmes originally designed for alcoholism in the late 1980s.

The treatment system in the United States now includes a broad array of public and private programme types. The proportion of privately funded alcohol and drug abuse treatment programmes increased during the 1980s. By the 1990s, drug abuse treatment was delivered in a wider variety of settings, including chemical dependency programmes (formerly exclusive alcohol treatment programmes), community mental health centres, as well as treatment programmes designed primarily for alcohol. The distinction between publicly funded and private treatment has become blurred. With the movement to a fee for service structure, substance abuse treatment clients may receive services from an even broader array of providers. Despite the multiple service need and the availability of community resources, the treatment of many clients in the traditional public treatment modalities has seldom been supported by public funds at a level that parallels annual inflation.

Effectiveness

The effectiveness of both alcohol and drug abuse treatment has been continually questioned. One of the major reasons for this is the difficulty of conducting broad-based epidemiological outcome studies or controlled clinical trials of sufficient scope to answer some of the major questions about treatment. In the United States, only one national study of alcohol treatment and three of drug abuse treatment have been successfully mounted in the past 30 years. Clinical trials based on unblinded random assignment have often failed because of limited compliance (Fuller et al. 1986) and retention (Bale et al. 1980) for sufficiently long periods of time to demonstrate the efficacy of any particular treatment approach.

Epidemiological outcome studies do indicate positive effects. The major clinical epidemiological study of alcohol treatment was conducted in the early 1970s with a sample of 593 clients followed 18 and 48 months after treatment (Armor et al. 1978; Polich et al. 1981). After 4 years, 21 per cent were abstinent for at least 1 year before the follow-up. A positive correlation was reported between those clients receiving five or more outpatient visits and those with more than 7 days worth of inpatient visits. Using a cost-offset framework in an analysis of health insurance data, Holder and Blose (1986) attributed substantial savings to alcohol treatment in health-care costs. Other follow-up studies of proprietary programmes reviewed by the Institute of Medicine (Committee to Identify Research Effectiveness in the Prevention and Treatment of Alcohol-Related Problems 1989) find abstinence rates between 40 and 60 per cent in the first year after treatment. Similar results were found in studies of state programmes (Hubbard et al. 1988) and proprietary programmes (Hoffman & Harrison 1987). Because of the often low rates of response to follow-up, the method of obtaining reports, imprecise measurement of treatment process, including continuing care and other methodological considerations, these rates of abstinence likely exaggerate the positive effects of treatment.

In contrast to these findings and those for drug abuse treatment reported below, the Institute of Medicine panel found little evidence supporting longer term treatment for alcohol abuse Reviews (Saxe et al. 1983; Annis 1986; Miller & Hester 1986), and a series of random assignment studies have found neither length of treatment nor intensity (inpatient versus outpatient) influenced outcome. In such unblinded research, however, the levels of severity of client problems likely interact with selection bias from compliance and attrition to confound the interpretation of results. Further, most alcohol treatment protocols tested, typically less than 3 months, may not be of sufficient duration or intensity to produce demonstrable effects. Controlled studies of alcohol treatment may need to focus more on comparison of different continuums of care to examine how inpatient and outpatient programmes can contribute to long-term compliance with aftercare and relapse prevention.

Such an approach has been implemented in a national multisite trial of three outpatient protocols for alcohol abuse based on 12-step, cognitive-behavioural, or motivational enhancement approaches (Project MATCH Research Group 1993). These studies demonstrated that in all three approaches, clients did achieve reductions in alcohol.

A series of studies conducted primarily over the past four decades has demonstrated the effectiveness of the publicly funded methadone maintenance and therapeutic community approaches (Tims 1981; Tims & Ludford 1984; Hubbard et al. 2008). Use of most drugs declines during and after treatment (Sells & Simpson 1976; Smart 1976; Sells 1979; Holland 1982; DeLeon 1984). Criminal activity is reduced among programme clients, particularly during treatment (Gorsuch et al. 1976; Nash 1976; McGlothlin et al. 1977; Dole & Joseph 1978).

In the late 1970s, a clinical epidemiological study of drug abuse treatments assessed outcomes for 10 000 methadone, residential, and outpatient drug-free clients up to 5 years after treatment (Hubbard et al. 1989). Substantial decreases in regular heroin, cocaine, and psychotherapeutic drug abuse, and diminished overall severity of drug abuse were apparent during and after treatment for clients treated over a period of at least 3 months. The prevalence of regular heroin use for methadone clients in the first year after treatment (17 per cent) was one-quarter of the pretreatment rate. For residential clients, the post-treatment prevalence of regular heroin (12 per cent) was one-third of the rate prior to treatment, and nonmedical psychotherapeutic drug use (9 per cent) was one-fifth of the rate prior to treatment; regular use of cocaine declined by half to 16 per cent in the post-treatment period. In the case of outpatient drug-free clients, prevalence of non-medical psychotherapeutic drug use was half the pretreatment rate. In any given year of followup, less than 20 per cent of former clients in any modality were regular users of drugs other than marijuana or alcohol. Reductions in criminal activity were maintained up to 5 years after leaving treatment.

All types of treatment did achieve statistically and clinically significant reductions for the drug usage they were designed to treat if a client stayed in a programme long enough. In multivariate analysis controlling for a variety of factors, including demographics, drug use patterns, prior treatment, and reason for seeking treatment, the risk of relapse was reduced three- to four-fold for those clients who stayed in treatment for 6 months or more, compared to those who left earlier. The authors conclude that although treatment does have a demonstrable effect, substantial improvement is needed. Programmes only attract a relatively low proportion of individuals who might benefit from treatment. Retention rates have been low, particularly for long-term treatment or continuum of care necessary. The increasingly complex problems of multiple drug usage and impairment require more trained and committed staff. Further, recovering addicts and abusers must also have access to an array of relapse prevention rehabilitation, habilitation, and support services in the community.

This research was replicated in the Drug Abuse Treatment Outcome Studies (DATOS) for a sample of 10 000 adults entering treatment between 1991 and 1993 (Flynn et al. 1997). The DATOS research in community-based treatment has replicated a number of major findings that have been consistently found in other studies. In addition to replication of major findings, the DATOS studies also found positive effects of treatment for adolescents (Hser et al. 2001) and for cocaine abusers (Simpson *et al.* 1999). The changes in behaviour and the influence of time in treatment were confirmed 5 years after termination of treatment (Hubbard *et al.* 2003), even after taking into account the characteristics of the persons and a variety of intervening events over the 5 years.

Another set of findings requires further examination, as studies have included a broader variety of programmes in complex, changing health care, social service, and criminal justice environments. There has been a broad array of programmes designed to meet the needs of substance abusers, including therapeutic community or long-term residential, outpatient drug-free, methadone, and short-term inpatient programmes. The range of options, however, appears to be diminishing, including the elimination of short-term inpatient rehabilitation and longer-term stays in therapeutic communities (Etheridge *et al.* 1997). Clients select and are selected for different modalities of treatment based on the type of drug use, the severity of related problems, and the resources to pay for treatment. Few clients are referred to methadone treatment by the criminal justice system, and increasing proportions of clients in other modalities are referred by the criminal justice system. The source of referral can result in longer stays (Joe *et al.* 1999).

The diverse modality and programme approaches to treatment can be described by the nature of core therapy for substance abuse and the comprehensive services for related problems. Over the decades of the 1970s and 1980s, core services have improved, particularly the integration of 12-step components, while comprehensive services have declined and are less likely to meet the needs of clients (Etheridge *et al.* 1997).

Treatment has been effective for the type of drug use for which it has been targeted; opioids in the 1960s and 1970s, multiple drug use in the 1980s, and cocaine in the 1990s. Stays of 90 days significantly reduce the probabilities of relapse to drug use within the first year following treatment. Involvement in self-help at least twice a week is related to further decreases in the probability of relapse to cocaine for those who stayed in treatment more than 90 days (Etheridge *et al.* 1999).

The effects of treatment (particularly time in treatment) on related problems are not as consistent, and appear to be diminishing with the erosion of comprehensive services. A 1-year stay in a therapeutic community has been consistently related to increases in the probability of post-treatment employment and decreases in the probability of illegal activity. However, the effects of treatment duration on illegal activity for methadone and outpatient drug-free clients in the follow-up year found in the 1970s–1980s have not been consistently replicated in more recent studies (Hubbard *et al.* 1997).

Economic analyses of benefits and costs consistently show that treatments in therapeutic communities, methadone, and outpatient drug-free treatment generate benefits in crime reduction during and after treatment that more than pay for the costs of treatments (Flynn *et al.* 1999). Clients in therapeutic communities, who have the highest crime rates, generate the greatest reduction in crime costs after treatment.

The NIDA Clinical Trial Network was implemented as a response to the concerns that clinical research did not address the gaps in knowledge in actual practice. A series of over 20 trials of pharmacological and psychosocial interventions have been undertaken. The major studies to date have demonstrated efficacy of the buprenorphine detoxification regimen (Amass *et al.* 2004) in community settings, identified a feasible approach to using incentives to encourage abstinence for stimulant users (Petry *et al.* 2005), determined that manual guided motivational interviewing led to greater retention (Carroll *et al.* 2006), and determined that post-residential programme discharge phone contact with patients increased the likelihood of subsequent attendance at community-based treatment (Hubbard *et al.* 2007). The trials have also focused on interventions for injecting drug users at risk for HIV/AIDS.

HIV/AIDS among injecting drug users

Over the last several decades, HIV infection among injecting drug users (IDUs) has become a worldwide public health problem. According to the most recent estimate, there are now 13 million IDUs in the world (Aceijas *et al.* 2006), of whom over 10 million live in developing and transitional countries. HIV has been spreading rapidly among IDUs in Eastern Europe and Asia. Approximately 10 per cent of all new HIV infections worldwide are among IDUs, and approximately 30 per cent of all new HIV infections outside of sub-Saharan Africa are among IDUs (UNAIDS/WHO 2006). HIV/AIDS clearly become the most dramatic example of the many health and social problems associated with illicit drug use.

Injection of illicit psychoactive drugs does not in itself transmit HIV; rather, it is the micro-transfusions of HIV-infected blood that transmit the virus when two or more persons use the same injection equipment. It is thus possible to reduce HIV transmission among IDUs not only by reducing illicit drug injection itself, but also by reducing the instances in which two or more IDUs use the same injection equipment. The urgent need to control HIV transmission among IDUs and the possibility that HIV can be prevented in persons who continue to inject illicit drugs have led to a number of programmes that would not have been considered prior to the emergence of HIV/AIDS, and to a new public health-oriented perspective on the problems of drug misuse.

The first HIV epidemic among IDUs almost occurred in New York City during the mid-1970s (Des Jarlais *et al.* 1994). During the 1980s, HIV then spread among IDUs in the rest of the United States and in Western Europe and Australia (Ball *et al.* 1998). During the late 1980s, HIV spread to IDUs in Asia, most notably in Thailand (Des Jarlais *et al.* 1992b), and also in Latin America. The spread of HIV among IDUs continued during the 1990s, particularly in Asia, and from the mid-1990s, onwards in Russia and Eastern Europe (Ball *et al.* 1998). Given the development of this pandemic of HIV transmission among IDUs, public health officials need to plan on continued diffusion of HIV among IDUs throughout the world.

In many areas, HIV has spread extremely rapidly among IDUs, with the HIV seroprevalence rate (the percentage of IDUs infected with HIV) increasing from less than 10–50 per cent or greater within a period of 1–2 years (Des Jarlais *et al.* 1992a; Stimson *et al.* 1998). Several factors have been associated with extremely rapid transmission of HIV among IDUs. First, a lack of awareness of HIV/AIDS as a local threat can contribute to rapid spread. Without an awareness of AIDS as a local threat, IDUs are likely to use each other's equipment very frequently. Indeed, prior to an awareness of HIV/AIDS, providing previously used equipment to another IDU is likely to be seen as an act of solidarity among IDUs, or as a service for which one may legitimately charge a small fee.

Second, situations that promote 'rapid partner change' among persons who share needles and syringes contribute to rapid transmission.

Not all types of sharing of injection equipment will lead to rapid transmission of HIV within population of IDUs. Rapid transmission requires sharing within settings that permit IDUs to share with large numbers of other IDUs within short time periods (rapid risk partner change). 'Shooting galleries' (places where IDUs can rent injection equipment, which is then returned to the gallery owner for rental to other IDUs) and 'dealer's works' (injection equipment kept by a drug seller, which can be lent to successive drug purchasers) are examples of situations that provide rapid, efficient mixing within an IDU population. 'Hit doctors', who administer injections to IDUs who have trouble injecting themselves, may use the same needle and syringe for many different clients. In these situations, many different IDUs may share the same needle and syringe within a short time period. Sharing in these types of settings can spread HIV across potential social boundaries, such as friendship groups, which otherwise might have served to limit transmission.

Third, persons who are recently infected with HIV ('acute HIV infection') also tend to be highly infectious (Wawer *et al.* 2005). This increases the possibility of extremely rapid HIV transmission if the virus should enter an IDU population structured to produce rapid partner change syringe sharing.

At present, there is no vaccine to prevent HIV infection. There is effective treatment to manage HIV infection, but this treatment is expensive, does not cure infection, and drug resistance frequently develops. Thus, while it is very important to provide treatment for HIV-infected IDUs, public health efforts to reduce morbidity and mortality related to HIV among IDUs must focus on modifying the risk behaviour of IDUs. We will review current knowledge of HIV prevention programmes for IDUs. In doing so, it will be useful to provide some historical context on the evolution of these efforts.

Early risk reduction among IDUs

The first evidence that IDUs would change their risk behaviour in response to information about AIDS came from several studies in New York City (Des Jarlais *et al.* 1985; Friedman *et al.* 1987; Selwyn *et al.* 1987). This risk reduction occurred due to the implementation of formal HIV prevention programmes for IDUs in the city. In all of these studies, the majority of drug users reported that they knew about AIDS, that they knew that it was transmitted through the sharing of needles and syringes, and that they had already made at least some changes in their injection behaviour (e.g. reduced sharing of injection equipment).

IDUs in New York had learned about AIDS through the mass media and through their own oral communication networks. Because of the relatively large number of cases of AIDS among IDUs in New York City, even in the early 1980s, there had been a considerable amount of mass media coverage. The relatively large number of cases of AIDS among IDUs in New York also meant that a substantial number of IDUs either knew someone first-hand who had developed AIDS, or knew someone who knew someone who had developed AIDS. An additional potentially important factor in this early behaviour change/risk reduction was the expansion of the illicit market in sterile injection equipment (Des Jarlais *et al.* 1985).

While early studies indicated that IDUs would learn about AIDS from the mass media and through oral communication networks, it became clear by the mid-1980s that there would be many additional advantages to having health workers provide face-to-face AIDS education for IDUs. Face-to-face education would permit transmitting more detailed information, using culturally appropriate terminology (that might not have been possible in mass media), answering any questions that the drug users might have, and adopting an emotional tone responsive to the IDUs participating in the immediate communication.

It is possible to provide AIDS education for drug users in drug abuse treatment programmes, and many treatment programmes did develop AIDS education efforts (Des Jarlais *et al.* 1992c). With the great majority of drug users, however, various types of 'community outreach' programmes were developed to provide AIDS education to active drug users. The earliest programmes were in New Jersey (Jackson & Rotkiewicz 1987) and San Francisco (Watters 1994). Outreach programmes have since become a primary method for preventing HIV transmission among IDUs in most countries throughout the world. Outreach programmes have become increasingly sophisticated in terms of the theories utilized to lead to risk reduction, the use of former or current drug users as health outreach workers, and provision of the means for behaviour change (sterile needles and syringes for safer drug injection and condoms for safer sexual behaviour).

Using psychological theories of health-related behaviour to prevent HIV among IDUs

While the earliest studies did show an effect of providing 'education' about AIDS in changing HIV risk behaviour among IDUs, it was also clear that simple 'information-only' prevention programmes were not likely to be very strong in producing long-term behaviour change. Knowledge of possible adverse consequences is rarely sufficient to change behaviour in the health field.

Various theories of health-related behaviour, including the Health Belief model (Becker & Joseph 1988), social learning theory (Bandura 1977), and the theory of reasoned action (Fishbein & Ajzen 1975) have been utilized in programmes. While there are differences among these theories, there are also more important similarities. All include elements of expectancy-value decision-making analyses. Thus, these theories tend to emphasize perceived probabilities (of getting or avoiding AIDS, of being able to successfully perform new behaviours) and subjective valuations of different outcomes (the seriousness of developing AIDS, social costs of performing new behaviours if one's injecting or sexual partners are resistant). With some variation in explicitness, these theories also consider social factors (role models, perceived social norms) and various 'barriers' to changing HIV risk behaviours.

Utilizing these psychological theories of health behaviour required more than the one-way communication possible in mass-media approaches and more than the usually brief conversations that occur between outreach programme workers and IDUs encountered in the streets. The National AIDS Demonstration Research/AIDS Targeted Outreach Model programme began in the United States in 1987, and eventually included 41 projects in nearly 50 different cities (Brown & Beschner 1993). In all of the cities, the NADR/ATOM project involved street outreach to IDUs not in treatment programmes. The eligibility requirements for subjects to be enrolled in the research component of the NADR/ATOM projects required that the person must have injected illicit drugs in the previous 6 months and must not have been in drug abuse treatment in the preceding month. Approximately 40 per cent of the more than 30 000 subjects enrolled in the NADR/ATOM projects reported that they had never been in drug abuse treatment. Many of the NADR/ATOM projects used experimental designs to test psychological theories of health behaviour change. All subjects were provided with a 'standard' intervention to reduce HIV risk behaviour, which included information about HIV and AIDS, a baseline risk assessment, and the option of HIV counselling and testing. Some of these subjects were then randomly assigned to an 'enhanced' condition that typically involved several additional hours of counselling/education/skills-training that incorporated components of the psychological theories of health behaviour. Subjects were followed at 6-month intervals to assess changes in HIV risk behaviours and the incidence of new HIV infections.

The NADR/ATOM projects provided a wealth of data about HIV risk behaviours among IDUs not in drug treatment programmes. With respect to changes in HIV risk behaviours, there were two strong and very consistent findings. First, almost all of the NADR/ATOM projects showed substantial reductions in injection risk behaviour from the baseline assessment to the follow-up interviews. For example, those reporting sharing needles declined from 54 to 23 per cent (Stephens et al. 1993).

The second consistent finding was that almost none of the different projects showed significant differences in risk reduction between the 'standard' intervention and the 'enhanced' interview. The general lack of differences between the 'standard' and the 'enhanced' interventions should not be interpreted as meaning that the psychological theories of health behaviour are not relevant to HIV risk reduction among IDUs; rather, these results suggest two other possible explanations. First, after provision of basic information about AIDS (as in the standard intervention), 2–8 h of additional education and counselling does little to further 'strengthen' anti-AIDS attitudes, perceptions and intentions.

A second explanation is that risk reduction among IDUs—again, after basic HIV/AIDS education—is primarily a function of social processes rather than the characteristics of individual IDUs.

Using social network theories to prevent HIV among IDUs

There is increasing evidence that social network processes, particularly peer influences, are important in HIV risk reduction among IDUs (Des Jarlais et al. 1994; Neaigus et al. 1994; Latkin et al. 1996). Almost all injection risk behaviours (sharing of injection equipment) and all sexual risk behaviours occur within social settings. Initiating and maintaining safer injection and sexual behaviours may require changes in the social relationships among IDUs and their sexual partners.

In an analysis of factors associated with risk reduction among IDUs in four of the cities (Bangkok, Glasgow, Rio de Janeiro, and New York City) participating in the World Health Organization's Multi-Centre Study of AIDS and Drug Injection, 'talking with drug-using friends' was significantly associated with risk reduction in all four cities (Des Jarlais et al. 1993a). Despite the substantial variation in the drugs injected in these cities (heroin in Bangkok, heroin and buprenorphine in Glasgow, cocaine in Rio de Janeiro, and heroin and cocaine in New York) and the obvious cultural differences

among IDUs in these cities, peer influence appeared to be an important component of risk reduction in all four cities.

Several of the NADR/ATOM models explicitly focused on peer influence and social change processes. The Chicago project (Wiebel et al. 1996) had its origins in the long tradition of ethnography, community research, and outreach to drug users by researchers at the University of Chicago. In this particular project, ex-addicts, under the supervision of trained ethnographers, conducted outreach for IDUs not in treatment. Specific efforts were made to enrol influential persons (indigenous leaders) within drug use networks into the project and have them act to influence other IDUs to practice safer injection. This project thus utilized the naturally occurring network structure among IDUs to change HIV risk behaviours. A cohort research design was used, with subjects followed for 5 years. The subjects reported dramatic reductions in injection risk behaviour. At the start of the project, 95 per cent of subjects reported engaging in injection risk behaviour, and this declined to only 15 per cent of the subjects reporting injection risk behaviour in the 5th year of the study. There was also a significantly lower HIV incidence among the IDUs who received the indigenous leader prevention compared to HIV incidence among IDUs who lived in a different neighbourhood and did not receive the intervention (Wiebel 1993).

One of the New York City NADR projects involved 'self-organization' among IDUs (Friedman et al. 1992, 1993). The Dutch 'Junkie Bonds'—one of which had initiated the first syringe-exchange programme in Holland—served as a model for how IDUs can act together to further their own health interests. In the New York City project, outreach workers recruited IDUs and assisted them in developing self-help groups to address HIV transmission and other issues of importance to them. In particular, the subgroup of commercial sex workers among IDUs had a number of common interests. Regular group meetings were held to discuss how the participants could change peer norms of injection and sexual risk behaviours. Attending the meetings was strongly associated with both the subjects' own risk reduction and efforts to change the behaviour of other IDUs (Friedman et al. 1993).

Broadhead and colleagues (1998) developed a 'peer-driven' outreach programme for IDUs. Individual IDUs are recruited into the study and provided with AIDS education. These initial subjects are then asked to recruit other IDUs into the study, and paid modest stipends for their recruiting efforts. The initial subjects are asked not only to recruit new subjects, but also to provide AIDS education to the new subjects. An AIDS information test is given to each of the peer-recruited subjects, and if the newly recruited subject passes the test, the original subject who did the recruiting and educating receives an increased stipend.

Latkin and colleagues (1996) developed an AIDS risk reduction programme that utilizes naturally occurring peer networks of IDUs. Existing peer networks or single network members are brought in for multiple sessions that not only provide information about HIV and AIDS, but also attempt to develop new social norms within the peer groups. These new norms emphasize practising safer injection and safer sex. These efforts have led to substantial reductions in risk behaviours.

Social network theories do not necessarily replace 'AIDS education' and psychological theories of health-related behaviour. Knowledge of HIV infection and AIDS and how to practice safer sex and safer injection are still important, as are perceptions of risk and a sense of efficacy in practising safer behaviours. Given the continuing developments in HIV/AIDS research (such as new therapies), AIDS education must also be done on a continuing basis.

Social network theories offer important additional power for reducing HIV risk behaviours, however. Influencing others to adopt new behaviours can also serve to strengthen the intentions of prevention programme participants to change their own risk behaviours. If social norms of injection and sexual behaviour can be changed, then it will be possible to change the behaviour of IDUs who do not directly participate in the prevention programme. Finally, the peer approval that comes with following the new norms can itself serve to reinforce safer injection and safer sex practices among IDUs.

Using social structural theory to prevent HIV among IDUs

Much recent theoretical work on HIV prevention for IDUs has centred on social structural interventions (Blankenship *et al.* 2000; Des Jarlais 2000; Sumartojo & Laga 2000). Structural invention theory often includes individual and social network components, but represents a major change in the focus for interventions. The focus in structural interventions is not on changing the individual IDU (increasing knowledge, motivation, skills) or changing social networks (changing social norms), but on changing the 'risk environment' in which drug injection occurs. The main problem to be addressed is not lack of knowledge or motivation among individual IDUs or inappropriate social norms among IDUs, but rather the many societal factors make it very difficult for IDUs to practice safer behaviours. There are a number of central ideas within the broad concept of structural interventions to reduce HIV transmission among IDUs, including: (1) providing the means for safer behaviours; (2) removing barriers to practising safer behaviours; (3) 'comprehensive' interventions; and (4) the amount of 'coverage' required.

1. Providing the means for behaviour change

While knowledge, motivation, skills, and social support are all important, having access to sterile needles and syringes is necessary for practising safer injection. Syringe exchange has become the prototype programme for HIV prevention for IDUs. As the name suggests, these programmes exchange new, sterile needles and syringes for used needles and syringes. Such exchange both provides IDUs with sterile injection equipment and removes the potentially HIV-contaminated needles and syringes from the community.

The first syringe exchange was set up in the city of Amsterdam in 1984. The exchange was implemented after a large pharmacy in the city centre stopped selling needles and syringes to drug users. The exchange was actually established to prevent hepatitis B, not HIV, transmission among IDUs in the city. In 1985, the HIV antibody test became available, and it became clear that many IDUs in the city (over 30 per cent) were already infected with HIV. This led to a rapid expansion of syringe exchange in Amsterdam and implementation of syringe exchanges in many other Dutch cities (Buning *et al.* 1988). In 1987, the United Kingdom implemented a nationwide system of syringe-exchange programmes (Stimson *et al.* 1988). In 1987, France repealed its laws requiring prescriptions for the sale of sterile injection equipment and set up a programme for encouraging pharmacists to sell injection equipment to IDUs

(Espinoza *et al.* 1988; Ingold & Ingold 1989). Australia repealed its prescription requirement laws in 1984, then established a system of syringe-exchange programmes (Wodak 1995). In many European countries, such as Italy, Germany and Spain, there were no legal restrictions on the sale and possession of injection equipment, and education programmes were implemented to educate and encourage IDUs to inject with sterile equipment. Almost all of these countries have since established syringe exchange programmes as a means for providing sterile needles and syringes to IDUs (Lurie *et al.* 1993).

In the United States, there was also some early consideration of providing legal access to sterile injection equipment as a method for reducing HIV transmission among IDUs (Des Jarlais & Hopkins 1985). Early exchanges were implemented by activists in the northeast and by community-based organizations in the northwest (see Lurie *et al.* 1993; Normand *et al.* 1995 for histories of early syringe exchange efforts in the United States). There were many impediments to providing legal access to sterile injection equipment for IDUs in the United States (Des Jarlais & Friedman 1992a; Lurie *et al.* 1993; Normand *et al.* 1995; Gostin 1998). The states with large numbers of IDUs (e.g. New York, California, Illinois) had laws requiring prescriptions for the sale of injection equipment, and almost all states had laws criminalizing the possession of equipment for injecting illicit drugs.

Efforts to increase access by IDUs to sterile injection equipment, either through changing laws and/or by implementing 'underground' syringe exchanges in defiance of existing statutes, often generated intense controversy over whether this would increase illicit drug use and/or represent official 'condoning' of illicit drug use (Lurie *et al.* 1993; Normand *et al.* 1995). In some areas, racial/ethnic group antagonisms compounded the controversies (Anderson 1991). In 1989, federal legislation was enacted that prohibited the use of any federal funds to support syringe exchanges or other distribution of sterile injection equipment to persons who inject illicit drugs, and this prohibition remains in effect. Despite lack of federal funds, syringe exchange has expanded in the United States from 68 programmes in 1994 to 185 programmes in 2005 (McKnight *et al.* 2007). This expansion has occurred with funding from state, county, and local governments and from private sources.

There are now a moderately large number of studies that have used HIV infection (either incidence or trends in prevalence) as an outcome measure for assessing syringe exchange programmes. Almost all studies have shown low HIV incidence associated with syringe exchange programmes, including studies in Tacoma, WA (Hagan *et al.* 1995); Lund, Sweden (Ljungberg *et al.* 1991); Glasgow, Scotland (Frischer *et al.* 1993), the United Kingdom (Stimson *et al.* 1991; Stimson 1995), Portland, OR (Oliver *et al.* 1994); New York, NY (Des Jarlais *et al.* 1996, 2005), Seattle (Hagan & Thiede 2000), Australia (Wodak 1996), and France (Emmanuelli & Desenclos 2005; Des Jarlais *et al.* 2007). Although it is not possible to draw a direct causal connection, the expansion of syringe exchange programmes in the United States has been followed by reductions in HIV incidence among IDUs. HIV incidence is currently approximately 1/100 person-years at risk. Injecting drug use may be the only transmission category for which HIV incidence has declined over the last decade in the United States (Des Jarlais *et al.* 2005).

While the great majority of the studies of syringe exchange programmes have shown low HIV incidence associated with the programmes, there are also several studies of syringe exchange programmes that clearly did not provide sufficient protection against HIV infection for either their participants or for other IDUs in the community. In both Montreal (Bruneau *et al.* 1994) and Vancouver (Strathdee *et al.* 1997), HIV incidence exceeded 10/100 person-years at risk among syringe exchange participants. The factors that most probably led to the very high HIV incidence in Montreal and Vancouver included the exchanges attracting very high-risk drug injectors and that the supplies of sterile injection equipment were not sufficient to protect against HIV transmission within the context of very frequent cocaine injection. In response to the outbreaks of HIV among IDUs in Montreal and Vancouver, the syringe exchanges were expanded, and HIV incidence did then decline (Tyndall *et al.* 2001, 2002).

There have been a series of summary evaluations of syringe exchange programmes, including ones conducted by the United States National Commission on AIDS (1991), the United States Government Accounting Office (1993), the University of California (Lurie *et al.* 1993), and the National Academy of Science (Normand *et al.* 1995) (Gibson *et al.* 2002; Ksobiech 2003; Committee on the Prevention of HIV Infection 2006). All of these evaluations have concluded that syringe exchange programmes do lead to reductions in injection risk behaviour and do not lead to increases in illicit drug use.

2. Removing barriers to practising safer behaviours: Reducing stigmatization

Effective structural interventions require not only implementing programmes for IDUs, but removing barriers to IDUs participating in the programmes. Stigmatization of persons with (or at risk for) HIV is a critical aspect of the social environment of HIV transmission. Stigmatization can have multiple adverse consequences. First, stigmatization clearly increases the suffering of persons with HIV and AIDS. Second, stigmatization of groups at risk for or with HIV/AIDS can reduce public support for both prevention and treatment services. Third, fear of stigmatization may lead persons at risk for HIV/AIDS to avoid using the programmes that have been implemented, leading to increased transmission of HIV. Finally, members of ethnic/racial minority groups are at higher risk for HIV/AIDS in the United States and in many other countries. Stigmatization of HIV/AIDS can thus be compounded with stigmatization based on racial/ethnic minority status, increasing the multiple adverse consequences.

Stigmatization of HIV/AIDS, of illicit drug use, and of racial/ethnic minority status can all be difficult to change. However, there are important steps that can be taken. Civil rights laws clearly do not end stigmatization of racial/ethnic minorities, but such laws can reduce harmful actions based on stigmatization. The Americans with Disabilities Act (ADA) similarly prohibits discrimination based on AIDS and a history of drug use. (The ADA does not prohibit discrimination based on current drug use.) It is also possible and important to work with specific groups to reduce stigmatization of IDUs at risk for HIV/AIDS. There have been a number of projects that have worked with pharmacists to increase sales of sterile injection equipment to IDUs (Emmanuelli & Desenclos 2005; Fuller *et al.* 2007). It is also possible to work with local law enforcement agencies to reduce potential police interference with IDUs participating in HIV prevention programmes (Hammett *et al.* 2007).

3. Comprehensive programming to prevent HIV among IDUs

Structural analyses also include consideration of multiple prevention services rather than a single programme for all IDUs. Any IDU population is likely to have considerable diversity in terms of frequency of injection, frequency of needle sharing, and frequency of sexual risk behaviour. Different IDUs will also have different other issues, such as lack of stable housing, unemployment, and psychiatric problems, which may need to be addressed in order to consistently practice HIV risk reduction. Thus, no single programme is likely to be able to meet all of the needs within an IDU population. Over time, syringe exchange programmes have become multi-service organizations. In the United States and in other industrialized countries, syringe exchange programmes often provide services such as condom distribution, HIV and hepatitis C virus counselling and testing, and sexually transmitted disease screening on-site. Additional services are often provided through referrals. One critical aspect of syringe exchanges is that the great majority of the programmes provide referrals to drug abuse treatment programmes. Thus, rather than syringe exchange programmes keeping drug users from entering treatment, syringe exchange programmes have become an important linkage into drug abuse treatment (McKnight *et al.* 2007).

The most recent review of HIV prevention for IDUs emphasizes provision of sterile injection equipment within 'comprehensive programming' (Committee on the Prevention of HIV Infection 2006). This reflects both practical aspects of HIV prevention; many drug users require more than access to sterile injection equipment in order to avoid HIV infection. It also reflects a basic ethical position—that societies have an ethical obligation to address needs of drug users beyond HIV prevention; in particular, societies have an ethical obligation to provide effective treatment to reduce drug abuse.

4. The amount of 'coverage' required

Pilot programmes do not stop HIV epidemics. A critical aspect of structural interventions is having interventions that are large enough to control HIV transmission in a population of IDUs. Knowing what level of 'coverage' is needed to control HIV transmission is of obvious importance in areas with limited resources for HIV prevention. Studying the amount of 'coverage' needed, however, is difficult, and consensus among expert opinions and mathematical modelling are the two most frequently used methods of estimating coverage requirements. Coverage of sterile injection equipment for the number of injections in IDU populations has received the greatest amount of attention. The 'ideal' for HIV prevention is that each drug user would use a new, sterile needle and syringe for each injection (Des Jarlais *et al.* 1995a). Depending upon sharing patterns (sharing limited within small groups is much less likely to lead to widespread HIV transmission than sharing in large groups of IDUs) and the number of times IDUs re-use their own needles and syringes (which can lead to bacterial infections, but does not transmit HIV), the current estimate/opinion is that syringe distribution should cover about 25 per cent of injections (Vickerman *et al.* 2006).

High coverage to reduce unsafe injections does not require extremely large numbers of IDUs personally attending syringe exchange programmes or personally purchasing sterile needles and syringes at pharmacies. Rather, individual IDUs may exchange for peers ('secondary exchange') or purchase for peers who do not want to attend exchanges or purchase from pharmacies, usually because of concerns over confidentiality. Effective structural interventions need to provide for secondary exchange and purchasing for peers, and avoid artificial limits on the numbers of syringes that can be exchanged or purchased at a single visit (Des Jarlais *et al.* 1995b).

The low incidence rates in areas with syringe exchange programmes may occur through both direct and indirect effects of syringe exchanges. Participants in the exchanges receive both supplies of sterile injection equipment and counselling and information about HIV. Since syringe exchanges tend to attract IDUs who would otherwise be at very high risk for HIV infection, reducing risk behaviour among the IDUs who come to syringe exchanges can have a partial 'herd immunity' effect that protects the local IDU population as a whole. Sterile injection equipment, information about HIV, and new social norms against sharing injection equipment may also diffuse outwards from IDUs who directly participate in syringe exchange programmes to other IDUs in the community. Thus, large-scale syringe exchange programmes should probably be considered as community-level interventions whose protective effect extends beyond the IDUs who participate directly in the programmes.

New challenges

As discussed earlier, HIV prevention has been quite successful overall in industrialized countries, with incidence rates of 1/100 person-years or less in most of the countries. Certainly implementation of public health scale prevention programmes for IDUs could have been accomplished much earlier, and this would have averted thousands of HIV infections (Lurie & Drucker 1997). But injecting-related HIV transmission can now be considered under public health control in industrialized countries. The current challenges in industrialized countries concern hepatitis C virus and sexual transmission of HIV among injecting and non-injecting drug users. Hepatitis C virus (HCV) is hyperendemic among IDUs in both industrialized and developing/transitional countries, with prevalence rates of 60 to 90+ per cent (Hagan *et al.* 2007). HCV is also much more easily transmitted than HIV, and thus programmes that dramatically reduce HIV transmission may or may not be effective in controlling HCV transmission. Reduction in needle-borne HIV transmission has led to emergence of sexual transmission as the leading cause of new HIV infections among IDUs in some areas (Kral *et al.* 2001; Strathdee *et al.* 2001; Strathdee & Sherman 2003).

As noted above, however, the current predominant issue is rapid transmission of HIV among IDUs in many developing and transitional countries. An estimated one-third of incident HIV infections outside of sub-Saharan Africa are occurring among IDUs, particularly in parts of Eastern Europe and Central and Southeast Asia (UNAIDS/WHO 2006).

Harm reduction

The emergence of HIV/AIDS among IDUs has been a profound challenge to public health systems. In some areas, there was a rapid response and potential HIV epidemics among IDUs were averted. In other areas, HIV epidemics occurred before effective public health responses, but the responses eventually brought the epidemics under control, and in still other areas, HIV epidemics are occurring among IDUs without any effective public health responses.

The HIV/AIDS crisis has furthered the development of a policy framework that provides a new perspective on the use of psychoactive drugs (both licit and illicit). This perspective has generally come to be known as 'harm reduction' (Berridge 1999; Buning 1991; see *Journal of Harm Reduction*).

It may be best to present Harm Reduction in the words of its practitioners (Harm Reduction Coalition 2007 [http://www.harm-reduction.org/]).

Harm reduction is a set of practical strategies that reduce negative consequences of drug use, incorporating a spectrum of strategies from safer use to managed use to abstinence. Harm reduction strategies meet drug users 'where they're at', addressing conditions of use along with the use itself.

Because harm reduction demands that interventions and policies designed to serve drug users reflect specific individual and community needs, there is no universal definition of or formula for implementing harm reduction. However, HRC considers the following principles central to harm reduction practice.

- Accepts, for better and for worse, that licit and illicit drug use is part of our world, and chooses to work to minimize its harmful effects rather than simply ignore or condemn them.

- Understands drug use as a complex, multi-faceted phenomenon that encompasses a continuum of behaviours from severe abuse to total abstinence, and acknowledges that some ways of using drugs are clearly safer than others.

- Establishes quality of individual and community life and well-being—not necessarily cessation of all drug use—as the criteria for successful interventions and policies.

- Calls for non-judgmental, non-coercive provision of services and resources to people who use drugs and the communities in which they live in order to assist them in reducing attendant harm.

- Ensures that drug users and those with a history of drug use routinely have a real voice in the creation of programmes and policies designed to serve them.

- Affirms drugs users themselves as the primary agents of reducing the harms of their drug use, and seeks to empower users to share information and support each other in strategies that meet their actual conditions of use.

- Recognizes that the realities of poverty, class, racism, social isolation, past trauma, sex-based discrimination, and other social inequalities affect both people's vulnerability to and capacity for effectively dealing with drug-related harm.

- Does not attempt to minimize or ignore the real and tragic harm and danger associated with licit and illicit drug use.

The two basic components of harm reduction are respecting the civil rights of drug users (Gilmore 1996; Elliott 2004; Wolfe & Malinowska-Sempruch 2004) and pragmatism—doing what works. Harm reduction is thus a particularly appropriate policy framework for incorporating scientific data into public health practice (Des Jarlais 1995).

References

Aaron, P. and Musto, D. (1981). Temperance and prohibition in America: a private historical overview. In *Alcohol and public policy: beyond the shadow of prohibition* (eds. M.H. Moore and D.R. Gerstein). National Academy Press, Washington, DC.

Aceijas, C., Friedman, S.R., Cooper, H.L.F., Wiessing, L., Stimson, G.V., and Hickman, M. (2006). Estimates of injecting drug users at the national and local level in developing and transitional countries, and gender and age distribution. *Sexually Transmitted Infections*, 82 (Suppl III), iii10–7.

Amass, L., Ling, W. et al. (2004). Bringing buprenorphine-nalozone detoxification to community treatment providers: the NIDA clinical trials network field experience. *American Journal of Addictions*, 13 (Suppl 1), S42–66.

American Psychiatric Association. (1994). *Diagnostic and statistical manual of mental disorders*, 4th edn. (DSM-IV). American Psychiatric Association, Washington, DC.

Anderson, W. (1991). The New York needle trial: the politics of public health in the age of AIDS. *American Journal of Public Health*, 81, 1506–17.

Aneshensel, C.S. and Huba, G.J. (1983). Depression, alcohol use, and smoking over one year: a four-wave longitudinal causal model. *Journal of Abnormal Psychology*, 92, 134–50.

Annis, H.M. (1986). Is inpatient rehabilitation of the alcoholic cost effective, Con position. *Advances in Alcohol and Substance Abuse*, 5, 175–90.

Armor, D.J., Polich, J.M., and Stambul, H.B. (1978). *Alcoholism and treatment*. Wiley, New York.

Babor, T.E. (ed.) (1986). *Alcohol and culture: comparative perspectives from Europe and America*. New York Academy of Sciences, New York.

Babor, T., Cooney, N., Hubbard, R. et al. (1988). The syndrome concept of alcohol and drug dependence: results of the secondary analysis project. In *Problems of drug dependence, 1987. Proceedings of the 49th Annual Scientific Meeting, The Committee on Problems of Drug Dependence, Inc.* Research Monograph Series 81 (ed. L.S. Harris). National Institute on Drug Abuse, Rockville.

Bachman, J.G., O'Malley, P.M., and Johnston, L.D. (1978). *Youth in transition Vol. VI: adolescence to adulthood—change and stability in the lives of young men*. Institute for Social Research, University of Michigan, Ann Arbor.

Bale, R.N., Van Stone, W., Kuldau, J.M., Engelsing, T.M.J., Elashoff, R.M., and Zarcone, V.P. (1980). Therapeutic communities vs. methadone maintenance. *Archives of General Psychiatry*, 37, 179–93.

Ball, A.L., Rana, S. et al. (1998). HIV prevention among injecting drug users: responses in developing and transitional countries. *Public Health Reports*, 113 (Suppl 1), 170–181.

Bandura, A. (1977). *Social learning theory*. Englewood; Prentice-Hall, Englewood Cliffs.

Becker, M.H. and Joseph, J.K. (1988). AIDS and behavioral change to reduce risk: a review. *American Journal of Public Health*, 78, 394–410.

Berridge, V. (1992). *Harm reduction: an historical perspective*. 3rd International Conference on Reduction of Drug-Related Harm, Melbourne.

Berridge, V. (1999). Histories of harm reduction: illicit drugs, tobacco, and nicotine. *Substance Use & Misuse*, 34, 35–47.

The Betty Ford Institute Consensus Panel (2007). What is recovery? A working definition from the Betty Ford Institute. *Journal of Substance Treatment*, 33, 221–8.

Blankenship, K., Bray, S., and Merson, M. (2000). Structural interventions in public health. *AIDS*, 14, S11–21.

Botvin, G.J. (1983). Prevention of adolescent substance abuse through the development of personal and social competence. In *Preventing adolescent drug abuse: intervention strategies* (eds. T.J. Glynn, C.G. Leukefeld, and J.P. Ludford), pp. 115–40. Research Monograph 47. National Institute on Drug Abuse, Rockville.

Brecher, E.M. and the Editors of Consumer Reports (1972). *Licit and illicit drugs: the Consumers Union report on narcotics, stimulants, depressants, inhalants, hallucinogens, and marijuana—including caffeine, nicotine, and alcohol*. Consumers Union, Mount Vernon.

Broadhead, R.S., Heckathorn, D.D. et al. (1998). Harnessing peer networks as an instrument for AIDS prevention: results from a peer driven intervention. *Public Health Reports*, 113 (Suppl 1), 42–57.

Brown, B.S. and Beschner, G.M. (eds.) (1993). *Handbook on risk of AIDS: injection drug users and sexual partners*. Greenwood Press, Wesport.

Bruneau, J., Lamothe, E, Lachance, N., Soto, J., and Vincelette, J. (1994). *HIV prevalence and incidence in a cohort of IDUs in Montreal, according to their needle exchange attendance, Abstract PD0496*. Presented at the Tenth International Conference on AIDS, Yokohama.

Brunswick, A.F. and Boyle, J.M. (1979). Patterns of drug involvement: developmental and secular influences on age at initiation. *Youth and Society*, 2, 139–62.

Bry, B.H. (1983). Empirical foundations of family-based approaches to adolescent substance abuse. In *Preventing adolescent drug abuse: intervention strategies* (eds. T.J. Glynn, C.G. Leukefeld, and J.P. Ludford), pp. 154–71. Research Monograph 47, National Institute on Drug Abuse, Rockville.

Buning, E.C. (1991). Effects of Amsterdam needle and syringe exchange. *International Journal of Addictions*, 26, 1303–11.

Buning, E.C., van Brussel, G.H.A. et al. (eds.) (1988). *Amsterdam's drug policy and its implications for controlling needle sharing. Needle sharing among intravenous drug abusers: national and international drug perspectives*. Research Monograph, National Institute on Drug Abuse, Rockville.

Cacciola, J. and Woody, G.E. (2005). Evaluation and early treatment. In *Substance abuse: a comprehensive textbook* (eds. J.H. Lowinson, P.Ruiz, R.B. Millman, and J.G. Langrod), pp. 559–63. Lippincott Williams & Wilkins, Philadelphia.

Carroll, K.M., Ball, S.A., Nich, C. et al. (2006). Motivational interviewing to improve treatment engagement and outcome in individuals seeking treatment for substance abuse: a multisite effectiveness study. *Drug and Alcohol Dependence*, 81, 301–12.

Chaisson, R.E., Osmond, D., Moss, A.R., Feldman, H.W., and Biernacki, P. (1987). HIV, bleach and needle sharing (letter). *Lancet*, 1, 1430.

Clayton, R.R. (1985). Cocaine use in the United States: in a blizzard or just being snowed? In *Cocaine use in America: epidemiologic and clinical perspectives* (eds. N.J. Kozel and E.H. Adams), pp. 8–34. Research Monograph Series 61, National Institute on Drug Abuse, Rockville.

Cloninger, R., Bohman, M., and Sigvardsson, S. (1981). Inheritance of alcohol abuse. *Archives of General Psychiatry*, 38, 861–8.

Committee on the Prevention of HIV Infection among Injecting Drug Users in High Risk Countries. (2006). *Preventing HIV infection among injecting drug users in high risk countries: an assessment of the evidence*. Institute of Medicine, Washington, DC.

Community Epidemiology Work Group. (2007). *Proceedings of the Community Epidemiology Work Group, January 2007*. National Institute on Drug Abuse, Rockville.

Cook, C.C.H. (1988). The Minnesota model in the management of drug and alcohol dependency: miracle, method, or myth? Part I. The philosophy and the programme. *British Journal of Addiction*, 83, 625–34.

Day, N.A., Houston-Hamilton, A., Deslondes, J., and Nelson, M. (1988). Potential for HIV dissemination by a cohort of black intravenous drug users. *Journal of Psychoactive Drugs*, 179–226.

DeLeon, G. (1984). *The therapeutic community: study of effectiveness*. National Institute on Drug Abuse, Rockville.

Des Jarlais, D.C. (1997). *Fifteen years of research on HIV and injecting drug use*. Fourth Science Forum: Research Synthesis Symposium on the Prevention of HIV in Drug Abusers., Flagstaff.

Des Jarlais, D.C. (2000). Structural Interventions to reduce HIV transmission among injecting drug users. *AIDS*, 14, S41–6.

Des Jarlais, D.C. and Hopkins, W. (1985). "Free" needles for intravenous drug users at risk for AIDS: current developments in New York City. *New England Journal of Medicine*, 313(23), 1476.

Des Jarlais, D.C. and Friedman, S.R. (1988). HIV infection among persons who inject illicit drugs: problems and prospects. *Journal of Acquired Immune Deficiency Syndromes*, 1, 267–73.

Des Jarlais, D.C. and Friedman, S.R. (1992a). The AIDS epidemic and legal access to sterile equipment for injecting illicit drugs. *Annals of the American Academy of Political and Social Science*, **521**, 42–65.

Des Jarlais, D.C. and Friedman, S.R. (1992b). AIDS prevention programs for intravenous drug users. In *AIDS and other manifestations of HIV infection.* (ed. G.P. Wormser) (2nd edn), pp. 645–j8. Raven Press, New York.

Des Jarlais, D.C., Friedman, S.R. et al. (1985). Risk reduction for the acquired immunodeficiency syndrome among intravenous drug users. *Annals of Internal Medicine*, **103**, 755–9.

Des Jarlais, D.C., Friedman, S.R., and Strug, D. (1986). AIDS and needle sharing within the intravenous drug use subculture. In *The social dimensions of AIDS: methods and theory* (eds. D. Feldman and T. Johnson), pp. 111–25. Praeger, New York.

Des Jarlais, D.C., Friedman, S.R., Novick, D. et al. (1989). HIV-1 infection among intravenous drug users in Manhattan. *Journal of the American Medical Association*, **261**, 1008–12.

Des Jarlais, D.C., Choopanya, K. et al. (1992a). Risk reduction and stabilization of HIV seroprevalence among drug injectors in New York City and Bangkok, Thailand. In *Science challenging AIDS.* (eds. G.B. Rossi, E. Beth-Giraldo, L. Chieco-Bianchi et al.), pp. 207–13. Karger, Basel.

Des Jarlais, D.C., Friedman, S.R. et al. (1992b). International epidemiology of HIV and AIDS among injecting drug users. *AIDS*, **6**, 1053–68.

Des Jarlais, D.C., Friedman, S.R., and Sotheran, J.L. (1992c). The first city: HIV among intravenous drug users in New York City. In *AIDS: the making of a chronic disease.* (eds. E. Fee and D. M. Fox), pp. 279–95. University of California Press, Berkeley.

Des Jarlais, D.C., Choopanya, K. et al. (1993a). Cross-cultural similarities in AIDS risk reduction among injecting drug users. 9th International Conference on AIDS, Berlin.

Des Jarlais, D.C., Friedman, S.R. et al. (1993b). Harm reduction: a public health response to the AIDS epidemic among injecting drug users. *Annual Review of Public Health*, **14**, 413–50.

Des Jarlais, D.C., Friedman, S.R. et al. (1994). Continuity and change within an HIV epidemic: injecting drug users in New York City, 1984 through 1992. *Journal of the American Medical Association*, **271**(2), 121–7.

Des Jarlais, D.C., Hagan, H.H., Friedman, S.R. et al. (1995a). Maintaining low HIV seroprevalence in populations of injecting drug users. *Journal of the American Medical Association*, **274**, 1226–31.

Des Jarlais, D.C., Paone, D., Friedman, S.R., Peyser, N., and Newman, R.G. (1995b). Regulating controversial programs for unpopular people: methadone maintenance and syringe exchange programs. *American Journal of Public Health*, **85**, 1577–84.

Des Jarlais, D.C., Marmor, M. et al. (1996). HIV incidence among injecting drug users in New York City syringe-exchange programmes. *The Lancet*, **348**, 987–91.

Des Jarlais, D.C., Perlis,T.P., Arasteh, K. et al. (2005). HIV incidence among injection drug users in New York City, 1990 to 2002: use of serologic test algorithm to assess expansion of HIV prevention services. *American Journal of Public Health*, **95**, 1439–44.

Des Jarlais, D.C., Kling, R., Hammett, T.M., Ngu, D., Liu, W., Chen, Y., Thanh Binh, K., and Friedmann, P. (2007). Reducing HIV infection among new injecting drug users in the China-Vietnam Cross Border Project. *AIDS*, **21** (Suppl 8), S109–14.

Dole, V.P. and Joseph, H. (1978). Long-term outcome of patients treated with methadone maintenance. *Annals of the New York Academy of Sciences*, **311**, 181–9.

Edwards, G., Gross, M.M., Keller, M., and Moser, J. (1976). Alcohol-related problems in the disability perspective. *Journal of Studies on Alcohol*, **37**, 1360.

Edwards, G., Arif, A., and Hodgson, R. (1981). Nomenclature and classification of drug and alcohol related problems: a WHO memorandum. *Bulletin of the World Health Organization*, **59**, 225.

Elliott, R. (2004). Drug control, human rights, and harm reduction in the age of AIDS. *HIV/AIDS Policy & Law Review*, **9**, 86–90.

Elliott, D.S., Huizinga, D., and Ageton, S.S. (1985). *Explaining delinquency and drug use.* Sage, Beverly Hills.

Emmanuelli, J. and Desenclos, J.C. (2005). Harm reduction interventions, behaviours and associated health outcomes in France, 1996–2003. *Addiction*, **100**(11), 1690–700.

Espinoza, P., Bouchard, I., Ballian, P., and Polo DeVoto, J. (1988). *Has the open sale of syringes modified the syringe exchanging habits of drug addicts.* Abstract 8522. Presented at the Fourth International Conference on AIDS. 12–16 June, Stockholm, Sweden.

Etheridge, R.M., Hubbard, R.L., Anderson, J., Craddock, S.G., and Flynn, P.M. (1997). Treatment structure and program services in the Drug Abuse Treatment Outcome Study (DATOS). *Psychology of Addictive Behaviors*, **11**(4), 244–60.

Etheridge, R.M., Craddock, S.G., Hubbard, R.L., and Rounds-Bryant, J.L. (1999). The relationship of counseling and self-help participation to patient outcomes in DATOS. *Drug and Alcohol Dependence*, **57**, 99–112.

Farrington, D.P. (1985). Predicting self-reported and official delinquency. In *Prediction in criminology* (eds. D.P. Farrington and R. Tarling), pp. 150–73. State University of New York Press, Albany.

Fishbein, M. and Ajzen, I. (1975*). Belief, attitude, intention and behavior.* Addison-Wesley, Reading.

Flay, B.R. and Sobel, J.L. (1983). The role of mass media in preventing adolescent substance abuse. In *Preventing adolescent drug abuse: intervention strategies.* (eds. T.J. Glynn, C.G. Leukefeld, and J.P. Ludford), pp. 535. Research Monograph 47, National Institute on Drug Abuse, Rockville.

Flynn, P.M., Craddock, S.G., Hubbard, R.L., Anderson, J., and Etheridge, R.M. (1997). Methodological overview and research design for the Drug Abuse Treatment Outcome Study (DATOS). *Psychology of Addictive Behaviors*, **11**, 230–47.

Flynn, P.M., Kristiansen, P.L., Porto, J.V., and Hubbard, R.L. (1999). Costs and benefits of treatment for cocaine addiction in DATOS. *Drug and Alcohol Dependence*, **57**, 167–74.

Friedman, S.R., Des Jarlais, D.C., Sotheran, J.L., Garbar, J., Cohen, G., and Smith, D. (1987). AIDS and self-organization among intravenous drug users. *International Journal of Addictions*, **22**, 201–9.

Friedman, S.R., Des Jarlais, D.C. et al. (1992). Organizing drug injectors against AIDS: preliminary data on behavioral outcomes. *Psychology of Addictive Behaviors*, **6**(2), 100–6.

Friedman, S.R., de Jong, W. et al. (1993). Community development as a response to HIV among drug injectors. *AIDS*, S263–9.

Friedman, S.R., Jose, B., Deren, S., Des Jarlais, D.C., Neaigus, A., and the National AIDS Research Consortium (1995). Risk factors for HIV seroconversion among out-of treatment drug injector in high and low seroprevalence cities. *American Journal of Epidemiology*, **142**, 864–74.

Frischer, M., Des Jarlais, D.C. et al. (1993). Modeling AIDS awareness and behavior change among IDUs in Glasgow and New York. 9th International Conference on AIDS, Berlin.

Fuller, R.K., Branchey, L., Brightwell, D.R. et al. (1986). Disulfiram treatment of alcoholism. *Journal of the American Medical Association*, **245**, 1449–55.

Fuller, C.M., Galea, S., Caceres, W., Blaney, S., Sisco, S., and Vlahov, D. (2007). Multilevel community-based intervention to increase access to sterile syringes among injection drug users through pharmacy sales in New York City. *American Journal of Public Health*, **97**, 117–24.

Gibson, D.R., Brand, B., Anderson, K., Kahn, J.G., Perales, D., and Guydish, J. (2002). Two- to sixfold decreased odds HIV risk behavior associated with use of syringe programs. *Journal of Acquired Immune Deficiency Syndromes*, **31**, 237–42.

Gilmore, N. (1996). Drug use and human rights: privacy, vulnerability, disability, and human rights infringements. *Journal of Drug Policy*, **14**, 155–69.

Goodstadt, M.S. (1980). Drug education—a turn on or a turn off? *Journal of Drug Education*, **10**, 89–93.

Goodstadt, M.S. (1981). Planning and evaluation of alcohol education programs. *Journal of Alcohol and Drug Education*, **26**, 1–10.

Goodwin, D.W. (1985). Alcoholism and genetics: the sins of the fathers. *Archives of General Psychiatry*, **6**, 171–4.

Gorsuch, R.L., Abbamonte, M., and Sells, S.B. (1976). Evaluation of treatments for drug users in the DARP: 1971–1972 admissions. In *The effectiveness of drug abuse treatment, Vol. 4. Evaluation of treatment outcomes for the 1971-1972 Admission Cohort* (eds. S.B. Sells and D.D. Simpson). Ballinger, Cambridge.

Gostin, L. (1998). The legal environment impeding access to sterile syringes and needles: the conflict between law enforcement and public health. *Journal of Acquired Immune Deficiency Syndromes and Human Retrovirology*, **18**(1), S60–70.

Grant, B.E., Harford, T.C., Chou, P. *et al.* (1991). Epidemiologic Bulletin No. 27: prevalence of DSM-III-R alcohol abuse and dependence: United States, 1988. *Alcohol Health Research*, **15**(1), 91–6.

Greenspan, S.I. (1985). Research strategies to identify developmental vulnerabilities for drug abuse. In *Etiology of drug abuse: implication for prevention* (eds. C.L. Jones and R.J. Battles). National Institute on Drug Abuse, Rockville.

Hagan, H., Des Jarlais, D.C. *et al.* (1995). Reduced risk of hepatitis B and hepatitis C among injecting drug users participating in the Tacoma syringe exchange program. *American Journal of Public Health*, **85**(11), 1531–7.

Hagan, H., McGough, J. *et al.* (1999). Syringe exchange and risk of infection with hepatitis B and C viruses. *American Journal of Epidemiology*, **49**(3), 203–13.

Hagan, H. and Thiede, H. (2000). Changes in injection risk behavior associated with participation in the Seattle needle-exchange program. *Journal of Urban Health*, **77**, 369–82.

Hagan, H., Des Jarlais, D.C., Stern, R., Lelutiu-Weinberger, C., Scheinmann, R., Strauss, S., and Flom, P.L. (2007). HCV synthesis project: preliminary analyses of HCV prevalence in relation to age and duration of injection. *International Journal of Drug Policy*, **18**, 341–51.

Hammett, T.M., Wu, Z., Duc, T.T., Stephens, D., Sullivan, S., Liu, W., Chen, Y., Ngu, D., and Des Jarlais, D.C. (2007). 'Social Evils' and harm reduction: the evolving policy environment for human immunodeficiency virus prevention among injection drug users in China and Vietnam. *Addiction*, **103**, 137–45.

Hanson, D. (1980). Drug education: does it work? In *Drugs and the youth culture* (eds. E Scarpitti and S. Batesman). Sage, Beverly Hills.

Hanzo, C., Chatterjee, A. *et al.* (1997). Reaching out beyond the hills: HIV prevention among injecting drug users in Manipur, India. *Addiction*, **92**(7), 813–20.

Harm Reduction Coalition. (2007). *Harm Reduction Coalition Website*. Retrieved 2007 (http://www.harmreduction.org/).

Harwood, H.J., Napolitano, D.M., Kristiansen, P.L., and Collins, J.J. (1984). *Economic costs to society of alcohol and drug abuse and mental illness: 1980*. Research Triangle Institute, Research Triangle Park.

Hawkins, J.D., Lishner, D.M., and Catalano, R.F. (1985). Childhood predictors and the prevention of adolescent substance abuse. In *Etiology of drug abuse: implications for prevention. Research Monograph 56* (eds. C.L. Jones and R.J. Battjes). National Institute on Drug Abuse, Rockville.

Hawkins, J.D., Lishner, D.M., Jenson, J.M., and Catalano, R.F. (1987). Delinquents and drugs: what the evidence suggests about prevention and treatment programming. In *Youth at risk for substance abuse* (eds. B.S. Brown and A.R. Mills), pp. 81–133. National Institute on Drug Abuse, Rockville.

Heather, N., Wodak, A. *et al.* (eds.) (1993). *Psychoactive drugs and harm reduction: from faith to science*. Whurr, London.

Hewitt, L.E. and Blane, H.T. (1984). Prevention through mass media communication. In *Prevention of alcohol abuse* (eds. P.M. Miller and T.D. Nirenberg), pp. 281–323. Plenum Press, New York.

Hilton, M.E. and Clark, W.B. (1987). Changes in American drinking patterns and problems, 1967–1984. *Journal of Studies in Alcohol*, **48**, 515–22.

Hoffman, N.G. and Harrison, P.A. (1987). *Chemical abuse treatment outcome registry, 1986 report: findings two years after treatment*. Comprehensive Assessment and Treatment Outcome Research (CATOR), St Paul.

Holder, H.D. and Blose, J.O. (1986). Alcohol treatment and total health care utilization and costs. *Journal of the American Medical Association*, **256**, 1456–60.

Holland, S. (1982). *Residential drug-free programs for substance abusers: the effect of planned duration on treatment*. Gateway Houses, Chicago.

Hser, Y., Grella, C.E., Hubbard, R.L., Hsieh, S.C., Fletcher, B.W., Brown, B.S., and Anglin, M.D. (2001). An evaluation of drug treatment for adolescents in four U.S. cities. *Archives of General Psychiatry*, **58**(7), 689–95.

Huba, G., Wingard, J., and Bentler, P. (1980). Applications of a theory of drug use to prevention programs. *Journal of Drug Education*, **10**, 25–38.

Hubbard, R.L., Bray, R.M., and Craddock, S.G. (1986). Issues in the assessment of multiple drug use among drug treatment clients. In *Strategies for research on drugs of abuse* (eds. M. Braude and H.M. Ginzburg), pp. 15–40. National Institute on Drug Abuse, Rockville.

Hubbard, R.L., Brownlee, R.F, and Anderson, R. (1988). Initiation of alcohol and drug abuse in the middle school years. *Elementary School and Guidance Counselling*, **23**, 118–23.

Hubbard, R.L., Marsden, M.E., Rachal, J.V., Harwood, H.J. Cavanaugh, E.R., and Ginzburg, H.M. (1989). *Drug abuse treatment: a national study of effectiveness*. UNC Press, Chapel Hill.

Hubbard, R.L., Craddock, S.G., Flynn, P.M., Anderson, J., and Etheridge, R.M. (1997). Overview of 1-year follow-up outcomes in the Drug Abuse Treatment Outcome Study (DATOS). *Psychology of Addictive Behaviors*, **11**(4), 261–78.

Hubbard, R.L., Craddock, S.G., and Anderson, J. (2003). Overview of 5-year follow-up outcomes in the Drug Abuse Treatment Outcome Studies (DATOS). *Journal of Substance Abuse Treatment*, **25**(3), 125–34.

Hubbard, R.L., Simpson, D.D., and Woody, G. (2008). *Journal of Drug Issues: Special Issue*.

Ingold, E.R. and Ingold, S. (1989). The effects of the liberalization of syringe sales on the behavior of intravenous drug users in France. *Bulletin on Narcotics*, **41**, 67–81.

Institute of Medicine, Committee to Identify Research Effectiveness in the Prevention and Treatment of Alcohol Related Problems (1989). *Prevention and treatment of alcohol problems*. National Academy Press, Washington, DC.

Jackson, J. and Rotkiewicz, L. (1987). *A coupon program: AIDS education and drug treatment*. Third International Conference on AIDS, Washington, DC.

Jaffe, J.H. (1979). The swinging pendulum: the treatment of drug users in America. In *Handbook on drug abuse* (eds. R.L. DuPont, A. Goldstein, and J. O'Donnell), pp. 3–16. National Institute on Drug Abuse, Rockville.

Jessor, R., Chase, J.A., and Donovan, J.E. (1980). Psychosocial correlates of marijuana use and problem drinking in a national sample of adolescents. *American Journal of Public Health*, **70**, 604–13.

Joe, G.W., Simpson, D.D., and Broome, K.M. (1999). Retention and patient engagement models for different treatment modalities in DATOS. *Drug and Alcohol Dependence*, **57**, 113–25.

Johnston, L.D., O'Malley, P.M., and Eveland, L. (1978). Drugs and delinquency: a search for causal connections. In *Longitudinal research on drug use. Empirical findings and methodological issues* (ed. D. Kandel), pp. 137–56. Wiley, New York.

Johnston, L.D., O'Malley, P.M., and Bachman, J.G. (1984). *Highlights from drugs and American high school students 1975–1983*. National Institute on Drug Abuse, Rockville.

Johnston, L.D., O'Malley, P.M., and Bachman, J.G. (1989). *Drug use, drinking, and smoking: national survey of results from high school, college, and young adult populations.* National Institute on Drug Abuse, Rockville.

Johnston, L.D., O'Malley, P.M., and Bachman, J.G. (1999). *National survey results on drug use from the monitoring the future study, 1975–1998, Vol. I: secondary school students (NIH Publication No. 99-4660).* National Institute on Drug Abuse, Rockville.

Johnston, L.D., O'Malley, P.M., Bachman, J.G., and Schulenberg, J.E. (2005). *Monitoring the future national survey results on drug use, 1975–2004. Vol. 1: secondary school students (NIH Publication No. 05-5727).* National Institute on Drug Abuse, Bethesda.

Kandel, D.B. (1980). Drug and drinking behavior among youth. *Annual Review of Sociology*, **6**, 235–85.

Kandel, D.B. (1982). Epidemiological and psychosocial perspectives on adolescent drug use. *Journal of American Academy of Clinical Psychiatry*, **21**, 328–47.

Kandel, D.B. and Logan, J.A. (1984). Patterns of drug use from adolescence to young adulthood: I. Periods of risk for initiation, continued use, and discontinuation. *American Journal of Public Health*, **74**, 660–6.

Kandel, D.B. and Raveis, V.H. (1989). Cessation of illicit drug use in young adulthood. *Archives of General Psychiatry*, **46**, 109–16.

Kandel, D.B., Kessler, R., and Margulies, R. (1978). Antecedents of adolescents' initiation into stages of drug use: a developmental analysis. In *Longitudinal Research in drug use: empirical findings and methodological issues* (ed. D.B. Kandel), pp. 73–99. Hemisphere-Wiley, Washington, DC.

Kandel, D.B., Simcha-Fagan, O., and Davies, M. (1986). Risk factors for delinquency and illicit drug use from adolescence to young adulthood. *Journal of Drug Issues*, **60**, 67–90.

Kaplan, H.B., Martin, S.S., and Robbins, C.A. (1982). Applications of a general theory of deviant behavior: self derogation and adolescent drug use. *Journal of Health and Science Behavior*, **23**, 274–94.

Kaplan, H.B., Martin, S.S., Johnson, R.J., and Robbins, C.A. (1986). Escalation of marijuana use: application of a general theory of deviant behavior. *Journal of Health and Social Behavior*, **27**, 44–61.

Kellam, S.G. and Brown, H. (1982). *Social adaptational and psychological antecedents of adolescent psychopathology ten years later.* Johns Hopkins University, Baltimore.

Kral, A.H., Bluthenthal, R.N., Lorvick, J., Gee, L., Bacchetti, P., and Edlin, B.R. (2001). Sexual transmission of HIV-1 among injection drug users in San Francisco, USA: risk-factor analysis. *Lancet*, **357**, 1397–401.

Ksobiech, K. (2003). A meta-analysis of needle sharing, lending, and borrowing behaviors of needle exchange program attenders. *AIDS Education and Prevention*, **15**, 257–68.

Latkin, C.M.W.V.D., Oziemkowska, M., and Celentano, D. (1996). People and places: behavioral settings and personal network characteristics as correlates of needle sharing. *Journal of Acquired Immune Deficiency Syndromes and Human Retrovirology*, **30**, 273–80.

Laudet, A.B. (2007). What does recovery mean to you? Lessons from the recovery experience for research and practice. *Journal of Substance Abuse Treatment*, **33**, 243–56.

Laundergan, J.C. (1982). *Easy does it: alcoholism treatment outcomes, Hazelden and the Minnesota Model.* Hazelden Foundation, Duluth.

Lewin Group. (2005). Comparative evaluation of Pennsylvania's HealthChoices program and fee-for-service program. Report prepared for the Coalition of Medical Assistance Managed Care Organizations.

Ljungberg, B., Christensson, B. *et al.* (1991). HIV prevention among injecting drug users: three years of experience from a syringe exchange program in Sweden. *JAIDS*, **4**, 890–5.

Lurie, P. and Drucker, E. (1997). An opportunity lost: HIV infections associated with lack of a national needle-exchange programme in the USA. *Lancet*, **349**, 604–8.

Lurie, P., Reingold, A.L., and Bowser, B. (eds.) (1993). *The public health impact of needle-exchange programs in the United States and abroad, Vol. I.* Centers for Disease Control and Prevention, Atlanta.

McAlister, A.L. (1983). Social-psychological approaches. In *Preventing adolescent drug abuse: intervention strategies* (eds. T.J. Glynn, C.G. Leukefeld, and J.P. Ludford), pp. 36–50. Research Monograph 47, National Institute on Drug Abuse, Rockville.

McCoy, C.B., Rivers, J.E. *et al.* (1994). Compliance to bleach disinfection protocols among injection drug users in Miami. *Journal of the Acquired Immune Deficiency Syndrome*, **7**, 773.

McGlothlin, W., Anglin, M., and Wilson, B. (1977). *An evaluation of the California Civil Addict Program, DHEW Publication No. ADM 78-558.* National Institute on Drug Abuse, Rockville.

McKnight, C., Des Jarlais, D.C., Perlis, T. *et al.* (2007). Syringe exchange programs – United States, 2005. *Morb Mort Wkly Rep MMWR*, **56**, 1164–7.

Meyer, R.E. (1989). Who can say no to illicit drug use? *Archives of General Psychiatry*, **46**, 189–90.

Miller, W.R. and Hester, R.K. (1986). Inpatient alcoholism treatment: who benefits? *American Psychologist*, **41**, 794–805.

Moskowitz, J.M. (1983). Preventing adolescent substance abuse through education, In *Preventing adolescent drug abuse: intervention strategies* (eds. T.J. Glynn, C.G. Leukefeld, and J.P. Ludford), pp. 233–49. Research Monograph 47. National Institute on Drug Abuse, Rockville.

Myers, J.K., Weissman, M.M., Tischler, G.L. *et al.* (1984). Six-month prevalence of psychiatric disorders in three communities. *Archives of General Psychiatry*, **41**, 959–67.

Nash, G. (1976). An analysis of twelve studies of the impact of drug abuse treatment upon criminality. In *Drug use and crime: report of the panel on use and criminal behavior, Appendix.* Research Triangle Institute, Research Triangle Park.

National Institute on Drug Abuse (1989). *Highlights from the National Household Survey on Drug Abuse: 1988.* National Institute on Drug Abuse, Rockville.

National Institutes of Health, U. S. (1997). *Interventions to prevent HIV risk behaviors.* NIH Consensus Statement, National Institutes of Health.

Neaigus, A., Friedman, S.R., Curtis, R. *et al.* (1994). The relevance of drug injectors' social and risk networks for understanding and preventing HIV infection. *Social Science & Medicine*, **38**(1), 67–78.

Newmeyer, J.A., Feldman, H.W. *et al.* (1989). Preventing AIDS contagion among intravenous drug users. *Medical Anthropology*, **10**, 167–75.

Normand, J., Vlahov, D. *et al.* (eds.) (1995). *Preventing HIV transmission: the role of sterile needles and bleach.* National Academy Press/National Research Council/Institute of Medicine, Washington, DC.

Office of National Drug Control Policy (2004). *The economic costs of drug abuse in the United States, 1992–2002.* Executive Office of the President (Publication No. 207303), Washington, DC.

Oliver, K., Maynard, H., Friedman, S.R., and Des Jarlais, DC. (1994). Behavioral and community impact of the Portland syringe exchange program. In *Proceedings of the workshop on needle exchange and bleach distribution programs*, pp. 35–9. National Academy Press, Washington, DC.

Pentz, M.A. (1983). Prevention of adolescent substance abuse through social skill development, In *Preventing adolescent drug abuse: intervention strategies* (eds. T.J. Glynn, C.G. Leukefeld, and J.P. Ludford), pp. 195–232. Research Monograph 47. National Institute on Drug Abuse, Rockville.

Pentz, M.A., Cormack, C., Flay, B., Hansen, W.B., and Johnson, C.A. (1986). Balancing program and research integrity in community drug abuse prevention: project STAR approach. *Journal of School Health*, **56**, 389–93.

Pentz, M.A., Dwyer, J.H., MacKinnon, D.P. *et al.* (1989). A multi-community trial for primary prevention of adolescent drug abuse. *Journal of the American Medical Association*, **261**, 3259–66.

Petrakis, P.L. (1985). *Alcoholism: an inherited disease*. DHHS Publication No. ADM 85-1426. National Institute on Alcohol Abuse and Alcoholism, Rockville.

Petry, N.M., Peirce, J.M., Stitzer, M.L. *et al.* (2005). Effect of prize-based incentives on outcomes in stimulant abusers in outpatient psychosocial treatment programs. *Archives of General Psychiatry*, **62**, 1148–56.

Polich, J.M., Armor, D.J., and Braiker, H.B. (1981). *The course of alcoholism*. Wiley, New York.

Project MATCH Research Group. (1993). Project MATCH: rationale and methods for a multisite clinical trial matching patients to alcoholism treatment. *Alcoholism Clinical and Experimental Research*, **17**, 1130.

Rachal, J.V., Guess, L.L., Hubbard, R.L. *et al.* (1982). Facts for Planning No. 4: alcohol misuse by adolescents. *Alcohol Health and Research World*, **6**, 61–8.

Reif, S., Geonnotti, K., and Whetten, K. (2006). HIV infection and AIDS in the Deep South. *American Journal of Public Health*, **96**(6), 970–3.

Robert-Guroff, M., Weiss, S.H., Giron, J.A. *et al.* (1986). Prevalence of antibodies to HTLV-1, -2, and -3 in intravenous drug abusers from an AIDS endemic region. *Journal of the American Medical Association*, **255**, 3133–7.

Robins, L.N. (1980). The natural history of drug abuse. Evaluation of treatment of drug abusers. *Acta Psychiatrica Scandinavica*, **284** (Suppl 62), 7–20.

Robins, L.N. and Przybeck, T.R. (1985). Age of onset of drug use and other disorders. In *Etiology of drug abuse: implications for prevention. Research Monograph 56* (eds. C.L. Jones, R.J. Battjes *et al*). National Institute on Drug Abuse, Rockville.

Robins, L.N., Helzer, J.E., Weissman, M.M. *et al.* (1984). Lifetime prevalence of specific psychiatric disorders in three sites. *Archives of General Psychiatry*, **11**, 949–58.

Roman, P.M., Ducharme, L.J., and Knudsen, H.K. (2006). Patterns of organization and management in private and public substance abuse treatment programs. *Journal of Substance Abuse Treatment*, **31**(3), 235–43.

Rounsaville, B. (2002). Experience with ICD-10/*DSM-IV* substance use disorders. *Psychopathology*, **35**, 82–8.

Rounsaville, B.J., Spitzer, R.L., and Williams, J.B. (1986). Proposed changes in DSM-III substance use disorders: description and rationale. *American Journal of Psychiatry*, **143**, 463–8.

Saxe, L., Dougherty, D., Esty, K., and Fine, M. (1983). *The effectiveness and costs of alcoholism treatment, Health Technology Case Study No. 22*. US Congress, Office of Technology Assessment, Washington, DC.

Schaps, E., DiBartolo, R., Moskowitz, J., Palley, C.S., and Churgin, S. (1981). A review of 127 drug abuse prevention program evaluations. *Journal of Drug Issues*, **11**, 17–43.

Schaps, E., Moskowitz, J., Malvin, J., and Schaeffer, G. (1984). *The Napa drug abuse prevention project: research findings*, DHHS Publication No. ADM 84-1339. National Institute on Drug Abuse, Rockville.

Schuckit, M.A. (1980). Self-rating of alcohol intoxication by young men with and without family histories of alcoholism. *Journal of Studies in Alcohol*, **41**, 242–249.

Scitovsky, A. and Rice, D. (1987). Estimates of the direct and indirect costs of acquired immunodeficiency syndrome in the United States, 1985, 1986, 1990. *Public Health Reports*, **102**, 5–17.

Sells, S.B. (1979). Treatment effectiveness. In *Handbook on drug abuse* (eds. R.L. DuPont, A. Goldstein, and John O'Donnell). National Institute on Drug Abuse, Rockville.

Sells, S.B. and Simpson, D. (1976). *The effectiveness of drug abuse treatment, Vols. 1–5*. Ballinger, Cambridge.

Selwyn, P.A., Schoenbaum, E.E. *et al.* (1987). *Natural history of HIV infection in intravenous drug abusers (IVDAs)*. Third International Conference on AIDS, Washington, DC.

Skinner, H.A. and Horn, J.L. (1984). *Guidelines for using the Alcohol Dependence Scale (ADS)*. Addiction Research Foundation, Toronto.

Simpson, D.D., Joe, G.W., Fletcher, B.W., Hubbard, R.L., and Anglin, M.D. (1999). A national evaluation of treatment outcomes for cocaine dependence. *Archives of General Psychiatry*, **56**, 507–14.

Sloboda, Z. (2008). Reflections on 40 years of drug abuse research. *Journal of Drug Issues*.

Smart, R.G. (1976). Outcome studies of therapeutic community and halfway house treatment for addicts. *International Journal of Addiction*, **11**, 143–59.

Spencer, B.D. (1989). On the accuracy of estimates of numbers of intravenous drug users. In *AIDS: sexual behavior and intravenous drug use* (eds. C.F. Turner, H.G. Miller, and L.E. Moses). National Academy Press, Washington, DC.

Spitzer, R.L. and Williams, J.P. (1987). *Diagnostic and statistical manual of mental disorders (3rd edn. revised)*. American Psychiatric Association, Washington, DC.

Stephens, R.C., Simpson, D.D., Coyle, S.L., McCoy, C.B., and the National AIDS Research Consortium (1993). Comparative effectiveness of NADR interventions. In *Handbook on risk of AIDS* (eds. B.S. Brown and G.M. Beschner), pp. 519–56. Greenwood Press, Westport.

Stimson, G.V. (1995). AIDS and injecting drug use in the United Kingdom, 1987–1993: the policy response and the prevention of the epidemic. *Social Science and Medicine*, **41**(5), 699–716.

Stimson, G.V., Alldritt, L.J., Dolan, K.A., Donoghoe, M.S., and Lart, R.A. (1988). *Injecting equipment exchange schemes: final report*. Monitoring Research Group, Goldsmith's College, London.

Stimson, G.V., Keene, J. *et al.* (1991). *Evaluation of the syringe exchange programme Wales, 1990–1991*. Final Report to the Welsh Office, The Centre for Research on Drugs and Health Behavior, University of London.

Stimson, G.V., Des Jarlais, D.C., and Ball, A. (1998). Drug injecting and HIV infection: global dimensions and local responses. UCL Press, London.

Strathdee, S.A. and Sherman, S.G. (2003). The role of sexual transmission of HIV infection among injection and non-injection drug users. *Journal of Urban Health*, **90**(4 Suppl 3), iii 7–14.

Strathdee, S., Patrick, D. *et al.* (1997). Needle exchange is not enough: lessons from the Vancouver injection drug use study. *AIDS*, **11**, F59–65.

Strathdee, S.A., Galai, N., Safaeian, M., Celentano, D.D., Vlahov, D., Johnson, L., and Nelson, K.E. (2001). Sex differences in risk factors for HIV seroconversion among injection drug users: a 10-year perspective. *Archives Internal Medicine*, **161**, 1281–8.

Substance Abuse and Mental Health Services Administration (1999). *Summary findings from the 1998 National Household Survey on Drug Abuse*. Office of Applied Studies, Rockville.

Substance Abuse and Mental Health Services Administration (2007). Results from the 2006 National Household Survey on Drug Use and Health: National Findings.

Sumartojo, E. and Laga, M. (eds.). (2000). Structural factors in HIV prevention. *AIDS*, **14**, S1–73.

Tims, F.M. (1981). *Effectiveness of drug abuse treatment programs. Treatment Research Report DHHS Publication No. ADM 84-1143*. National Institute on Drug Abuse, Rockville.

Tims, E.M. and Ludford, J.P. (1984). Drug abuse treatment evaluation: strategies.

Titus, S., Marmor, M., Des Jarlais, D.C., Kim, M., Wolfe, H., and Beatrice, S. (1994). Bleach use and HIV seroconversion among New York City injection drug users. *Journal of Acquired Immune Deficiency Syndromes*, **7**, 700–4.

Tobler, N.S. (1986). Meta-analysis of 143 adolescent drug prevention programs: quantitative outcome results of program participants compared to a control or comparison group. *Journal of Drug Issues*, **16**, 537–67.

Turner, C.E, Miller, H.G., and Moses, L.E. (eds.) (1989). AIDS: sexual behavior and intravenous drug use. National Academy Press, Washington, DC.

Tyndall, M., Johnston, C., Craib, K. *et al.* (2001). HIV incidence and mortality among injection drug users in Vancouver – 1996–2000. *Canadian Journal of Infectious Diseases,* **12,** 69B.

Tyndall, M.W., Bruneau, J., Brogly, S., Spittal, P., O'Shaughnessy, M.V., and Schechter, M.T. (2002). Satellite needle distribution among injection drug users: policy and practice in two Canadian cities. *Journal of Acquired Immune Deficiency Syndromes,* **31**(1), 98–105.

UNAIDS/WHO. (2006). AIDS epidemic update: December 2006. Geneva: Joint United Nations Programme on HIV/AIDS (UNAIDS) and World Health Organization (WHO).

United States General Accounting Office (1993). *Needle exchange programs: research suggests promise as an AIDS prevention strategy.* Report to the Chairman, Select Committee on Narcotics Abuse and Control, House of Representatives. US House of Representatives, Washington, DC.

United States National Commission on AIDS (1991). *Twin epidemics of AIDS and substance abuse.* Government Report, Washington, DC.

Vickerman, P., Hickman, M., Rhodes, T., and Watts, C. (2006). Model projections on the required coverage of syringe distribution to prevent HIV epidemics among injecting drug users. *Journal of Acquired Immune Deficiency Syndromes,* **42,** 355–61.

Vlahov, D., Astemborski, J. *et al.* (1994). Field effectiveness of needle disinfection among injecting drug users. *Journal of the Acquired Immunodeficiency Syndromes,* **7,** 760–6.

Watters, J.K., Estilo, M.J., Clark, G.L., and Lorvick, J. (1994). Syringe and needle exchange as HIV/AIDS prevention for injection drug users. *Journal of the American Medical Association,* **271**(2), 115–20.

Wawer, M.J., Gray, R.H., Sewankambo, N.K. *et al.* (2005). Rates of HIV-1 transmission per coital act, by stage of HIV-1 infection, in Rakai, Uganda. *Journal of Infectious Diseases,* **191**(9), 1403–9.

Westat. (2003). *Evaluation of the national youth anti-drug media campaign: 2003 report of findings executive summary.* National Institute on Drug Abuse, Rockville.

Wiebel, W. (1993). *The indigenous leader outreach model: intervention manual.* National Institute on Drug Abuse, Rockville.

Wiebel, W.W., Jimenez, A. *et al.* (1996). Risk behavior and HIV seroincidence among out-of-treatment injection drug users: a four-year prospective study.

Wodak, A. (1995). Needle exchange and bleach distribution programmes: the Australian experience. *International Journal of Drug Policy,* **6,** 46–56.

Wolfe, D. and Malinowska-Sempruch, K. (2004). *Illicit drug policies and the Global HIV epidemic effects of UN and National Government approaches.* Open Society Institute, New York.

World Health Organization. (1992). *Tenth revision of the international classification of disease (ICD-10).* World Health Organization, Geneva.

10.3

Alcohol[1]

Robin Room

Abstract

This chapter begins with a discussion on alcohol, its uses, and its effects, both positive and negative, followed by a review of the recent research on its cumulative adverse effects on health. The history of alcohol as a public health issue is also briefly reviewed. The temperance movements of the nineteenth and early-twentieth centuries were succeeded by an impulse to deflate alcohol's adverse effects and, in turn, by a 'new public health' approach. Although this approach gained ground among researchers from the 1970s onwards, it has often been resisted in the policy process. Seven main strategies to prevent or control alcohol problems are described, and their effectiveness briefly assessed. The chapter concludes with an account of alcohol policy in a globalizing world. An international convention on alcohol control has been called for to counter the influence of trade agreements and the globalization of alcohol production, distribution, and promotion.

Alcohol and its effects

Alcoholic beverages have been consumed in most, if not all, human societies since the beginning of recorded history. Beverages containing ethanol (C_2H_5OH) can be fermented from a large number of organic materials that comprise carbohydrates, and in one part of the world or another, these products are prepared from fruits, berries, various grains, plants, honey, or milk. Under most circumstances, such fermented beverages can contain up to 14 per cent ethanol. The most widely commercialized fermented beverages are beer prepared from barley or other grains (usually 3–7 per cent ethanol), apple and other fruit ciders (usually 3–7 per cent ethanol), and grape wine (usually 8–14 per cent ethanol). Other fermented beverages are also common in particular cultures, often from home production or in commercial form: For example, sorghum or millet beers in Eastern and Southern Africa, palm wine toddy in West Africa and the Indian subcontinent, pulque (prepared from the maguey cactus) in Mexico, and rice wine (sake) in Eastern Asia.

Distilled beverages, in which ethanol is concentrated by evaporation and condensation from a fermented liquid, were a Chinese invention, which came to Europe *via* Arabia in the Middle Ages. In Europe, at first, their use was primarily medicinal, but by the 1600s, popular use as a social beverage spread rapidly. Distilled beverages can be made up of almost-pure ethanol, but those sold for drinking contain between 25 per cent and 50 per cent ethanol. Distilled alcohol is also added to wine, producing 'fortified wines' with about 20 per cent ethanol. Because distilled beverages and fortified wines do not readily spoil, they could be shipped over long distances, even before refrigeration and airtight packaging became available, and played a particularly important part in commerce and exploitation in the age of the European empires. Different cultures consume varying strengths of alcoholic beverages, often with water or a 'mixer' being added to distilled beverages and, in some cultures, also to wine and other fermented beverages.

Use-values of alcohol

Ethanol has many uses in human life. These include non-beverage uses as a fuel and as a solvent. Important beverage-related use-values include use as a medicine, as a religious sacrament, as a foodstuff, and as a thirst-quencher (Mäkelä 1983). But, alcoholic beverages have received special attention as a public health hazard because of their psychoactive properties. These properties carry with them another set of use-values: In terms of psychopharmacology, ethanol is a depressant, and alcoholic beverages have long been used to affect mood and feelings. With enough consumption, alcohol becomes an anodyne and, indeed, an anaesthetic; distilled spirits were used as an anaesthetic in surgical practice before the mid-nineteenth century. Many drinkers seek and appreciate the levels of intoxication, which lie between mild mood alteration at one end of the spectrum and being comatose at the other.

The decisions to drink and how much to drink are, however, often not made by the individual in isolation. Drinking is usually a social act, and the pace and level of drinking are frequently subject to collective influence, with drinking together being seen as an expression of solidarity and community. Although drunkenness may be sought to relieve misery or loneliness, it is more commonly associated with sociable celebration.

Adverse effects

Alcohol consumption can have a variety of adverse effects, some of which are acute effects associated with the particular drinking event.

---

[1] Author's note: Portions of this chapter have been adapted from 'Prevention of alcohol-related problems' in the *New Oxford Textbook of Psychiatry*. Oxford University Press.

Drinking progressively impairs physical coordination, cognition, and attention, resulting in an increased risk of accidents and injury. Above a threshold level, drinking can also affect intention and judgement, so intoxication potentially plays a causal role in violent behaviour and crime (Graham *et al.* 1998). This relation appears to be culturally mediated, because there is a substantial variation between cultures in the association of intoxication with violence and crime (MacAndrew & Edgerton 1969). A sufficient amount of alcohol may result in a potentially fatal overdose, by interrupting various autonomic bodily functions.

Other adverse effects of alcohol consumption are chronic effects related to a repeated pattern of drinking. Alcohol consumption can adversely affect nearly every organ of the body, although some effects are not common. Chronic conditions in which alcohol is implicated as an important cause include liver cirrhosis; cancers of the upper digestive tract, liver, and breast; cardiomyopathy; and gastritis and pancreatitis (Rehm *et al.* 2004). Through a variety of mechanisms, alcohol is also implicated in the incidence and course of infectious diseases (NIAAA 1997).

Repeated heavy drinking can also adversely affect mental health; specific neurological disorders are associated with sustained heavy drinking. More common concomitants include depression and affective disorders. Alcoholism—the experience of loss of control over drinking, along with other psychological and physical sequelae—has also been considered a mental disorder in modern times. In current nosologies, alcoholism has been replaced by the terms *alcohol dependence* (in *Diagnostic and Statistical Manual of Mental Disorders* [DSM-IV] terminology) and the *alcohol dependence syndrome* (in the *International Classification of Diseases* [ICD-10]).

The impairment of coordination and judgement produced by drinking potentially affects bystanders and the drinkers' acquaintances, friends, and family, as well as themselves: The effects can be through impairment of coordination or judgement during the drinking event, resulting in injury or distress, or through impairment of performance in family, friendship, work, and other social roles as a result of recurring drinking episodes. The actual and potential adverse effects on others have historically been the primary justification for alcohol controls and other societal responses to problematic drinking (Room 1996); the effects on the adult drinker's own health have been of much less importance in determining public policy on alcohol.

Positive effects

For the drinker, and sometimes for those around, alcohol consumption can have positive effects. We have already mentioned the different use-values of alcohol—which mean that drinkers are usually willing to pay more than just the cost of production and distribution of the beverage. Apart from its valued effects on mental state, alcohol use has some positive outcomes on health. By far, the most important of these, in terms of public health, is its potential for preventing cardiovascular disease (CVD). A fairly consistent finding in studies in several societies is that drinking at moderate levels protects against CVD (Klatsky 1999), although controversy about the existence and extent of this effect remains (e.g. Fillmore *et al.* 2006). The findings on the upper limit of drinking for such protection vary. Taken together, it appears that most of the protective effect can be gained with as little as one drink of an alcoholic beverage every second day (Maclure 1993). About half of this effect seems to come from inhibiting the build-up of plaque in arteries,

whereas the other half seems to result from a relatively immediate effect of diminishing the likelihood of blood clots. To the extent this is true, irregular or occasional drinking is likely to have a less protective effect.

Although it has been argued that this protection comes primarily from red wine constituents (particularly resveratrol) rather than from the ethanol, the balance of evidence favours an ethanol effect (Klatsky 1999). However, relatively little is known about how this effect interacts with or overlaps other risk and protective factors for chronic heart disease (CHD), such as regular exercise, diet, or taking aspirin (acetyl salicylic acid [ASA]) or other pharmaceuticals (Criqui *et al.* 1998). The protective effect of alcohol appears to be higher for cigarette smokers than for non-smokers (Kozlowski *et al.* 1994).

Drinking is also often bad for the heart (Poikolainen 1999; Chadwick & Goode 1998). Studies have found that a pattern of intermittent heavy drinking, such as getting drunk every weekend, is associated with an elevated rate of coronary death (Kauhanen *et al.* 1997), probably through mechanisms such as heart arrhythmias (Kupari & Koskinen 1998; McKee & Britton 1998). Data from countries in the former Soviet Union, where a pattern of intermittent intoxication is common, support the strong adverse effect of binge drinking on heart disease mortality. During a period of deliberate restriction of alcohol supplies, the estimated per-capita consumption in Russia, including the illicit alcohol market, fell from 14.2 litres in 1984 to 10.7 litres in 1987 (Shkolnikov & Nemtsov 1997)—a fall of 25 per cent. The death rate from ischemic heart disease among males fell by 10 per cent in the same period (Leon *et al.* 1997). This rate rose again when the restrictions lapsed, although this time, unlike between 1985 and 1988, other risk factors also changed.

Research on cumulative effects of alcohol

Effects on the drinker's health

In most studies, the relationship between amount of drinking and overall mortality is a J-shaped curve, with abstainers, and often, very light drinkers showing a higher mortality than those drinking a little more. This may be because, in these findings, a substantial part of the study population were older adults, and thus were at risk of mortality from CVD. Studies limited to younger cohorts typically found a monotonic relationship between amount of drinking and mortality (Andréasson *et al.* 1991; Rehm & Sempos 1995). Such an association might also be expected in any population, such as in some developing countries, that has a low rate of CVD.

The pattern of drinking is also a potentially important factor in mortality due to alcohol. Although this has long been obvious in casualty deaths, there is growing recognition of its significance in other causes of death, as implied by the earlier-mentioned Russian data. However, until recently, there have been only few measurements of this pattern in studies on alcohol and overall mortality. Variations among cultures in drinking habits may partly explain why the J-curve relation of volume of drinking to mortality shows different low-points in different cultures.

The risks and potential benefits associated with a given level of drinking, thus, vary with the age and sex of the drinker, and possibly with other sociocultural characteristics, as well as with the pattern and circumstances related to drinking. This variation has posed a considerable challenge because of political demand in a number of countries for advice on 'low-risk drinking' or 'safe drinking' guidelines (Hawks 1994). Whereas earlier guidelines were inclined to be stated only in terms of the volume of drinking, in line with the measurement methods of medical epidemiology literature, more recent guidelines have also emphasized limits on the amount consumed on a given occasion or day (Bondy *et al.* 1999).

Current literature on the cumulative effects of drinking on health relies substantially on summations of prospective epidemiological literature, following the tradition set up by English *et al.* (1995). Using meta-analysis on studies of the relationship between volume of drinking and specific causes of death in which alcohol was either a risk or protective factor, the studies following this tradition derive attributable fractions for different levels of the volume of drinking and apply these fractions to segments of the population at each level in order to arrive at estimates on total lives and life-years lost and gained. In the WHO's estimation of the global burden of disease (GBD) for 2000, drinking patterns were also taken into account for injuries and heart disease, and the estimations were extended to cover all regions of the world (Rehm *et al.* 2004). In these estimates, the projected protective effects of alcohol are subtracted from the negative burden. In addition to life-years lost, the study's most comprehensive indicator, disability-adjusted life years (DALYs), includes a projection of the burden of disability attributable to alcohol.

According to GBD estimates, 4.0 per cent of the total burden of disease globally (as measured in DALYs) is attributable to alcohol (Ezzati *et al.* 2002). This compares with 4.1 per cent for tobacco and 0.8 per cent for illegal drugs. The alcohol share of the burden is highest in high-income societies, including Eastern Europe and Northern Asia, as well as in Latin America. The relative position of alcohol among risk factors is actually highest in middle-income countries, where it ranks first; although the alcohol share of all DALYs is lower in other developing regions, this fraction is calculated on the basis of a higher total burden of disease and disability in these countries.

Effects at the population level

So far, we have dealt with estimates of alcohol's effects at the individual level. The methodological difficulties in the studies underlying these estimates extend beyond those we have already discussed (Edwards *et al.* 1994). The estimates rely primarily on prospective epidemiological studies in which alcohol consumption is measured at one point in time; such a measurement is, at best, a poor surrogate for either of the main aspects of alcohol consumption as a risk factor—chronic effects of cumulated alcohol consumption or acute effects of intoxication at a specific event. In these studies, the effects of possible confounders are dealt with by statistically controlling for them in the analysis. But this can be problematic if drinking and the potential confounder are causally intertwined, as is true in the case of hypertension or tobacco smoking. Consider, for instance, a person who only smokes when under the influence of alcohol; controlling for that person's smoking behaviour potentially limits some of the alcohol effect.

From a public health perspective, it is the effects at the population level, rather than the individual level, that are the main concern. If drinking was entirely a matter of individual choice and behaviour, and if the effects of drinking happened only to the drinker, then effects at the population level would be a simple aggregation of the effects at the individual level. But neither of these conditions is applicable. Drinking is by and large a social activity, and the drinking behaviour of a person is likely to influence and be influenced by those around that person. In a given population, the amounts drunk by infrequent or light drinkers and by heavy drinkers tend to move up and down in concert. Thus, if there is some health gain when those at the lower end of the spectrum increase their consumption, there will also be health losses from an increase in consumption for those at the top end of the spectrum. In view of this, it has been argued that the level of per-drinker consumption where the balance of health benefits and losses is optimized in a population is likely to be considerably lower than the optimum level of consumption for the individual drinker (Skog 1996). For instance, Skog (1996) argued that the optimum level of alcohol consumption with respect to mortality was likely to be lower than the present-day per-capita consumption of any nation in western Europe. His argument is supported by findings of a generally positive relationship of the level of alcohol consumption with total mortality in time-series analysis of differenced data in a number of high-income countries (Norström & Ramstedt 2005).

By their design, the prospective studies typically used for investigations of alcohol's effects on mortality or morbidity do not measure the effects of drinking on others. Other types of individual-level studies, such as studies of the effects of drinking–driving (Perrine *et al.* 1989) or studies of homicide and other crimes (Wolfgang 1958), document the importance of such effects in terms of death or injury. But the strongest evidence of the magnitude of these effects comes from aggregate-level studies of the covariation of changes over time in a given society or place. Differenced time-series analyses in European societies have suggested that a 1 litre change in per capita alcohol consumption produces about a 1 per cent change in the overall mortality rate (Norström 1996; Her & Rehm 1998). Here again, however, drinking patterns and social circumstances are likely to make a difference. For instance, the drop in Russian total mortality during the alcohol restrictions of 1985–88 imply a decline of about 2.7 per cant in age-standardized mortality for each 1 litre drop in per capita consumption (calculated from Shkolnikov & Nemtsov 1997, and Leon *et al.* 1998). Even specifically for heart disease, any protective effects from changes in low-level drinking seem to be outbalanced in the population as a whole by negative effects from changes at high-consumption levels, levels of consumption typical in high-income societies. Thus, time-series analyses of differenced data on alcohol consumption and on CHD mortality in 14 European countries found no evidence of net protective effects and some evidence of net adverse effect (Hemström 2001; Ramstedt 2006).

Alcohol as an issue in public health

Shifting societal responses to problematic drinking

Efforts to control problematic drinking date back to the beginning of recorded history. These efforts have been many-sided, including informal responses in the family and community, as well as governmental controls. Religious teachings and movements have often been directed against drinking or intoxication: Moslems are forbidden by their faith to drink at all, and drinking is also discouraged or forbidden in at least some branches of all the major world religions.

In the last few centuries, European and Europe-derived societies have been hosts to conflicting trends in terms of alcohol issues. The production of alcoholic beverages became an important part of European economies and of imperial domination and trade in the age of European colonization. Alcohol production and exports took on political importance not only in the wine cultures of Southern Europe, but also in such countries as the Netherlands and Britain. In the British colonies as well as in America, in the late-eighteenth century, distilled spirits was the only profitable way to get grain to market (Rorabaugh 1979). In recent decades, alcohol beverage industries have become increasingly internationalized and concentrated (Jernigan 1997), and multinational companies, mostly based in Europe or North America, have pressed with considerable success to open up global markets for alcohol.

Starting in the early 1800s, there were substantial waves of popular, and eventually, governmental response to the problems that were resulting from the very heavy consumption of alcoholic beverages in English-speaking and Northern European societies (Blocker 1989; Levine 1991). As a culmination of decades of popular temperance movements, in the early-twentieth century, alcohol prohibition was adopted in several of these countries and stringent controls on the availability of alcohol in others. Although alcohol's impact on public order and morals and on family life were more central to the temperance movement thinking than the public health issues, mainstream thought in medicine and public health acknowledged the substantial adverse impacts of alcohol on health (Emerson 1932), and prohibition or an alternative, stringent controls on the availability of alcohol (Catlin 1931), were often identified with the public health interest.

In the United States, and other societies which had adopted alcohol prohibition, there was a strong reaction against it by the early 1930s, with middle-class youth in the lead (Room 1984a, 1984b). In this cultural–political context, as the new generation moved into professional and research positions, adverse effects of alcohol were downplayed or denied (Herd 1992; Katcher 1993), and alcohol issues almost disappeared from public health textbooks and discourse. Any problems with drinking were seen as attributable to a relatively small cadre of alcoholics, unable to control their drinking because of a mysterious predisposing factor. As late as 1968, the main emphasis of the American Public Health Association was on building treatment capacity for alcoholism (Cross 1968).

The 'new public health' approach

The last three decades of the twentieth century saw the rise of what has been termed in the alcohol literature the 'new public health' approach (Beauchamp 1976; Tigerstedt 1999) to alcohol issues. This approach brought together several strands of research and philosophy. In contrast to a concept in terms of 'alcoholism', the approach was premised on a disaggregated approach: There was a diversity of alcohol-related problems, fairly widely distributed among the drinking population (Knupfer 1967; World Health Organization, Expert Committee on Problems Related to Alcohol Consumption 1980). It was noted that for many problems, the heaviest drinkers accounted for only a minority, because there were so many more drinking at somewhat lower levels (Moore & Gerstein 1981); picking up Rose's (Rose 1981) phrase, Kreitman (Kreitman 1986) termed this the 'preventive paradox'. Attention was, therefore, paid not only to the heaviest drinkers, but also to the whole range of drinking levels, and indeed, to the distribution of consumption in the population (Ledermann 1956; De Lint 1968). What happens with moderate drinkers, it was argued, influences the social climate for heavy drinking, because drinking is largely a social activity, marked by mutual influences and norms of reciprocity

(Bruun et al. 1975a; Skog 1985). In a given population, it was found that rates of alcohol-related problems tend to rise and fall with changes in the level of consumption (Seeley 1960). Controls on the availability of alcohol, including taxes, affect the level of consumption, and thus, also the rates of alcohol-related problems (Seeley 1960; Terris 1967; Popham et al. 1976). The level of alcohol consumption in a population, and controls on alcohol availability, is thus seen as a public health concern, and part of a society's overall 'alcohol policy' (Bruun et al. 1975a).

In enumerating the elements of the new public health approach, we have given references for early statements of each element. It will be seen that the strands of this approach were woven together gradually over a period of some years. A 1975 report by an international group of researchers (Bruun et al. 1975a) became a pivotal document for the approach. A few years later, the approach was given an authoritative endorsement in the United States by a committee of the National Academy of Sciences (Moore & Gerstein 1981). The most recent restatement of the approach by an international group of scholars appeared in 2003 (Babor et al. 2003), with a somewhat parallel analysis oriented to the developing world (Room et al. 2002).

The approach has had considerable influence on WHO programmes in the field of alcohol (Room 2005; World Health Organization 2007). At national levels, there has been a considerable variation in its influence on policy. In Sweden, where it is known as the Total Consumption Model, it attained dominance as the basis for official policy (Sutton 1998). However, policies based on this approach have been eroded as a consequence of Sweden's accession to the European Union (Holder et al. 1998). The approach also has had considerable backing in other Nordic countries.

In English-speaking countries, it has encountered substantial resistance in the cultural–political realm. Those allied with the alcoholic beverage industry have strongly attacked the approach, both in analyses and polemics (e.g. Mott 1991; Grant & Litvak 1998) and through direct political action to remove official proponents (Room 1984c). An approach that contemplates government regulation and influencing of private consumer choices is also unwelcome to those committed to consumer sovereignty and the primacy of individual choice (e.g. Peele 1987). Often, proponents of approaches seeking to 'domesticate' drinking—to reduce problems from drinking by integrating it into everyday life—have portrayed the new public health approach as antithetical to this (Olsson 1990), although some researchers have noted that there is no necessary antithesis (Whitehead 1979).

In terms of its influence on policy, the approach has undoubtedly had some effect in strengthening the defence of existing control structures and regulations. But efforts to get the approach adopted as the practical base for policy have met with resistance and failure in a number of countries (Baggott 1990; Hawks 1993). One response to this resistance has been some calls for an alternative approach (Stockwell et al. 1997), arguing that policy measures directed at heavy and problematic drinkers are more politically acceptable than measures directed at all drinkers.

The policy approach offered as an alternative is a focus on harm reduction, primarily by reducing instances of intoxication or insulating the drinkers from harm (Plant et al. 1997; Stimson et al. 2007). However, there is in fact usually no conflict between approaches aimed at total consumption and approaches aiming to reduce harm from heavy drinking. As Stockwell et al. (1997) noted, 'aggregate consumption levels are in fact likely to fall if effective (harm reduction) strategies are introduced'. Conversely, many measures that affect the whole drinking population—taxation being a good example—are especially hard on heavier drinkers. Nor are targeted harm reduction measures necessarily more politically acceptable than measures that affect all drinkers. Old systems of rationing and individual buyer surveillance (Järvinen 1991), which were directed specifically at restraining heavy drinking, are now politically unacceptable in any high-income society, although rationing, at least, was highly effective as a targeted prevention measure (Norström 1987).

Beyond its specific features, the controversy over the new public health approach replicates familiar patterns of controversy over public health approaches in general, particularly when those approaches impinge on familiar and valued patterns of behaviour, with substantial economic interests at stake. At the level of the knowledge base, the approach has had considerable success: The empirical evidence underlying the approach has considerably strengthened since the approach was first put forward. At a political level, however, the approach has had only limited success, and primarily in areas peripheral to its main focus—that is, in drinking–driving and minimum-age limits for drinkers.

Strategies of prevention and control and their effectiveness

Simplifying them, there are seven main strategies to minimize alcohol problems. One strategy is to educate or persuade people not to use alcohol or about ways to use it so as to limit harm. A second strategy, a kind of negative persuasion, is to deter drinking-related behaviour with the threat of penalties. A third strategy, in the positive direction, is to provide alternatives to drinking or to drink-related activities. A fourth strategy is in one way or another to insulate the user from harm. A fifth strategy is to regulate availability of alcohol or the conditions of its use; prohibition of supply may be regarded as a special case of such regulation. A sixth strategy is to work with social or religious movements oriented to reducing alcohol problems. And, a seventh strategy is to treat or otherwise help people who have in trouble with their drinking habits. We will consider, in turn, these strategies and the evidence on their effectiveness.

Education and persuasion

In principle, education can be offered to any segment of the population in a variety of venues, but it is usually education of youth in schools that first comes to mind in the prevention of alcohol problems. Community-based prevention programmes, which are often also directed at adults, also may include an educational component.

Education offers new information or ways of thinking and leaves it to the listener to draw conclusions concerning beliefs and behaviour. However, most alcohol education programmes go beyond this. Commonplace in North American evaluative literature on alcohol education is that 'knowledge-only' approaches do not result in changes in behaviour (Botvin 1995). School-based alcohol education has, thus, usually had a persuasional element, aiming to influence students in a particular direction.

Persuasion is directly concerned with changing beliefs or behaviours, and may or may not also offer information. Mass-media campaigns aimed at persuasion have been a very common component of prevention programmes for alcohol-related problems, but this can also be pursued through other media and modalities.

In most societies, public-health-oriented persuasion about alcohol must compete with a variety of other persuasive messages, including those intended to sell alcoholic beverages. The evidence that alcohol advertising influences teenagers and young adults towards increased drinking and problematic drinking is becoming stronger (Wyllie et al. 1998a, b; Casswell et al. 2002). Even where alcohol advertising is not allowed in the mass media, these messages are often conveyed to consumers and potential consumers in a variety of other ways.

Evidence on effectiveness

The literature on effectiveness of educational approaches is dominated by studies on school-based education from the United States. This means that alcohol education has usually been in the context of drug and tobacco education and that the emphasis has been on abstention (Beck 1998) or at least on delaying the start of drinking, in cultural circumstances where the median age of actually starting to drink is about 13 years although the minimum legal drinking age is 21 years. In general, despite the best efforts of a generation of researchers, this literature has had difficulty showing substantial and lasting effects (Foxcroft et al. 2003; Gorman et al. 2007). There is a good argument from general principles for alcohol education in the context of consumer and health, but there is little evidence from the formal evaluation literature at this point of its effectiveness beyond the short term.

Persuasive media campaigns have also been a favourite modality in many places in recent decades. In general, evaluations of such campaigns have been able to demonstrate impacts on knowledge and awareness about substance use problems, but show little success in affecting attitudes and behaviours (Babor et al. 2003). As with school education approaches, there are hints in literature that more success may come from influencing the community around the drinker—in terms of attitudes of significant others or popular support for alcohol policy measures—than from directly persuading the drinker himself or herself. Thus, media messages can be effective as agenda-setting mechanisms in the community, increasing or sustaining public support for other preventive strategies (Casswell et al. 1989).

Deterrence

In its broadest sense, deterrence means simply the threat of negative sanctions or disincentives for behaviour—a form of negative persuasion. Criminal laws deter in two ways: By general deterrence, which is the effect of the law in preventing a prohibited behaviour in the population as a whole; and specific deterrence, which is the effect of the law in discouraging those who have been caught from doing it again (Ross 1982). A law will have a greater preventive effect and be cheaper to administer to the extent it has a strong general deterrence effect.

Prohibitions on driving after drinking more than a specified amount are now in effect in most nations (World Health Organization 2004). In many societies, there have also been laws against public drunkenness (being in a public place while intoxicated) and against obnoxious behaviour while intoxicated. Other common prohibitions are concerned with producing or selling alcoholic beverages outside state-regulated channels and with aspects of drinking under a specified minimum age.

Evidence on effectiveness

Drinking–driving legislation, such as 'per-se' laws outlawing driving while at or above a defined blood-alcohol level, has been shown to be effective in changing behaviour and reducing rates of alcohol-related problems (Babor *et al.* 2003; Ross 1982; Hingson 1996). The effect is through both general and specific deterrence. The quickness and certainty of punishment as well as its severity are important in the deterrent value (too much severity tends to undercut the quickness and certainty). Drinking–driving is an ideal area for applying general deterrence, as the gains from breaking the law are limited and automobile drivers typically have something to lose by being caught.

Many English-speaking and Scandinavian countries have had a tradition of criminalizing drinking in public places or public drunkenness as such. The trend in the 1970s and following was to decriminalize public drunkenness, although in many places it remains illegal. In the 1990s and following, there has been some trend to criminalize drinking in specific public places (Edwards *et al.* 1994). Although there are few specific studies, criminalization of such behaviours has some effect in moving behaviour around, but is probably not very effective in changing the behaviour of marginalized heavy drinkers who have little to lose.

Providing and encouraging alternative activities

Another strategy, in principle involving positive incentives, is to provide and seek to encourage activities that are an alternative to drinking or to activities closely associated with drinking. This includes initiatives such as making soft drinks available as an alternative to alcoholic beverages, providing locations for sociability as an alternative to taverns, and providing and encouraging recreational activities as an alternative to leisure activities involving drinking. Job creation and skill development programmes are other examples.

Evidence on effectiveness

'Boredom' and 'because there's nothing else to do' are certainly among the reasons given by some for drinking. And, there are often good reasons of general social policy for providing and encouraging alternative activities. But as has been noted, the problem with alternatives to drinking is that drinking combines so well with many of them. Soft drinks are indeed an alternative to alcoholic beverages for quenching thirst, but they may also serve as a mixer in an alcoholic drink. Involvement in sports may go along with drinking as well as replace it. The few evaluation studies of providing alternative activities, again from a restricted number of societies, have generally not shown lasting effects on drinking behaviour (Moskowitz *et al.* 1983; Norman *et al.* 1997), although they undoubtedly often serve a general social purpose in broadening opportunities for the disadvantaged (Carmona & Stewart 1996).

Insulating use from harm

A major social strategy for reducing alcohol-related problems in many societies has been measures to separate the drinker, and particularly heavy drinkers, from potential harm. This separation can be physical (in terms of distance or walls), it can be temporal, or it can be cultural (e.g. defining the drinking occasion as 'time out' from normal responsibilities). These 'harm-reduction' strategies, as they are called in the context of illicit drugs, are often built into cultural arrangements around drinking, but can also be the object of purposive programmes and policies (Moore & Gerstein 1981), such as promotion of 'designated drivers', where one person in a social group is chosen to abstain and drive in the particular social situation (DeJong & Hingson 1998).

A variety of modifications to the driving environment positively affect casualties associated with drinking and driving, along with other casualties. These include mandatory use of seat belts, airbags, and improvements in the safety of vehicles and roads. Many other practical measures to separate intoxication episodes from casualties and other adverse consequences have been put into practice, although usually without formal evaluation.

Evidence on effectiveness

Drinking–driving countermeasures are a prime example of an approach in terms of insulating drinking behaviour from harm, as they seek to reduce alcohol-related traffic casualties without necessarily stopping or reducing alcohol use (Evans 1991). There is substantial evidence on the success of a range of such countermeasures, including environmental change approaches as well as deterrence (DeJong & Hingson 1998; Forsyth 1996). Some environmental measures that reduce traffic casualties in general—such as requiring the wearing of seat belts in cars or providing sidewalks separated from the road—may prevent casualties associated with intoxication even more than other casualties.

Regulating the availability and conditions of use

In terms of the substantial harm to health and public order they can cause, alcoholic beverages are not ordinary commodities. Governments have, thus, often actively intervened in the markets for such beverages, far beyond usual levels of state intervention in markets for commodities.

Total prohibition can be viewed as an extreme form of regulation of the market. In this circumstance, where no one is licensed to sell alcohol, the state has no formal control over the conditions of the sales that occur nevertheless and there are no legal sales interests, controlled through licensing, to cooperate with the state in market regulation.

With a general prohibition, typically, the consumption of alcohol does fall in the population, and there are also declines in the rates of the direct consequences of drinking such as cirrhosis or alcohol-related mental disorders (Moore & Gerstein 1981; Teasley 1992). But prohibition also brings with it characteristic negative consequences, including the emergence and growth of an illicit market and the crime associated with this. Partly for this reason, prohibition is now not a live option in any high-income society, although it still is in some other societies and local areas.

The features of alcohol control regimes that regulate the legal market in alcohol vary greatly. Special taxes on alcohol are very common, imposed often as much for revenue as for public health considerations. Many societies have minimum-age limits forbidding sales to underage customers and regulations forbidding sales to the already intoxicated. Often, the regulations include limiting the number of sales outlets, restricting hours and days of sale, and limiting sales to special stores or drinking places. Rationing of alcohol purchases—limiting the amount individuals can buy in a given time period—has also been used as a means of regulating availability. Regulations restricting or forbidding advertising of alcoholic beverages attempt to limit or channel efforts by private interests to increase demand for particular alcoholic beverages.

Such regulations potentially complement education and persuasion efforts. State monopolization on sales of some or all alcoholic beverages at the retail and/or wholesale level has also been commonly been used as a mechanism to minimize alcohol-related harm (Room 1993).

Effectiveness of specific types of regulation on availability

The decades since the 1970s have seen the development of a burgeoning literature on the effects of alcohol control measures. Reference guides for communities, summarizing the research evidence and attuned to particular national or regional conditions, are becoming available (e.g. Grover 1999; Neves *et al.* 1998). Specific types of regulation of the alcohol market, and the evidence on their effectiveness, are discussed as follows:

Minimum-age limits: A minimum-age limit is a partial prohibition, applied to one segment of the population. There is a strong evaluation literature showing the effectiveness of establishing and enforcing minimum-age limits in reducing alcohol-related problems (Babor *et al.* 2003). However, this literature is mostly based on North America, focusing mostly on youthful driving casualties and evaluating reduction from and increases to age 21 years as the limit, a minimum-age limit higher than in most societies. There is limited evidence on the applicability of the literature's findings in other societies and where youth cultures may be less automobile-focused (but see Møller 2002; Kypri *et al.* 2006).

Taxes and other price increases: Generally, consumers show some response on the price of alcoholic beverages, as on all other commodities. If the price goes up, the drinker will drink less; data from high-income societies suggests this is at least as true of the heavy drinker as of the occasional drinker (Babor *et al.* 2003). Studies have found that alcohol tax increases reduce the rates of traffic casualties, of cirrhosis mortality, and of incidents of violence (Cook 1981; Cook & Moore 1993).

Limiting sales outlets, and hours and conditions of sale: A substantial body of literature shows that levels and patterns of alcohol consumption, and rates of alcohol-related casualties and other problems, are influenced by such sales restrictions, which typically make the purchase of alcoholic beverages slightly inconvenient or influence the setting of and after drinking (Babor *et al.* 2003). Enforced rules influencing 'house policies' in drinking places on not serving intoxicated customers, for example, have also been shown to have some effect (Saltz 1997).

Monopolizing production or sale: Studies of the effects of privatizing retail alcohol monopolies have often shown some increase in levels of alcohol consumption and problems, in part because the number of outlets and hours of sale typically increase with privatization (Her *et al.* 1999) and partly also because the new private interests typically exert political influence for further increases in availability. From a public health perspective, it is the retail level that is important, although monopolization of the production or wholesale level may facilitate revenue collection and effective control of the market.

Rationing sales: Rationing the amount of alcohol sold to an individual potentially directly impacts on heavy drinkers and has been shown to reduce levels both of intoxication-related problems such as violence and of drinking-history-related problems such as cirrhosis mortality (Norström 1987; Schechter 1986). But, although a form of rationing—the medical prescription system—is well accepted in most societies for psychoactive medications, it has proved politically unacceptable nowadays for alcoholic beverages in high-income societies.

Advertising and promotion restrictions: Many societies have regulations on advertising and other promotion of sales of alcoholic beverages (World Health Organization 2004). Although it is well accepted that advertising can strongly affect consumer choices on products in the market, it has proved difficult to measure the effects of advertising on demand for alcoholic beverages as a whole, partly because the effects are likely to be cumulative and long-term, making them difficult to measure. However, the evidence on the effects of advertising and promotion on overall demand has become somewhat stronger in recent literature (Casswel 1995; Saffer 1998; Casswell & Zhang 1998).

Social and religious movements and community action

Substantial reductions in alcohol-related problems have often been the result of spontaneous social and religious movements, which put a major emphasis on quitting intoxication or drinking. In recent decades, efforts have also been made to form partnerships between state organizations and non-governmental groups to work on alcohol problems, often at the level of the local community. There has been an active tradition of community action projects on alcohol problems, often using a range of prevention strategies (Giesbrecht *et al.* 1990; Greenfield & Zimmerman 1993; Holmila 1997; Holder 1998). School-based prevention efforts have also moved increasingly to try to involve the community, in line with general perceptions that such multifaceted strategies will be more effective (Paglia & Room 1999).

Although some of the biggest historical reductions in alcohol problem rates have resulted from spontaneous and autonomous social or religious movements, support or collaboration from a government can easily be perceived as official co-optation or manipulation (Room 1997). Thus, there is considerable question about the extent to which such movements can or should become an instrument of government prevention policies.

Evidence on effectiveness

In the short term, movements of religious or cultural revival can be highly effective in reducing levels of drinking and of alcohol-related problems. Alcohol consumption in the United States fell by about half in the first flush of temperance enthusiasm in 1830–45 (Moore & Gerstein 1981). Rates of serious crime are reported to have fallen for a while to a fraction of their previous level in Ireland in the wake of Father Mathew's temperance crusade (Room 1983). The enthusiasm that sustains such movements tends to decay over time, although they often leave behind new customs and institutions of much longer duration. For instance, although the days when the historic temperance movement in English-speaking societies was strong are long gone, the movement had the long-lasting effect of largely removing drinking from the workplace in these societies.

Particularly in the developing world, religious or cultural renewal movements oriented to reducing or prohibiting drinking are often a strong avenue of preventive action (Room *et al.* 2002). A reform movement among poor indigenous people in a region of Ecuador touched off in 1987 by religious renewal movements and an earthquake appears to have had lasting effects on popular sobriety (Butler 2006).

Treatment and other help

Providing effective treatment or other help for drinkers who find they cannot control their drinking can be regarded as an obligation of a just and humane society. The help can take several forms: A specific treatment system for alcohol problems, professional help in general health or welfare systems, or non-professional assistance in mutual-help movements. To the extent such help is effective, it is also a means of preventing or reducing future alcohol-related problems in the person helped, although less clearly on a population basis.

Treatments for alcohol problems need not be complex or expensive. The evaluation literature suggests that brief outpatient interventions aimed at changing cognitions and behaviour around drinking are as effective in most circumstances as longer and more intensive treatment (Finney & Monahan 1998; Long *et al.* 1998). Positive results from such interventions in primary health-care settings were shown in a WHO study that included a number of countries (Babor & Grant 1994).

Evidence on effectiveness

In terms of the effects of treatment on those who come for it, there is good evidence on the effectiveness of treatment for alcohol problem. Typically, the improvement rate from a single episode of treatment is about 20 per cent higher than the no-treatment condition: Further treatment episodes are often needed. Brief treatment interventions or mutual-help approaches usually result in net savings in social and health costs associated with the heavy drinker (at least where health care is not self-paid), as well as improving the quality of life (Holder *et al.* 1992; Holder & Cunningham 1992).

The effectiveness of providing treatment as a strategy for reducing rates of alcohol problems in a society is more equivocal. In a North American context, it has been argued that the steep increase in alcohol problems treatment provision and mutual-help group membership in recent decades has contributed to reducing alcohol problems rates (Smart & Mann 1990). But the strength of the evidence for this contention is disputed (Holder 1997; Smart & Mann 1997). A treatment system for alcohol problems is an important part of an integrated national alcohol policy, but as an instrument of prevention—of reducing societal rates of alcohol problems—it is probably not very cost-effective.

Building integrated alcohol policies

Alcohol policy at a community or societal level

Often, the different strategies for preventing alcohol problems appear to be synergic in their effects (DeJong & Hingson 1998). For instance, controls on availability are more likely to be adopted, continued, and respected when the public has been successfully persuaded of their effects and effectiveness. But strategies can also work at cross-purposes: A prohibition policy, for instance, makes it difficult to pursue measures that insulate drinking from harm.

In a society where alcohol is a regular item of consumption, in view of the resulting rates of alcohol-related social and health problems, there is a strong justification for adopting a comprehensive policy concerning alcohol, taking into account production, marketing, and consumption, and the prevention and treatment of alcohol-related problems. In recent years, the idea that there should be an integrated alcohol policy at community or national levels, reaching across the many sectors of government and civil society that deal with alcohol issues, has become a common public health aim, although accomplishing this has often proved difficult (Smart & Mann 1997; Crombie *et al.* 2007).

In terms of strategies we have reviewed for managing and reducing the rates of alcohol problems in the society, there is a clear evidence for effectiveness and cost-effectiveness of measures regulating the availability and conditions of use, and measures which insulate use from harm. With respect to some aspects of alcohol problems, notably drinking–driving, deterrence measures also fall in the same category. Despite their perennial popularity, evidence of the effectiveness of education or persuasion and treatment strategies in reducing societal rates of problems is limited at best. Education and treatment are good things for a society and a government to be doing about alcohol problems, but they do not constitute in themselves a public health policy on alcohol. These strategies will nevertheless be pursued in most societies, and they can best pursued with attention to using cost-effective methods, and to integrating targets and messages with other aspects of alcohol policy.

Alcohol policy in a global perspective

Apart from agreements made a century ago among the European colonial powers about control of the spirits trade in Africa (Bruun *et al.* 1975b), there is little tradition of collaboration on alcohol policy at the international level. It has been largely up to each nation to cope on its own with the serious social and health problems associated with drinking. Although alcohol smuggling has a long history, the nation-state could usually rely on distances and traditional trade barriers to keep alcohol issues largely a matter within its borders, in terms of the supply as well as of the problems.

Since the 1980s, an accelerated rate of economic globalization has been seen, which has increasingly rendered obsolete the assumption that alcohol issues are local issues. This globalization affects alcohol issues in three main ways. The first of these is the influence of a global ideology of free markets. In its sweep, this ideology has caught up and dismantled a variety of market arrangements that served to hold down and to structure alcohol consumption. State and provincial alcohol monopolies in North America were weakened or dismantled (Her *et al.* 1999). In Eastern Europe and the countries in transition, alcohol monopolies were swept away along with most other governmental intrusions in the market (Moskalewicz 1993). Many of the municipally-run beer halls in Southern African countries were privatized (Jernigan 1997). In line with the general ideology, privatization of alcohol production and distribution has been often suggested, abetted or imposed on developing countries by international development agencies (White & Batia 1998).

Secondly, trade agreements, trade dispute mechanisms, and the growth of new sales media have effectively reduced the ability of national and subnational governments to control their local alcohol markets. The influence of trade agreements and trade dispute decisions in breaking down alcohol controls, including control of price through taxation, has been most fully documented for North America (Room *et al.* 2006) and Europe (Holder *et al.* 1998; Tigerstedt 1990), but these mechanisms also operate in the developing world. For instance, average taxes on alcoholic beverages in South Korea were lowered in 2000 as a result of complaints to the World Trade Organization by the European Union and the United States (Kim 2000). Sales of alcoholic beverages through the Internet have become a fast-growing threat to national or local control of alcohol markets (Apple 1999).

Third, alcohol production, distribution, and marketing became increasingly globalized (Jernigan 1997; Room *et al.* 2002). Transnational alcohol companies expanded rapidly into the developing world and the countries in transition in search of new markets, benefiting from weak policy environments and the sweeping tide of market liberalization. Although most alcoholic beverages are still produced in the country in which they are sold, industrially produced beverages were increasingly produced in plants owned, co-owned, or licensed by multinational firms. To promote increased sales, these firms have been able to transform and step up the marketing techniques used in the national market, bringing forth all the marketing resources and expertise they have developed in other markets.

In light of these converging trends, there is a growing need for mechanisms to express public health interests in alcohol issues at the international level, both in trade agreements and settlements of trade disputes, and in creating mutual obligations for one nation to back up rather than subvert the alcohol regulations and policies of another. There are growing calls for a framework convention on alcohol control to be negotiated under the WHO auspices or otherwise, on the model of the tobacco convention (Room 2006; A framework convention on alcohol control 2007).

Conclusion

The comparative risk analysis in the WHO's estimation of the global burden of disease has underlined the substantial role of alcohol in death and disability, particularly in high-income and middle-income countries. Over the last 30 years, sufficient literature has emerged, which allows a differentiation of prevention strategies and policies in terms of their effectiveness. Some strategies—for example, school education, public information campaigns, and provision of alternatives—are often politically popular but have limited or no effect. A few strategies that have proved effective—notably, drinking–driving countermeasures—have been applied in a number of countries. Other effective strategies—especially, controls on price and availability—have been widely resisted in the political process. In a globalized world, control of the alcohol market in the interest of public health is needed not only at the local and national level, but also internationally. This need has led to calls for a framework convention on alcohol control, which would also provide an impetus and template for actions at national and subnational levels.

References

A framework convention on alcohol control [editorial]. *Lancet* 2007 Sep 29;**370**(9593):1102.

Andréasson S., Romelsjö A., Allebeck P. Alcohol, social factors, and mortality among young men. *British Journal of Addiction* 1991;**86**:877–87.

Apple R.W. Zinfandel by mail? New York Times 1999 May 19.

Babor T., Caetano R., Casswell S. *et al. Alcohol: no ordinary commodity – research and public policy.* Oxford: Oxford University Press; 2003.

Babor T.F., Grant M. *et al.* Randomized clinical trial of brief interventions in primary health care: summary of a WHO project (with commentaries and a response). Addiction 1994;**89**:657–78.

Baggott R. *Alcohol, politics, and social policy.* Aldershot, UK: Avebury; 1990.

Beauchamp D. Exploring new ethics for public health: developing a fair alcohol policy. *Journal of Health Politics, Policy, and Law* 1976; **1**:338–54.

Beck J. 100 years of 'just say no' versus 'just say know'. *Evaluation Review* 1998;**22**:15–45.

Blocker J. *American temperance movements: cycles of reform.* Boston (MA): Twayne Publishers; 1989.

Bondy S.J., Rehm J., Ashley M.J. *et al.* Low-risk drinking guidelines: the scientific evidence. *Canadian Journal of Public Health* 1999;**90**:272–6.

Botvin G.J. Principles of prevention. In: Coombs RH, Ziedonis D, editors. *Handbook on drug abuse prevention: a comprehensive strategy to prevent the abuse of alcohol and other drugs.* Boston (MA): Allyn and Bacon; 1995. p. 19–44.

Bruun K., Edwards G., Lumio M. *et al. Alcohol control policies in public health perspective.* Helsinki: Finnish Foundation for Alcohol Studies; 1975a. FFAS Vol. 25.

Bruun K., Rexed I., Pan L. The gentlemen's club. Chicago (IL): University of Chicago Press; 1975b.

Butler B.Y. Holy intoxication to drunken dissipation: alcohol among Quichua speakers in Otavalo, Ecuador. Albuquerque (NM): University of New Mexico Press; 2006.

Carmona M., Stewart K. *Review of alternative activities and alternatives programs in youth-oriented prevention.* Rockville (MD): Center for Substance Abuse Prevention; 1996. CSAP Technical Report 13.

Casswell S. Does alcohol advertising have an impact on public health? *Drug and Alcohol Review.* 1995;14:395–404.

Casswell S., Gilmore L., Maguire V. *et al.* Changes in public support for alcohol policies following a community-based campaign. *British Journal of Addiction* 1989;**84**:515–22.

Casswell S., Pledger M., Pratap S. Trajectories of drinking from 18 to 26 years: identification and prediction. *Addiction* 2002;**97**(11): 1427–37.

Casswell S., Zhang J.F. Impact of liking for advertising and brand allegiance on drinking and alcohol-related aggression: a longitudinal study. *Addiction* 1998;**93**:1209–17.

Catlin G.E.G. *Liquor control.* London: Thornton Butterworth; 1931.

Chadwick D.J., Goode J.A., editors. Alcohol and cardiovascular diseases. Chichester, UK: John Wiley & Sons; 1998.

Cook P. Effect of liquor taxes on drinking, cirrhosis, and auto accidents. In: Moore M.H., Gerstein D.R., editors. *Alcohol and public policy: beyond the shadow of prohibition.* Washington (DC): National Academy Press; 1981. p. 255–85

Cook P.J., Moore M.H. Violence reduction through restrictions on alcohol availability. *Alcohol Health and Research World* 1993;**17**:151–6.

Criqui M. *et al.* Discussion. In: Chadwick D.J., Goode J.A., editors. *Alcohol and cardiovascular diseases.* Chichester, UK: John Wiley & Sons; 1998. p. 122–4.

Crombie I.K., Irvine L., Elliott L. *et al.* How do public health policies tackle alcohol-related harm? A review of 12 developed countries. *Alcohol and Alcoholism* 2007;**42**(**5**):492–9.

Cross J.N. *Guide to the community control of alcoholism.* New York (NY): American Public Health Association; 1968.

De Lint J., Schmidt W. The distribution of alcohol consumption in Ontario. *Quarterly Journal of Studies on Alcohol* 1968;**29**:968–73.

DeJong W., Hingson R. Strategies to reduce driving under the influence of alcohol. *Annual Review of Public Health* 1998;**19**:359–78.

Edwards G., Anderson P., Babor T.F. *et al. Alcohol policy and the public good.* Oxford: Oxford University Press; 1994.

Emerson H., editor. *Alcohol and man: the effects of alcohol on man in health and disease.* New York (NY): Macmillan; 1932.

English D.R., Holman C.D.J., Milne E. *et al. The quantification of drug caused morbidity and mortality in Australia* (2 vol.). Canberra: Australian Government Publishing Service; 1995.

Evans L. *Traffic safety and the driver.* New York (NY): Van Nostrand Reinhold; 1991.

Ezzati M., Lopez A.D., Rodgers A. *et al.* and the Comparative Risk Assessment Collaborating Group. Selected major risk factors and global and regional burden of disease. *Lancet* 2002;**360**(9343):1347–60.

Fillmore K.M., Kerr W.C., Stockwell T. *et al.* Moderate alcohol use and reduced mortality risk: systematic error in prospective studies. *Addiction Research and Theory* 2006;**14**(2):101–32.

Finney J.W., Monahan S.C. Cost-effectiveness of treatment for alcoholism: a second approximation. *Journal of Studies on Alcohol* 1998;**57**:229–43.

Forsyth I. Alcohol and drugs: the role of insurance in promoting effective countermeasures. In Proceedings of the Conference on Road Safety in Europe and Strategic Highway Research Program (SHRP). Linköping, Sweden: Swedish National Road and Transport Safety Institute; 1996. VTI Conferens No. 4A. Part 3. p. 45–63.

Foxcroft D.R., Ireland D., Lister-Sharp F.J. *et al.* Longer-term primary prevention for alcohol misuse in young people: a systematic review. *Addiction* 2003;**98** Suppl 4:397–411.

Giesbrecht N., Conley P., Denniston R. *et al.* editors. *Research, action and the community: experiences in the prevention of alcohol and other drug problems.* Rockville (MD): Office of Substance Abuse Prevention; 1990. DHHS Publication No. (ADM) 89–1651.

Gorman D.M., Conde E., Huber Jr. J.C. The creation of evidence in 'evidence-based' drug prevention: a critique of the Strengthening Families Program Plus Life Skills Training evaluation. *Drug and Alcohol Review* 2007;**26**(6):585–93.

Graham K., Leonard K.E., Room R. *et al.* Current directions in research on understanding and preventing intoxicated aggression. *Addiction* 1998;**93**:659–76.

Grant M., Litvak J. Introduction: beyond per capita consumption. In: Grant M, Litvak J, editors. *Drinking patterns and their consequences.* Washington (DC): Taylor and Francis; 1998. p. 1–4.

Greenfield T., Zimmerman R., editors. *Experiences with community action projects: new research in the prevention of alcohol and other drug problems.* Rockville (MD): Center for Substance Abuse Prevention; 1993. DHHS Publication No. (ADM) 93–1976.

Grover P.T., editor. *Preventing problems related to alcohol availability— environmental approaches: reference guide.* Washington (DC): Center for Substance Abuse Prevention; 1999. DHHS Publication No. SMA 99–3298. Available from: http://text.nlm.nih.gov/ftrs/dbaccess/csap

Hawks D. A review of current guidelines on moderate drinking for individual consumers. *Contemporary Drug Problems* 1994;**21**:223–37.

Hawks D. The formulation of Australia's National Health Policy on Alcohol. *Addiction* 1993;**88** Supplement:19S–26S.

Hemström Ö. Per capita alcohol consumption and ischaemic heart disease mortality. *Addiction* 2001;**96** Suppl 1:93–112.

Her M., Giesbrecht N., Room R. *et al.* Privatizing alcohol sales and alcohol consumption: evidence and implications. *Addiction* 1999;**94**:1125–39.

Her M., Rehm J. Alcohol and all-cause mortality in Europe 1982–1990: a pooled cross-section time-series analysis. *Addiction* 1998;**93**:1335–40.

Herd D. Ideology, history, and changing models of liver cirrhosis epidemiology. *British Journal of Addiction* 1992;**87**:179–92.

Hingson R. Prevention of drinking and driving. *Alcohol Health and Research World.* 1996;20;219–26.

Holder H.D. *Alcohol and the community: a systems approach to prevention.* Cambridge, UK: Cambridge University Press; 1998.

Holder H. Can individually directed interventions reduce population-level alcohol-involved problems?. *Addiction* 1997;**92**:5–7.

Holder H.D., Cunningham D.W. Alcoholism treatment for employees and family members: its effect on health care costs. *Alcohol Health and Research World* 1992;**16**:149–53.

Holder H.D., Kühlhorn E., Nordlund S. *et al. European integration and Nordic alcohol policies.* Aldershot, UK: Ashgate; 1998.

Holder H.D., Lennox R.D.L., Blose J.O. Economic benefits of alcoholism treatment: a summary of twenty years of research. *Journal of Employee Assistance Research* 1992;**1**:63–82.

Holmila M., editor. *Community Prevention of Alcohol Problems.* Basingstoke, UK: Macmillan; 1997.

Järvinen M. The controlled controllers: women, men, and alcohol. *Contemporary Drug Problems* 1991;**18**:389–406.

Jernigan D.H. *Thirsting for markets: the global impact of corporate alcohol.* San Rafael (CA): Marin Institute for the Prevention of Alcohol and Other Drug Problems; 1997.

Katcher B.S. The post-repeal eclipse in knowledge about the harmful effects of alcohol. *Addiction* 1993;**88**:729–44.

Kauhanen J., Kaplan G.A., Goldberg D.E. *et al.* Beer bingeing and mortality: results from the Kuopio ischaemic heart disease risk factor study, a prospective population-based study. *British Medical Journal* 1997;**315**:846–51.

Kim H-R. Revised liquor taxes leave soju makers in lurch. Korea Herald 2000 Mar 13.

Klatsky A.L. Moderate drinking and reduced risk of heart disease. *Alcohol Research and Health* 1999;**23**(1):15–23.

Knupfer G. The epidemiology of problem drinking. *American Journal of Public Health* 1967;**57**:973–86.

Kozlowski L.T., Heller D.A., Pillitteri J.L. *et al.* Tobacco use, the health effects of moderate alcohol drinking, and the assessment of their interaction. *Contemporary Drug Problems* 1994;**21**:81–9.

Kreitman N. Alcohol consumption and the preventive paradox. *British Journal of Addiction* 1986;**81**:353–63.

Kupari M., Koskinen P. Alcohol, cardiac arrhythmias and sudden death. In: Chadwick DJ, Goode JA, editors. *Alcohol and Cardiovascular Diseases.* Chichester, UK: John Wiley & Sons; 1998. p. 68–79.

Kypri K., Voas R.B., Langley J.D. *et al.* Minimum purchasing age for alcohol and traffic crash injuries among 15- to 19-year-olds in New Zealand. *American Journal of Public Health* 2006;**96**(1):126–31.

Ledermann S. *Alcool, Alcoolisme, Alcoolisation.* Paris: Presses Universitaires de France. INED Cahier No. 29; 1956.

Leon D.A., Chenet L., Shkolnikov V.M. *et al.* Huge variation in Russian mortality rates 1984–94: artefact, alcohol, or what?. *Lancet* 1997;**350**:383–8.

Levine H.G. Temperance cultures: concern about alcohol problems in Nordic and English-speaking cultures. In: Lader M, Edwards G, Drummond DC, editors. *The nature of alcohol and drug related problems.* Oxford: Oxford University Press; 1991. p. 15–36.

Long C.G., Williams M., Hollin C.R. (1998) Treating alcohol problems: a study of program effectiveness and cost-effectiveness according to length and delivery of treatment. *Addiction;***93**:561–71.

MacAndrew C., Edgerton R.E. *Drunken Comportment.* Chicago (IL): Aldine; 1969.

Maclure M. Demonstration of deductive meta-analysis: ethanol intake and risk of myocardial infarction. *Epidemiologic Reviews* 1993;**15**:328–51.

Mäkelä K. The uses of alcohol and their cultural regulation. *Acta Sociologica* 1983;**26**:21–31.

McKee M., Britton A. The positive relationship between alcohol and heart disease in Eastern Europe: potential physiological mechanisms. *Journal of the Royal Society of Medicine* 1998;**91**:402–7.

Møller L. Legal restrictions resulted in a reduction of alcohol consumption among young people in Denmark. In: Room R, editor. *The effects of Nordic alcohol policies: what happens to drinking when alcohol controls change?* Helsinki: Nordic Council for Alcohol and Drug Research; 2002. NAD Publication 42 p. 93–100. Available from: http://www.nad.fi/pdf/NAD_42.pdf

Moore M.H., Gerstein D.R. (1981) (eds) *Alcohol and Public Policy: Beyond the Shadow of Prohibition.* Washington (DC): National Academy Press; 1981.

Moskalewicz J. Privatization of the alcohol arena in Poland. *Contemporary Drug Problems* 1993;**20**:63–275.

Moskowitz J.M., Mailvin J., Schaeffer G.A. *et al.* Evaluation of a junior high school primary prevention program. *Addictive Behaviors* 1983;**8**:393–401.

Mott G. The anti-alcohol network. *Moderation Reader* 1991;**5**(5):6–20.

Neves P., de Pape D., Giesbrecht N. *et al.* (1998) Communities take action! A practical guide for municipalities, enforcement agencies, community groups, and others concerned about the impact of alcohol on public health and safety. Toronto: Addiction Research Foundation.

NIAAA. *Alcohol and the Immune System*. In the 9th special report to the US Congress on alcohol and health. Rockville (MD): National Institute on Alcohol Abuse and Alcoholism; 1997. p. 163–9. NIH Publication No. 97–4017.

Norman E., Turner S., Zunz S.J. *et al.* Prevention programs reviewed: what works? In: Norman E, editor. *Drug-free Youth: A Compendium for Prevention Specialists.* New York (NY): Garland Publishing; 1997. p. 22–45.

Norström T. Abolition of the Swedish rationing system: effects on consumption distribution and cirrhosis mortality. *British Journal of Addiction* 1987;**82**:633–41.

Norström T. Per capita consumption and total mortality: an analysis of historical data. *Addiction* 1996;**91**:339–44.

Norström T., Ramstedt M. Mortality and population drinking: a review of the literature. *Drug and Alcohol Review* 2005;**24**(6)**537–47**. Available from: http://www.informaworld.com.ezproxy.lib.unimelb.edu.au/ smpp/title~content=t713412284~db=all~tab=issueslist~branches=24 - v24

Olsson B. Alkoholpolitik och alkoholens fenomenologi: uppfattningar som artikulerats i pressen [Alcohol policy and the phenomenology of alcohol: concepts articulated in the press]. *Alkoholpolitik* 1990;**7**: 184–95.

Paglia A., Room R. Preventing substance use problems among youth: a literature review and recommendations. *Journal of Primary Prevention* 1999;**20**:3–50.

Peele S. The limitations of control-of-supply models for explaining and preventing alcoholism and drug addiction. *Journal of Studies on Alcohol* 1987;**48**:61–77.

Perrine M.W., Peck R.C., Fell J.C. Epidemiologic perspectives on drunk driving. In: *Surgeon General's Workshop on Drunk Driving: Background Papers.* Washington (DC): US Department of Health and Human Services; 1989. p. 35–76.

Plant M., Single E., Stockwell T., editors. *Alcohol: Minimizing the Harm— What Works?* London and New York (NY): Free Association Books; 1997.

Poikolainen K. It can be bad for the heart, too—drinking patterns and coronary heart disease. *Addiction* 1999;**93**:1757–9.

Popham R., Schmidt W., de Lint J. The effects of legal restraint on drinking. In: Kissin B., Begleiter H., editors. *The Biology of Alcoholism: vol. 4. Social Aspects of Alcoholism.* New York (NY) and London: Plenum; 1976. p. 579–625.

Ramstedt M. Is alcohol good or bad for Canadian hearts? A time-series analysis of the link between alcohol consumption and IHD mortality. *Drug and Alcohol Review* 2006;**25**(**4**):315–20.

Rehm J., Room R., Monteiro M. *et al.* Alcohol use. In: Ezzati M., Lopez D., Rodgers A., Murray C.J.L., editors. *Comparative quantification of health risks. Global and regional burden of disease attributable to selected major risk factors: volume 1.* Geneva: World Health Organization; 2004. p. 959–1108.

Rehm J., Sempos C.T. Alcohol consumption and all-cause mortality. *Addiction* 1995;**90**:471–80.

Room R. A 'reverence for strong drink': the lost generation and the elevation of alcohol in American culture. *Journal of Studies on Alcohol* 1984b;**45**:540–6.

Room R. Alcohol and crime: behavioral aspects. In: Kadish S, editor. *Encyclopedia of crime and justice.* Vol. 1. New York (NY): Free Press; 1983. p. 35–44.

Room R. Alcohol and the World Health Organization: the ups and downs of two decades. *Nordisk Alkohol- & Narkotikatidskrift* 2005;**22** (English suppl):146–162.

Room R. Alcohol consumption and social harm—conceptual issues and historical perspectives. *Contemporary Drug Problems* 1996; **23**:373–88.

Room R. Alcohol control and public health. *Annual Review of Public Health* 1984a;**5**:293–317.

Room R. Former NIAAA directors look back: policy makers on the role of research. *Drinking and Drug Practices Surveyor* 1984c;**19**:38–42.

Room R. International control of alcohol: alternative paths forward. *Drug and Alcohol Review* 2006;**25**:581–95.

Room R. The evolution of alcohol monopolies and their relevance for public health. *Contemporary Drug Problems* 1993;**20**:169–87.

Room R. The idea of alcohol policy. *Nordic Studies on Alcohol and Drugs* 1999;**16** (English Suppl):7–20.

Room R. Voluntary organizations and the state in the prevention of alcohol problems. *Drugs and Society* 1997;**11**:11–23.

Room R., Giesbrecht N., Stoduto G. Trade agreements and disputes. In: Giesbrecht N, Demers A, Ogborne A *et al.* editors. *Sober reflections: commerce, public health, and the evolution of alcohol policy in Canada, 1980–2000.* Montreal and Kingston: McGill-Queen's University Press; 2006. p. 74–96.

Room R., Jernigan D., Carlini-Marlatt B. *et al. Alcohol and developing societies: a public health approach.* Helsinki: Finnish Foundation for Alcohol Studies; 2002.

Rorabaugh W.J. *The alcoholic republic.* New York (NY): Oxford University Press; 1979.

Rose G. Strategy of prevention: lessons from cardiovascular disease. *British Medical Journal* 1981;**282**:1847–51.

Ross H.L. Deterring the drinking driver: legal policy and social control. Lexington (MA): Lexington Books; 1982.

Saffer H. Economic issues in cigarette and alcohol advertising. *Journal of Drug Issues* 1998;**28**:781–93.

Saltz R.F. Prevention where alcohol is sold and consumed: server intervention and responsible beverage service. In: Plant M., Single E., Stockwell T., editors. *Alcohol: minimizing the harm—what works?* New York (NY): Free Association Books; 1997. p. 72–84.

Schechter E.J. Alcohol rationing and control systems in Greenland. *Contemporary Drug Problems* 1986;**13**:587–620.

Seeley J.R. Death by liver cirrhosis and the price of beverage alcohol. *Canadian Medical Association Journal* 1960;**83**:1361–6.

Shkolnikov V.M., Nemtsov A. The anti-alcohol campaign and variations in Russian mortality. In: Bobadilla J.L., Costello C.A., Mitchell F., editors. *Premature death in the new independent states.* Washington (DC): National Academy Press; 1997. p. 239–61.

Skog O-J. The collectivity of drinking cultures: a theory of the distribution of alcohol consumption. *British Journal of Addiction* 1985;**80**:83–99.

Skog O-J. Public health consequences of the J-curve hypothesis of alcohol problems. *Addiction* 1996;**91**:325–37.

Smart R.G., Mann R.E. Are increased levels of treatment and Alcoholics Anonymous large enough to create the recent reduction in liver cirrhosis?. *British Journal of Addiction* 1990;**85**:1385–7.

Smart R.G., Mann R.E. Interventions into alcohol problems: what works? *Addiction* 1997;**92**:9–13.

Stimson G., Grant M., Choquet M. *et al.* editors. *Drinking in context: patterns, interventions, and partnerships.* New York (NY) and Abingdon, Oxfordshire: Routledge; 2007.

Stockwell T., Single E., Hawks D. *et al.* Sharpening the focus of alcohol policy from aggregate consumption to harm and risk reduction. *Addiction Research* 1997;**5**:1–9.

Sutton C. Swedish alcohol discourse: constructions of a social problem. *Acta Universitatis Upsaliensis, Studia Sociologica Upsaliensia.* 1998;45.

Teasley D.L. Drug legalization and the 'lessons' of Prohibition. *Contemporary Drug Problems* 1992;**19**:27–52.

Terris M. Epidemiology of cirrhosis of the liver: national mortality data. *American Journal of Public Health* 1967;**57**:2076–88.

Tigerstedt C. Alcohol policy, public health, and Kettil Bruun. *Contemporary Drug Problems* 1999;**26**:209–35.

Tigerstedt C. The European Community and the alcohol policy dimension. *Contemporary Drug Problems* 1990;**17**:461–79.

White O.C., Batia A. *Privatization in Africa.* Washington (DC): World Bank; 1998.

Whitehead P.C. Prevention of alcoholism. In: Robinson D, editor. *Alcohol problems*. New York (NY): Holmes and Meier; 1979.

Wolfgang M.E. *Patterns in criminal homicide*. Philadelphia (PA): University of Pennsylvania Press; 1958.

World Health Organization, Expert Committee on Problems Related to Alcohol Consumption. Problems related to alcohol consumption. Geneva: World Health Organization; 1980. Technical Report Series 650.

World Health Organization, Expert Committee on Problems Related to Alcohol Consumption. Second Report. Geneva: World Health Organization; 2007. Technical Report Series 944. Available from: http://www.who.int/substance_abuse/activities/expert_comm_alcohol_2nd_report.pdf

World Health Organization. *Global status report: alcohol policy*. Geneva: World Health Organization; 2004.

Wyllie A., Zhang J.F., Casswell S. Positive responses to televised beer advertisements associated with drinking and problems reported by 18- to 29-year-olds. *Addiction* 1998a;**93**:749–60.

Wyllie A., Zhang J.F., Casswell S. Responses to televised advertisement associated with drinking behaviour of 10–17-year-olds. *Addiction* 1998b;**93**:361–71.

10.4

Injury prevention and control: The public health approach

Corinne Peek-Asa and Adnan A. Hyder

Abstract

Injuries are among the leading causes of death and disability throughout the world, and injury rates are highest among middle- and low-income countries. Efforts in injury prevention have high potential gain for society because they disproportionately reduce death and disability to the young. Many opportunities to implement injury prevention strategies exist, and a systematic approach to injury prevention can help identify the most effective and efficient approaches. Building capacity for injury prevention activities in low- and middle-income countries is an important public health priority.

Introduction

Injuries are a leading contributor to the disease burden worldwide. They contribute significantly to premature life lost and years lived with disability for all countries, all regions of the world, and all age groups. Injuries cause over 5 million deaths per year, with approximately 1.2 million of these due to road traffic injuries (Krug *et al.* 2000; Peden *et al.* 2002; World Health Organization 2004). For children under 14 years of age, road traffic crashes, drowning, fires, poisoning, interpersonal violence, and war are all in the leading 10 causes of death. Deaths represent just a small proportion of the many injuries that cause serious injury and potentially life-long disability, and injuries also cause significant psychological trauma and financial loss. The burden of traumatic injuries necessitates that injury prevention be considered an international public health priority.

Because the majority of us will suffer multiple minor injuries throughout our lives, most of which cause only minor discomfort or inconvenience, we may be lulled into believing that injuries are just part of life. However, a serious injury or the traumatic death of a loved one can completely change the course of the lives of those affected. Many of these severe and fatal injuries can be prevented, and global investment in traumatic injury prevention will have significant long-term health and financial benefits.

For developed countries, progress has been made in reducing the toll of traumatic injuries. In the United States, for example, road traffic crashes per million vehicle miles travelled decreased nearly 90 per cent from the 1930s into the twenty-first century (Institute of Medicine 1999). Mortality rates have decreased for deaths from drowning, residential fires, homicide, poisoning, among others. However, these rates remain unacceptably high knowing that many effective prevention strategies have not yet been widely implemented.

The burden of traumatic injury worldwide is disproportionately concentrated in lower-income countries (Hofman *et al.* 2005; Ameratunga *et al.* 2006). The World Health Organization (WHO) anticipates that, if current trends continue, road traffic injuries, interpersonal violence, war, and self-inflicted injuries will all be among the leading 15 causes of disability-adjusted life years lost by the year 2020. Road traffic crashes, which in 1990 ranked as the ninth leading cause of disability-adjusted life years lost, is predicted to reach the rank of three in 2020 (Peden *et al.* 2002). Operations of war will rise from the rank of 16 in 1990 to 8 by 2020, and interpersonal violence will rise from rank 19 to 12. Despite some successes in many areas of injury prevention, new risks, changing environments, and increasing population size constantly challenge injury control efforts.

Effective injury prevention strategies will require organization of the public health response and increased integration of professionals from many backgrounds. Modern injury control research combines ideas and skills from public health, biomechanics, engineering, behavioural sciences, law, law enforcement, medicine, and urban planning, among others. Research that identifies how effective interventions in high-income countries can be translated in low- and middle-income settings is a priority, but injury prevention strategies will need to be appropriate for local environments. Injury prevention activities that integrate multiple approaches within an organized public health response have a stronger chance of success.

This chapter will present the current state of knowledge regarding the burden of injuries and will introduce the basic concepts of building injury prevention infrastructure and capacity.

Causal model of injuries

Injuries are generally divided into the two broad categories of intentional and unintentional. Intentional injuries are those in which there was an intent to commit harm, either to oneself or someone else. Unintentional injuries occur without a direct intent to commit harm, even if gross negligence was involved. For example, a motor vehicle occupant death caused by a drunk driver would be considered an unintentional injury even though in many countries the driver could be prosecuted for a crime.

Injuries are further classified by their cause, such as motor vehicle occupant injuries, drowning, suicide/attempted suicide, homicide/assault, or residential fire injuries. Until the late 1990s, cause and intent were coded together, so that, for example, a poisoning death would not be distinguished as intentional or unintentional. In the 1990s, a collaboration between the US Centers for Disease Control and Prevention and the American Public Health Association recommended that cause and intent be considered as separate components of describing an injury, and most data are now coded accordingly (Centers for Disease Control and Prevention 1997). Through this collaboration, a matrix to code injuries by intent and cause using the International Classification of Diseases, 9th revision, was developed. This matrix served as a template to create codes for injury cause and intent that are now included in the 10th revision of this coding system.

Injury causes are very broad and represent a diverse range of physical harm. What, therefore, is the uniting feature that defines an injury? The traditional epidemiologic model for infectious diseases provides a framework for the epidemiologic study of traumatic injury (Fig. 10.4.1). At the centre of the causal pathway for injuries is the agent-host interaction. The agent, which in the case of injuries is energy, is absorbed by the host to cause injury. Energy can take many forms, such as mechanical, electrical, chemical, radiation, and thermal. An example of an agent-host relationship is a motor vehicle crash, in which the energy exerted on the individual is mechanical. The reservoir is the place in the environment where the agent is found. The potential for energy transfer exists everywhere, but its potential to cause injury is limited to specific conditions. For instance, the potential energy in a motor vehicle exists only when the car is being driven, and causes injury only when the vehicle crashes.

Vehicles and vectors are mechanisms which transport energy from the reservoir to the host. A vehicle is an inanimate object, such as a motor vehicle; a vector is animate, such as a dog biting a child. For many injury causes, vehicles and vectors are both involved in energy transfer, such as when one individual (vector) stabs another with a knife (vehicle). The injury outcome is the trauma or injury sustained by the individual, and is influenced by host responses to the energy. Only energy transmitted beyond a host's tolerance causes an injury, and therefore not all exposures to energy result in noticeable injury. A human has some resistance to energy which can be increased through exercise or protective devices, or reduced through changes in intrinsic factors such as existing medical conditions or age and through extrinsic factors such as fatigue and alcohol.

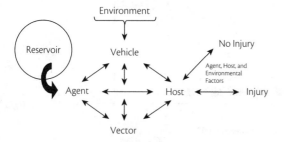

Fig. 10.4.1 Causal model of injury.

This causal model is important when considering injury prevention strategies. Injury prevention aims to prevent energy transfer or to reduce the amount of energy that is transferred. Prevention activities can focus on the host, on the environment, on vehicles or vectors, or combine all of these components. A theoretical approach to injury prevention based on this model is presented later in this chapter.

Data sources

Data that describe injury events and that provide information related to injuries can be found from a wide variety of sources, both within and outside of the health sector (Hyder & Morrow 2006). Data sources within the health sector include some that capture a wide range of health conditions, such as health information systems, vital registration systems and hospital discharge data. Other sources are specific to injuries, such as emergency medical services data and trauma registries. Sources outside the health sector cover a wide spectrum, including data from police, the transportation sector, legal records, and insurance company claims. Sources such as newspaper articles and consumer reports have also been used to describe injury incidence and risk. This diversity of data sources makes the field of injuries and violence unique in terms of the inter-sectoral nature of the information (Norton et al. 2006).

In many instances, data sources need to be linked together to provide a complete description of the injury. Motor vehicle crash injuries, for example, often require data from traffic enforcement to describe the cause and nature of the crash and data from the health sector to describe the injuries and their severity. Linking these data sources can be impeded by issues of privacy and access to identifying information for linkage, as well as data quality issues. In low- and middle-income countries these data systems, if they exist at all, are often not computerized and have never been evaluated for quality, making such linkages even more challenging. However, information from multiple sources is often necessary to examine causal hypotheses about injuries.

The Global Burden of Disease study attempted to collect consistent and internationally comparable data (Murray & Lopez 1996; WHO 2002). This global data has several limitations in regard to injuries. For example, burn data include deaths from fire-related burns only, and exclude scalds, and drowning deaths exclude drowning deaths due to floods. However, this data is the most comprehensive source for describing the global burden of injuries, especially in relation to other health conditions, and it is thus very useful for public health purposes.

Generally, mortality data has the highest quality, and most high- and middle-income countries have some vital statistics systems that capture the majority of deaths and their causes. Population-based data that describe the causes and types of non-fatal injuries and their outcomes are more challenging to collect and far less available, especially in the developing world. The public health infrastructure and routine collection of health information in the developing world has been fragile, especially in regions such as sub-Saharan Africa and South Asia. It is thus not surprising that there has been little tradition of developing specific information sources for injuries. Population-based studies from low- and middle-income countries, though, consistently conclude that the injury burden is higher than reported in national official statistics and that injuries are significantly underreported in these regions.

One of the important developments over the past decades in the field of health information systems has been the development of summary measures of population health (Hyder & Morrow 2006). The sentinel work of the Ghana Health Assessment Team in the development of the days of life lost indicator evolved into the launch of the disability adjusted life year (DALY) by the World Bank and WHO (WDR 1993; Hyder *et al.* 1998). The DALY combines the loss of healthy life from premature mortality and that lost from life lived with disability in the uni-dimensional measure of time (Murray & Lopez 1996). This allows deaths, morbidity, disability—both fatal and non fatal health outcomes—from a disease to be measured (Fig. 10.4.2). The combination of years of life lost (premature deaths) and years lived with disability in summary measures of population health (like DALY) is important for injuries which cause both types of health outcomes. Technical details of the DALY and other measures are available elsewhere (Murray and Lopez 1996; www.who.int).

Global burden of injury

Over 5 million deaths occur from all injuries worldwide each year (Table 10.4.1), of which nearly 85 per cent are in low–middle income countries (LMIC) (World Health Organization 2002). Nearly 25 per cent of these deaths are caused by road traffic injuries, with self-inflicted injuries and violence comprising a further 17 and 11 per cent of deaths respectively (Fig. 10.4.3). Injury death rates are highest for road traffic injuries, followed by 'other' unintentional injuries, self-inflicted injuries and violence; similar patterns are observed for non-fatal health outcomes using DALY rates (Table 10.4.2).

Road traffic injuries (RTIs) alone kill over 1 million people every year, qualifying these types of injuries as the tenth leading cause of death worldwide (World Health Organization 1999). According to the Global Burden of Disease study, death and disability from road traffic injuries are projected to rise substantially in future years to become the third leading cause of disability-adjusted life years lost worldwide by 2020 (Murray & Lopez 1996). Globally, the majority of those killed are from low- or middle-income countries. The absolute number of fatalities and the mortality rate resulting from road traffic injuries vary considerably across countries, and although all age groups are affected young adults, particularly males, are most at risk of loss of life. Since this age group corresponds to the most economically productive segment of the population, road traffic injuries have serious implications for national economies.

The WHO estimates that there are over 3 million cases of acute poisoning resulting in over 300 000 deaths each year. More males die from poisoning and over 90 per cent of these events occur in LMIC. Non-fatal, unintentional poisoning resulted in a loss of over 7.5 million DALYs globally. Falls cause more than 350 000 deaths worldwide with a mortality rate of 6 per 100 000 globally. They result in more than 15 million DALYs lost per year (2 DALYs per 1000 population)—signifying the important contribution of morbidity and disability from falls. The global burden from falls is also disproportionately high in low- and middle-income countries. Over 300 000 deaths are caused by fire burns resulting in more than 10 million DALYs lost; however, unlike other injuries, more females than males died from fires (male to female ratio of 0.6:1.00). Causing an estimated 400 000 deaths each year, drowning is the second leading cause of unintentional injury death globally, with 97 per cent of these deaths in low- and middle-income countries. (These data include only 'accidental drowning and submersion and exclude drowning due to floods [cataclysms], boating and water transport'.) One-third of drowning occurs in the Western Pacific Region, though Africa has the highest drowning fatality rate. Overall, the male rate of drowning is more than twice that for females.

Self-inflicted injuries, including suicides, attempted suicide, self-destructive behaviours and self-mutilation, cause the deaths of over 850 000 people globally, resulting in more than 20 million DALYs lost. Interpersonal violence disproportionately affects low- and middle-income countries with an estimated rate of 32 per 100 000 people, compared to 14.4 per 100 000 in high-income countries

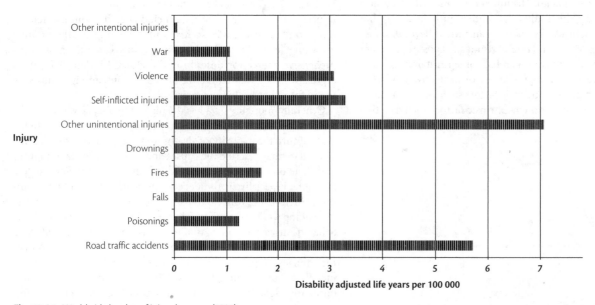

Fig. 10.4.2 Worldwide burden of injury by cause (2001).

Table 10.4.1 Deaths from injuries worldwide, 2001

	Total	Males	Females
All injuries	5 185 745	3 482 854	1 702 891
Unintentional injuries	3 534 562	2 296 318	1 238 244
Road traffic accidents	1 189 417	866 871	322 547
Poisonings	349 460	225 797	123 664
Falls	387 477	233 661	153 816
Fires	309 740	118 583	191 157
Drowning	384 666	263 145	121 521
Other unintentional injuries	913 802	588 262	325 539
Intentional injuries	1 651 183	1 186 536	464 647
Self-inflicted injuries	874 533	547 017	327 516
Violence	556 272	442 137	114 136
War	207 589	187 128	20 461
Other intentional injuries	12 788	10 253	2 534

(Krug *et al.* 2002). Surveys indicate that up to 8 per cent of women (over 16 years) report experiencing sexual violence within the past 5 years, while up to 27 per cent report experiencing sexual violence from an intimate partner in the past year (Krug *et al.* 2002). An estimated 200 000 youth homicides are committed globally varying from 1 in high-income countries to 36 per 100 000 in Latin America. It is estimated that for every youth homicide, there are up to 40 victims of non-fatal youth violence receiving hospital treatment (Krug *et al.* 2002).

Surprisingly, the burden of homicide is found in children under 5 years of age as well; the rate of homicides are 2.2 per 100 000 for boys and 1.8 per 100 000 for girls in high-, and 6.1 and 5.1 per 100 000 for boys and girls, respectively, in low-income countries (Krug *et al.* 2002). Abuse of the elderly occurs in the home and institutions and there is a lack of global data on this issue; however,

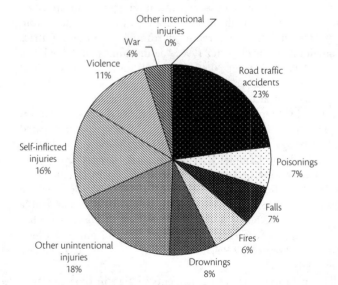

Fig. 10.4.3 Distribution of injury deaths in low- and middle-income countries, 2001.

surveys in the developed world indicate a prevalence of 4–6 per cent of abuse of older persons (Krug *et al.* 2002). War is also an important form of collective violence and was estimated by WHO to cause more than 200 000 direct deaths worldwide in 2001.

Disparity in injury morbidity and mortality

South Africa reported drowning as the 2nd leading cause of injury mortality for children less than 15 years (Kibel *et al.* 1990) and demonstrated an increasing trend in drowning deaths for all ethnic groups in the 1980s and 1990s (Cywes *et al.* 1990; Kibel *et al.* 1990). A review of more than 300 paediatric deaths (0–14 years) in the United Arab Emirates revealed that drowning was the 2nd leading cause of death for both genders (Bener *et al.* 1998). Drowning is also the second leading cause of death for the 10–19 year age group in Taiwan; while it remains the number one cause for males aged 10–14 years (Lu *et al.* 1998). China and India—the world's most populous nations—contribute 43 per cent of the world drowning deaths and 41 per cent of the total DALYS attributed to drowning globally (World Health Organization 2003).

Recent work from South Asia explores police data in Pakistan, and provides a unique picture of trends in suicides over 15 years (1985–1999). During this period, there were 2568 reported suicides, 71 per cent in men and 39 per cent in women. While firearms are the leading method of suicide in the United States, in Pakistan, the leading method was organophosphates followed by hanging (Khan & Hyder 2006).

The true extent of intimate partner violence is largely unknown but surveys in Paraguay and the Philippines reveal that 10 per cent of women surveyed reported being assaulted by an intimate partner compared to 22 per cent in the United States, 29 per cent in Canada, and 34 per cent in Egypt (Krug *et al.* 2002). Other studies show that 3 per cent of women in Australia, the United States and Canada had been assaulted by a partner in the previous 12 months, compared to 27 per cent in Nicaragua, 38 per cent in South Korea, and 53 per cent in West Bank and Gaza (Krug *et al.* 2002). Country comparisons are difficult because data is sparse and because of varying definitions of what constitutes abuse. Furthermore, cultural norms may lead to very different reporting tendencies. Women in countries who have conducted programmes to screen and respond to intimate partner violence, including victim's assistance programmes and social marketing campaigns against intimate partner violence, may be less inhibited to divulge their experiences with violence.

Economic and societal burden

The average annual cost of road crashes has been estimated at about 1 per cent of the gross national product in developing countries, 1.5 per cent in countries in economic transition, and 2 per cent in highly motorized countries. The annual economic cost of road traffic injuries globally is about US$518 billion. In low- and middle-income countries, the annual cost of road traffic crashes is about US$65 billion, exceeding the total annual amount received by these countries in development assistance (Jacobs 2000). Studies exploring the economic and social costs of road traffic injuries in low-income countries show that males who provided the majority of the household income in India and Bangladesh were the most common victims of road traffic fatalities; and the consequences included reduced household income and reduced food consumption for the victim's family

Table 10.4.2 The Haddon matrix for motor vehicle safety (illustrative)

Phases	Factors			
	Human	**Vehicle**	**Physical environment**	**Sociocultural environment**
Pre-injury	Reduce alcohol intoxication, programmes to increase defensive driving and decrease road rage	Increase vehicle stability, increased visibility	Improvements in road structure and traffic controls, traffic calming measures	Support safety programmes and increase consumer awareness of safety issues
Injury	Use of seat belts and car seats, proper placement of car seats, booster seats	Increase energy absorbed by the vehicle frame, safety features such as air bags, head rests, shatterproof windshields, and collapsible steering columns	Install energy-absorbing guard rails	Programmes to provide car seats, educational programmes about car seat installation and placement
Post-injury	Stabilize serious injuries, reduce bleeding and other complications	Design for easier extrication	Enhanced emergency medical systems and field care	Support infrastructure of trauma care, including 911 system, emergency and trauma care, and rehabilitation services

(Aeron-Thomas *et al.* 2004). In addition, the poor were found to spend a much greater proportion of their income on funeral and/or medical costs than the non-poor (Aeron-Thomas *et al.* 2004).

Estimates of the cost of violence the United States reach over 3 per cent of the gross domestic product. In England and Wales, the total costs from violence amount to an estimated US$40 billion annually. The economic effects of interpersonal violence are expected to be more severe in poorer countries, and yet, there is a scarcity of studies on the costs of violence in low- and middle-income countries (Waters *et al.* 2004). However, estimates from low- and middle-income countries indicate that the overall costs of violence are substantial, ranging up to 25 per cent of annual gross domestic product. Comparisons with high-income countries are complicated by the fact that economic losses related to productivity tend to be undervalued in lower-income countries. Child abuse results in US$94 billion in annual costs to the US economy (1 per cent of GDP) and intimate partner violence costs the US economy nearly US$13 billion (0.1 per cent of GDP); this can be compared to 1.6 per cent of GDP in Nicaragua and 2 per cent of GDP in Chile. The cost of gun violence also has been calculated at US$155 billion annually in the United States.

Risk factors for injuries

Motorization rates rise with income (Kopits & Cropper 2003), and in a growing number of LMIC where economies are experiencing growth, there has been a corresponding increase in the numbers of motor vehicles (Ghaffar *et al.* 1999). Data obtained from routinely collected police reports in a number of LMIC show that speed is a leading causal factor in road traffic crashes (Afukaar 2003; Odero 2003; Wang *et al.* 2003), accounting for up to 50 per cent of all crashes. Alcohol is associated with an increased risk of road crashes (Peden *et al.* 2004) and in studies conducted in LMIC alcohol has been shown to be present in up to 69 per cent of fatally-injured drivers (Odero & Zwi 1995). A study from China showed a two-fold increased risk of car crash associated with driver chronic sleepiness (Liu *et al.* 2003); while surveys of commercial road transport in African countries have shown that drivers often

work unduly long hours and go to work when exhausted (Mock *et al.* 1999; Nafukho & Khayesi 2002). A significant risk factor for increased injury severity is non-use or inappropriate use of safety devices such as motorcycle helmets (Kulanthayan *et al.* 2000; Liu *et al.* 2004), and seat belts (Peden *et al.* 2004).

Risk factors for falls in older people include: Low bone density; poor nutritional status; low body mass index; low calcium intake; co-morbid conditions (hypertension, diabetes); poor performance in activities of daily living; poor cognitive function; poor vision; environmental factors affecting balance; family history of hip fracture; and alcohol consumption (Cummings *et al.* 1995; Dargent-Molina *et al.* 1996; Clark *et al.* 1998; Boonyaratavej *et al.* 2001). A study in Thailand suggested that features associated with poor socioeconomic status may also be risk factors, for example, lack of electricity in the house and living in Thai huts (Jitapunkul *et al.* 2001). In younger ages, falls from balconies, apartment windows, beds, nursery equipment, and playground equipment are commonly reported in high-income nations. In addition, falls from roof tops and trees are reported from developing countries (Bangdiwala & Anzola-Perez 1990; Adesunkanmi *et al.* 1999; Kozik *et al.* 1999; MacGregor 2000; Raja *et al.* 2001; Istre *et al.* 2003; Dedoukou *et al.* 2004).

Women appear to be at greater risk of fire-related burn injuries compared with men, and burn-related injuries account for a much higher proportion of injuries in young children when compared with other age groups (Jie & Ren 1992; Liu *et al.* 1998). In addition, place of residence, smoking, alcohol use, lack of water supply, low-income, crowding, presence of a pre-existing impairment in a child, sibling death from a burn, clothing of manmade fabrics, cooking equipment within reach of children, storage of a flammable substance in the home, and lack of temperature controls for hot water have also been identified as risk factors for burns (Forjuoh *et al.* 1995; Werneck & Reichenheim 1997; Warda *et al.* 1999; Jaye *et al.* 2001).

The majority of drowning incidents in high-income countries are associated with recreational or occupational activities, while in most LMIC they are associated with everyday activities near natural bodies of water (Celis 1997; Kobusingye *et al.* 2001; Brenner 2003; Hyder *et al.* 2003). Children aged 1–4 years, males, those living in rural areas, alcohol use, number of children in the family, presence of a well in the home, and lack of child supervision are additional risk factors for drowning (Kibel *et al.* 1990; Celis 1997; Ahmed *et al.* 1999; Kozik *et al.* 1999; Carlini-Cotrim & da Matta Chasin 2000; Kobusingye *et al.* 2001; Brenner 2003; Driscoll *et al.* 2004). Several studies have shown that young age, residential mobility, limited adult supervision of children, previous poisoning, the use of non-standard containers for storage (e.g. Coca-Cola bottles); and the storage of poisons at ground level are risk factors for childhood poisoning (Azizi *et al.* 1993; Chatsantiprapa *et al.* 2001; Soori 2001). Access to prescription drugs is also a frequent cause of poisoning.

A number of factors have been associated with an increased risk of suicide. Depression, schizophrenia, anxiety disorders and alcohol and drug abuse play a significant role in increasing risk (Krug *et al.* 2002). In addition, a previous suicidal attempt, family history of suicide, painful current illness, personal loss, interpersonal conflict, social isolation, place of residence (rural), unemployment, immigration status, religious affiliation, and poor economic conditions have been shown to pose a higher risk for suicide (Krug *et al.* 2002; Khan & Hyder 2006). Risk factors for violence, in general, have been identified in various studies including being male and young, abuse of alcohol and drugs, being a victim of child abuse, low socio-economic status, marital discord, parental conflict, and low access to medical care (Krug *et al.* 2002). In addition, macro-risk factors for violence in the literature include rapid social change, economic inequality, poverty, weak economic safety nets, corruption, gender inequalities, and high firearm availability. Previous victimization, having many sexual partners, and involvement in sex work have also been shown to be associated with increased levels of sexual violence in particular.

Theoretical basis for injury prevention

The causal model for injuries allows the injury process to be categorized into distinct phases which are important for prevention (Haddon 1970, 1972). The *pre-injury* phase is the period prior to the energy transfer, the *injury* phase is the often millisecond period in which the energy is transferred to the host, and the *post-injury* phase is the period of recovery and rehabilitation. Prevention approaches affect the injury process in one of these three injury phases.

Primary injury prevention includes prevention strategies that aim to prevent the transfer of injury to the host, and thus act in the pre-injury phase. Examples of successful primary prevention strategies include roadway designs that reduce motor vehicle collisions (Graham 1993), child-resistant caps on medication bottles to prevent ingestion and poisoning (Poison Prevention Technical Advisory Committee 1971), and pool fences to prevent submersion and drowning (Thompson & Rivara 2007).

Secondary injury prevention includes strategies that reduce the amount of energy that is transferred to the host. While these strategies are often put in place long before the injury event, their function acts to reduce energy transferred during the injury phase. Examples of secondary prevention strategies include seat belts and air bags (Evans 1995), motorcycle and bicycle helmets (US General Accounting Office 1991; Thomas *et al.* 1994). Seat belts and helmets do not prevent the crash itself, but they reduce the amount of energy transmitted to the host during the crash. Secondary prevention strategies might not prevent injury completely. For example, lower extremity injuries are not prevented by either seat belts or helmets. However, studies have consistently shown that when these devices are present, the risk for mortal injury is much less and injury severity is reduced.

Tertiary prevention strategies act in the post-injury phase to help with recovery and rehabilitation once an injury has occurred. One example is the development of trauma systems, which help with triage and transport of an injured individual to reduce the time between injury and definitive medical care (Mann *et al.* 1999; Nathens *et al.* 2000). Optimizing resources to enable recovery and rehabilitation does not prevent the injury or reduce the amount of energy transfer, but tertiary prevention strategies can have enormous impact on improving survival, function and quality of life following an injury.

The Haddon Matrix is a framework that combines these injury phases with the major components of the injury causal model to help identify prevention approaches (Fig. 10.4.1). This matrix, developed by Dr. William Haddon in the United States, was the foundation for the study of motor vehicle crashes and countermeasures for highway safety and continues to be an applicable theoretical framework for injury prevention (Haddon 1972). Using the three injury phases, Haddon categorized prevention approaches into those that affect the host, vehicles and vectors, the physical environment, and the socio-cultural environment. An example of the Haddon Matrix with examples from motor vehicle occupant protection is included in Table 10.4.2.

The Haddon Matrix provides a framework for identifying individual approaches to injury prevention. However, one single intervention strategy is unlikely to be highly effective. Multiple collaborative approaches need to be combined to maximize success. For example, the success of seat belt use in reducing motor vehicle occupant fatalities in the United States required a combination of engineering, education, policy, and enforcement that led to the current use rate of 80 per cent (National Highway Traffic Safety Administration 2007). Although seat belts were developed and available from the early 1900s, they were not required to be a standard feature on passenger cars in the United States until 1968. The steps to getting seat belts installed as a regular feature in passenger cars required considerable advocacy and policy initiatives. However, once the seat belts were installed, use rates without any occupant incentive or education were about 11 per cent. Efforts in the areas of legislation, enforcement, and public education were necessary to achieve the high use rates currently observed. Stricter legislation, for example, is associated with higher use, as evidenced by the higher use rates consistently observed among states with primary (not wearing a seat belt is by itself a citable offence) compared with secondary (not wearing a seat belt can be cited only along with another citation) laws in the United States (National Highway Traffic Safety Administration 2007).

Successful injury prevention strategies

It cannot be emphasized strongly enough that success in reducing injuries will depend on multi-faceted and comprehensive efforts. As demonstrated through the Haddon Matrix, injuries occur as a complex interplay between individuals and their physical and socio-cultural environments. Injury rates have very clear patterns within both individuals and geographic areas. Understanding these patterns within the context of the environment is essential to reducing the global burden of injuries. Below are some examples of successful injury prevention efforts.

Trends in road traffic injuries throughout the world provide a case study of how an integrated approach can lead to successful prevention. Over the last several decades, developed countries have experienced decreases in motor vehicle occupant death rates, even while the total miles driven, and thus exposure to the roadway, have dramatically increased. In contrast, developing countries have experienced large increases in the rate of road traffic fatality rates. For example, developed countries experienced a cumulative decrease in the number of road traffic fatalities of nearly 40 per cent between 1968 and 1985, while Asian countries experienced an increase of over 150 per cent and African countries an increase of over 300 per cent (Transport and Road Research Laboratory 1991; WHO 2004). Nearly 90 per cent of road traffic deaths now occur in low- or middle-income countries (WHO 2004).

The main reason for success in developed countries has been a comprehensive approach to intervention which has included environmental, engineering, legislative, and educational approaches. In the United States, The National Highway Traffic Safety Administration and the Federal Highway Safety Administration estimate that 243 000 lives were saved between 1966 and 1990 as a result of highway, traffic, and motor vehicle safety programmes (Institute of Medicine 1999). Road modifications mandated by the Federal Highway Traffic Safety Act of 1966 led to a shift from two-lane rural roads to interstate freeways. Although vehicle volume and speed are highest on interstate highways, the number of crashes per mile travelled on interstate highways is the lowest of all roadway types. Safety features built into interstate roads are numerous, and include: Divided highways that separate traffic flow in different directions, avoiding lane crossings and decreasing the risk for head-on crashes; graded curves; crash-absorbing barriers that reduce the risk of cars running off the road, especially in areas where roadside hazards exist; skid-resistant surfaces that reduce loss of traction while braking; and, lighted signage to increase visibility and reduce distraction (Graham 1993).

At the same time, changes to the motor vehicle itself increased the likelihood of survival in a crash. In addition to the implementation of seat belts and then air bags, legislation required modifications that improved vehicle crash worthiness. Some examples of these modifications include shatter-resistant windshields, collapsible steering columns, crash-friendly dashboard surfaces, frames that are resistant to passenger space intrusion, increased strength of the vehicle frame, seat, and doors, lap and shoulder belts, and air-bags (Haddon & Baker 1981). Studies have found that these safety improvements to the motor vehicle led to a 24–40 per cent decrease in fatal crashes and saved over 9000 lives each year (Robertson 1981; Institute of Medicine 1999).

Most of these changes were due in part to legislative efforts, and these efforts were themselves collaborative in nature. For example, the successful modification of the roadway and vehicle environments was facilitated by the establishment of the National Highway Traffic Safety Administration (NHTSA) through the Federal Highway Act of 1966. NHTSA was established as the lead United States federal agency to identify and respond to road traffic hazards, and its establishment was due largely to advocacy efforts that educated the general public and legislators about the scope and potential to prevent roadway fatalities.

Additional legislative approaches that have contributed to motor vehicle occupant safety include laws to require seat belt use, driver training, speed limits, and laws that aim to reduce drunk driving. These laws were all introduced because of successful education of legislators. However, their effectiveness varies dramatically. For example, most countries have laws against drinking and driving, yet countries have wide variation in the rate of alcohol-involved crashes as well as the number of drinking drivers, drivers cited for drinking and driving, and punished for drinking and driving. While this variation has much to do with factors associated with patterns of alcohol consumption, access to transportation, and the driving culture, this variation is also due to factors associated with the laws themselves. The effectiveness of legislative approaches depends on the level of enforcement that accompanies them and on the perception that the legislated consequences will actually occur (Mann et al. 2003). The effectiveness of drinking and driving laws is influenced by the level of enforcement, the ability of courts to impose penalties, and that the nature of the penalties serves as a deterrent.

Historically, many developed countries have focused much of their efforts on protecting vehicle occupants, and these efforts have shown many successes. However, the focus on motor vehicle occupants without concomitant integration of urban planning, sustainable transportation, and pedestrian and bicycle safety may be problematic in the long run. More recently, countries throughout Europe as well as Australia and the United States have introduced an approach called 'traffic calming' that aims to control motor vehicle traffic and speed in neighbourhoods, and thus increase safety and walkability in communities (Ewing 1999; Richter et al. 2006). The concept of traffic calming dates back to the Dutch city of Delft in the 1960s, when residents angry with fast-moving cars cutting through their local streets blocked them with gardens, social areas, and play grounds (Ewing 1999). Modern traffic calming involves a variety of approaches to reduce traffic volume and speed in residential areas using visually appealing strategies.

Success in reducing road traffic deaths has depended on the development of an infrastructure that can identify and respond to road hazards, and a wide variety of approaches to address these hazards. In some developed and many developing countries, the car culture is growing without concomitant safety efforts (Bishai et al. 2003). Highway design standards are often outdated or translated too directly from an industrialized country, and insufficient resources for roadway maintenance are available (Transport and Road Research Laboratory 1991). Poorly designed and maintained roadways are even further stressed by an ever-increased number and variety of vehicles. In addition to a growing number of passenger cars and a high proportion of commercial vehicles and buses, developing countries' roadways include animal-powered vehicles, small engine vehicles (such as scooters and motorcycles) that carry multiple people, bicycles, human-powered transport vehicles (such as a rickshaw), and pedestrians. This complex mix of vehicles contributes to increased deaths on the road.

In order to avert the growing toll of road traffic deaths, the WHO has called for a 'systems approach' in which the interaction between vehicles, roads, road users and their physical, social, and economic environments form the basis for a multi-sectoral response (WHO 2004).

Road traffic crashes provide one example of the potential for injury prevention success, the necessity for an integrated approach, and the need for building capacity for injury prevention. Throughout the world, general capacity for conducted injury prevention activities is limited. Growing awareness of the burden of traumatic injury coupled with a growing evidence base of successful injury prevention approaches bode well for increasing injury prevention activities in many countries.

Resources to identify successful injury prevention programmes

In addition to information to measure the scope, burden, and cost of injuries, several good resources are available to identify evidence-based injury prevention approaches. Two international collaborative efforts provide structured and systematic reviews of existing literature.

The Cochrane Collaboration provides scientific evidence-based reviews of health care interventions through the Cochrane Library (Bero & Rennie 1995; Alderson *et al.* 2004). The library has more than 100 reviews on the prevention, treatment, and rehabilitation of traumatic injuries, including topics such as fall-related injuries to older persons, pool fencing to prevent drowning in children, and interventions for promoting smoke alarm ownership and function. Abstracts are available free of charge (http://www.cochrane.org/reviews/index.htm) and full reviews are available by subscription, with most major libraries holding subscriptions. Cochrane reviews are highly weighted towards evidence from randomized controlled trials, which excludes many of the observational evaluations conducted for injury interventions. The search strategy protocol requires inclusion of international findings as well as unpublished data, and when sufficient data are present meta-analyses are conducted. Thus, these reviews are meant to be applicable to an international audience.

The Campbell Collaboration, begun in 1999, includes systematic reviews of social service programmes, divided into the categories of education, crime and justice, and social welfare (Davies & Boruch 2001). The goal of the collaboration is to provide evidence for policy decisions regarding social issues. While the majority of injury prevention-related reviews are found within the crime and justice reviews, many reviews in the other categories are strongly related to injury and violence prevention. The Campbell Collaboration includes evidence from all types of study designs, and has methods groups to ensure systematic interpretation of findings. Methods groups include experimental methods, quasi-experimental methods, and process and quantitative methods. Campbell reviews can be accessed free of charge (http://www.campbellcollaboration.org/frontend.asp).

Another source of recommendations for injury prevention strategies is *The Guide to Community Preventive Services: Systematic Reviews and Evidence-Based Recommendations* (the *Guide*). This system was developed by the Task Force on Community Preventive Services, established by the United States Centers for Disease Control and Prevention (Pappaioanou & Evans 1998). The *Guide's* recommendations are primarily based on evidence of effectiveness, including the suitability of the study design, but they also assess the applicability of the intervention to other populations or settings, the economic impact, barriers observed in implementing the interventions, and if the intervention had other beneficial or harmful effects (Briss *et al.* 2000). The *Guide* then provides a recommendation as to whether the approach is 'strongly recommended', 'recommended', has 'insufficient evidence' or is 'discouraged'. The Guide has injury-related reviews in the categories of alcohol, motor vehicle, physical activity, substance abuse, worksite, mental health, social environment, and violence. Reviews are available free of charge at http://www.thecommunityguide.org/default.htm.

In addition there are more global sources of information that provide help and guidance on a variety of injury issues. The Department of Violence and Injuries Prevention of the WHO (www.who.int) offers a diversity of guidelines and manuals that provide assistance in implementing programmes or conducting research. Examples include guidelines for establishing injury surveillance systems, conducting community based surveys and evaluating prehospital care. International non-governmental organizations also offer a variety of assistance and expert members on specific issues. Examples include the International Society for Child and Adolescent Injury Prevention (www.iscaip.net), the Road Traffic Injuries Research Network (www.rtirn.net), and the International Society for Violence and Injury Prevention (www.isvip.org).

Another source of recent estimates of the burden of injuries and cost-effectiveness of interventions is the Disease Control Priorities for Developing Countries Project (www.dcp2.org). This project worked on both intentional and unintentional injuries as well as emergency care to present a consistent set of estimates for the global burden of injuries and their impact in low- and middle-income countries. In addition, using a consistent set of guidelines, the project worked out the cost-effectiveness of interventions to reduce the burden of injuries across the world.

Building capacity for injury prevention

In order to implement the comprehensive strategies for injury prevention that are most effective, countries, states, and local communities need to develop the infrastructure and capacity to conduct the essential activities needed for an injury prevention programme. Infrastructure includes the identification of agencies to oversee essential injury control activities and the integration of these activities. Capacity includes the availability of human, financial, relational, and structural resources.

Most important of these is the development of a critical mass of trained injury professionals in a country to understand the local environment, develop, implement, and evaluate prevention programmes. Because there is a lack of trained injury prevention professionals in low- and middle-income countries, capacity development should focus on the developing world. In order to facilitate training of injury prevention professionals, the WHO developed a training programme called Teach Violence and Injury Prevention—TeachVIP (http://www.who.int/violence_injury_prevention/capacitybuilding/teachvip/en/print.html)This programme provides teaching materials to introduce the major topics of the field of injury and violence prevention, and is an important tool for trainers. The WHO has also identified priorities for global reduction in the two leading causes of injury death: Motor vehicle injuries and violence. These priorities are listed in Box 10.4.1. Capacity-building efforts are best organized around the public health framework of surveillance, prevention/evaluation, and treatment.

Box 10.4.1 WHO's priorities for the future of injury prevention

Continued success in the prevention and control of injuries will depend on systematic and organized efforts. Worldwide, much progress has been made, and it is important to find efficient methods to share and adapt successful approaches. The World Health Organization has developed reports on two of the leading causes of injury mortality and morbidity: Road traffic injuries and violence. Below, the priorities that were identified in these reports are summarized.

Priorities from the World Report on Road Traffic Injury Prevention:[a]

1. Identify a lead agency in government to guide national road traffic safety efforts

2. Assess the problems, policies, institutional settings and capacity relating to road traffic injury

3. Prepare a national road traffic safety strategy and plan for action

4. Allocate financial and human resources to address the problem

5. Implement specific actions to prevent road traffic crashes, minimize injuries and their consequences, and evaluate these efforts

6. Support the development of national capacity and international collaboration

Priorities from the World Report on Violence and Health:[b]

1. Create, implement, and monitor a national action plan for violence prevention

2. Enhance capacity for collection of data on violence

3. Define priorities for, and support research on, the causes, consequences, costs and prevention of violence

4. Promote primary prevention responses

5. Strengthen responses for victims of violence

6. Integrate violence prevention into social and educational policies, and thereby promote gender and social equality

7. Increase collaboration and exchange of information on violence prevention

8. Promote and monitor adherence to international treaties, laws, and other mechanisms to protect human rights

9. Seek practical, internationally agreed responses to the global drug trade and the global arms trade

Sources:
[a] World Health Organization. *World Report on Road Traffic Injury Prevention.* (http://www.who.int/violence_injury_prevention/publications/road_traffic/world_report/en/index.html)
[b] World Health Organization. *World Report on Violence and Health.* (http://www.who.int/violence_injury_prevention/violence/world_report/en/index.html)

Surveillance

One of the most important priorities for injury prevention worldwide is the development of dependable local injury surveillance systems. These systems are necessary to identify and explain the nature of the injury problem, and also to track changes over time as interventions are implemented and new risks emerge. Surveillance efforts need to focus on two priorities: Enhanced data quality and the establishment of registry systems to track injury trends.

Several efforts to collect international injury mortality data have found that differences in death certification systems, methods of data collection, and definitions of variables severely challenge international comparisons (Krug *et al.* 2000; Fingerhut 2004; Hofman *et al.* 2005; Polinder *et al.* 2007). As mentioned in the previous section on data sources, many countries have an insufficient infrastructure to accurately enumerate and code traumatic injury deaths. The International Collaborative Effort on Injury Statistics, undertaken by the US National Center for Health Statistics as a multi-country exercise, was the first effort to compare international mortality rates (Fingerhut 2004). This collaboration has undertaken several projects to improve data compatibility between countries, such as the Barell injury diagnosis matrix that provides guidance for coding injury diagnoses by body region and nature of injury. Other efforts have been undertaken by the WHO and the European Union, among others (Krug *et al.* 2000; Polinder *et al.* 2007). These efforts consistently identify data quality as a major impediment.

The burden of traumatic injury is disproportionately born by low- and middle-income countries, and these countries are also the least likely to have established surveillance systems to monitor injury trends (Hofman *et al.* 2005). Surveillance systems are needed to identify and track trends in injuries for research and prevention efforts, and are also necessary to attract the attention of policymakers and community leaders. Data registries need to be developed using methods that are not highly resource-intensive, such as adding injuries to existing medical reporting systems for conditions such as infectious diseases. In order to be effective, minimum data elements with standard definitions need to be employed. If possible, surveillance should be developed to provide some benefit to the agencies responsible for collecting the data. One method of accomplishing this is to integrate measurable quality indicators into the data collection so that agencies can use the data systems to monitor their own performance.

Investment in data infrastructures will be critical to the long-term sustainability of injury prevention efforts. Data will be necessary to monitor changes over time, to evaluate new efforts, and to continue to engage new partners in injury control efforts. Guidelines for injury surveillance and surveys have been released by the WHO (www.who.int).

Prevention and evaluation

Effective and cost-beneficial injury prevention programmes are needed worldwide. In developed countries, a growing number of programmes are emerging, but far too many are not evaluated. Among approaches that are evaluated and found to be effective and adaptable to wider populations, few are the subject of wide-spread dissemination.

The wide-spread dissemination of injury prevention programmes takes concerted effort. For example, smoke alarms have been shown to reduce the risk of dying in a house fire by half (Hall 1994). When smoke alarms were first introduced, few homes had them, and currently, the majority of homes do not install them effectively (Harvey *et al.* 1998; Peek-Asa *et al.* 2005). In order to increase the number of homes with operational smoke alarms, several agencies in the United States, such as the National Fire Protection Agency and the Centers for Disease Control and Prevention, initiated national campaigns to educate consumers about smoke alarms, to change building codes to require smoke alarms, and to engage public health agencies in the dissemination and installation of alarms (Ballesteros et al. 2005). These efforts appear to be effective, and currently, nearly 90 per cent of US homes have at least one operational smoke alarm (Harvey et al. 1998).

Although a number of successful strategies for injury prevention have been identified, these have primarily been developed in high-income countries. Existing strategies will have varying success in different environments. For example, random breath alcohol screening for drivers has been an effective policy/enforcement method to reduce drinking and driving in Australia, especially when combined with social marketing campaigns raising awareness of the risks of drinking and driving, and bringing attention to the likelihood and penalties of being caught. However, random driver screening is not adaptable to the United States because law enforcement lacks the authority to randomly stop drivers without cause (Peek-Asa et al. 1999). Policy efforts need to work within the authorities of the local agencies as well as the local economic, political, and cultural environments. Without an understanding of the local environment, it is unlikely that translation of existing strategies will be effective.

Thus, injury prevention efforts can occur at multiple levels (national, regional, and local), but are most effective when integrated within the local environments. When developing a new approach to an injury problem, it is important to identify the scope of the problem, the populations that are at highest risk, the causal mechanisms of the injury, and the environment in which the injuries occur. For example, one could propose to address a high incidence of dog bites to children through an educational campaign focused on dog owners and veterinarians. However, if most of the bites are caused by feral dogs that have no owner and are unlikely to see a veterinarian, this educational campaign is unlikely to make any difference.

Priority should be placed on adapting proven interventions from high-income countries to low- and middle-income countries (Peden et al. 2004). Growing evidence supports this approach. Data from a controlled study undertaken in South Africa has shown that the free distribution of child resistant containers appears to be a highly effective means of preventing poisoning in children (Krug et al. 1994). Increased supervision of children around bodies of water, and use of barriers have also been proposed as measures that might reduce drowning in developing countries (Hyder et al. 2003).

There are many factors to consider when either developing a new strategy or adapting an existing strategy to a new community. Some of these factors are obvious, such as the cost of the programme, the existence of an agency or group of individuals to conduct the work, and good evidence that the strategy is effective when implemented correctly. Other considerations are equally important but less obvious. These include issues such as acceptance of the strategy by the community, equity or perceived equity, and the potential to stigmatize the affected community (Runyan 1998).

An international panel assembled by the Fogarty Center of the US National Institutes of Health recognized that, in addition to lack of data, the trained workforce to develop injury prevention programmes was lacking in most low- and middle-income countries (Hofman et al. 2005). In particular, the proportion of the trained public health workforce that focuses on injury prevention and safety issues is relatively small when compared to health conditions of equal magnitude. And, ironically, many health care professionals cannot mobilize to conduct prevention activities because they are overwhelmed in treating the injuries and illnesses of the individuals who are in need of the prevention services. In addition to a paucity of trained injury prevention professionals, funding to conduct injury prevention activities is scarce, if existent at all. Although resources are scarce, the potential of pooling resources among multiple agencies offers promise. Building sufficient infrastructure to bring the necessary stakeholders together will help identify better uses of existing resources, while also increasing the number of individuals who can move programmes forward. This, in turn, will help leverage increased resources to sustain efforts that can be proven effective.

Treatment

Many injuries lead to death because of inadequate emergency and trauma care, although an organized trauma response system can dramatically reduce deaths from injuries (Mann et al. 1999; Hofman et al. 2005). For example, one study reported up to 58 per cent pre-hospital mortality for intentional injuries in Pakistan (Chotani 2002), while in a comparative study trauma mortality was 65 per cent in resource poor settings compared with 55 per cent and 35 per cent in moderate and good resource settings (Mock 1998).

However, many countries lack trained medical personnel, equipment, and infrastructure (Kobusingye 2005). An evaluation of trauma care capabilities in Mexico, Vietnam, India, and Ghana indicated that even when a sufficient number of health care professionals were trained, 'brain drain' from rural to urban and from low- to higher-income communities led to widespread provider shortages (Mock et al. 2006). In order to develop a stronger trauma response system, improvements must be made in the areas of increased human resources, physical resources, security for health care personnel, transportation systems to get patients to definitive treatment, and administrative infrastructure (Kobusingye 2005; Mock et al. 2006).

Although many of these improvements require new resources, system-wide changes are possible through effective planning even in the absence of significantly increased resources. For example, several low-cost trauma training programmes have been developed and used effectively in low-income countries, and these have contributed to decreased injury mortality (Kobusingye 2005). Administrative changes, such as making necessary diagnostic equipment available for critical trauma cases, are also low-cost. However, identifying and implementing low-cost strategies cycles back to the need for data. Finding the low-cost strategies that will work in a health care facility will be enhanced by data systems that can track trends in patient treatment and be used for quality assurance. These systems are lacking in many health care organizations throughout the world.

Improving emergency medical systems and trauma treatment capacity could greatly reduce injury mortality worldwide, and also reduce the physical, emotional, and financial consequences of severe injuries. These efforts need to be in collaboration with general worldwide efforts to improve access to public health and medical services. Over the past few years, WHO has released guidelines for pre-hospital and trauma care with a special focus on low- and middle-income countries (www.who.int). In addition, an evaluation of interventions for emergency care has been evaluated and checklists developed to identify potentially useful approaches in the developing world (Kobusingye *et al.* 2006).

Necessary elements to sustainable injury programmes

Resources are the biggest challenge to implementing needed surveillance, prevention, and treatment components; although these needed resources come in a variety of forms. A review of the Swedish Safe Communities programme concluded that no single type of resource or programme component is sufficient to sustain injury prevention efforts (Nilsen *et al.* 2005). The Swedish Safe Communities model, adopted in many variations throughout the world, encourages communities to establish grassroots efforts to address local safety and injury prevention issues. Each local community identifies its own priorities, methods to address the priorities, and methods to integrate with regional and national safety efforts. The evaluation identified financial resources as necessary but not sufficient for sustainability, and, furthermore, that reliance on several key individuals was not predictive of sustainability. Sustainable efforts required financial, human, relational, and structural resources that bring together people with many different skills and capabilities to work together. This is a challenge in any community, but particularly challenging in a community with already limited public health and medical resources.

Conclusion

Despite the high burden of injuries throughout the world, investment in safety and injury prevention infrastructure has been low. In low-income countries such as Pakistan and Uganda, approximately US$0.07 per capita was devoted to safety. In every country, the amount invested in prevention is far surpassed by the amount spent on the treatment of traumatic injuries, and thus studies that focus on cost-benefits are badly needed. International assistance has also not prioritized safety or injury prevention. External assistance to the health sectors of low income countries was US$2–3 per DALY lost to infectious diseases, but only US$0.06 per DALY lost to injuries (Mock *et al.* 2004).

Since 90 per cent of the world's population lives in low- and middle-income countries, and the burden of injuries is predicted to increase in these countries, it is imperative that future research and development activities focus especially on their needs. Basic research to describe the existing burden, causes, and distribution of injuries is still needed in LMIC. Trials of injury interventions have largely not been conducted in LMIC, and there is a great need to modify, adapt and test existing, as well as new interventions in these specific settings (Peden *et al.* 2004). More work is also required to assess barriers to implementation of such interventions globally.

The role of international organizations (such as WHO and the World Bank) and national agencies (such as ministries of health or medical research councils) needs to be emphasized in moving ahead the injury prevention agenda. The international movements currently underway for violence prevention and road traffic injuries prevention as promulgated through the two World Reports are examples of how joint global-national partnerships are needed for making change.

Progress will also be supported if a growing number of professionals become advocates for safety. Professionals from public health, medicine, engineering, social services, urban planning, law and law enforcement, among others, can all have a strong voice in raising awareness for safety programmes and to encourage individuals to make safe choices.

Key points

- Injuries and violence are a leading cause of mortality and morbidity worldwide.
- Injuries disproportionately affect young and vulnerable populations, and injury rates are disproportionately high among low- and middle-income countries.
- Prevention of injuries is very feasible and works best with a multidisciplinary and integrated approach.
- Building capacity for injury prevention should be a priority for all countries, but is an urgent need for low- and middle-income countries.
- Improvement in global injury prevention efforts would be aided by increased capacity in data systems, building an evidence base for successful approaches, trauma care delivery, and trained injury prevention professionals.

References

Adesunkanmi, A. R., Oseni, S. A., & Badru, O. S. 1999, 'Severity and outcome of falls in children', *West African Journal of Medicine*, vol. 18, no. 4, pp. 281–5.

Aeron-Thomas, A., Jacobs, G. D., Stexon, B., Gururaj, G., & Rahmann, F. 2004, 'The involvement and impact of road crashes on the poor: Bangladesh and India case studies', *Published Project Report PRP 010*. Crowthorne: Transport Research Laboratory LTD.

Afukaar, F. K. 2003, 'Speed control in LMICs: Issues, challenges and opportunities in reducing road traffic injuries', *Injury Control and Safety Promotion*, vol. 10, no. 1–2, pp. 77–81.

Ahmed, M. K., Rahman, M., & van Ginneken, J. 1999, 'Epidemiology of child deaths due to drowning in Matlab, Bangladesh', *International Journal of Epidemiology*, vol. 28, no. 2, pp. 306–11.

Alderson, P., Green, S., & Higgins, J. P. T. (eds.) 2004, *Cochrane Reviewers Handbook 4.2.2.* Retrieved 3/07 from http://www.cochrane.org/resources/handbook/hbook.htm.

Ameratunga, S., Hijar, M., & Norton, R. 2006, 'Road traffic injuries: Confronting disparities to address a global health problem', *Lancet*, vol. 367, pp. 1533–40.

Anonymous. Bulletin of the Clearinghouse National Poison Control Centers Poisoning Prevention Technical Advisory Committee, 1971, *Poisoning Prevention Packaging Act of 1970*, May–June, 1–2.

Azizi, B. H., Zulkifli, H. I., & Kasim, M. S. 1993, 'Risk factors for accidental poisoning in urban Malaysian children', *Annals of Tropical Paediatrics*, vol. 13, no. 2, pp. 183–8.

Ballesteros, M., Jackson, M., & Martin, M. W. 2005, 'Working towards the elimination of residential fire deaths: CDC's Smoke Alarm Installation and Fire Safety Education (SAIFE) Program', *Journal of Burn Care and Rehabilitation*, vol. 26, no. 5, pp. 434–9.

Bangdiwala, S. I., & Anzola-Perez, E. 1990, 'The incidence of injuries in young people: II. log-linear multivariable models for risk factors in a collaborative study in Brazil, Chile, Cuba and Venezuela', *International Journal of Epidemiology*, vol. 19, no. 1, pp. 125–32.

Bener, A. K., Al-Salman, M., & Pugh, R. N. H. 1998, 'Injury mortality and morbidity among children in the United Arab Emirates', *European Journal of Epidemiology*, vol. 14, pp. 175–8.

Bero, L., & Rennie, D. 1995, 'The Cochrane Collaboration. Preparing, maintaining, and disseminating systematic reviews of the effects of health care', *Journal of the American Medical Association*, vol. 274, pp. 1935–8.

Bishai, D., Hyder, A. A., Ghaffar, A., Morrow, R. H., & Kobusingye, O. 2003, 'Rates of public investment for road safety in developing countries: Case studies of Uganda and Pakistan', *Health Policy and Planning*, vol. 18, no. 2, pp. 232–5.

Boonyaratavej, N., Suriyawongpaisal, P., Takkinsatien, A., Wanvarie, S., Rajatanavin, R., & Apiyasawat, P. 2001, 'Physical activity and risk factors for hip fractures in Thai women', *Osteoporosis International*, vol. 12, no. 3, pp. 244–8.

Brenner, R. A. 2003, 'Prevention of drowning in infants, children and adolescents', *Pediatrics*, vol. 112, no. 2, pp. 440–5.

Briss, P. A., Zaza, S., Pappaioanou, M. *et al.* 2000, 'Developing an evidence-based guide to community preventive services-methods', *American Journal of Preventive Medicine*, vol. 19, no. 1S, pp. 35–43.

Carlini-Cotrim, B., & da Matta Chasin, A. A. 2000, 'Blood alcohol content and death from fatal injury: A study in metropolitan area of Sao Paulo, Brazil', *Journal of Psychoactive Drugs*, vol. 32, no. 3, pp. 269–75.

Celis, A. 1997, 'Home drowning among preschool age Mexican children', *Injury Prevention*, vol. 3, no. 4, pp. 252–6.

Centers for Disease Control and Prevention and the Injury Control and Emergency Health Services Section of the American Public Health Association. 1997, 'Recommended framework for presenting injury mortality data', *MMWR Recomm Rep.*, vol. 46, no. RR-14, pp. 1–30. http://www.cdc.gov/mmwr/preview/mmwrhtml/00049162.htm

Chatsantiprapa, K., Chokkanapitak, J., & Pinpradit, N. 2001. 'Host and environment factors for exposure to poisons: A case control study of preschool children in Thailand', *Injury Prevention*, vol. 7, no. 3, pp. 214–7.

Clark, P., de la Pena, F., Gomez Garcia, F., Orozco, J. A., & Tugwell, P. 1998, 'Risk factors for osteoporotic hip fractures in Mexicans', *Archives of Medical Research*, vol. 29, no. 3, pp. 253–7.

Cummings, S. R., Nevitt, M. C., Browner, W. S. *et al.* 1995, 'Risk factors for hip fracture in white women', *New England Journal of Medicine*, vol. 332, 12, pp. 767–73.

Cywes, S., Kibel, S. M., Bass, D. H., Rode, H., Millar, A. J. W. & De Wet, J. 1990, 'Paediatric trauma care', *South African Medical Journal*, vol. 78, pp. 413–8.

Dargent-Molina, Favier, P. F., Grandjean, H. *et al.* 1996, 'Fall-related factors and risk of hip fracture: The EPIDOS Prospective Study', *Lancet*, vol. 348, no. 9021, pp.145–9.

Davies, P., & Boruch, R. 2001, 'The Campbell Collaboration does for public policy what Cochrane does for health', *British Medical Journal*, vol. 323, no. 7308, pp. 294–5.

Dedoukou, X., Spyridopoulos, T., Kedikoglou, S., Alexe, D. M., Dessypris, N., & Petridou, E. 2004, 'Incidence and risk factors of fall injuries among infants: A study in Greece', *Archives of Pediatric and Adolescent Medicine*, vol. 158, no. 10, pp. 1002–6.

Driscoll, T. R., Harrison, J. A., & Steenkamp, M. 2004, 'Review of the role of alcohol in drowning associated with recreational aquatic activity', *Injury Prevention*, vol. 10, no. 2, pp. 107–13.

Evans, L. 1995, 'Restraint effectiveness, occupant ejection from cars, and fatality reductions', *Accident Analysis and Prevention*, vol. 22, pp. 167–75.

Ewing, R. H. 1999, 'Traffic calming: State of the practice', *Federal Highway Administration* FHWA-RD-99-135. Washington D.C., (http://www.ite.org/traffic/tcstate.htm#tcsop).

Fingerhut, L. A. 2004, 'International collaborative effort on injury statistics: 10 year review', *Injury Prevention*, vol. 10, pp. 264–7.

Forjuoh, S. N., Guyer, B., Strobino, D. M., Keyl, P. M., Diener-West, M., & Smith, G. S. 1995, 'Risk factors for childhood burns: A case-control study of Ghanaian children', *Journal of Epidemiology and Community Health*, vol. 49, no. 2, pp. 189–93.

Ghaffar, A., Hyder, A. A., Mastoor, M. I., & Shaikh, I. 1999, 'Injuries in Pakistan: Directions for future health policy', *Health Policy and Planning*, vol. 14, no. 1, pp. 11–17.

Graham, J. D. 1993, 'Injuries from traffic crashes: Meeting the challenge', *Annual Review of Public Health*, vol. 14, pp. 515–43.

Haddon, W., Jr. 1970, 'On the escape of tigers: An ecologic note', *American Journal of Public Health*, vol. 60, pp. 2229–34.

Haddon, W., Jr. 1972, 'A logical framework for categorizing highway safety phenomena and activity', *Journal of Trauma*, vol. 12, pp. 193–207.

Haddon, W., & Baker, S. P. 1981, *Injury Control*, eds. D. W. Clark & B. McMahaon, Preventive and Community Medicine, 2nd edn, pp. 109–40, Little, Brown, and Company, Boston, Massachusetts.

Hall, J. R., Jr. 1994, 'The U.S. experience with smoke detectors: Who has them? How well do they work? When don't they work?' *National Fire Protection Association Journal*, pp. 36–46.

Harvey, P. A., Sacks, J. J., Ryan, G. W., & Bender, P. F. 1998, 'Residential smoke alarms and fire escape plans', *Public Health Report*, vol. 113, pp. 459–464.

Hofman. K., Primack, A., Keusch, G., & Hrynkow, S. 2005, 'Addressing the growing burden of trauma and injury in low- and middle-income countries', *American Journal of Public Health*, vol. 95, pp. 13–17.

Hyder, A. A., Arifeen, S., Begum, N., Fishman, S., Wali, S., & Baqui, A. H. 2003, 'Death from drowning: Defining a new challenge for child survival in Bangladesh', *Injury Control and Safety Promotion*, vol. 10, no. 4, pp. 205–10.

Hyder, A. A., & Morrow, R. H. 2006, *Measures of Health and Disease in Populations*, eds. R. B. Black, M. Merson & A. Mills, International Public Health: Diseases, Programs, Systems and Policies, 2nd edn, Jones & Bartlett Publishers, Boston, MA.

Hyder, A. A., Rotllant, G., & Morrow, R. H. 1998, 'Measuring the burden of disease: Healthy life years', *American Journal of Public Health*, vol. 88, no. 2, pp. 196–202.

Institute of Medicine 1999, *Reducing the Burden of Injury: Advancing Prevention and Treatment*. Bonney, R. J., Fulco, C. E., & Liverman, C. T., eds, Washington, D.C. National Academy Press.

Istre, G. R., McCoy, M. A., Stowe, M. *et al.* 2003, 'Childhood injuries due to falls from apartment balconies and windows', *Injury Prevention*, vol. 9, no. 4, pp. 349–52.

Jaye, C., Simpson, J. C., & Langley, J. D. 2001, 'Barriers to safe hot tap water: Results from a National Study of New Zealand Plumbers', *Injury Prevention*, vol. 7, pp. 302–6.

Jie, X., & Ren, C. B. 1992, 'Burn injuries in the Dong Bei area of China: A study of 12,606 cases', *Burns*, vol. 18, no. 3, pp. 228–32.

Jitapunkul, S., Yuktanandana, P., & Parkpian, V. 2001, 'Risk factors of hip fracture among Thai female patients', *Journal of the Medical Association of Thailand*, vol. 84, no. 11, pp. 1576–81.

Khan, M. M., & Hyder, A. A. 2006, 'Suicides in the developing world: Case study from Pakistan', *Suicide & Life Threatening Behavior*, vol. 36, no. 1, pp. 76–81.

Kibel, S. M., Joubert, G., & Bradshaw, D. 1990, 'Injury-related mortality in South African children, 1981–1985', *South African Medical Journal*, vol. 78, no. 7, pp. 398–403.

Kobusingye, O. C. 2005, 'Emergency medical systems in low- and middle-income countries: Recommendations for action', *Bull World Health Organisation*, vol. 83, no. 8, pp. 626–31.

Kobusingye, O., Guwatudde, D., & Lett, R. 2001, 'Injury patterns in rural and urban Uganda', *Injury Prevention*, vol. 7, no. 1, pp. 46–50.

Kobusingye, O. C., Hyder, A. A., Bishai, D., Joshipura, M., Hicks, E. R., & Mock, C. 2006. Emergency Medical Services. *Disease Control Priorities in Developing Countries*, 2nd edn, Jamison, D. *et al.*, eds., Disease Control Priorities in Developing Countries, 1261–9.Oxford University Press and the World Bank, New York, NY.

Kopits, E., & Cropper, M. 2003, *Traffic Fatalities and Economic Growth*, Policy Research Working Paper 3035, World Bank, Washington, DC.

Kozik, C. A., Suntayakorn, S., Vaughn, D. W., Suntayakorn, C., Snitbhan, R., & Innis B. L. 1999, 'Causes of death and unintentional injury among schoolchildren in Thailand', *Southeast Asian Journal of Tropical Medicine and Public Health*, vol. 30, no. 1, pp. 129–35.

Krug, E. G., Dahlberg, K. L., Mercy, J. A., Zwi, A. B., & Lozano, R, (eds.) 2002, *World Report on Violence and Health*, Geneva, World Health Organisation.

Krug, A., Ellis, J. B., Hay, I. T., Mokgabudi, N. F., & Robertson, J. 1994, 'The impact of child-resistant containers on the incidence of paraffin (kerosene) ingestion in children', *South African Medical Journal*, vol. 84, no. 11, pp. 730–4.

Krug, E. G., Sharma, G. K., & Lozano, R. 2000, 'The global burden of injuries', *American Journal of Public Health*, vol. 90, pp. 523–6.

Kulanthayan, S., Umar, R. S., Hariza, H. A., Nasir, M. T., & Harwant, S. 2000, 'Compliance of proper safety helmet usage in motorcyclists', *Medical Journal of Malaysia*, vol. 55, no. 1, pp. 40–4.

Liu, G. F., Han, S., Liang, D. H. *et al.* 2003, 'Driver sleepiness and risk of car crashes in Shenyang, a Chinese Northeastern city: Population-based case-control study', *Biomedical and Environmental Sciences*, vol. 16, no. 3, pp. 219–26.

Liu, B., Ivers, R., Norton, R., Blows, S., & Lo, S. K. 2004, 'Helmets for preventing injury in motorcycle riders', *Cochrane Database of Systematic Reviews*, vol. 4, CD004333.

Liu, E. H., Khatri, B., Shakya, Y. M., & Richard, B. M. 1998, 'A 3 year prospective audit of burn patients treated at the Western Regional Hospital of Nepal', *Burns*, vol. 24, no. 2, pp. 129–33.

Lu, T. H., Lee, M. C., & Chou, M. C. 1998, 'Trends in injury mortality among adolescents in Taiwan, 1965–94', *Injury Prevention*, vol. 4, pp. 111–5.

MacGregor, D. M. 2000, 'Injuries associated with falls from beds', *Injury Prevention*, vol. 6, no. 4, pp. 291–2.

Mann, N., Mullins, R, MacKenzie, E. *et al.* 1999, 'A systematic review of published evidence regarding trauma system effectiveness', *Journal of Trauma*, vol. 47, pp. S25–33.

Mann, R. E., Smart, R. G., Stoduto, G. *et al.* 2003, 'The effects of drinking-driving laws: A test of the differential deterrence hypothesis', *Addiction*, vol. 98, no. 11, pp. 1531–6.

Mock, C., Amegashi, J., & Darteh, K. 1999, 'Role of commercial drivers in motor vehicle related injuries in Ghana', *Injury Prevention*, vol. 5, no. 4, pp. 268–71.

Mock, C., Nguyen, S., Quansah, R., Arreola-Risa, C., Viradia, R., & Joshipura, M. 2006, 'Evaluation of trauma care capabilities in four countries using the WHO-IATSIC Guidelines for Essential Trauma Care', *World Journal of Surgery*, vol. 30, pp. 946–56.

Mock, C., Quansah, R., Krishnan, R., Arreola-Risa C., & Rivara, F. 2004, Strengthening the prevention and care of injuries worldwide, *Lancet*, vol. 363, pp. 2172–9.

Murray, C., & Lopez, A. 1996, *Global Burden of Disease and Injuries*, Harvard University Press, Cambridge, MA.

Nafukho, F. M., & Khayesi, M. 2002, 'Livelihood, conditions of work, regulation, and road Safety in the small-scale public transport sector: A case of the Matatu mode of transport in Kenya', in Urban Mobility for All, ed X. Godard and I. Fatonzoun, pp. 241–5, Proceedings of the Tenth International CODATU Conference, Lome, Togo, 12–15 November 2002, Lisse, The Netherlands.

Nathens, A., Jurkovich, G., Cummings, P., Rivara, F., & Maier, R. 2000, 'The effeect of organised systems of trauma care on motor vehicle crash mortality', *The Journal of the American Medical Association*, vol. 283, pp. 1990–4.

National Highway Traffic Safety Administration. 2007, 'Seat belt use in 2006 – Use rates in states and territories', *Traffic Safety Facts*. DOT-HS-810-960. January, 2007. (http://www-nrd.nhtsa.dot.gov/pdf/nrd-30/NCSA/RNotes/2007/810690.pdf).

Nilsen, P., Timpka, T., Nordenfelt, L., & Lindqvist, K. 2005, 'Towards improved understanding of injury prevention program sustainability', *Safety Science*, vol. 43, pp. 815–33.

Norton, R., Hyder, A. A., & Gururaj, G. 2006, *Unintentional Injuries and Violence*, R. B. Black, M. Merson, A. Mills, eds., International Public Health: Diseases, Programs, Systems and Policies, 2nd edn., Jones & Bartlett Publishers, Silver Boston, Massachusetts.

Odero, W. O., & Zwi, A. B. 1995, *Alcohol-Related Traffic Injuries and Fatalities in LMICs: A Critical Review of Literature*, C. N. Kloeden & A. J. McLean, eds., In Proceedings of the 13th International Conference on Alcohol, Drugs and Traffic Safety, pp. 713–20. Road Accident Research Unit, Adelaide.

Peden, M., McGee, K., & Sharma, G. 2002, *The Injury Chart Book: A Graphical Overview of the Global Burden of Injuries*, World Health Organisation, Geneva.

Peden, M., Scurfield, R., Sleet, D. *et al.* (eds.) 2004, *World Report on Road Traffic Injury Prevention*, World Health Organisation, Geneva.

Peek-Asa, C., Allareddy, V., Yang, J., Taylor, C., Lundell, J., & Zwerling, C. 2005, 'When one is not enough: Prevalence and characteristics of homes not adequately protected by smoke alarms', *Injury Prevention*, vol. 11, no. 6, pp. 364–8.

Polinder, S., Meerding, W. J., Mulder, S. *et al.* 2007, *Assessing the Burden of Injury in Six European Countries*, Bulletin of the World Health Organisation vol. 85, no. 1, pp. 27–34.

Pappaioanou, M., & Evans, C., Jr. 1998, 'Development of the Guide to Community Preventive Services: A U.S. Public Health Service initiative', *Journal of Public Health Management & Practice*, vol. 4, no. S2, pp. 48–54.

Raja, I. A., Vohra, A. H., & Ahmed, M. 2001, 'Neurotrauma in Pakistan', *World Journal of Surgery*, vol. 25, no. 9, pp. 1230–7.

Richter, E. D., Friedman, L. S., Berman, T., & Rivkind, A. 2006, 'Death and injury from motor vehicle crashes: A tale of two countries', *American Journal of Preventive Medicine,* vol. 30, no. 5, pp. 440–9.

Robertson, L. S. 1981, 'Automobile safety regulations and death reductions in the United States', *American Journal of Public Health*, vol. 71, no. 8, pp. 818–22.

Runyan, C. W. 1998, 'Using the Haddon Matrix: Introducing the third dimension', *Injury Prevention*, vol. 4, pp. 302–7.

Soori, H. 2001, 'Developmental risk factors for unintentional childhood poisoning', *Saudi Medical Journal*, vol. 22, no. 3, pp. 227–30.

Thomas, S., Acton, C., Nixon, J., Battistutta, D., Pitt, W. R., & Clark, R. 1994, 'Effectiveness of bicycle helmets in preventing head injury in children: Case-control study', *British Medical Journal*, vol. 308, pp. 173–7.

Thompson, D. C., & Rivara, F. P. 2007, *Pool Fencing for Preventing Drowning in Children*, The Cochrane Database of Systematic Reviews, Issue 1.

Transport and Road Research Laboratory. 1991, *Towards Safer Roads in Developing Countries: A Guide for Engineers and Planners*, Overseas Development Administration, ISBN 1-851221-176-5, Berkshire, England.

U.S. General Accounting Office. 1991, *Motorcycle Helmet Laws Save Lives and Reduce Costs to Society*, Washington, DC: U.S. General Accounting Office, GAO/RCED-91-170.

Wang, S., Chi, G. B., Jing, C. X., Dong, X. M., Wu, C. P., & Li, L. P. 2003, 'Trends in road traffic crashes and associated injury and fatality in the People's Republic of China, 1951–1999', *Injury Control and Safety Promotion*, vol. 10, no. 1–2, pp. 83–7.

Warda, L., Tennebein, M., & Moffatt, M. E. K. 1999, 'House fire injury prevention update, Part I: A review of risk factors for fatal and non-fatal house fire injury', *Injury Prevention, vol.* 5, no. 3, pp. 145–50.

Waters, H., Hyder, A. A., & Rajkotia, Y. Basu, S., Rehwinkel, J. A., & Buchchart, A. 2004, *The Economic Dimensions of Interpersonal Violence*, World Health Organisation, Geneva.

Werneck, G. L., & Reichenheim, M. E. 1997, 'Pediatric burns and associated risk factors in Rio de Janeiro, Brazil', *Burns*, vol. 23, no. 6, pp. 478–83.

World Bank. 1993, *World Development Report 1993: Investing in Health*, 1993 World Health Organisation, Oxford University Press, New York. Available at www.who.int.

World Health Organisation. 2002, *The World Health Report 2002: Reducing Risks, Promoting Health Life*, World Health Organisation, Geneva.

World Health Organisation. 1999, *Injury: A Leading Cause of the Global Burden of Disease*, World Health Organisation, Geneva.

World Health Organisation. 2003, *Drowning Fact Sheet*, World Health Organisation, Geneva.

10.5

Interpersonal violence prevention: A recent public health mandate

Deborah Prothrow-Stith

Introduction

This chapter on public health presents approaches to prevent inter-personal violence in response to the epidemic of adolescent and young adult homicide in the United States, and the growing international attention and concerns about this problem. The chapter provides a short history of the efforts within public health to address violence, a definition and description of the problem, and a discussion of examples of public health approaches to violence prevention. While several types of violence are briefly discussed, the focus of the chapter is youth violence and the increase in youth homicide in the United States. The 1987 United States homicide rate for 15–24-year-old men of 22 per 100 000 was the highest among industrialized countries not at war in 1986/1987 (Fig. 10.5.1). By 1991, it had increased to 37 per 100 000, but declined to 20 per 100 000 in 2004, still the highest among industrialized nations. While high homicide rates also plagued South Africa at the same time, the political instability and violent freedom struggle make it an exception. For further details on international issues, we recommend the 2003 WHO report, *World Report on Violence and Health* (Krug 2002) and the WHO website, http://www.who.int/violence_injury_prevention/en/ (WHO).

The public's demand for solutions to violence in the United States has generated increased multidisciplinary attention, expanding the traditional criminal justice responses of punishment and deterrence to include public health and other health and human service disciplines. In the past 25 years, we have witnessed a dramatic effort by public health professionals to prevent violence in the United States. National leadership has emerged from the Centers for Disease Control (CDC) and the US Surgeon General's office. In addition, many state and local health department leaders have embraced the issue, creating offices of violence prevention within their departments. There are several international meetings, initially geared towards discussion of peace and ending war, which have included interpersonal violence prevention on their conference agendas.

The Centers for Disease Control and Prevention established the Violence Epidemiology Branch in 1983, for the study of homicide

and suicide, and the early data fuelled the violence prevention efforts in public health. Initial Morbidity and Mortality Weekly Reports revealed that homicide is the leading cause of death for black men between 15 and 24 and 25 to 44 years, and that for all adolescents, homicide is the second leading cause of death (CDC 1982; CDC 1983; CDC 2007a). Additional information concerning the characteristics of homicides was published for public health audiences, indicating that 58 per cent of the victims knew their assailants, 47 per cent were precipitated by an argument, and only 15 per cent were as a result of another felony (burglary, drug trafficking, etc.) (CDC 1983). The application of basic epidemiology and reporting techniques became the impetus for public health professionals across the country to confront the issue.

In October 1985, C. Everett Koop convened an invitational meeting, the Surgeon General's Workshop on Violence and Public Health, in Leesburg, Virginia, in the United States. The interdisciplinary meeting focused on assault and homicide, child abuse, rape and sexual assault, domestic violence, elder abuse, and suicide. The disproportionate impact of homicide among young black men in the United States was addressed at the workshop, and a classroom-based violence prevention education programme designed for that population was presented (Prothrow-Stith 1985). The workshop and published proceedings continue to fuel public health professionals' efforts to frame violence as a mainstream public health problem. Over the next decade, the dramatic increase in public health attention to the problem that followed the Surgeon General's conference led to the establishment of the National Center for Injury Prevention and Control at the CDC in 1994. Every Surgeon General since Koop has encouraged the public health community to use its strategies to better understand and prevent violence. Into the new millennium, public health professionals' endeavours to understand and prevent violence have continued to grow with increasingly more programmes, publications, and presentations.

Public health efforts to prevent violence utilizing standard epidemiology, community outreach, screening, community-based programmes, health education, behaviour modification, public

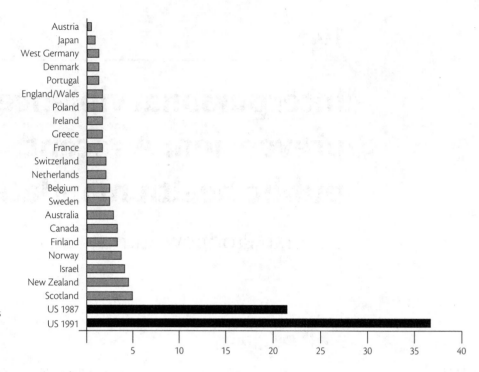

Fig. 10.5.1 International comparisons of homicide rates per 100 000 population (males, aged 15–24) in the years 1986 or 1987.

awareness, and education campaigns continue to involve every aspect of the United States Public Health Service. These efforts are based upon similar multidisciplinary efforts to prevent lung cancer deaths, heart disease, and fatal car crashes.

Consisting of thousands of local programmes scattered across the country, the dramatic increase in interpersonal violence prevention activities has the potential for the same level of success that public health professionals have had with reducing smoking and drunk-driving in the United States. The analogy between violence prevention and other public health problems is not flawless, yet over two decades of experience employing comparable techniques and strategies indicates enough similarity for success. In addition, a number of efforts to train health and public health professionals have been developed and disseminated (Sege & Hoffman 2005).

Definition and classification

The National Center for Injury Prevention and Control at the US Centers for Disease Control classifies both unintentional injuries (accidents) and intentional injuries (violence) as public health problems, as illustrated in Fig. 10.5.2. Intentional injuries are divided into self-directed violence (suicides and suicide attempts) and interpersonal violence (assaults and homicides) (Fig. 10.5.3). Violence is defined by the CDC, as 'the threatened or actual use of physical force or power against another person, against oneself, or against a group or community that either results or is likely to result in injury, death, or deprivation'.

Suicide, a more traditional problem for health and public health professionals, has several commonalities with interpersonal violence. Both often it involves alcohol and other drugs, and the risk for both increases with the presence of a firearm. Media and entertainment values appear to have an impact on both. Adolescent suicide and homicide rates rose dramatically during the early 1980s. While suicide remains an important public health concern, recent efforts

using public health strategies to address interpersonal violence have proliferated.

There are at least four reasons why interpersonal violence became an important concern for public health professionals in the United States: (1) the magnitude and persistence of the problem; (2) the characteristics of and contributing risk factors for violence; (3) the contact health professionals and other professionals in the field of public health have with the victims and perpetrators of violence; and (4) the applicability of public health strategies to both understanding and preventing violence.

Public health professionals have offered a unique comprehensive and prevention-oriented approach to violence that has yielded significant contributions and offers further promise.

Violence is preventable

Perhaps not all of the violence is preventable, but it is clear from the literature and from history that much of it is. The United States and other countries that have similar youth violence problems have a preventable problem; a problem they do not have to have. Evidence that violence is a preventable problem comes from many sources. The comparisons of homicide rates for young men in industrialized countries published by the WHO demonstrate a 5–70-fold difference in rates. If homicide were a genetic or inevitable part of the human condition, one would expect rates from country to country to be fairly similar. The wide discrepancy in rates illustrated in Fig. 10.5.1 indicates a preventable problem. In addition, the changes and variability within US rates among different groups and at different times suggest a preventable problem. For example, the recent increases in the arrest rates for girls in the United States indicate that change is possible. What goes up can come down. In Boston, the significant reduction from 1996 to 2000 in the murder of children 16 or younger illustrated in Fig. 10.5.4 is further indication that violence is preventable. The Boston reduction was celebrated by many and some called it 'the Boston Miracle'. Boston, along with

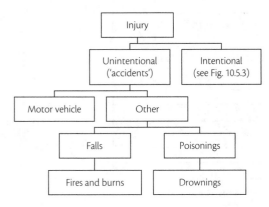

Fig. 10.5.2 Classifications of injury in public health.

most US urban settings, has experienced a recent increase in youth homicide. What goes down can go back up. An inverse relationship between youth homicide rates and resources appears to emerge. In Boston (Fig. 10.5.4), declines in youth homicide appear to be associated with increases in resources and programmes, and the recent increases with a retreat of resources. This appears to also hold true for the success of prevention efforts on a national scale.

The end of a former, rather ubiquitous, practice of duelling (often to the death) among elite white gentlemen of the 1800s in the United States (and many European countries for that matter) is further indication that violence is preventable. Peaking in the United States around 1850, duelling claimed the lives of many, including politicians, journalists, and even physicians, who were recorded as duelling over the proper treatment for a patient. Though illegal, this practice often drew crowds and became a public event. Harriet Martineau, a New Orleans-based journalist, wrote that there were 2–3 duels a day, and as many as 15 on the weekend in New Orleans. Women were advised not to marry a man unless he had proven himself with the blade. Duelling pistols were created to allow 'fairness' in the duels. The Code Duello (originally written in Ireland) was revised and published in 1838 in the United States by a former governor of South Carolina, John Lyde Wilson. Alexander Hamilton, signer of the US Constitution and the first Secretary of the Treasury in the United States, was killed in a duel in 1804. His son, Phillip Hamilton, was killed in a duel 3 years prior. Alexander Hamilton kept a diary, and the entry the night before he was killed in a duel with Aaron Burr is a powerful reminder of the role culture and social norms play in human behaviour (Fig. 10.5.5).

In the case of duelling, culture trumped laws for nearly 100 years. Today, in the United States, we are up against similar cultural forces that encourage children to fight and indicate that it is the strong superhero who justifies a wrong with violence. The extent to which the entertainment media propagate these messages corresponds to the extent to which the US exports them to a broader international community.

Data sources

There are several sources of data on violence in America which are accessible to the public or through community partnerships with academic institutions. The National Center for Education Statistics (NECS) and the Bureau of Justice Statistics (BJS) are the primary federal entities for collecting, analysing, and reporting data related to education and crime, respectively, in the United States and other nations. The Department of the Treasury, Bureau of Alcohol, Tobacco and Firearms (ATF) publication, *Commerce in Firearms in the United States*, is an annual report of activities relating to the regulation of firearms. The Youth Crime Interdiction Initiative (YCGII), *Crime Gun Trace Analysis Reports: The Illegal Youth Firearms Market in 27 Communities*, brings together federal, state, and local law enforcement officials to improve information about the illegal sources of guns recovered from juveniles and adult criminals.

The Uniform Crime Reports (UCR), published by the Federal Bureau of Investigation, is the most frequently cited source of national information on violent crime. These annual reports date back to 1930. The UCR use police data that are submitted to the FBI and which are aggregated into a national data source. Homicides are manditorily reported in these data sets, but other crimes (including non-fatal violent assaults) are reported voluntarily and therefore inconsistently. The reports give cursory information on homicides and assaults, including victim and perpetrator relationship, weapons used, location of the violent episode, and races of victim and perpetrator.

More recently, the National Violent Death Reporting System was established by the US Centers for Disease Control and Prevention (CDC) in 2002 and seeks to provide detailed information concerning each violent death in the United States. The system is organized and run on the state level, and includes data from vital statistics, medical, and criminal justice sources. Although the programme is planned to include the entire country, as of this writing, 17 states are contributing data.

Since 1991, behavioural risk factors reported by high school students in the United States have been measured every other year to the present in the YRBSS (Youth Risk Behavioral Surveillance System).

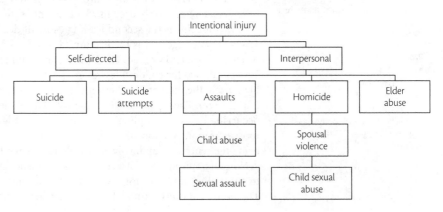

Fig. 10.5.3 Classifications of intentional injury.

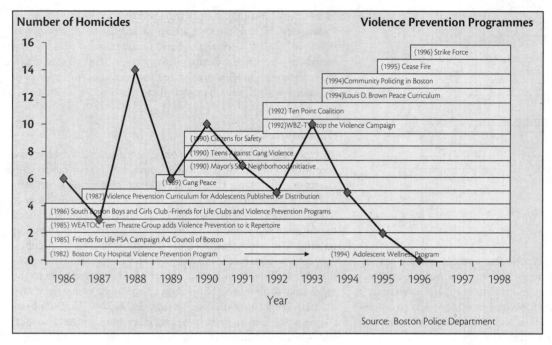

Number of Homicides   **Violence Prevention Programmes**

(1996) Strike Force
(1995) Cease Fire
(1994)Community Policing in Boston
(1994)Louis D. Brown Peace Curriculum
(1992) Ten Point Coalition
(1992)WBZ-TV Stop the Violence Campaign
(1990) Citizens for Safety
(1990) Teens Against Gang Violence
(1990) Mayor's Safe Neighborhood Initiative
(1989) Gang Peace
(1987) Violence Prevention Curriculum for Adolescents Published for Distribution
(1986) South Boston Boys and Girls Club -Friends for Life Clubs and Violence Prevention Programs
(1985) WEATOC Teen Theatre Group adds Violence Prevention to it Repertoire
(1985) Friends for Life-PSA Campaign Ad Council of Boston
(1982) Boston City Hospital Violence Prevention Program ———→ (1994) Adolescent Wellness Program

Year

Source: Boston Police Department

Fig. 10.5.4 Boston Violence Prevention Movement. The number of children under 17 murdered with guns and violence prevention programme examples by start date in Boston 1986–1996.

These data are collected nationally, with local- and state-enhanced collection where contracted. Violent behaviour, weapon carrying, and exposure to violence are measured along with many other health risk factors (drug use, smoking, exercise, etc.). YRBSS data are available on-line on a user-friendly website that facilitates several levels of analysis. In addition to being a site for researchers, the website has generated youth-run research activities. A similar survey of adults, the BRFSS (Behavioral Risk Factor Surveillance System), is on-line accessible as well. Both the YRBSS and the BRFSS are conducted by CDC.

The magnitude of the problem

The United States Federal Bureau of Investigation estimates that 1.8 million Americans are victims of violence each year. Adolescents are more likely than any other age group to be victims of violence, mostly from their peers (same race, from the same neighbourhood). A complete representation of the magnitude of violence is unavailable because of the unreliable and inconsistent measures of non-fatal episodes of violence. Homicides, the tip of the iceberg, are most accurately measured, as reporting is mandatory, as noted

above. Other countries have made their homicide rates available through the World Health Organization.

The magnitude of the problem of homicide in the United States was mind-boggling when compared to that of other industrialized nations not at war. Not only was the United States homicide rate 10–25 times higher than most industrialized nations, but the homicide rates rivalled some less-developed countries facing war or considerable social, political, and economic turmoil (Wolfgang 1986). An international study of 1985 homicide rates in industrialized countries showed that the United States rate for both sexes, ages 1–19, was more than three times that of the next highest rate, Canada (Williams & Kotch 1990). Little has changed with respect to these international comparisons over the past several decades.

In 2006, of the 14 990 murder victims, 50 per cent were black and 47 per cent were white. In 45 per cent of the murders, the relationships between the victim and perpetrator were not known; in 30 per cent, they were friends or acquaintances, in 13 per cent, they were in the same family, and in 12 per cent, they were strangers. In addition, 93.2 per cent of black victims were killed by black offenders and 82.9 per cent of white murder victims were killed by white offenders. Firearms were used in 73.4 per cent of the murders (FBI 2007). Homicide is the second leading cause of death for persons 15–24 years of age and is the leading cause of death for African–American men and women. The United States' child homicide rate, 2.6 per 100 000 for children less than 15 years of age, is five times higher that the rates of 25 other industrialized countries combined (CDC 1997). These patterns continue with fatal violence primarily occurring between people of the same race, handguns being the most common weapon of fatality, and youth and young adults being the central group involved in violence-related fatalities.

Non-fatal episodes of violence and assaults are not always reported to the police, and are not always treated in emergency rooms. Therefore, data sets on non-fatal violence are often inconsistent.

Cons
- I have a wife and children whom I love.
- I am deeply in debt and should not leave this burden to my family.
- I have no ill-will for Burr.
- Dueling is illegal in NY.
- Dueling is condemned by Christianity, my religion.

Pros
- There is a pressing necessity not to decline the call.
- Not dueling will cost me political support.
- Dueling is essential to my ability to be useful in the future.

Fig. 10.5.5 Hamilton's pros and cons.

Police are often unaware of numerous, sometimes serious violent injuries and events. Emergency rooms capture a much larger number of the assaults. In 2004, 5292 youth aged 10 years were murdered, while an estimated 721 000 were treated in hospital emergency departments for violence-related injury—a ratio of approximately 120:1 (CDC 2007b). This ratio is a comparable to that in the Northeast Ohio Trauma Study, in which for each single homicide, there were 20 assaults reported to the police and 100 reported to the emergency rooms in one standard metropolitan statistical area in northeast Ohio. Furthermore, many episodes of violence, particularly those occurring among friends and family, are not reported to either the police or the emergency rooms.

The epidemic of youth violence in the United States is not limited to homicide. Arrest rates reported by police reveal an increase in nonfatal episodes of adolescent violence, despite the limitations of the data set. The decade of 1980–1990 saw the juvenile violent crime arrest rate for black adolescents increase by 19 per cent; for white adolescents, it increased 44 per cent, while the other race categories, despite a large increase in Asian youth, declined 53 per cent (FBI 1992). Although minors accounted for less than 14 per cent of the US population, in 1995, 37 per cent of homicide arrests, 28 per cent of rape arrests, and 51 per cent of robbery arrests were committed by minors. In 1982, 390 youth aged 13–15 were arrested for homicide. By 1992, this figure had nearly doubled. Although these rates dropped between 1994 and early 2000, they are starting to increase in most urban areas in the United States. The escalation of adolescent violent crime rates in the last several decades cuts across race, class, and geographic location, despite a common misconception that it is an urban black problem. More recently, the United States has experienced dramatic increases in violent crime rates involving girls as both perpetrators and victims, reflecting a growing involvement of girls in the epidemic of violence.

Adolescent violence

Violence involving youth has persisted at alarming levels in the United States. In 2003, the National Center for Health Statistics reported that homicide was the second leading cause of death for the 15–19-year age group (second only to motor vehicle accidents), at almost twice the rate of the overall United States population (CDC 2006). In 1997, 6146 people aged 15–24 years were victims of homicide. This amounts to an average of 17 youth homicide victims per day in the United States. Since then, the rate of youth homicide has dropped to 14 deaths per day (5085 total deaths). Homicide has remained the second leading cause of death for persons (men and women) 15–24 years of age (crude rate 12.8/100 000 for the period 1999–2007) and the leading cause of death for African–Americans, with 2004 rates still astronomically high: 77.2 per 100 000 for males, 8.8 for females.

Furthermore, adolescent mortality rate trends indicate that although overall death rates and death rates due to motor vehicle crashes both decreased for persons aged 10–24 years from 1979 to 1988, death rates for homicide increased by 6.7 per cent. In eight US states, firearm-related deaths surpassed automobile crashes as the leading cause of death for this age group (Centers for Disease Control and Prevention 1994). Since the peak in the late 1990s, these same rates have seen a modest decline of 5.6 per cent in the period 1999–2004.

Even for non-fatal violent victimizations, the 1990 National Crime Survey found that age was one of the most important single predictors of an individual's risk, which peaks at age 16–19 for both

men (95 per 1000) and women (54 per 1000) (Bureau of Justice Statistics 1992, 1993). This was a dramatic change from several decades earlier, when the mean age of victims of violence was approximately 10 years older. Clearly, our nation's youth are at high risk for experiencing violence.

Dating violence is a form of adolescent and young adult violence that is often overlooked, even within discussions of domestic violence. Very little research has been done, and the general awareness of the problem of dating violence is relatively recent. A survey within a college population found that 21 per cent of the students admitted being in violent relationships and 62 per cent personally knew of someone affected by a violent relationship (Makepeace 1981). Several studies since then have indicated that between 12 and 19 per cent of high school students are involved in dating violence, either as a victim or as a perpetrator. As with domestic violence, women are more often the victims.

School violence

School suspension data offer another measure of the violence occurring, yet there are several limitations. Suspension numbers may vary within a school depending upon the persons responsible for collecting the data. There are not standard criteria within or between school systems as to what behaviour results in student suspension. There are also disincentives to reporting incidents of violence in schools, as this information may lead to negative consequences for school personnel themselves.

Violence in schools is not new, but it has become more severe and occasionally lethal. In the 2005 YRBSS, amongst students in the 9th to 12th grade in the 50 states, including the District of Columbia and Virgin Islands, 18.5 per cent reported carrying a weapon 30 days prior to the survey, and 5.4 per cent reported that they had carried a gun. Among students nationwide, 25.9 per cent had been in a physical fight one or more times during the 12 months preceding the survey (CDC 2007), and 3.6 per cent had required medical treatment for fighting-related injuries.

The CDC survey also revealed that 6 per cent of the students said that they missed at least 1 day of school in a month before because they felt unsafe at school (CDC 2007). In 1989, the United States Department of Justice found that 6 per cent of students report having to avoid certain places in school or on the way to or from school because they were afraid of being attacked. A poll conducted by Metropolitan Life showed that only 23 per cent of the students said they never saw violent incidents at school. A Louis Harris Associates Poll of youth and guns conducted in 1993 of 2500 students in the 6th to 12th grades showed that 15 per cent carried a handgun to school in the past year. Fifty-nine per cent said they could get a handgun if they wanted one. The addition of weapons to the typical school brawl has contributed significantly to the greater severity and mortality of school fights.

The CDC, the United States Department of Education, and the National School Safety Center conducted a study of actual deaths in schools. Data show that 105 school-associated violent deaths occurred in the school years 1992–1993 and 1993–1994, including 81 homicides, 19 suicides, and 5 unintentional firearm-related deaths. Sixty-six per cent of these occurred on school property and 75 per cent were committed with a firearm (Satcher 1985).

While the arrest rates for overall crime and violent crime are significantly lower for young women than young men, recent increases in girls' arrests have narrowed the gap. From 1981 to 1995, there was a 129 per cent increase in the violent crime arrest rate for young women when compared to a 56 per cent increase over the same time period for young men. Currently, girls account for over 25 per cent of juvenile arrests for violent crime, unheard of two decades ago. More girls are entering the juvenile justice system and doing so at younger ages; there has been a 10 per cent increase in the numbers of 13- and 14-year olds coming into juvenile court.

Some experts, including Meda Chesney-Lind (1998) at the University of Hawaii, believe that there really has not been a significant increase in the proportion of young women committing crimes. Rather, 'we're criminalizing a lot of schoolyard scuffles where, in the past, we'd call it a cat fight, we'd giggle and keep walking. Now we're calling the cops'.

Chesney-Lind and others also point to changes and biases within the juvenile justice system that they believe explain the increased number of girls arrested. For example, girls are twice as likely as boys to be detained, with the detention period lasting five times longer for girls than their male counterparts. Girls are more likely than boys to be charged with status offences, which if committed by an adult, would not be considered a crime (e.g. running away from home, truancy, incorrigibility), and are more likely to be incarcerated for these offences than males.

However, it is important to note that more recent increases in arrests for girls involve violent crimes, not status offences. Furthermore, these increases are occurring at the same time that arrest rates for boys for various categories of violent crime are either declining or barely increasing. With severely limited juvenile facilities and detention spaces for girls, police actually have a disincentive to arrest girls, as there is no place to take them.

Suicide

Historically, suicide in the United States was viewed as primarily a problem of older adult white men with clinical depression or other mental disorders; thus, suicide prevention involved identifying and treating mental illness. A steady rise in the adolescent and young adult (15–24-year old) suicide rates from 4.5 per 100 000 in 1950 to 10.1 per 100 000 in 1999–2004 created the need for new prevention strategies (CDC 1998). The rise was alarming, particularly as research indicated that only one out of three of those who committed suicide fit the criteria for clinical depression or other mental illness (Shaffer *et al.* 1988).

Race and gender disparities in suicide rates are striking. The rates for adolescent girls and women have remained relatively stable over the last 30 years, and the rates for white men have levelled since 1988. However, there has been a dramatic rise in the suicide rates for young black males (15–24-year old) since 1986 (Shaffer *et al.* 1994). While the suicide rates for white males remain higher than those for black males in each age cohort, the rates among black males increased at a faster rate than any other group. Male rates of completed suicide reflect their choice of rapidly lethal means (firearms and hanging), compared to females who more commonly choose ingestions resulting in high rates of non-lethal suicide attempts.

The CDC convened a panel of experts and conducted a study of youth suicide prevention programmes. The study reviewed the existing programmes and delineated eight suicide prevention strategies:

1. School gatekeeper training. This type of programme is directed at school staff to help them identify and defer students at risk of suicide and to organize the response in case of a suicide.

2. Community gatekeeper training. This type of programme provides the same service to community staff, clergy, police, merchants, etc.

3. General suicide education. These programmes are school-based education on suicide, often incorporating self-esteem building or social competency exercises.

4. Screening programmes. Screening involves administering an instrument to identify high-risk youth in order to provide services.

5. Peer support programmes. School- or community-based programmes to help adolescents develop competency in relationships and to help each other.

6. Crisis centres and hotlines. These programmes provide 24-h emergency counselling.

7. Means restriction. Strategies to restrict access to firearms, drugs, or other means of committing suicide.

8. Intervention after a suicide. Commonly called postvention, these programmes are designed to help survivors and prevent suicide clusters.

Miller and colleagues have published compelling evidence demonstrating the tragic role of firearms availability in youth suicide rates (Miller *et al.* 2006). As a result, suicide prevention recommendations now strongly support controlling access to firearms, as well as improved identification of depression and access to mental health services (AAP 2007).

Domestic violence

Domestic violence or partner violence is defined as violence between those involved in an intimate relationship. According to Department of Justice, approximately 4.8 million women and 2.9 million men were victims of intimate partner violence (Tjaden 2000). It involves physical abuse, sexual assault, threats of violence, and emotional abuse. Coercive control through degradation, malicious enforcement of petty rules, intermittent rewards and isolations are examples of the methods employed to demonstrate and maintain power.

However, in family situations, children under 12 years of age represent 62 per cent of all victims. Juveniles aged 12–17 comprise 30 per cent of the victims in overall offences, and 23 per cent in family occurrences. Females are most frequently the victims of family and overall offences, comprising 74–76 per cent of the victims of family and overall offences, respectively (Uniform Crime Reports 1998).

In 1998, 27 per cent of victims of family-related violence were reported to have been related to one or more of their offenders. A higher percentage of victims of family violence are over the age of 18 than the victims of overall crimes of violence (80 vs. 76 per cent). Additionally, victims of family violence are overwhelmingly female (71 per cent for family violence and 58 per cent for overall violence) (Uniform Crime Reports 1998).

Rape and sexual assault

The Federal Bureau of Investigation in the 1993 Uniform Crime Reports recorded 104 806 rapes in 1993, with a national rate of 79 per 100 000. The National Crime Victimization Survey indicates women report approximately 133 000 rapes each year, with half saying they reported them to the police and 55 per cent indicating that they knew the assailant.

Rape accounts for slightly less than 1 per cent of all violent offences. In particular, children under 12 years of age comprise a larger proportion of victims of family rape than all victims of rape (36 vs. 12 per cent) (FBI 1998).

Additional information is available from a national sample, the National Women's Study (Kilpatrick *et al.* 1992), suggesting a higher incidence and prevalence. According to this study, an estimated 683 000 women are raped each year, with 60 per cent being younger than 18 years old. The perpetrator was a stranger in only 22 per cent of the cases. This study estimates that 12.1 million American women are raped at some point in their lives. Only 16 per cent of them report the rape to the police.

Economic costs

In 2000, the total economic cost of violence in the United States from non-fatal injuries and death were over US$70 billion (Corso *et al.* 2007). Each year, US citizens pay about US$53.5 billion for criminal justice interventions for violence, and an additional US$158 billion for cost of lifetime care for victims of violence (medical treatment, rehabilitation, and lost productivity). These figures reflect only the monetary costs of violence, not the pain, suffering, and lost quality of life for victims. They do not reflect the cost for safety measures—the inability of children and adults to walk or play in their own neighbourhood, the cost of guard dogs and guns for 'protection', and an immeasurable sense of fear of crime victimization. In considering the impact of violence on society, it is also important to note the costs of violent crimes.

A framework model developed by Miller and colleagues (1993) was used to quantify costs of violent crime; it incorporated direct losses other than property losses (medical, mental health, and emergency services, insurance administration), productivity losses (wages, fringe benefits, housework), and non-monetary losses (pain, suffering, lost quality of life). Costs to victims of crimes resulting in injury were estimated to be US$110 000 for rape survivors, and US$23 000 for assault survivors (in 1993 dollars). Moreover, the lifetime costs of criminal victimizations for a person aged 12 and older was estimated to be US$10 billion for rape, US$96 billion for assault, and US$48 billion for murder (Miller *et al.* 1993).

Furthermore, these figures do not include property losses incurred during violent acts, nor the mammoth costs incurred by collective society's reactive response to violence, including law enforcement, adjudication, victim services, and correctional expenditures.

In 1993, the cost of direct medical spending, emergency services, and claims processed for the victims of gun violence nationwide totalled approximately US$3 billion. Average hospital charges for treating one child wounded by gunfire were more than US$14 000.

Taxpayers pay for gun violence. The average cost (including medical treatment and the prosecution and incarceration of the shooter) of one gunshot wound patient (all age groups) can be up to US$1.79 million (Lengel 1997). Approximately 80 per cent of patients who suffer from violence are uninsured and/or eligible for government medical care assistance. A study of all direct and indirect costs of gun violence, including medical, lost wages, and security costs, estimates that gun violence costs the nation US$100 billion a year (Cook 2000). The average total cost of one gun crime can be as high as US$1.79 million, including medical treatment and the prosecution and imprisonment of the shooter (Rice 1993). At least 80 per cent

of the economic costs of treating firearm injuries are paid by taxpayer dollars (Wintemute 1992).

The characteristics of violence

Contrary to the stereotype of violence as predominantly stranger-related or occurring in the context of criminal behaviour such as racial harassment, robbery, or drug-dealing, much of the violence experienced in the United States is intimate and occurs in the context of personal relationships (FBI 2006). A typical homicide involves two people who know each other, who are under the influence of alcohol and get into an argument that escalates in the presence of a gun. Only 15 per cent of homicides occur in the course of committing a crime, as compared with over 50 per cent that stem from arguments among acquaintances (CDC 1982). This 50 per cent takes place in family relationships (e.g. child abuse, elder abuse, spouse abuse) or friends (interpersonal peer violence). In the remaining 35 per cent, the relationship between victim and perpetrator is unknown.

The perpetrators and victims of violence share many traits. They are likely to be young and male and of the same race. They are likely to be poor and to have been exposed to violence in the past, especially family violence. They may be depressed and use alcohol and/or other drugs (Prothrow-Stith & Weissman 1991). This incongruity between public perception and actual circumstances has resulted in demands for resources and solutions that address only part—possibly the smaller part—of the problem. While certainly not discarding established anti-crime and anti-violence strategies, we must recognize the diversity of violent circumstances that exist and must build a broader base of efforts that not only responds to violent events, but also focuses on preventive services as well.

A closer look at the demographic characteristics reveals certain noteworthy factors contributing to a complex picture of adolescent violence. Breaking down the 10–24 years of age spectrum further, 1997 homicide rates (deaths per 100 000) were considerably higher among 20–24-year-olds (19) and 15–19-year-olds (11.7) compared with 10–14-year-olds (1.7)—yet, it is still important to note that the rates increased among all three groups from 1979 to 1988 (CDC 1998). In terms of gender, males greatly exceed females in the number of violent victimizations, with the exception of sexual assault and are also more likely to be violent offenders and witnesses to violence.

Contact that health professionals have with victims and perpetrators

The regular contact physicians and nurses have with victims of violence, particularly in emergency departments, has caused many to begin to address this problem. The American College of Emergency Physicians has included violence prevention on the agenda of their annual meetings. The Journal of the American Medical Association has dedicated two special issues to the topic of violence, concurrent with the American Medical Associations publication of manuals for health providers on domestic violence, child abuse, and rape and sexual assault.

The Northeast Ohio Trauma Study illustrates the need for greater data from emergency departments in showing that five times the number of assaults reported to the police was reported to hospital emergency departments. Not only are non-fatal violent episodes inadequately measured with police data, but the greater contact health providers have with victims provides an opportunity to offer public health prevention and intervention strategies in the emergency department. Such programmes have been started at Boston City Hospital (now the Boston Medical Center and no longer a government hospital), Cook County Hospital in Chicago, Harborview Hospital in Seattle, and the Washington and Grady Memorial Hospital in Atlanta, Georgia, in the United States.

There is a substantial body of research which suggests that crime rates reflect 'community social disorganization'. The social disorganization theory was originally developed by the Chicago School researchers, Clifford Shaw and Henry McKay, in their classic work, *Juvenile Delinquency and Urban Areas* (1942). Shaw and McKay demonstrated that the same socioeconomically disadvantaged areas in 21 US cities continued to exhibit high delinquency rates over a span of several decades, despite changes in their racial and ethnic composition, indicating the persistent contextual effects of these communities on crime rates, regardless of what populations experienced them. This observation led them to reject individualistic explanations of delinquency and to focus instead on community processes such as disruption of local community organization and weak social controls, which lead to the apparent trans-generational transmission of criminal behaviour. In general, social disorganization is defined as the 'inability of a community structure to realize the common values of its residents and maintain effective social controls' (Sampson & Groves 1989). The social organizational approach views local communities and neighbourhoods as complex systems of friendship, kinship, and acquaintanceship networks, as well as formal and informal associational ties rooted in family life and ongoing socialization processes (Sampson 1995). From the perspective of crime control, a major dimension of social disorganization is the ability of a community to supervise and control teenage peer groups, especially gangs. Thus, Shaw and McKay (1942) argued that residents of cohesive communities were better able to control the youth behaviours that set the context for gang violence. Examples of such controls include 'supervision of leisure-time youth activities, intervention in street-corner congregation, and challenging youth who seem to be up to no good'. Socially disorganized communities with extensive street-corner peer groups are also expected to have higher rates of adult violence, especially among younger adults who still have ties to youth gangs' (Sampson 1995).

Application of public health strategies

Public health professionals have applied traditional public health strategies to violence prevention. They have brought a different perspective and orientation to bear on the problem. Applying public health techniques and strategies complements and strengthens the criminal justice approach.

Public health brings an analytic approach to problems by concentrating on identifying risk factors as well as factors that influence resiliency that could become the focus of preventive interventions. It also brings a record of accomplishment in controlling 'accidental' (unintentional) injuries through both environmental manipulations (for example, seat belts and childproof caps on medicines) and behavioural change (for example, laws and educational campaigns to reduce drunk-driving).

Identification of risk factors

Public health strategies have added to the literature on the understanding of violence and its risk factors. In combination with the work from other disciplines, major risk factors for youth violence have been identified. These factors can be broadly categorized into environmental and psychological risk factors. The major environmental risk factors include firearms, alcohol and other drugs, and cultural factors; being a victim of child abuse, witnessing family violence, exposure to media violence, and exposure to high levels of peer and community violence. A consistent and strong environmental risk factor for homicide is poverty. The mechanism for this interaction is not completely understood, but may include: (1) the anger and frustration associated with not having money and essential commodities; (2) the experience of classism; (3) the likely absence of adult male role models; (4) the scarcity of recreational, extracurricular, and after-school activities; and (5) more time spent watching television.

Corporal punishment is a controversial environmental factor that may be related to risk for violence. Certainly, in its extreme form, abuse, there is an evidence to suggest that it increases the risk of delinquency. Efforts to improve parenting and to reduce child abuse often focus on alternative disciplinary strategies. Other environmental risk factors for adolescents include peer pressure, the crack cocaine epidemic, and policing practices.

Race and poverty

There appear to be extremely large racial differences in violence rates among young Americans. In 1991, homicide was the number one cause of death for black youth aged between 15 and 24; the homicide rate for black youth (both sexes) was eight times the rate for white youth aged between 15 and 24 (90 per 100 000 vs. 10.8 per 100 000, respectively). National statistics concerning other ethnic minority groups, such as Latin Americans, Asian–Americans, and Native Americans, are scant.

The racial data are not indicative of any biological or genetic factor, because they are confounded by socioeconomic status, urban living, gun availability, and racism. Using family income as the primary indicator of socioeconomic status, the National Crime Survey found an inverse relationship between income and the risk of violent victimization (Bureau of Justice Statistics 1992). In 1988, the risk of victimization was found to be 2.5 times higher for people in low-income families (under US$7500 per year) when compared to high-income families (US$50 000 per year).

It is important to note, however, that the relationship of violence and social factors is complex and still unclear. For example, multivariate studies have shown a complicated interaction between race and socioeconomic status. That is to say, at low socioeconomic levels, black individuals have a higher risk of homicide compared to white individuals. At higher socioeconomic levels, however, the difference disappears. William Julius Wilson's work on neighbourhood poverty offers a possible explanation. Poor black people are much more likely than poor white people to live in neighbourhoods, where the majority of the people are poor. Although it appears that race is a significant social predictor in certain studies, multivariate studies show a more complex situation.

Other studies have suggested that, in fact, socioeconomic status is the major predictor, and race is merely a marker. One study that used several markers for poverty, including number of people per square foot of housing, disaggregated the race and socioeconomic variables. In this study, overcrowded white people had the same high domestic homicide rates as overcrowded black people.

Less-crowded members of both groups had the same lower rates (Centerwall 1984, 1993). In 1987, the homicide rate for young black men in the military was 1/12th of their national rate, strongly indicating the influence of social, structural, cultural, and economic factors.

Child neglect and abuse

Child abuse and neglect are general terms used to encompass many harmful behaviours toward children. Verbal, emotional, and sexual abuse are included, as well as failure to meet a child's needs, and outright physical violence. Child sexual abuse is most often considered separately, yet each state has its own definition and guidelines for protective custody.

Because child abuse has been a reportable crime for many years, better statistics are available. An annual 50-state survey estimated two million reports of child abuse and neglect in 1986. Over the decade of the 1980s, the number of reports increased by 184 per cent (Daro & Mitchel 1987). The number of child sexual abuse reports increased dramatically as well, a 12-fold increase within the decade. It is obvious that researchers have the same problem documenting both child abuse and child sexual abuse as they do documenting other forms of violence—unreliable data sources, under-reporting by victims, inconsistent definitions, and failure to recognize an event as precipitated by violence.

With child abuse, reporting biases work in both directions, both to inflate or deflate the numbers. Episodes of child abuse occurring in families of middle-class and professional parents are less likely to be reported, even with mandatory reporting laws, which diminish prevalence estimates. Yet, greater awareness and sensitivity to child abuse and the advent of mandatory reporting no doubt increase the numbers. There is a struggle among child health and human service professionals to determine the way to maintain mandatory reporting and improve the effectiveness of the state protective services. An over-reliance on foster care without adequate attention to family preservation seems to have been the rule in the past.

The cycle of violence

The relationship between child abuse, neglect, and witnessing violence to adolescent and adult violence has been demonstrated in several studies. Existing studies suggest that there is a greater likelihood of abuse by parents if they were abused as children. Estimates of the percentages of abusive parents who were abused as children ranged from 7 per cent (Gil 1973) to 70 per cent (Egeland & Jacobvitz 1984). Among adults who were abused, up to one-third of them abuse their children (Straus & Gelles 1990).

A retrospective look at violent juvenile delinquents compared with non-violent juvenile delinquents showed a significantly higher rate of physical child abuse. Both interviews with the delinquents and medical chart reviews yielded evidence of greater victimization, skull fractures, emergency trauma visits, and other physical injuries.

A cohort study of abused or neglected children demonstrated a greater risk for delinquency, adult criminal behaviour, and violent criminal behaviour, even though the majority of such children do not demonstrate these behaviours. The abused children had a number of offences, and began delinquent behaviour at earlier ages, regardless of race and gender (Widom 1989).

For black adolescents aged 11–19 living in or around an urban housing project, the self-reported use of violence was associated with exposure to violence and personal victimization, hopelessness, depression, family conflict, and previous corporal punishment. Those with a higher sense of purpose in life and less depression were better able to handle the exposure to violence in the home and community (Durant et al. 1994).

Children and exposure to media violence

The association between childhood exposure to media violence and subsequent aggressive behaviour has been firmly established over the past four decades. The American Psychological Association collected these data and decided unequivocally to pronounce the negative influence of entertainment media violence on children in a report (American Psychological Association Commission on Violence and Youth 1993). They expected the report to have an impact on parents and policy makers. Other reviews of the literature have been done with similar conclusions (Dietz & Strasburger 1991; Sege & Dietz 1994).

Pre-school children exposed to violent activity in a controlled setting were observed to imitate and repeat the violent behaviours (Bandura et al. 1963). It involved an actor appearing on screen attacking a Bobo-the-clown doll. Following this attack, in three separate video sequences, the actor was praised, ignored, or punished. The pre-school-aged viewers who saw the violent behaviour rewarded onscreen were more likely than the other two groups to repeat the violent actions when shown a Bobo-the-clown doll themselves. This experiment demonstrated that children can learn violent behaviours from television, and are especially likely to do so when these activities are depicted as socially acceptable.

Older children's behaviour is also heavily influenced by exposure to media violence. Meta-analysis of a series of experiences demonstrates conclusively that school-aged boys have more fights in the days following exposure to violent mainstream movies that they do in the days following exposure to less-violent movies (Turner et al. 1986; Wood et al. 1991).

In a landmark cohort study involving children raised in Pennsylvania, Huesmann and Eromn showed that preference for violent television programmes at age eight, as well as total hours of television viewing, predicted the severity of violent criminal convictions by age 30 (Huesmann et al. 1984). This effect should, however, be modified by parental interventions (Huesmann et al. 1983; Liebert 1988; Austin et al. 1990; Weaver & Barbour 1992; Sang et al. 1993).

Centerwall has shown that in three different countries (the United States, Canada, and South Africa), homicide rates doubled approximately 10–12 years after the introduction of English-language television (Centerwall 1992). In the United States, homicide rates doubled first among those portions of the population exposed to television first (white urban dwellers), and only later among those segments of the population who received television later. He attributes approximately 10 000 deaths annually in the United States as the results of exposure to media violence.

Taken together, we believe that these studies meet most of the criteria for causality set forth in the Surgeon General's 1964 report on smoking and health (United States Department of Health, Education, and Welfare 1964), and established that exposure to media violence places children at risk for subsequent violence.

Public debate flourishes concerning the roles of video games and violence-oriented musical lyrics in encouraging violence. Currently, however, no definitive data are available on these issues.

Firearms

The United States has more firearms than any other industrialized nation not at war, and the following facts, extracted from the well-referenced 2007 website of the Brady Campaign to Prevent Gun Violence, are astounding:

- There are approximately 192 million privately owned firearms in the United States—65 million of which are handguns.

- Currently, an estimated 39 per cent of US households have a gun, while 24 per cent have a handgun.

- In 1998 alone, licensed firearms dealers sold an estimated 4.4 million guns, 1.7 million of which were handguns. Additionally, it is estimated that one to three million guns change hands in the secondary market each year, and many of these sales are not regulated.

- In 2004, 29 569 people in the United States died from firearm-related deaths—11 624 (39 per cent) of those were murdered, 16 750 (57 per cent) were suicides, 649 (2.2 per cent) were accidents, and for 235 (0.8 per cent), the intent was unknown. In comparison, 33 651 Americans were killed in the Korean War and 58 193 Americans were killed in the Vietnam War.

- In 2004, firearms were used to murder 56 people in Australia, 184 people in Canada, 73 people in England and Wales, 5 people in New Zealand, and 37 people in Sweden. In comparison, firearms were used to murder 11 344 people in the United States.

- In 2005, there were only 143 justifiable homicides by private citizens using handguns in the United States.

- In 2004, nearly eight children and teenagers aged 19 and under were killed with guns each day.

- In 2004, firearm homicide was the second leading cause of injury death for men and women 10–24 years of age, second only to motor vehicle crashes.

- In 2004, firearm homicide was the leading cause of death for black males aged 15–34 years.

- From 1999 through 2004, an average of 916 children and teenagers took their own lives with guns each year.

- For each time a gun is used in a home in a legally justifiable shooting, there are 22 criminal, unintentional, and suicide-related shootings.

- The presence of a gun in the home triples the risk of homicide in the home.

- The presence of a gun in the home increases the risk of suicide five-fold. A gun in the home is 43 times more likely to kill a family member or friend than it is to be used in self-defence.

- In the United States, in 2006, firearms were used in 67.9 per cent of murders, 42.2 per cent of robbery offences, and 21.9 per cent of aggravated assaults.

- In 2002, 1830 children in the United States under the age of 19 years died from gunshot wounds; 167 of these children were shot accidentally.

Teenage and young adult homicides are uniquely American problems. This high rate of youth homicide in the United States has been attributed to the much higher rate of gun ownership in the United States. An international study of gun ownership and homicide found positive correlations between the rates of household gun ownership and the national rates and proportions of gun-related homicide (Lester 1988; Killias 1993).

Handgun availability appears to be playing an increasingly important role in youth homicides. As an example, the increasing trend seen in the total homicide rate among 15–19-year-olds from 1979 to 1989 is solely attributable to the increase in firearm homicides; the firearm-related homicide rate increased 61 per cent (6.9–11.1 per 100 000), while, at the same time, the non-firearm-related homicide rates actually decreased by 29 per cent (3.4–2.4 per 100 000) (Fingerhut et al. 1992). From 1980 to 1989, over 65 per cent of the 11 000 homicides committed by high-school aged youth were firearm-related.

Handguns are widely accessible to adolescents in the United States. The national 2005 Youth Risk Behavior Survey found that about 5.4 per cent of high school students had carried a firearm at least once in the 30 days preceding the survey. The incidence was higher among males, 9.9 per cent (Centers for Disease Control and Prevention 2006). In another study of inner-city youths, as many as 35 per cent of males carried a gun outside of school (Sheley et al. 1992).

Firearms contribute to both the violent victimization of youth and to the violent offences committed by youth. The presence of a weapon in the home is associated with a three-fold increase in the likelihood of homicide, compared with matched controls drawn from the neighbourhood surrounding the victim (Kellerman et al. 1993).

Comparisons of two cities (Seattle and Vancouver) with similar demographic characteristics showed that Seattle's excess homicide rate is entirely attributable to firearm homicides (Sloan et al. 1988) (Fig. 10.5.6). Another study designed to look at the effect of implementation of gun control legislation showed a positive effect of the enactment of tougher gun control laws in the District of Columbia compared with both neighbouring states (Loftin et al. 1991).

All of these studies demonstrate that availability of firearms is strongly correlated with increased homicide rates. Logically, this result coincides with the earlier observation that most homicides result from conflicts among people who know each other well, including friends and acquaintances, as well as relatives and spouses.

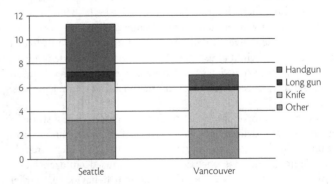

Fig. 10.5.6 Comparison of homicide rates in cities of similar demographics.

In a situation of passionate conflict, handgun availability appears to increase the likelihood of serious injury or death.

Psychological and behavioural factors

In pioneering studies conducted in the late 1980s, Slaby and Guerra (1988) demonstrated that adolescents involved in violence have habits of thought that lead them into violent confrontations. They examined the responses of three groups of teenaged boys to a specific scenario. One group of boys were in custody for the commission of violent crimes, a second group was identified by their teachers as being violence-prone, and a third group was identified by their teachers as not being violence-prone. Each boy was presented with the same scenario: They were going after school to work on their batting so that they could make the baseball team. As a boy arrived, another boy took the last bat. In understanding this scenario, the more violence-prone boys were more likely to assign malicious intent to the boy who took the bat than the less-violent boys. In imagining ways to resolve this scenario, these boys could envisage fewer alternative means towards resolution.

Slaby and Guerra concluded from this study that the more violence-prone boys got into more fights because they were more likely to see harmful intent in a given situation, and, having seen such intent, were less likely to come up with a peaceful way to resolve the situation. These results have been confirmed with a larger-scale study conducted in the New York City schools (Center for Disease Control and Prevention 1993). Boys who reported having been in serious fights were more likely to suggest that carrying a weapon or threatening to use a weapon were good ways to stay out of fights than the general school population; they were also far less likely to say that one could avoid fighting by apologizing compared with the overall population.

Witnessing violence

In addition to the young people directly injured by violence, increasing attention is being given to the scores more young people who are affected indirectly as witnesses to violent acts or by exposure to chronic violent environments (Groves et al. 1993). Pynoos and colleagues (1987) examined the appearance of post-traumatic stress disorder (PTSD) symptoms in children who experienced a fatal sniper attack on their elementary school, and reported a correlation between the type and number of post-traumatic stress disorder symptoms and proximity to the violent incident, as well as more severe symptoms in children who knew the deceased child.

In addition to acute incidents, other studies relate findings of correlations between exposure to chronic violence and distress symptoms (Fitzpatrick & Boldizar 1993; Freeman et al. 1993; Lorion & Saltzman 1993; Martinez & Richters 1993; Osofsky et al. 1993). In addition, Lorion and Saltzman (1993) described anecdotal reports from their research participants, including reports from teachers and administrators about children who lived in violent settings arriving at school in distress, who were unable to concentrate or maintain appropriate behaviour in class, and who hid in the classroom and were afraid to return home or take the bus. Clearly, there is a need to address not only the physical threat of violence, but also the potential for psychopathological and/or emotional disturbances in both victims and bystanders (Emde 1993; Durant et al. 1994).

Approaches to violence prevention and control

Historically, society has relied almost exclusively on the criminal justice system both to respond to and prevent violence. This tactic is rooted in the beliefs that violence is criminal, that those who commit violence should be punished, and that the threat of punishment is a potential deterrent to violent acts. A large, elaborate set of institutions has been developed to achieve these goals, which includes police, prosecutors, public defenders, judges, probation officers, and prison guards. It is principally designed to respond to crimes after they have been committed by identifying, apprehending, prosecuting, punishing, and controlling the violent offender. It is guided not only by the practical goals of reducing crimes of all types (including violence), but also by the normative goal of assuring justice to victims and the accused.

The public health and criminal justice systems historically have been separate in their conceptualization of approaches to violence and the development of activities to reduce or prevent violence. The public health field has approached the issue through efforts to identify the risk factors related to violent behaviour. The field comes to this issue in reaction to the magnitude of intentional injuries that are present in health care settings. The criminal justice system has approached the issue through efforts to identify and assign blame for criminal behaviour, maintain public safety, and remove violent offenders from the community.

Viewed from the perspective of those interested in reducing violence, the criminal justice system's responses have had only limited success. Part of the reason is inherent limitations in the overall approach of the criminal justice system. First, it is more reactive than preventive in its basic orientation. True, deterrence may produce some preventive results. True too, the criminal justice system has sought to rehabilitate offenders through special programmes in prisons, and to prevent children from becoming violent offenders through the development of the juvenile justice system, whose most fundamental goal is to prevent future criminal activity by children. Nonetheless, the criminal justice system comes into play only after a crime episode occurs.

Second, the criminal justice system, and particularly the police, is focused primarily on the predatory violence that occurs among strangers on the street. The violence that emerges from nagging frustrations and festering disputes and takes place in intimate settings is far more difficult for the criminal justice system to deal with than stranger-inflicted violence that arises from greed or desperate need, and takes place in the open. Robbery and burglary and their associated violence are more traditional and central to the criminal justice system's business (and consciousness) than aggravated assaults that spring up among friends in bars, lovers in bedrooms, or teenagers at dances.

Public health and criminal justice: Interdisciplinary challenges

Unfortunately, the collaboration of public health and criminal justice in the area of violence prevention has not reached its full potential. This may partially arise from a basic failure in effectively reducing the problem of violence that has put both disciplines on the defensive—criminal justice for its failure to bring the problem under control and meet societal expectations, and public health for the slowness with which it has recognized and taken on the problem. However, much of this tension probably comes from the divergence of perspective of the two disciplines and the fact that there are inadequate resources directed to addressing violence, which has forced the disciplines to compete rather than collaborate.

Public health is primarily focused on identifying causality (or its approximation) and intervening to control or reduce the risk factors; it has little interest in assigning blame or meting out punishment and does not discriminate between victim and offender. The public health community may agree that justice must be done, but is not professionally committed to the process. The criminal justice system, on the other hand, is deeply and morally rooted in 'justice' and criminal offenders being properly identified and punished. In this field, there is less emphasis on the precursors or factors that may have led to the violent event. The criminal justice system is less likely to consider external factors that might have motivated the offender to engage in violence, because it sees these issues as largely irrelevant to judgement of guilt and innocence. At worst, the claim that these other factors were causally important in the particular instance seems like a rationalization or an apology for what was a criminal deed. This rift is further exacerbated by the fact that the criminal justice profession continues to develop preventive agendas, such as first offender programmes and community policing initiatives, and probably feels that their 'thunder' and leadership are in jeopardy of being stolen by the entry of another professional player onto their turf.

This tension is clearly unproductive. It threatens effective collaboration and frustrates the opportunity to pool resources and expertise at a time when resources are seriously inadequate and the problem is increasing. Healing this rift requires a more collaborative spirit from both disciplines. The public health 'purists' must get beyond their science and recognize the invaluable contributions and practical experiences of the criminal justice professionals. The criminal justice 'moralists' must in turn recognize the limitations of a primary agenda of assigning blame and assuring justice is done.

If we are to get past these initial reactions and successfully exploit the complementary qualities of these two approaches to violence, it is essential to put aside professional jealousies. More importantly, we must better define the perspective, roles, and expertise both groups bring to the issue. This will not only lead to a more creative process, but will also establish productive working relationships.

Primary, secondary, and tertiary prevention

A conceptual framework that can alleviate professional tension, facilitate definitions of roles in addressing the problem, and assist in developing a broader perspective on programmatic strategies involves breaking the spectrum of violence into levels that reflect different points of intervention (Fig. 10.5.7). This framework, used frequently in public health circles, structures approaches to problems into three stages: Primary prevention, secondary prevention (or early intervention), and tertiary prevention (or treatment/rehabilitation). More recently, in public health, these levels have been labelled universal (primary), selected (secondary), and targeted (tertiary) (Prothrow-Stith & Weissman 1991; Guterman 2004). However, the most user-friendly label emerged from a group of young people working on the Blueprint for a Safer Philadelphia: Up-Front (primary), In-the-Thick (secondary), and After-the-Fact (tertiary). Labels aside, these three levels have proven to be valuable

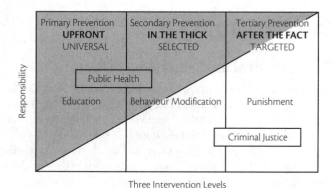

Fig. 10.5.7 Three levels of violence prevention: Public health and criminal justice.

in understanding a spectrum of intervention efforts. Their boundaries are not rigid or discrete; the same prevention activity for an adolescent or young adult 'in-the-thick' might actually be 'up-front' for a younger brother/sister or son/daughter. Tertiary prevention is distinguished from secondary and primary prevention in which it lies on the opposite side of the violent event than the other two. Its focus is on trying to reduce the negative consequences of a particular event after it has occurred, or on trying to find ways to use the event to reduce the likelihood of similar incidents occurring in the future. Thus, one might think of improved trauma care on the one hand, and increased efforts to rehabilitate or incapacitate violent offenders on the other hand, as tertiary prevention instruments in the control of or the response to violence.

Primary prevention, which by definition addresses the broadest level of the general public, might seek to reduce the level of violence that is shown on television or to promote gun control. This would be an effort directed towards dealing with the public values and attitudes that may promote or encourage the use of violence.

Secondary prevention is distinguished from primary prevention in that it identifies relatively narrowly defined subgroups or circumstances that are at high risk for being involved in or occasioning violence, and focuses its attention on them. Thus, secondary prevention efforts might focus on poor urban young men who are at particularly high risk for engaging in or being victimized by violence, and educating them in non-violent methods of resolving disputes or displaying competence and power.

The relative risk level of groups or circumstances is a continuum, with some people and circumstances at very high risk (a person who has been victimized by violence in his or her own home, also surrounded by violence in school, entering a bar in which members of a rival gang are drinking), and others at relatively low-risk (e.g. a happily married professor who owns no weapon more lethal than a screwdriver, writing on her computer at home). Moreover, it is generally true that the higher risk groups are smaller than the lower risk groups.

Primary prevention instruments are those that can affect larger and larger populations, ideally at relatively low cost. Indeed, the need to reach very large populations requires primary prevention efforts to be low cost per individual reached. Thus, primary prevention instruments tend to be those providing information and education on the problem of violence through the popular media; for example, the recruitment of Bill Cosby to the cause of using the media to prevent adolescent violence, or Sarah Brady's efforts to advocate for gun control laws and educate the public about the risks of handguns, rather than providing non-violence training to the entire population. There are, of course, the ultimate long-term primary prevention goals that have to do with eliminating some of the root causes of violence, such as social injustice and discrimination.

This public health model can be very useful when applied specifically to the issue of interpersonal violence. In the past, the criminal justice system has addressed each of the three points of intervention to varying degrees as represented, yet the bulk of the efforts have focused on the response to serious violent behaviour, with moderate attention to early identification and intervention and limited efforts in the area of primary prevention.

The major activities of the criminal justice system have historically involved the roles of the police, the courts, and the prison system in responding to criminal or violent events. Most resources have been directed to investigating and punishing criminal behaviour. Tertiary prevention has generally involved incarceration. In the area of secondary prevention, the police have focused efforts on 'situated' crime prevention, and the juvenile justice system has made attempts at early intervention with youthful offenders, although youth were frequently ignored by the courts and probation system until their criminal behaviour reached a relatively high level of concern. Primary prevention efforts have focused on elementary school drug and violence prevention education by the police, as well as on controlling 'criminogenic' commodities such as drugs, guns, and alcohol.

With the more recent involvement of the public health system, attention has been broadened, with enhanced efforts in the prevention arena. The public health agenda has focused primarily on prevention and early intervention, playing only a small role in the treatment of individuals with serious violence-related problems. The roles and activities of the public health system are newer, less extensive, and therefore less evolved than that of the criminal justice system.

Traditionally, public health responded by treating the violence-related injury in the emergency setting. Today, a new generation of committed health practitioners, community violence-prevention practitioners, social workers, and community activists have devised numerous intervention programmes to serve medium- to high-risk adolescents. At the primary prevention level, efforts have focused on gun control and safety, and enhanced public awareness of risk factors and the true characteristics of most violence to dispel myths and modify societal values around the use of violence. Additionally, some educational interventions (e.g. violence prevention curricula) have been applied to broader, less high-risk settings. Again, much of this work is relatively recent, and therefore has not yet established a long track record to fully assess its effects. Finally, public health has applied its analytical expertise to greatly enhance the understanding of risk factors, allowing for a broader vision in the planning and development of preventive approaches (Prothrow-Stith & Spivak 2004).

Recently published information regarding the effectiveness of school-based primary prevention (universal) programmes was encouraging for practitioners (Hahn et al. 2007; Prothrow-Stith 2007). Robert Hahn and colleagues, in a meta-analysis, demonstrated an average of 15 per cent reduction in fighting in those schools employing a universal programme, regardless of the grade level of the school, the socioeconomic status of students, or other related factors. One can conclude from these data that every US school should have an 'up-front' violence prevention programme for all students.

In the area of secondary prevention, public health has been involved in the development of educational interventions specifically focused on behaviour modification of high-risk individuals, particularly children and youth. A number of curricula are currently in use addressing both the risks of violence in solving problems and conflict resolution techniques (Prothrow-Stith & Spivak 2004).

It is important to note that the criminal justice system has more recently increased its involvement with primary and secondary prevention efforts. For example, some criminal justice professionals have become increasingly involved in gun control initiatives. In 1974, the Juvenile Justice and Delinquency Prevention Act was passed and it gave a primary responsibility to the Justice Department for delinquency prevention programmes. The Office of Juvenile Justice and Delinquency Prevention was designed in part to encourage the development of model delinquency prevention programmes. One such programme is the Boys Clubs of America Targeting Programs for Delinquency Intervention. Other community groups refer at-risk boys to the programme, who are then recruited. Early evaluations of these programmes seem promising. Data indicate that 39 per cent of the boys did better in school and 93 per cent of those who completed the programme have not been re-involved with the juvenile system (Boys Clubs of America 1986). These types of interventions reflect an important interface between the criminal justice and public health professions. With further attention and the dedication of resources of the public health system to this issue and the broadening vision of criminal justice, a more reasonable balance between prevention and treatment can be achieved in the future. Efforts can be broadened to reflect more fully the range of efforts needed to reduce both the extent of violent behaviour and respond to the violence that does occur. The emphasis of the public health system will be on prevention, with the criminal justice system prioritizing the response to violence, but with both disciplines working together across the spectrum.

Cigarette smoking reduction: A model for intervention

To illustrate the advantages of this approach, it is useful to the review how it has worked successfully in other areas. One example, which on the surface appears to be a considerable stretch from violence, is the multidisciplinary approach that has been developed to deal with tobacco use. It is important to note that while this example illustrates a collaboration between public health and the medical care system, it represents a useful analogy to the possible collaboration between public health and criminal justice.

Smoking is a major contributing factor to death and disability in the United States. Significant inroads have been made in turning the tide on this major health threat. What was once a valued, sexy, and socially acceptable behaviour is now viewed as a disgusting, unhealthy, and socially unacceptable behaviour. Heroes in the media used to smoke all the time; now they rarely do. Nationally, the number of people who smoke has declined dramatically, although smoking was and still is a learned behaviour; one that can be unpleasant or distasteful when starting, but is extremely difficult to stop.

The strategy to deal with smoking involved a three-pronged approach: Primary prevention for those not yet smoking to teach the reasons for not starting and to support the decision not to start; secondary prevention to encourage stopping or reducing use for those who had already started smoking (often this involves helping individuals to identify alternative behaviours to replace the smoking behaviour); and treatment in the form of surgery or chemotherapy and other medical interventions for those smokers who have developed cancer or other health consequences of their behaviour. Broad public initiatives to alter the societal values that encouraged smoking were also established to support the above efforts. This has been done through legislation (package labelling, advertising constraints, restrictions on sales to minors, establishment of smoke-free environments), public education, and pressure on media to change images and role models. Although, as stated earlier, this is an example of a public health/medical care interface, it represents an important success that has value in looking at the possibilities of a public health and criminal justice collaboration in addressing violence.

A similar approach could and should be taken with respect to violence. Primary prevention strategies and more targeted secondary prevention efforts need to be applied that proactively value and teach non-violent behaviours in response to anger and conflict. This is particularly important when the growing evidence that violence is a learned behaviour is given (Bandura *et al.* 1963; Liebert *et al.* 1973; Slaby & Quarfoth 1980; Allen 1981; Eron & Huesmann 1984; Straus 1991; Vissing *et al.* 1991; Prothrow-Stith & Spivak 2004; Prothrow-Stith & Spivak 2005). Well-child health visits in neighbourhood health centres provide an ideal window of opportunity for early intervention. Peter Stringham, a paediatrician at the East Boston Neighborhood Health Center, incorporates a violence prevention protocol for families, from newborn visits through the teenage years. Social skills are as important to teach our children as the academic subjects which we now emphasize in our society. This will in no way eliminate the underlying societal stresses that influence violent behaviour, but can affect and direct responses to these stresses toward a pro-social and productive outcome. Curricula that place emphasis on decision-making, non-violent conflict resolution, and self-esteem development currently exist, but are terribly under-utilized and viewed as an 'add on' in academic settings rather than a basic component. A move to place more emphasis on the use of such curricula, with enhanced investment in social and support services for families and youth, will be an important step in countering the learned use of violence by our youth. Such a move would also require that the education, human services, and public health institutions play major roles in effecting these changes in our communities.

Indeed, the recognition that education designed to teach non-violent behaviours might be an important part of a combined public health/criminal justice response to the problem of violence helps to remind us that the modern view of how the law operates on behaviour in the society has become far more narrow that it once was. In our modern conceptions of the law, we imagine it operating on individual behaviour primarily through its incentive effects—the promise of punishment for misconduct made concrete and credible through individual prosecutions.

In the classic writings on laws, however, a great deal of attention was devoted not only to the passage of laws and to their application to individual cases, but also to their promulgation throughout society (Friedman 1975). Extensive efforts to explain and educate citizens as to why the laws were necessary helped to ensure both their justice and their efficacy. Unless citizens knew about the law—its

spirit as well as its letter—they could not reasonably be held accountable for failures to obey it. If the purpose of the law is not made clear, voluntary compliance—which is crucial to the law's effect—could not be counted upon.

The public health community's interest in non-violence education can be viewed as the modern rediscovery of the importance of explaining to and educating the public about violence, as well as simply having laws and applying them. It also incorporates an important modern discovery about the promulgation of obligations; it is often far easier to persuade people to comply with an important obligation when one can show individuals that it is in their best interests to do so, and when one can help them comply with the law. Persuasion and assistance are often more effective tools than accusation and blame. Still, it often helps in persuading and assisting if there is a broad social rule against violence that becomes part of the context for the education. Thus, behavioural change may depend on a combination of education and laws that were previously known as promulgation.

Gun control legislation efforts represent an important example of the interconnection between education and laws. Although there is growing support for increased handgun ownership restrictions as a primary prevention strategy, legislation alone is unlikely to create great change in violent injury rates in the foreseeable future. With over 60 million handguns in circulation in the United States (Bureau of Alcohol, Tobacco & Firearms 1991), understanding and acceptance of the risks of handgun ownership and carrying is as important as legislative restrictions to reduce intentional handgun injuries.

Secondary level strategies require a more targeted effort. They require early identification of individuals at high risk for or already beginning to exhibit violent behaviour and the development of treatment services for these individuals. This area represents an important interface between the human services and the criminal justice systems, because early identification of individuals at high risk for violence requires considerable collaboration. Points of early identification occur in schools, health facilities, police departments, courts, and a variety of other community institutions. Professional training in early identification and appropriate evaluation and treatment is necessary. This is not an easy process. Professional definitions and institutional boundaries have been established that encourage limited one-dimensional approaches.

Treatment interventions (tertiary prevention) for the most seriously affected individuals represent a key focal point for the criminal justice system. Violent behaviour cannot be condoned; punishment is an appropriate response to violent crimes or episodes, and some individuals with serious pathology are not able to live in the general society. While it is essential that we understand how violent behaviour evolves, we must deal with it firmly to maintain safety within communities.

Although tertiary prevention falls most extensively into the criminal justice realm, with incarceration as the major strategy, public health needs to work along with the prison system in the area of rehabilitation. Without increased attention to rehabilitative efforts, including supportive services for those returning from prison to the community, most of them will continue to leave the prison system without the skills to avoid violence in the future. Public health must advocate for and support drug and alcohol treatment services, job training efforts, conflict resolution and violence prevention skills, as well as the development of more extensive behavioural change interventions. To date, successful rehabilitative efforts are limited, further reinforcing the need for more attention focused on this area as well.

Promising prevention programmes using public health strategies

Researchers Joy G. Dryfoos and Lisbeth Schorr both agree that the most effective programmes must be comprehensive, family- and community-oriented, and collaborative in nature. Some schools, communities, social agencies, and politicians around the country have incorporated this formula for success and have developed strategies to help children and their families prevent or cope with violence. These programmes offer the opportunity to learn from their successes and failures.

Peace zone: An elementary school programme for emotional intelligence

Peace Zone is an elementary school-based programme (ages 4–11 years) that is designed to increase students' ability to make positive decisions, avoid risk-taking behaviour, and heal from trauma and loss. A secondary goal of the PZ programme is to assure that the adults are able to reinforce the core concepts with children, both at home and in school. 'Two Approaches to Violence Prevention' are integrated into Peace Zone. The programme combines classroom activities that build social skills with those that promote healing from trauma, grief, and loss. Psychomotor expressive activities (visual arts, music, dance, etc.) and community service shape the key healing activities. The programme includes a School Climate Change Module and six classroom-based units:

◆ The Louis D. Brown Story

◆ Pledge for Peace

◆ Trying Your Best

◆ Self-Control

◆ Thinking and Problem Solving

◆ Cooperation

Each unit contains four 30-min lessons and takes approximately 1 week to complete. The last lesson of each unit links the topic to a community service activity. The entire programme can be presented in 6 weeks; however, it should be continued and reinforced throughout the school year with supplemental booster activities. Full implementation of the programme includes lead teachers at each grade level, a half-time school counsellor to support both classroom- and school-wide activities, and a commitment to consistent utilization of the common Peace Zone language throughout the school.

A strong theoretical foundation supports the Peace Zone programme, which was created by an experienced, diverse, academic-practitioner partnership (comprised of Harvard Youth Violence Prevention Center, the Lesson One Company, the Louis D. Brown Peace Institute, and the Boston Public Schools). The programme is based upon social cognitive theory and the research of Howard Gardner (*Frames of Mind*), who advances the concept of developing 'emotional intelligence' to enhance a child's ability for personal adjustment and resiliency throughout life.

Positive evaluation data and a substantial developmental process underlie the efforts to adapt and disseminate Peace Zone. In 1998, the partners received a multi-million dollar competitive grant from the US Department of Education to create Peace Zone. The programme qualified for the maximum full 5 years of funding by demonstrating positive impact data. Pre- and post-surveys were conducted in grades 3–5 in experimental and comparison schools. Paired *t*-tests were conducted to assess changes in outcomes relevant to the programme in three intervention schools. Both boys and girls reported significant reductions in being victimized by other children at school. Boys reported a decrease in perpetration of violence, and there were remarkable reductions in mild to severe depression reported by both boys and girls.

Resolving Conflict Creatively Program— school-based conflict resolution programme in New York, California, and Alaska

The 'Resolving Conflict Creatively Program', a holistic school-based conflict resolution programme, works with the entire school structure to create safe schools. The K-12 curriculum, developed and refined since 1986, requires support from school administration, although it does not mandate that every teacher should be trained. Each of the 32 school districts in New York City that use the curriculum maintains a certain autonomy, leaving decision-making to the school community. After an intense 40-h training on the curriculum, teachers incorporate the methods into their classrooms.

The programme invites and encourages the participation of parents in training. Both teachers and administrators in these schools document fewer fights and a sense of peace. Students become peer mediators and receive special training to negotiate and mediate arguments that break out during school hours.

The programme provides a win–win situation. Not only do students develop leadership skills and a sense of responsibility for peace and respect, but teachers and administrators find practical use for conflict resolution skills in their lives. The programme also offers regular advanced training sessions in such topics as helping students deal with death and grief.

A walk through the hallways of the Satellite Academy High School in the Bronx gives the sense that despite unsafe surroundings, the school offers an oasis of safety, a place of mutual respect—a place where learning takes place. Programme evaluations show that both teachers and students notice a positive change in the schools. A more comprehensive programme evaluation was recently funded through a grant from the Centers for Disease Control and Prevention.

Louis D. Brown Peace Institute (LDBPI) and survivors of violence for prevention

The Louis D. Brown Peace Institute was founded in 1994 to continue the peacemaking legacy of a 15-year-old youth leader named Louis D. Brown. The following seven principles are the core of this work: Love, unity, faith, hope, courage, justice, and forgiveness. The LDBPI is a unique organization in the City of Boston and in the nation. Founded to assist and support the families of homicide victims, the LDBPI rapidly grew into a model agency offering shelter and services to families in the most difficult times of their lives and a model for nonviolence to the city that Louis D. Brown called home.

The LDBPI has now developed a fully integrated curriculum for all elementary, middle- and high-school students that prepares them to deal with trauma and grief, build nonviolence and conflict resolution skills, and commit themselves to peace work in their families and their communities. These skills are also taught in workshops for community-based groups throughout the Commonwealth.

Policy advocacy is an ongoing effort of the Peace Institute. The LDBPI has successfully advocated for a state-wide calendar of events related to violence prevention, and worked with the state legislators to establish a Survivors of Homicide Victims Awareness Month, from November 20 to December 20 every year. The LDBPI staff and volunteers have also testified against the death penalty. The LDBPI is committed to restorative justice and building sustainable peace in our home communities. To perform this, the LDBPI works hand-in-hand with young men who have been defined as 'the problem' to build peace block by block in the communities of Dorchester. Following the lead of these young men, mothers who have lost their sons to murder or to prison have reached out to each other to form the Massachusetts Mothers on the Move (Memo's).

The LDBPI works to create and promote an environment where families can live in peace and unity. It is committed to restorative justice practices and struggles together with the members of our communities to create and promote an environment, where young people and their families are valued for their peacemaking efforts. The goals are to develop programmes and activities that teach and instil the values of peace and enrich the lives of young people; to assist/empower survivors of homicide victims with tools that not only rebuild their lives but also their communities through education, collaboration, and policy advocacy; and to inform and educate the public about the causes and the consequences of violence on the individual, the family and the community, while transforming the community.

School-based management—Comer method schools

More than 300 schools from around the country have adopted an educational model designed by Yale University's James P. Comer. Comer, a psychiatrist, began his school-based work in one of New Haven's most troubled schools in 1968. He designed a multidisciplinary approach to school management. The programme stresses that a partnership between educators and parents is critical to a school's success. Its philosophy is based on the premise that each child is special and that schools should be places of learning.

Comer's model is also based on the premise that the initial relationship between schools and disadvantaged parents is too often wrought with mistrust and alienation. Comer schools require parental representation on all levels, including the school's management team. These parents also work to increase the involvement of other parents in the school's mission to educate all children.

Blueprint for a safer Philadelphia

In 2006, State Representative Dwight Evans of Philadelphia, Pennsylvania, in the United States, culminated several years of community organizing and partnership building activities by kicking off a 10-year initiative to end youth violence in Philadelphia, The Blueprint for a Safer Philadelphia. The Blueprint's mission is to use proven, research-based public health methods to develop and implement a long-term strategy to help reduce gun violence and end youth homicides in Philadelphia by the year 2016. The multi-tiered Blueprint for a Safer Philadelphia Initiative includes influencing attitudes and changing community norms surrounding youth violence, and uses social, cultural, and educational programmes as a way to prevent violence before it begins.

The *Blueprint* Campaign has more than 400 community partners citywide that have pledged their support. Community partners, including community-based organizations, schools, churches, recreation centres, clinics, etc., receive information and updates about various Blueprint events, meetings, and activities.

Created to stop rising gun and youth violence, the Blueprint for a Safer Philadelphia Initiative is a unique and innovative approach that augments the traditional criminal justice response with a public health prevention model.

The public health initiative is disseminating pro-social messages to both youth and adults through a variety of traditional and non-traditional communications channels. All elements of the violence prevention campaign are culturally relevant, street-credible, and audience-tested.

Over the next decade, the Blueprint Initiative will work to:

◆ Heighten public awareness of alternatives to violence.

◆ Provide youth and their families with access to support and resources, along with options for changing their lives.

◆ Empower local community-based organizations to address the root needs of the area youth.

Harvard Youth Violence Prevention Center (HYVPC)

The Harvard Youth Violence Prevention Center (HYVPC) is a multidisciplinary violence prevention centre dedicated to *working collaboratively to build community capacity for youth violence prevention in Boston*. Located at the Harvard School of Public Health, the Center activities are based on the premise that effective prevention evolves from mutually respectful, reciprocal relationships between community members, researchers, and policy-makers. HYVPC has an outstanding multidisciplinary staff with expertise in survey research, programme evaluation, youth violence prevention, social capital, and interactive collaborations with community agencies and organizations. Other important, inter-related issues addressed by the centre include injury and suicide prevention, collective efficacy and community capacity-building, safety for children and youth, and youth development.

HYVPC collaborates with 11 Grassroots Community Partners in Boston, as well as with the Boston Mayor's Office, Boston Centers for Youth and Families, Boston Public Schools, Boston After School and Beyond, Boston Redevelopment Authority, Boston Police Department, and the Boston Foundation. HYVPC's primary goals are to work collaboratively across multiple levels of community to: (1) define the problem of youth exposure to, victimization by, and perpetration of violence; (2) identify risk and protective factors for youth experiences with violence; (3) develop and test youth violence prevention strategies; and (4) assure widespread adoption of strategies shown to be effective. Central to this effort, HYVPC is creating a multi-layered data gathering and analysis system for youth violence in Boston that includes: (1) a comprehensive representative biennial survey of public and private high-school and middle-school students; (2) a concurrent biennial community-based telephone survey of adults in Boston households conducted in parallel with the youth survey; (3) GIS integration and mapping of city, state, and federal data on neighbourhood characteristics, city trends, and initiatives that affect youth and communities; and (4) an Emergency Department Surveillance System on violence-related injuries to youth serious enough to result in hospital visits. These data will be used to determine individual and community risk and resiliency factors, track the changing needs of Boston's youth and communities, supporting HYPV's Community Partners, develop evidence-based prevention programmes and track their effectiveness, and evaluate the impact of city and community policies on youth violence and well-being.

The Youth Violence Prevention Center also works with Boston's Office of Community Partnerships on the Annual Youth Development Symposium, and conducts a biannual Boston Peace Party to honour community members who have made significant contributions in violence reduction. Finally, the Center recognizes that research and programmatic support must be supplemented by training. The Center provides Community Partner agencies and community members with training in programme evaluation and works with Center Partners to create local- and city-wide community action plans to reduce violence. The Center also provides formal training to graduate students, residents, and other physicians, community leaders, and injury control personnel in State Health Departments. Through its emphasis on research, practice, and collaboration, the HYVPC is continuing the Boston tradition of developing, implementing, and evaluating cutting-edge violence prevention strategies.

A programme for students who exhibit emotional disturbances—Montgomery County, MD, public schools

A 20-member committee that included principals, teachers, and support services representatives in Montgomery County, Maryland, in the United States, developed an interagency plan to serve students who exhibit violent behaviour. The cooperating agencies include public schools, departments of social services, the juvenile justice system, police, family resource services, recreation departments, drug, alcohol and mental health services, the state's attorney office, and the Office of Management and Budget.

The school district, mandated to serve students under the age of 16, has traditionally placed violent students in home instruction and provided 6 h of instruction per week. The new plan includes creating centres that have school days longer than 8 h and a half-day Saturday session. The longer school days, coupled with the mandated Saturday sessions, are meant to encourage students to return to public school.

The programme employs a case management approach. First, an assessment team evaluates the student to determine individual and family needs. The intense interagency programme is then implemented according to each student's identified needs. The school instructional day includes science and mathematics, life-skills-building, physical education, group counselling, and English and social studies. The day also includes meetings with students, teachers, case managers, and counsellors. By coordinating existing resources and redirecting existing funds, the programme requires only a moderate budget increase.

'Overcoming Obstacles'

The Los Angeles-based 'Overcoming Obstacles' is an education, jobs, and entrepreneurship programme that teaches young people the skills needed to: (1) succeed in education; (2) find jobs; (3) develop entrepreneurial skills; and (4) involve themselves in the community. It is an example of business partnering with a community programme to give students a chance to succeed.

This three-phased programme includes course work to:

- Improve self-esteem
- Develop a sense of personal responsibility
- Instil a sense of pride in community
- Set realistic goals
- Develop communications and conflict resolution skills
- Gain employment-seeking and retention skills

An evaluation demonstrated positive behaviour change in successful students during the school year and after graduation.

After the first educational phase, high-school students move to a job placement phase. Through a network, part-time and summer employment is secured for students, while full-time employment is offered for programme graduates. One example is a special programme with ARCO Product Company/Prestige Stations, Inc. Students working for this company receive a salary subject to increases and bonuses based on performance and have the opportunity to attend college paid for by ARCO.

Phase three encourages students to learn to become managers and owners of a business. Presently, funding has been provided for several businesses designed and managed by graduates of Overcoming Obstacles.

Survivors for Violence Prevention, Inc. (SVP)

The Harvard School of Public Health (HSPH) convened the first SVP Inc. forum, with a gathering of approximately 150 parents and family members who had loved ones killed or injured as a result of violence. Participants recognized the need for the creation of a survivor-led initiative. The organizational goals became increasing education and effecting public policy regarding survivorship. SVP Inc. was created to provide extensive information dissemination, communication, training, and technical assistance around survivorship issues. Advisory board members were identified and came together the following year. Advisory board members included practitioners who typically provide services to survivors and victims at both individuals- and community-based organizations, located in the cities of Boston, Atlanta, Rochester, Detroit, Columbus, Minneapolis, San Diego, Seattle, and Orange County, CA. From 1998 through 2004, SVP Inc. convened six annual conferences in partnership with the HSPH, violence practitioners and survivors, along with community activists and committed systems change advocates supportive of survivor and victim services.

The mission of SVP Inc. is to provide a powerful, united voice for survivors of victims of a violent crime and homicide. SVP Inc. informs thought and encourages debate regarding national public policy for the purpose of reducing violence in the United States.

Urban Networks to Increase Thriving Youth Through Violence Prevention (UNITY)

Urban Networks to increase Thriving Youth Through Violence Prevention is a CDC-funded cooperative agreement awarded in 2005 to a partnership comprised of the Prevention Institute, Deborah Prothrow-Stith of the Harvard School of Public Health, and Billie Weiss from the University of California at Los Angeles Southern California Injury Prevention Research Center.

The goal of UNITY is to strengthen urban youth violence prevention, build national support for necessary resources and policies, and develop tools and framing to ensure long-term sustainability of youth violence prevention efforts. To accomplish this, UNITY aims to engage youth and representatives of the 45 largest cities, along with national violence prevention advocates and leaders, in a National Consortium to shape the US strategy for urban youth violence prevention. UNITY will provide tools, training, and technical assistance to help cities to be more effective in preventing youth violence.

Development of this programme is supported by the Centers for Disease Control and Prevention (CDC). Its contents are solely the responsibility of the authors and do not necessarily represent the official views of the US Department of Health and Human Services or the Centers for Disease Control and Prevention (CDC).

Co-coordinating coalitions

The Contra Costa County California Health Department is widely known for its efforts to develop comprehensive programmes harnessing existing resources to alleviate poor health outcomes. Rather than designing and implementing their own stand-alone projects, Contra Costa County Program, CCCP, coordinates and develops existing programmes to meet identified community needs. It serves as a lead agency for a number of health-related issues, including violence prevention. Some CCCP premises are that coalitions:

◆ Offer more resources for less money

◆ Can reach more people than a single organization

◆ Provide greater credibility than single organizations

◆ Offer more political clout

◆ Serve a community networking function

◆ Offer more diverse opinions and talents

The CCCP defines eight steps to building effective coalitions. An initial planning group should: (1) analyse programme objectives and decide if a coalition is needed; (2) recruit relevant and effective organizations/community representatives; (3) develop preliminary objectives and activities; and (4) convene the group. By using the input from the planning group, the coalitions should: (5) develop a budget and structure; (6) maintain coalition vitality (communications, public relations); (7) evaluate programmes; and (8) based on evaluation offer recommendations to improve programmes.

A guide further defining the eight-step process is available from the Contra Costa County Health Department.

A school-based planning model: Pittsburgh safe schools project

The Safe Schools Project of the Pittsburgh Public Schools is a model for multidisciplinary violence prevention coalition. Members of the Pittsburgh Public Schools, the Jewish Healthier Foundation, the Western Psychiatric Institute and Clinic, the Center for Injury Research and Control at the University of Pittsburgh, and the Boys and Girls Club of Western Pennsylvania formed a working group that produced a Blueprint for Violence Reduction in Pittsburgh Public Schools. It is an action plan based on sound theoretical framework, data collection and analysis, a commitment to understand the causes of violence and an analysis of state-of-the-art school violence prevention programmes.

The blueprint contains a review of the project's components and discusses each step in a thorough manner which lends itself to replication in other school districts. The blueprint also includes a set of valuable guiding principles for school-based programme implementation:

◆ Violence prevention must be a long-term priority for the school district.

◆ Adequate resources should be focused on very young children, particularly those at risk for developing aggressive lifestyles.

◆ Developmentally appropriate programmes should be integrated in a comprehensive approach for all grade levels.

◆ Students, teachers, and parents should participate in planning and assessing violence prevention activities.

◆ Activities should be culturally and racially appropriate.

◆ Prevention efforts should include home, school and community coordination.

◆ Programme evaluation measures should be integrated into the programme design.

◆ New programmes should be built upon successful existing programmes.

Conclusions

The contributions made by public health professionals towards efforts to prevent violence have been tremendous. The continued application of public health strategies to the understanding and prevention of violence assures success. The public health campaign to reduce smoking took 30 years after the first Surgeon Generals' report to reduce smoking. Violence reduction can be expected to take at least as long and require as many, if not more diverse strategies.

References

Allen, N.H., (1981). Homicide prevention and intervention. *Suicide and Life Threatening Behavior*, **11**, 167.

American Academy of Pediatrics (2007). Suicide and suicide attempts in adolescents. *Pediatrics*, **120**, 669–76.

American Psychological Association Commission on Violence and Youth (1993). *Violence and Youth: Psychology's Response*.

Austin, E.W., Roberts D.F., and Nass, C.I. (1990). Influences of family communication on children's television-interpretation processes. *Communication Research*, **4**, 545–65.

Bandura, A., Ross, D., and Ross, S.A. (1963a). Imitation of film-mediated aggressive models. *Journal of Abnormal Social Psychology*, 3–11.

Bandura, A., Ross, D., and Ross, S.A. (1963b). Vicarious reinforcement and imitative learning. *Journal of Abnormal Psychology*, **63**, 601–7.

Blueprint for a Safer Philadelphia. Campaign information on website: http://www.phillyblueprint.com/ Last checked December 2007.

Boys Clubs of America (1988). *Targeted Outreach Newsletter*, Vol. II-1.

Brady Campaign to Prevent Gun Violence. Firearms Facts on the website: http://www.bradycampaign.org/facts/factsheets/pdf/firearm_facts.pdf Last checked December 2007.

Bureau of Alcohol, Tobacco and Firearms (1991). *Firearm Census Report*. U.S. Treasury Department, Washington, DC.

Bureau of Justice Statistics (1992). *Criminal victimization in the United States, 1991*. U.S. Department of Justice, Washington, DC.

Bureau of Justice Statistics (1993). *Highlights from 20 Years of surveying crime victims: The national crime victimization survey, 1972–1992*. U.S. Department of Justice, Washington, DC.

Bureau of Justice Statistics (1994). *Violence between inmates*. NCJ-149259. Office of Justice Programs, U.S. Department of Justice, Washington, DC.

CDC (Centers for Disease Control) (1982a). Homicide. *Morbidity and Mortality Weekly Report*, November 12, **31**, 594.

CDC (Centers for Disease Control) (1982b). Homicide – United States. *Morbidity and Mortality Weekly Report*, **31**, 599–602.

CDC (Centers for Disease Control) (1983a). Violent deaths among persons 15–24 years of age – United States, 1970–1978. *Morbidity and Mortality Weekly Report*, September 9, **32**, 453.

CDC (Centers for Disease Control) (1983b). *Homicide surveillance, high risk racial and ethnic groups – Blacks and Hispanics, 1970–1983*. U.S. Department of Health and Human Services, Public Health Service, Washington, DC.

CDC (Centers for Disease Control) (1990). Homicide among black males – United States, 1978–1987. *Morbidity and Mortality Weekly Report*, **39**, 869–72.

CDC (Centers for Disease Control) (1992). *Youth suicide prevention program: A resource guide*. Department of Health and Human Services, Public Health Service, Centers for Disease Control, National Center for Injury Prevention and Control, Atlanta.

CDC (Centers for Disease Control) (1993). *Advance report of final mortality statistics, 1991, Monthly vital statistics report*. August, Atlanta.

CDC. (1997). Rates of homicide, suicide, and firearm related deaths among children–26 industrialized countries. *Morbidity & Mortality Weekly Report*, **46**, 101–5.

CDC, National Center for Injury Prevention and Control, Office of Statistics and Programming. Web-based Injury Statistics Query and Reporting System (WISQARS). Online at http://www.cdc.gov/ncipc/wisqars/ Accessed September 2007a.

CDC. *Facts at a glance: Youth violence*. Summer 2007. Online at http://www.cdc.gov/ncipc/dvp/YV_DataSheet.pdf Accessed December 2007b.

Centers for Disease Control and Prevention (1991). Weapon carrying among high school students – United States, 1990. *Morbidity and Mortality Weekly Report*, **40**, 681–4.

Centers for Disease Control and Prevention (1993). Violence-related attitudes and behaviors of high school students – New York City, 1991. *Morbidity and Mortality Weekly Report*, **40**, 773–7.

Centers for Disease Control and Prevention (1994). Deaths resulting from firearm- and motor-vehicle-related injuries – United States, 1968–1991. *Morbidity and Mortality Weekly Report*, **3**, 37–42.

Centers for Disease Control and Prevention (CDC) (2006). Youth risk behavior surveillance—United States, 2005. *Morbidity & Mortality Weekly Report*, **55** (SS-05), 1–108.

Centerwall, B.S. (1984). Race, socio-economic status, and domestic homicide, Atlanta, 1971–1972. *American Journal of Public Health*, **8**, 813–15.

Centerwall, B.S. (1992). Television and violence: The scale of the problem and where to go from here. *Journal of the American Medical Association*, 3059–63.

Centerwall, B.S. (1993). Race, socio-economic status, and domestic homicide in New Orleans. The Second World Conference on Injury Control.

Cook, P.J., and Ludwig, J. (2000). *Gun violence: The real costs*. Oxford University Press, New York.

Corso, P.S., Mercy, J.A., Simon, T.R., Finkelstein, E.A., and Miller, T.R. (2007). Medical costs and productivity losses due to interpersonal violence and self-directed violence. *American Journal of Preventive Medicine*, **32**(6), 474–82.

Daro, D., and Mitchel, L. (1987). *Deaths due to maltreatment soar: The results of the 1986 annual fifty state survey*. National Center on Child Abuse Prevention Research, National Committee for Prevention of Child Abuse, Chicago.

Dietz, W.H., and Strasburger, V.C. (1991). Children, adolescents and television. *Current Problems in Pediatrics*, **1**, 8–31.

Durant, R. Pendergast, R., and Cadenhead, C. (1994). Exposure to violence victimization and fighting behavior by urban black adolescents. *Journal of Adolescent Health*, **4**, 311–8.

Egeland, B., and Jacobvitz, D. (1984). *Intergenerational continuity of parental abuse: Cases and consequences*, presented at the conference on the Bio Social Perspectives on Abuse and Neglect, New York.

Emde, R.N. (1983). The horror! The horror! Reflection on our culture of violence and its implication for early development and morality. *Psychiatry*, **1**, 119–23.

Eron, L., and Huesman, L.R. (1984). Television violence and aggressive behavior. In *Advances in clinical child psychology* (eds. B. Lahey and A. Kardin). Plenum Press, New York.

FBI (Federal Bureau of Investigation) (2006). *Uniform crime report: Crime in the United States*. U.S. Department of Justice, Washington, DC. Online at http://www.fbi.gov/ucr/cius2006/offenses/expanded_information/homicide.html.

Fingerhut, L.A., and Kleinman, J.C. (1990). International and interstate comparisons of homicide among young males. *Journal of the American Medical Association*, **24**, 3292–4.

Fingerhut, L.A., Ingram, D.D., and Feldman, J.J. (1992). Firearm and non-firearm homicide among persons 15 through 19 years of age. *Journal of the American Medical Association*, **22**, 3048–53.

Fitzpatrick, K.M., and Boldizar, J.P. (1993). The prevalence and consequences of exposure to violence among African-American youth. *Journal of the American Academy of Child and Adolescent Psychiatry*, **2**, 424–30.

Freeman, L., Mokros, H., and Poznanski, E. (1993). Violent events reported by normal urban school-aged children: Characteristics and depression correlates. *Journal of the American Academy of Child and Adolescent Psychiatry*, **2**, 419–23.

Friedman, L.M. (1975). *The legal system: A social science perspective*, pp. 56–66. Russell Sage Foundation, New York City.

Gil, D. (1973). *Violence against children: Physical child abuse in the United States*. Harvard University Press, Cambridge.

Groves, B.M. *et al.* (1993). Silent victims: Children who witness violence. *Journal of the American Medical Association*, **2**, 262–4.

Guterman, N.B. (2004). Advancing prevention research on child abuse, youth violence and domestic violence: Emerging strategies and issues. *Journal of Interpersonal Violence*, **19**(3), 299–321.

Hemenway, D. (2005). Private guns, public health. Insert Publisher.

Huesmann, L.R. *et al.* (1983). Mitigating the imitation of aggressive behaviors by changing children's attitudes about media violence. *Journal of Personality and Social Psychology*, 899–910.

Huesmann, L.R. *et al.* (1984). Stability of aggression over time and generations. *Developmental Psychology*, 1120–34.

Kellerman, A.L. *et al.* (1993). Gun ownership as a risk factor for homicide in the home. *New England Journal of Medicine*, **15**, 1084–91.

Kellermann, A.L. *et al.* (1998). Injuries and deaths due to firearms in the home. *The Journal of Trauma*, **45**, 263–7.

Killias, M. (1993). International correlations between gun ownership and rates of homicide and suicide. *Canadian Medical Association*, **10**, 1721–5.

Kilpatrick, D.G., Edmunds, C.N., and Seymour, A.K. (1992). *Rape in America: A report to the Nation*. National Victim Center, Arlington.

Krug, E.G. *et al.*, eds. (2002). *World report on violence and health*. World Health Organization, Geneva.

Wintemute, G.J., and Wright, M.A. (1992). Initial and subsequent hospital costs of firearm injuries. *The Journal of Trauma*, **34**, 556–60.

Lester, D. (1988). Firearm availability and the incidence of suicide and homicide. *Acta Psychiatrica*, 387–93.

Liebert, R.M. (1988). *Early window: The effects of television on children and youth*, 6th edition. Allyn and Bacon, Needham.

Liebert, R., Neale, J., and Davidson, E. (1973). *Early window: The effects of television on children and youth*. Pergamon Press, New York.

Loftin, C. *et al.* (1991). Effects of restrictive licensing of handguns on homicide and suicide in the District of Columbia. *The New England Journal of Medicine*, **23**, 1615–20, 1647–9.

Lorion, R.P., and Saltzman, W. (1993). Children's exposure to community violence: Following a path from concern to research to action. *Psychiatry*, **1**, 55–65.

Makepeace, J.M. (1981). Courtship violence among college students. *Family Relations*, **30**, 97–102.

Martinez, P., and Richters, J. (1993). The NIMH community violence project: II. Children's distress symptoms associated with violence exposure. *Psychiatry*, February, 22–35.

Miller, T.R., Cohen, M.A., and Rossman, S.B. (1993). Datawatch: Victim cost of violent crime resulting injuries. *Health Affairs*, Winter, 187–97.

Miller *et al.* (1996). *Victim costs and consequences: A new look*. National Institute of Justice, U.S. Department of Justice, Washington, DC. Online at http://www.ncjrs.org/pdffiles/victcost.pdf.

Miller, M., Azrael, D., Hepburn, L., Hemenway, D., and Lippmann, S.J. (2006). The association between changes in household firearm ownership and rates of suicide in the United States, 1981–2002. *Injury Prevention*, **12**, 178–82.

Osofsky, J. *et al.* (1993). Chronic community violence: What is happening to our children? *Psychiatry*, February, 36–45.

Prothrow-Stith, D. (1985). *Prevention of interpersonal violence and homicide in black youth*. Report of the Surgeon General's Workshop on Violence and Public Health, Leesburg, October 27–29. *Public Health Reports* No. HRS-D-MC 86-1, 35–43. U.S. Government Printing Office, Washington, DC.

Prothrow-Stith, D., and Weissman, M. (1991). *Deadly consequences: How violence is destroying our teenage population and a plan to begin solving the problem*, pp 1–203. Harper Collins Publishers, New York.

Pynoos, R.S. *et al.* (1987). *Life threat and post traumatic stress in school-age children*. *Archives of General Psychiatry*, December, 1057–63.

Rice, M. (1993). Shooting in the dark: Estimating the cost of firearm injuries. *Health Affairs*, **12**, 171–85.

Sang, F., Schmitz, B., and Tasche, K. (1993). Developmental trends in television coviewing of parent-child dyads. *Journal of Youth and Adolescence*, **5**, 531–43.

Satcher, D. (1985). *The Public Health Approach to Violence*. National Education Association National Conference, Los Angeles, California, April 8.

Sege, R., and Dietz, W. (1994). Television viewing and violence in children: The pediatrician as agent for change. *Pediatrics*.

Sege, R., and Hoffman, J. (2005). Training health professionals in youth violence prevention. *American Journal of Preventive Medicine (supplement)*, **29**(5S2), 175–81.

Shaffer, D., Garland, A., Gould, M., Fisher, P., and Trautman, P. (1988). Preventing teenage suicide: A critical review. *Journal of the American Academy of Child and Adolescent Psychiatry*, **27**, 673–87.

Shaffer, D., Garland, M., and Hicks, R. (1994). Worsening suicide rate in black teenagers, Brief Reports. *American Journal of Psychiatry*, **151**, 12.

Sheley, J., McGee, Z., and Wright, J. (1992). Gun-related violence in and around inner-city schools. *Journal of Diseases of Childhood*, June 677–82.

Slaby, R.G., and Guerra, N.G. (1988). Cognitive mediators of aggression in adolescent offenders: 1. Assessment. *Developmental Psychology*, **4**, 580–8.

Slaby, R., and Quarfoth, G. (1980). Effects of television on the developing child. *Advanced Behavioral Pediatrics*, **1**, 225–66.

Sloan, J.H. *et al.* (1988). *Handgun regulations, crime, assaults, and homicide: A tale of two cities*. *New England Journal of Medicine*, **19**, 1256–62.

Spivak, H., Prothrow-Stith, D., and Hausman, A. (1988). Dying is no accident: Adolescents, violence, and intentional injury. *Pediatric Clinics of North America*, **35**, 1339–47.

Straus, M. (1991). Discipline and deviance: Physical punishment of children and violence and other crime in adulthood. *Social Problems*, **38**, 137–54.

Straus, M., and Gelles, R. (1990). How violent are American families? Estimates from the National Family Violence Resurvey and other studies. In *Physical violence in American families: Risk factors and adaptations to violence in American families: Risk factors and adaptations to violence in 8,145 families* (eds. M. Straus and R. Gelles). Transaction, New Brunswick.

Tjaden, P., and Thoennes, N. (2000). Extent, nature, and consequences of intimate partner violence: Findings from the National Violence Against Women Survey. U.S. Department of Justice, Washington DC. Publication number 181867.

Turner, C.W., Hesse, B.W., and Peterson-Lewis, S. (1986). *Naturalistic studies of the long-term effects of television violence*. *Journal of Social Issues*, 51–73.

United States Department of Health, Education, and Welfare (1964). *Smoking and health*. Report of the Advisory Committee to the Surgeon General, Public Health Service, Washington, DC.

Vissing, Y., Straus, M., Gelles, R., and Harrop, J. (1991). Verbal aggression by parents and psychological problems of children. *Child Abuse and Neglect*, **15**, 223–38.

Weaver, B., and Barbour, N. (1992). Mediation of children's televiewing. Families in Society. *The Journal of Contemporary Human Services*, **4**, 236–43.

Widom, C.S. (1989). The cycle of violence. *Science*, April 14, **244**, 160–6.

Williams, B.C., and Kotch, B.J. (1990). Excess injury mortality among children in the United States: Comparison of recent international statistics. *Pediatrics* (Supplement), 1067–73.

Wolfgang, M. (1986). Homicide in other industrialized countries. *Bulletin of the New York Academy of Medicine*, **62**, 400.

Wood, W., Wong, F.Y., and Chachere, J.G. (1991). Effects of media violence on viewer's aggression in unconstrained social interaction. *Psychological Bulletin*, 3371–83.

World Health Organization (2007). Online at http://www.who.int/violence_injury_prevention/en/ Last checked August 18, 2007.

Collective violence: War

Victor W. Sidel and Barry S. Levy

Abstract

Three types of violence—self-directed, interpersonal, and collective—have been defined by the World Health Organization (WHO) in its efforts to urge public health workers to consider violence prevention as an important public health issue. This chapter deals with collective violence, which includes war, terrorism, and their health consequences, and suggests public health approaches to prevention of collective violence and promotion of justice and peace. These approaches include the following: Conducting research on the health and environmental consequences of collective violence; educating public health workers, the public, and decision makers on the impact of collective violence on health and environment; intervening to prevent collective violence or to end it; and advocating for changes in attitudes and policies on the public health aspects of collective violence.

Public health workers have a responsibility to promote four levels of prevention of collective violence as well as to promote peace and justice. Pre-primary prevention consists of alleviating the underlying causes of armed conflict. Primary prevention consists of preventing specific conflicts from turning into collective violence. Secondary prevention is minimizing the health consequences of collective violence and ending the violence. Tertiary prevention is the rehabilitation and reintegration of victims of the violence into society, the remediation of the physical, social, cultural, and economic damage, and the prevention of recurrence of the collective violence.

Collective violence as threat to public health

In 1966, the World Health Assembly declared violence 'a major and growing public health problem across the world' (World Health Assembly 1996). The World Report on Violence and Health, published by WHO in 2002, was the first comprehensive report by WHO on violence as a public health problem (Krug 2002). The WHO report presents a typology of violence that defines three broad categories based on the characteristics of those committing the violent acts: Self-directed violence, interpersonal violence, and collective violence. Other chapters in the textbook cover the first two categories of violence, and this chapter will deal primarily with war, an important component of collective violence.

Collective violence has been characterized as 'the instrumental use of violence by people who identify themselves as members of a group—whether this group is transitory or has a more permanent identity—against another group or set of individuals in order to achieve political, economic, ideological, or social objectives'. Collective violence includes armed conflict (such as war and genocide), state-sponsored violence (such as genocide, repression, disappearances, and torture), and organized violent crime (such as gang warfare and banditry).

The Report gives examples of collective violence: 'Violent conflicts between nations and groups, state and group terrorism, rape as a weapon of war, the movement of large numbers of people displaced from their homes, and gang warfare'. As the Report notes, 'all of these occur on a daily basis in many parts if the world' and 'the effects of these different types of events on health in terms of deaths, physical illness, disabilities, and mental anguish are vast'. Also included in this chapter is limited information on what has been termed *terrorism* and the *war on terror*, as Chapter 10.8 covers *bioterrorism*. This chapter will not cover the topic of *gang warfare*, which is covered in Chapter 10.5 ('Interpersonal violence prevention: A recent public health mandate').

The health impacts of collective violence

Direct consequences of war and military operations

Armed conflicts in the twenty-first century largely consist of the civil wars (conflicts within countries, to which other countries sometimes contribute military troops) that continue to rage in many parts of the world. For example, at the beginning of 2007, it was reported that there were 15 significant armed conflicts (1000 or more reported deaths) and another 21 'hot spots' that could slide into or revert to war (Smith 2007). During the post-Cold War period of 1990–2001, there were 57 major armed conflicts in 45 locations—all but three of which were civil wars (Stockholm International Peace Research Institute 2002).

Some of the impacts of war on public health are obvious, whereas others are not. The direct impact of war on mortality and morbidity is apparent. Many people, including an increasing percentage of civilians, are killed or injured during war. An estimated 191 million people died directly or indirectly as a result of conflict during the twentieth century, more than half of whom were civilians (Rummel 1994). The exact figures are unknowable because of the generally poor record keeping in many countries and its disruption in time of conflict.

War has direct, immediate, and deadly impact on human life and health. The 'body counts' and the data on those with war-caused injuries and disabilities, both physical and psychological, although woefully incomplete, document the many people tragically killed and wounded as a direct result of military activities. Through the early twentieth century up to the start of World War II, the vast preponderance of the direct casualties of war were uniformed combatants, usually members of national armed forces. Although non-combatants suffered social, economic, and environmental consequences of war and may have been the victims of what is now termed *collateral damage* of military operations, 'civilians' were generally not directly targeted and were largely spared direct death and disability resulting from war (Levy & Sidel 2008).

However, since 1937, when Nazi forces bombed the city of Guernica, a non-military target in the Basque region of Spain, military operations have increasingly killed and maimed civilians through purposeful targeting of non-military targets. The use of 'carpet bombing' and the collateral damage of heavy attacks on military targets have caused many civilian casualties. The percentage of civilian deaths as a proportion of all deaths directly caused by war has therefore increased dramatically. Many of these civilian deaths may have been indirectly rather than directly caused by war.

Since September 11, 2001, there has been increasing concern in the United States and other countries about violence conducted by individuals and groups to create fear and advance a political agenda—a form of violence commonly called *terrorism*. We believe that there needs to be a balanced approach to strengthening systems and protecting people in response to the threat of terrorism, an approach that strengthens a broad range of public health capacities and preserves civil liberties (Levy & Sidel 2007). Terrorism is often defined in a partisan fashion: Those called *terrorists* by one side in a conflict may be viewed as 'patriots', 'freedom fighters', or 'servants of God' by the other. We have defined terrorism as, 'politically motivated violence or the threat of violence, especially against civilians, with the intent to instil fear'. This definition includes violent acts conducted by nation-states against civilians with the intent to instil fear as well as acts committed by individuals and subnational groups. The term *terrorism* has considerable overlap with the term *war* and many actions conducted during war fit our definition of terrorism. The initiation of a 'war on terror', in contrast to use of education, law enforcement, economic aid, and other methods to prevent such acts, has led some analysts to include this war on terror as an example of collective violence.

Indirect effects of war and other military activities

Along with the direct impacts of war and other military activities on health, collective violence may also cause serious health consequences through its impact on the physical, economic, social, and biologic environments in which people live. The environmental damage may affect people not only in nations directly engaged in collective violence but also in all nations. Much of the morbidity and mortality during war, especially among civilians, has been the result of devastation of societal infrastructure, including destruction of food and water supply systems, health-care facilities and public health services, sewage disposal systems, power plants and electrical grids, and transportation and communication systems. Destruction of infrastructure has led to food shortages and resultant malnutrition, contamination of food and of drinking water and the resultant foodborne and waterborne illness, and health-care and public health deficiencies and resultant disease (Levy & Sidel 2008).

Preparation for war also can adversely affect human health. Some of the impacts are direct, such as injuries and deaths during training exercises, and others are indirect. As with war itself, preparation for war can divert human, financial, and other resources that otherwise might be used for health and human services.

Damage to the physical environment—water, land, air, and space—and use of non-renewable resources may be the result of preparation for war as well as war itself. Lakes, rivers, streams and aquifers, land masses, and the atmosphere may be polluted through testing and use of weapons. Outer space could be damaged by placement of weapons. Non-renewable resources may be used in weapons production, testing, and use.

The economic environment may also be adversely affected by the diversion of resources from education, housing, nutrition, and other human and health services to military activities and through an increase in national debt and/or taxation. These economic impacts affect both developed and developing countries.

Governmental and societal preoccupation with preparation for wars—often known as *militarism*—may lead to massive diversion and subversion of efforts to promote human welfare. This preoccupation may lead to policies that promote 'pre-emptive war' (when an attack is allegedly imminent) and to 'preventive war' (when an attack may be feared sometime in the future). Diversion of resources to war is a problem worldwide, but is especially important in developing countries. Many developing countries spend substantially more on military expenditures than on health-related expenditures; for example, in 1990, Ethiopia spent US$16 per capita for military expenditures and only US$1 per capita for health, and Sudan spent US$25 per capita for military expenditures and only $1 per capita for health.

The social environment may be affected by increasing militarism, by encouragement of violence as a means for settling disputes, and by infringement on civil rights and civil liberties. In addition, preparation for war, like war itself, can promote violence as a means for settling disputes.

Another indirect impact of war is the creation of many refugees and internally displaced persons: Many of the world's 12 million refugees have left their native countries as a result of war. Refugees often flee to neighbouring less-developed countries, which often face significant challenges in addressing the public health needs of their own populations. In addition, the vast majority of the 22–25 million internally displaced persons worldwide have left their homes to escape war. These internally displaced persons are often worse off than refugees who have left their countries because they frequently do not have easy access to food, safe water, health care, shelter, and other necessities. Approximately 8 million of these internally displaced persons live in the Democratic Republic of Congo, Uganda, and Sudan—all in Africa. In West Darfur, Sudan, more than 700 000 people have been internally displaced and more than 250 000 people have fled to refugee camps in neighbouring Chad as a result of bitter ethnic conflict. Refugees and internally displaced persons experience much higher rates of mortality and morbidity, much of it due to malnutrition and infectious diseases.

The vast majority of refugees and internally displaced persons as a result of war are women, children, and elderly people who may be highly vulnerable not only to disease and malnutrition, but also to threats of their security.

The environment may be disrupted during war or the preparation for war. Conventional weapons may damage the environment such that the health-supporting infrastructure—systems of food and water supply, sewage disposal, medical care, transportation, and communication—is severely disrupted or destroyed. Malnutrition of the affected population may increase the frequency and severity of infectious diseases. The biological environment may also be disrupted by the production, testing, and use of biological weapons. Ionizing radiation from the production, testing, use, and disposal of nuclear weapons and radioactive materials, such as depleted uranium, may also disrupt and damage the environment. So may toxic substances by the release of hazardous substances from damaged industrial facilities or from the production, testing, use, and disposal of chemical weapons.

Hazardous wastes from military operations represent potential contaminants of air, water, and soil. For example, groundwater was contaminated with trichloroethylene (TCE), a probable human carcinogen, and other toxins at the Otis Air Force Base in Massachusetts; 125 chemicals were dumped over a period of 30 years at the Rocky Mountain Arsenal in Colorado; and benzene, a definite human carcinogen, was found in extremely high concentrations at the McChord Air Force Base in the State of Washington (Renner 2000).

Both during war and the preparation for war, military forces consume huge amounts of fossil fuels and other non-renewable materials. Energy consumption by military equipment can be substantial. For example, an armoured division of 348 battle tanks operating for one day consumes more than 2.2 million L of fuel and a carrier battle group operating for one day consumes more than 1.5 million L of fuel. In the late 1980s, the US military annually consumed 18.6 million tons of fuel (more than 44 per cent of the world's total) and emitted 381 000 tons of carbon monoxide, 157 000 tons of oxides of nitrogen, 78 000 tons of hydrocarbons, and 17 900 tons of sulphur dioxide (Renner 2000).

Weapons systems

Conventional weapons

Conventional weapons consist of explosives, incendiaries, and weapons of various sizes, ranging from 'small arms and light weapons' to heavy artillery and bombs. Small arms and light weapons (SALW), which include pistols, rifles, machine guns, and other hand-held or easily transportable weapons, are the weapons most often used in wars. Although some restrictions have been placed on their use in war, such as the outlawing of the use of 'dum-dum bullets' (which cause extensive injuries when striking a human), there has been little effective effort to outlaw their use. In the Millennium Report of the UN Secretary-General to the General Assembly, Kofi Annan stated that small arms could be described as weapons of mass destruction (WMD) because the fatalities they produce 'dwarf that of all other weapons systems—and in most years greatly exceed the toll of the atomic bombs that devastated Hiroshima and Nagasaki'.

Conventional weapons have accounted for the overwhelming majority of adverse environmental consequences due to war. During World War II, for example, extensive carpet bombing of cities in Europe and Japan accounted not only for many deaths and injuries, but also for widespread devastation of urban environments. During the Persian Gulf War, the more than 600 oil fires in Kuwait accounted for widespread environmental devastation as well as for acute, and possibly chronic, respiratory ailments among people who were exposed to the smoke from these fires. The bombing of mangrove forests during the Vietnam War led to destruction of these forests, and the resultant bomb craters remain several decades afterward, often filling with stagnant water that serves as a breeding ground for mosquitoes transmitting malaria and other mosquito-borne diseases.

Nuclear weapons

Nuclear weapons have been increasingly widespread since their development in the 1940s. There are now an estimated 20 000 nuclear warheads in at least eight nations—the United States, Russia, the United Kingdom, France, China, Israel, India, and Pakistan—and possibly also in North Korea (Sutton & Gould 2007). The historic high in the explosive capacity of the world nuclear weapons stockpiles was reached in 1960 with an explosive capacity equivalent to 20 000 megatons (20 billion tons or 40 trillion pounds) of trinitrotoluene (TNT), equivalent to that of 1.4 million of the nuclear bombs dropped on Hiroshima (Yokoro & Kamada 2000). In the United States in 1967, the nuclear stockpile had reached approximately 32 000 nuclear warheads of 30 different types. In 2003, the US stockpile was about 10 400 warheads, totalling about 2000 megatons—equivalent to 140 000 Hiroshima-size bombs. Five thousand of the nuclear weapons in the United States, Russia, and possibly other countries are on 'hair-trigger' alert, ready to fire on a few minutes notice.

The detonation of nuclear bombs over Hiroshima and Nagasaki in August 1945 during World War II led to the immediate deaths of approximately 200 000 people, primarily civilians, as well as to lasting injury and later death of many others, with massive devastation—and widespread radioactive contamination—of the environment in these two cities (Yokoro & Kamada 2000). Atmospheric testing of nuclear weapons by the United States, the Soviet Union, and other countries has also led to environmental contamination, with increased rates of leukaemia and other cancers among populations who were downwind from these tests. The effects of exposure to iodine-131 (a radioactive isotope of iodine produced by the testing) on children has been well-documented (Institute of Medicine, National Research Council 1999). In addition to the potential for use of nuclear weapons by national armed forces, such as that described in the recent US Nuclear Posture Review, which threatened use of nuclear weapons under a wider range of circumstances, there is an increasing threat of their use by individuals and groups.

From 1945 to 1990, the United States produced approximately 70 000 nuclear weapons; other nations also produced many of these weapons. Production of nuclear weapons has led to major environmental contamination (Levy & Sidel 2005). For example, the area around Chelyabinsk in Russia has been heavily contaminated with radioactive materials from the nuclear weapons production facility in that area. The level of ambient radiation in and near the Techa River in the area has been documented to be as high as 28 times the normal background radiation level (Burmistrov *et al.* 2006). Another example is the leakage of radioactive materials from the storage of wastes from nuclear weapons production at Hanford, along the Columbia River in Washington State, leading to extensive radioactive contamination (Renner 2000).

The dismantling and disposal of nuclear weapons has also led to environmental contamination. The primary site for the disassembly of US nuclear weapons is the Pantex Plant, located 17 miles northeast of Amarillo in the Texas panhandle (Levy & Sidel 2005). Overall, the United States has dismantled about 60 000 nuclear warheads since the 1940s; during the 1990s, 11 751 warheads were dismantled. More than 12 000 plutonium pits (hollow shells of plutonium encased in steel or another metal that are essential components of nuclear weapons) are stored in containers at Pantex (Levy & Sidel 2005). Plutonium, an element first produced in the Manhattan Project in 1942, has a half-life of 24 000 years. Plans are underway to produce as many as 80 new pits annually at Los Alamos National Laboratory, and the Bush administration advocates building a modern pit facility capable of producing 250–900 pits annually by 2018 (Levy & Sidel 2005).

Radiologic weapons

'Dirty bombs', consisting of conventional explosive devices mixed with radioactive materials, or attacks on nuclear power plants with explosive weapons could widely scatter highly radioactive materials. Another example of a radioactive substance used in weapons is depleted uranium (DU), uranium from which the uranium isotope usable for nuclear weapons or as fuel rods for nuclear power plants has been removed (Depleted Uranium Education Project 1997). DU is used militarily as a casing for armour-penetrating shells. An extremely dense material, uranium used as a casing increases the ability of the shell to penetrate the armour of tanks; uranium is also pyrophoric and bursts into flames on impact. DU-encased shells were used by the United States during the Persian Gulf War and the Iraq War as well as the war in Kosovo; similar shells were used by the United Kingdom in the Iraq War. DU, which is both radioactive and extremely toxic, has been demonstrated to cause contamination of the soil and groundwater. Use of DU is considered legal by the nations using it, but its use is considered by others to be illegal under the Geneva Conventions and other international treaties.

Chemicals

A variety of chemical weapons and related materials have the potential for direct health effects during collective violence and also for contaminating the physical environment during war and the preparation for war. The potential for exposure exists not only for military and civilian populations, who may be exposed during the use of chemical weapons in wartime, but also for workers involved in the development, production, transport, and storage of these weapons and for community residents living near facilities where these weapons are developed, produced, transported, and stored. In addition, disposal of these weapons, including their disassembly and incineration, can be hazardous.

During the Vietnam War, the US military used defoliants on mangrove forests and other vegetation, which not only defoliated and killed trees and other plants, but may also have led to excessive numbers of birth defects and cases of cancer among nearby residents (Levy & Sidel 2005). In addition, development and production of conventional weapons involve the use of many chemicals that are toxic and can contaminate the environment. Furthermore, there is now a plausible threat of non-state agents using chemical

weapons; a Japanese cult, Aum Shinrikyo, used sarin in the subway system of two Japanese cities in the mid 1990s, accounting for the death of 19 people and injuries to thousands (Spanjaard & Khabib 2007).

The Chemical Weapons Convention (CWC), which came into force in 1997, prohibits all development, production, acquisition, stockpiling, transfer, and use of chemical weapons. It requires each state party to destroy its chemical weapons and chemical weapons production facilities, as well as any chemical weapons it may have abandoned on the territory of another state party. The verification provisions of the CWC affect not only the military sector but also the civilian chemical industry worldwide through certain restrictions and obligations regarding the production, processing, and consumption of chemicals that are considered relevant to the objectives of the convention. These provisions are to be verified through a combination of reporting requirements, routine onsite inspection of declared sites, and short-notice challenge inspections. The Organization for the Prohibition of Chemical Weapons (OPCW) in The Hague, established by the CWC, ensures implementation of the provisions of the CWC. The disposal of chemical weapons required by the CWC has raised controversy about the safety of two different methods of disposal: Incineration and chemical neutralization. The controversy about safety and protection of the environment has delayed completion of the disposal by the date required by the CWC.

Biological agents

These consist of bacteria, viruses, other microorganisms, and their toxins, which can not only directly produce illness in humans, but can also be used against other animals or plants, thereby adversely affecting human food supplies or agricultural resources and indirectly affecting human health. Biological agents have been used relatively infrequently during warfare, but there has long been a potential for their use. These agents have been used as weapons, albeit sporadically, since ancient times. In the sixth century BC, Persia, Greece, and Rome tried to contaminate drinking water sources with diseased corpses. In AD 1346, Mongols besieging the Crimean seaport of Kaffa placed cadavers of plague victims on hurling machines and threw them into Kaffa. In the mid-eighteenth century, during the French and Indian War, a British commander sent blankets infected with smallpox to Native Americans. During World War I, Germany dropped bombs containing plague bacteria over British positions and used cholera in Italy. During the 1930s, Japan contaminated the food and water supplies of several cities and sprayed the cities with cultures of microorganisms.

Gruinard Island, off the coast of Scotland, was contaminated in 1942 by a test use of anthrax spores by the United Kingdom and the United States (Harris & Paxman 1962). During the 1950s and 1960s, secret large-scale open-air tests at the US Army Dugway Proving Ground may have introduced the microorganisms that cause Q fever and Venezuelan equine encephalitis into the deserts of Western Utah (Cole 1988). In 1979, the accidental release of anthrax spores near Sverdlovsk in the Soviet Union resulted in at least 77 cases of inhalation anthrax and at least 66 deaths (Meselson 1994).

There is concern that biological agents could be used as terrorist weapons. In the fall of 2001, anthrax spores were disseminated through the US mail, causing 23 cases of inhalational and skin anthrax, 5 of which were fatal. The Centers for Disease Control and

Prevention has identified three categories of diseases caused by biological agents, according to its level of concern that they may be used as terrorist weapons. Category A consists of the agents that cause anthrax, botulism, plague, smallpox, tularaemia, and several viral haemorrhagic fevers. Category B consists of the agents that cause brucellosis, glanders, melioidosis, psittacosis, Q fever, and food safety threats (such as salmonella and shigella species, and *Escherichia coli* O157:H7), as well as epsilon toxin of *Clostridium perfringens*, ricin toxin from castor beans, and staphylococcyl enterotoxin B. Category C consists of the agents that cause emerging infectious diseases such as Nipah virus and hantavirus (Centers for Disease Control and Prevention 2007).

Antipersonnel landmines

Approximately 80 million landmines are still deployed worldwide in at least 78 countries. These landmines have been termed 'weapons of mass destruction, one person at a time'. They have mostly been placed in rural areas, posing a threat to residents of these areas and often disrupting farming and other activities. Civilians are the most likely to be injured or killed by landmines, which continue to injure and kill 15 000–20 000 people annually; more than 90 per cent of landmine victims are civilians, primarily poor people living in rural areas. One-fourth of landmine victims are children, putting landmines among the six most preventable major causes of death to children throughout the world. It is estimated that half of all landmine victims die of their injuries before they reach appropriate medical care. Although a mine may cost as little as US$3 to produce, it may cost as much as a US$1000 to remove and its adverse economic impact on human health and well-being is substantially higher. Mines, in addition to maiming and killing people, also make large areas of land uninhabitable. Remaining in place for many years, they pose long-term threats to people, including refugees and internally displaced persons returning to their homes after long periods of war. Since the entry into force of the Anti-Personnel Landmine Convention in 1997, production of landmines has been markedly reduced and a number of those that had been implanted in the ground have been removed (International Campaign to Ban Landmines 2006). Many of the mines are still buried and additional resources will be required to continue unearthing and destroying them, tasks that pose inherent risks to demining personnel (Sirkin *et al.* 2008).

Weapons in space

The deployment of weapons in space represents another risk of weapons systems igniting armed conflict or adding to its potential health consequences. Attempts by the 65-member United Nations Conference on Disarmament in Geneva to limit weapons in space have failed. UN Secretary-General Ban Ki-moon opened the 2008 session of the Conference by urging progress. In early 2008, the Russian and Chinese delegates to the Conference presented a draft treaty banning weapons in space, but the United States opposed such a treaty. The risk of an arms race of weapons in space continues.

The role of public health in addressing war

War and the preparation for war have enormous adverse impact on humans and their environment. Public health has an important part to play in response to war. As the World Health Assembly declared in 1981, 'the role of health workers in promoting and preserving peace is a significant factor for achieving health for all' (World Health Assembly 1981).

Prevention of war

The health and environmental problems created by collective violence can appear to be overwhelming. However, standard public health principles and implementation measures can be successfully applied in addressing these problems. The following subsection of this chapter highlights three standard public health approaches that can be developed and implemented in addressing these environmental problems: (a) surveillance and documentation, (b) education and raising awareness, and (c) advocacy for sound policies and programmes.

Surveillance and documentation

Much can be accomplished by undertaking surveillance and other activities to document the problems caused by war. Although the numbers of deaths, injuries, and diseases among uniformed combatants are generally well-documented, deaths, injuries, and diseases among civilians are more difficult to document. Household cluster surveys have been used during the Iraq War to estimate the civilian casualties. Technical approaches to surveillance can include environmental monitoring as well as biological monitoring, the latter to document and assess the human burden of environmental contaminants and their adverse health consequences. Non-technical approaches can include information from physician reports, reports in the mass media, and assessments by government agencies.

Education and raising awareness

Much can also be accomplished by educating and raising the awareness of health professionals, policy makers, and the general public about the problems caused by war. A multifaceted approach that incorporates publications by citizens' groups and professional organizations, communications of the mass media, and personal communication is often valuable. In addition, efforts should be made to assist people in distinguishing between accurate and inaccurate information and in setting priorities.

Advocacy for sound policies and programmes

Finally, much can also be accomplished by advocating for improved policies and programmes that help prevent collective violence and minimize its public health impact.

Levels of prevention

Those concerned with the promotion and protection of health classify preventive measures into four basic categories: Primordial prevention (a recent addition, which in this chapter will be called *pre-primary prevention*), primary prevention, secondary prevention, and tertiary prevention. Pre-primary prevention consists of measures to prevent adverse health consequences by removing the conditions that lead to them. Primary prevention consists of measures to prevent the health consequences of a specific illness or injury by preventing its occurrence in a specific individual or among a specific group. Secondary prevention consists of measures to prevent or limit the health consequences of an illness or injury, or to limit the spread of an infectious disease to others, after the disease process has begun. Tertiary prevention consists of efforts to rehabilitate those injured and to reintegrate them into society or, in the case of prevention of collective violence, to prevent the resumption of violence.

Prevention of scurvy may be used as an example. Policies that assure that a population has information about and access to an adequate diet that includes vitamin C are examples of pre-primary prevention. Provision of foods containing vitamin C to ensure an adequate intake of this vitamin among a group that does not otherwise have access to it is an example of primary prevention; James Lind, a pioneer of public health in the 1700s, provided limes to sailors on British warships to prevent scurvy (Lind 2006). To use prevention of smallpox as another example, elimination of small-pox virus in the ecosphere is pre-primary prevention and vaccination against smallpox before exposure is primary prevention. Vaccination may also be used after exposure to smallpox has occurred to prevent the disease and its spread to others, an example of secondary prevention.

Pre-primary prevention

In general, pre-primary prevention requires political and social will. Pre-primary and primary prevention may be difficult to accomplish because the causes of the disease or injury may be unknown and, when they are known, the preventive methods may be difficult to implement technically or politically. As measures for pre-primary or primary prevention are usually more effective and rarely have negative consequences, they are generally considered preferable to secondary prevention even when implementation is difficult or expensive. Secondary prevention is usually easier to implement politically and technically but, because such methods are often ineffective or only partially effective, they may create a false sense of security and encourage risk taking, can be more expensive than primary prevention, and more likely than pre-primary or primary prevention methods to have adverse consequences. The health consequences of war and the aftermath of war can be prevented or reduced through primordial prevention. This generally requires cooperation among civil society (non-governmental) organizations, governmental agencies, and organizations of health professionals.

The underlying causes of collective violence include poverty, social inequities, adverse effects of globalization, and shame and humiliation. Some of the underlying causes of war and militarism are becoming more prevalent or worsening.

Persistence of socioeconomic disparities and other forms of social injustice are among the leading underlying causes of war. The rich–poor divide is growing. In 1960, in the 20 richest countries, the per-capita gross domestic product (GDP) was 18 times that of the 20 poorest countries; by 1995, this gap had increased to 37 times. Between 1980 and the late 1990s, inequality increased in 48 of the 73 countries for which there are reliable data, including China, Russia, and the United States (Marmot & Bell 2006). Inequality is not restricted to personal income, but includes other important areas of life, such as health status, access to health care, education, and employment opportunities. In addition, abundant national resources, such as oil, minerals, metals, gemstones, drug crops, and timber, have fuelled many wars in developing countries.

Globalization is similarly a two-edged sword. Insofar as globalization leads to good relations among nation-states and reductions in poverty and disparities within and among nations, it may play a powerful role in prevention of collective violence. Conversely, if globalization leads to exploitation of people, of the environment, and of other resources, it may be among the causes of war.

The Carnegie Commission on Preventing Deadly Conflict has identified the following factors that put nations at risk of violent conflict, including:

- Lack of democratic processes and unequal access to power, particularly in situations where power arises from religious or ethnic identity and leaders are repressive or abusive of human rights.
- Social inequality characterized by markedly unequal distribution of resources and access to these resources, especially where the economy is in decline and there is, as a result, more social inequality and more competition for resources.
- Control by one group of valuable natural resources, such as oil, timber, drugs, or gems.
- Demographic changes that are so rapid that they outstrip the capability of a nation to provide basic necessary services and opportunities for employment.

The United States and other nations must increase funding for humanitarian and sustainable development programmes that address the root causes of collective violence, such as hunger, illiteracy, and unemployment.

Promoting multilateralism

Since its founding in 1946, the UN has attempted to live up to the goal stated in its charter: 'To save succeeding generations from the scourge of war'. Its mandate, along with preventing war, includes protecting human rights, promoting international justice, and helping the people of the world to achieve a sustainable standard of living. Its affiliated programmes and specialized agencies include, among many others, the United Nations Children's Fund (UNICEF), the World Health Organization (WHO), the Food and Agriculture Organization (FAO), the International Labour Organization (ILO), the United Nations Development Programme (UNDP), and the Office of the UN High Commissioner for Refugees (UNHCR). These UN-related organizations, and the UN itself, have made an enormous difference in the lives of people.

The resources allocated to the UN by its member states are grossly inadequate. The annual budget for the core functions—the Secretariat operations in New York, Geneva, Nairobi, Vienna, and five required commissions—is far less than New York City's annual budget and far less than annual worldwide military expenditures. Indeed, the world's military expenditures for one year would pay for the annual core functions of the United Nations for close to a century. This is about 4 per cent of New York City's annual budget—and nearly a billion dollars less than the yearly cost of Tokyo's Fire Department. The entire UN system (excluding the World Bank and International Monetary Fund) spends US$12 billion a year. By comparison, annual world military expenditures—$1 trillion—would pay for the entire UN system for more than 65 years.

The UN has no army and no police. It relies on the voluntary contribution of troops and other personnel to halt conflicts that threaten peace and security. The United States and other member states on the Security Council decide when and where to deploy peacekeeping troops. Long-term conflicts, such as those in the Sudan and Kashmir and the Israeli–Palestinian conflict, fester while conflicting national priorities deadlock the UN's ability to act. In fact, if stymied by the veto, the organization has little power beyond the bully pulpit. The United States and the United Kingdom have severely weakened the UN by their unauthorized and illegal invasion of Iraq in 2003. The United States also failed to support the International War Crimes Tribunal through signature and ratification of the Statute of the International Criminal Court.

Ending poverty and social injustice

Poverty and other manifestations of social injustice contribute to conditions that lead to collective violence. Growing socioeconomic and other disparities between the rich and the poor within countries, and between rich and poor nations, also contribute to the likelihood of armed conflict. By addressing these underlying conditions through policies and programmes that redistribute wealth within nations and among nations, and by providing financial and technical assistance to less-developed nations, countries such as the United States can minimize poverty and other forms of social injustice that lead to collective violence.

Creating a culture of peace

Workers in the health and environment sectors can do much to promote a culture of peace, in which non-violent means are utilized to settle conflicts. A culture of peace is based on the values, attitudes, and behaviours that form the deep roots of peace. They are in some ways the opposite of the values, attitudes, and behaviours that reflect and inspire collective violence, but should not be equated with just the absence of war. A culture of peace can exist at the level of the family, workplace, school, and community as well as at the level of the state and in international relations. Health and environment professionals and others can play important roles in encouraging the development of a culture of peace at all these levels.

The Hague Appeal for Peace Civil Society Conference was held in 1999 on the 100th anniversary of the 1899 Hague Peace Conference. The 1899 conference, attended by governmental representatives, was devoted to finding methods for making war more humane. The 1999 conference, attended by 1 000 individuals and representatives of civil society organizations, was devoted to finding methods to prevent war and to establish a 'culture of peace'. The document adopted at the 1999 conference, the Hague Appeal for Peace and Justice for the 21st Century, has been translated by the United Nations into all its official languages and distributed widely around the world. Its ten-point action agenda addressed education for peace, human rights, and democracy; the adverse effects of globalization; sustainable and equitable use of environmental resources; elimination of racial, ethnic, religious, and gender intolerance; protection of children; reduction of violence; and other issues.

Primary prevention

Primary prevention includes preventing specific elements of collective violence and sharply reducing preparation for war, as follows.

Strengthening of nuclear weapons treaties

Unlike the implementation of treaties banning chemical weapons and biological weapons, there is no comprehensive treaty banning the use or mandating the destruction of nuclear weapons. Instead, a series of overlapping incomplete treaties have been negotiated. The Partial Test Ban Treaty (PTBT) of 1963, promoted in part by concerns about radioactive environmental contamination, banned nuclear tests in the atmosphere, under water, and in outer space. The expansion of the PTBT, the Comprehensive Nuclear Test Ban Treaty (CTBT), a key step towards nuclear disarmament and preventing proliferation, was opened for signature in 1996 but has not yet received sufficient signatures or ratifications to enter into force.

It bans nuclear explosions, for either military or civilian purposes, but does not ban computer simulations and subcritical tests, which some nations rely on to maintain the option of developing new nuclear weapons. As of early 2008, the CTBT had been signed by 178 nations and ratified by 144. Entry into force requires ratification by the 44 nuclear-capable nations, of which 35 had ratified it by early 2008. The United States has not yet ratified the CTBT.

The Treaty on the Non-Proliferation of Nuclear Weapons (the 'Nuclear Non-Proliferation Treaty', or NPT) was opened for signature in 1968 and entered into force in 1970. By early 2008, a total of 189 states parties (nations) had ratified the treaty. The five nuclear weapon states recognized under the NPT—China, France, Russia, the United Kingdom, and the United States—are parties to the treaty. The NPT attempts to prevent the spread of nuclear weapons by restricting transfer of certain technologies. It relies on a control system carried out by the International Atomic Energy Agency (IAEA), which also promotes nuclear energy. In exchange for the non-nuclear weapons states' commitment not to develop or otherwise acquire nuclear weapons, the NPT commits the nuclear weapon states to good-faith negotiations on nuclear disarmament. Every five years since 1970 the states parties have held a review conference to assess implementation of the treaty. The review conference in 2000 identified and approved practical steps towards the total elimination of nuclear arsenals. The International Court of Justice (the World Court) in 1996 in an advisory opinion urged that the nations possessing nuclear weapons move expeditiously toward nuclear disarmament, as is required by Article VI of the NPT.

The Anti-Ballistic Missile (ABM) Treaty between the United States and the Soviet Union was signed and entered into force in 1972. The ABM Treaty, by limiting defensive systems that would otherwise spur an offensive arms race, has been seen as the foundation for the strategic nuclear arms reduction treaties. In late 2001, President Bush announced that the United States would withdraw from the ABM Treaty within six months and gave formal notice, stating that it 'hinders our government's ability to develop ways to protect our people from future terrorist or rogue-state missile attacks'. The United States in 2007 announced plans to establish a ballistic missile defence system in Eastern Europe, which led Russia to threaten to increase its arsenal of nuclear weapons.

The United States should help stop the spread of nuclear weapons by actively supporting and adhering to these treaties, and by setting an example for the rest of the world by renouncing the first use of nuclear weapons and the development of new nuclear weapons. It should work with Russia to dismantle nuclear warheads and increase funding for programmes to secure nuclear materials so that they will not fall into the hands of individuals and groups.

Increasing attention is being focused on the elimination of nuclear weapons. Policy makers, such as former US Secretaries of State Henry Kissinger and George Shultz and former military leaders, have called for measures towards the elimination of these weapons (Shultz *et al.* 2007). One measure that may accomplish this is a nuclear weapons convention comparable to the Chemical Weapons Convention, the Biological and Toxin Weapons Convention, and the Anti-Personnel Landmine Convention. A model nuclear weapons convention has been drafted by an international coalition of civil society and professional organizations, and has been presented by Costa Rica to the United Nations.

Strengthening the chemical weapons convention

The Chemical Weapons Convention (CWC) is the strongest of the arms control treaties outlawing a single class of weapons. Inspection and verification of compliance with its provisions lies in the hands of the Organization for the Prohibition of Chemical Weapons (OPCW) in The Hague, established by the CWC (Spanjaard & Khabib 2003). Controversies about safety and protection of the environment during the disposal of chemical weapons required by the CWC have delayed completion of the disposal, and large stockpiles still remain in a number of the world's nations that pose a continuing threat to health and to the environment. The United States has failed to fully support the OPCW in its difficult tasks of inspection and in urging nations to comply with the CWC.

Strengthening the biological and toxin weapons convention

Although the development, production, transfer, or use of biological weapons was prohibited by the 1975 Biological and Toxin Weapons Convention (BWC), several nations are believed to retain stockpiles of such weapons. The verification measures included in the BWC are weak and attempts to strengthen them have been unsuccessful. During 2002, the United States blocked attempts to strengthen the verification measures of the BWC, announcing that such measures might lead to exposure of US industrial or military secrets. The United States must be urged to reverse its rejection of the international community's attempts to develop strong inspection and verification protocols for the BWC. Efforts must be made to convince all nations to support strengthening of the BWC and all nations must refrain from secret activities, often termed *defensive*, that may fuel a biological arms race.

Perhaps even more important, global public health capacity to deal with all infectious disease must be strengthened. The best individual and collective efforts at diagnosing and treating disease outbreaks can be overwhelmed by any natural or intentionally induced epidemic. Consequently, support for strong global preventive public health capabilities provides the best ultimate defence against ever-evolving threats. The significant vulnerabilities to persistent global reservoirs of endemic illness in impoverished and underserved populations can provide the source of future pandemics. For example, in India during 1999, there were 2 million new cases of tuberculosis, causing about 450 000 deaths. An investment of $30 million annually over a few years, compared to the current US contribution to India of US$1 million for this purpose, could virtually wipe out the disease. In addition, the United Nations has estimated that US$10 billion invested in safe water supplies could cut by up to one-third the current 4 billion cases of diarrhoea worldwide that result in 2.2 million annual deaths.

Promoting the support of the Anti-Personnel Landmine Convention

As of April 2008, a total of 158 nations had signed or acceded to the 1997 Land Mines Convention. Of these, 156 nations had formally ratified. Regrettably, 37 nations had neither signed nor ratified, including China, India, Iran, Iraq, Israel, Russia, and the United States. Resources are desperately needed to clear the landmines currently deployed. All the nations of the world must be urged to contribute more resources to this task.

Secondary prevention

The consequences of collective violence can also be prevented or diminished by secondary prevention if war occurs, by preventing casualties among military personnel and civilians, by preventing environmental destruction, and by seeking an end to the war.

Secondary prevention methods include strengthening adherence to the Geneva Conventions and other treaties that lessen the effects of war; reducing military activities, including preparation for war; and negotiating effective treaties to lessen environmental damage.

Tertiary prevention

Efforts after the end of an armed conflict to rehabilitate and reintegrate those living with disabilities due to the conflict, to repair the damage to the physical, social, cultural and economic environments, and thereby to prevent new conflicts and new collective violence are extremely important. Tertiary prevention methods include programmes for physical and social rehabilitation for individuals, groups and communities; provision of appropriate aid to communities and nations damaged by collective violence, such as the Marshall Plan after World War II; assurance of environmental remediation after the armed violence has ended; and the establishment of truth and reconciliation commissions, such as the highly successful commission set up in South Africa by President Nelson Mandela.

The role of non-governmental organizations

Important roles for public health workers in the prevention and alleviation of the consequences of collective violence lie in work with non-governmental organizations (NGOs). These organizations are increasingly being called *civil society organizations*, and focus on war from a medical and public health perspective in a variety of ways:

- Intervening to mitigate the consequences of armed conflict
- Researching the effects of war
- Educating the public and decision makers about its impact on health and the environment
- Advocating for changes in global attitudes and policies towards war and the most dangerous weapons and practices of war (Loretz 2008)

Other non-governmental organizations provide direct humanitarian assistance to the victims of collective violence. These organizations generally participate in secondary and tertiary prevention but some, such as the International Committee of the Red Cross, have also in recent years begun to play a role in primary prevention. Humanitarian assistance organizations may also play a role in primary prevention of specific acts of violence and atrocities. They may be strong advocates on behalf of civilian populations among whom they live and for whom they provide humanitarian assistance (Waldman 2008).

Acknowledgement

Parts of this chapter are modified from a background paper on 'Collective Violence: Health Impact and Prevention' for the Workshop on Violence Prevention in Low- and Middle-Income Countries conducted by the Institute of Medicine in 2007, which was published as an appendix in the Workshop Summary (Sidel & Levy 2008).

References

Burmistrov D., Kossenko M., Wilson R. *Radioactive contamination of the Techa River and its effects*. Cambridge (MA): Harvard University; 2006.

Available from: http://phys4.harvard.edu/~wilson/publications/pp747/techa_cor.htm. [Accessed 2006 Mar 8].

Centers for Disease Control and Prevention. Bioterrorism agents/diseases. Centers for Disease Control and Prevention; 2007. Available from: http://www.bt.cdc.gov/agent/agentlist-category.asp. [Accessed 2007 Jun 9].

Cole L.A. Clouds of secrecy: the Army's germ warfare tests over populated areas. Totowa (NJ): Rowman & Littlefield; 1988.

Depleted Uranium Education Project. *Metal of dishonor: depleted uranium.* New York (NY): International Action Center; 1997.

Harris R., Paxman J. A higher form of killing: the secret story of chemical and biological weapons. New York (NY): Hill and Wang; 1962.

Institute of Medicine, National Research Council. Exposure of the American people to iodine-131 from Nevada nuclear-test: review of the National Cancer Institute report and public health implications. Washington (DC): National Academy Press; 1999. p. 193.

International Campaign to Ban Landmines [Online]. Available from: www.icbl.org. [Accessed 2008 July 29].

Krug E.G. *et al.*, editors. 2002 *world report on violence and health.* Geneva: World Health Organization. Available from: http://www.who.int/violence_injury_prevention/violence/world_report/en/full_en.pdf

Levy B.S., Sidel V.W., editors. Terrorism and public health: a balanced approach to strengthening systems and protecting people. Updated ed. New York (NY): Oxford University Press; 2007.

Levy B.S., Sidel V.W., editors. *War and public health.* 2nd ed. New York (NY): Oxford University Press; 2008.

Levy B.S., Sidel V.W. War. In: Frumkin H, editor. *Environmental health: from local to global.* New York (NY): Jossey-Bass; 2005. p. 269–87.

Loretz J. The role of nongovernmental organizations. In: Levy B.S., Sidel V.W., editors. *War and public health.* 2nd ed. New York (NY): Oxford University Press; 2008. p. 381–92.

Marmot M., Bell R. The socioeconomically disadvantaged. In: Levy B.S., Sidel V.W., editors. *Social injustice and public health.* New York (NY): Oxford University Press; 2006. p. 25–45.

Meselson M., Guillemin J., Hugh-Jones M. *et al.* The Sverdlovsk anthrax outbreak of 1979. *Science* 1994;**266**:1202–8.

Renner M. Environmental and health effects of weapons production, testing, and maintenance. In: Levy B.S., Sidel V.W., editors. *War and public health.* Updated ed. Washington (DC): American Public Health Association; 2000. p. 117–36.

Rummel R.J. *Death by government: genocide and mass murder since 1900.* New Brunswick (NJ), London: Transaction Publications; 1994.

Securing our survival: the case for a nuclear weapons convention. Cambridge (MA): International Physicians for the Prevention of Nuclear War; 2007.

Shultz G.P., Perry W.J., Kissinger H.A. *et al.* A world free of nuclear weapons. Wall Street Journal 2007 Jan 4;Sect. A:15.

Sidel V.W., Levy B.S. Collective violence: health impact and prevention. In: Institute of Medicine (IOM). *Violence prevention in low- and middle-income countries.* Washington (DC): National Academies Press; 2008. p. 171–99.

Sirkin S., Cobey J.C., Stover E. Landmines. In: Levy B.S., Sidel V.W., editors. *War and public health.* 2nd ed. New York (NY): Oxford University Press; 2008. p. 102–16.

Smith D. World at war. *The Defense Monitor* 2007;**36**(1):1–9.

Spanjaard H., Khabib O. Chemical Weapons. In: Levy B.S., Sidel V.W., editors. *Terrorism and public health: a balanced approach to strengthening systems and protecting people.* Updated ed. New York (NY): Oxford University Press; 2007. p. 199–219.

Stockholm International Peace Research Institute. *SIPRI yearbook 2002: armaments, disarmament, and international security.* New York (NY): Oxford University Press; 2002.

Sutton P.M., Gould R.M. Nuclear, radiological, and related weapons. In: Levy B.S., Sidel V.W., editors. *Terrorism and public health: a balanced approach to strengthening systems and protecting people.* Updated ed. New York (NY): Oxford University Press; 2007. p. 220–42.

Waldman R. The roles of humanitarian assistance. In: Levy B.S., Sidel V.W., editors. *War and public health.* 2nd ed. New York (NY): Oxford University Press; 2008. p. 369–80.

World Health Assembly. Resolution WHA34.38 Geneva: World Health Organization; 1981.

World Health Assembly. Resolution WHA49.25 on prevention of violence: a public health priority. Geneva: World Health Organization; 1996.

Yokoro K, Kamada N. The health effects of the use of nuclear weapons. In: Levy BS, Sidel VW, editors. *War and public health.* Updated ed. Washington (DC): American Public Health Association; 2000. p. 65–83.

10.7

Urban health in low- and middle-income countries

Mark R. Montgomery

Abstract

Over the next 30 years, low- and middle-income countries will cross an historic threshold, becoming for the first time more urban than rural. This chapter explores the implications for urban public health. To date, health research and policy discussions have been overly concerned with urban–rural differences in health, which generally favour urban areas except for human immunodeficiency virus (HIV)/acquired immunodeficiency syndrome (AIDS), and insufficient attention has been paid to the wide disparities in health that exist within urban areas. Empirical studies show clearly that the urban poor—especially those who live in slums, without adequate drinking water, sanitation, and housing—face health risks that are similar to and sometimes markedly worse than the risks facing rural villagers.

The private sector is a more prominent element of the urban than the rural health system, and the monetary costs of care often cause the urban poor to delay or forgo needed treatment. In addition, although high-quality health care is in principle available in large cities, the quality of the basic health-care services accessible to the urban poor can be abysmally low. It is not so much the physical distance to services that matter for them, but the social, informational, and economic costs of access. A number of urban health risks warrant more attention: Women's mental health, which is doubtless a key determinant of self-efficacy and thus health-seeking behaviour; the incidence of intimate-partner violence and the risks of crime faced by the urban poor; injuries and deaths due to motor vehicles, typically ranking near the top of the urban burden of disease; tuberculosis and malaria (in sub-Saharan Africa and parts of Southeast Asia); the health threats posed by indoor and outdoor air pollution; and the risks that climate change will present for the cities of low- and middle-income countries, which are likely to experience increases in extreme weather in the coming decades. As national governments and health systems continue to decentralize, the health needs of smaller, secondary cities cannot continue to be neglected—it is in these smaller cities where the majority of urbanites live in most countries. To meet the health challenges of an urban era, the public health sector must engage in what Harpham (2007) terms 'joined-up government', forging partnerships with other urban agencies and sectors at the municipal and regional as well as the national level.

Introduction

Sometime in the next 30 years, if United Nations (UN) projections prove to be on the mark, the populations of poor countries will cross an historic threshold, becoming for the first time more urban than rural (United Nations 2005). In public health, as in other fields, the full implications of this urban transition are only beginning to be appreciated. Part of the difficulty is that the term *urban* refers to a bewildering variety of environments. The health circumstances of small cities and towns differ in many ways from those of larger cities. Within any given city, some residents live in secure, gated communities having all the amenities of Europe or the United States, whereas others—especially those who live in slums—exist in grim Dickensian settings lacking the most basic of human needs such as water supply, sanitation, and housing. The health systems of cities in low- and middle-income countries are also astonishingly varied.

An urban system will often present the full array of health providers, ranging from traditional healers, purveyors of drugs in street markets, ill-equipped pharmacists and chemists operating from ramshackle storefronts, and so on up the scale to the most highly-trained surgeons. Among all urban providers, a high percentage is likely to be engaged in private practice, whether on a full- or part-time basis, and for this reason, urban health care is more monetized than rural care. In urban areas, unlike rural, it is not so much the distance to services that presents a barrier to their use, but rather the social, informational, and economic costs of access.

To be sure, the urban–rural contrast should not be overdrawn. Many residents of the developing world live on the peripheries of cities in locations that are arguably neither urban nor rural; circular migration and other social linkages have long connected the two sectors, and the multiplicity of contacts provides opportunities for communicable diseases to pass between them. Although urban health cannot be separated out and studied apart from rural, it may nevertheless be useful to consider the features of urban health environments and behaviour that have a distinctive quality.

To convey the scale of the urban health challenge that lies ahead, we first provide a sketch of the demographic forces that are reshaping the landscape of low- and middle-income countries. The next section then summarizes the urban health differentials that can be identified in data from internationally comparable sample surveys.

Here, we begin by documenting urban–rural differences and proceed to give closer attention to the within-urban inequalities in health. Next, we draw out the salient features of the supply side of urban health, with particular emphasis on the money costs and quality of health care. Following this, we turn to a description of urban health risks that have not been sufficiently appreciated, or which, to be effectively addressed, would require an expansive conception of the role of the public health system. Finally, we provide a conclusion.

The demographic context

The urban population of the developing world, estimated by the United Nations Population Division to have been 1.97 billion persons in the year 2000, is projected to increase to 3.90 billion by 2030 and to 5.26 billion by 2050 (United Nations 2005). These additions to the cities and towns of poor countries will account for nearly 90 per cent of all world population growth over this period. By 2050, according to the projections, fully two-thirds of the inhabitants of poor countries will live in urban areas, with the number of large cities in these countries reaching historically unprecedented levels.

In 1950, there were only two metropolitan areas in the world—the Tokyo and the New York–Newark agglomerations—with populations of 10 million or more. (Cities of this size are commonly called megacities.) By 2025, according to the UN forecasts, the low- and middle-income countries alone will contain 21 cities of this size. Even more striking is the number of cities in the 1–5 million range. In 1950, only 33 such cities were found in the developing world, whereas by 2025, the UN projects a total of no fewer than 431 cities in this range.

Forecasts such as these seem to have fostered the impression that most urban-dwellers in poor countries live in huge urban agglomerations. This is simply not the case. As Fig. 10.7.1 shows, among all developing-country urbanites in cities of 100 000 and above, only 12 per cent live in megacities—about 1 in 8 of these urban residents.

Twice as many people live in the small cities ranging from 100 000 to a half-million in size. As the Panel on Urban Population Dynamics (2003) has argued, such smaller cities warrant much more attention than they have been given.

These cities are generally less well-provisioned than larger places with basic services such as improved sanitation and adequate supplies of drinking water. Rates of malnutrition and the risks of infant and child mortality in small cities differs only little from what is seen in the countryside. Yet, the municipal governments of such cities seldom possess the range of health expertise and managerial talent that can be found in the governments of larger places. As low- and middle-income countries continue to decentralize their political and administrative systems—transferring more responsibilities for service delivery and revenue-raising from national governments and health ministries to the local tiers of government and the local ministry offices—the thinner resources and weaker capabilities of smaller cities will need careful attention (Panel on Urban Population Dynamics 2003). The preoccupation with the largest of developing-country cities in health-policy discussions, and the general neglect of small cities, has left unaddressed a wide array of important health concerns.

The urban burden of disease: Overview

Because very few low- and middle-income countries maintain reliable vital statistics systems, sample surveys provide much of what is known of urban health in these countries.[1] The two major ongoing survey programmes are the Demographic and Health Survey (DHS), which has fielded and put into the public domain over 150 surveys

---

[1] See the WHO report (*World health statistics* 2007. Geneva: World Health Organization 2007c), which indicates that, of the 115 countries reporting to the WHO on the quality of cause-of-death statistics, only 29 (representing a mere 13 per cent of world population) were judged to have adequate records.

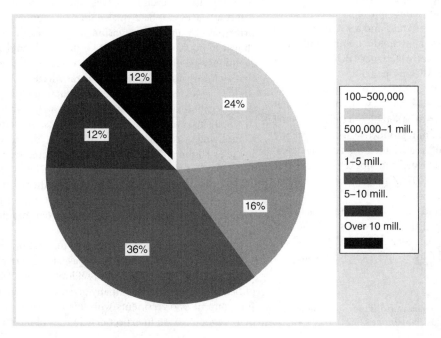

Fig. 10.7.1 Distribution of urban population by city size, population of 100 000 or more, in low- and middle-income countries in 2000.
Source: United Nations. *World urbanization prospects: the 2005 revision population database.* New York [NY]: Department of Economic and Social Affairs, Population Division, United Nations (2005).

Table 10.7.1 Health data routinely collected in the Demographic and Health Surveys (DHSs) and the Multiple Indicator Cluster Surveys (MICSs)

Demographic group	Health data	Gaps
Infants and children	Survival, approximate age at death Vaccination status Recent experience of fever, cough, diarrhoea Height and weight for age (in many surveys)	No reliable cause-of-death information No detailed account of health-seeking behaviour
Adolescents and women of reproductive age	Knowledge of reproduction, contraception, HIV/AIDS, and sources of contraception and health care Detailed data on use of contraception For recent births, nature and timing of prenatal care, place of delivery and attendance	Induced abortion and aftermath not studied Maternal mortality examined indirectly via 'sisterhood' methods No exploration of asymptomatic health conditions unless biomarkers are collected
Sources of care	Knowledge of sources of contraception and health care in some cases supplemented with an urban 'community questionnaire'	No systematic inventory of health providers Not obvious whether geographic boundaries effectively define urban accessible care

since the mid-1980s, and the Multiple Indicator Cluster Survey (MICS), for which some 50 surveys are now available.[2] The DHS and MICS are nationally representative, and are designed to provide reliable estimates for the urban sector as a whole. However, the sample sizes are too small to yield reliable health estimates at the level of individual cities. These programmes have broad data collection agendas in which health is only one among many areas of inquiry. This breadth is both a weakness and a strength: It enables health measures to be linked to household economic and social variables, allowing some investigation of the social determinants of health (Marmot 2005; Marmot & Wilkinson 2005).

The surveys have focused mainly on women of reproductive age and their children. Men are not always interviewed, and even when they are, it is uncommon for a man to be sought out unless he is the partner of an interviewed woman of reproductive age. Nor are the elderly eligible to be interviewed. As a result, cross-national comparisons of the health of the urban elderly are not yet possible (but see Wong *et al.* 2006; Hu *et al.* 2007; Zimmer & Kwong 2004; Kaneda *et al.* 2005; and WHO 2007a).

Table 10.7.1 summarizes the health data that are routinely gathered in the course of a DHS and MICS. This table presents only the core measures that are almost always collected; a number of surveys have been far more ambitious than the list in this table would suggest.

---

[2] For more information, see http://www.measuredhs.com/aboutdhs for the DHS and http://www.childinfo.org/index.htm for the MICS.

There are well-known limits on what can be learned about health in a survey interview. When they are led through their reproductive histories by a skilled interviewer, women can supply reliable information on infant and child survival, but they are unlikely to give medically meaningful accounts of the causes of death. Adult mortality also presents difficulties for the DHS and MICS instruments, given that the women who are the primary respondents are generally no older than 50 years of age themselves. (Ingenious attempts have been made to measure maternal mortality via the 'sisterhood' method (Graham *et al.* 1989), and the DHS and MICS could, in theory, do more along these lines.)

Obviously, asymptomatic conditions cannot be identified in the course of an interview unless blood or tissue samples are collected or the interviewee undergoes a physical examination. (Collection of biomarker data is becoming more common in the DHS programme, but is not yet the norm.) Even reports on symptomatic morbidities and conditions may be clouded by local understandings of what constitutes a disease. The measurement of health-seeking behaviour is also difficult via general-purpose surveys. Although instruments can be designed to retrace the steps leading from problem recognition to treatment, relatively few such surveys of this type have been fielded.

Averages and inequalities

It is commonly believed that in modern-day populations, rural levels of health are worse than urban, and this belief is supported by good scientific evidence. In its analysis of 90 surveys from the DHS programme, the Panel on Urban Population Dynamics (2003) found that, on average, the urban populations of poor countries exhibit lower levels of child mortality than rural populations, and similar urban–rural differences were evident across a range of health indicators. HIV/AIDS presents the large exception to the general rule of urban health advantage. As will be discussed, although the epidemic is penetrating rural areas and may be driving up incidence rates there, prevalence continues to be higher in urban areas, often substantially so. Apart from HIV/AIDS, however, in most low- and middle-income countries, the urban advantage in terms of average health levels is too well-documented to dispute.

But averages can be a misleading basis on which to set health priorities. Upon disaggregation, urban health averages can be shown to mask wide within-city differentials, and when these are examined, the urban poor are often discovered to face health risks that are nearly as bad as those of rural villagers and are sometimes decidedly worse. To see the urban situation clearly, two types of disaggregation are needed at a minimum: The urban poor must be distinguished from other urban residents; and among the poor, those living in communities of concentrated deprivation—slums, in the usual shorthand—need to be considered separately from the poor who live elsewhere (Montgomery & Hewett 2005). It is also important to distinguish cities from each other on the basis of their health institutions and personnel, and in terms of the strength of oversight and management that is exercised by municipal and other tiers of government.

The data needed to explore these distinctions are not always available. Demographic surveys will usually allow a country's urban poor to be studied as a group, but seldom provide reliable estimates of health among the poor in any given city, to say nothing of the subgroup of poor residents who live in a city's slums. Although there is good reason to expect deficiencies of health personnel and services in the smaller and less-advantaged cities, the empirical evidence on this point is still very thin. The comprehensive review provided by Dussault and Franceschini (2006) emphasizes urban–rural imbalances in health personnel, but does not differentiate among types of urban areas.

The urban poor

Intra-urban health inequalities—which are all too often overlooked by health and development agencies—are clearly apparent in household survey data. Using the 90 DHSs mentioned earlier, the Panel on Urban Population Dynamics (2003) estimated all-cause infant mortality for the urban poor, other urban households, and all rural households. The results are summarized in Table 10.7.2. As can be seen, the urban poor face significantly greater mortality risks than other urban residents, although as a rule, rural-dwellers face even higher levels of risk. In a survey-by-survey comparison of the poor urban and rural infants, this study found that the risks facing the urban poor were significantly lower in about two-thirds of the surveys. However, in 29 per cent of the surveys, poor urban infants faced significantly higher mortality risks than their rural counterparts. (In the remaining surveys, there was no significant difference between poor urban and rural infants.) Even the generalization that urban infant mortality is lower than rural needs to be carefully qualified; much depends on whether the urban poor are separated out in the urban–rural comparisons.

The evidence available does not yet permit broad pronouncements to be made about the relative risks of the urban poor and rural-dwellers that apply irrespective of health measure. The National Research Council study analysed children's height for age—an indicator that summarizes a child's history of nutrition and disease—obtaining the results shown in Table 10.7.3 for children in the age range of 3–36 months. (The table's entries are Z-scores, with a value of −100 indicating that a child is one standard deviation shorter, given its age and sex, than the median height of an international reference population.) The urban poor are again seen to exhibit worse health than other urban children. When the heights of poor urban and rural children were compared, in almost all surveys (60 of the 67 examined) the poor urban children were found to be significantly taller for their age than were rural children.

Table 10.7.2 Infant mortality estimates for urban poor, urban non-poor, and rural, by region

DHSs (in region)	Rural	Urban	
		Poor	Non-poor
North Africa	81	60	43
Sub-Saharan Africa	103	89	74
Southeast Asia	59	53	27
South, Central, West Asia	74	69	49
Latin America	69	62	39
Total	86	75	56

Rates expressed per 1000 births.
Source: Panel on Urban Population Dynamics. In: Montgomery MR et al., editors. *Cities transformed: demographic change and its implications in the developing world.* Washington (DC): National Academies Press (2003).

Table 10.7.3 Height-for-age **Z**-scores among children 3–36 months of age, by residence and poverty status

DHSs (in region)	All rural	Urban	
		Poor	Non-poor
North Africa	−155.00	−122.35	−86.53
Sub-Saharan Africa	−184.60	−153.64	−125.86
Southeast Asia	−139.01	−106.46	−48.18
South, Central, West Asia	−176.78	−157.95	−120.31
Latin America	−157.09	−130.28	−80.61
Total	−173.51	−145.43	−109.37

Values are Z-scores, with a value of −100, indicating that a child is 1 SD shorter for its age and sex than the median height of an international reference population.
Source: Panel on Urban Population Dynamics. In: Montgomery MR et al, editors. *Cities transformed: demographic change and its implications in the developing world.* Washington (DC): National Academies Press ;(2003).

In the height-for-age measure, evidence of an urban advantage persists even for the urban poor.

As is well known, poor urban-dwellers are exposed to substantial risks when their neighbourhoods lack the public health infrastructure needed to safeguard water supply and assure sanitary disposal of waste (UN-Habitat 2003a, 2003b) The WHO (WHO 2002) estimates that in 2001, diarrhoeal diseases accounted for some 2 million deaths, almost all of which took place in low- and middle-income countries, with unsafe water, inadequate sanitation, and poor hygiene implicated as the possible causes in a large percentage of these. In its examination of data from the DHSs, the Panel on Urban Population Dynamics (2003) showed that urban poverty is associated with a lack of access to piped drinking water and with inadequate sanitation. Table 10.7.4 presents selected findings from this study, again comparing poor urban households with other urban and also rural households. As the table shows, the urban poor are markedly ill-served in comparison with other urban households. Rural households receive even less than poor urban households by way of water and sanitation services, although they benefit to an extent from lower population densities, which offer a form of natural protection against some communicable diseases.

Investments in public health infrastructure require the mobilization of substantial financial sums, and although public health authorities can help publicize needs and exert pressure, the key decision makers are generally located elsewhere in the political–bureaucratic system.[3] There are, however, complementary initiatives that lie squarely within the purview of public health. As McGranahan (2007) argues, citing Cairncross and Valdmanis (2006) among others, the literature on water and sanitation has tended to give too little attention to the hygienic and storage behaviours that cause

---

[3] See Evans (Evans B. Understanding the urban poor's vulnerabilities in sanitation and water supply. Paper presented at *Innovations for an Urban World*, the Rockefeller Foundation's *Urban Summit*; 2007; Bellagio, Italy) on recent innovations in financing improvements in urban water supply, sanitation, and housing.

Table 10.7.4 Percentages of poor urban households with access to services, compared with rural households and the urban non-poor

DHSs (in region)		Piped water on premises	Water in neigh- bourhood	Flush toilet	Pit toilet
North Africa	Rural	41.6	37.3	41.3	17.5
	Urban poor	67.3	27.8	83.7	8.5
	Urban non-poor	90.8	7.8	96.3	2.6
Sub-Saharan Africa	Rural	7.8	55.7	1.1	47.6
	Urban poor	26.9	61.6	13.0	65.9
	Urban non-poor	47.6	45.8	27.4	67.2
Southeast Asia	Rural	18.6	53.7	55.5	24.3
	Urban poor	34.0	53.7	61.8	22.9
	Urban non-poor	55.8	40.1	89.0	9.4
South, Central, West Asia	Rural	28.1	53.6	4.3	55.4
	Urban poor	58.0	36.3	39.8	34.1
	Urban non-poor	80.2	17.7	64.0	23.2
Latin America	Rural	31.4	36.4	12.6	44.0
	Urban poor	58.7	35.2	33.6	47.0
	Urban non-poor	72.7	24.9	63.7	31.6
Total	Rural	18.5	50.7	7.5	46.6
	Urban poor	41.5	49.4	28.3	51.7
	Urban non-poor	61.5	34.0	48.4	46.5

Source: Panel on Urban Population Dynamics. In: Montgomery MR *et al.*, editors. *Cities transformed: demographic change and its implications in the developing world.* Washington (DC): National Academies Press (2003).

water to be contaminated after it has been drawn from the pipes. Important faecal–oral routes for contamination can be addressed through domestic hygiene interventions, including an emphasis on hand-washing especially after defecation, control of flies, and encouragement of safer practices in food preparation and water storage. Cairncross and Valdmanis (2006) assembled evidence showing that behavioural interventions in these areas can achieve substantial reductions in diarrhoeal diseases.

Other important health risks also arise in or near the homes of the poor, with the risks presented by indoor air pollution being increasingly recognized. Recent estimates suggest that, worldwide, more than 2 billion people rely on solid fuels, traditional stoves, and open fires for their cooking, lighting, and heating needs (Larson & Rosen 2002). These fuels generate hazardous pollutants—including suspended particulate matter, carbon monoxide, nitrogen dioxide, and other harmful gases—that are believed to substantially raise the risks of acute respiratory infections and chronic obstructive pulmo- nary disorders. Such fuels are often used by the urban poor, who must cook in enclosed or inadequately ventilated spaces. The health burdens associated with indoor air pollution are likely to fall heavily upon women, who spend much of their time cooking and tending fires, and also afflict the children who accompany them.

The spatially concentrated urban poor

It is not surprising that when poor city-dwellers live in close prox- imity to each other without the benefit of safe drinking water and

adequate sanitation, they face elevated risks from water-, air-, and food-borne diseases. This much has been known since the eight- eenth century in the West, well before the mechanisms of transmis- sion were understood (Woods 2003). It remains difficult, however, to divide the overall risks facing slum-dwellers into the risks attrib- utable to household poverty, and the additional risks produced by the spatial concentration of poverty in slum neighbourhoods and communities.

Although not definitive on this score, Fig. 10.7.2 is suggestive of the impact of concentrated poverty on child mortality in Nairobi, Kenya. In the slums of Nairobi, child mortality rates, at 150 per 1000 births, are substantially above the rates seen elsewhere in that city; slum mortality rates are high enough even to exceed rural Kenyan mortality. The addition to risk evident in these slums may be due to multiple factors: The poor quality and quantity of water and sanitation in these communities; inadequate hygienic practices; poor ventilation and dependence on hazardous cooking fuels; the city's highly monetized health system, which for the poor delays or prevents access to modern health services; and the transmission of disease among densely settled slum-dwellers.

There are additional factors of a social epidemiological character that are worth considering. Facing health threats from their unpro- tected physical environments—with the lack of services being a con- stant reminder of social exclusion—and lacking the incomes needed to counteract these daily threats, the urban poor may well feel una- ble to take effective action to safeguard their health. Poor individuals and families may thus lack the sense of self-efficacy needed to ener- gize their health-seeking behaviour in such difficult environments. Poor communities may be reminded by the absence of basic services that the community as a whole is socially excluded and lacks the political voice needed to bring attention to its plight. At the individ- ual and family level, as we will discuss, social exclusion combined with the daily stresses of poverty may bring on paralyzing fatigue, anxiety, low-level depression, and other expressions of mental ill- health. At the community level, the symptoms may be expressed in the weaknesses and fragilities of local community organizations; that is, in the lack of what has been termed 'bonding' social capital.

The urban health system

The concept of 'health system' is a very broad one and bringing definition to it is especially difficult in urban areas, within which a disparate set of health providers serves what is typically a highly diverse population, with core health needs arising in part from the many ways in which the population's subgroups come into contact. The urban health system is itself situated within larger political– economic frames at the country level. In the structural adjustment era of the 1980s and early 1990s, a number of low- and middle-income countries introduced user fees into public-sector care as they under- took broad health sector reforms (Harpham 2007). As discussed earlier, in many of these countries, the process of decentralization— a transformation of governance that accelerated in the mid-1990s, and which is in its way as profound as the urban transformation—is reshaping relationships between national, regional, and local gov- ernments, with important implications for health service planning, finance, and service delivery. These developments provide the con- text for our discussion of urban health systems.

A distinguishing feature of urban health systems is the promi- nence of the private sector. Not surprisingly, given the higher average

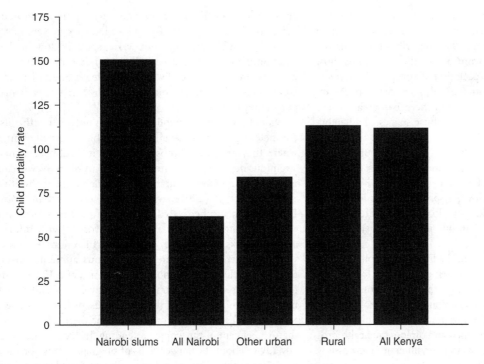

Fig. 10.7.2 Comparison of child mortality rates ($_5q_0$) in the Nairobi slums sample with rates for Nairobi, other cities, rural areas, and Kenya as a whole.
Source: African Population and Health Research Center. *Population and health dynamics in Nairobi's informal settlements: report of the Nairobi cross-sectional slums survey [NCSS] 2000.* Nairobi: African Population and Health Research Center (2002).

levels of income in urban populations and the income diversity that establishes market niches, private services tend to be much more developed in cities than in rural areas, especially in the larger cities (Dussault & Franceschini 2006). Fee-for-service arrangements are generally characteristic of urban health care, whereas rural services are often ostensibly provided free of cost (or made available for nominal fees) at public health posts and clinics.[4]

In the more monetized urban economy, the urban poor without cash on hand can find themselves unable to gain entry to the modern system of hospitals, clinics, and well-trained providers. They may then seek care in other niches of the urban system where less-trained providers make drugs and diagnoses available for affordable fees, and may also pursue traditional practitioners, who can adjust the level and type of payment to the needs of their poor clients.

As the Islam *et al.* (2006) study has documented for Manila and Indore, India, urban health providers are well aware of the effects of monetization on the health-seeking behaviour of the poor. They see poor clients who, having endured their illnesses until care cannot be put off any longer, finally present themselves in a more debilitated condition than they would otherwise have been. Health providers realize that the poor are likely to abandon courses of prescribed medication to save on the costs of purchasing medicines, or may economize by buying less than what was prescribed. They are not really surprised when the poor fail to return as requested for follow-ups and assessments of progress.

In only very few low- and middle-income countries is it possible for the urban poor to receive subsidized care from for-profit private

providers, and generally such subsidies are available only through the private non-profit and public-sector clinics and hospitals. Manila's public-sector subsidy programme provides one instructive example. In this health system, subsidies are made available for the purchase of medicines but supplies are not similarly covered. As one physician said in exasperation: 'Sometimes, they say they can ask for discounts or even for free medicines, depending on the [income] class. But in supplies, they cannot. So, for instance, they get antibiotics for free [but] if you do not have syringe, how can you provide it? We still ask them to buy syringe to provide the vaccines'.

As this quotation suggests, stockouts of medicines and basic supplies such as syringes occur frequently in Manila's public-sector facilities. When they occur, it is left to the patient to find the funds to seek out prescribed medicines and supplies at private pharmacies or other sources. In Manila, the lowest tier of the public health system—the barangay health centre—is a vital component of the system for the poor because, for various reasons, the barangay centres are more likely to hold small stocks of some of the subsidized medicines.

As the Manila example illustrates, subsidies for the urban poor often depend on an unsystematic set of arrangements, requiring poor patients and their families to spend time searching and negotiating with what must be a bewildering variety of personnel at scattered locations. As they engage in this form of health-seeking behaviour, the poor can be discouraged by the difficulties of finding affordable transport, inconvenient hours of operation at clinics or health centres, the frequent absence of key staff, and long waits to receive care. In effect, the poor are being asked to substitute the costs of their time for the prospect of reduced costs of medicines. In a full-cost sense, a subsidy for the poor that exists in theory may prove to be no subsidy at all.

We have emphasized the monetary costs of health care, which clearly discourage the urban poor, but they can also be driven away

---

4 Even in Latin America, where health-insurance systems are more inclusive than in other low- and middle-income regions, only 20 per cent of the urban poor are covered by insurance. (Fay M, editor. *The urban poor in Latin America*. Washington [DC]: The World Bank; 2005.)

from the modern health system by the indifference or abuse that they anticipate at the hands of formal sector health workers. A study of urban Zimbabwe (Bassett *et al.* 1997) describes the nature of interactions between nurses and women from the community thus:

'To community women, the expectation of abrupt or rude treatment was the main complaint about the health services. Community complaints were voiced most strongly in the urban areas, where accusations of patient neglect and even abuse suggested a heightened hostility between the clinic and community in the urban setting. Several explanations for nurse behaviour were put forward, chief among them was elitism ... it is in urban areas that class differentiation is most advanced. [The perspective of nurses differed. For them] overwork and low pay promote the adoption of the attitude of an industrial worker—to do what is required and no more. Most nurses work more than one job, not to get rich but to survive'.

As this quotation suggests, much of the literature emphasizes the social distance between providers and their patients, the formal language that providers can use to reinforce their own status, and the possibilities for rude or abusive behaviour on part of the staff towards poor patients. But the literature has not much stressed how difficult it is, even for the most well-intentioned and diplomatic health provider, to get basic information across to poor, illiterate, and possibly intimidated patients. As a Manila obstetrician–gynaecologist explained (Islam *et al.* 2006):

'I guess, for 90 per cent of our patients, it is us who tell them things. Although there are some who are really inquisitive, especially those who have had some education. [But among the urban poor?] They just accept everything we tell them. They rarely ask questions. And sometimes it is difficult to relate to them. They have a hard time understanding what we are saying, even if we use the most basic words or terms. Like for instance, sometimes, we tell them, this is the right way to take the medicine; to make sure that they understand us, we ask them to demonstrate. [Are they receptive to that?] Some, yes. But the others just don't care. They don't know anything, they don't even know when was their last period, family history, nothing. It's really frustrating'.

When the poor do succeed in receiving formal health care, is that care likely to be of sufficient quality to make an effective difference to their health? A recent urban quality-of-care study in New Delhi raises serious doubts on this score (Das & Hammer 2007a, 2007b). The study was set in both slum and non-slum neighbourhoods, covering a range of income levels. A full inventory was made of the health providers who serve these neighbourhoods; it revealed that a 15-minute walk would bring a typical neighbourhood resident within reach of 70 health providers of some sort. Even for the poor, access in the sense of geographic distance was not the problem in this case; and if anything, the Delhi poor tended to seek care for illness at least as often as the non-poor. The study assessed the quality of health-care provision in two ways: Via a series of vignettes measuring provider knowledge of the steps to take in making a diagnosis and prescribing treatment or referral (rating the provider responses in relation to examination protocols); and by a follow-up in which many of the same providers were observed as they interacted with patients.

The study found that the quality of care available in the poor neighbourhoods was so low that the authors could fairly describe it as 'money for nothing'. Both public-sector and private providers serve the poor neighbourhoods of Delhi, and both know less about appropriate care than the providers who practice in better-off neighbourhoods. (Levels of provider knowledge were low across all study neighbourhoods, but were especially low in the poor neighbourhoods.) When later observed as they interacted with patients, providers generally asked even fewer questions and exerted even less effort in examinations than their vignettes had suggested they would.

Evidently, the Indian public sector does not see to it that its more competent providers are allocated to the poor neighbourhoods where they are needed most. In short, it would seem that even strenuous health-seeking efforts on the part of the New Delhi poor would bring them no assurance of reasonable quality health care.

Mayank *et al.* (2001), who studied poor urban women in Dakshinpuri, another New Delhi slum, found that local antenatal clinics did little to provide pregnant women with information about the risks of pregnancy and childbirth. A number of pregnant women suffered from potentially serious ailments—over two-thirds were clinically diagnosed as anaemic, and 12 per cent were found to be seriously anaemic. Yet, relatively few understood that high fevers and swelling of the face, hands, or feet might be symptoms of conditions that could endanger their pregnancy. Fewer than 10 per cent of the women attending the local clinic were given any advice about the danger signs of pregnancy. It is not altogether surprising that the maternal mortality rate in this urban sample was estimated at 645 deaths per 100 000, a rate not much different from that prevailing in rural India.

Figure 10.7.3 shows that low quality of care is generally characteristic of urban India (Fig. 10.7.3a) and is also a concern in the urban areas of the Philippines (Fig. 10.7.3b). The figure depicts the percentage of women who, in one or more prenatal care visits, were warned of the complications of pregnancy. Among poor urban Indian women, not even 40 per cent are told during prenatal visits of the danger signs of pregnancy. Although the percentages are somewhat higher in urban Philippines, less than half of the poor women are informed of the risks and fewer still are told where to seek care if signs of danger surface.

Urban health risks and risk factors

In this subsection, we turn attention to specific urban risks and causes of mortality and morbidity. Several themes unite this material. First among them is the importance of disaggregation of urban health conditions and risk factors by poverty and place. A second and closely-related theme is that of urban social epidemiology, with emphasis on the concepts of individual and collective efficacy in health seeking. A third theme in the discussion concerns health conditions or risks that are sometimes overlooked, or which are not as well-integrated as they might be in urban public health policies. Mental health is perhaps the leading example of such a condition. It is closely associated with poverty and with the health threats that arise from violence and alcohol abuse, which place disproportionate burdens on women. Other examples include the burdens of illness and death stemming from road traffic accidents and outdoor air pollution. In many countries, HIV/AIDS already occupies a prominent place on the urban health agenda, whereas urban tuberculosis and malaria receive less attention. Only the most expansive public health programmes in low- and middle-income countries have conceived of the field of action in such broad terms as to encompass all these areas.

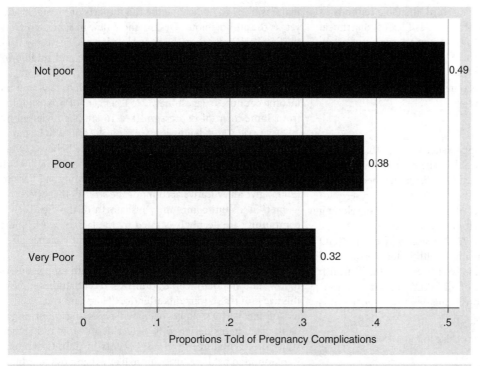

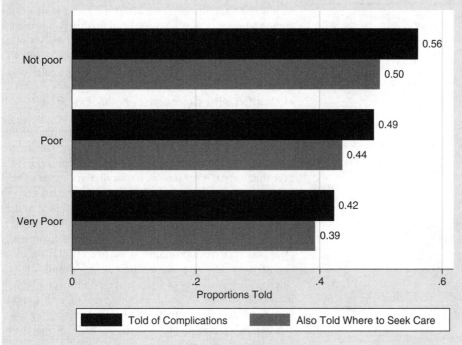

Fig. 10.7.3 Information on pregnancy complications given during prenatal care, by relative poverty, women with one or more visits, in urban India and urban Philippines:
(a) Women informed of complications and their danger signs during pregnancy, urban India; (b) Women informed of complications and danger signs during pregnancy, and told where to seek care if these appear, urban Philippines.
Source: Islam M, Montgomery MR, Taneja S. *Urban health and care-seeking behavior: a case study of slums in India and the Philippines.* Bethesda [MD]: PHRPlus Program, Abt Associates (2006).

To bring some order to a wide-ranging discussion, we begin with an overview of urban causes of death and disability, drawing upon data from Mexico, one of the few low- and middle-income countries that can provide reliable information. With this as background, we then present a series of remarks on the specific features of urban health that warrant closer study.

The urban burden of disease

Table 10.7.5 shows the 15 leading causes of disability-adjusted life years (DALYs) lost in rural and urban areas for Mexico. Several lessons can be extracted from this table. First, urban areas do not necessarily present health profiles that are wholly distinct from those of rural areas. In Mexico, the causes of DALYs lost are much the same in urban and rural areas, although they follow a different rank order. Of the top five causes in Mexico's urban areas, three (deaths related to motor vehicles, homicide and violence, and cirrhosis) are also found among the top five in rural areas. Second, interventions to address two of the most important causes of death and disability in urban Mexico—those related to violence, and to traffic-related deaths and injuries—would in many countries be considered outside the scope of the public health system. Third, the table reminds us that even in a middle-income country such as Mexico, diarrhoeal disease and pneumonia continue to be important causes of urban death and disability—here as elsewhere, an epidemiological transition is underway whereby the burden of disease is tilting towards non-communicable causes, but this transition is evidently far from being complete.

Mental health

Mental health, as such, makes no appearance in Table 10.7.5, but it is arguably a central factor in the health of the urban poor, and one whose contribution to the urban burden of disease has been under-appreciated. Over the past decade, the WHO has issued a series of reports emphasizing the importance of mental health in developing as well as developed countries (WHO 1996, 2001, 2005a).

In a recent review, Prince *et al.* (2007) summarize the WHO burden-of-disease estimates for mental health in low-income and middle-income countries. In these countries, mental ill-health accounts for roughly 24 per cent of all DALYs lost due to non-communicable diseases. For reasons to be described shortly, this

Table 10.7.5 Disability-adjusted years of life lost in Mexico, by cause and area of residence

Cause	Rural	Rural rank	Urban	Urban rank	Rural urban
Diarrhoea	12.0	1	2.8	9	4.28
Pneumonia	9.3	2	3.9	7	2.39
Homicide and violence	9.2	3	7.4	2	1.23
Motor vehicle-related deaths	7.9	4	8.3	1	0.95
Cirrhosis	7.5	5	6.3	4	1.19
Anaemia and malnutrition	6.8	6	2.4	11	2.86
Road traffic accidents	5.5	7	6.8	3	0.81
Ischaemic heart disease	5.1	8	5.3	6	0.96
Diseases of the digestive system	4.7	9	1.7	15	2.74
Diabetes mellitus	4.1	10	5.7	5	0.72
Cerebrovascular disease	3.0	11	3.0	8	1.02
Alcohol dependence	3.0	11	1.9	13	1.56
Accidents (falls)	2.8	13	2.6	10	1.09
Chronic lung disease	2.6	14	1.9	13	1.39
Nephritis	2.2	15	2.2	12	1.01

1991 estimates, expressed per 1000 population.

Source: Lozano R, Murray C, Frenk J. El peso de las enfermedades en Mexico. In: Hill K, Morelos JB, Wong R, editors. *Las consecuencias de las transiciones demografica y epidemiológical en América Latina.* Mexico City: El Colegio de México (1999).

figure is likely to understate the full impacts of mental health. And yet, as the authors note, 'Despite these new insights, ten years after the first WHO report on the global burden of disease, mental health remains a low priority in most low-income and middle-income countries'.

Community-based studies of mental health in low- and middle-income countries suggest that 12–51 per cent of urban adults suffer from some form of depression (see 16 studies reviewed by Blue 1999). Anxiety and depression are typically found to be more prevalent among urban women than men and are believed to be more prevalent in poor than in non-poor urban neighbourhoods (Almeida-Filho *et al.* 2004). In a study of Mumbai, Parkar *et al.* (2003) give an evocative account of the stresses that affect men and women in a slum community just north of the city. Men in this community are deeply frustrated by the lack of work, and this is reflected in a high incidence of alcoholism and violence directed at their wives.

Although less is known about mental health among adolescents in low- and middle-income countries, recent studies indicate that this age group also warrants attention. Harpham *et al.* (2004) made use of the WHO's short-form, self-reporting questionnaire—a bank of 20 items designed to detect depression and anxiety—to study the mental health of adolescents in Cali, Colombia. Girls were found to be three times more likely than boys to exhibit signs of ill-health (as Prince *et al.* 2007, note, the female–male ratio among adults is typically 1.5–2.0) and further multivariate analysis showed that low levels of schooling, within-family violence, and perceptions that violence afflicts the community were all significantly associated with mental ill-health among adolescents.

There are two avenues by which an individual's mental ill-health might affect other dimensions of health. First, it has been hypothesized that socioeconomic stress undermines the physiological systems that sustain health. Prince *et al.* (2007) emphasize the effects of depression on serotonin metabolism, cortisol metabolism, inflammatory processes, and cell-mediated immunity; they also note that mental disorders are implicated in a range of behaviours (e.g. smoking, poor diet, obesity) that raise the risks of other diseases. Boardman (2004), McEwen (1998), Steptoe and Marmot (2002), and Cohen *et al.* (2006) provide supportive evidence, although Hu *et al.* (2007) are sceptical of the hypothesized link from poverty to socioeconomic stress to cortisol metabolism, finding little evidence for it in their large sample of Taiwanese elderly. The possibility of such adverse spill-over effects from an individual's mental ill-health to other areas of health, and the need for a full accounting of these effects in calculating the disease burden stemming from mental disorders, is the principal theme of the comprehensive review by Prince *et al.* (2007).

The second avenue needing exploration also involves spill-over effects, but in this case the posited linkage would connect women's mental health to the health-seeking energies they can deploy on behalf of their children and other family members. To judge from the review by Prince *et al.* (2007), very little research has been conducted on how mental health affects women's health-seeking behaviour. A few studies have linked mental ill-health to the difficulties that individuals face in adhering to their own treatment regimens, especially the demanding protocols required in antiretroviral therapies for HIV/AIDS and directly observed short-course treatments for tuberculosis. A bit more attention has been given to the associations between a woman's mental health and her reproductive health, and between the health status of pregnant women and their children's birth weight, with the latter possibly involving health-seeking behaviour. But almost nothing seems to have been written on whether and how mental ill-health undermines the sense of self-efficacy that motivates a woman to seek health-care for others in her family. This is a surprising gap in the literature, especially in view of the well-documented role that women play in protecting the health of their families and the equally common finding that mental ill-health is more common among women than men.[5]

Intimate-partner violence and alcohol abuse

Violence in urban areas takes a variety of forms, ranging from political and extra-judicial violence to gang violence, local violent crime, and abuse taking place within the home. Moser (2004) develops a framework within which these complex forms of violence can be analysed and describes the points of intervention within the judicial, public health, and other urban systems (also see Winton 2004). Garrett and Ahmed (2004) have developed a module for measuring aspects of crime, violence, and physical insecurity that could be adapted for use in surveys, so that these problems can be better documented than they are at present. Our discussion is mainly concerned with intimate-partner violence and its links to alcohol abuse and women's mental health.

Heise *et al.* (1994) reviewed community-based data for eight urban areas from different regions of the developing world, finding that mental and physical abuse of women by their partners was common, with damaging consequences for women's physical and psychological well-being. Using data collected from a module included in several DHSs, Kishor and Johnson (2004) examined

whether women had ever been beaten by a spouse or partner. In Cambodia, 18 per cent of women had been beaten, and the percentages in the other study countries were also high: Colombia (44 per cent), Dominican Republic (22 per cent), Egypt (34 per cent), Haiti (29 per cent), India (19 per cent), Nicaragua (30 per cent), Peru (42 per cent), and Zambia (48 per cent). In seeking to understand why women who were the victims of violence did not seek help from the authorities or others outside the home, this study found that embarrassment was a major reason given by women, as well as the belief that it would be futile to seek care or that partner violence was simply a part of life. In some countries (but not in all), poor women were more likely than other women to have experienced violence at the hands of their spouses or partners. Where the connection could be explored, strong links were also found between spousal alcohol abuse and violence.

These findings were echoed in the WHO (2005b) study, summarized in Fig. 10.7.4, which covered both urban and rural study sites. The WHO analysis also documented a close association between the experience of violence and women's mental health. As Fig. 10.7.5 shows, among the women who had been abused by their partner in this study's Bangladeshi urban site (left-most bars), some 21 per cent had had thoughts of suicide, against only 7 per cent of the women who had not been abused. In all but one of the sites in the study, the difference in this measure of mental health was statistically significant, and as can be seen in the figure, the ratios are on the order of 2:1 or higher.

Other forms of urban violence also merit attention. Crime is particularly prevalent in Latin America's large cities, where it disproportionately victimizes men living in low-income neighbourhoods (Barata *et al.* 1998; Grant 1999; Heinemann & Verner 2006). Data collected between 1991 and 1993 in São Paulo suggested that men aged 15–24 years in low-income areas were over five times likelier to fall victim to homicide than were men of the same age in

---

[5] See Montgomery & Ezeh (2005b) for further discussion with attention to social capital and collective efficacy.

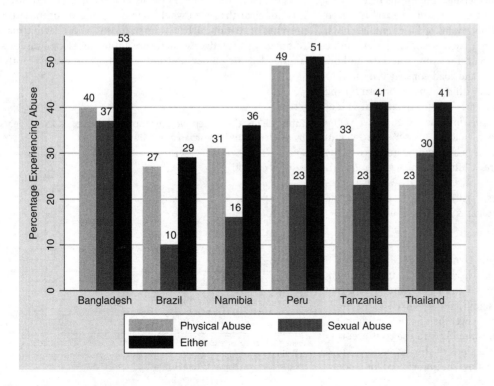

Fig. 10.7.4 Experience of physical or sexual violence by an intimate partner since age 15, among ever-partnered urban women.
Source: WHO. *WHO multi-country study on women's health and domestic violence against women: summary report of initial results on prevalence, health outcomes and women's responses.* Geneva: World Health Organization (2005b).

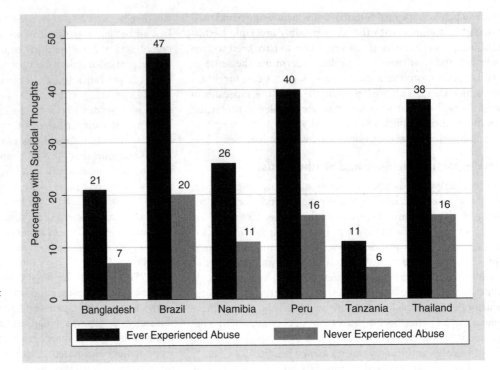

Fig. 10.7.5 Percentage of ever-partnered urban women reporting suicidal thoughts, according to their experience of physical or sexual violence, or both, by an intimate partner.
Source: WHO. *WHO multi-country study on women's health and domestic violence against women: summary report of initial results on prevalence, health outcomes and women's responses.* Geneva: World Health Organization (2005b).

higher-income areas (Soares *et al.* cited in Grant 1999). South African cities also exhibit extraordinarily high rates of violent crime (Stone 2006).

A need exists for systems that can provide women and the poor with some protection from the varied forms of urban violence to which they are vulnerable within and outside the home. To create such systems will require new partnerships linking agencies across urban sectors. In the transport sector, for example, there is a need to make safe the areas where the poor wait for buses and jeepneys; the health sector also has a role to play in security, in that public latrines can be places of risk especially for women; and the authorities responsible for electrification and road construction need to attend to the unlit paths and lanes within slums, a concern for the poor who must commute in the early morning hours or late at night. Effective partnerships against crime and violence involve the formulation of community-driven violence-prevention strategies and the initiation of dialogue between community groups and the police. (The police may initially resist efforts to involve them in this way, complaining of having to be 'social workers' as well as policemen.) Creation of safe spaces is especially high on the policy agenda for adolescent girls and boys (Erulkar & Matheka 2007).

Reproductive health

The Panel on Urban Population Dynamics (2003) provides a lengthy discussion of reproductive health among urban women; here, we select only a few points for emphasis. Among all urban women, those who are poor are significantly less likely to use modern contraception to achieve control over their family-building (see Table 10.7.6). They are generally more likely to use contraception than rural women, but in some regions of the developing world there is little to separate the two groups. The unmet need for modern

contraception—this is measured by the proportion of women in a reproductive union who say that they want to prevent or delay their next birth, believe themselves to be capable of conceiving, and yet do not make use of modern contraception to achieve their stated aims—is markedly higher among poor urban than other urban women.

As the Panel on Urban Population Dynamics (2003) discusses, it is not clear that even when they use modern contraception to prevent conception, urban women do so in an effective manner. Although quantitative estimates are limited to selected case studies, unintended pregnancy and induced abortion are evidently not

Table 10.7.6 Contraceptive use among women aged 25–29 years, by residence, and for urban areas, by poverty status

DHSs (by region)		Urban	
	All rural	Poor	Non-poor
North Africa	0.26	0.37	0.48
Sub-Saharan Africa	0.08	0.13	0.22
Southeast Asia	0.44	0.40	0.47
South, Central, West Asia	0.33	0.35	0.44
Latin America	0.32	0.37	0.47
Total	0.22	0.26	0.35

Source: Panel on Urban Population Dynamics. In: Montgomery MR *et al.*, editors. *Cities transformed: demographic change and its implications in the developing world.* Washington (DC): National Academies Press (2003).

uncommon for urban women.[6] To cite a few examples: Women in three squatter settlements in Karachi, Pakistan, were estimated to have a lifetime rate of 3.6 abortions per woman (Jamil & Fikree 2002). Another study found abortion to be widespread in Abidjan, Côte d'Ivoire, where abortion is illegal yet nearly one-third of the women surveyed who had ever been pregnant had had one (Desgrées du Loû et al. 2000). A recent study of Ouagadougou, Burkina Faso by Rossier (2007) estimated an annual abortion rate of 4 per cent among women aged 15–49 years, suggesting that over a reproductive lifetime, a woman would have 1.4 abortions on average. Calvés (2002) studied women in their twenties living in Yaoundé, Cameroon; of these young women, 21 per cent reported having had an abortion, with just over 8 per cent having had more than one. Once again, the fact that modern contraceptive services are available in urban areas does not imply that women, especially poor women, have the knowledge and the social and economic wherewithal to make effective use of the methods.

Maternal mortality risks offer another revealing view of urban reproductive health. Because it is difficult to predict whether life-threatening problems will emerge in the course of a woman's pregnancy, delivery, and the aftermath, the prevention of maternal mortality depends crucially on fast access to emergency care.

---

6   The Alan Guttmacher Institute (AGI. *Sharing responsibility: women, society, and abortion worldwide*. New York [NY]: Alan Guttmacher Institute; 1999) provides an excellent overview of induced abortion, a generally hidden and difficult-to-study area of health. See *International Family Planning Perspectives*, which is a good source of information on this topic; available from: http://www.guttmacher.org/pubs. The journal *Studies in Family Planning* is another helpful source; available from: http://www. blackwell-synergy.com/loi/sifp.

It might be thought that cities, which offer many more transport options than do rural areas, would exhibit much lower levels of maternal mortality. The cases in which the expected urban advantage does not emerge are therefore instructive about the circumstances of the urban poor.

Fikree *et al.* (1997) compared maternal mortality rates in the low-income communities of Karachi with rates in six rural districts elsewhere in Pakistan. Estimates of maternal mortality ratios (MMRs), together with their confidence bands, are shown in Fig. 10.7.6. Although the MMR estimate for Karachi is the lowest among all these sites, the rural estimates are significantly higher than Karachi's only for the remote districts of Loralai and Khuzdar. It appears that Karachi's poor suffer from maternal health disadvantages not unlike those that afflict Pakistan's rural-dwellers.

Why did the urban health advantage not prove greater in this case? In the poor communities of Karachi, some 68 per cent of the births are delivered at home and 59 per cent are attended by traditional birth attendants (TBAs). Yet, rural women are even more likely to deliver at home and to have family members or TBAs in attendance. Another study of Karachi slums (Fikree *et al.* 1994) identified the core of the problem: When acute pregnancy and delivery complications arise in these communities, there can be critical delays in locating male decision makers and obtaining their consent to hospital care. (It has not been customary for husbands or other men to be present at the time of childbirth.) Delays in initiating the search for care are compounded by the tendency for poor Karachi families to pursue local care first, going from place to place in the neighbourhood before making an effort to reach the modern health facilities located outside the neighbourhood. Fikree *et al.* (2004) have illustrated similar care-seeking patterns in a study of postpartum morbidities in the Karachi slums.

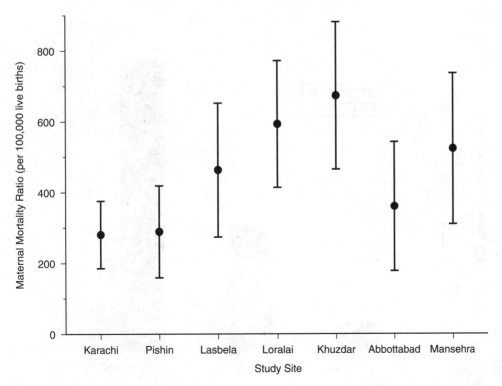

Fig. 10.7.6 Maternal mortality ratios in Karachi, Pakistan, and six rural sites. *Source:* Fikree FF, Midhet F, Sadruddin S et al. Maternal mortality in different Pakistani sites: ratios, clinical causes, and determinants. *Acta Obstetricia et Gynecologica Scandinavica* 1997;**76**:637–45.

HIV/AIDS

An enormous literature is now available on the social epidemiology of HIV/AIDS in both developing and developed countries. Despite the quantities of research underway on HIV/AIDS, much remains to be learned about its social components. Indeed, although HIV/AIDS is commonly thought to be more prevalent in urban than rural areas, until recently the scientific basis for this belief has been thin (UNAIDS 2004). In only a few low- and middle-income countries are community-based studies of prevalence now available that can quantify the urban–rural differences.[7]

Figure 10.7.7 presents findings from several nationally representative community-based studies in which prevalence is estimated from blood samples taken in connection with a DHS. In these three cases—Mali, Kenya, and Zambia—urban prevalence rates are clearly much higher than rural rates. Where HIV/AIDS is concerned, there is little evidence of the 'urban advantage' that is seen in other domains of health. However, circular and urban-to-rural migration is contributing to the spread of disease in rural areas (UNAIDS 2004), and many observers foresee an era of rising rural incidence and prevalence.

Because the community-based studies are relatively recent, the role played by urban poverty in the risks of HIV/AIDS in low- and middle-income countries is only beginning to be studied. Using the community surveys conducted under the DHS programme,

---

[7] See Dyson (Dyson T. HIV/AIDS and urbanization. *Population and Development Review* 2003;**29**:427–42.) Country profiles are available from http://www.census.gov/ipc/www/hivaidsn.html, but these profiles are worked up from the reports of selected clinics and various sentinel sites, which do not necessarily yield statistically representative portraits for urban or rural populations.

Mishra *et al.* (2007) found that contrary to expectation, HIV prevalence is higher among the better-off families. These families were more likely to live in urban areas, which accounts for a part of the association, and other risk factors (including sexual risk-taking, use of condoms, and male circumcision) tended to mask the association between living standards and prevalence. Even with statistical controls for such factors in place, a positive association between living standards and HIV prevalence persisted.

In studies of urban adolescents and other selected socioeconomic groups, however, poverty has been linked to higher HIV prevalence as well as to a number of contributing risk factors, including earlier sexual initiation and more reported forced or traded sex, which would seem to place poor women at higher risk of contracting the virus (Hallman 2004). In short, the association with living standards is still a matter of dispute.

Tuberculosis

Tuberculosis is even today among the leading causes of death for adults in low- and middle-income countries, killing an estimated 1.6 million people worldwide in 2005 (WHO 2007b). As in the nineteenth century, urban crowding increases the risk of contracting tuberculosis (van Rie *et al.* 1999), and high-density low-income urban communities may face elevated levels of risk. The interactions between HIV/AIDS and tuberculosis, and the spread of multi-drug-resistant strains of the disease, have generated fears of a global resurgence of tuberculosis and have caused WHO to expand its programme beyond DOTS as such.

The concept of urban collective efficacy is directly relevant to the DOTS strategy, the core of WHO's treatment strategy. In a study of tuberculosis in urban Ethiopia, Sagbakken *et al.* (2003) showed how the local social resources of urban communities (organized in 'TB clubs') can be marshalled to reduce the stigma associated with

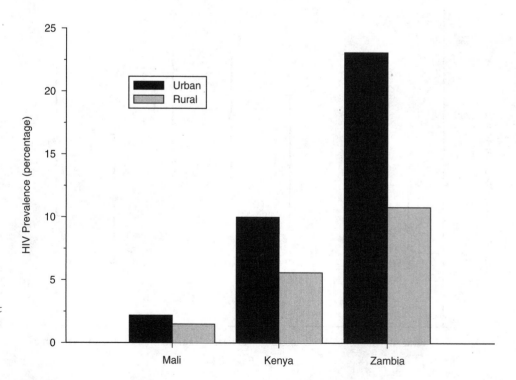

Fig. 10.7.7 Estimates of urban and rural prevalence of HIV from the Demographic and Health Surveys in Mali, 2001; Kenya, 2003; and Zambia, 2001–2002.
Source: Mali Ministère de la Santé. *Enquête Démographique et de Santé Mali 2001.* Mali; Calverton [MD]: Ministère de la Santé, ORC Macro; 2002; Kenya Central Bureau of Statistics. *Kenya Demographic and Health Survey 2003: preliminary report.* Nairobi, Kenya: Central Bureau of Statistics; 2003; Zambia Central Statistical Office. *Zambia Demographic and Health Survey 2001–2002.* Zambia; Calverton [MD]: Central Statistical Office, Central Board of Health; ORC Macro (2003).

the disease and encourage patients to adhere to the demanding short-course regimen of treatment. Similar interventions have been fielded in urban India, as described by Barua and Singh (2003), using community health volunteers to identify local residents with symptoms of tuberculosis and refer them to hospitals for diagnosis; local health workers attached to the hospitals then provide follow-up care and lend support during treatment.

An elaborate system of care, involving multiple urban community and health-service associations in Lima, Peru, is described in Shin *et al.* (2004) As reported in a WHO (2007b) report, Bangladesh has made urban DOTS a focus in a programme that links non-governmental organizations, private practitioners, medical colleges, and the corporate sector. As the country profiles presented in this report make clear, a number of countries have yet to reach WHO's treatment success rate target of 85 per cent of identified patients, and although data are scarce, it is very likely that detection rates of tuberculosis among the urban poor are well below rates for other urban residents.

Urban malaria

Although malaria has often been regarded as a problem afflicting rural populations, and rural rates of transmission are known to be markedly higher than urban rates, there is clear evidence that malaria vectors have adapted to urban conditions in sub-Saharan Africa (Modiano *et al.* 1999), and some evidence suggestive of urban risks has emerged for parts of Asia as well. As Hay *et al.* (2004) argue, urban population growth in Southeast Asia, as well as sub-Saharan Africa, may be contributing substantially to the global burden of malaria morbidity.

Keiser *et al.* (2004) calculate that in urban sub-Saharan Africa, some 200 million city-dwellers face appreciable risks of malaria, and they estimate that 25–100 million clinical episodes of the disease occur annually in this region's cities and towns. Indirect estimates suggest wide variations in prevalence by site, even within small geographic areas, with higher prevalence in the suburbs and city peripheries (especially when these are adjacent to wetlands) than in city centres.[8]

Pictet *et al.* (2004) describe a recent urban intervention programme mounted in Ouagadougou, Burkina Faso's capital, which aimed to make use of the social resources of urban communities to provide care in uncomplicated cases of child malaria. Inspired by a rural programme that yielded good results, this urban programme enlisted local community residents ('health agents'), gave them training in the recognition of malarial symptoms in young children, and supplied the agents with packets of chloroquine and paracetamol in age-appropriate doses. (In Ouagadougou, a high fraction of malaria cases still respond to chloroquine, although the parasite's resistance is evidently growing.)

In cases of childhood fevers, it has been common practice for residents of the Ouagadougou slums to buy chloroquine tablets (or drugs that have a similar appearance) in local markets, using these

to medicate their ill children. Preliminary research showed, however, that the residents had little knowledge of the dosages or lengths of treatment appropriate for children. Hence, when judged against the medication practices that were already prevalent in these communities, the programme intervention was expected to improve the standard of malaria care.

When pilot-tested in two communities in Ouagadougou, the malaria intervention showed the expected positive results in the lower-income community, which was located on the fringes of the city and somewhat isolated from sources of modern health care. Of the two study communities, this was the more homogeneous in social and economic terms, and it exhibited evidence of greater 'neighbourliness' and other forms of social interaction through which information about the intervention might have circulated. In the other pilot community, however, easier access was already available to modern health clinics and reputable pharmacies, and more residents could afford to pay for their own care. In this middle-income site it proved difficult to sustain community interest in the intervention. As this Ouagadougou example shows, urban health interventions can be designed so as to tap the social energies and social organization of local neighbourhoods and communities, but the design may need to be tailored to fit the specific circumstances of each such community.

Traffic-related injuries and deaths

We now broaden the discussion to encompass sectors that have not always been linked to or carefully integrated with urban public health programmes, yet which have significant implications for health; injuries and deaths from traffic accidents are a case in point. Table 10.7.5 for Mexico showed just how important these are among all-urban causes of death and disability, but the great range of factors involved—touching on engineering concerns, and urban planning and land-use policies, as well as individual behaviour—seem in many countries to have inhibited the public health sector from taking action. The scale of this public health problem is enormous: The WHO (2004) estimates that road traffic injuries lead to 1.2 million deaths annually and an additional 20–50 million non-fatal injuries, the majority of which occur in low- and middle-income countries.

To elucidate the factors involved, Híjar *et al.* (2003) conducted a detailed analysis of pedestrian injuries in Mexico City, where pedestrian death rates are estimated at three times those of Los Angeles. Using a mix of spatially coded quantitative data and qualitative methods, these authors developed portraits of drivers and victims that underscore the importance of several mutually reinforcing risk factors: Poverty; a lack of understanding of how drivers are apt to react to pedestrians; inattention by drivers and pedestrians alike to risky conditions; insufficient public investment in traffic lights and road lighting; and dangerous mixes of industrial, commercial, and private traffic. Bartlett (2002) draws on hospital- and community-based studies to show how poverty and gender affect the risks, and how the time pressures on urban parents limit the effort they can devote to closely supervising their children.

In seeking to raise the public health profile of these important causes, the WHO (2004, 2007d) has given particular emphasis to the risks that are faced by adolescents and young adults, among whom road traffic injuries rank (worldwide) in the top three causes of death in the ages of 5–25 years. In the WHO's Africa region, it is pedestrians (especially children 5–9 years old) who face the greatest

---

[8] A detailed, time-series study of Dar es Salaam, Tanzania (see Caldas de Castro M, Yamagata Y, Mtasiwa D *et al.* Working paper on integrated urban malaria control: a case study in Dar es Salaam, Tanzania. Office of Population Research, Princeton University; 2004), which relies on an unusual combination of high-resolution aerial photography and extensive ground validation, depicts the micro-zones of high malaria risk within this city.

risks, whereas in Southeast Asia, the deaths occur disproportionately among riders of bicycles and motorized two-wheelers, who are aged 15–24 years.

Figure 10.7.8 shows how in poor countries of Asia, it is the vulnerable road users—pedestrians, bicyclists, and operators of motorized two-wheelers—who bear a greater share of the injury burden than the occupants of cars, vans, and buses. Among adolescents, young adults, and children, males face greater risks than females.

The full package of interventions known to be effective in high-income countries has typically not been implemented in low-income countries. The interventions include behavioural interventions—the promotion through media campaigns and other public-health communication outlets of seat belt use for adolescents and adults, appropriate restraints for infant and child passengers, and encouragement for bicycle and motorcycle riders to wear helmets—as well as traffic engineering concerns, such as the need to remove 'unforgiving' roadside objects, properly maintain existing roads, and situate new ones so that high-speed traffic is not routed through densely settled communities or placed near busy markets, schools, and children's play spaces.

In many low- and middle-income countries, only meagre resources are allotted to traffic control and enforcement of speed and road safety laws. Public health planners will also need to assess the priority that has been given to emergency rescue services (which may involve connections between the health system and the police) and the availability of pre-hospital care and in-hospital trauma centres.

Outdoor air pollution

Traffic and vehicular regulation are also key factors in outdoor air pollution. The Latin-American literature is especially rich in scientific analyses of outdoor urban air pollution and its effects on respiratory illness via the intake of airborne particulates and other pollutants emitted by industry and vehicles. Ribeiro and Alves Cardoso (2003) provide a thorough review of such studies for São Paulo; for Mexico City, Santos-Burgoa and Riojas-Rodríguez (2000) have assembled and reviewed a great range of studies.

There is increasing interest in the problem in India, China, and other rapidly developing countries of Asia, where the effects of economic growth are readily apparent in the levels and severity of outdoor air pollution.[9] In Delhi, a crucial public health intervention was recently made by the Supreme Court in a decision that mandated conversion to compressed natural gas (CNG) for bus, taxi, and other fleets of vehicles. There is reason to think that on a per-vehicle basis, this intervention has been effective; however, because the total volume of traffic has increased in Delhi, it is not yet obvious that the total volume of particulates and other pollutants has decreased (Kumar 2007; Narain & Krupnick 2007).

Future risks from climate change

Although much remains to be done to clarify the health implications of climate change, enough is already known to sketch the core

---

9   For an overview of air pollution issues in Asia, see http://www.healtheffects.org/Asia/papasan-overview.htm.

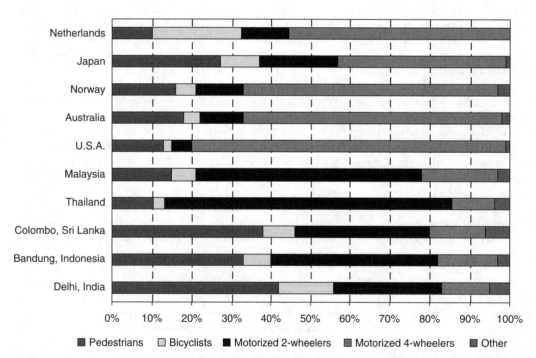

Fig. 10.7.8 Composition of road traffic injuries, by type, in selected high-income countries and Asian low- and middle-income countries.
Source: WHO. World report on road traffic injury prevention: main messages and recommendations. Geneva: World Health Organization; 2004. Available from: http://www.who.int/violence_injury_prevention/publications/road_traffic%'/world_report/whd_presentation.pdf

elements of an urban adaptation strategy for low- and middle-income countries (Huq *et al.* 2007; McGranahan *et al.* 2007; Satterthwaite *et al.* 2007). According to current estimates, gradual increases in sea level are now all but inevitable over the coming decades, and this will place large coastal urban populations under threat. Alley *et al.* (2007) forecast rises in sea level of between 0.2 m and 0.6 m by 2100, which will be accompanied by periods of exceptionally high precipitation, more intense typhoons and hurricanes, and episodes of severe thermal stress. (The health effects of heat waves have not been much studied in the low- and middle-income countries, but the effects in Europe and the United States have been well-documented.)

In Asia, many of the region's largest cities are located in the flood plains of major rivers (the Ganges–Brahmaputra, Mekong, and Yangtze rivers) and in coastal areas that have long been cyclone-prone. Mumbai saw massive floods in 2005, as did Karachi in 2007. Flooding and storm surges also present a threat in coastal African cities (e.g. Port Harcourt, Nigeria, and Mombasa, Kenya) and in Latin America (e.g. Caracas, Venezuela). Figure 10.7.9 depicts one of the major low-elevation coastal zones of China near Shanghai and Tianjin, two of the world's fastest-developing economic regions, in which increasing numbers of urban dwellers will be placed at risk.

Urban flooding risks in poor countries stem from a number of factors: The predominance of impermeable surfaces that cause water run-off; the general scarcity of parks and other green spaces to absorb these flows; rudimentary drainage systems that are often clogged by waste and which in any case are quickly overloaded with

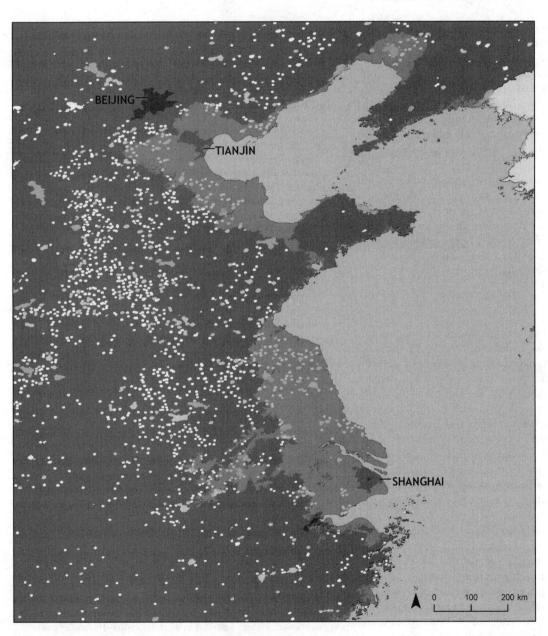

Fig. 10.7.9 Yellow Sea region of China, areas within 10 m of sea level.
Source: McGranahan G, Balk D, Anderson B. The rising tide: assessing the risks of climate change to human settlements in low-elevation coastal zones. *Environment and Urbanization* 2007;**19**:17–37.

water; and the ill-advised development of marshlands and other natural buffers. When urban flooding takes place, faecal and other hazardous materials contaminate flood waters and spill into open wells, elevating the risks of water-borne disease. The urban poor are often more exposed to these environmental hazards than others, because the housing they can afford tends to be located in the riskier areas.

As Revi (2008) discusses in a detailed analysis of urban adaptation needs in India, governments from the local to national levels and their public health systems will need to anticipate increases in extreme-weather events. The Indian Ocean tsunami of 2005 heightened attention to coastal zone management in India and the region, but to judge from Revi's account, the responsibilities for urban adaptation and disaster management have been strewn across the bureaucratic landscape and are not yet organized in any coherent manner.

He puts special emphasis on what is termed the 'lifeline' infrastructure needed to cope with extreme events: The roads, bridges and other transport systems; water, sewer, and gas pipelines; infrastructure for coastal defences and drainage; the power and telecommunications infrastructure that are of vital importance during disasters; arrangements made with local non-governmental and relief agencies for alerting populations to imminent threats and responding to disaster; and the hospitals, fire and police stations, schools, military forces and other first-responders involved during the onset and aftermath of such disasters (McGranahan 2007; Satterthwaite et al. 2007). In short, to plan adequately for the upcoming era of climate change, the urban public health system must engage with partners across a broad range of urban agencies. Many of the priority areas needing attention are already areas of concern on other counts—for instance, improvements in water and sanitation systems for the urban poor—but the prospects of climate change adds a new element of urgency to them.

Conclusions

The preceding sketch of urban health in low- and middle-income countries is no substitute for the full treatment that these issues deserve, but it may at least suggest where further basic scientific and programme intervention research is most needed. A theme running through the discussion is the need for concerted action, with the public health sector working in tandem with other local government agencies. Public health professionals cannot by themselves mandate the provision of safe water and adequate sanitation for the urban poor, with all the attendant financial costs; nor can they, acting alone, rise to meet the challenges of mitigating urban air pollution, reorganizing traffic and pedestrian activities to reduce deaths and injuries, and readying cities to adapt to the threats that will be posed by climate change.

What is needed is what Harpham (2007) terms 'joined-up government', whereby public health agencies join with concerned actors in other sectors of municipal, regional, and national governments. Because the urban health system is dauntingly complex, with private for-profit and private non-profit care being a significant presence in most cities, effective partnerships are also likely to require engagement with the private sector. With political and administrative decentralization now well underway in many low- and middle-income countries, the arena in which creative partnerships are forged will increasingly be the local and municipal level.

Much remains to be learned about how health expertise, which is now situated in national ministries of health, and the international funding and technical assistance that has also been directed to national ministries, can be redeployed effectively to meet the many health needs of cities and their neighbourhoods.

Author's note: To draw out the distinctions of urban health environments and behaviour with proper care and nuance would, of course, require a book-length treatment. For those seeking more comprehensive accounts of urban health than can be provided in this chapter, I would like to direct attention to the recent US National Research Council report (Panel on Urban Population Dynamics 2003), to documents by Montgomery and Ezeh (2005a, 2005b), and especially, to papers by Harpham (2007), Mercado et al. (2007), and McGranahan (2007) for up-to-date reviews.

References

Alley R.B., Bertsen T., Bindoff N.L. et al. Summary for policymakers: contribution of Working Group I to the Fourth Assessment Report. Intergovernmental Panel on Climate Change; 2007. Available from: http://www.ipcc.ch [accessed 2007 Nov 7]

Almeida-Filho N., Lessa I., Magalhães L. et al. Social inequality and depressive disorders in Bahia, Brazil: Interactions of gender, ethnicity, and social class. Social Science and Medicine 2004;59:1339–53.

Barata R.B., Ribeiro M.C., Guedes M.B. et al. Intra-urban differentials in death rates from homicide in the city of São Paulo, Brazil, 1988–1994. Social Science and Medicine 1998;47:19–23.

Bartlett S.N. The problem of children's injuries in low-income countries: A review. Health Policy and Planning 2002;17:1–13.

Barua N., Singh S. Representation for the marginalized—linking the poor and the health-care system. Lessons from case studies in urban India. Draft paper, New Delhi. World Bank; 2003.

Bassett M.T., Bijlmakers L., Sanders D.M. Professionalism, patient satisfaction, and quality of health care: Experience during Zimbabwe's structural adjustment programme. Social Science and Medicine 1997;45:1845–52.

Blue I. Intra-urban differentials in mental health in São Paulo, Brazil. Ph.D. thesis. London: South Bank University; 1999.

Boardman J.D. Stress and physical health: the role of neighborhoods as mediating and moderating mechanisms. Social Science and Medicine 2004;58:2473–83.

Cairncross S., Valdmanis V. Water supply, sanitation, and hygiene promotion. In: Jamison D.T. et al. editors. Disease control priorities in developing countries. Washington (DC): World Bank; Oxford University Press; 2006. 2nd ed. p. 771–92.

Calvés A.E. Abortion risk and decision-making among young people in urban Cameroon. Studies in Family Planning 2002;33:249–60.

Cohen S., Doyle W.J., Baum A. Socio-economic status is associated with stress hormones. Psychosomatic Medicine 2006;68:414–20.

Das J., Hammer J. Location, location, location: residence, wealth, and the quality of medical care in Delhi, India. Health Affairs 2007a; 26:w338–51.

Das J., Hammer J. Money for nothing: the dire straits of medical practice in Delhi, India. Journal of Development Economics 2007b;83:1–36.

Desgrées du Loû A., Msellati P., Viho I. et al. The use of induced abortion in Abidjan: a possible cause of the fertility decline. Population 2000;12:197–214.

Dussault G., Franceschini M.C. Not enough there, too many here: understanding geographic imbalances in the distribution of the health workforce. Human Resources for Health 2006;4:1–16. Available from: http://www.human-resources-health.com

Erulkar A.S., Matheka J.K. Adolescence in the Kibera slums of Nairobi, Kenya. New York (NY); Nairobi: Population Council; 2007.

Fikree F.F., Gray R.H., Berendes H.W. *et al.* A community-based nested case-control study of maternal mortality. *International Journal of Gynecology & Obstetrics* 1994;**47**:247–55.

Fikree F.F., Midhet F., Sadruddin S. *et al.* Maternal mortality in different Pakistani sites: ratios, clinical causes, and determinants. *Acta Obstetricia et Gynecologica Scandinavica* 1997;**76**:637–45.

Fikree F.F., Ali T., Durocher J.M. *et al.* Health service utilization for perceived postpartum morbidity among poor women living in Karachi. *Social Science and Medicine* 2004;**59**:681–94.

Garrett J., Ahmed A. Incorporating crime in household surveys: a research note. *Environment and Urbanization* 2004;**16**:139–52.

Graham W., Brass W., Snow R.W. Estimating maternal mortality: the sisterhood method. *Studies in Family Planning* 1989;**20**:125–35.

Grant E. State of the art of urban health in Latin America. European Commission funded concerted action: 'Health and human settlements in Latin America'. London: South Bank University; 1999.

Hallman K. Socio-economic disadvantage and unsafe sexual behaviors among young women and men in South Africa. New York (NY): Population Council; 2004. Policy Research Division Working Papers, No. 190.

Harpham T., Grant E., Rodriguez C. Mental health and social capital in Cali, Colombia. *Social Science and Medicine* 2004;**58**:2267–77.

Harpham T. Background paper on improving urban population health. Paper presented at Innovations for an Urban World, the Rockefeller Foundation's Urban Summit; 2007; Bellagio, Italy.

Hay S.I., Guerra C.A., Tatem A.J. *et al.* The global distribution and population at risk of malaria: past, present, and future. *The Lancet. Infectious Diseases* 2004;**4**:327–36.

Heinemann A., Verner D. Crime and violence in development: a literature review of Latin America and the Caribbean. Washington (DC): World Bank; 2006. World Bank Policy Research working paper no. 4041.

Heise L.L., Raikes A., Watts C.H. *et al.* Violence against women: a neglected public health issue in less developed countries. *Social Science and Medicine* 1994;**39**:1165–79.

Híjar M., Trostle J., Bronfman M. Pedestrian injuries in Mexico: A multi-method approach. *Social Science and Medicine* 2003;**57**:2149–59.

Hu P., Wagle N., Goldman N. *et al.* The associations between socio-economic status, allostatic load, and measures of health in older Taiwanese persons: Taiwan Social Environment and Biomarkers of Aging study. *Journal of Biosocial Science* 2007;**39**:545–56.

Huq S., Kovats S., Reid H. *et al.* Reducing risks to cities from climate change: an environmental or a development agenda? *Environment and Urbanization* 2007: Brief no. 15.

Islam M., Montgomery M.R., Taneja S. Urban health and care-seeking behavior: a case study of slums in India and the Philippines. Bethesda (MD): PHRPlus Program, Abt Associates; 2006.

Jamil S., Fikree F.F. Determinants of unsafe abortion in three squatter settlements of Karachi. Karachi, Pakistan: Department of Community Health Sciences, Aga Khan University; 2002.

Kaneda T., Zimmer Z., Tang Z. Socio-economic status differentials in life and active life expectancy among older adults in Beijing. *Disability and Rehabilitation* 2005;**27**:241–51.

Keiser J., Utzinger J., Caldas de Castro M. *et al.* Urbanization in sub-Saharan Africa and implications for malaria control. Working paper. Office of Population Research, Princeton University, Swiss Tropical Institute; 2004.

Kishor S., Johnson K. Profiling domestic violence: a multi-country study. Measure DHS+. Calverton (MD): ORC Macro; 2004.

Kumar N. Spatial sampling for demography and health survey. Paper presented at the 2007 Annual Meetings of the Population Association of America. New York (NY): Department of Geography, University of Iowa; 2007.

Larson B.A., Rosen S. Understanding household demand for indoor air pollution control in developing countries. *Social Science and Medicine* 2002;**55**:571–84.

Marmot M.G., Wilkinson R.G., editors. *Social Determinants of Health*. London: Oxford University Press; 2005. 2nd ed.

Marmot M.G. Social determinants of health inequalities. *Lancet* 2005;**365**:1099–104.

Mayank S., Bahl R., Rattan A. *et al.* Prevalence and correlates of morbidity in pregnant women in an urban slum of New Delhi. *Asia-Pacific Population Journal* 2001;**16**:29–44.

McEwen B.S. Protecting and damaging effects of stress mediators. *New England Journal of Medicine* 1998;**338**:171–9.

McGranahan G., Balk D., Anderson B. The rising tide: assessing the risks of climate change to human settlements in low-elevation coastal zones. *Environment and Urbanization* 2007;**19**:17–37.

McGranahan G. Evolving urban health risks in low- and middle-income countries: from housing, water, and sanitation to cities and climate change. Paper presented at Innovations for an Urban World, the Rockefeller Foundation's Urban Summit; 2007; Bellagio, Italy.

Mercado S., Havemann K., Nakamura K. *et al.* Responding to the health vulnerabilities of the urban poor in the 'new urban settings' of Asia. WHO Centre for Health Development, Alliance for Healthy Cities, and Southeast Asian Press Alliance. Paper presented at Innovations for an Urban World, the Rockefeller Foundation's Urban Summit; 2007; Bellagio, Italy.

Mishra V., Bignami S., Greener R. *et al.* A study of the association of HIV infection and wealth in sub-Saharan Africa. Calverton (MD): Macro International; 2007. DHS Working Papers, No. 31.

Modiano D., Sirima B., Sawadogo A. *et al.* Severe malaria in Burkina Faso: urban and rural environment. *Parassitologia* 1999;**41**:251–4.

Montgomery M.R., Ezeh A.C. The health of urban populations in developing countries: an overview. In: Galea S., Vlahov D., editors. *Handbook of Urban Health: Populations, Methods, and Practice.* New York (NY): Springer; 2005a.

Montgomery M.R., Ezeh A.C. Urban health in developing countries: insights from demographic theory and practice. In: Galea S., Vlahov D., editors. *Handbook of Urban Health: Populations, Methods, and Practice.* New York (NY): Springer: 2005b.

Montgomery M.R., Hewett P.C. Urban poverty and health in developing countries: household and neighborhood effects. *Demography* 2005;**42**:397–425.

Moser C. Urban violence and insecurity: an introductory roadmap. *Environment and Urbanization* 2004;**16**:3–16.

Narain U., Krupnick A. The impact of Delhi's CNG program on air quality. Washington (DC): Resources for the Future; 2007. Discussion Paper 07–08.

Panel on Urban Population Dynamics. In: Montgomery M.R. *et al.*, editors. *Cities Transformed: Demographic Change and its Implications in the Developing World.* Washington (DC): National Academies Press; 2003.

Parkar S.R., Fernandes J., Weiss M.G. Contextualizing mental health: gendered experiences in a Mumbai slum. *Anthropology and Medicine* 2003;**10**:291–308.

Pictet G., Kouanda S., Sirima S. *et al.* Struggling with population heterogeneity in African cities: the urban health and equity puzzle. Paper presented to the 2004 Annual Meetings of the Population Association of America; 2004; Boston (MA).

Prince M., Patel V., Saxena S. *et al.* No health without mental health. *Lancet* 2007;**370**:859–77.

Revi A. Climate change risk: an adaptation and mitigation agenda for Indian cities. *Environment and Urbanization* 2008;**20**:207–229.

Ribeiro H., Alves Cardoso M.R. Air pollution and children's health in São Paulo (1986–1998). *Social Science and Medicine* 2003;**57**:2013–22.

Rossier C. Attitudes towards abortion and contraception in rural and urban Burkina Faso. Paris: Institut National d'Etudes Démographique; 2007.

Sagbakken M., Bjune G., Frich J. *et al.* From the user's perspective—a qualitative study of factors influencing patients' adherence to medical treatment in an urban community, Ethiopia. Paper presented at the conference 'Urban Poverty and Health in Sub-Saharan Africa', African Population and Health Research Centre, Nairobi. Norway: Faculty of Medicine, University of Oslo; 2003.

Santos-Burgoa C., Riojas-Rodríguez H. Health and pollution in Mexico City Metropolitan Area: a general overview of air pollution exposure and health studies. Presentation to the Panel on Urban Population Dynamics, U.S. National Research Council; 2000; Mexico City.

Satterthwaite D., Huq S., Pelling M. *et al.* Building climate change resilience in urban areas and among urban populations in low- and middle-income nations. Paper prepared for Innovations for an Urban World, the Rockefeller Foundation's Urban Summit; 2007; Bellagio, Italy.

Shin S., Furin J., Bayona J. *et al.* Community-based treatment of multi-drug-resistant tuberculosis in Lima, Peru: 7 years of experience. *Social Science and Medicine* 2004;**59**:1529–39.

Steptoe A., Marmot M. The role of psychobiological pathways in socioeconomic inequalities in cardiovascular disease risk. *European Heart Journal* 2002;**23**:13–25.

Stone C. Crime, justice, and growth in South Africa: toward a plausible contribution from criminal justice to economic growth. Cambridge (MA): Harvard University; 2006. Center for International Development working paper no. 131.

UNAIDS. 2004 report on the global AIDS epidemic. New York (NY): UNAIDS; 2004.

UN-Habitat. *The Challenge of Slums: Global Report on Human Settlements 2003.* London: Earthscan; 2003a.

UN-Habitat. *Water and Sanitation in the World's Cities: Local Action for Global Goals.* London: Earthscan; 2003b.

United Nations. World urbanization prospects: the 2005 revision population database. New York (NY): Department of Economic and Social Affairs, Population Division, United Nations; 2005.

van Rie A., Beyers N., Gie R.P. *et al.* Childhood tuberculosis in an urban population in South Africa: burden and risk factor. *Archives of Disability in Children* 1999;**80**:433–7.

WHO. Global age-friendly cities: a guide. Geneva: World Health Organization; 2007a.

WHO. Global tuberculosis control: surveillance, planning, financing. Geneva: World Health Organization; 2007b.

WHO. Investing in health research and development: report of the ad hoc committee on health research relating to future intervention options. Geneva: World Health Organization; 1996.

WHO. Mental health: facing the challenges, building solutions. Report from the WHO European Ministerial Conference; Copenhagen, Denmark. World Health Organization Regional Office for Europe; 2005a.

WHO. *The World Health Report 2001. Mental Health: New Understanding, New Hope.* Geneva: World Health Organization; 2001.

WHO. *The World Health Report 2002. Reducing Risk, Promoting Healthy Life.* Geneva: World Health Organization; 2002.

WHO. WHO multi-country study on women's health and domestic violence against women: summary report of initial results on prevalence, health outcomes and women's responses. Geneva: World Health Organization; 2005b.

WHO. World report on road traffic injury prevention: main messages and recommendations. Geneva: World Health Organization; 2004. Available from: http://www.who.int/violence_injury_prevention/publications/road_traffic%'/world_report/whd_presentation.pdf

WHO. Youth and road safety. Geneva: World Health Organization; 2007d.

Winton A. Urban violence: a guide to the literature. *Environment and Urbanization* 2004;**16**:165–84.

Wong R., Peláez M., Palloni A. *et al.* Survey data for the study of aging in Latin America and the Caribbean. *Journal of Aging and Health* 2006;**18**:157–79.

Woods R. Urban-rural mortality differentials: an unresolved debate. *Population and Development Review* 2003;**29**:29–46.

Zimmer Z, Kwong J. Socio-economic status and health among older adults in urban and rural China. *Journal of Aging and Health* 2004;**16**:44–70.

10.8

Public health aspects of bioterrorism

Manfred S. Green

Introduction

Biological warfare

While deliberate infliction of injury, other than in self-defence, runs contrary to almost all social norms, there is a special kind of abhorrence and dread associated with the use of biological agents. Many possible reasons for this can be suggested. The agents are 'invisible', they can cause injury indiscriminately and not only to those targeted and they can inflict disease and death in numbers quite out of proportion to the resources expended. Furthermore, their effects may only be experienced long after exposure and they may cause large outbreaks through person-to-person spread. Prior to the twentieth century, there were documented instances of crude attempts to use biological agents as weapons of war. For example, there are several reports of bodies of plague victims being hurled into the enemy ranks in order to infect their forces. There is also some evidence to suggest that European colonists in the Americas either actually used, or intended to use, 'smallpox' infected blankets to infect the native populations, who were previously unexposed (Patterson & Runge 2002).

Early in the twentieth century, rapid progress in the field of microbiology was accompanied by an increased interest in the use of biological weapons. This became evident during World War I, when German agents used glanders bacteria (*Burkholderia pseudomallei*) to infect horses, mules, and cattle being sent from the United States to the allied forces in Europe. As a result, several hundred soldiers became ill (Centers for Disease Control 2006). In 1918, the modern version of biological warfare became institutionalized when the Japanese established a biological weapons unit in their army. Due to growing concern about the potential military use of biological agents, in 1925 an international agreement to prohibit the use of biological weapons was signed by 132 countries. This agreement, 'the Geneva Protocol', did not limit development or production of such weapons. Despite the agreement, in 1931, the Japanese army began to experiment with biological weapons in Manchuria, including exposing prisoners to aerosolized anthrax spores. During World War II, other major powers, such as Germany, the United States, the Soviet Union, and the United Kingdom, initiated bioweapons programmes as part of their strategies to stockpile weapons of mass destruction.

In 1969, President Nixon ended the United States offensive bioweapons programme. Three years later, the 'Biological Weapons

Convention' was signed by 171 countries. Article 1 of the convention states that 'each party to this convention undertakes never in any circumstances to develop, produce, stockpile or otherwise acquire or retain microbial or other biological agents, or toxins whatever their origin or method of production, of types and in quantities that have no justification for prophylactic, protective or other peaceful purposes'. The document also specifies a ban on the production of weapons, equipment or means of delivery designed to use such agents or toxins for hostile purposes or in armed conflict.

In 1985, the 'Australia Group' was formed to address the regulations governing exportation of materials necessary to manufacture chemical and biological weapons. It now has a membership of 40 countries plus the European Commission. The 'Wassenaar Arrangement', which regulates the control of exports of 'dual-use technologies' which could be applied to weapons of mass destruction, was confirmed in 1994 by more than 40 countries.

The emergence of bioterrorism

One of the earliest instances of the use of the term 'terrorism' in a political context, was during the French revolution (1789–1799). During the 1960s, cross-border terrorism became a major international issue. In general, terrorist objectives are considered to include the desire 'to promote nationalist or separatist objectives, to retaliate or take revenge for a real or perceived injury or to protest government policies' (Tucker 1999). While terrorism may be state-sponsored, terrorist groups usually commit their acts outside of formal government agencies and in most countries terrorism is defined as a criminal act. Terrorist groups tend to claim that they resort to illegal or illegitimate methods to achieve political or social change, because they have been excluded from, or frustrated by regular legal and diplomatic processes (Hoffman 2007).

Initially, conventional thinking held that biological weapons were so morally unacceptable and the means of production and dissemination so complex, that they would not be included in the armaments of terrorist groups. In the late 1990s, warnings began to appear in the professional literature about the potential use of biological agents by terrorist groups and the term 'bioterrorism' was coined (Franz *et al.* 1997; Henderson 1998). Several major events brought into focus the potential emergence of bioterrorism as a major threat to public security and health.

In the 1990s, it became evident that the Soviet Union had failed to adhere to the Biological Weapons Convention, and continued to develop biological weapons. In the early 1990s, investigations revealed that in 1979, anthrax spores were accidentally released from a military facility in Sverdlovsk (now Yekaterinburg), Russia, resulting in an outbreak of respiratory anthrax, with at least 70 deaths (Meselson *et al.* 1994). There was also evidence that a major facility in Novosibirsk, Siberia, housed a large programme to weaponize agents such as the smallpox and viral haemorrhagic fever viruses and anthrax spores (Henderson 1998). The breakup of the former Soviet Union increased concern that the biological agents that had been weaponized and the expertise acquired by the scientists, would fall into the hands of terrorist groups. There was also evidence that other countries were continuing to develop biological weapons (Zilinskas 1997).

Weaponizing biological agents is not trivial and generally requires a high level of technology and skill. However, state-sponsored biological weapons programmes could supply the necessary technology to terrorist groups. In 2001, the terrorist attacks on the Twin Towers in New York and the Pentagon in Washington renewed concern that international terrorist groups would attempt to expand their armaments to biological weapons.

A bioterrorist attack has been defined by the United States Centers for Disease Control (CDC) as 'the deliberate release of viruses, bacteria, or other germs (agents) used to cause illness or death in people, animals, or plants' (Centers for Disease Control 2006). This definition relates primarily to the physical impact of the attack. However, others have stressed the psychological impact, and defined bioterrorism as 'the use, or threatened use, of biological agents to promote or spread fear or intimidation upon an individual, a specific group, or the population as a whole for religious, political, ideological, financial, or personal purposes'. (Arizona Department of Health Services 2005). Since contagious agents are invisible, the threat of infection may be perceived to be ubiquitous with almost no way of avoiding it. Thus, while the potential physical impact is of major concern, the psychological impact may be much broader and longer-lasting than physical injury.

Four factors have been delineated as the basis for the assessment of the bioterrorism threat. They are the intent of the groups or individuals and willingness to use weapons of mass destruction, the technical capabilities of the groups, the attributes of the pathogens/toxins, and the range of possible targets for an attack (Zilinskas *et al.* 2004).

Contemporary incidents of bioterrorism and biocrimes

Until 2001, the only modern instance of bioterrorism recognized in the United States by the Federal Bureau of Investigation, occurred in 1984. The Bhagwan Shree Rajneesh sect deliberately contaminated salads with *Salmonella typhimurium* in salad bars in Oregon, with the intention of disrupting local elections and several hundred people became ill (Torok 1997). Bioterrorism attempts have been documented in other countries. For example, in 1980, a group called the Red Army Faction was reported to have used botulinum toxin against government officials in West Germany. In 1995, a Japanese cult, Aum Shinrikyo, produced quantities of anthrax spores, Q fever bacteria, botulinum toxin, and Ebola viruses and attempted to disseminate them (Sugishima 2003). Fortunately, there were no casualties.

Despite the paucity of actual events, there have been a number of bioterrorism threats. Among the most prominent occurred in the early 1970s when an extremist group in the United States, the 'Weather Underground', threatened to contaminate the urban water supplies with biological agents. In addition, there have been a number of so-called 'biocrimes' where biological agents have been used against individuals without a defined ideological motive. For example, in 1997, a disgruntled worker deliberately used *Shigella dysenteriae* type 2 bacteria to contaminate food served to co-workers (Kolavic *et al.* 1997).

The 'anthrax letters' incident in the United States, in 2001, dramatically demonstrated the potential for bioterrorism. During approximately three months, six envelopes contaminated with anthrax spores in powder form were identified in the regular mail and 22 people were infected. Half suffered from inhalation anthrax and the others from the cutaneous form (Jernigan *et al.* 2002). Recently, the United States Federal Bureau of Investigation announced that they had evidence to suggest that a scientist from a United States Army Medical Research laboratory may have been responsible for sending the letters (Federal Bureau of Investigation 2008). Since no clear motive has been established, this incident may be an example of either bioterrorism or a biocrime. There was major disruption of government offices and the mail services. Thousands of workers received prophylactic therapy, and there was a large-scale programme to decontaminate affected buildings. The cost of managing the incident may have exceeded one billion dollars. In addition, other countries also instituted safety measures and many suspected cases were investigated.

Confronting the threat of bioterrorism

Bioterrorism may be viewed from the perspective of the biological agents that pose the greatest danger, the potential impact on society and the likelihood that biological agents would be employed as terrorist weapons. Preparedness for a bioterrorism attack is multifaceted and includes prevention, detection, diagnosis, treatment, pre- and post-exposure prophylaxis, and risk communication. Prevention ranges from attempting to address the root causes of terrorism, implementation of deterrence measures and control of access to potentially dangerous pathogens to protection of food supplies and drinking water. Early detection of an incident will depend on effective human, environmental, and animal surveillance, rapid and accurate diagnoses, and comprehensive epidemiological investigations.

In order to deal effectively with an actual incident, countries will need to allocate substantial resources to develop contingency plans and training programmes. They will have to expand their infrastructure to ensure prompt diagnosis and treatment of patients and implement pre- and post-exposure prophylactic measures for both contagious and non-contagious diseases. Preparedness measures include stockpiling of medications, vaccines, and special protective equipment, and developing plans for non-pharmacological interventions in order to reduce spread of the disease. The possible need for decontamination of the environment following the incident will require prior investment in specialized equipment and supplies. Methods for risk communication and education of both health professional and the public will have to be tailored to the threat of bioterrorism. In addition, the special legal and ethical aspects must be resolved. This chapter addresses the above issues.

Biological weapons

General characteristics of bioterrorism agents

Biological weapons have features which make them particularly attractive for terrorist acts. They can be extremely difficult to detect in the environment and their effects are not felt for several hours to days. Both the agents and hardware for their production and dissemination are relatively easy to conceal. Thus, the perpetrators could produce and disseminate the agents and escape during the incubation or latent period before any illness is detected.

While the biological agents could be disseminated through food, human carriers or infected insects, aerosol spread will maximize the number of people exposed and produce the most damage. Since most of the potential agents do not transmit naturally as aerosols, their use in bioterrorism attacks may produce disease with shorter incubation periods and different manifestations of clinical disease. Furthermore, surreptitious and simultaneous aerosol dissemination of a contagious agent could produce an inordinately large number of second- and later-generation cases. The effects of each agent are likely to depend on the exposure dose and host factors such as age, sex, underlying illnesses, and immune status.

Classification of potential bioterrorism agents

Almost all potential bioterrorism agents occur naturally as known pathogens, although many are zoonoses that do not normally infect humans. The genetic composition of the biological agents may be modified to make them more virulent and increase their resistance to medications or vaccines.

In 1999, the United States CDC classified the potential agents for bioterrorism into three categories, A, B, and C (Tables 10.8.1 and 10.8.2), depending on how easily they can be spread, the severity of illness they might cause and the death rates that may result (Rotz *et al.* 2002). The highest priority is given to the category A agents

Table 10.8.1 CDC categorization of biological agents that may be used as weapons (http://www.bt.cdc.gov/agent/agentlist-category.asp)

Category A

High-priority agents include organisms and toxins that pose the highest risk to the public and national security

- They can be easily disseminated or transmitted from person to person.
- They result in high death rates and have the potential for major public health impact.
- They are likely to cause public panic and social disruption.
- They require special action for public health preparedness.

Category B

Second-highest-priority agents

- They are moderately easy to spread.
- They result in moderate illness rates and low death rates.
- They require specific enhancements of laboratory capacity and enhanced disease monitoring.

Category C

Third-highest-priority agents include emerging pathogens that could be engineered for mass spread in the future

- They are easily available.
- They are easily produced and spread.
- They have potential for high morbidity and mortality rates and major health impact.

Table 10.8.2 Examples of bioterrorism agents by category (http://www.bt.cdc.gov/agent/agentlist-category.asp)

Category A

Infectious and contagious diseases

- Smallpox (variola major)
- Plague (*Yersinia pestis*)
- Viral haemorrhagic fevers (filoviruses [e.g. Ebola, Marburg] and arenaviruses [e.g. Lassa, Machupo])

Infectious but not contagious diseases

- Anthrax (*Bacillus anthracis*)
- Tularaemia (*Francisella tularensis*)

Toxins

- Botulism (*Clostridium botulinum* toxin)

Category B

- Brucellosis (*Brucella* species)
- Epsilon toxin of *Clostridium perfringens*
- Food safety threats (*Salmonella* species, *Escherichia coli* 0157, *Shigella*)
- Glanders (*Burkholderia mallei*)
- Meliodosis (*Burkholderia pseudomallei*)
- Psittacosis (*Chlamidia psittaci*)
- Q fever (*Coxiella burnetii*)
- Ricin toxin from *Ricinus communis* (castor beans)
- Staphylococcal enterotoxin B
- Typhus fever (*Rickettsia prowazekii*)
- Viral encephalitis (alphavirus—e.g. Venezuelan equine encephalitis, eastern equine encephalitis, western equine encephalitis)
- Water safety threats (e.g. *Vibrio cholerae, Cryptosporidium parvum*)

Category C

- Emerging infectious diseases such as Nipah virus and hantavirus

which are considered the greatest risk to the public and national security. These agents can be classified into three types: Those that are both infectious and contagious, those that are infectious but not usually contagious and toxins. Category B includes diseases that are considered an intermediate risk to the public, since the causative agents are moderately easy to spread and the diseases result in moderately high death rates. Category C agents include emerging pathogens which have the potential to be engineered to spread and cause high rates of morbidity and mortality.

Characteristics of category A bioterrorist agents

Since the category A biological agents are of greatest concern, they will be described in some detail.

Diseases which are both infectious and contagious
Smallpox (Henderson et al. 1999)

Smallpox is a severe, systemic illness caused by a large, brick-shaped, DNA virus from the orthopoxvirus genus. Prior to its eradication in 1978, it was endemic in many countries. The case-fatality rate for variola major in unvaccinated subjects was estimated at around 30 per cent. The infectious dose is unknown but may be as low as a few virions. There is evidence that smallpox may have been weaponized by the Soviet Union during the 1980s (Henderson 1998). The long period since cessation of universal vaccination, combined with the severity of the disease, has made smallpox one of the most feared potential bioterrorist agents.

After the virus enters the respiratory tract, it multiplies in the lymph nodes, and three to four days later produces an asymptomatic viremia. On about the eighth day, there is a second viremia accompanied by fever and toxemia. The virus then localizes in small blood vessels of the dermis and beneath the oral and pharyngeal mucosa. In addition to fever, the patient suffers from symptoms such as malaise, headache, backache, occasional abdominal pain, and delirium.

Macular-papular lesions appear on the mucosa of the mouth and oro-pharynx and the patient becomes infectious. Later the rash appears on the face, forearms, and legs and the lesions become vesicular, round, rubbery, and pustular. Scabs begin to form around the eighth day of the rash and following their separation, the person is no longer infectious. Overall, the patient may be infectious for an average of 16 days. The haemorrhagic and flat types of smallpox are less common, but more severe, with case-fatality rates approaching 80–90 per cent. The haemorrhagic type has a shorter incubation period and is more difficult to diagnose clinically. Pregnant women are particularly susceptible to these forms (Kiang & Krathwohl 2003).

Following the initial cases arising from the aerosolized virus, secondary cases may occur through droplet spread, usually over a distance of less than two meters, or through contact with the virus from the skin lesions or body fluids (Kiang & Krathwohl 2003). There are rare reports of apparent airborne transmission, such as in an outbreak in Germany in 1970. A single hospitalized patient, with severe cough, infected seventeen other patients on three floors in the hospital, probably through the ventilation system (Wehrle et al. 1970).

The spread of smallpox is likely to be slower than for diseases such as chickenpox and measles and pandemic influenza, since the reproduction number is smaller and the generation time longer. In addition, transmission of the disease only occurs after onset of the rash, at which stage patients are seriously ill and tend to remain at home or in healthcare facilities. Thus, family members and healthcare workers are at greatest risk.

Plague (Prentice & Rahalison 2007)

Plague is caused by a Gram-negative bacillus, *Yersinia pestis*, which is an enzootic infection of rodents and is transmitted by infected fleas.

The natural disease begins as a blood-borne infection of the lymph nodes resulting in 'bubonic plague'. If the patient develops pneumonia, the disease is termed 'pneumonic plague' and can be transmitted by droplets. Weaponization of the plague bacillus was attempted during the United States programme and probably accomplished by Soviet scientists (Ingelsby *et al.* 2002).

Inhaled, aerosolized plague bacilli cause primary pneumonic plague. The incubation period may be as short as 24 h, but symptoms usually occur two to four days after exposure. The disease presents with fever, cough, and dyspnoea, sometimes with bloody, watery or purulent sputum. Occasionally there may be gastrointestinal symptoms including nausea, vomiting, abdominal pain, and diarrhoea. The subsequent clinical picture of primary pneumonic plague is similar to any type of severe, rapidly progressive pneumonia.

Untreated pneumonic plague has a case-fatality rate approaching 100 per cent, and the time from exposure to death has been found to be around 2–6 days. Since pneumonic plague can spread from person-to-person through droplets, several generations of the disease can occur. Appropriate isolative precautions are effective in preventing transmission. The epidemic curve for a simulated, point-source outbreak of pneumonic plague is shown for illustrative purposes in Fig. 10.8.1, where diagnosis is established at day four. The initial cases are due to exposure at source and treated appropriately once the cause is known. The second wave is due to secondary spread prior to control of the epidemic.

Viral haemorrhagic fevers (Borio et al. 2002)

The viral haemorrhagic fevers are illnesses associated with fever and bleeding diathesis caused by small RNA viruses belonging to the families, Filovioridiae, Arenaviridae, Bunyaviridae, and Flaviviridae. The filoviruses and arenaviruses have been weaponized by the former Soviet Union, Russia, and the United States. In particular, the Soviet Union is reported to have produced quantities of Marburg, Lassa, Ebola, Junin and Machupo viruses.

The incubation period varies from 2 to 21 days. Clinical manifestations include fever, myalgias, rash, and encephalitis. Patients display a non-specific prodrome of high fever, headache, malaise, arthralgias, myalgias, nausea, abdominal pain, and non-bloody diarrhoea, which may last about a week. Most have cutaneous flushing or a skin rash. Later patients show signs of haemorrhagic disease. Second and later generations of disease can occur through direct contact with body fluids of the patients, which are highly infectious. Healthcare workers are at the greatest risk.

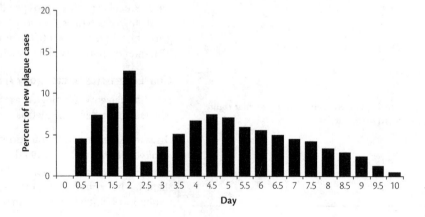

Fig. 10.8.1 Epidemic curve for a simulated point-source outbreak of pneumonic plague, with diagnosis on day four after exposure and appropriate treatment given to cases. *Source*: Scheulen, J., Latimer, C., and Brown, J. (2006). Electronic Mass Casualty Assessment and Planning Scenarios (EMCAPS). Johns Hopkins University. Available at: http://www.hopkins-cepar.org/EMCAPS/EMCAPS. Accessed July 14, 2007.

Diseases that are infectious but not contagious
Anthrax (Ingelsby et al. 2002)

Anthrax is caused by Gram-positive, aerobic, spore-forming, rod-shaped bacteria (*Bacillus anthracis*). It was one of the leading agents in the biological weapons programmes due to its stability and virulence. The vegetative spores are easily disseminated, resistant to drying and highly infectious. In addition, since the disease is not contagious, its effects can be restricted to the target population. There are three clinical manifestations of the disease: Cutaneous, gastrointestinal, and inhalation. The cutaneous form is not uncommon in nature, mainly among people occupationally exposed while handling domestic animals. Gastrointestinal anthrax is much less common and occurs as a result of the consumption of contaminated meat. Inhalation anthrax is exceedingly rare and has been reported mainly among woolsorters and workers exposed to contaminated animal hides and bones.

Aerosol dissemination of the spores, which is the likely scenario in a bioterrorist attack, causes inhalation anthrax (Ingelsby *et al.* 2002). Anthrax spores are about 1 μm in size and in order to enter the lung alveoli, the spore-bearing particles must be in the range of 1–5 μm. Thus, in order to weaponize the organism, the spore-bearing particles must be of the appropriate size and remain suspended in the air long enough to be inhaled. Once the spores penetrate the lung alveoli, they are ingested by macrophages, enter the lymphatic system and settle in the mediastinal lymph nodes, where they germinate. They cause disease by producing three factors called protective antigen, oedema factor and lethal factor. These combine to form two toxins, lethal toxin and oedema toxin. Protective antigen allows the binding of lethal and oedema factors to the cell membrane and facilitates their transport across it. To achieve full virulence, the bacteria must have an intact capsule together with the three toxin components.

The initial symptoms include fever, chills, sweats, fatigue, malaise, cough, nausea, and dyspnoea. This stage lasts from hours to a few days and is often accompanied by a brief period of recovery. The second stage is characterized by sudden fever, dyspnoea, dyaphoresis and shock. Cyanosis and hypotension progress rapidly, followed by death in a few hours. The disease is a sepsis syndrome with a haemorrhagic mediastinitis and many patients develop haemorrhagic meningitis. Alveolar pneumonia is not a major clinical feature. Untreated, the case-fatality rate is essentially 100 per cent.

Mathematical models based on the Sverdlovsk accident have been used to predict the incubation period and the dose-response of inhalation anthrax (Brookmeyer *et al.* 2001). The incubation period is estimated at 1–6 days but can be longer than 40 days, and is probably related to the exposure dose. For illustrative purposes, a possible epidemic curve for a simulated point-source outbreak of inhalation anthrax is shown in Fig. 10.8.2.

In fatal cases, the time between onset of symptoms and death in untreated cases has been found to be an average of three days (Ingelsby *et al.* 2002). The severity of the disease appears to be related to the exposure dose and it is possible that this is age-dependent. The spores can survive in the environment for many years, although once they are on the ground, they will tend to produce cutaneous anthrax.

Tularemia (Dennis et al. 2001)

Tularemia is a febrile illness caused by a small, non-motile, aerobic, Gram-negative, spore-forming coccobacillus, *Francisella tularensis*. It was initially identified in rodents and subsequently in humans exposed to infected animals. The agent has the potential for causing waterborne outbreaks and early on was described as a hazard for laboratory workers. Tularemia has been weaponised in biowarfare programmes.

The onset of the disease is usually abrupt with fever (38–40°C), headache, chills, rigors, generalized body aches, coryza, and sore throat. A pulse-temperature disassociation has been noted in many patients. There is often a dry or slightly productive cough. Inhalation tularaemia causes haemorrhagic inflammation of the airways early on in the course of the disease, which may progress to bronchopneumonia. Untreated, the fatality rates could be between 30–60 per cent. There is no secondary person-to-person spread.

Toxins
Botulism (Arnon et al. 2001)

Botulism is caused by a 150 Kd toxin which is produced by *Clostridium botulinum*, a spore-forming, obligate, anaerobic bacteria. Sporadic cases occur naturally such as through consumption of improperly canned foods. It is one of the most potent neurotoxins known and has been weaponized in biowarfare programmes. In a bioterrorist incident, it could be disseminated either through food or by aerosol.

After ingestion or inhalation of the toxin, an endopeptidase blocks acetylcholine-containing vesicles from fusing with the terminal membrane of the motor neurons. The incubation period for inhalational botulism is unknown for humans, but in animal experiments it was between 12 and 80 h. The main clinical manifestation is an acute, afebrile, symmetric, descending flaccid paralysis which

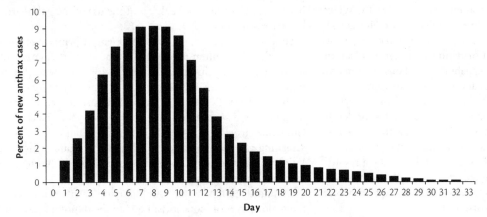

Fig. 10.8.2 Epidemic curve for a simulated point-source outbreak of inhalation anthrax, without intervention.
Source: Scheulen, J., Latimer, C., and Brown, J. (2006). Electronic Mass Casualty Assessment and Planning Scenarios (EMCAPS). Johns Hopkins University. Available at: http://www. hopkins-cepar.org/EMCAPS/EMCAPS. Accessed July 14, 2007.

begins in the bulbar musculature. The main presenting symptoms are difficulty in seeing, speaking, and swallowing with neurological signs such as ptosis, diplopia, blurred vision, enlarged or slow reacting pupils, dysarthria, dysphonia, and dysphagia. There are no significant sensory changes. In untreated cases, death occurs due to airway obstruction and inadequate tidal volume.

The patient is not contagious at any stage of the disease. Since aerosol spread of botulinum toxin does not occur in nature, the lethal dose is not known, but has been estimated at 0.70–0.90 µg.

Estimating the extent of a bioterrorist incident

Contagious diseases

The three major epidemiological factors affecting the spread of a contagious disease are the number of people initially exposed, the secondary reproduction rate and the generation time. The reproduction rate is defined by R_0, which is a measure of the average number of people who will be infected by each sick person. If it is less than one, transmission is not sustainable. The reproduction rate is not static and can change with the progression of the epidemic. $R(t)$ is the reproduction rate at a certain point in time t and is likely to drop following the introduction of control measures. For pneumonic plague, R_0 has been estimated at around 1.3 (Gani & Leach 2004). The R_0 for smallpox is larger and has been estimated as between 5 and 10, although it is likely to be closer to 5 (Leach 2007).

Estimates have been made of the extent of a smallpox incident under various bioterrorism scenarios, where the virus is disseminated by human vectors, in a building and in an airport (Bozzette et al. 2003). Since the number of initial cases will vary from tens to thousands, the total number of cases could be small or reach hundreds of thousands. Clearly, if vaccination is instituted early, the numbers could be reduced accordingly.

Infectious but not contagious diseases

Estimates have been made of the potential size of inhalation anthrax outbreaks under varying circumstances of the population exposed and the timing of antibiotic prophylaxis (Walden & Kaplan 2004). Since the disease is not contagious, the final total number of cases will only be a proportion of the number initially exposed. There could be some secondary cases of inhalation anthrax from reaerosolization of spores. However, most of the secondary cases are likely to be cutaneous anthrax.

Preparedness—general guidelines

During the 1990s, many countries began to actively prepare for the possibility of a bioterrorist event (Bonin 2007). In 2004, the WHO published bioterrorism preparedness guidelines (WHO 2004). They include threat analysis, pre-emption of an attack, preparing to respond, preparing public information and communication packages, validation of response capabilities, response before any overt release of biological agents, and potential consequences. In 2001, the 54th World Health Assembly requested the Director-General 'to provide technical support to member states for developing or strengthening preparedness and response activities against risks posed by biological agents, as an integral part of their emergency management programmes'. This was followed by a resolution in 2002, which requested the Director-General to continue to issue international guidance and technical information on public health measures related to bioterrorism.

In 2000, the United States CDC published a strategic plan for preparedness and response to biological and chemical terrorism (Khan et al. 2000). The strategic plan focused on five areas: Preparedness and prevention, detection and surveillance, diagnosis and characterization of biological and chemical agents, response and communication. In the preparedness area, the United States CDC undertook to provide public health guidelines and technical support to local and state public health agencies.

Prevention

The public health approach to the prevention of bioterrorism includes identifying the causes of terrorism and evaluating appropriate preventive strategies at the most basic level. The causes are likely to be multi-factorial. Political elements frequently dominate and the distinction between terrorist and 'freedom-fighter' is often blurred. There is no generic cause of terrorism. Poverty and deprivation can provide fertile ground for recruiting members to a terrorist organization. In addition to reducing ethnic and religious tensions, an international goal should be to ensure that there are adequate processes for non-violent resolution of differences. At a government level, there needs to be a clear, universal condemnation of terrorism as a means of achieving change. Rather emphasis should be placed on searching for common ground between groups.

Currently, the prevention of bioterrorism incidents remains largely in the hands of the security forces and intelligence agencies. At the international level, Interpol has established a special training programme to combat cross-border bioterrorism. Since bioterrorism will impact primarily on the health of the population, it is now considered to be an important public health issue. Coordination between professionals from various disciplines is needed to prepare for and manage an incident. They include specialists in epidemiology, infectious diseases, microbiology, vaccinology, general public health, medical informatics, emergency medicine, environmental health, food safety, veterinary medicine, health law, risk communication and management of health services.

Primary prevention of a bioterrorist incident is the first priority. This should be based on close cooperation between security authorities and international collaboration. The incentive for bioterrorism can be reduced if there are effective means to deal with a possible attack. Abuse of biological agents can be reduced by restricting access and good intelligence. The threat of bioterrorism has called into question some of the dogmas related to programmes to eradicate diseases such as poliomyelitis and measles. For example, if polio is successfully eradicated, universal vaccination may have to continue due to the threat of the use of the polio virus as a bioterrorism agent.

Food safety is an important component of primary prevention. Other than botulinum toxin, agents that are particularly suitable for dissemination through food are mainly in category B. Some potential agents include salmonella, Escherichia coli and shigella (Sobel et al. 2002). Other bacteria, such as streptococci, have also been proposed as potential bioterrorist agents (Kaluski et al. 2006). Guidelines have been issued by the United States CDC regarding screening and monitoring of food handlers in public institutions. Vulnerability assessments need to be carried out including controls and checks on importation of foods.

Contamination of water with biological agents is unlikely to be the major target of bioterrorism due to the diluting factor and the need for large quantities of the agent in order to cause significant outbreaks. Nevertheless, the cryptosporisium outbreak in Milwaukee, United States, in 1993, is an example of the large number of people that can be affected by a waterborne outbreak. Thus, the potential threat exists and should not be underestimated (Meinhardt 2005). In the United States, the Environmental Protection Agency addresses water security in three areas: Vulnerability assessments, emergency/incident planning and security enhancements.

Secondary prevention can be achieved by detection of the bioterrorist event in the early stages, in order to institute appropriate measures such as post-exposure pharmacological and non-pharmacological prophylaxis. Thus, comprehensive surveillance will be a cornerstone of secondary prevention. Tertiary prevention will include early treatment and rehabilitation of those people who contract the disease and public information campaigns to reduce the long-term psychological impacts of the incident.

Surveillance and early detection

The purpose of surveillance

The objectives of surveillance for bioterrorism incidents are two-fold. The first is early detection of cases in order to facilitate prompt treatment of people already ill, identification of the exposure source and rapid introduction of prophylaxis for those who have been exposed or are at risk of exposure. If the disease is contagious, early detection will assist in limiting spread of the disease by ensuring isolation of cases and enforcing quarantine, where necessary. The second objective is monitoring the progress of the outbreak to assist the authorities in deciding to upgrade and redistribute health services and provide reliable and timely information for the media.

There are four main limitations of traditional surveillance systems for the detection and monitoring of bioterrorism incidents. Firstly, diagnosis of the early cases may be missed due to a failure to suspect or report unusual diseases. Secondly, there may be a considerable delay in reporting due to the lag time between clinical diagnosis and laboratory confirmation. Thirdly, since the flow of information in traditional surveillance systems tends to be relatively slow, there may be a substantial delay in alerting public health authorities. Finally, access to timely, processed information during the epidemic may be seriously limited.

Syndromic surveillance

Principles of syndromic surveillance

Most infectious diseases have prodromal periods characterized by non-specific symptoms and signs. As a result, surveillance of symptoms and signs of disease, or 'syndromic surveillance', was proposed as a more sensitive method for early detection and monitoring of an outbreak. Although syndromic surveillance is a relatively new term, surveillance for 'influenza-like illness' (ILI) is well-established for monitoring the incidence of influenza itself. Any system based on non-specific signs and symptoms will require balancing of sensitivity, specificity, and positive predictive value. Systems that are highly sensitive will tend to have low specificity and positive predictive value, with many false alarms.

The roles of syndromic surveillance

There are basically three potential roles for syndromic surveillance. These are detection of the first cases of the outbreak, detection of the outbreak at an early stage and management of the outbreak.

Theoretically, syndromic surveillance could be successful in detecting the first cases of a slowly evolving outbreak. However, for bioterrorist scenarios, it is probably more realistic to describe the role of syndromic surveillance as detection of cases at an early stage of the outbreak. This would complement the reporting of the first cases clinically diagnosed by individual physicians. The system could be used to confirm the outbreak and help estimate its location. For this purpose, the syndromic surveillance system needs to be maintained and analysed periodically. In the event of a report of a suspicious or confirmed case, focused analysis of the data base could determine whether there are changes in the pattern of non-specific disease rates, relevant to the diagnosed cases reported.

Syndromic surveillance can also play a major role in the management and control of the outbreak. During large infectious disease outbreaks, occurring under emergency conditions, laboratory diagnosis of individual cases is likely to be limited and often not done at all. In addition, the transmission of information on diagnosed cases will often be delayed. Thus, once an outbreak has been confirmed, syndromic surveillance systems would provide timely and detailed data on the location and evolution of the outbreak. The system can also provide important, current information on general disease patterns in the total population so as to place the outbreak in perspective.

Sources of data

Syndromic surveillance has been facilitated by electronic reporting and the Internet. The sources of the data include visits to primary care physicians and emergency rooms, occasionally supplemented by medication prescription data. Since not all patients will visit a physician, surrogates of symptoms such as sales of the over-the-counter medications could also be used. In addition, other more crude indices of increased disease incidence could include hospital bed occupancy, mortality rates and the numbers of blood cultures requested. Syndromic surveillance could be complemented by special reporting systems such as PulseNet and FoodNet, which were established to monitor food-borne diseases. International data sharing will be essential for detecting cross-border bioterrorism.

Syndromic surveillance systems usually have statistical computing capabilities to determine whether there are unusual changes in either time or space or both (Kaufman et al. 2007; Rolka et al. 2007). Analytic tools, such as time series analysis and the cusum method, can be used to detect temporal changes in disease patterns. Detection of clusters, both in time and place, can be facilitated by the use of Geographic Information Systems (GIS), combined with statistical analysis tools. If a bioterrorist attack occurs in a public place, home addresses of the patients will not be helpful in detecting the location of the exposure. Clusters may be identified when only residential addresses are available if the communities surrounding a public place are overrepresented among people gathering at a public place (Green & Kaufman 2005). Other approaches that could be useful include searching for clusters in families or in age distributions. Once the outbreak has been identified, the syndromic surveillance data source should include a question on the location of the patient at the time of the attack.

Responding to alarms

A syndromic surveillance system must be accompanied by a response mechanism. It should include procedures to be followed in the event that an incident is suspected. In traditional surveillance, when a notifiable disease or obvious outbreak is diagnosed or suspected, the procedure to be followed is usually well-defined. For syndromic surveillance, it may not be clear which irregularities should be reported and investigated. This should include who should receive the report and what kind of investigation should be pursued. Since many of the systems use anonymized data, the investigation will need to be carried out together with those supplying the source data. Privacy issues should also be addressed. Unless there is a very large deviation from the expected incidence rates, each investigation is likely to be complex and time-consuming.

Syndromic surveillance systems

Guidelines for developing syndromic surveillance systems have been published by the United States CDC. They require that the goals of the system be detailed and include specifications of the kind of information that is expected. Syndromic surveillance systems are currently operating in a number of centres, mainly in the United States (Bravata *et al.* 2004a). One of the earliest systems was developed in the New York City Department of Health. Since 1999, they have been actively monitoring hotline calls on a daily basis to identify temporal or geographic increases in respiratory illnesses that might represent a potential bioterrorist event (Heffernan *et al.* 2004). The Health Department also developed systems to monitor community-based gastrointestinal outbreaks. The United States CDC is developing a national surveillance system called Biosense (Bradley *et al.* 2005).

Evaluation of syndromic surveillance systems

The surveillance system must be evaluated for each biological agent separately. The factors most likely to determine the success of the system have been listed as simplicity, flexibility, data quality, acceptability, sensitivity, predictive value, representativeness, timeliness, and stability (Centers for Disease Control 2001). Technical factors that should be considered include methods of collecting data, amount of follow-up, method of managing the data, methods for analysing and disseminating the data, staff training and time spent on maintaining the system.

Since there are essentially no actual bioterrorist events, evaluations of surveillance systems must be based on simulations. There is evidence that syndromic surveillance will identify influenza outbreaks earlier than sentinel surveillance based on laboratory isolates. However, since a bioterrorism incident is likely to be a point-source outbreak, it is questionable whether the efficacy of a system for detecting influenza outbreaks can be extrapolated to bioterrorism scenarios.

Benefits of syndromic surveillance

An appropriate surveillance system serves as the cornerstone of the information base at all stages of the outbreak. The benefits of electronic syndromic surveillance are primarily in the reduction in the lag time between early symptoms and clinical and laboratory, timeliness of the reports and reduced reliance on individual physicians to complete forms. This is of particular relevance in emergency situations. The system can provide current, updated information to decision-makers at the national or regional disease control centre. This information will be critical for confirming the outbreak, guiding decisions on intervention and monitoring the impact of control measures.

Limitations of syndromic surveillance

Despite the widespread implementation of syndromic surveillance systems, primarily in the United States, their contribution to the early detection of bioterrorism events has been questioned (Reingold 2003).

There are two main criticisms. The first is the contention that early cases with clear clinical signs are likely to be detected in hospital emergency rooms earlier or at the same time as the outbreak is detected by syndromic surveillance. The second, and perhaps more dominant criticism, is that there is a real danger that an abundance of false reports could desensitize and paralyse the system. Thus, it is not at all clear whether these surveillance systems will play a significant role in early detection, and whether they can function efficiently in the long term, without overburdening the public health services.

The role of animals as sentinels

Where they have an enhanced sensitivity to the disease, illness in both domestic and wild animals could provide early warnings of exposure to biological agents (Rabinowitz *et al.* 2006). This could be relevant for anthrax, plague and tularaemia. Sheep and cattle could be sentinels for anthrax due to their sensitivity to the organism and the fact that they are largely outdoors. They may become ill quicker and at lower doses. For example, in the Sverdlovsk outbreak, sheep and cows began to die three days after the release of the aerosol, up to 50-km downwind from the point of release (Meselson *et al.* 1994). The incubation period for plague in cats may be as short as 1–2 days, compared with 1–6 days in humans. Rodents are sensitive to tularaemia and may become ill before humans. It is not known whether animals will be affected by aerosols of the haemorrhagic fevers. While the botulinum toxin type that would affect humans does not generally affect animals when transmitted by food, this does not exclude possible toxic effects if exposure is through the respiratory system.

Environmental and food surveillance

Bravata *et al.* (2004b) reviewed systems for environmental detection of biological agents and found that in many cases, the sensitivity and specificity of the systems had not been evaluated. The detection systems included particulate counters or biomass indicators that detect an increase in particles in aerosol samples, systems designed to rapidly detect biological agents collected from environmental, human, animal or agricultural samples and systems that integrate the collection, identification, and communication of the results. Autonomous detection systems for detecting anthrax spores are being developed particularly for use in the workplace (Meehan *et al.* 2004). Wherever any system installed, there should be detailed response plans in the event of a positive signal.

Current status of surveillance for bioterrorist incidents

Despite the increased sophistication of the surveillance systems, early identification of deliberately caused diseases will depend largely on the ability of primary care and emergency room physicians to identify and immediately report typical cases. The diagnosis of uncommon diseases may be missed by physicians who have rarely or never seen cases of the disease. Thus, medical personnel, particularly in hospital emergency rooms, should be updated regularly on the clinical manifestations of diseases which may result from bioterrorism.

The epidemiological investigation

In many respects, the epidemiological investigation of a bioterrorist incident is similar to any outbreak investigation. The main objectives are to identify and characterize the outbreak and predict its course.

For bioterrorism, the investigators should have specialized knowledge of the possible biological agents and the natural history of the diseases they produce. This will require a multi-disciplinary team led by specialists in infectious disease epidemiology. It will also require close cooperation with law enforcement authorities, risk communicators and the media. Where appropriate, those interviewing patients will need personal protective equipment (PPE).

There are likely to be three distinct phases of the investigation. The first is when an outbreak is suspected without a definitive diagnosis, the second is when the diagnosis has been confirmed and the third is when it is concluded that the outbreak was intentional. Clear, operational protocols for all phases, including agreed upon definitions of cases and contacts, and appropriate questionnaires, should be available for all potential agents. Data should be meticulously collected on each patient, including the date and time of onset of symptoms, the nature of the signs and symptoms, a history of all public places visited during a period compatible with the incubation periods of the suspected agents, details of personal acquaintances or knowledge of other patients with similar symptoms and contacts since the onset of symptoms. All relevant results of the medical examination should be recorded, including treatment received prior to presentation at a health care facility and that prescribed by the treating physician. The natural history of the disease should be described, including changes in the condition of the patient. A detailed history of previous vaccinations should be recorded. All relevant contacts of the patients need to be identified and interviewed.

Diagnosis in bioterrorist outbreaks

Most of the biological agents can be easily grown and diagnosed with high accuracy in hospital laboratories. However, some may require more specialized laboratories and there is a need for international collaboration. New technologies, especially those based on DNA technology, are being developed to speed up the pathogen recognition process. Concern for the safety of laboratory workers requires investment in safety equipment.

The clinical diagnosis of smallpox is based on the course of the disease and the typical rash (Henderson *et al.* 1999). The diagnosis is confirmed by electron microscopy. Recently, a real-time PCR method was described to identify the variola virus (Scaramozzino *et al.* 2007). The clinical diagnosis of anthrax is classically based on symptoms and chest X-ray findings which are usually abnormal, but can be confused with pneumonic plague (Ingelsby *et al.* 2002). There are not usually signs of classical bronchopneumonia, but later there is evidence of a widened mediastinum, pleural effusions, air bronchograms, necrotizing pneumonic lesions, and consolidation. The basic diagnostic tests for B anthracis are available in hospital laboratories and rapid tests are being developed. The confirmatory tests such as immuno-histochemical staining, gamma phage, and PCR assays are carried out in special reference laboratories.

The clinical diagnosis of plague is based on a finding of severe pneumonia and sepsis (Ingelsby *et al.* 2002; Prentice & Rahalison 2007). The index of suspicion is likely to be low unless there is a cluster of patients with fever, cough, shortness of breath, chest pain and a fulminant course. Gram stain may reveal Gram-negative bacilli or cocco-bacilli. A Wright, Giemsa or Wayson stain will often show bipolar staining and direct fluorescent antibody testing could be positive. Cultures of sputum, blood or lymph node aspirate should demonstrate growth approximately 24–48 h after inoculation. Up to 72 h may be required to identify the organism.

Since inhalation tularaemia presents with acute, non-specific, respiratory symptoms, the clinical diagnosis is difficult and usually, only a cluster of cases is likely to arouse suspicion (Dennis *et al.* 2001). The X-ray findings include atypical pneumonia, pleuritis and hilar lymphadenopathy, and routine microbiological tests may not be successful in identifying the bacteria. Diagnosis is made using direct examination of secretions, exudates and biopsy specimens using direct fluorescent antibody or immunohistological stains or blood cultures. Tests results can be obtained from reference laboratories within a few hours.

Botulism presents classically with a symmetric descending paralysis (Arnon *et al.* 2001). The electromyogram can sometimes help in the diagnosis. The CSF is unchanged in botulism. Laboratory testing for botulism is only obtainable at selected laboratories. The laboratory test is based on a mouse bioassay using serum, faeces, gastric aspirate. For food-transmitted botulism, vomitus and suspected foods can be tested. Suspected contaminated food should be refrigerated until tested. The mouse bioassay yields results within one to two days.

The clinical presentation of the viral haemorrhagic fevers varies widely and requires a high index of suspicion (Borio *et al.* 2002). Only specialized laboratories can currently make rapid diagnoses. The laboratory methods include antigen and antibody capture ELISA, RT-PCR, and viral isolation. Virus isolation requires a BSL-4 facility. Although a rise in antibody titre is diagnostic, antibodies appear late in the disease and are of limited value for early diagnosis.

Treatment of patients in bioterrorist incidents

Preparedness for bioterrorism will require an infrastructure that is capable of dealing with a variety of biological agents and clinical surge capacity. For contagious diseases such as smallpox, plague, and haemorrhagic fever, special precautions, such as patient isolation, will be necessary. Guidelines for isolation precautions for patients in healthcare facilities, have recently been published by the United States CDC (Siegel *et al.* 2007). The needs of special groups such as the paediatric population, pregnant women, and people with immunological disorders will need to be addressed.

For smallpox, standard, contact, and airborne precautions must be instituted. Therapy comprises supportive therapy and antibiotics for secondary infections. No drug has been found to be effective in modifying the course of the disease. There is some evidence of the potential efficacy of the thiosemicarbazones, but this is still under study. Patients with pneumonic plague must be managed using standard and droplet precautions. Streptomycin and gentamicin have been found to be effective in treatment. There is some evidence of the development of multiple, antimicrobial resistance in plague (Welch *et al.* 2007). For tularaemia, isolation of the patients is not necessary and standard precautions should be employed. The antibiotics, streptomycin, and gentamicin have been found to be effective. For the haemorrhagic fevers, initially standard, contact, and airborne precautions should be implemented until diagnosis has been confirmed. Subsequently, droplet can be used in place of airborne precautions. The treatment consists of supportive care and treatment of secondary infections. No drug has been found effective in modifying the course of the disease. There are no anti-viral drugs approved, although ribavirin may be effective.

Patients with inhalation anthrax need to be treated early (Ingelsby *et al.* 2002). Protective respirators (N95) and clothing should be used by healthcare personnel. Clothing of patients should undergo decontamination and thorough handwashing procedures should be enforced. Following the appearance of respiratory signs, the prognosis is very poor, even with treatment. In addition to supportive therapy, antibiotics such as ciprofloxacin, doxycycline, and ampicillin have been found to be effective. However, since the bacteria may have been engineered to be resistant to some of the antibiotics, the actual treatment regimen (Meselson *et al.* 1994) will dependent on the results of sensitivity testing. For symptomatic patients, antibiotics are given intravenously until the patient is stable, followed by oral therapy. In the event of a large number of casualties, intravenous therapy may not be feasible and only oral therapy will be used.

Patients with botulism do not need to be isolated and standard precautions should be maintained. Therapy includes supportive care and passive immunization with equine antitoxin. The licensed antitoxin contains types A, B, and C. There is also an investigational heptavalent (ABCDEFG) antitoxin held by the United States army. The dose is a single vial by slow intravenous infusion. Hypersensitivity reactions may occur. The rates of serum sickness or urticaria appear to be about 2 per cent and milder signs occur at rates as high as 18 per cent.

Handling of dead patients and burial procedures

The handling of dead patients should be carried out with the same barrier precautions as for live patients, according to the biological agent involved. Usually, post-mortem examinations should be kept to a minimum and should be carried out by staff appropriately protected and where necessary, given medications and/or vaccines. The burial procedures also have to be carried out using protective clothing which must be disposed in biohazard bags. At all times, the religions and traditions of the community involved should be respected.

For diseases such as smallpox, other than valuables, clothing and disposable medical equipment should be buried with the body. The body should be double-wrapped in sealed polyethylene bags. Some have proposed that quicklime should be added both inside the wrapping and in the grave itself. Care should be taken to bury the dead at places that are not near underground water sources, residential areas, agricultural sites or concentrations of animals.

Pharmacologic prophylaxis

Pre- and post-exposure prophylaxis

There are basically two modes of pharmacalogical prophylaxis, depending on the biological agent. Pre-exposure prophylaxis is given prior to the incident to people at increased risk of exposure. Post-exposure prophylaxis is given after known or suspected exposure to the biological agent. The first mode is generally confined to vaccines, whereas the second mode may combine the use of both antibiotics and vaccines. Antivirals and immunoglobulins are currently considered only for treatment and not for prophylaxis.

The role of vaccines

As part of primary prevention of bioterrorism, vaccines are one of the most effective means of protecting the public. Improved preparedness for bioterrorism will be heavily dependent on the development of new vaccines. Currently, vaccines are only relevant for smallpox and anthrax. If adverse events associated with these vaccines can be reduced to negligible levels, it is conceivable that some countries may consider including them in the infant vaccination schedules. For some of the other potential bioterrorist agents, vaccines are in various stages of development.

Smallpox

As a result of a world-wide campaign by the WHO, global eradication of smallpox was achieved in 1978 (Henderson *et al.* 1999). Since 1972, routine vaccination has been phased out and in most countries, more than 50 per cent of the population has never been vaccinated. Antibody titres have been shown to decline markedly after 5–10 years, although there is some evidence that residual immunity persists for many years (Eichner 2003). In such cases, even if the disease is not prevented, it is likely to be much milder. On the one hand this may reduce transmission (Nishiura & Eichner 2006), but on the other hand, milder cases may circulate in the community increasing the risk of spread (Kerrod *et al.* 2005).

The current vaccine is based on the established live, attenuated form of the vaccinia virus (Henderson *et al.* 1999). Some of the current vaccine stocks in the United States were produced during the 1970s using the New York City Board of Health (NHYBH) strain. Other types of smallpox vaccines include the Lister strains in the United States, LC16m8 in Japan and the modified Ankara strain (MVA) in Germany. Some 200 million doses of a cell-line vaccine are currently held by the United States government. New smallpox vaccines are currently being developed (Wiser *et al.* 2007).

The potential adverse effects of vaccination with vaccinia include post-vaccinial encephalitis, vaccinia necrosum, eczema vaccinatum, generalized vaccinia and accidental infection. The rates of life-threatening complications of post-vaccinia encephalitis and vaccinia necrosum in primary vaccinees are estimated as at least 3 and 1 per million, respectively (Aragon *et al.* 2003), although adverse effects may be higher for some strains. Rare, adverse effects on the cardiovascular system have been reported. The rates of adverse events may be substantially higher in areas where immunodeficiency is common.

Vaccinia immune globulin (VIG) is hyperimmune globulin produced from sera of previously vaccinated subjects. It is used under two circumstances. When a patient with relative contraindications to the vaccine is at high risk of contracting the disease, the smallpox vaccine is given together with VIG. In the event that a vaccinee experiences a severe adverse event, VIG is given intravenously and if the response is inadequate, it can be repeated after 72 h.

Smallpox pre-exposure prophylaxis

Most pre-exposure prophylaxis strategies call for vaccinating subgroups such as the military, healthcare workers, ambulance crews and police. Opinions vary on how large the portion of the population should be encouraged to be vaccinated. Healthcare workers have shown some resistance to vaccination due to concern about adverse effects and the perception that there is a low risk of a bioterrorist incident using smallpox.

Smallpox post-exposure prophylaxis

The method of post-exposure prophylaxis has been debated widely. There are data from the beginning of the twentieth century suggesting that vaccination within several days of exposure provides protection against clinical disease (Mortimer 2003). Since the incubation period for smallpox is around seven to fourteen days, if the identification of the first cases is the earliest indication of exposure, post-exposure vaccination will be too late to influence the outcome of those exposed at the site of the incident. It will therefore be relevant only for contacts.

Two approaches have been proposed for post-exposure prophylaxis. 'Ring vaccination', entails intensive tracing and vaccination of all primary contacts immediately following diagnosis of a case. This is followed by vaccination of the secondary contacts in the second ring. This approach was used successfully in the eradication of naturally occurring smallpox (Henderson et al. 1999). An alternative approach is to carry out mass vaccination of the population, following diagnosis of the first cases. Using mathematical modelling, some have favoured ring vaccination (Riley & Ferguson 2006) whereas others have found that rapid mass vaccination of the population is most effective (Kaplan et al. 2002). Ring vaccination accompanied by mass vaccination of affected regions (Hall et al. 2007), followed by countrywide mass vaccination, appear to be the most practical approach.

Anthrax

In the United States, the current vaccine is made from the cell-free filtrate of a non-encapsulated attenuated strain of Bacillus anthracis. It was licensed in 1970 to be given in a series of six doses. The United Kingdom produces a vaccine based on the same principles, where the protective antigen is the most important immunogen. Live spore vaccines from an attenuated strain have been produced in Russia and China. Pre-exposure prophylactic vaccination with the United States vaccine was shown to be protective in animal challenge studies. In a follow-up of vaccines, no unexpected local or systemic events were reported (Martin et al. 2005). Compliance may be a problem, due to factors such as concern about the safety of the vaccine. For post-exposure prophylaxis, the vaccine series, initiated together with antibiotics, has been shown to be the most cost-effective strategy (Fowler et al. 2005).

Vaccines for other category A agents

There are essentially no effective vaccines available for use in bioterrorist incidents for the other category A agents. The previous licensed, formalin-inactivated, whole bacilli, plague vaccine was not effective against primary pneumonic plague. Research continues in this area. A live, attenuated vaccine against tularaemia for high risk military personnel is held as an investigational new drug by the United States military. The vaccine has not been used widely for pre-exposure prophylaxis and does not appear to have any place in post-exposure prophylaxis.

A multivalent vaccine for some of the types of botulism is available at the CDC, but it is impractical to use in a bioterrorist incident. In the United States, an investigational pentavalent (ABCDE), botulinum toxoid is provided by the CDC for laboratory workers at high risk of exposure to botulinum toxin and by the military for protection against attack. Botulinum toxoid takes several months to produce immunity and has no value for post-exposure prophylaxis. New botulism vaccines are under development. As regards viral haemorrhagic fevers, with the exception of the yellow fever live attenuated 17D vaccine and Hunin virus vaccine, there are no licensed vaccines. Some progress appears to have been made in developing a vaccine for post-exposure prophylaxis of Ebola infection (Feldmann et al. 2007).

The role of medications in post-exposure prophylaxis

Antibiotics have a role in post-exposure prophylaxis mainly for anthrax and plague. Ciprofloxacin, doxycycline, and ampicillin should be effective against anthrax, depending on the sensitivity of the organism, and are recommended for a period of up to 60 days. Mild adverse events may be common, but serious reactions and hospitalizations are rare (Shephard et al. 2002). Since the response to antibiotics deteriorates rapidly following the onset of symptoms, prophylactic therapy should be provided as soon as possible to those who have been exposed. Due to the need to take the medications for a long period, compliance becomes a major problem. It may be possible to shorten the duration of antibiotic therapy, if vaccine is given concurrently.

Post-exposure prophylaxis for plague should be provided using appropriate antibiotics for a shorter period than required for anthrax. There is currently no effective vaccine for use under these circumstances.

It has been shown that antivirals, such as cidofovir or a related acyclic nucleoside phosphonate analogue, are more effective than post-exposure smallpox vaccine in preventing mortality, in monkeys experimentally infected with monkeypox virus (Stittelaar et al. 2006). This suggests that antivirals may have an important place in planning for a smallpox outbreak. For viral haemorrhagic fevers, ribavirin may have some efficacy in post-exposure prophylaxis.

National and international stockpiles of vaccines and medications

A number of countries have established national stockpiles of pharmaceuticals and vaccines, for use in the event of biological or chemical attacks or for serious diseases that may achieve epidemic proportions. The United States maintains the Strategic National Stockpile (SNS) of antibiotics, chemical antidotes, antitoxins, vaccines, life-supporting medications and emergency medical equipment. The operation of the SNS, in the event of an emergency, is based on 'push packages' that can be deployed to the designated sites within 12 h. The model is based on the 'Dispensing/Vaccination Centers' (DVCs). Either medications and vaccines will be taken directly to people's homes, or individuals will attend DVCs to receive medications or be vaccinated. The stocks in the SNS programme are rotated and kept within potency shelf-life limits.

NATO has initiated a programme to develop a deployable laboratory and biological defence stockpiles. In 2005, at least 40 countries had stockpiles of smallpox vaccine, varying from amounts sufficient to vaccinate the whole population to enough for only a proportion of the population (Arita 2005). The global inventory reported at that time was in excess of 800 million doses with a total global production potential of more than 400 million doses. Since some of the vaccines can be diluted at least one to five without losing potency (Couch et al. 2007), globally, the total number of doses potentially available in the event of an emergency may be in excess of three billion, with a production capacity in excess of two billion doses annually. International stockpiles of smallpox vaccine are held by the WHO with about 200 million doses being held under agreement by selected donor states, to be supplied to countries in need, in the event of an outbreak.

National vaccination programmes

Some countries have carried out active vaccination programmes against smallpox in the military and 'first-responders'. Since 2001, in the United States, more than half a million military personnel and about 40 000 healthcare workers have been vaccinated (Arita 2005). In addition, United States military personnel are now routinely vaccinated against anthrax and in the United Kingdom, the vaccine is offered to military personnel.

Non-pharmaceutical prophylaxis

Non-pharmacological prophylaxis is an important means of reducing the spread of the contagious diseases, smallpox, plague and the haemorrhagic fevers. These include strict isolation and barrier nursing procedures when treating patients, and public actions such as quarantine, social distancing, and the use of face masks, to reduce exposure in the community.

Isolation of sick patients

The first action to reduce propagation of contagious diseases, is to isolate sick patients. Isolation is defined as 'the separation and confinement of individuals known or suspected to be infected with a contagious disease to prevent them from transmitting the disease to others' (Barbera *et al.* 2001). This includes the transfer of patients to healthcare facilities. Once hospitalized, the highest level of isolation comprises special units with appropriate negative pressure air filtration. Simpler isolation with strict barrier nursing would represent a lower level of isolation. If the number of cases is large and overwhelms isolation facilities in hospitals, it may be necessary to establish isolation facilities at alternative locations. In addition, a policy of voluntary isolation could be implemented, where sick patients are encouraged to be treated at home.

Quarantine (curfews)

A second measure to limit spread of contagious diseases, is to quarantine those who may have been exposed. The definition of quarantine is: 'compulsory physical separation, including restriction of movement of populations or groups of healthy people who have been potentially exposed to a contagious disease, or to efforts to segregate them within specified geographical areas' (Barbera *et al.* 2001). The term 'cordon sanitaire' applies to restriction of movement of people and materials, and community-wide intervention strategies. The enforcement of quarantine is generally in the hands of the law-enforcement authorities. Since the quarantined population contains both people who have been exposed but are not yet ill, and others who were suspected of having been exposed but in fact were not, there is increased risk of disease transmission in the quarantined population.

Factors that contribute to imposing quarantine include the size of the exposed population and the severity and contagiousness of the disease (Barbera *et al.* 2001). Decisions have to be made regarding who should be quarantined and for how long. Border closure is a sensitive issue and will need special attention, according to the disease in question. The commercial consequences need to be recognized. Good risk communication is likely to improve compliance.

Social distancing

Social distancing has been proposed as an important non-pharmacalogical means of reducing the spread of transmissible diseases such as influenza. It includes measures such as closing of schools, limiting crowding in workplaces and other public places and reducing use of public transport. The possible impact on diseases caused by bioterrorism agents is less clear. Using mathematical modelling, there is evidence that social distancing could reduce the spread of smallpox (Kress 2005).

Masks and personal protective equipment (PPE)

There are clear, agent-specific, guidelines for the use of masks and PPE by healthcare personnel and the public health and emergency workers coming into contact with sick patients or moving in contaminated areas. The issue of whether the public should be encouraged to use masks during an outbreak of a contagious disease is less clear. The efficacy of the masks remains questionable and the type of masks to be used is not clear. Surgical masks may be adequate for droplet spread, but N95 type masks would be necessary to protect against aerosols. The N95 mask is more expensive, more complicated to use, requires special fitting and is uncomfortable to use for long periods of time.

Public education and risk communication

The goal of the terrorist has been described as 'an attempt to produce fear, magnified by an exaggerated sense of risk . . . and perpetuated by misinformation and rumors' (Shine 2001). The novel and largely unpredictable characteristics of biological weapons are likely to increase the uncertainty surrounding a bioterrorism incident. This uncertainty can reduce public trust in the ability of the authorities to control the incident. Public education and effective risk communication are essential in order to bolster public confidence and improve cooperation with the authorities.

Structured education programmes should be directed at healthcare personnel, other first responders and the general public. Clinicians and public health personnel should have access to up-to-date emergency information, which requires a solid infrastructure for rapid and reliable communication (Khan *et al.* 2000). The general public needs to have access to non-technical descriptions of the potential diseases that may be encountered and simple instructions on how to act in an emergency situation.

Risk communication plays a critical role in mitigating public panic responses and encouraging rational behaviour during an emergency. While there is a considerable literature on risk communication, relatively little has dealt with bioterrorism (Covello *et al.* 2001). Nevertheless, the general approaches that have been developed are relevant for a bioterrorism incident. Since the public's perception of risk may be somewhat different from the true risk, this is a critical component of risk communication (Slovic 1987). There are frequently misconceptions about what information should and should not be presented to the public. One approach is to encourage open discussion of the risk.

Due to the inherent uncertainty in a bioterrorism incident, the authorities may possess very little factual information. The impression may be that information is being withheld and the public may respond with hostility towards the authorities. In such situations, Sandman (2003) has proposed that 'one should not over-reassure, acknowledge uncertainty and share dilemmas'. Over-reaction or panic should be anticipated when new information about the risk is made public, although this is often complicated when rumours of ineffective and expensive solutions are propagated (Taig 1999).

As a convenient conceptual and operational framework, risk communication associated with a bioterrorist event may be divided into five stages—prior to the event, on suspicion of an event, on confirmation of the event, during the event and following the event. At each stage, the public is likely to ask questions relevant to that stage.

The main questions that are likely to be raised prior to a bioterrorist incident are whether in fact it can occur, and are the authorities well-prepared. On suspicion of an event, the public will want to know how likely it is that a bioterrorist incident has occurred. On confirmation of an incident, people will want to know where is it located, when did it start, is it contagious, are they at risk and is there a cure. During the event, there will be questions about the efficacy of the treatment, whether the disease is spreading, who is at risk and when will the event end. The questions after the event focus on whether the event has really ended and is there still a risk of exposure. The ability of the authorities to respond adequately to these questions depends on their access to good information. Timely and reliable surveillance data will be an important resource.

Problems that may be encountered during an outbreak

During an outbreak, the epidemiological investigation team should anticipate the numerous problems that may arise. These include atypical presentation of cases and varying responses to treatment. Unexpected laboratory difficulties are often more the rule than the exception and unexpectedly high percentages of false positive and negative diagnoses may be encountered. There are likely to be reports of side-effects of the medications and vaccines. In addition, there may be instances of vaccine or medication prophylaxis failure, which will reduce the trust of the public in the intervention procedures recommended.

Reports of the appearance of suspected new exposure foci are likely. A sense of mistrust may occur when disease is reported in apparently unexposed people. There may be incidences of inadequate isolation of patients and a breakdown of the implementation of quarantine regulations. It is possible that untried, new treatments will be proposed, often by professionals or lay persons not included among those handling the outbreak. Finally, unexpected changes in established policy may occur.

International cooperation (Bonin 2007)

The International Health Regulations (IHR) were first initiated in 1969 to 'prevent, protect against, control and provide a public health response to the international spread of disease in ways that are commensurate with and restricted to public health risks, and which avoid unnecessary interference with international traffic and trade'. The regulations were updated in 2005 and taken into account the increased threat of bioterrorism. They took effect in June 2007.

The WHO has established the Global Outbreak Alert and Response Network (GOARN) for international collaboration for the identification, confirmation and response to outbreaks with international implications. The Epidemic and Pandemic Alert and Response (EPR) component supports member states in epidemic preparedness in the context of the IHR. It includes training for preparedness and response, developing standardized approaches for readiness and response to major epidemic diseases, strengthening biosafety, biosecurity, and preparedness for outbreaks of diseases caused by dangerous pathogens and developing a global platform to support outbreak response.

The European Union also has a programme to improve cooperation between member states on preparedness and response to biological and chemical agent attacks (BICHAT). They operate the Early Warning and Response System (EWRS) for outbreaks of communicable diseases. A number of research activities are funded within the European Framework programmes and NATO funds activities such as Advanced Research Workshops where one of the major programme areas is bioterrorism preparedness.

Tabletop exercises

Tabletop exercises have been carried out, largely in the United States, to test the preparedness of the authorities in dealing with a bioterrorist attack. The 'Dark Winter' exercise in 2001, simulated a covert smallpox attack on the United States (O'Toole et al. 2002) and the TOPOFF exercise in 2000 simulated a simultaneous radiological, chemical and biological attack with Yersinia pestis (Ingelsby et al. 2001), They revealed serious deficiencies in the management of such incidents and provided impetus to the improvement of bioterrorism preparedness programmes. In 2005, the 'New Watchman' exercise, initiated by the European Commission, was conducted to evaluate European preparedness for a deliberate smallpox outbreak (Health Protection Agency 2007). Serious limitations were revealed in communications between member states, compatibility of response plans, countermeasures and adequacy of resources. In addition to recommendations on measures to overcome these limitations, it was stressed that similar exercises should be carried out as part of a routine programme.

Post-incident actions

Decontamination

Decontamination issues are relevant, mainly for anthrax and smallpox, in the general environment of an aerosol attack and places where patients were treated. This should including bedding, clothing and equipment. Methodologies for decontamination of the general environment from anthrax have been evaluated (Canter et al. 2005). Formaldehyde solution was effective in inactivating anthrax spores on the island of Gruinard, contaminated experimentally during the British biowarfare programme (Manchee et al. 1994). Hypochlorite solution is also effective.

Low humidity and temperature prolong survival of the smallpox virus in the environment (Kiang & Krathwohl 2003). Viruses on scab material can remain viable for as long as 12 weeks (Huq 1976). There are detailed procedures for sterilizing bedding and clothing and disinfecting the immediate environment of the patients.

Long-term consequences of bioterrorism incidents

Following a bioterrorist incident, residual public fear and anxiety is likely to persist. In a five-year follow-up of victims of the terrorist incident in the Tokyo subway attack, post-traumatic stress disorder symptoms were observed (Ohtani et al. 2004). There will inevitably be questions about the extent to which the authorities were able to control the incident, criticism of actions taken or not taken, and general recriminations. Part of the preparedness planning should include public education of the public on lessons learned from the incident and actions taken to address deficiencies.

Legal and ethical aspects

Bioterrorism preparedness requires the necessary legislation to enable the public health authorities to carry out measures with adequate legal backing. Laws that are of particular importance relate to closing buildings, taking over hospitals and ordering isolation and quarantine. Other issues that require regulation are active surveillance of presumed infected individuals and their contacts.

The authorities may have to exercise unusual powers to control the outbreak, which will require information campaigns. Civil liberties may be compromised. Questions that frequently arise relate to who enforces a quarantine, who detains an infected or exposed person and how civil liberties are protected. There will be a need for ethical review of surveillance procedures, but there is also 'an ethical mandate to undertake surveillance that enhances the well-being of the population' (Fairchild & Bayer 2004).

Agroterrorism

Agroterrorism includes the deliberate infection of livestock or crops with biological agents (Cupp *et al.* 2004). A number of countries, including the United States and the Soviet Union, had agricultural bioweapons programmes during the twentieth century. As previously noted, glanders was used against horses and mules in World War I, and it is alleged that Japan considered use of anthrax and rinderpest in World War II. The potential deliberate damage to crops or livestock will require special vigilance.

Conclusions

Bioterrorism falls into the category of low risk but high impact public health emergencies. Deterrence remains the prime goal, and delegitimization of the use of biological agents as weapons should be carried out at every level. The BioWeapons Prevention Project (BWPP) is an initiative based in Geneva with the objective of strengthening the opposition to the use of biological weapons. In addition, good preparedness for a bioterrorist incident both serves the goal of deterrence and ensures that the public health system and the society will deal effectively with the incident.

Questions have been raised about the justification for investing considerable resources in what is perceived to be a low risk event, possibly at the expense of the general public health services (Cohen *et al.* 2004). The United States CDC has defined 'ten essential services for public health' to respond to bioterrorism (CDC 2006). In summary, they recommend developing greater capacity to monitor health status and rapidly detect, diagnose, and investigate infectious disease and environmental health problems. The means to inform and educate people about health threats should be improved. Partnerships should be mobilized and policies and plans developed to respond to public health emergencies and enforce laws and regulations that protect health. Finally there is a need to develop a competent and trained public health workforce, evaluate the effectiveness, accessibility and quality of health services for emergencies and promote research for new and innovative solutions to health problems.

All these actions will serve public health in general, stressing the dual-benefit concept. An excellent example of such dual-benefit is the role played by of the United States military in developing new vaccines to protect the troops (Artenstein *et al.* 2005). This has resulted in vaccines for diseases affecting the general public, such as yellow fever, pneumococcal disease, hepatitis A and B and Japanese encephalitis. Preparedness for bioterrorism will benefit preparedness for disease outbreaks in general and other public health emergencies.

References

Aragon, T.J., Ulrich, S., Fernyak, S., and Rutherford, G.W. (2003). Risks of serious complications and death from smallpox vaccination: a systematic review of the United States experience, 1963–1968. *BMC Public Health*, **3**, 26–37.

Arita, I. (2005). Smallpox vaccine and its stockpile in 2005. *Lancet Infectious Diseases*, **5**, 647–52.

Arizona Department of Health Services. (2005). Bureau of Emergency Preparedness and Response. Bioterrorism. Available at: http://www.azdhs.gov/phs/edc/edrp/es/bthistor1.htm. Accessed July 1, 2007.

Arnon, S.S., Schechter, R., Ingelsby, T.V. *et al.* (2001). Botulism toxin as a biological weapon. Medical and public health management. *Journal of the American Medical Association*, **285**, 1059–70.

Artenstein, A.W., Opal, J.M., Opal, S.M., Tramont, E.C., Peter, G., Russell, P.K. (2005). *Military Medicine* **170**(4 Suppl):3–11.

Barbera, J., Macintyre, A., Gostin, L. *et al.* (2001). Large-scale quarantine following biological terrorism in the United States: scientific examination, logistic and legal limits, and possible consequences. *Journal of the American Medical Association*, **286**, 2711–8.

Bonin, S. (2007). In *International Biodefense Handbook. An inventory of national and international biodefense practices and policies* (series eds. A. Wegner, V. Mauer, and M. Dunn). *Center for Security Studies at ETH, Zurich*.

Borio, L., Ingelsby, T., Peters C.J. *et al.* (2002). Hemorrhagic fever viruses as biological weapons. *Journal of the American Medical Association*, **287**, 2391–405.

Bozzette S.A., Boer, R., Bhatnagar, V. *et al.* (2003). A model for a smallpox vaccination policy. *New England Journal Medicine*, **348**, 416–25.

Bradley C.A., Rolka, H., Walker, D., and Loonsk, J. (2005). BioSense: implementation of a national early event detection and situational awareness system. *Morbidity and Mortality Weekly Report*, **54**(Suppl), 11–9.

Bravata D.M., McDonald K.M., Smith W.M. *et al.* (2004a). Systematic review: surveillance systems for early detection of bioterrorism-related diseases. *Annals of Internal Medicine*, **140**, 910–22.

Bravata D.M., Sundaram, V., McDonald K.M. *et al.* (2004b). Evaluating detection and diagnostic decision support systems for bioterrorism response. *Emerging Infectious Diseases*, **10**, 100–8.

Brookmeyer, R., Blades, N., Hugh-Jones, M., and Henderson D.A. (2001). The statistical analysis of truncated data: application to the Sverdlovsk anthrax outbreak. *Biostatistics*, **2**, 233–47.

Canter D.A., Gunning, D., Rodgers, P., O'connor, L., Traunero, C., and Kempter C.J. (2005). Remediation of *Bacillus anthracis* contamination in the U.S. Department of Justice mail facility. *Biosecurity and Bioterrorism*, **3**, 119–27.

Centers for Disease Control and Prevention. (2001). Updated guidelines for evaluating public health surveillance systems. *Morbidity and Mortality Weekly Report*, **50**(RR13), 1–35.

Centers for Disease Control and Prevention. (2006). Bioterrorism overview. February 28, 2006. Available at: www.bt.cdc.gov/bioterrorism. Accessed July 1, 2007.

Cohen H.W., Gould R.M., and Sidel V.W. (2004). The pitfalls of bioterrorism preparedness: the anthrax and smallpox experiences. *American Journal of Public Health*, **94**, 1667–71.

Couch R.B., Winokur, P., Edwards K.M. *et al.* (2007). Reducing the dose of smallpox vaccine reduces vaccine-associated morbidity without reducing vaccination success rates or immune responses. *Journal of Infectious Diseases*, **195**, 826–32.

Covello V.T., Peters R.G., Wojtecki J.G., and Hyde R.C. (2001). Risk communication, the West Nile virus epidemic, and bioterrorism: responding to the communication challenges posed by the intentional or unintentional release of a pathogen in an urban setting. *Journal of Urban Health*, **78**, 382–91.

Cupp OS, Walker DE 2nd, Hillison J. Agroterrorism in the U.S.: key security challenge for the 21st century. (2004). *Biosecurity and Bioterrorism* **2**:97–105.

Dennis D.T., Ingelsby T.V., Henderson D.A. *et al.* (2001). Tularemia as a biological weapon. Medical and public health management. *Journal of the American Association*, **285**, 2763–73.

Eichner, M. (2003). Analysis of historical data suggests long-lasting protective effects of smallpox vaccination. *American Journal of Epidemiology*, **158**, 717–23.

Fairchild A.L., and Bayer, R. (2004). Public health. Ethics and the conduct of public health surveillance. *Science*, **303**, 631–2.

Federal Bureau of Investigation. Headline Archives. Anthrax investigation. Closing a chapter. Available at: http://www.fbi.gov/page2/august08/amerithtrax080608.html. Accessed October 1, 2008.

Feldmann, H., Jones S.M., Daddario-DiCaprio K.M. *et al.* (2007). Effective post-exposure treatment of Ebola infection. *PLOoS Pathogens*, **3**, 54–60.

Fowler R.A., Sanders G.D., Bravata D.M. *et al.* (2005). Cost-effectiveness of defending against bioterrorism: a comparison of vaccination and antibiotic prophylaxis against anthrax. *Annals of Internal Medicine*, **142**, 601–10.

Franz D.R., Jahrling P.B., Friedlander A.M. *et al.* (1997). Clinical recognition and management of patients exposed to biological warfare agents. *Journal of the American Medical Association*, **278**, 399–411.

Gani, R. and Leach, S. Epidemiologic determinants for modeling pneumonic plague outbreaks. (2004). *Emerging Infectious Diseases* **10**:608–614.

Green M.S. and Kaufman, Z. (2005). Syndromic surveillance for early location of terrorist incidents outside of residential areas. Morbidity and Mortality Weekly, **54** (Suppl), 189. Available at http://www.cdc.gov/mmwr/preview/mmwrhtml/su5401a35.htm. Accessed July 14, 2007.

Hall I.M., Egan J.R., Barrass, I., Gani, R., and Leach, S. (2007). Comparison of smallpox outbreak control strategies using a spatial metapopulation model. *Epidemiology and Infection*, **135**, 1133–44.

Health Protection Agency. Exercise New Watchman. A Smallpox exercise for the European Union. Serial 5.1. Final Report, March 2006. Available at: http://ec.europa.eu/health/ph_threats/com/watchman.pdf. Accessed October 6, 2007.

Heffernan, R., Mostashari, F., Das, D., Karpati, A., Kulldorff, M., and Weiss, D. (2004). Syndromic surveillance in public health practice, New York City. *Emerging Infectious Diseases*, **10**, 858–64.

Henderson D.A. (1998). Bioterrorism as a public health threat. *Emerging Infectious Diseases*, **4**, 488–92.

Henderson D.A., Ingelsby T.V., Bartlett J.G. *et al.* (1999). Smallpox as a biological weapon. Medical and public health management. *Journal of the American Medical Association*, **281**, 2127–37.

Hoffman, B. (2007). In "Terrorism". Microsoft Encarta Online Encyclopedia. Available at: http://encarta.msn.com. Accessed July 14, 2007.

Huq, F. (1976). Effect of temperature and relative humidity on variola virus in crusts. *Bulletin of the World Health Organisation*, **54**, 710–2.

Ingelsby T.V., Grossman, R., and O'Toole, T. (2001). A plague on your city: observations from TOPOFF. *Clinical Infectious Diseases*, **32**, 436–45.

Ingelsby T.V., O'Toole, T., Henderson D.A. *et al.* (2002). Anthrax as a biological weapon, 2002. Updated recommendations for management. *Journal of the American Medical Association*, **287**, 2236–52.

Jernigan D.B., Raghunathan, P.I., Bell B.P. *et al.* (2002). Investigation of bioterrorism-related anthrax, United States, 2001: epidemiologic findings. *Emerging Infectious Diseases*, **8**, 1019–28.

Kaluski D.N., Barak, E., Kaufman, Z. *et al.* (2006). A large food-borne outbreak of group A streptoccocal pharyngitis in an industrial plant: potential for deliberate contamination. *Israel Medical Association Journal*, **8**, 824.

Kaplan E.H., Craft D.L., and Wein L.M. (2002). Emergency response to a smallpox attack: the case for mass vaccination. *Proceedings of the National Academy of Sciences USA*, **99**, 10935–40.

Kaufman, Z., Wong W.K., Peled-Leviathan, T. *et al.* (2007). Evaluation of a syndromic surveillance system using the WSARE algorithm for early detection of an unusual, localized summer outbreak of influenza. Implications for bioterrorism surveillance. *Israel Medical Association Journal*, **9**, 3–7.

Kerrod, E., Geddes A.M., Regan, M., and Leach, S. (2005). Surveillance and control measures during smallpox outbreaks. *Emerging Infectious Diseases*, **11**, 291–7.

Khan A.S., Morse, S., and Lillibridge, S. (2000). Public-health preparedness for biological terrorism in the USA. *Lancet*, **356**, 1179–82.

Kiang K.M., and Krathwohl M.D. (2003). Rates and risks of transmission of smallpox and mechanisms of prevention. *Journal of Laboratory Clinical Medicine*, **142**, 229–38.

Kolavic S.A., Kimura, A., Simons S.L., Slutsker, L., Barth, S., and Haley C.E. (1997). An outbreak of Shigella dysenteriae type 2 among laboratory workers due to intentional food contamination. *Journal of the American Medical Association*, **278**, 396–8.

Kress, M. (2005). The effect of social mixing controls on the spread of smallpox—a two-level model. *Health Care Management Science*, **8**, 277–89.

Leach, S. (2007). Some public health perspectives on quantitative risk assessments for bioterrorism. In *Risk assessment and risk communication strategies in bioterrorism preparedness* (eds. M.S. Green, J. Zenilman, D. Cohen, I. Wiser, and R.D. Balicer). *NATO Security through Science Series – A: Chemistry and Biology*. Springer, The Netherlands.

Manchee R.J., Broster M.G., Stagg A.J., and Hibbs S.E. (1994). Formaldehyde solution effectively inactivates spores of Bacillus anthracis on the Scottish island of Gruinard. *Applied Environmental Microbiology*, **60**, 4167–71.

Martin S.W., Tierney B.C., Aranas, A. *et al.* (2005). An overview of adverse events reported by participants in CDC's anthrax vaccine and antimicrobial availability program. *Pharmacoepidemiology and Drug Safety*, **14**, 393–401.

Meehan P.J., Rosenstein N.E., Gillen, M. *et al.* (2004). Responding to detection of aerosolized Bacillus anthracis by autonomous detection systems in the workplace. *Morbidity and Mortality Weekly Report*, **53**(RR07),1–12.

Meinhardt, P.L. (2005). Water and bioterrorism: preparing for the potential threat to U.S. water supplies and public health. *Annual Reviews of Public Health*, **26**, 213–37.

Meselson, M., Guillemin, J., Hugh-Jones, M. *et al.* (1994). The Sverdlovsk anthrax outbreak of 1979. *Science*, **266**, 1202–8.

Mortimer, P.P. (2003). Can postexposure vaccination against smallpox succeed? *Clinical Infectious Diseases*, **36**, 622–8.

Nishiura, H., and Eichner, M. (2006). Estimation of the duration of vaccine-induced residual protection against severe and fatal smallpox based on secondary vaccination failure. *Infection*, **34**, 239–40.

Ohtani, T., Iwanami, A., Kasai, K., Yamasue, H., Kato, T., Sasaki, T., and Kato, N. (2004). Post-traumatic stress disorder symptoms in victims of Tokyo subway attack: a 5-year follow-up study. *Psychiatry Clinical Neuroscience*, **58**, 624–9.

O'Toole, T., Mair, M., and Ingelsby T.V. (2002). Shining light on "Dark Winter". *Clinical Infectious Diseases*, **34**, 972–83.

Patterson K.B., and Runge, T. (2002). Smallpox and the native American. *American Journal of Medical Sciences*, **323**, 216–22.

Prentice M.B., and Rahalison, L. (2007). Plague. *Lancet*, **369**, 1196–207.

Rabinowitz, P., Gordon, Z., Chudnov, D. *et al.* (2006). Animals as sentinels of bioterrorist agents. *Emerging Infectious Diseases*, **12**, 647–52.

Reingold, A. (2003). If syndromic surveillance is the answer, what is the question? *Biosecurity and Bioterrorism*, **1**, 1–5.

Riley, S., and Ferguson N.M. (2006). Smallpox transmission and control: spatial dynamics in Great Britain. *Proceedings of the National Academy of Sciences*, **103**, 12637–42.

Rolka, H., Burkom, H., Cooper G.F., Kulldorff, M., Madigan, D., and Wong, W.-K. (2007). Issues in applied statistics for public health bioterrorism surveillance using multiple data streams: research needs. *Statistics in Medicine*, **26**, 1834–56.

Rotz L.D., Khan A.S., Lillibridge S.R., Ostroff S.M., and Highes J.M. (2002). Public health assessment of potential biological terrorism agents. *Emerging Infectious Diseases*, **8**, 225–230.

Sandman, P.M. (2003). Bioterrorism risk communication policy. *Journal of Health Communication*, **8** (Suppl 1), 146–7; discussion 148–51.

Scaramozzino, N., Ferrier-Rembert, A., Favier A.L. *et al.* (2007). Real-time PCR to identify variola virus or other human pathogenic orthopox viruses. *Clinical Chemistry*, **53**, 606–13.

Shephard C.W., Soriano-Gabarro, M., Zell E.R. *et al.* (2002). CDC adverse events working group. Antimicrobial post-exposure prophylaxis for anthrax: adverse events and adherence. *Emerging Infectious Diseases*, **8**, 1124–32.

Shine, K. (2001). "For a Hearing on Risk Communication: National Security and Public Health" (testimony presented to the Subcommittee on National Security, Veterans Affairs, and International Relations, House Committee on Government Reform, Washington, D.C.: November 29, 2001). Available at: http://www7.nationalacademies.org/ocga/testimony/Risk_Communication_Natl_Security_Public_Health.asp. Accessed July 1, 2007.

Siegel J.D., Rhinehart, E., Jackson, M., Chiarello, L. and the Healthcare Infection Control Practices Advisory Committee. (2007). Guideline for isolation precautions: preventing transmission of infectious agents in healthcare settings. pp. 119–24. Available at: http://www.cdc.gov/ncidod/dhqp/pdf/isolation2007.pdf. Accessed July 22, 2007.

Slovic, P. (1987). Perception of risk. *Science*, **236**, 280–5.

Sobel, J., Khan A.S., and Swerdlow D.L. (2002). Threat of a biological terrorist attack on the US food supply: the CDC perspective. *Lancet*, **359**, 874–80.

Stittelaar K.J., Neyts, J., Naesens, L. *et al.* (2006). Antiviral treatment is more effective than smallpox vaccine in monkeypox virus infection. *Nature*, **439**, 745–48.

Sugishima, M. (2003). Aum Shinrikyo and the Japanese law on bioterrorism. *Prehospital Disaster Medicine*, **18**, 179–83.

Taig, T, (1999). Benchmarking in government: case studies and principles. In *Risk Communication and Public Health* (eds. P. Bennett and K. Calman), pp. 117–32. Oxford University Press, Oxford.

Torok, T., Tauxe R.V., Wise R.P. *et al.* (1997). A large community outbreak of Salmonella caused by intentional contamination of restaurant salad bars. *Journal of the American Medical Association*, **278**, 389–95.

Tucker, J.B. (1999). Historical trends related to bioterrorism: an empirical analysis. *Emerging Infectious Diseases*, **5**, 498–504.

Walden, J., and Kaplan E.H. (2004). Estimating time and size of bioterror attack. *Emerging Infectious Diseases*, **10**, 1202–5.

Wehrle, P., Posch, J., Richter, K., and Henderson, D, (1970). An airborne outbreak of smallpox in a German hospital and its significance with respect to other recent outbreaks in Europe. *Bulletin of the World Health Organisation*, **43**, 669–79.

Welch, T.J., Fricke, W.F., McDermott, P.F. *et al.* (2007). Multiple antimicrobial resistance in plague: an emerging public health risk. *PloS ONE*, **2**(3), e309. doi:10.1371/journal.pone.0000309.

Wiser, I., Balicer, R.D., and Cohen, D. (2007). An update on smallpox vaccine candidates and their role in bioterrorism related vaccination strategies. *Vaccine*, **25**, 976–84.

World Health Organization. (2004). Public health response to biological and chemical weapons: WHO guidance. Available at: http://www.who.int/csr/delibepidemics/biochemguide/en/print.html. Accessed July 1, 2007.

Zilinskas, R.A. (1997). Iraq's biological weapons. *Journal of the American Medical Association*, **278**, 418–24.

Zilinskas, R.A., Hope, B., North, D.W. (2004). A discussion of findings and their possible implications from a workshop on bioterrorism threat assessment and risk management. *Risk Analysis*, **24**, 901–8.

SECTION 11

Public health needs of population groups

The changing family

Julien O. Teitler

Abstract

Families are dynamic, heterogeneous entities that vary by size and age, gender, and generational compositions, and in political, social, and technological contexts. Thus, families can affect the health of its members in complex, indirect, and potentially overlapping ways. This chapter presents a broad overview of the micro- and macro-level processes by which families affect the health of individuals and highlights issues that are likely to be salient over the next several decades.

Introduction

How families affect health is a very broad area of inquiry, for several reasons: Families are dynamic, heterogeneous entities that vary by size and have different age, gender, and generational compositions. The political, social, and technological contexts that influence family structure and processes vary across place and over time. Families can affect health in a myriad of complex, indirect, and potentially overlapping pathways. Health itself is a broad construct that encompasses a variety of physical and mental health conditions, with varying degrees of severity. This chapter presents a broad overview of the micro- and macro-level processes by which families affect the health of individuals. It paints with broad strokes, emphasizing breadth over depth and offering salient examples rather than a detailed review of the complex pathways by which families can affect health.

The first section focuses on how processes within families affect health. The second section describes macro-level contexts that have influenced, and have been influenced by, family processes that are related to health. There is considerable overlap between these two sections, as the multidimensional topic of how families affect health cannot be divided neatly into categories. The third section will highlight issues related to family and health that will likely be at the forefront of future policy, legal, and ethical debates.

Within-family (micro) processes

Resource distribution

Perhaps the most central manner in which families affect health is through the distribution of resources. Families, as institutions, allocate resources both within and across generations. Family resources are usually fixed in quantity, so allocating them to one member of the family comes at the expense of another. Within-family resource allocation decisions can affect health directly through nutrition and healthcare. Parents' investments of resources in their children can also affect their children's health indirectly—through the children's educational attainment and future income, both of which are strongly associated with health and mortality.

Kinship systems and gender roles in societies define authority relationships within families, which determine who makes decisions of resource allocation and how they are made. Individuals whose status in the family is relatively low (typically based on sex, age, or birth order) tend to receive fewer resources. Examples of how expenditures, care, and food allocation to family members vary by status within the family abound. To give just a few examples: In the United States, parents allocate fewer resources to step-children than to their biological children (Case *et al*. 1999). In eighteenth and nineteenth century Bosnia, maternal mortality rates were higher among women married to husbands who were junior among brothers than among those married to oldest brothers (Hammel & Gullickson 2004). In China, where there are strong preferences for male children, infant mortality is higher among girls than boys and selective abortion favouring males is high (Coale & Banister 1994). In Egypt, where son preference is also present, infant mortality is higher among girls than boys, and girls receive lower-quality healthcare (Yount 2003). At the extreme, sex preferences can lead to infanticide or abandonment. Although this practice is uncommon today, studies continue to uncover differences in resource allocation by gender, even in the most economically advanced countries.

The health consequences of inequalities within families may not always benefit those who have higher status. For example, patriarchy appears to be associated not only with higher female mortality, but also with higher male mortality (Stanistreet *et al*. 2005). One explanation is that constructions of masculinity in patriarchal societies encourage males to engage in unhealthy behaviours (Courtenay 2000).

Resources may not always be directed disproportionately to family members who are healthy. While some parents may invest disproportionately in their healthy children, whom they may consider to have the best chance of achievement, others may invest more in children who are in poor health because of their greater needs, diverting resources away from healthy children.

Socialization

Families can affect children's health by modelling behaviours. Parents can shape tastes and health habits—including eating habits and food preferences, levels of physical activity, and standards of hygiene.

Some of the preferences and health behaviours that are transmitted to children have cultural origins. As such, families act as agents of socialization in ways that can have profound health consequences (positive and negative) that can reproduce across generations. For example, women of Mexican descent in the United States have birth outcomes on par with those of non-Hispanic whites despite being much poorer on average. Some have hypothesized that the Mexican-origin advantage is due to cultural factors, such as healthful diets and low rates of substance use.

Family gender roles determine whether and how much time women spend working in the paid labour force versus on childrearing and housework. Changes in women's social and economic status in many countries have had complicated implications for resource allocation and health. The greater earnings and increased status of women have given them more control over resources, but they also have contributed to large increases in the divorce rate from 1960 to 1980 in most industrialized countries as well as to increases in rates of non-marital childbearing. Both of these trends have resulted in increased poverty among women and children. Also, despite working more outside, the home than in the past, women continue to bear most of the childrearing and housework responsibilities (Hochschild & Machung 1989). Having dual responsibilities can result in overburden and role strain, taking a toll on women's physical and mental health and potentially having ripple effects on other members of the family. Of course, the net effects of female labour force participation depend on the family's unique circumstances and the characteristics of the individuals within those families.

Cultural variations (intra and cross-nationally, as well as over time) also shape gender norms, which affect health practices. One area in which gender norms play an important role is reproductive behaviour: Fertility decisions, contraception, and protection from sexually transmitted infections. In places with high levels of gender inequality, rates of contraception and condom use tend to be relatively low and fertility tends to be relatively high, though there are many exceptions to this pattern (McDonald 2000). Moreover, women often find ways to control their fertility even in regions with low levels of gender equality. Finally, changes in fertility over time, in turn, can affect gender equality and gender relations (Behrman et al. 2002).

Increases in gender equality may affect relationships and risks associated with sexual activity, even at very early ages. One illustrative example involves the timing of sexual initiation across European countries. As female labour force participation increased and the gender wage gap diminished during the second-half of the twentieth century, boys' and girls' age at sexual initiation converged (the age for boys decreased only slightly while that for girls decreased dramatically), teen fertility rates decreased, and condom use increased (Bozon & Kontula 1998; Teitler 2002).

Marriage may socialize health behaviours. Being married is associated with better health compared to not being married (Waite & Gallagher 2000). This 'marriage advantage' may reflect behavioural changes (i.e. refraining from engaging in risky behaviours) induced by social expectations of married individuals. It could also result from a more stable lifestyle with lower levels of stress. Or, it may simply reflect the people who get married (i.e. those who are healthier may be more likely to choose to get married). Despite numerous attempts to ascertain the reasons for the marriage advantage in health, the reasons remain very much an open question.

Social support

Families, including extended kin, can be a source of financial, social, and emotional support to the individuals within them. Support of these types can mitigate the negative effects of adverse shocks in life circumstances, which can be financial in nature (such as losing a job) or health-related (such as having an accident or experiencing a major illness). The more wealth a family has, the greater its ability to assist members through difficult times. In addition to the direct and immediate benefits that family and extended kin may offer in times of crisis, the security of having a resource buffer may make individuals more inclined to invest in education or training. Both the peace of mind that comes from social support and the accumulated wealth that may result from human capital investment that it affords can translate into improved immediate and longer-term physical and mental health.

There is a potential downside to having strong family or social support, which is that its obligations are usually reciprocal. Being on the receiving end of family support provides advantages, but at a cost to those providing the support—especially if family resources are relatively scarce. The fewer financially secure members in the family, the more taxing within-family support obligations will be to those members. Reciprocal obligations among family members may be particularly strong among low-income populations, which could explain why, in the United States, the returns to investments in education and training are smaller among African–Americans (who are more likely to be first-generation middle class with connections to large numbers of low-income kin) than Whites (whose families are more homogeneously middle class). In sum, more extensive family ties in disadvantaged communities can play very important safety net roles, but may also burden economically mobile members when public assistance programmes do not offset demands of their kin.

Kin obligations are likely to increase as family composition in the United States and some other countries further diversifies due to increased rates of union dissolution, re-partnering, and other changes in family structure described later. Recent studies are just beginning to examine the competing resource demands in complex families and their consequences for family members' well-being, but at the present time, very little about this topic is known.

Reciprocal effects

Not only can families affect individuals' health, but the health of individuals can also impact their families. Ill family members can draw resources away from others, and because care giving responsibilities can interfere with regular work hours, limit their ability to maintain stable employment. For example, stress from hardships associated with the care of ill or disabled children can lead to relationship strains and, in extreme cases, to parental separation or divorce (Reichman et al. 2004).

Macro-level processes

Demographic factors

Fertility and mortality

An indirect way that resources become allocated across family members is by parents regulating their fertility. The more children parents have, the fewer the resources available to each child. When total resources are limited, additional births can impact nutrition by reducing the per-person availability of food. The same is true for resources allocated to healthcare (both preventive care and treatments) and education. Larger families can affect children negatively for this reason, but can benefit parents later in life if they depend on their children for financial or emotional support. Support from children is particularly important in societies that do not have institutionalized income redistributive programmes (e.g. public retirement programmes) and among low-income families who are unable to accumulate sufficient financial reserves to achieve self-sufficiency later in life.

Two demographic changes have had large effects on fertility. One is the decline in infant and child mortality that began in the mid-1800s in industrialized countries and in the late 1900s in developing countries. The expectation that children would survive into adulthood increased their value to parents. As the perceived value of children increased for individual sets of parents, so too did the collective valuation of children by society at large—leading to greater investments on the part of social welfare institutions and expansions of legislative protections, including the enactment of child labour and compulsory education laws (Zelizer 1994). The lower child mortality rates and increased perceived value of children led to a reduction in the average number of children per family, which in turn increased the resources available to individual family members.

In sum, the shift from high mortality and high fertility to low mortality and low fertility, often referred to as the 'first demographic transition', profoundly reduced the size of families and increased the value of children, which in turn increased family and institutional investments in children, further benefiting their health.

Patterns of fertility declines, both caused by and positively affecting health, were observed throughout the nineteenth and most of the twentieth century (Coale & Watkins 1986). However, declines beyond replacement levels (approximately 2.1 children per woman) have the potential to negatively affect the health of both children and adult family members. Again, the reasons have to do with the supply and allocation of resources. Fertility declines below replacement level cause the population to age, meaning that the proportion of old people relative to young people increases. When fertility declines are accompanied by increases in longevity and delays in entry into the labour force, as was the case in many Western European countries during the latter part of the twentieth century, the ageing of the population can be highly consequential. One reason is that the healthcare costs for the elderly are high relative to those for other age groups because the elderly disproportionately have chronic expensive-to-treat health problems. Another is that the fraction of the population paying into programmes that support the elderly (e.g. health insurance and pensions) decreases.

Italy exemplifies how low fertility rates can burden the working-aged population. The total fertility rate in that country declined from 2.7 children per woman in 1965 to 1.2 children per woman in 2000. As a result, the working-aged population is expected to decline from 39 million in 1995 to 22 million in 2050. Life expectancy also increased in the latter half of the twentieth century and young adults have remained in school longer, delaying entry into the labour force and remaining financially dependent on their parents until later ages. Two indicators—the old age dependency ratio and the ratio of pensioners to workers—indicate the extent to which the burden placed on workers has increased and will continue to increase. The old age dependence ratio is the number of people over 65 divided by the number of people aged 15–64. In Italy, this ratio has been increasing rapidly and is projected to triple by 2050. The ratio of pensioners to workers is currently 0.8 and is projected to increase to 1.6 in 2050 (Bongaarts 2004), meaning that, in 2050, there will be 1.6 times more people drawing on pensions than there are workers paying into them. Italy is not the only extreme example and the ageing of the population is not unique to the West. Old age dependence ratio projections for Japan are similar to those for Italy.

Divorce and non-marital childbearing

Since the 1960s, most of the industrialized countries have experienced a series of demographic changes that have had profound impacts on family structure and the well-being of individuals within families. These changes include delays in marriage and childbearing, increases in non-marital cohabitation, increases in divorce, and increases in non-marital childbearing. These relatively recent trends are not confined to industrialized countries; Age at marriage and age at first birth have increased in much of the world in the past 50 years. In the United States, age at marriage rose from means of about 20 years for women and 23 years for men in 1950 to 25 years for women and 27 years for men in 2000. It rose about 3 years in Indonesia over the same period. Even African countries, which typically have very early ages at marriage, have experienced significant increases over the last decade.

Among Western industrialized countries, the proportion of marriages ending in divorce more than doubled between 1960 and 1980, reaching about 1 in 2, and has since stabilized. Divorce rates rose to similar levels in Russia and Cuba. And, though overall rates are comparatively low in Asia, the rates of increase in divorce in many Asian countries have been higher than in Western countries. For example, the divorce rate in China tripled between 1980 and 2000. Marriage delays and increased divorce rates have resulted in adults and children spending an increasing amount of time outside marital unions and in reconstituted families.

The impact of divorce (and family disruption more generally) on health can be direct or indirect. Parental separation, parental conflict, and changes in living environments and schools that often ensue can lead to emotional, behavioural, and academic problems among children, though, for most children, the effects are short-term (Hetherington 2002). In some instances, parental separation can have positive effects on the health of spouses and children if it ends physical or emotional abuse. Separation generally reduces material resources available to women and children (whose economic well-being tends to decline more than that of men after family disruption), which can negatively impact educational and occupational trajectories.

Rates of non-marital fertility have increased dramatically in all Western industrialized countries. In the United States, the proportion of births born to unmarried mothers increased from 5 per cent in 1960 to one-third in 2000. And the United States is not an outlier in this regard as shown in Fig. 11.1.1. Non-marital childbearing is now more common in the United Kingdom, France, Iceland, and Scandinavian countries than in the United States. About half of all births in Scandinavian countries and about two-thirds of births in Iceland are to unmarried parents. In the United States and United Kingdom, non-marital fertility is strongly associated with poverty, whereas elsewhere (e.g. France, the Netherlands, and Scandinavian countries), it crosses social strata,

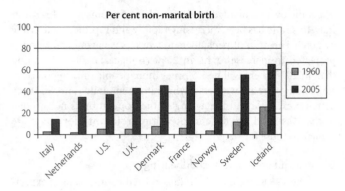

Fig. 11.1.1 Per cent non-marital birth.
Sources: NCHS Vital Statistics Reports, **48**(16). NCHD Births: Preliminary Data for 2005. Eurostat demographic trends 2005.

is not associated with single parenthood or poor child outcomes, and often leads to marriage of the biological parents.

Increases in cohabitation, divorce, and non-marital childbearing have resulted in large increases in multi-partner fertility (women bearing children with different fathers and men fathering children with more than one woman). One recent study estimates that close to one-third of low-income mothers in the United States had children with more than one partner, and over one-third of fathers had children with more than one partner (Meyer *et al.* 2005). The complexity of family structures and parental obligations that multi-partner fertility creates can increase resource strains.

The impact of the changes in family structure described above has not been uniform across country or socioeconomic status. Among highly educated women, delays in childbearing and expanded labour market opportunities have increased resources available for themselves and their children. Among less-educated women, rising rates of union dissolution and non-marital childbearing have led to increased poverty. The divergent trends have increased socioeconomic disparities in the conditions of children, particularly in the United States (McLanahan 2004). In most European countries, where cohabiting unions are more stable and family support policies provide greater supports to children than in the United States, increases in non-marital fertility are likely to be less consequential in terms of health-related resources available to children.

Maternal age

The age at which women give birth impacts their health and that of their children. In terms of children's health, there is a U-shaped association between maternal age and infant health as measured by birth weight (a risk factor for long term health and developmental outcomes). Rates of low birth weight are highest at very young and older ages. Since childbearing tends to begin earliest among low-income populations, the already higher risks of low birth weight for those groups may be compounded by early fertility.

Teen childbearing has costs for mothers as well as children. Women who have children before age 18 often interrupt their schooling. Though many eventually return to school or obtain high school equivalency diplomas, their academic achievement and attainment, on an average, suffers. The strong associations between

socioeconomic status, income, and health—within and across generations—underscores the importance of fertility decisions on the health of parents and their dependents.

Rates of teen childbearing in most industrialized countries have decreased substantially since the 1960s, as shown in Fig. 11.1.2. The decline in teen pregnancy has been accompanied by an increase in the mean age of childbearing. In the United States, the mean age at first birth increased from 22 years in the 1950s to 25 years in 2000. In the Netherlands, the mean age increased from about 23 to 29 years over the same period. More recently, childbearing ages have been increasing in less-developed countries as well. The trend towards later childbearing may have positive implications for the health of children and their families.

The decoupling of sex and marriage

Across all social classes and most countries, the age of sexual initiation has been decreasing since 1960 as the age of marriage has been increasing. Consequently, men and women now spend many more years in short-term relationships than they did 50 years ago and have a greater number of sexual partners, both of which are associated with increased risks of sexually transmitted infections.

The middle generation squeeze

Increases in longevity, which were discussed earlier in terms of their impact on population-level resource allocation, also have consequences at the family level. As life expectancy increases, individuals experience more years of their adult lives with living parents, whose caretaking and financial needs may divert resources from other family members.

At the earlier end of the life cycle, transitions to adulthood are lengthening. Young adults are delaying marriage and childbearing, spending more years in school, and relying on parental support for longer periods of time (Settersten *et al.* 2005). Increasing delays in leaving the parental home have been observed in the most-developed countries (Fernández Cordon 1997; Corijn & Klijzing 2001), with Italian men representing an extreme example—leaving home at age 27, on an average (Billari *et al.* 2001).

Over the past 30 years, as longevity has increased, the period of schooling has lengthened, and the transition to adulthood has occurred at older ages, the costs of raising children have risen

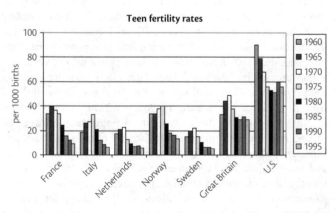

Fig. 11.1.2 Teen fertility rates.
Sources: Eurostat and US Vital Statistics Reports.

considerably (Schoeni & Ross 2004). Institutional supports have not kept pace with these changes. Consequently, many working age adults have been burdened with the support of both younger and older generations. Little is known about the extent to which the time, emotional, and financial costs of caring for both their parents and children have affected the allocation of resources or health in 'sandwich generation' families.

Technological factors

Contraception

Fertility regulation has been facilitated by modern, effective contraception. Most notably, the birth control pill has been available since the early 1960s. More recently, contraceptive patches, implants, and hormone shots offer protection for weeks or months at a time, making dose compliance much easier than in the past. These improvements in contraceptive technology have greatly reduced unplanned pregnancies. Additionally, newly available 'emergency contraception' provides women with the ability to end pregnancies up to 72 h after having sex. The increased efficacy of condoms has also improved fertility planning, while providing protection against sexually transmitted infections.

Neonatal care

Recent advances in neonatal care technology have led to the survival of infants born very preterm, who only decades ago would not have survived their first year (Reichman 2005). The tremendous benefits of saving lives are undisputable, but this progress has come with a big price tag because the technology is expensive and because modern medicine has lagged in terms of preventing chronic and disabling health conditions that arise from being born with an underdeveloped biological systems. Substantial costs are borne by healthcare systems, third-party payers, and families. Coping with the long-term needs of these 'new survivors' can create substantial financial and emotional hardships for families, which could take a toll on all family members' health.

Assisted reproduction

The benefits of assisted reproductive technology are clear. Medical advances over the past 20 years have allowed many couples, who would not have been able to do so in the past, to have children. These new opportunities, however, come with health related costs as well. One is an ageing parent population since the new technologies offset natural declines in women's ability to bear children. Another is an increase in the rate of multiple births. Because multiples are much more likely than singleton infants to be born low birth weight, assisted reproductive technology may be increasing chronic health problems among children.

Prenatal care

Advances in prenatal care technology provide information about the health and gender of foetuses (through genetic testing, ultrasound technology, or amniocentesis), creating opportunities for parents to selectively abort foetuses with unwanted traits. For example, parents can choose to terminate pregnancies if there are indications that the child will have Down Syndrome, abnormally developed organs, or be of the undesired sex. The ability to selectively abort can reduce hardships for family members, reduce the number of children with chronic health problems, and increase the proportion of 'wanted' children. However, selective abortions raise a host of complex ethical considerations that do not have easy answers.

Economic and political factors

Female labour force participation

Increases in female labour force participation, as discussed earlier, have had profound effects on organization of families. Mothers spending more time outside the home means that childcare is more likely to be delegated to others (childcare centres, relatives, children, and, less frequently, fathers). Housework, too, is either contracted out or reduced. Increased employment among women and entry into higher status occupations has obvious advantages for families in terms of household income. However, the health consequences of this change are not clear. For example, evidence of maternal employment on children's cognitive development is mixed (Waldfogel 2006).

Abortion laws

The criminalization of abortion in many countries can affect fertility control, the wantedness of children, and the health (and sometimes the life) of women who seek illegal and unregulated abortions. Worldwide, abortions are very common regardless of legality. The estimated number of abortions, in 1995 was 46 million. Abortion rates are no lower in places where they are restricted by law. 20 million of the 46 million abortions that took place in 1995 were illegal (Henshaw et al. 1999). Though some countries have at times increased restrictions on abortions, the overall trend has been toward liberalization. Most industrialized countries, Eastern European countries, China, and India legalized abortion between the 1950s and 1980s. Developing countries, overall, have been slower to legalize abortion, but many do not actively treat it as a crime (Henshaw 1994).

Gay marriage and civil unions

A few countries recognize unmarried same and opposite sex couples who are living together as families and confer legal rights to partners. It is not known whether legal recognition of alternative family forms will dissuade partners from marrying or encourage same sex unions or what effect either would have on individual well-being. While most research finds that many gay parent families are similar to heterosexual parents in terms of parenting, it is difficult to generalize from existing studies because of methodological limitations (Meezan & Rauch 2005). Evidence on domestic partnerships and civil unions is stronger and suggests that parents who cohabit are more likely to separate than those who are married (Manning et al. 2004). However, differences in dissolution rates by type of union vary by country, with smaller differences in countries where cohabitation is more prevalent (Liefbroer & Dourleijn 2006). Additionally, because individuals who enter different types of unions may be different in any number of ways, it is difficult to draw conclusive causal inferences about the effects of alternative family forms on individuals' health and well-being.

Future challenges

Across the world, families are becoming smaller, older, more complex, and more diverse. All of these changes have consequences for individuals' well-being and are likely to lead to important health related issues and ethical challenges in years to come. Several key issues at the nexus of family and health that will be at the forefront of ethical, legal, and policy debates are highlighted below:

♦ Legislation redefining parental rights and the acceptable scope of scientific research will need to be drafted as science increasingly makes it possible to screen foetuses for genetic predispositions to health and physical traits and to clone living organisms.

♦ In countries where non-marital fertility is both increasing and strongly associated with single-mother households, such as the United States and United Kingdom, social policies will need to adapt to declines in economic and social support that mothers and children receive from fathers.

♦ Legal definitions of family for the purposes of property and inheritance rights, child guardianship, and health insurance coverage will need to be revised. This will become increasingly necessary as complexities in family structure evolve. Some European countries provide legal status to non-marital domestic partnerships, but with only very specific and limited rights. In the United States, same-sex domestic partnerships are sometimes recognized for health insurance eligibility.

♦ Retirement systems will need to be adapted to an ageing population. This is a pressing challenge for developed countries. Either contributions into pension systems will have to increase (by increasing premiums or easing immigration restrictions) or disbursements will have to decrease (by reducing pension payments or delaying the retirement age). The interests of working and retired constituents will compete.

♦ End of life issues that arise because of advancing medical technologies will need to be debated. As families become more complex, the question of whose right and responsibility it is to make end of life decisions will become a particularly salient issue.

Acknowledgement

I am grateful to Nancy Reichman for her many helpful substantive and editorial comments.

References

Behrman, J.R., Kohler, H.-P., and Watkins, S.C. (2002). Social networks and changes in contraceptive use over time: evidence from a longitudinal study in rural Kenya. *Demography*, **39**(4), 713–38.

Billari, F.C., Philipov, D., and Baizán, P. (2001). Leaving home in Europe: the experience of cohorts born around 1960. *International Journal of Population Geography*, **7**(5), 339–56.

Bongaarts, J. (2004). Population aging and the rising cost of public pensions. *Population Council Working Paper* no. 185.

Bozon, M. and Kontula, O. (1998). Sexual initiation and gender in Europe. In *Sexual behavior and HIV/AIDS in Europe* (eds. M. Hubert, N. Bajos, and T. Sandfort), pp. 37–67. UCL Press, London.

Case, A., Lin, I., and McLanahan, S. (1999). Household resource allocation in stepfamilies: Darwin reflects on the plight of Cinderella. *The American Economic Review*, **89**(2), 234–8.

Coale, A.J. and Watkins, S.C. eds. (1986). *The decline of fertility in Europe*. Princeton University Press, Princeton.

Coale, A.J. and Banister, J. (1994). Five decades of missing females in China. *Demography*, **31**(3), 459–79.

Corijn, M. and Klijzing, E. (Eds.). (2001). *Transitions to Adulthood in Europe*. Kluwer Academic Publishers: Dordrecht.

Courtenay, W.H. (2000). Constructions of masculinity and their influence on men's well-being: a theory of gender and health. *Social Science & Medicine*, **50**, 1385–401.

Fernández Cordon, J.A. (1997). Youth residential independence and autonomy: a comparative study. *Journal of Family Issues*, **16**(6), 567–607.

Hammel, E.A. and Gullickson, A. (2004). Kinship structures and survival: maternal mortality on the Croatian-Bosnian border 1750–898. *Population Studies - A Journal of Demography*, **58**(2), 145–59.

Henshaw, S.K. (1994). Recent trends in the legal status of induced abortion. *Journal of Public Health Policy*, **15**(2), 165–72.

Henshaw, S.K., Singh, S., and Haas, T. (1999). The incidence of abortion worldwide. *International Family Planning Perspectives*, **25**, S30–8.

Hetherington, E.M. (2002). *For better or for worse: divorce reconsidered*. W.W. Norton & Co., New York.

Hochschild, A. and Machung, A. (1989). *The second shift: working parents and the revolution at home*. Viking Penguin, New York.

Liefbroer, A.C. and Dourleijn, E. (2006). Unmarried cohabitation and union stability: testing the role of diffusion using data from 16 European countries. *Demography*, **43**(2), 203–21.

Manning, W., Smock, P., and Majumdar, D. (2004). The relative stability of cohabiting and marital unions for children. *Population Research and Policy Review*, **23**(2), 135–59.

McDonald, P. (2000). Gender equity in theories of fertility transition. *Population and Development Review*, **26**(3), 427–39.

McLanahan, S. (2004). Diverging destinies: how children are faring under the second demographic transition. *Demography*, **41**(4), 607–27.

Meezan, W. and Rauch, J. (2005). Gay marriage, same-sex parenting, and America's children. *The Future of Children*, **15**(2), 97–115.

Meyer, D.R., Cancian, M., and Cook, S.T. (2005). Multiple-partner fertility: incidence and implications for child support policy. *Social Service Review*, **79**(5), 577–601.

Reichman, N.E. (2005). Low birth weight and school readiness. *The Future of Children*, **15**(1), 91–116.

Reichman, N.E., Corman, H., and Noonan, K. (2004). Effects of child health on parents' relationship status. *Demography*, **41**(3), 569–84.

Schoeni, R. and Ross, K. (2005). Material assistance received from families during the transitions to adulthood. In *On the frontier of adulthood: theory, research and public policy* (eds. R.A. Settersten, F.F. Furstenburg, and R.G. Rumbaut). The University of Chicago Press, Chicago.

Settersten, R.A., Furstenburg, F.F., and Rumbaut, R.G., eds. (2005). *On the frontier of adulthood: theory, research and public policy*. The University of Chicago Press, Chicago.

Stanistreet, D., Bambra, C., and Scott-Samuel, A. (2005). Is patriarchy the source of men's higher mortality? *Journal of Epidemiology and Community Health*, **59**, 873–6.

Teitler, J.O. (2002). Trends in youth sexual initiation and fertility in developed countries: 1960–1995. *The Annals of the American Academy of Political and Social Science*, **580**, 134–52.

Waite, L.J. and Gallagher, M. (2000). *The case for marriage: why married people are happier, healthier, and better off financially*. Doubleday, New York.

Waldfogel, J. (2006). *What children need*. Harvard University Press, Cambridge.

Yount, K.M. (2003). Gender bias in the allocation of curative health care in Minia, Egypt. *Population Research and Policy Review*, **22**(3), 267–99.

Zelizer, V.A. (1994). *Pricing the priceless child: the changing social value of children*. Princeton University Press, Princeton.

Women, men, and health

Sarah Payne and Lesley Doyal

Abstract

This chapter explores the ways in which sex and gender influence health. Figures for mortality and life expectancy reveal important differences between men and women in their risk of death and in the causes of death. In virtually every country around the world, men have a lower life expectancy than women, although the gap in life expectancy is narrower in low-income countries. Similarly, women and men have different patterns of ill health, and again, the gap varies between countries. Both sex and gender play a part in these variations. Sex, or biological factors, influences women's and men's risks of different diseases and health conditions, including reproductive disorders and diseases affected by the immune system and genetic factors, as well as survival following diagnosis. However, socially constructed gender-linked factors are also important. Gender affects behaviours such as smoking and alcohol use, which increase the risk of certain conditions, and also affects exposure to social and environmental risk factors, including paid and unpaid work, caring responsibilities, poverty and poor environmental conditions, and the risk of sexual and physical violence.

Introduction

This chapter explores the ways in which sex and gender influence health. It discusses variations in health between women and men across the life course, examines differences in male and female patterns of illness and premature death, and explores related differences in experiences of health care. It asks how far we can explain these differences with reference to biological sex and socially constructed gender.

Although the main determinants of health for a woman agricultural worker in rural China may be the same as those for a female office worker in New York or Sydney, the impact of different determinants will vary. Both women will be affected to some extent by their sex—by biological factors which increase or reduce the risk of particular health problems, including those associated with reproduction. However, social factors such as gender also play an important part in shaping morbidity and mortality. Key influences on the health of each woman may include whether or not she has children, the paid and unpaid work she performs, her access to material resources and to health care, and the levels of social support she receives.

But the impact of these influences on her health is also related to each woman's particular circumstances, which are in turn shaped by geographical, social, and cultural factors. The rural farm worker in China will have great difficulty accessing health care, particularly specialist services; she may have more access to familial support but experience greater stress from family relationships; and she may have little money in her own right and little say over the work she does, either inside the house or outside it. The office worker in New York, on the other hand, may have easier access to health care, depending on her insurance status and level of income, and she will almost certainly live closer to these services. She may have less family support, especially if she has moved to New York to find employment, but may have better sources of support from close friends. She may have money in her own right. In her employment, although she too may have little control over her work and it may offer little in terms of satisfaction, she will be less at risk from some forms of accidental injury and less exposed to noxious chemicals than the woman in agricultural work.

Both these women will be affected by their diet and by behaviours which impact on health, but again the effects are likely to be very different. The Chinese woman may be undernourished through lack of an adequate food supply combined with heavy physical work, whereas the woman in New York may be obese due to lack of exercise and overconsumption of a highly calorific diet. The two women will also probably show significant differences in their use of substances such as tobacco and alcohol.

If we compare the influences on men in the same location as these women, the main determinants of their health will again be the same for both men—the nature of work and paid employment, access to material resources, physical hazards encountered in daily life, health behaviour, and social support for example. But, as with the women, the relative importance and impact of these influences will vary between rural China and New York. And if we then compare the factors affecting the health of the man and woman in each location, there will be further differences between them reflecting gendered distributions of power, resources, and role expectations, associated with cultural and socioeconomic factors. This suggests that the roles of sex and gender in the health of men and women are complex and relational, reflecting various factors which come into play in different ways, with various intensities, and at different points in time.

In the following subsections, we will explore in detail some of the explanations for these differences between women and men in their experiences of health and health care, and their likelihood of developing specific diseases. We begin with an overview of the key differences between male and female mortality and morbidity, before turning to look at the part played by sex and gender in shaping these variations. The model of causality that will emerge from this exploration is not one by which the simple differences between women and men can provide a total explanation of variations in health outcomes. The next subsection will, therefore, look in more detail at the complex links between sex and gender and other determinants of heath such as geographical location, poverty, and socioeconomic status. This will be done by examining specific conditions, including coronary heart disease and HIV and AIDS. We finish this chapter with a discussion of the way gender differentials impact on the appropriateness and availability of health care.

Men, women, and mortality

Mortality data are widely available and relatively reliable, especially when looking at overall rates. These figures suggest that women have an advantage over men in terms of life expectancy and can expect to live longer than their male counterparts in virtually every country in the world. In 2004, for example, male life expectancy at birth was higher than female life expectancy in only 5 out of the 192 countries covered in the World Health Organization's (WHO) Annual Health Report (World Health Organization 2006). There were five countries where men and women had the same life expectancy. In all of the others—182 countries—women could expect to live longer than men.

The countries showing the narrowest gap between women and men are those in which life expectancy is low overall. These are also countries which are among the poorest in the world, notably those in the sub-Saharan region of Africa. For example, in Cameroon, women had only one year's advantage over men, whereas in Somalia and South Africa, women's life expectancy was two years higher than that of men. A number of influences are involved in creating health chances for women and men, but it is especially significant that in these countries where there is only a narrow gap there has been a reversal in both male and female life expectancy in recent years as a result of the increasing burden of HIV and AIDS together with persistent poverty.

Countries with gaps in life expectancy between women and men of five or more years are more diverse in terms of economic status, level of development, and culture: For example, Australia, Finland, Sri Lanka, and Cambodia (World Health Organization 2006). However, the countries showing the greatest divergence between male and female life expectancy are clustered in Eastern Europe, notably those countries which were formerly part of the Soviet Union. In the Russian Federation, for example, women might expect to live up to 13 years longer than men.

In these Eastern European countries, the gap between women and men in life expectancy has widened in recent years following the rapid rise in poverty and deprivation in the post-communist era, combined with high levels of unemployment and changing patterns of alcohol and substance use. This highlights not only the importance of socioeconomic factors in health experience but also the vulnerability of health gains to adverse conditions. In addition, it illustrates gender differences in the impact of socioeconomic

Table 11.2.1 Differences in male and female life expectancy, 2004—selected countries

Country	Male life expectancy at birth (2004)	Female life expectancy at birth (2004)	Difference
Russian Federation	59	72	−13
Estonia	66	78	−12
Republic of Korea	73	81	−8
Cambodia	51	58	−7
Sri Lanka	68	75	−7
Finland	75	82	−7
Czech Republic	73	79	−6
Cote D'Ivoire	41	47	−6
United States of America	75	80	−5
Australia	78	83	−5
United Kingdom	76	81	−5
China	70	74	−4
Egypt	66	70	−4
Angola	38	42	−4
Iceland	79	83	−4
Samoa	66	70	−4
Sierra Leone	37	40	−3
India	61	63	−2
Somalia	43	45	−2
South Africa	47	49	−2
Pakistan	62	63	−1
Cameroon	50	51	−1
Nepal	61	61	0
Niger	42	41	+1
Kenya	51	50	+1

Source: WHO. *World health report 2006: working together for health*. Geneva: WHO; 2006. World Health Report Annex 1. Reproduced with permission from WHO.

change, as the widening gap between women and men reflects a dramatic reduction in life expectancy particularly for men in these countries (Macintyre 2001).

These variations in the gap between women and men across different cultures, time periods, locations, and levels of development suggest that the underlying reasons for such differences do not simply reflect economic factors or specific cultural factors but are explained by more complex influences involving both biological and social causes.

An alternative way of exploring the gap in mortality is through deaths in early childhood. Males and females have different risks of dying before their fifth birthday, and slightly fewer countries show a female advantage. There are 12 countries where girls under five have a higher mortality risk than boys, including China, India, Niger, Somalia, and Nepal, whereas in the majority of countries,

Table 11.2.2 Under-5 male and female mortality rates, 2004—
selected countries

Country	Male under-5 mortality rate per 1000 population (2004)	Female under-5 mortality rate per 1000 population (2004)	Male: female ratio (male rate as proportion of female)
Republic of Korea	5	7	0.7
China	27	36	0.8
India	81	89	0.9
Nepal	75	79	0.9
Somalia	222	228	1.0
Niger	256	262	1.0
Egypt	36	36	1.0
Pakistan	102	100	1.0
Angola	276	243	1.1
Sierra Leone	296	269	1.1
Cameroon	156	143	1.1
United States of America	8	7	1.1
Australia	6	5	1.2
Cambodia	154	127	1.2
South Africa	72	62	1.2
Kenya	129	110	1.2
United Kingdom	6	5	1.2
Czech Republic	5	4	1.2
Russian Federation	18	14	1.3
Sri Lanka	16	12	1.3
Cote D'Ivoire	225	162	1.4
Iceland	3	2	1.5
Finland	5	3	1.7
Estonia	10	6	1.7
Samoa	42	17	2.5

Source: WHO. *World health report 2006: working together for health.* Geneva: WHO; 2006. World Health Report Annex 1. Reproduced with permission from WHO.

more boys under five die than girls, including Angola and Cote D'Ivoire where male children have an especially high risk of such early death (World Health Organization 2006).

These differences between countries are explained by a mixture of social, cultural, and biological influences, including gender differences, which affect the treatment of girl and boy children. For example, the male advantage in some countries is partly explained by cultural factors including the practice of breastfeeding male children for longer, and giving boys more food and better access to health care in comparison with girls (Ravindran 2000).

It is also important to consider differences between women and men in causes of death. Overall, men and women have very similar patterns. Globally, around one-third of both men and women die

from communicable diseases such as respiratory infections, tuberculosis, or HIV and AIDS (World Health Organization 2004b); similarly, around 60 per cent of both men and women die from non-communicable diseases, including cardiovascular disease and cancer. If we look in more detail at the major causes of death, there is a degree of consistency in this pattern: The top three causes of male deaths worldwide are ischaemic heart disease (13 per cent of total male deaths), cerebrovascular disease (8 per cent), and accidental injury (8 per cent) (World Health Organization 2004b). For women, the top two causes of death are the same as those for men—ischaemic heart disease (12 per cent of female deaths) and cerebrovascular disease (11 per cent)—but fewer women die from accidental injury, whereas deaths from lower respiratory infections are the third most common cause of female deaths (7 per cent).

However, although the key causes of death for women and men are similar, a main difference between them for the major mortality causes is age at death. Women tend to be older than men when they die of cardiovascular disease and cancer, and this reflects both biological and gendered differences, as we shall see.

One important cause of female deaths in many countries is maternal mortality. Although this accounts for less than 2 per cent of all female deaths worldwide, it is a relatively modifiable cause of death, in that improved health care before conception, during pregnancy, and in childbirth can dramatically reduce the risk of death. As such, maternal mortality figures are also important in explanations of the ways in which the ratio of male to female deaths varies over time and between countries.

Overall, more than half a million women die each year as a result of complications following pregnancy and childbirth, including problems arising from miscarriage and terminations (World Health Organization 2005a). Maternal mortality figures also include deaths among women that follow from a reduced immunity to some diseases during pregnancy or in which they suffer a deterioration in pre-existing illness as a result of pregnancy or childbirth.

The risk of such death varies widely, with very low rates in high-income countries and very high rates in low-income countries. For example, in 2000, the maternal mortality rate in Sierra Leone was 2000 deaths per 100 000 live births, compared with 6 in Australia and 11 in the United Kingdom (World Health Organization 2005a).

The relative risk of maternal mortality in different countries reflects social and economic differences rather than biological ones and is particularly associated with the availability of care, as well as maternal age and the number of previous pregnancies. In Sierra Leone, three-fifths of births are not attended by skilled health personnel; similarly, in Niger, a country with a maternal mortality rate of 1600 per 100 000 live births in 2000, only 11 per cent of women received skilled health care during childbirth.

A second major difference between women and men in terms of mortality risk is the higher male mortality rate for both accidental and non-accidental injury. For example, in the Russian Federation, four times many men as women die from injury, and in Thailand, male mortality from such causes is around three and a half times as high as female mortality.

More men than women die each year as a result of homicide, especially among younger age groups. In 2000, for example, global figures show that men aged 15–44 years were five times as likely to be the victims of homicide as women (World Health Organization 2003c). There are also gender differences in the perpetrators of such violence: Women are more at risk of being killed by close family, notably partners, whereas more men are killed by people outside their circle of family and acquaintances (Hemenway *et al.* 2002).

Men are similarly much more likely than women to die or be injured as a result of conflict, with more than 90 per cent of deaths in conflicts among men (World Health Organization 2004b). This reflects the ratio of men to women both in formal military organizations and in informal or paramilitary organizations, as well as the roles played by them in such organizations. However, conflicts also increase the risk of poor health for women, as a result of causes such as infectious diseases, accidental death, and sexual violence (World Health Organization 2003c). In addition, displacement among civilian populations due to conflict combined with the loss of employment, land, or source of income creates economic insecurity and poverty, leading to high risks of poor mental health and malnutrition among such people, a majority of whom are female.

Overall, women have longer life expectancies than men, although the gap varies between countries and there are differences between women and men for some causes of death. The following subsection explores an alternative indicator of the differences between women and men, focusing on measures of morbidity or illness.

Men, women, and morbidity

Figures for death are useful for broad comparisons between women and men but they also have limitations. Most importantly, they do not accurately capture health experience across the life course. Some causes of death are not usually associated with a period of ill health beforehand—for example, accidental injury. Other causes of death may have produced relatively short periods of illness, and still others may be associated with poor health and low quality of life for some years before death occurs. These considerations are important when exploring health differences between women and men as it is possible that excess male mortality does not equate to a similar disadvantage in terms of health enjoyed during a lifetime.

An alternative measure of health is morbidity, which refers to illness, both short-term acute periods of ill health and also longer-term or chronic illness. It has long been assumed that women experience poorer health during their lives in comparison with men—the suggestion that 'women get sicker but men die quicker' (Lorber 1997). But the true picture of the gap between women and men is more complex. The health of women and men varies across the life course and the gap widens or narrows reflecting different age-related patterns of health. Similarly, although women report more of some conditions (such as arthritis), men are more at risk of others, including respiratory diseases. There are also other variations in health status—for example, between socioeconomic groups and different ethnic groups—that may affect the health gap between women and men.

One of the reasons why there is no simple story to tell in terms of the burden of ill health among women and men is that morbidity can be measured in a number of ways, and each measure is potentially different in terms of how well it captures the experiences of men and women. The main indicators include self-reported health, which is based on individuals' judgements of their own health as either 'poor', 'good', or 'excellent'; data based on use of health-care services, including inpatient and community-based services; and composite indicators of health at population level, including measures of healthy life expectancy (HALE) and measures of disability-adjusted life years (DALYs). With each of these measures, there is a range of differences between women and men which varies across the life course, between different demographic groups, and also, between countries.

Self-reported health

In most countries, women report their health to be poorer, in comparison with men. In the WHO's *World Health Survey 2005*, for example, figures from China, France, India, Malawi, the Russian Federation, Pakistan, and Portugal all revealed that more women reported their health as either bad or very bad, whereas more men reported their health as either good or very good (World Health Organization 2005).

The gap between women and men in these countries also varies. One of the widest differences in self-reported health is found in the Russian Federation where nearly a quarter of women reported their health as either bad or very bad, compared with 13 per cent of men (World Health Organization 2005). When this finding is compared with the low male life expectancy in Russia discussed earlier, the data support the argument that in this country at least women report more illness while men have less chance of a long life.

However, women do not always report poorer health than men. In Australia, for example, national survey data for 2004–2005 show that slightly more women than men to say their health is either very good or excellent and, that in every age group other than young adults, more women than men report their health as either very good or excellent (ABS 2006). In the United Kingdom, similar numbers of men and women report their health as bad and although in the United States more men than women report good health, the gap between them is very narrow (ONS 2006; Schiller & Bernadel 2004).

These differences are difficult to interpret. They might reflect variations in the wording of survey questions and some are also influenced by whether or not the data are age-standardized. They might also reflect class or income differences as poorer health is reported by those in lower-income groups, which may include a greater proportion of women in some countries.

As these differences are based on a subjective measure, the findings specifically tell us about how men and women perceive themselves, rather than their objective health status. Variations among countries in terms of whether it is men or women who are more likely to report ill health might also suggest that cultural differences are important in shaping perceptions of health status.

However, the variations, particularly the relatively narrow gap between women and men in richer countries compared with the wider gap found in poorer countries, might also reflect the fact that men in some societies do enjoy better health than women.

One indication of the extent to which these self-reported measures reflect more objective indicators of health comes from evidence in the United States that men who report poor health more often die prematurely than those reporting themselves as being in good health (Benjamins *et al.* 2004). However, there is less evidence of such an association for women, which may mean that self-report surveys are measuring different things for women and men. One factor that affects self-reported health is the extent to which individuals make this judgement not only on any symptoms of illness, but also on the basis of their knowledge about their own behaviours (such as smoking, alcohol use, and diet) that might affect health risks.

Given the difficulties presented by self-report data on morbidity, especially in the context of whether there are gender differences in the measures used, we need to also look at other measures of health experience in order to understand the gap between women and men.

Use of health services

Another way in which health differences between women and men have been measured is through data on consultation with health professionals. Again, these figures are likely to be influenced by more than health status and symptoms alone. A number of issues affect the use of health care, including economic factors such as whether an individual has health insurance or the means to pay user fees in countries where access to health care requires payment; the ability to take time off from either paid employment or caring responsibilities to visit health facilities; and the availability of appropriate services and transport to reach them.

Of course these factors are themselves influenced by gender. For example, women are more often responsible for the care of children and vulnerable dependents, and this can limit their ability to seek help when faced with health symptoms. They are also less likely to be able to finance health consultations—for example, if they do not have command over household expenditure or when they earn less than men and are less able to afford user fees and charges. In some countries, women also need to be accompanied when using services and are therefore dependent on someone being available and willing to take them (Baghadi 2005).

Data from the *World Health Survey 2005* (World Health Organization 2005) shows that there are differences between women and men in their use of health-care services, with the pattern varying among countries and for different kinds of care. For example, in France, India, the Russian Federation, and China, more men than women reported using ambulatory services in the past 12 months, including primary care from general practitioners, community services, and outpatient care. In the United Kingdom and Portugal, similar percentages of men and women used this kind of care. More women than men reported receiving inpatient treatment in Portugal, Malawi, and China, but in France and the United Kingdom, more men reported such treatment. However, in all of these countries, more men than women reported not using any form of health care in the previous twelve months.

National survey data from the United Kingdom reveal that women consult more often than men throughout the health-care system and also take more prescribed medication. Similar gendered patterns of consultation are also found in the United States and Australia (Payne 2006).

There are further differences between women and men in terms of what they are treated for. For example, in general practice in the United Kingdom, more women than men are treated for hypertension, depression, and anxiety, whereas their male compatriots are more often treated for coronary heart disease and diabetes (ONS 2000). The difference in treatment for depression is particularly wide, with more than twice as many women receiving such a diagnosis in general practice.

Overall, data on consultation suggests that women do consult more often than men and are more likely to use health care, although patterns vary between countries and also in response to other factors including age. However, gender-linked influences, including financial or cultural constraints, limit their use of services in some countries and may help explain variations in the gap between women and men.

Composite health indicators

The third way in which we can assess the health gap between women and men is through composite indicators of health at population level. One of the best known of these is the estimate of healthy life expectancy (HALE) produced by the WHO. HALE is a measure that begins with life expectancy at birth and is then adjusted downwards to reflect an estimate of time spent during the life course in poor health (World Health Organization 2004b). This estimate is carried out for each of the WHO's member countries, using a range of survey statistics and other measures to calculate the adjustment separately for men and women.

HALE figures for 2002 revealed that, in 14 out of 192 countries, males had either the same or a better HALE than females. In the remaining 178 countries, women could expect to live a longer time in full health (World Health Organization 2004b). However, as with mortality and life expectancy, the extent of female advantage varies. In the Russian Federation, for example, female HALE was over 11 years greater than male HALE. In France, Spain, and Portugal, females had more than 5 years advantage, whereas in the United Kingdom, the advantage shrank to under three years. Again, it is useful to compare these figures with self-reported health—especially those which show that in the Russian Federation less women than men describe themselves as having good health.

However, if we look not at years spent in healthy life but at the proportion of overall life expectancy that is lost due to poor health, women appear to do rather less well. For the same 192 countries, there were only 4 countries in 2002 where men lost a greater proportion of their life expectancy to illness and disability; in the remaining countries, the proportion of life expectancy lost due to ill health was higher for women (World Health Organization 2004b).

An alternative measure of health, using disability-adjusted life years (DALYs), highlights the distribution of the burden of disease and combines data on death with data on poor health and disability. DALYs are based on calculations of the value of years of disability-free life that are lost as a result of either premature death or the onset of disability (Lopez *et al.* 2006). DALYs can be used in relation to specific conditions as well as to overall health and may also be used to indicate the value of particular interventions which reduce mortality or disability. For example, the number of DALYs gained through reductions in disease following health promotion or clean water policies can be measured. Worldwide, an estimated 1.5 billion DALYs are lost annually due to various health conditions (World Health Organization 2004b). Nearly 25 per cent of these are because of infectious and parasitic diseases, including HIV and AIDS (which accounts for almost 6 per cent of the total), and diarrhoeal diseases (which account for 4 per cent) (World Health Organization 2004b). Mental health problems account for between 12 and 15 per cent of the total number of DALYs lost each year, injuries account for 12 per cent, and heart disease contributes nearly 10 per cent.

Overall, there is only a narrow gap between women and men in their experience of morbidity using this measure: Men comprise 52 per cent of total DALYs lost per annum and women comprise the remaining 48 per cent (World Health Organization 2004b). However, men are much more likely than women to suffer illness or disability as a consequence of accidental and non-accidental injury, as well as from heart disease, alcohol-use disorders, and some cancers. Males also have higher risks of perinatal disabilities. Healthy years lost by women are most likely to result from complications of pregnancy and childbirth, depression, sensory disorders such as cataracts, and sexually transmitted infections.

For example, reproductive conditions including maternal deaths, disability arising from pregnancy and childbirth, sexually transmitted infections, and cancers of the reproductive organs account for between 5 and 15 per cent of all DALYs worldwide. There is a wide gap between men and women in the burden of disease associated with reproductive health and these conditions account for only 3 per cent of the male burden of disease compared with 22 per cent of female DALYs (Dejong 2006).

However, DALYs only measure a limited number of illnesses and health problems relating to reproduction and almost certainly undercount the poor health experienced by women due to various reproductive disorders. For example, infections of the reproductive tract that are not sexually transmitted—such as candidiasis—are not included, neither are menstrual disorders and psychosocial problems associated with difficulties conceiving or with sexuality (AbouZahr & Vaughan 2000). Similarly, mental health aspects of rape and sexual violence are not counted by the DALYs approach. Overall, the failure to include a range of health difficulties suggests that the burden of disease in relation to reproductive health is underestimated for women.

DALYs have also been criticized for their focus on economic rather than social costs of disease and poor health—the loss of income or the costs of care rather than suffering, stigma, and individual well-being (Sen & Bonita 2000). In addition, some have argued that because the severity of the impact of a disease was estimated by experts in the field rather than individuals with the condition, DALYs fail to measure the full burden of a disease, especially those illnesses with wider social costs affecting quality of life (Dejong 2006). This needs to be borne in mind when using DALYs to assess the gender gap in health, as there may well be variations between women and men in the social impact of different diseases.

For example, obstetric fistulae are highly debilitating conditions, which arise as a result of prolonged or obstructed labour, often in women who have undergone female genital mutilation (FGM). There are a number of serious health consequences for the women who are affected, including infection, ulcers, and incontinence. Fistulae are also highly stigmatizing and create enormous social problems for the women involved including, for some women, loss of home and economic security following marital breakdown. But this stigma and the consequences are not counted as part of the burden of DALYs, leaving the social and functional disabilities facing many women undercounted (Dejong 2006).

Summary—differences between women and men in morbidity

Taken together, the various ways of counting morbidity or ill health between women and men suggest that there is a complex relationship between sex, gender, and health, which is mediated by age. Other factors, including socioeconomic status and ethnicity, will also play a part. Although the picture for mortality is relatively straightforward, with most countries showing poorer life expectancy and higher death rates among men, morbidity data suggest that patterns of ill health vary for men and women around the world. On the whole, women report poorer health, use services more, particularly where health care is relatively accessible, and experience more of some conditions, notably those associated with chronic ill health. However, men experience higher levels of illness

and disability from those conditions which also contribute to their higher mortality rates.

Sex and gender influences on health are central to explanations of these differences. First we need to define these terms and explore the ways in which each might affect health and health outcomes before going on to consider how sex and gender contribute to specific diseases.

Sex, gender, and health

In order to understand the ways in which sex- and gender-linked factors might influence health, it is important to clarify what is meant by these terms and particularly the differences between them. Despite increasing recognition of the various ways in which sex and gender can impact on the health of men and women, the terms are still sometimes used wrongly. Specifically, although the term *gender* is found more often than in the past in biomedical literature, it is often used interchangeably for *sex* rather than as a distinct concept with a very different meaning (Krieger 2003; Doyal 2001).

Sex and health

Sex refers to biological influences including not only differences between women and men based on the reproductive system, but also those reflecting genetic and hormonal factors. For many years reproductive differences between women and men were seen as the most significant sex-linked influence on health. However, more recent studies have widened our understanding of the complexity of sex-linked factors on men's and women's health.

The Committee on Understanding the Biology of Sex and Gender Differences, set up by the Institute of Medicine in the United States in 1999, produced an important review of the evidence relating to biological factors and their effects on health. The final report concluded that 'sex matters' (Wizeman & Pardue 2001). That is, the health of men and women is influenced in important ways by 'genetic, biochemical, physiological, and physical' elements, as well as those which are social in origin (Wizeman & Pardue 2001). Although hormonal and reproductive factors play a part in patterns of health and vulnerability to different conditions, this review also highlighted the significance of genetic and molecular factors, and important differences between men and women in gene expression. The report concluded with a number of recommendations for further research in the field stressing that genetic factors are not fully understood as yet.

The range of sex-linked influences on health

Sex-linked factors play a key part in human health throughout the life course. Males are more vulnerable to mortality than females at every age, from conception onwards (Waldron 1985). For example, studies of foetal mortality—deaths in the womb at any gestational age—reveal higher rates of mortality among males than females (MacDorman *et al.* 2007). Indeed, the higher rate of male deaths before birth is an important indication of the part played by biological factors in male excess mortality.

Hormones play a key role in differences in health experience between women and men. Female sex hormones appear to protect women against a range of conditions including ischaemic heart disease (Waldron 1985; Kane 1991). One explanation for this advantage is that oestrogen increases the flexibility of the female circulatory system, and that high blood pressure is less damaging for premenopausal women (Bird & Rieker 1999). Also, oestrogen affects cholesterol, increasing HDL cholesterol levels and decreasing LDL cholesterol, and improves the functioning of the heart (Wizeman & Pardue 2001).

Hormones are also implicated in irritable bowel syndrome, another condition demonstrating a female excess. Women are up to four times as likely to suffer from this chronic painful condition. Although this reflects gender-linked factors such as stress and anxiety, there is also evidence that men may receive protection from testosterone whereas female hormones may increase the severity of the symptoms experienced (Heitkemper *et al.* 2003).

Hormonal changes across the menstrual cycle also appear to affect health outcomes for women in the context of interventions as diverse as smoking cessation and surgery for breast cancer (Wizeman & Pardue 2001). Further evidence of biological influences comes from research on alcohol-related damage. Women and men have different patterns of risk from alcohol consumption. Women suffer the adverse effects of alcohol in terms of brain and liver damage more quickly than men do and are more likely to suffer health damage at the same level of consumption as men. These differences are partly due to differences in metabolism and hormonal factors, which means that women's bodies process alcohol differently (Redgrave *et al.* 2003).

There are also differences in male and female immune systems, which in turn are related to reproductive factors, especially the capacity of women to conceive and carry a child. These differences mean that women's immune systems are more at risk from autoimmune disorders (Bird & Rieker 1999). Changes in the immune system of pregnant women, particularly, put them at higher risk of some communicable diseases ranging from measles to malaria (Wizeman & Pardue 2001). However, other pregnancy-related changes such as the tendency for autoimmune diseases (such as rheumatoid arthritis) to go into remission highlight the complexity of the relationship between sex and the immune system.

Recent research has also suggested important sex differences in gene expression, contributing to women's higher risks for some forms of cancer. For example, among smokers, women appear to be more at risk of lung cancer than men at the same level of smoking, and lung cancer is also more common among non-smoking women than non-smoking men (Keohavong *et al.* 2003). This has been related to gene expression. Expression of genes related to lung cancer may be greater among women than men due to the location of the expressed gene on the X chromosome, leading to an increased risk of this cancer as well as shaping the type of lung cancer which women develop (Haugen 2002; Shields 2002; Payne 2001).

In addition, there is increasing evidence of sex differences in the way the brain is organized, including the use of language and verbal abilities. For example, women tend to recover more language ability than men following a left-hemisphere stroke (Wizeman & Pardue 2001). There are also differences between women and men in the way the brain responds to noxious stimuli, which in turn affect experiences of symptoms such as pain. Women have higher prevalence rates for what are often described as 'pain conditions', including headache, abdominal, and facial pain (Bradley & Alarcon 1999; LeResche 1999). Although this reflects the fact that the expression of pain is culturally more sanctioned for women than men, biological factors also play a part, especially differences between women and men, in particular certain neurological pathways (Yunus 2002).

However, we must be wary of attributing too much to biology. For example research on the relationship between parity and some health conditions, notably non-reproductive carcinomas such as colorectal cancer, has suggested that there might be a relationship in women between pregnancy and subsequent health risks. But recent studies have also revealed a similar relationship between parity and cancer for men, implying that social factors such as stress, access to resources, and expectations associated with having children may be more significant than biological factors in this association (Kravdal 1995).

Wizeman and Pardue (Wizeman & Pardue 2001) point out the limitations in this area of knowledge. Despite many years of research on the ways in which biology impacts on health, conclusive evidence and clear understanding of the pathways concerned remain scarce. There are various reasons for this, including a lack of research which is disaggregated for men and women and the fact that negative research findings which fail to find a difference between women and men are often not published, despite the fact that such results also advance our understanding.

What remains clear, however, is that biology or sex-linked factors interact with environmental factors, including gender, and the health of women and men is also shaped in a number of ways by socially constructed gender differences.

Gender and health

Gender refers to socially constructed differences between women and men; that is, the conventions, roles, and expectations of men and women that are culturally ascribed (Krieger 2003). Gendered influences on health include access to health promoting resources, exposure to health damaging and health promoting factors in daily life, and different expectations of behaviour such as drinking alcohol, risk taking, and the use of health care. In addition, gender impacts on health through the ways in which health services are organized and delivered, especially when such services operate in gender-insensitive ways.

One of the key differences between sex and gender is the extent to which they are fixed, or can change over time. Sex—male or female—is assigned to a child at birth on the basis of external genitalia and is fixed, other than for a minority of people undergoing medical sex reassignment. Gender is generally ascribed on the basis of biological sex, although what is meant in any one society or culture by gender may vary over the years and between social or other groupings. Thus, a child is identified at birth as either male or female and this in turn leads to the categorizations embedded in masculinity or femininity in that society.

Gender is an important influence on the health of men and women, both alone and in the interaction between gender and biology. Krieger and Zierler (Krieger & Zierler 1995) describe such interactions in terms of *the biologic expression of gender* and the *gendered expression of biology*. The biologic expression of gender refers to the ways in which gender becomes embodied. For example, in many societies, gender is constructed to mean that women see themselves, and are seen by others, as weaker than men. This in turn may result in women taking less exercise or choosing less strenuous forms of activity, which in turn affect the female body. The gendered expression of biology refers to the ways in which biological understandings of women and men lead to gendered differentiations, which often take the form of discrimination. So, for example, women's reproductive capacity is used to justify their exclusion from some forms of paid work on the basis that it is unsafe. Similarly, their exclusion from medical research is said to be justified on the basis that it may cause harm to an unborn child. This exclusion, in turn, strengthens social constructions of gender in which women are seen as less able to undertake some forms of paid work, or less vulnerable to some forms of disease.

For many writers, gender is seen as something that is 'performed' in various ways, in exchange with other people. That is, we 'do' gender in our daily lives—in our paid work, in relationships, in leisure activities, and so on (Courtenay 2000). This view of gender allows us to see how it changes over time and across societies, and also how individuals might 'do' gender differently at different times and in different settings. In addition, it highlights the fact that what is appropriate gendered behaviour for one group may not be so for another—for example, gender roles vary according to class and ethnicity. Finally, it allows for the possibility that individuals might choose to adopt gender roles that are not commensurate with their biological sex. But, although various gender roles may be available, it is also the case that in all societies some forms of masculinity and femininity are more sanctioned than others and this may impact on health in negative or positive ways.

Many writers have observed that in most (if not all) cultures, masculinity is privileged over femininity, but it is also true that all men are not equally advantaged. The term *hegemonic masculinity* has been used to refer to the most privileged form of masculinity, typically occupied by white middle-class men (Connell & Messerschmidt 2005). Men occupying different class positions may experience masculinity in a range of ways, with associated health benefits and/or risks. Similarly, women can experience gender in a number of ways, again with varying impacts on their health.

Gender affects the health of both men and women in numerous interlocking ways. Firstly, gender mediates the effect of physical and psychological risks encountered in daily life. There is substantial evidence, for example, that material factors such as poverty and social exclusion, socioeconomic status, poor housing and environmental disadvantage, and occupation and unpaid work all impact on health in varying ways and to varying degrees (Leon & Walt 2001; Krieger & Higgins 2002). And, men and women may face differential risks of experiencing these adverse effects, because of their gender. Secondly, gender roles and expectations are closely associated with individual behaviour, which in turn may impact on the health of women and men.

Socioeconomic determinants of health and gender

Material factors influence the health of women and men in complex ways through aspects of daily life such as paid work and employment status, household work and domestic labour, income, caring responsibilities, living arrangements, and experiences of conflict, stress, and violence. The extent to which men and women are exposed to these risk factors, and how they impact on their health, varies in relation to geographical location, socioeconomic status, and cultural differences.

Paid employment exerts numerous effects on health. There are a range of hazards associated with particular jobs, including exposure to unsafe chemicals, hazardous work environments, and dangers inherent in the nature of the work itself. The gender division of labour, which sees men more often employed in certain sectors and in certain occupations within sectors, creates a gendered division of occupational risk. Men typically work in industries and in jobs with a higher mortality risk, including construction, transport, and the emergency services.

However, in recent years, the occupational injury gap between women and men has narrowed, following a rise in the numbers of women in the labour force, and there has been a corresponding increase in some forms of injury-related mortality among women (Waldron et al. 2005). Other work-related hazards affect the risk of poor health, such as repetitive strain injury (RSI) from keyboard work and some production processes in manufacturing. Such injuries are more common among women partly as a result of the jobs they occupy and partly because the design of workstations is often based on male rather than female physiology (De Zwart et al. 2001; Lacerda et al. 2005).

Gender differences in occupational risk are compounded by differences outside the workplace and particularly by gender differences in domestic work. Women still carry out most household chores. For example, in the United Kingdom, despite their increasing participation in paid work, women still spend on average twice as many hours per day as men in housework and childcare (ONS 2003). In addition, even where men take on some of the work, women retain overall responsibility for domestic labour—for planning, organizing, and ensuring it is done (Hunt & Annandale 1993). Domestic labour carries further implications for health, including the stress of managing responsibilities combined with lack of reward, loneliness, and isolation, as well as lack of an independent income and low status for those women who are not also employed. Women working at home are notably vulnerable to mental health problems in comparison with those who have paid work, but the strain of juggling two roles and the dual burden of paid work and domestic labour also puts women who enter the labour market at risk of poor mental health (Doyal 1995).

Daily life brings pronounced health risks when either men or women are living in poverty or social exclusion. However, there are gender differences in the risk of such poverty, with women in most parts of the world being more likely to be poor. This is due to lower wages, reduced access to paid work as a result of caring responsibilities, and (in some countries) cultural restrictions, and also reflects the fact that women may not always share equally in household resources. Poverty is often especially severe among older women whose health is already frail (World Health Organization 2003a).

Exposure to violence creates further risks including poor mental health, post-traumatic stress disorders, and physical injuries. Violence is one of the most important causes of death for younger age groups (World Health Organization 2002c), but there are marked gender differences not only in the level of risk from violence but also in the source. Although both women and men are at risk from interpersonal violence, violence against men is more common in the public domain and they are more at risk from strangers. On the other hand, women are more often exposed to violence in the home, from partners and members of their family (World Health Organization 2002c). Women are at particular risk from sexual violence both in the home and elsewhere, and the consequences for their health can include pregnancy and sexually transmitted infections as well as mental health problems. Although sexual violence against men is less common, it may be especially damaging for their mental health due to feelings of stigma and shame (Ganju et al. 2004).

Taken together, these material aspects of daily life can create particular health stresses, which are often different for men and women.

To these health risks, we can add those associated with 'doing gender'—the ways in which social constructions of masculinity and femininity are associated with the increased risk of particular behaviours, which further impact on health.

'Doing gender'—masculinity, femininity, and health

Behaviour has long been seen as the leading gendered explanation for men's poorer health and premature mortality. In the seventeenth century, John Gaunt (quoted in Ciocco [1940]) suggested that women lived longer than men despite their experiences of illness because, 'Men, being more intemperate than women, die as much by reason of their vices, as women do by the infirmity of their sex'. There are still important differences between women and men in behaviours such as smoking, alcohol and substance use, physical activity, diet, risk taking, and the use of health-care services including preventive care and screening. These differences taken together are a key part of the explanation for men's higher mortality; a number of writers in this area have highlighted the extent to which masculinity accounts for the greater mortality risks experienced by men across a range of cultural settings (Courtenay 2000).

One of the most damaging behaviours—smoking and tobacco use—has a strongly gendered history. More men than women die each year from smoking-related diseases; lung cancer, for example, killed twice as many men as women worldwide in 2002 (World Health Organization 2004b). This reflects the gender ratio in smokers: Throughout the world more men than women smoke, and in countries where the epidemic is relatively new, the great majority of those using tobacco are male (World Health Organization 2002b). In Malaysia, for example, 53 per cent of men smoke compared with less than 3 per cent of women; in Malawi, 25 per cent of men and 6 per cent of women smoke; and in India, the comparable figures are 42 per cent and 9 per cent.

However, more developed regions where smoking has a longer history have seen increasing numbers of women beginning to use tobacco, to the point where in some countries similar proportions of women and men are smokers, such as in Norway and Sweden (World Health Organization 2002b). In the United States, 23 per cent of men and 19 per cent of women smoke, compared with 27 per cent of men and 24 per cent of women in the United Kingdom (Schiller & Bernadel 2004; GHS 2004). However, in the United Kingdom, female smokers have outnumbered males in recent years in younger age groups and there are also more women smokers than men in some minority ethnic groups, particularly those described as mixed race (GHS 2004).

Alcohol and substance use also have gendered profiles. Excessive consumption of alcohol on a regular basis is associated with an increased risk of a number of diseases, including liver cirrhosis and other liver disease, some forms of coronary heart disease, and oral cancers (World Health Organization 2004a). Other forms of alcohol consumption, including what is sometimes referred to as 'binge drinking' in which high levels of alcohol are consumed over a short period of time, also lead to an increased risk of violence and accidental injury, as well as self-harm and suicide (World Health Organization 2004a).

In surveys of national and international data, more women than men are described as 'abstainers', that is, as non-drinkers. The extent of the gender gap varies: In the Philippines, for example, women are seven times more likely than men to be abstainers, whereas in Iceland, the ratio of female to male abstainers is nearly equal (World Health Organization 2004a).

In many countries, more men than women are defined as heavy drinkers; that is, they consume a high number of units of alcohol on a weekly basis and/or have a high daily intake. Figures for Argentina, for example, show that over 11 per cent of male drinkers compared with 2 per cent of women are defined as consuming high levels of alcohol on a daily basis; similarly, 52 per cent of male drinkers in Colombia compared with 21 per cent of female drinkers are defined as heavy consumers; and 23 per cent of male drinkers in Japan compared with only 5 per cent of female drinkers are defined as having a problematic intake (World Health Organization 2004a). However, in some countries (including Australia, Nigeria, and the United Kingdom), more women than men are defined as drinking over recommended daily limits.

If we look at binge drinking rather than daily consumption, this remains much more common among men than women around the world, despite fears in some countries that such behaviour is increasing among younger women. Such drinking is highest among males in Finland where nearly half of male drinkers report very high consumption on single occasions compared with 14 per cent of women, although there are also high levels of binge drinking among men in Mexico, Nigeria, and Iceland. In Nigeria, nearly 40 per cent of female drinkers reported binge drinking at least once a month (World Health Organization 2004a).

Diet is also an important, modifiable contributor to health risks. The influence of diet on health is becoming increasingly clear, with growing evidence suggesting that a diet which is rich in fruit, vegetables, and fibre and low in fat may reduce the risk of various health problems including cancer and heart disease (Thune & Furberg 2001). Gender differences in what we eat may therefore play an important role in explaining different patterns of health for men and women. Men are more likely than women to die from colorectal cancer, for example, and part of the explanation for this seems to stem from differences in diet (Steinemetz & Potter 1991).

On the whole, men's diets are less healthy than those of women, especially in high-income countries, where men more often consume inadequate amounts of vegetables and fruit and also eat higher than recommended amounts of red meat (Payne 2006; Courtenay 2000). However, in low- and middle-income countries, notably those where food is scarce, women and girls are less likely than men to be eating adequate levels of fruit and vegetables. For example, in Malawi, 42 per cent of women and 37 per cent of men have diets with less than the recommended amount of fruit and vegetables. In other low-income countries (such as in Pakistan, India, Swaziland, and Kenya), a large majority of both men and women report diets insufficient in fruit and vegetables, and the differences between them are slight (World Health Organization 2006). In these countries, where there is a high risk of food insecurity, there are important gender differences in the distribution of food within households, in expectations about what men and women will eat, and also in what will be given to male and female children.

However, food intake and diet also need to be set against energy requirements, and again there are important gender differences both in levels of physical activity and in kinds of activity.

In high-income countries, lack of physical activity is a health concern that has increased in prominence in recent years. Physical activity can have a positive effect on health: It helps to protect against heart disease and may play a part in reducing vulnerability to other conditions, including some cancers and mental health problems (Thune & Furberg 2001). WHO estimate that around 2 million deaths and 19 million DALYs each year are associated with insufficient physical activity (World Health Organization 2002a). Physical activity levels in most communities are different for men and women, although the size of the gap varies in relation to other factors including employment-related activity levels and available leisure time.

Data on activity levels are complex and not always comparable. Some surveys refer to total physical activity including that associated with work and travel (e.g. cycling and walking) as well as leisure activities such as sport. One of the problems with this data is that physical domestic work, mainly carried out by women, is often not included in such measures (O'Brien 2005). This means that some figures (based on total activity), principally those from low- and middle-income countries, overestimate the extent to which women are leading sedentary lives. Data based on leisure activities alone, however, might also miss out some activities that are more frequent among women, such as dancing (O'Brien 2005).

Data from the West often focus on leisure activity rather than total activity, making it difficult to compare findings with poorer countries. However, in high-income countries, there is a gap between men and women in time spent in physical activity, with men tending to be more active. Figures from the United States, for example, show that a higher proportion of men participate regularly in physical activity (Schiller & Bernadel 2004). Similarly, in England, more men than women take part in such activity, with the widest gap among young adults between 16 and 24 years of age (NatCen 2003).

Figures for total physical activity in low- and middle-income countries suggest that men might be more likely than women to have active lifestyles, although this possibly reflects a failure to count some aspects of women's activities. In Kenya, for example, although less than 10 per cent of adults report physical activity levels that are too low (in terms of health benefit), slightly more women than men report insufficient time spent in physical activity (World Health Organization 2006). Similarly, in Malawi, few people have low levels of activity, but activity levels are lower among women than men. Activity levels are slightly lower in Pakistan, where women are twice as likely as men to report insufficient activity; and in India and China, fewer women than men report sufficient levels of activity.

However, in these countries it is also important to consider activity, or energy expenditure, alongside diet and calorie intake. In the poorest countries, women experience health risks because of activity levels that are high in the context of too little food. These problems are especially severe for pregnant and breastfeeding women, and carry long-term implications both for their health and that of their child. Jackson and Palmer-Jones (Jackson & Palmer-Jones 1998) talk of an 'energy trap' resulting from development policies that aim to increase various kinds of work in order to reduce poverty but which fail to take account of the increased need for food created by increased levels of activity. Gender differences in food allocation and access to calories, as well as in work carried out, mean this is an acute problem for women (Jackson & Palmer-Jones 1998; Standing 2002).

Diet and activity levels in high-income countries are also connected to a further measure of health risk: Obesity. Obesity is associated with various diseases including coronary heart disease, some forms of cancer, and diabetes. Obesity, defined as a body mass index (BMI) over 30, is more common among women than men although this varies between countries, whereas more men than women are defined as overweight (with a BMI of between 25 and 30) (Zaninotto *et al.* 2006; ASSO 2005). In older age groups and in lower-income groups in particular, women are more likely than men to be defined as obese (World Health Organization 2003a; NatCen 2003).

A final aspect of behaviour that is gendered and which affects health and mortality risk is the use of preventive services and health care. We have earlier discussed gender differences in consultation as a measure of morbidity, and economic factors play a part in the use of health care, but it is also important to consider the ways in which men and women differ in help-seeking behaviour. A number of studies have suggested that men are reluctant to seek medical help and attend services less readily than women. As one man put it, 'I don't go to the doctor unless something scares the hell out of me' (Stibbe 2004:36). Men describe themselves as unwilling to make a fuss or waste the time of health professionals (O'Brien *et al.* 2005). Although there are a number of variations in data on health-service use, such as those reflecting differences in age, in socioeconomic status, and for specific symptoms, men do appear less willing to see themselves as in need of health care. Similarly, men are more difficult to engage in health-promotion activities including screening, leading some health-care providers to devise various gender-sensitive strategies to increase take-up among men, such as placing clinics and information points in workplaces and bars (Alt 2002; Malterud & Okkes 1998). Overall, gender differences in roles, expectations, and behaviour combine to increase the risk of premature mortality for men and the risk of chronic health problems for women. Masculinity, insofar as it involves risk taking and unhealthy behaviours, increases risks of accidental and non-accidental injury, and of non-communicable diseases associated with smoking, alcohol, and substance use. Masculine practices also increase some health risks for women, notably the risks associated with male violence and sexually-transmitted infections.

Female gender roles and expectations may lead to reduced risks for some conditions because of lower rates of smoking, alcohol, and substance use, better diets, and less risk-taking, although the lower rates of physical activity more common among women will also affect their health risks. In poorer countries, however, women have different problems associated with insufficient food for the work they are expected to carry out. There are also pressures on both men and women arising from the stress of gender role expectations, especially in relation to failure to meet these expectations.

In order to illustrate these different influences and the complex associations between sex and gender, we now look at specific health problems: Cardiovascular diseases, cancer, HIV and AIDS, mental health difficulties, and malaria.

The impact of sex and gender on specific health problems

Cardiovascular diseases

Cardiovascular diseases include coronary heart disease (CHD) and stroke. Taken together, cardiovascular diseases account for around one-tenth of the global burden of disease, with more men than women affected. CHD is the major contributor to this burden, particularly among men, whereas strokes account for similar levels of illness among men and women. These conditions are also important in overall mortality: More men than women die as a result of CHD but more women die from a stroke (World Health Organization 2004b). One of the key differences between women and men in these illnesses is the age at which risk increases: Men are more likely than women to die prematurely from CHD and the male to female ratio is greatest in mid-life. On average, women with CHD die ten years later than men (Wizeman & Pardue 2001). In the United Kingdom, the male mortality rate for CHD is around five times the female rate between 45 and 54 years, whereas the male–female ratio has reduced to 1.4 to 1 by the age of 80 (Khaw 2006). Although trends in CHD have changed over time, men worldwide experience the greater risk of premature death and illness associated with this condition (Khaw 2006).

Why do men than women have higher risks for CHD at an early stage in the life course? In the aetiology of CHD, raised blood pressure and blood cholesterol are significant risk factors, and behaviours that are more common among men than women—notably poor diet and smoking—are important underlying explanations. Although women gain protection from heart disease due to female hormones, men increase their risks through the adoption of risky behaviours. The later age at which women appear to be at risk of CHD has led to speculation that until menopause female hormones might offer women some degree of protection. However, most recent research has failed to support this suggestion. For example, women's CHD risk does not increase immediately following menopause but some years later, suggesting that other factors may be important instead of, or alongside, female hormones. In addition, hormone replacement therapy does not appear to offer women protection from CHD (Khaw 2006).

However, there are also concerns over possible differences between women and men in the recognition and treatment of CHD. Because heart disease is seen as primarily a male condition, women may be less likely to have their illness diagnosed or to be offered appropriate treatment (Lockyer & Bury 2002). This topic is dealt with in a later subsection.

Cancer

Overall mortality from cancer is higher among men, and although both men and women are vulnerable to reproductive-related cancers, more men than women also die from cancers related to lifestyle and behaviours associated with an increased risk of cancer. Although cancers of the reproductive organs lead to more deaths among women than among men, the difference does not compensate for the male excess cancer mortality stemming from factors such as tobacco use, poor diet, and alcohol consumption.

Lung cancer, for example, accounts for more than twice as many deaths among men as among women, as well as for a large proportion of illnesses (World Health Organization 2004b). The main cause of lung cancer for both men and women is tobacco use, and in countries where tobacco use remains a predominantly male habit, the male–female ratio is especially high. In Thailand, for example, the ratio of men to women for lung cancer mortality is around 2.3:1, whereas in Denmark, where equal numbers of men and women now smoke, the ratio has reduced to 1.4 to 1 in recent years (World Health Organization).

However, research suggests that the risk of lung cancer is different for women and men irrespective of absolute levels of tobacco use.

These differences stem from gendered differences in patterns of tobacco use—such as the type of cigarettes smoked and the depth of inhalation—and from biological factors. Women have a greater biological vulnerability to lung cancer due to genetic factors and their higher use of low-tar cigarettes leads to an increased risk of one form of lung cancer—adenocarcinoma. However, although lung cancer is a particularly fatal form of cancer with very low one-year and five-year survival rates, women appear to have better prospects for survival in comparison with men, which is also related to biological differences between women and men.

Thus, sex- and gender-linked factors interact to produce different risks of cancer for women and men, reflecting hormonal and genetic influences and the impact of certain behaviours.

Mental health and illness

Among chronic and debilitating conditions, the most significant in terms of numbers affected and the impact on daily living are those associated with mental illness. Mental health problems, including depression, anxiety, substance use, and schizophrenia, account for around 12 per cent of the global burden of disease (World Health Organization 2003b). Around 450 million people worldwide experience mental illness of one kind or another at any one time. There are important differences between women and men in their risks of different kinds of mental health problems or disorders. More women are diagnosed as suffering from depression and anxiety-related conditions, and in community-based surveys, more women are found to be suffering from symptoms of these illnesses (Payne 2006). This gender gap is found throughout the world: The *World Health Survey* (World Health Organization 2005) for 2005 found that in countries as diverse as Malawi, India, Portugal, Pakistan, and the Russian Federation more women than men were diagnosed with depression. It is estimated that worldwide women are almost twice as likely as men to experience an episode of depression in a twelve-month period (World Health Organization 2003b).

Men, on the other hand, are more frequently treated for mental health difficulties associated with alcohol and substance use, including harmful use, dependence, and psychosis (Payne 2006). Men are also more likely to commit suicide than women in every country in the world apart from China. In contrast, more women than men are involved in acts of deliberate self-harm.

Although there is some evidence that biological influences play a part in shaping mental health—especially in relation to specific conditions such as postnatal depression—most research suggests that gendered factors play the more significant role. These include stress-linked factors such as those associated with poverty, parenting, employment, exposure to the threat of violence, and gendered expectations, as well as the extent to which gender stereotyping in mental health services affects the delivery of care by increasing diagnoses of depression among women (Blair-West et al. 1999).

HIV and AIDS

In many parts of the world, HIV/AIDS is one of the most significant threats to the health of women and men. More than 39 million people worldwide were living with HIV in 2006, with over 4 million new infections and nearly 3 million deaths (UNAIDS 2006). Most of those who are HIV positive (nearly 25 million) live in sub-Saharan Africa, and most of the world's AIDS deaths occur in this region. Not surprisingly, HIV/AIDS accounts for a large proportion of illness worldwide and was the fourth largest contributor to the global burden of disease in 2001 (Lopez *et al.* 2006).

One of the main features of the pandemic is the increasing numbers of women affected in parts of the world where prevalence is highest. For example, in sub-Saharan Africa, women comprise nearly 60 per cent of adults living with HIV, compared with 26 per cent in North America (UNAIDS 2006). Increasing numbers of women are also being infected in Asia, Eastern Europe, and South American countries, with the proportion likely to rise in future years. In the Russian Federation, women now comprise 40 per cent of new infections (UNAIDS 2006).

Women are vulnerable to HIV/AIDS due to a mixture of biological and gender-linked factors. In unprotected vaginal intercourse, women are at greater risk than men because the absorbent vaginal wall is exposed to seminal fluid and because semen carries a higher viral load than other bodily fluids. However, women are also less able to negotiate sexual relationships—such as to demand protection—and may be forced or coerced into unprotected sex. Female sex workers in particular are at risk, especially when sex without condoms offers the opportunity for more money. Women in insecure situations, such as forced migrants, may also be pressurized into unsafe sex in order to gain protection or resources. For example, a recent study of HIV infection rates among displaced persons in North Uganda found that women living outside protected camps had higher risks of infection than those living inside such camps (UNAIDS 2006).

HIV and AIDS have severe consequences for the health of both women and men. For both, there is an increased risk of opportunistic infection, and levels of malaria, tuberculosis, and some forms of cancer are higher among people living with HIV and AIDS. Both also experience reduced fertility. However, although all of those living with HIV and AIDS are at risk of premature mortality without access to essential medicines, women are at risk of pelvic inflammatory disease, recurrent yeast infections, cervical cancer, and problems in pregnancy and childbirth, all of which complicate treatment (National Institute of Allergy and Infectious Diseases 2004). Men also have increased risks of some associated diseases, particularly Kaposi's sarcoma (a type of skin cancer), which can lead to weight loss, fever, and painful swelling especially in the legs, groin area, or skin around the eyes.

Thus, sex and gender again intertwine, both in terms of men's and women's vulnerability to infection and in the consequences of the disease.

Malaria

Between 350 and 500 million people become ill each year with malaria, and over 1 million people (mainly children) die from this disease (World Health Organization 2005b). The vast majority of those affected live in sub-Saharan Africa. The global impact of malaria on the burden of illness has been calculated at more than 46 million DALYs per annum (World Health Organization 2004b).

Reduction of the incidence of malaria has been included in the eight Millennium Development Goals (MDGs) and has been a key focus of the WHO's work in recent years. Incidence of malaria has been growing over the past decade for a variety of reasons, including increasing resistance to the drugs used to treat the disease and resistance to the insecticides used to prevent transmission. In addition, the disease burden has worsened due to an increase in the lack of access to necessary medicine and preventive measures, notably among those in poorer countries, and due to deforestation in some areas creating wider vectors of transmission.

There is an important difference between women and men in the risk of malaria, with more women being infected and dying from this disease. Biology plays a key part in this difference, as women have a much greater risk of contracting malaria when pregnant due to temporary changes in their immune system brought about by the pregnancy. However, gender factors also increase their risks of malaria. In many parts of the world (including those where malaria is rife), women have less access than men to preventive measures such as bed nets treated with insecticide, because of the household division of resources. In addition, women's responsibility for work, such as water collection and some agricultural labour, increases their exposure to mosquitoes and the risk of being bitten. Further, studies have found women to be less well-informed than men about the risks of malaria and the means of protection, and are less able to access health care when infected because of less control over household resources and, in many cultures, the need to be chaperoned when attending health services (Tanner & Vlassoff 1998). When they do seek help, research has also suggested that they are often blamed by health professionals for not attending earlier, and they feel poorly treated by such professionals and by being stigmatized in their communities (Tanner & Vlassoff 1998).

Gender and the delivery of health care

The final way in which gender impacts on health is through the delivery of health care. In addition to material circumstances and behaviour, the health of both men and women is also associated with the way in which health care is provided and we need to ask if health services are equally available for both, if they are accessible, and if they are appropriate.

Gender differences in availability and accessibility

Gender affects access to health in a number of ways. Most importantly perhaps, it affects the resources that are necessary in order to use health services. Around the world, women earn less than men, and, where health insurance is related to paid work, are more often in jobs without insurance cover (Collins *et al.* 1999).

In many low- and middle-income countries, although both men and women experience difficulty in obtaining health care due to the location of services and the need to meet the costs of user fees, women are more disadvantaged because of a lack of independent income or a say in how household resources are used (Ravindran 2000; Benjamins *et al.* 2004).

In addition to access, there may be further differences in availability. Where services are only open during the day, they are less available to those with paid work who cannot take time off or to those whose caring responsibilities prevent attendance. Although more men are prevented from using daytime services due to employment, they are also more often in jobs where time off for medical appointments is sanctioned. For women juggling full-time or part-time work with childcare, seeking medical help may be especially difficult.

Similarly, some cultures require women to consult with female health professionals, who may not always be available. Even where it is not culturally prescribed, more women report a preference for a female clinician, particularly when consulting about intimate health problems. For example, women are more likely to prefer a female colonoscopist when being screened for bowel cancer, but the lack of women in this profession means that their preferences are often not met, potentially delaying detection of bowel cancer among women (Menees *et al.* 2005).

Gender differences in the quality of care

The second way in which gender impinges on health care is through differences in the quality of care offered to men and women. One important factor affecting this is medical knowledge. Medical research has for some time been criticized for failing to disaggregate findings for women and men, and also for failing to include women in studies of health problems affecting both sexes (Doyal 1998). This focus on male subjects is problematic when it is assumed that findings can be extended to female populations as though there is no difference. Both symptom recognition and treatment based on men may fail women—for example, women metabolize pharmaceuticals differently to men and prescribed drugs may be more or less effective, or carry different risks for women if the research was conducted only on men (Wizeman & Pardue 2001). Similarly, risk factors affecting women's health tend to have been less intensively studied: The mental and physical risks associated with housework, for example, are relatively unexplored compared with some traditionally male occupations (Ruiz & Verbrugge 1997).

In the United States, the National Institutes of Health have required (since 1994) research funded by them to include sufficient numbers of men and women, and members of minority ethnic groups, as well as to provide separate analyses and reporting of results. Despite this, some evidence shows that a number of studies still either focus on men alone or fail to disaggregate findings for men and women (Vidaver *et al.* 2000). In countries without such guidelines, the bias is even greater.

Studies have also explored the different ways in which services respond to the health needs of women and men. For example, women are less likely to have heart conditions recognized by their primary physician because they often present with atypical symptoms including fatigue, shortness of breath, and cold sweats. Men, on the other hand, are seen as candidates for heart complaints by themselves, by their families, and by health care workers, and the symptoms they typically present with have become the norm (Lockyer & Bury 2002). In addition, chest pain, a key symptom of heart disease, will often have other causes for women and this also leads to an underdiagnosis of heart disease. Not surprisingly, women are less often referred for tests and for treatment, and tend to be at a more advanced stage of illness when they are treated, with more severe symptoms and the risk this implies (Lockyer & Bury 2002).

Equally, men are less likely than women to have mental health problems such as depression recognized (Blair-West *et al.* 1999). Underdiagnosis and undertreatment of depression in men contribute to higher rates of male suicide mortality; where there have been increases in prescriptions of antidepressants among men, suicide rates have fallen (Gunnell *et al.* 2003).

In addition, health care may not be sensitive to more subtle gender differences in health needs. Some services are gender-blind and unknowingly discriminate against men or women by failing to identify their specific needs. For example, most smoking cessation interventions do not highlight gender differences in successful strategies, including the fact that women and men appear to smoke for different reasons and may take up smoking again in response to different stress factors (Samet & Yoon 2001). In addition, women metabolize nicotine differently to men and have more adverse reactions to withdrawal compared with men (Perkins 2001). Women and men also may need different kinds of support, both from friends or family and from health services (Gritz *et al.* 1996).

Conclusion

What we have seen in this chapter is that both sex and gender play an important part in shaping the health of men and women, alongside other forms of diversity. Sex, or biology, is more than reproduction. The health of both men and women is also affected by hormonal differences, and by genetic factors, which impact on their vulnerability to different diseases as well as the chances of recovery and survival.

Gender, or socially constructed difference, also affects health—by increasing the chances of exposure to specific risk factors, such as poverty, or by helping to shape the behavioural choices made by men and women—the way we 'do' masculinity or femininity. Gender is also important in the way health services are delivered— from how research is conducted and how medical knowledge is constructed and disseminated to health policy and planning, which shape the availability of medical care, access to care, and how appropriately it meets the needs of men and women. All of these factors combine at the level of the individual to shape their health experience and their need for care, and that care itself needs to be planned and delivered in such a way that both men and women are able to benefit.

Key points

◆ Both sex and gender play a part in women's and men's health.

◆ Sex or biological factors affect incidence, and also, survival for various diseases.

◆ Gender is socially constructed and affects exposure to risk factors, as well as influencing health behaviours.

◆ Gender also affects the delivery of health care, access to care, and how well this care meets the needs of women and men.

References

AbouZahr C., Vaughan J.P. Assessing the burden of sexual and reproductive ill-health: questions regarding the use of disability-adjusted life years [online]. *Bulletin of the World Health Organization* 2000;**78**(5):655–66.

Alt R. Where the boys are not: a brief overview of male preventive health. *Wisconsin Medical Journal* 2002;**287**:337–43.

Australian Bureau of Statistics (ABS). *National health survey 2004–5.* Canberra: Australian Bureau of Statistics; 2006.

Australian Society for the Study of Obesity (ASSO). *Obesity in Australian adults: prevalence data.* Sydney: Australian Society for the Study of Obesity; 2005.

Baghadi G. Gender and medicines: an international public health perspective. *Journal of Women's Health* 2005;**14**:82–6.

Benjamins M., Hummer R., Eberstein I. *et al.* Self-reported health and adult mortality risk. *Social Science and Medicine* 2004;**59**:1297–306.

Bird C.E., Rieker P.P. Gender matters: an integrated model for understanding men's and women's health. *Social Science and Medicine* 1999;**48**:745–55.

Blair-West G.W., Cantor C.H., Mellsop G.W. *et al.* Lifetime suicide risk in major depression: sex and age determinants. *Journal of Affective Disorder* 1999;**55**:171–8.

Bradley L., Alarcon G. Sex-related influences in fibromyalgia. In: Fillingham B.D., editor. *Sex, gender, and pain*. Seattle (WA): IASP Press; 1999. p. 281–307.

Ciocco A. Sex differences in morbidity and mortality. *The Quarterly Review of Biology* 1940;**15**:59–73.

Connell R., Messerschmidt J.W. Hegemonic masculinity: rethinking the concept. *Gender and Society* 2005;**19**:829–59.

Courtenay W. Constructions of masculinity and their influence on men's well-being: a theory of gender and health. *Social Science and Medicine* 2000;**50**:1385–401.

De Zwart B., Frings-Dressen M., Kilbom A. Gender differences in upper extremity musculoskeletal complaints in the working population. *International Archives of Occupational and Environmental Health* 2001;**74**:21–30.

Dejong J. Capabilities, reproductive health, and well-being. *The Journal of Development Studies* 2006;**42**:1158–79.

Division for the Advancement of Women (DAW). *Gender equality, development, and peace for the twenty-first century: the feminization of poverty*. New York (NY): Division for the Advancement of Women, United Nations; 2000. Available from: http://www.un.org/womenwatch/daw/followup/session/presskit/fs1.htm [Accessed 24 April 2007].

Doyal L. *Gender and health technical paper*. Geneva: World Health Organization; 1998. WHO/FRH/WHD/98.16.

Doyal L. Sex, gender, and health: the need for a new approach. *British Medical Journal* 2001;**323**:1061–3.

Doyal L. What makes women sick? Gender and the political economy of health. Basingstoke, UK: Macmillan; 1995.

Ganju D., Jejeebhoy S., Nidadavoluand V. *et al*. *Sexual coercion: young men's experiences as victims and perpetrators*. New Delhi: Population Council; 2004.

General Household Survey (GHS). *Living in Britain: results from the 2002 general household survey*. London: The Stationery Office; 2004.

Gritz E.R., Nielsen I.R., Brooks L.A. Smoking cessation and gender: the influence of physiological, psychological, and behavioural factors. *Journal of American Medical Women's Association* 1996;**51**:35–42.

Gunnell D., Middleton N., Whitley E. *et al*. Why are suicide rates rising in young men but falling in the elderly? A time-series analysis of trends in England and Wales, 1950–1998. *Social Science and Medicine* 2003;**57**:595–611.

Haugen A. Women who smoke: are women more susceptible to tobacco-induced lung cancer? *Carcinogenesis* 2002;**23**:227–9.

Heitkemper M., Jarrett M., Bond E. *et al*. Impact of sex and gender on irritable bowel syndrome. *Biological Research for Nursing* 2003; **5**:56–65.

Hemenway D., Shinoda-Tagawa T., Miller M. Firearm availability and female homicide victimization rates among 25 populous high-income countries. *Journal of American Women's Medical Association* 2002;**57**:100–4.

Hunt K., Annandale E. Just the job? Is the relationship between health and domestic and paid work gender-specific? *Sociology of Health and Illness* 1993;**15**:632–64.

Jackson C., Palmer-Jones R. *Work intensity, gender, and well-being*. United Nations Research Institute for Social Development; 1998 Oct. Discussion Paper Number 96.

Kane P. *Women's health from womb to tomb*. London: St Martins Press; 1991.

Keohavong P., Lan Q., Gao W.M. *et al*. K-ras mutations in lung carcinomas from nonsmoking women exposed to unvented coal smoke in China. *Lung Cancer* 2003;**41**:21–7.

Khaw K-T. Epidemiology of coronary heart disease in women. *Heart* 2006;**92**:2–4.

Kravdal O. Is the relationship between childbearing and cancer incidence due to biology or lifestyle? Examples of importance of using data on men. *International Journal of Epidemiology* 1995;**24**:477–84.

Krieger J., Higgins D. Housing and health: time again for public health action. *American Journal of Public Health* 2002;**92**:758–68.

Krieger N., Zierler S. Accounting for the health of women. *Current Issues in Public Health* 1995;**1**:251–6.

Krieger N. Genders, sexes, and health: what are the connections—and why does it matter? *International Journal of Epidemiology* 2003;**32**:652–7.

Lacerda E., Nacul L., da S Augusto L. *et al*. Prevalence and associations of symptoms of upper extremities, repetitive strain injuries (RSI), and 'RSI-like condition': a cross-sectional study of bank workers in Northeast Brazil. *BMC Public Health* 2005;**5**:107.

Leon D., Walt G., editors. *Poverty, inequality, and health: an international perspective*. Oxford: Oxford University Press; 2001.

LeResche L. Epidemiological perspectives on sex differences in pain. In: Fillingham B.D, editor. *Sex, gender, and pain*. Seattle (WA): IASP Press; 1999. p. 233–49.

Lockyer L., Bury M. The construction of a modern epidemic: the implications for women of the gendering of coronary heart disease. *Journal of Advanced Nursing* 2002;**39**:432–40.

Lopez A.D., Mathers C.D., Ezzati M. *et al*. Measuring the global burden of disease and risk factors, 1990–2001. In: Lopez AD, Mathers CD, Ezzati M, Jamison DT, Murray CJH, editors. *Global burden of disease and risk factors*. New York (NY): World Bank; Oxford: Oxford University Press; 2006. p. 1–13.

Lorber J. Gender and the construction of illness. London: Sage; 1997.

MacDorman M., Hoyert D., Martin J. *et al*. Fetal and perinatal mortality, United States, 2003. *National Vital Statistics Reports* 2007;**55**(6):1–18.

Macintyre S. Inequalities in health: is research gender blind? In: Leon D., Walt G., editors. *Poverty, inequality, and health: an international perspective*. Oxford: Oxford University Press; 2001.

Malterud K., Okkes I. Gender differences in general practice consultations: methodological challenges in epidemiological research. *Family Practice* 1998;**15**:404–10.

Menees S.B., Inadomi J.M., Korsnes S. *et al*. Women patients' preference for women physicians is a barrier to colon cancer screening. *Gastrointestinal Endoscopy* 2005;**62**(2):219–23.

National Centre for Social Research (NatCen). *Health survey for England 2003: summary of key findings*. London: National Centre for Social Research; 2003.

National Institute of Allergy and Infectious Diseases. *HIV infection in women*. Rockville (MD): National Institute of Allergy and Infectious Diseases; 2004.

O'Brien Cousins S., Gillis M.M. 'Just do it … before you talk yourself out of it': the self-talk of adults thinking about physical activity. *Psychology of Sport and Exercise* 2005;**6**:313–34.

O'Brien R., Hunt K., Hart G. 'It's caveman stuff, but that is to a certain extent how guys still operate': men's accounts of masculinity and help seeking. *Social Science and Medicine* 2005;**61**:503–16.

Office for National Statistics (ONS). *2001 census data: focus on health*. London: Office for National Statistics; 2006. Available from: http://www.statistics.gov.uk/cci/nugget.asp?id=1325

Office for National Statistics (ONS). *Key health statistics from general practice 1998*. London: Office for National Statistics; 2000.

Office for National Statistics (ONS). *UK 2000 time use survey*. London: Office for National Statistics; 2003.

Payne S. Smoke like a man, die like a man? A review of the relationship between sex, gender, and lung cancer. *Social Science and Medicine* 2001;**53**:1067–80.

Payne S. *The health of men and women*. Cambridge: Polity; 2006.

Perkins K. Smoking cessation in women: special considerations. *CNS Drugs* 2001;**15**:391–411.

Ravindran T.K.S. Engendering health. Seminar 489: *Unhealthy trends (a symposium on the state of our public health system)*; 2000 May. Available from: http://www.india-seminar.com/2000/489/489%20ravindran.htm

Redgrave G.W., Swartz K.L., Romanoski A.J. Alcohol misuse by women. *International Review of Psychiatry* 2003;**15**:256–68.

Ruiz M.T., Verbrugge L.M. A two-way view of gender bias in medicine. *Epidemiology and Community Health* 1997;**51**:106–9.

Samet J., Yoon S-Y. Women and the tobacco epidemic: challenges for the 21st century. Geneva: World Health Organization; 2001.

Schiller J., Bernadel L. *Summary health statistics for the US population: national health interview survey*. Washington (DC): National Centre for Health Statistics; 2004. Washington Vital Health Stat Series 10 Number 22.

Sen K., Bonita R. Global health status: two steps forward, one step back. *Lancet* 2000;**356**:577–82.

Shields P. Molecular epidemiology of smoking and lung cancer. *Oncogene* 2002;**21**:6870–6.

Standing H. Understanding the links between energy, poverty, and gender. *Boiling Point* 2002;**48**:11. Available from: http://practicalaction.org/docs/energy/docs48/bp48_pp11.pdf

Steinemetz K.A., Potter J.D. Vegetables, fruit, and cancer. I. Epidemiology. *Cancer Causes and Control* 1991;**2**:325–57.

Stibbe A. Health and the social construction of masculinity in men's health magazine. *Men and Masculinities* 2004;**7**:31–51.

Tanner M., Vlassoff C. Treatment-seeking behaviour for malaria: a typology based on endemicity and gender. *Social Science and Medicine* 1998;**46**:523–32.

Thune I., Furberg A. Physical activity and cancer risk: dose-response and cancer, all sites and site-specific. *Medicine and Science in Sports and Exercise* 2001;**33**:S530–50.

UNAIDS. *AIDS epidemic update*. Geneva: World Health Organization, UNAIDS; 2006.

Vidaver R., Lafleur B., Tong C. *et al.* Women subjects in NIH-funded clinical research literature: lack of progress in both representation and analysis by sex. *Journal of Women's Health and Gender-based Medicine* 2000;**9**:495–504.

Waldron I., McCloskey C., Earle I. Trends in gender differences in accidents mortality. *Demographic Research* 2005;**13**:415–54.

Waldron I. What do we know about the causes of sex differences in mortality? *Population Bulletin of United Nations* 1985;**18**:59–76.

Wizeman T., Pardue M. *Exploring the biological contributions to health: does sex matter?* Washington (DC): National Academy Press; 2001.

World Health Organisation *WHOSIS World Health Organisation Health Statistics and Information System* Geneva at: http://www.who.int/whosis/database/core/core_select.cfm

World Health Organization. *Gender, health, and ageing*. Geneva: World Health Organization; 2003a.

World Health Organization. *Global status report on alcohol*. Geneva: World Health Organization; 2004a.

World Health Organization. *Investing in mental health*. Geneva: World Health Organization; 2003b.

World Health Organization. *Myths about physical activity*. Geneva: World Health Organization; 2002a.

World Health Organization. *Tobacco atlas*. Geneva: World Health Organization; 2002b.

World Health Organization. *World health report 2004: changing history*. Geneva: World Health Organization; 2004b.

World Health Organization. *World health report 2005: make every mother and child count*. Geneva: World Health Organization; 2005b.

World Health Organization. *World health report 2006: working together for health*. Geneva: World Health Organization; 2006.

World Health Organization. *World health survey 2005*. Geneva: World Health Organization; 2005. Available from: http://www.who.int/healthinfo/survey/en

World Health Organization. *World malaria report 2005*. Geneva: World Health Organization; 2005a.

World Health Organization. *World mortality database: tables*. Geneva: World Health Organization. Available from: http://www.who.int/healthinfo/morttables/en/index.html

World Health Organization. *World report on violence and health*. Geneva: World Health Organization; 2003c.

World Health Organization. *World report on violence and health*. Geneva: World Health Organization; 2002c.

Yunus M. Gender differences in fibromyalgia and other related syndromes. *Journal of Gender Specific Medicine* 2002;**5**:42–7.

Zaninotto P., Wardle H., Stamatakis E. *et al. Forecasting obesity to 2010*. London: Department of Health; 2006.

11.3

Child health

Elizabeth Mason, Olivier Fontaine,
Bernadette Daelmans, Rajiv Bahl,
Cynthia Boschi-Pinto, and Jose Martines

Abstract

This chapter focuses on the health status of children, particularly those less than five years of age—the main health risks faced by this age group and the interventions that promote their survival, growth, and development.

The under-five mortality rate (U5MR) is one of the most sensitive indicators of the socioeconomic status and well-being of a society, and has been chosen to monitor the global and national achievements of the Millennium Development Goal (MDG) 4 of reducing, between 1990 and 2015, the under-five mortality rate by two-thirds. The Global U5MR burden remains unacceptably high. Moreover, progress in reducing under-five mortality is not equally distributed across countries and regions. Poverty and its consequences are directly or indirectly associated with most of the poor outcomes in child health.

Most children suffer and die from a small number of conditions—the main causes of morbidity being highly correlated with the major causes of death. Likewise, child growth, nutritional status, and development are intertwined. Strikingly, even in the poorest settings, a significant proportion of these outcomes could be prevented with a few interventions that are well-known, feasible, deliverable without complex technology, and affordable. These interventions are in the following areas: Essential newborn care and case management of newborn illness, infant and young child feeding and case management of malnutrition, and the prevention and management of diarrhoea, pneumonia, malaria and HIV infection.

Strengthening the health system and integrating the interventions into packages of care that can be delivered at all levels during pregnancy, childbirth, neonatal period, and childhood—from home to hospital—will be key to increasing the coverage of health interventions. Achievement of the MDG of reducing child mortality will require significant acceleration in investments on child survival.

The situation of children in the world

The Convention of the Rights of the Child defines children as, 'all persons below the age of 18 years, unless under the law applicable to the child, majority is attained earlier'. The life-course approach to health care recognizes the continuum from birth through childhood, adolescence, and adulthood, reflecting the principle that care provided to children at birth, or even before it occurs, will affect their immediate well-being and will also have an impact on their health and development in later years (Fig. 11.3.1).

In the life-course approach, the period of life before attaining adulthood is divided into three age subgroups based on epidemiology and health-care needs: The first five years (under-five children), the next five years (older children), and the second decade of life (adolescents). The first five years of life are further subdivided into neonatal period, infancy, and preschool years.

This chapter focuses on the health of under-five children and touches upon the health of older children. Chapter 11.4 deals with adolescent health. The most important indicators of the health status of the under five relate to their mortality, morbidity, growth, and development.

Mortality in under-five children

The U5MR and infant mortality rate are broadly recognized as two of the most sensitive indicators of a country's socioeconomic situation and quality of life. The 1980s saw an acceleration of large-scale health programmes focused on immunization, control of diarrhoeal diseases, acute respiratory infections (ARIs), and nutrition in low- and middle-income countries, with an associated decline in U5MR. However, the progress has slowed down since the 1990s. During the first five years of the twenty-first century, the decline in U5MR was 17 per cent, from 94 per 1000 live births in the year 2000 to 78 per 1000 live births in 2004 (analysis based on the WHO mortality database (World Health Organization), available on request). The result is that about 9.7 million children less than five years of age continue to die in a year (World Health Organization 2005b). This figure corresponds to more than twofold the number of all individuals dying in the same period from HIV infection or AIDS and tuberculosis combined.

When are under-five deaths occurring?

The risk of death is the highest closest to birth and then decreases over the subsequent days, months, and years. Almost 4 million of the 9.7 million under-five deaths occur in the first 28 days after birth, 3.3 million deaths occur in the following 11 months, and roughly the same number happen over the next four years (World Health Organization 2005b). Analysis of data from 39 demographic and health surveys (DHSs) shows that within the first month of life, about

Child Health

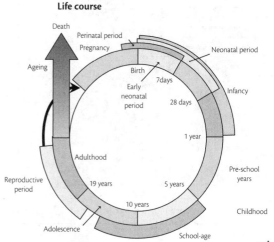

Life course

Age subgroups as defined by the World Health Organization	
Terminology	**Definition/Interval***
Under-five	*0–4 years*
Neonatal period	0–27 days
Early neonatal period	0–6 days
Post-neonatal period	28 days to 11 months
Infancy	0–11 months
Preschool	1–4 years
Older child	*5–9 years*
Adolescent	*10–19 years*

* *The upper limit of the interval refers to completed days, months, or years.*

World Health Organization

Fig. 11.3.1 The life course and respective age subgroups. *Source:* Adapted from World Health Organization. *Strategic directions for improving the health and development of children and adolescents.* Geneva: World Health Organization; 2002. WHO/FCH/CAH/02.21. Available from: http://www.who.int/child-adolescent-health/publications/OVERVIEW/CAH_Strategy.htm.

27 per cent of deaths occur on the day of birth, 45 per cent during days 0 and 1, and more than 70 per cent in the first week of life.

Where and why are under-five deaths occurring?

About three-quarters of all under-five deaths are clustered in just two regions of the world: Africa and Southeast Asia (Fig. 11.3.2). Although Africa has only about 20 per cent of the world's population, it accounts for 45 per cent of the global under-five deaths; in contrast, only 2 per cent of under-five deaths take place in the European region and 4 per cent in the region of the Americas. Similarly, most neonatal deaths occur in Africa and Southeast Asia, with about 30 per cent of all neonatal deaths in the African region and about 35 per cent in the Southeast Asian region. It is noteworthy that 90 per cent of the under-five deaths take place in just 40 countries, and even more striking is the fact that 50 per cent of all these deaths are concentrated in six countries: India, Nigeria, China, Democratic Republic of Congo (DRC), Ethiopia, and Pakistan.

Although the absolute number of deaths provides important information regarding the global magnitude of the problem, it does not take into account the size of the population at risk, and hence, it does not reflect the risk of death. For instance, although China is ranked third in the absolute number of under-five deaths, its under-five mortality rate is about 30 per 1000 live births, compared with several countries that have rates above 200 per 1000 (Afghanistan, Angola, Burkina Faso, DRC, Guinea-Bissau, Liberia, Mali, Niger, Sierra Leone, and Somalia).

Beyond inter-country inequities, further critical inequities are present within countries, where children from the poorest families living in rural areas and whose mothers are less educated are those more likely to die. Data from the DHSs, nationally representative household surveys with large sample sizes (usually between 5000 and 30000 households), have been used in Fig. 11.3.3 to illustrate these important equity differentials within countries.

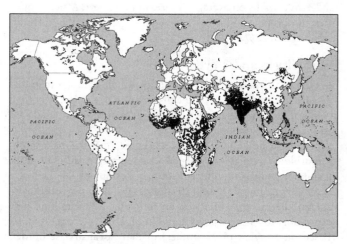

Percentage of under-five deaths by region
African region: 45%
Southeast Asian region: 28%
Eastern Mediterranean region: 14%
Western Pacific region: 7%
Region of the Americas: 4%
European region: 2%

Fig. 11.3.2 World distribution of under-five deaths—each dot represents 5000 deaths. (From Black RE, Morris SS, Bryce J. Where and why are 10 million children dying every year? *Lancet* 2003;**361**:2226–34. Reprinted with permission from Elsevier.)

Wealth quintiles

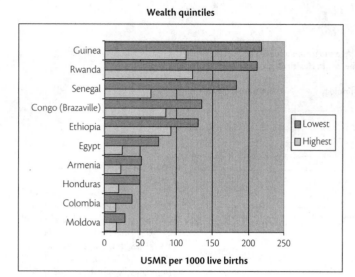

Level of mother's education

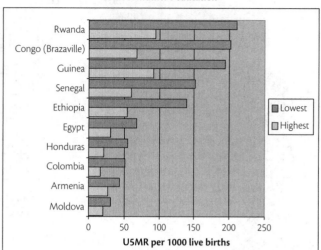

Fig. 11.3.3 Inequities in under-five mortality according to wealth and level of mother's education.
Source: Institut National de la Statistique du Rwanda (INSR), ORC Macro. *Rwanda demographic and health survey 2005*. Calverton (MD): Institut National de la Statistique du Rwanda, ORC Macro; 2006; Ndiaye S, Mohamed A. *Enquête Démographique et de Santé au Sénégal 2005*. Calverton (MD): Sénégal Centre de Recherche pour le Développement Humain, ORC Macro; 2006; National Institute of Public Health, National Institute of Statistics, ORC Macro. *Cambodia demographic and health survey 2005*. Phnom Penh, Cambodia, Calverton (MD): National Institute of Public Health, National Institute of Statistics, ORC Macro; 2006; National Institute of Population Research and Training (NIPORT), Mitra and Associates, ORC Macro. *Bangladesh demographic and health survey 2004*. Dhaka, Bangladesh: National Institute of Population Research and Training; 2005; Moroc Ministère de la Santé, ORC Macro, Ligue des États Arabes. *Enquête sur la population et la santé familiale (EPSF) 2003-4*. Calverton (MD): Ministère de la Santé, ORC Macro; 2005; Badan Pusat Statistik-Statistics Indonesia (BPS), ORC Macro. *Indonesia demographic and health survey 2002-3*. Calverton (MD): Badan Pusat Statistik-Statistics Indonesia (BPS), ORC Macro; 2003; El-Zanaty F, Way A. *Egypt demographic and health survey 2005*. Cairo, Egypt: Ministry of Health and Population, National Population Council, El-Zanaty and Associates, ORC Macro; 2006; National Statistics Office (NSO), ORC Macro. *National demographic and health survey 2003*. Calverton (MD): National Statistics Office (Philippines), ORC Macro; 2004; National Statistical Service, Ministry of Health, ORC Macro. *Armenia demographic and health survey 2005*. Calverton (MD): National Statistical Service, Armenian Ministry of Health, ORC Macro; 2006; Secretaría de Salud (SS), Instituto Nacional de Estadística (INE), Macro Internacional. *Encuesta nacional de salud y demografía 2005-6*. Tegucigalpa, Honduras, Calverton (MD): Secretaría de Salud, Instituto Nacional de Estadística, Macro International; 2006; National Scientific and Applied Center for Preventive Medicine (NCPM), ORC Macro. *Moldova demographic and health survey 2005*. Calverton (MD): National Scientific and Applied Center for Preventive Medicine, Moldova Ministry of Health and Social Protection, ORC Macro; 2006.

What are neonates and children dying from?

Poverty, low levels of maternal education, and poor quality health care are underlying determinants of most under-five deaths. However, most neonates and children eventually die from only a small number of disease conditions. Estimates of the distribution of direct causes of neonatal and under-five deaths are shown in Fig. 11.3.4. Most of these deaths are preventable by well-known and affordable interventions. Equally important is the fact that undernutrition directly or indirectly contributes to more than half of post-neonatal deaths in children under five years of age.

The relative importance of the different causes of under-five deaths varies across regions of the world, although the major causes remain the same. Deaths in the neonatal period represent about 45 per cent of child deaths in all regions, except in the African region where the lower proportion of 26 per cent reflects the high number of post-neonatal deaths.

The African region has, in general, the highest burden of global child mortality: 90 per cent of all under-five deaths attributable to malaria and to HIV and AIDS, 50 per cent of deaths from pneumonia, and 40 per cent of deaths from diarrhoea (World Health Organization 2005b). However, within the African region, the distribution of the burden of mortality attributable to HIV and to malaria differs substantially across countries. For example, in East African countries, HIV and AIDS contribute to 15 per cent of the under-five deaths on average, whereas in Southern African countries, this proportion increases to about 40 per cent (World Health Organization 2007).

Morbidity in under-five children

Because the measurement of morbidity is more complex than that of mortality, information on the distribution of morbidity burden among under-fives is scarce. Usual sources of morbidity data are national surveys or published studies.

Despite the limitations of data, it is known that the main causes of morbidity are highly correlated with the major causes of death in children under five. A recent study has estimated the incidence of clinical pneumonia to be 0.29 episodes per child per year in low- and middle-income countries, an estimated 150.7 million new pneumonia cases every year (Rudan *et al.* 2004). Recent estimates (based on a review of 27 studies) of diarrhoeal disease burden show a median of 3.2 episodes per child per year, with the highest incidence recorded in the African region (Kosek *et al.* 2003).

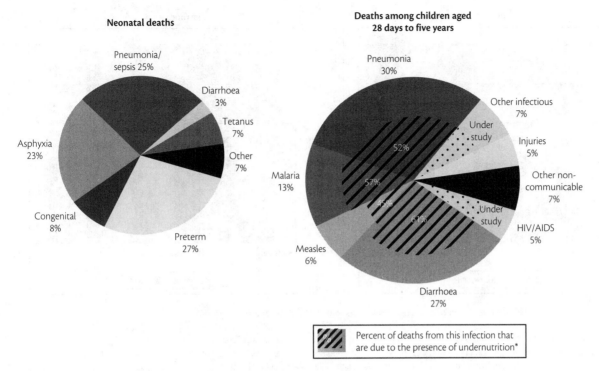

Fig. 11.3.4 Distribution of the main causes of death among neonates and children aged 28 days to 5 years in the year 2000.
Sources: World Health Organization (WHO 2005b), Caulfield *et al.* (2003).
* Recent estimates published by Black *et al.* (2008) indicate that nutrition-related factors are responsible for about 35% of all under-five deaths, but recent estimates of nutrition-related deaths by cause are not yet available.

An important consequence of persistently high rates of diarrhoea morbidity is a negative effect on child growth and development.

For both pneumonia and diarrhoeal diseases, morbidity rates are consistently higher in the first year of life, gradually decreasing from the second to the fifth year. The prevalence of pneumonia and diarrhoea can be more than twice as high among the poorest children as among the richest ones. Poor children are usually more exposed to health risks and less resistant to disease. Differences within and between countries are illustrated in Fig. 11.3.5.

Nutritional status of under-five children

Low weight at birth can be either the result of a birth that occurred too early (before 37 weeks of gestation) or of restricted growth during gestation. Low birth weight (LBW) is closely associated with increased risks of neonatal morbidity and mortality, cognitive problems, and chronic diseases during later periods in life. Every year, more than 20 million babies are born with LBW worldwide, the largest number of them in Africa and Southeast Asia (United Nations Children's Fund, World Health Organization 2004).

The nutritional status of under-five children is usually assessed through three standard indicators: Stunting, wasting, and underweight. A stunted child is a child who is too short for his or her age. Stunting is usually a result of chronic undernutrition or nutritional deprivation over a lengthy period of time. A child is considered wasted when the weight is too little for the child's height. Wasting usually reflects an acute nutritional deficiency, because of reduced food consumption or acute weight loss during an illness. Finally, a child is said to be underweight if his or her weight is too low for his or her age. This can be a result of stunting, wasting, or both.

It is estimated that 30 per cent of under-five children in the world are moderately or severely stunted, 9 per cent are moderately or severely wasted, and 25 per cent are underweight. In sub-Saharan Africa, these proportions are 37 per cent, 9 per cent, and 28 per cent, respectively (United Nations Children's Fund 2006). Poor nutritional status of a child is strongly correlated to his or her vulnerability to diseases, to delayed physical and mental development, and to an increased risk of mortality. As described for morbidity and mortality, underweight is usually associated with fewer years of mother's education and low levels in other indicators of well-being.

Development status of under-five children

The same biomedical risk factors, such as malnutrition and exposure to infectious diseases and to environmental contaminants, that threaten the survival of young children living in poverty in low- and middle-income countries also threaten their cognitive, motor, and socio-emotional development.

Currently, no global data on the status of early child development are available. Given the strong association of poor development with chronic growth retardation and poverty, to estimate the number of young children who are at risk for deficits in early development, country-level data on childhood chronic growth retardation (stunting, defined as length-for-age < −2SD) and living in absolute poverty (family income of less than US$1 per day) have been used to estimate the number of young who are at risk for deficits in early development (Grantham-McGregor *et al.* 2007). This estimate indicates that there are over 219 million, or 39 per cent of all children under five years of age, who are not fulfilling their developmental potential. Most of these children (89 million) live in South Asia. Ten countries (Bangladesh, China, DRC, Ethiopia,

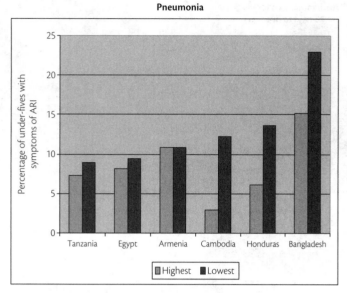

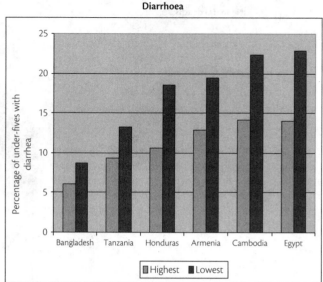

Fig. 11.3.5 Inequities in under-five morbidity due to pneumonia and diarrhoea (illness prevalence in the two weeks preceding the interview), according to wealth quintiles.

Source: National Bureau of Statistics, ORC Macro. *Tanzania demographic and health survey 2004-5.* Dar es Salaam, Tanzania: National Bureau of Statistics, ORC Macro; 2005; El-Zanaty F, Way A. *Egypt demographic and health survey 2005.* Cairo, Egypt: Ministry of Health and Population, National Population Council, El-Zanaty and Associates, ORC Macro; 2006; National Statistical Service, Ministry of Health, ORC Macro. *Armenia demographic and health survey 2005.* Calverton (MD): National Statistical Service, Armenian Ministry of Health, ORC Macro; 2006; National Institute of Public Health, National Institute of Statistics, ORC Macro. Cambodia demographic and health survey 2005. Phnom Penh, Cambodia, Calverton (MD): National Institute of Public Health, National Institute of Statistics, ORC Macro; 2006; Secretaría de Salud (SS), Instituto Nacional de Estadística (INE), Macro Internacional. *Encuesta nacional de salud y demografía 2005-6.* Tegucigalpa, Honduras, Calverton (MD): Secretaría de Salud, Instituto Nacional de Estadística, Macro International; 2006; National Institute of Population Research and Training (NIPORT), Mitra and Associates, ORC Macro. *Bangladesh demographic and health survey 2004.* Dhaka, Bangladesh: National Institute of Population Research and Training; 2005.

India, Indonesia, Nigeria, Pakistan, Tanzania, and Uganda) account for 145 million (66 per cent) of these 219 million disadvantaged children in the developing world (Grantham-McGregor *et al.* 2007).

Health status of the older child (children 5–9 years)

There is a considerably greater gap in knowledge of the epidemiology of health conditions and evidence for interventions for this age group as compared to under-five children. Although these children have survived the critical period of 0–59 months, when most deaths occur, many carry with them the consequences of a number of conditions suffered during their earlier years. Moreover, they are still exposed to additional health hazards during the 5–9 year period. Some of the main health problems related to this age group are as follows:

Poor growth and nutrition: Although the risk of acute clinical malnutrition is lower at this age, the accumulated consequences of poor diet and growth may significantly affect the school performance of these children.

Communicable diseases: Communicable diseases lead to considerable morbidity in this age group and, in some cases, to long-term disability. Major diseases that contribute to mortality and disability at this age are ARIs, diarrhoea, malaria, and tuberculosis, as well as nutritional deficiencies, particularly iron-deficiency anaemia.

Accidents, injuries, and violence: The older child has a higher risk of accidents, injuries, and violence than younger age groups. Children 5–9 years of age are primarily affected by poisoning, drowning, burns, and maltreatment by caregivers. Intentional injuries resulting from child maltreatment are associated with physical and cognitive deficits. Poor children, who commonly live in unsafe environments, are exposed to risks that increase their likelihood of being injured. Subgroups particularly at risk include those suffering abuse, exploitive labour, and also, street and orphaned children. Injury rates and patterns differ from country to country and from urban to rural areas. For example, in rural areas, injuries are related mainly to farming activities, pesticide poisoning, and drowning. In urban areas, most injuries in small children are traffic-related, linked to gadgets and electrical appliances, or to falls or poisonings resulting from the ingestion of household chemicals and pharmaceuticals.

Other conditions: Other main issues and conditions related to this age group are blood disorders, cardiac and respiratory diseases such as asthma and rheumatic cardiac disease, skin problems, and sensory and neurological diseases or impairment.

Child health in higher-income countries

The World Bank classifies countries into income group according to their growth national income (GNI) per capita. High-income countries (HIC) are those with a GNI per capita of US$10726 or more (World Bank 2007), and account for approximately 10 per cent of the world under-five population and to less than 1 per cent of under-five deaths. In general, children living in the 56 countries in this group have the lowest U5MR (average of 7 per 1000 live births) and benefit from better health and development than children elsewhere.

Upper-to-middle-income economies include 40 countries that have a GNI per capita between US$3466 and US$10725 (World Bank 2007). These countries have been experiencing a transition in child health epidemiology—transformation of the patterns of diseases and/or causes of death. These changes require prompt adjustments in national programmes and strategies to conform to the emerging new epidemiological profile.

Main challenges

The so-called 'epidemiological transition' has a complex and dynamic course and reflects the changes in various domains such as demographic, socioeconomic, cultural, biological, technological, and environmental factors. A major recent factor that has caused important changes in child health and survival patterns in high- and upper-middle-income economies was the emergence of HIV infection.

The beginning of HIV epidemics in Western European countries resulted in a threateningly large number of paediatric infections. Once interventions to prevent mother-to-child transmission became available, there was an impressive reduction in the transmission rates, which decreased from an initial level of 15–20 per cent to 2 per cent or less in more recent years. Nowadays, the HIV epidemics among infants in Western Europe can be considered mostly controlled, with only 149 reported cases of new infections among infants and young children in 2002 (World Health Organization 2004d).

However, Eastern Europe witnessed a dramatically growing rate of HIV infection over the same period. Following the collapse of the USSR, there was a large increase in injectable drug use and in the number of new HIV infections. Although there was an average decrease of more than 45 per cent in mother-to-child transmission in Western and Central European countries from 2002 to 2005, Eastern European countries faced an increase of 453 per cent during the same period. In the Russian Federation, for example, the number of infants born to HIV-positive mothers increased from 81 in 1998 to 2777 in 2002 (Euro HIV 2006).

Another example of the changing profile is illustrated by the increasing prevalence of overweight or obesity in high- and low-income countries. The number of children affected by these disorders continues to rise at an alarming rate. The current prevalence of childhood obesity is ten times higher than it was in the 1970s. In several countries of Western Europe, such as Greece, Malta, Spain, Sweden, and the United Kingdom, the prevalence of overweight children reached more than 15 per cent in 2002. Childhood obesity is associated with the premature burden of non-communicable diseases such as diabetes and cardiovascular disorder (World Health Organization 2005a).

The major challenge that wealthier nations face is the increasing socioeconomic inequities within their societies. Income inequalities are associated with poorer health and higher child mortality, regardless of the country's level of development. Gaps between and within countries have been widening in the last decade. Sometimes, differences between subgroups of the population within countries are so remarkable that these differences can constitute a contributory factor to social instability (United Nations Children's Fund 2005).

In a recent study, Collison et al. (2007) investigated the relationship between under-five mortality and income inequalities among the 24 countries that comprise the Organization for Economic Co-operation and Development (OECD). Most of these countries have achieved near-universal basic health care and education for children. Nevertheless, the investigators found a strongly significant association between the two variables examined. A recent review found an increase in the percentage of children living in relative poverty (households with income below 50 per cent of the national median income) in these same OECD countries in the last decade (United Nations Children's Fund 2005). According to this review, the proportion of children living below national poverty lines was lowest in the Scandinavian countries (2–4 per cent), ranged between 10 and 15 per cent in Australia, Austria, Canada, Greece, Germany, Japan, Netherlands, Spain, and the United Kingdom, and was as high as 22 per cent in the United States.

The impact of such inequities goes beyond child mortality and is likely to affect every stage of childhood development. For example, (1) overweight is more prevalent in children from lower income settings of industrialized countries than in those from higher income groups; (2) children from poor families are more likely to suffer injuries from road accidents or in the home than those from better-off families; (3) poor growth patterns are present in lower income groups in the United Kingdom; (4) poverty is closely associated with harmful environmental factors such as exposure to lead, poor housing, poor air quality, and undernutrition; and (5) there is strong evidence that poor diet, smoking, alcohol use, and lack of physical activity are all associated with lower socioeconomic conditions (World Health Organization 2004d).

Effective interventions for addressing major causes of child deaths

It is estimated that more than 60 per cent of under-five deaths can be prevented with universal coverage of a small set of known, effective interventions that do not require expensive technology (Jones et al. 2003). These interventions are reviewed in the following text for each of the major causes of under-five mortality and summarized in Table 11.3.1.

Newborn conditions

Improving newborn health and survival requires a continuum of care (World Health Organization 2005b) from pregnancy, childbirth, and the newborn period, into childhood and adolescence. Newborn health interventions can be classified into those relevant for all mothers and newborns, and those relevant only for newborns with conditions that require additional care.

Care for all mothers and newborns

The health and well-being of women and their children are closely associated with the education, nutrition, and health care they receive throughout the life cycle. Newborn health and survival requires empowerment (particularly of girls and women) and health promotion throughout life, which includes nutrition and education, prevention of harmful practices such as female genital mutilation, delay in sexual debut, prevention and treatment of sexually transmitted infections, and support for optimal timing and spacing of pregnancies.

Table 11.3.1 Summary of key interventions to address major causes of child deaths

Important causes of under-five mortality	Preventive interventions	Case management interventions
Newborn conditions	<ul><li>Antenatal care</li><li>Skilled care during labour and birth</li><li>Care at the time of birth (warmth, resuscitation, cord care, and early initiation of breastfeeding)</li><li>Care during the first days and weeks after birth (exclusive breastfeeding, warmth, hygienic skin and cord care, and prompt care-seeking for illness)</li></ul>	<ul><li>Additional care of LBW infants (particularly feeding and warmth)</li><li>Treatment of local eye, skin, and umbilical infections</li><li>Treatment of neonatal sepsis</li></ul>
Diarrhoea	<ul><li>Exclusive breastfeeding up to 6 months; continued breastfeeding with safe and appropriate complementary feeding at least up to 2 years</li><li>Immunization against measles, rotavirus (candidates being evaluated in efficacy trials), and shigella (under development)</li><li>Water and sanitation, hand washing</li></ul>	<ul><li>Oral rehydration therapy, including use of the new low-osmolarity ORS</li><li>Zinc for 10–14 days during diarrhoea</li><li>Antibiotics for dysentery and cholera</li><li>Continued feeding during diarrhoea</li></ul>
Pneumonia	<ul><li>Immunization against measles, diphtheria, tetanus, and pertussis, *Haemophilus influenzae*, and pneumococcus</li><li>Exclusive breastfeeding up to 6 months; continued breastfeeding with safe and appropriate complementary feeding at least up to 2 years</li><li>*Pneumocystis jiiroveci* pneumonia prophylaxis in HIV-exposed and HIV-infected infants</li><li>Reduction in environmental risk factors—e.g. indoor air pollution</li></ul>	<ul><li>Treatment of non-severe pneumonia with oral co-trimoxazole or amoxicillin</li><li>Treatment of severe pneumonia with parenteral antibiotics, and oxygen and other supportive treatment</li></ul>
Malaria	<ul><li>Vector control</li><li>Use of ITNs</li></ul>	<ul><li>Treatment of non-severe malaria with an oral antimalarial recommended for the area</li><li>Treatment of severe malaria.</li></ul>
HIV/AIDS	<ul><li>Primary prevention of HIV and of unintended pregnancies in HIV-infected women</li><li>Antiretrovirals—treatment of pregnant women when indicated, prophylaxis for others</li><li>Safer infant feeding options—exclusive breastfeeding for 6 months if replacement feeding is not acceptable, feasible, affordable, sustainable, and safe; otherwise replacement feeding</li></ul>	<ul><li>Co-trimoxazole prophylaxis for HIV-exposed and HIV-infected children</li><li>ART for children who are eligible for it</li></ul>
Malnutrition	<ul><li>Early initiation of breastfeeding</li><li>Exclusive breastfeeding up to 6 months of age</li><li>Continued breastfeeding with safe and appropriate complementary foods up to at least 2 years</li><li>Preventing vitamin A, iron, iodine, and zinc deficiency through supplementation, food fortification, or dietary diversification</li></ul>	<ul><li>Community-based management of children with severe malnutrition without complications</li><li>Hospital management of children with severe malnutrition with complications</li></ul>

Care during pregnancy is important for newborn survival. Antenatal care provides a platform to promote healthy lifestyles, including hygiene, nutrition, and family planning, and for integrating programmes that address malnutrition, HIV and AIDS, sexually transmitted infections, malaria, and tuberculosis. Interventions of proven benefit for newborn health provided during antenatal care include tetanus immunization, screening for and treatment of syphilis and HIV, and prevention and treatment of malaria. Antenatal care provides the basis for continued care during and after childbirth by planning for birth with a skilled attendant and preparing for unforeseen complications, and by helping the family prepare for good mother and newborn care practices, such as early initiation of and exclusive breastfeeding.

Box 11.3.1 Basic newborn care at the time of birth and in the days and weeks after birth

Care at the time of birth

- Birth in a warm room
- Resuscitation, if required
- Drying the baby thoroughly immediately after birth
- Keeping the baby in skin-to-skin contact with the mother
- Hygienic cord care
- Eye care
- Early initiation of breastfeeding as soon as the mother and the baby are ready (usually within the first hour of birth)

Care during the first days and weeks

- Initiation of breastfeeding, if not already initiated
- Exclusive breastfeeding
- Keeping the newborn warm
- Hygienic cord and eye care
- Vaccination
- Prompt recognition of danger signs (not feeding well, reduced activity, fast or difficult breathing, fever or low body temperature, or convulsions) and care seeking by the family

---

Skilled care at childbirth is needed for all women and babies without exception because the complications that may occur during and immediately following childbirth (for both mothers and babies) cannot be predicted and may very rapidly become fatal. This means that skilled childbirth care in first-level health facilities, with the backup of a hospital that can manage complications, should be available 24 hours a day, every day. For a home birth, it is crucial to have access to a skilled attendant and a companion who can stay with the mother and baby for the first 12–24 hours. For a woman and her family who cannot have access to a skilled attendant in a home birth, it is essential to ensure that they have knowledge of maternal and newborn danger signs (*see* Box 11.3.1), and a plan for a clean delivery and early care-seeking if problems arise.

Care for all newborns at the time of birth and during the days and weeks that follow includes several relatively simple and effective interventions that do not require advanced technology (Box 11.3.1). The most critical time to deliver these interventions is immediately after birth. Also important are the first 12–24 hours after birth, the period during which a large proportion of maternal and neonatal deaths occur (World Health Organization 2006c). Thereafter, at least one additional contact with a health provider within the first week, preferably on the second or third day of life, is required.

Management and care of newborn conditions

Additional care of LBW infants is critical for improving newborn survival because 60–80 per cent of neonatal deaths occur in these infants. Identification of LBW infants within the first hours after birth should be a part of the basic newborn-care package. In settings where birth weight measurement is not feasible, such as for home births, all newborns perceived to be 'small' should receive additional care.

In addition to basic newborn care, LBW infants need more attention for warmth, feeding, hygiene, early detection of infections, and growth monitoring. Kangaroo mother care or skin-to-skin care is the best way to keep them warm and to encourage breastfeeding. Mothers who cannot breastfeed directly should be taught to express breast milk and to feed from a cup. Much of this additional care can be provided at home and in first-level health facilities. However, care for babies weighing less than 1500 g, who may not be able to feed, or for a baby with any danger sign is best provided in a hospital. It is recommended that LBW infants have more contacts with health providers than envisaged for newborns who are not LBW. These may include one additional contact in the first week and weekly contacts thereafter until the infant is feeding and growing well.

Management of newborn illness in a prompt and appropriate manner can reduce neonatal mortality by about half. Community- and health-facility-based activities to support families in identifying the danger signs and seeking timely and appropriate care are therefore very important. The first step in the WHO Integrated Management of Childhood Illness (IMCI) for 0–2 month old infants is the assessment and classification for severe disease (World Health Organization 2006b). The next step is the assessment and treatment of eye, skin, and umbilical infections, diarrhoea, and feeding problems. The last step is giving advice on home care for sick newborns, including advice on feeding, keeping the young infant warm, and when to return. Newborns with severe disease (including those who have suffered from severe birth asphyxia, are very premature or have very LBW, or who have a severe infection), who require referral, should receive intravenous fluids or alternative feeding methods and other supportive therapy such as oxygen and parenteral antibiotics in a hospital.

Diarrhoea

Diarrhoea remains a leading cause of death in under-five children in low- and middle-income countries. Strategies for the control of diarrhoeal diseases have remained substantially unchanged since the initiation of the Diarrhoeal Diseases Control Programme in the early 1980s (Jamison *et al.* 2006).

Prevention

Exclusive breastfeeding, which means that no food or drink (not even water) other than breast milk (with the exception of vitamin and mineral supplements or necessary medicines), is recommended for the first six months of life. A review of studies shows that breast-fed children under six months of age are 6.1 times less likely to die of diarrhoea than non-breastfed infants (World Health Organization 2004b). Exclusive breastfeeding protects infants from diarrhoeal disease because breast milk contains both immune and non-immune antimicrobial factors, and because exclusive breastfeeding eliminates the intake of potentially contaminated food and water.

Sequential diarrhoeal disease leads to a vicious cycle of increasing nutritional deterioration, impaired immune function, and greater susceptibility to infection. The cycle may be broken by interventions to decrease infection or by improving nutritional status. Safe and appropriate complementary foods introduced at six months of age and continued breastfeeding for at least up to two years can improve nutritional status of infants and young children.

Almost all infants acquire rotavirus diarrhoea early in life. Rotavirus accounts for at least one-third of severe and potentially fatal watery diarrhoea episodes, primarily in low- and middle-income countries, where an estimated 440 000 vaccine-preventable rotavirus deaths per year occur. Two licensed rotavirus vaccines, derived from human or bovine rotavirus, are being marketed in a few countries (85 per cent protective efficacy against severe diarrhoea), and other candidate vaccines are undergoing field trials in low- and middle-income countries.

For cholera, the two oral vaccines licensed offer reasonable protection, but for only a limited period of time (60–65 per cent protective efficacy for about six months). There are no licensed vaccines against shigella. Although scientific interest in a cholera vaccine remains high, its public health priority is less than a vaccine for rotavirus or shigella. Measles is known to predispose to diarrhoeal disease secondary to measles-induced immunodeficiency; thus, measles vaccine also protects against post-measles diarrhoea.

Human faeces are the primary source of diarrhoeal pathogens. Poor sanitation, lack of accessible clean water, and inadequate personal and domestic hygiene are responsible for an estimated 90 per cent of childhood diarrhoeal cases. Hand-washing promotion reduces incidence of diarrhoea by an average of 33 per cent, and is best when part of a package of behaviour-change interventions. However, the required behaviour change is complex and significant resources are needed, the most important of which is access to water.

Case management

Most deaths from diarrhoea occur because of dehydration associated with acute diarrhoea, and because of dysentery (bloody diarrhoea). Management of diarrhoea includes:

- Treating dehydration with oral rehydration salts (ORS) solution, or with an intravenous electrolyte solution in cases of severe dehydration

- Continuing or increasing breastfeeding during and increasing feeding after the diarrhoeal episode

- Providing children with 20 mg per day of zinc for 10–14 days

- Using antibiotics only when appropriate (i.e. bloody diarrhoea) and not administering antidiarrhoeal drugs

- Advising mothers of the need to increase fluids and continue feeding during future episodes

Two recent advances are noteworthy in managing acute diarrhoea: Newly formulated ORS containing lower concentrations of glucose and salts, and zinc supplementation.

The ORS formulation recommended by UNICEF and WHO has proved safe and effective in the prevention and treatment of dehydration. However, mothers' and health workers' acceptance of standard ORS has been suboptimal because watery stools persist and the duration of diarrhoea is not reduced. Efforts over the past 20 years have led to the development of a new ORS formulation. Compared with standard ORS, this lower sodium and glucose ORS reduces stool output, vomiting, and the need for intravenous fluids (Hanh *et al.* 2001). The new ORS is safe and effective in both non-cholera diarrhoea and cholera in children and adults. WHO and UNICEF now recommend the use of ORS containing 75 meq of sodium and 75 mmol of glucose per litre (total osmolarity of 245 milliosmols per litre) everywhere (World Health Organization and United Nations Children's Fund 2004).

A review of all relevant clinical trials indicates that zinc supplements given during an episode of acute diarrhoea reduces both the duration and severity, and could prevent 300 000 deaths in children each year (Fontaine 2001). WHO and UNICEF now jointly recommend that all children with acute diarrhoea be given zinc in some form for 10–14 days during and after diarrhoea (10 mg per day for infants younger than six months of age and 20 mg per day for those over six months). Pilot studies in several countries show that including zinc routinely in the management of acute diarrhoea has two programmatically important effects: (1) use-rates of ORS increase and (2) use of antidiarrhoeals and antimicrobials decreases significantly.

The primary treatment for shigellosis—the most common and severe cause of bloody diarrhoea—is the use of antimicrobials. The choice of effective, safe, oral, and inexpensive drugs for use in low- and middle-income countries has, however, become problematic because of the increasing prevalence of antimicrobial drug resistance to several commonly used antibiotics. Because of its effectiveness, safety, ease of administration by the oral route, short course, and low cost (US$0.10 for a 3-day course for a 15-kg child), ciprofloxacin is the current drug of choice for shigellosis; however, ciprofloxacin-resistant strains are already appearing. Increasing antimicrobial resistance has made development of a vaccine for shigella a high priority.

ARIs

ARIs, particularly pneumonia, are a major cause of under-five child mortality in low- and middle-income countries. Interventions to control ARIs can be divided into preventive interventions such as immunization against specific pathogens, improvements in nutrition, and safer environments, and case management interventions (Jamison *et al.* 2006).

Prevention

Widespread use of vaccines against measles, diphtheria, pertussis, *Haemophilus influenzae* (Hib), pneumococcus, and influenza has the potential to substantially reduce the incidence of ARIs in children in low- and middle-income countries. Two particularly important vaccines are those against Hib and pneumococcus, pathogens responsible for about half of all cases of pneumonia.

The use of Hib conjugate vaccines in developed countries has resulted in the virtual elimination of invasive Hib disease (meningitis and bacteraemic pneumonia) because of immunity in vaccinated children and a herd effect in those not vaccinated. Studies in Bangladesh, Brazil, Chile, and the Gambia have shown that Hib vaccine reduced the incidence of radiological pneumonia by 20–30 per cent, but the results of a large study in Indonesia were inconclusive with regard to the effect of this vaccine on pneumonia. Several Hib conjugate vaccines are available; all are effective when given in early infancy and have virtually no side effects except occasional temporary redness or swelling at the injection site. To reduce the number of injections, Hib vaccine is sometimes given in combination with other vaccines, such as DTP and hepatitis B. Two to three doses are recommended depending on the manufacturer. The three-dose schedule is delivered at 6, 10, and 14 weeks of age.

Two types of pneumococcal vaccines are currently licensed for use: A polysaccharide vaccine effective against 23 different strains of pneumococcus and protein-conjugated vaccines effective against 7 strains. The polysaccharide vaccine is not recommended for use in children aged less than two years. A randomized controlled trial in the Gambia found a protein-conjugated vaccine with 9 strains to have a 77 per cent efficacy against vaccine-type pneumococcal invasive disease, 35 per cent reduction in radiologically confirmed pneumonia, and 16 per cent reduction in all-cause mortality. A similar study in South Africa showed that this vaccine was efficacious against vaccine-type invasive pneumococcal disease in both HIV-negative and HIV-positive children. One of the problems with the currently licensed protein-conjugated vaccine is that the serotypes included cover only 65–80 per cent of serotypes associated with pneumococcal disease among young children in Western industrialized countries, and this proportion may be lower in many low- and middle-income countries. Other pneumococcal conjugate vaccines with wider serotype coverage are in late stages of development.

Interventions that reduce the prevalence of LBW, malnutrition, and non-breastfeeding can reduce the incidence of pneumonia. Exclusive breastfeeding in the first six months of life and continued breastfeeding with complementary feeding up to at least two years of age reduce the incidence and severity of ARIs (Victora et al. 1999).

In a recently completed trial in Guatemala, environmental interventions to reduce exposure to indoor air pollution have been shown to reduce the incidence of severe respiratory infections in children. Therefore, wide use of interventions such as non-smoke stoves has the potential to substantially reduce pneumonia disease burden.

Case management

The simplification and standardization of ARI case management have enabled first-level health workers to provide effective treatment to millions of children in low- and middle-income countries. WHO clinical guidelines for ARI case management, which are part of IMCI, rely on two simple clinical signs: Fast breathing to identify children with ARI who need antibiotic therapy and lower chest wall in-drawing to identify children with severe pneumonia (World Health Organization 2006b). The latter sign requires referral and treatment in a hospital with parenteral antibiotics. Additionally, presence of audible stridor when calm and any of the general danger signs such as lethargy or unconsciousness, inability to feed and drink, or convulsions are also indications for referral to a hospital.

Fast breathing, defined by WHO as a respiratory rate of 60 or more for infants younger than 2 months, 50 or more for infants of 2–11 months, and 40 or more for children 1–4 years of age, detects about 85 per cent of pneumonia patients. The specificity of fast breathing is 70–80 per cent, which means that 20–30 per cent of children with ARI who do not need antibiotics will receive them. However, the use of this sign makes decision making by first-level health workers simple and, therefore, has increased the proportion of children with pneumonia who receive antibiotics. Children with fast breathing should be given an oral antibiotic (e.g. co-trimoxazole or amoxicillin) twice daily. It has been shown that oral antibiotic therapy for three days is as effective as that for five days (Qazi 2005).

Chest in-drawing is the inward movement of the lower chest wall when a child breathes in. WHO currently recommends that children with chest wall in-drawing should be referred to a hospital and treated with parenteral antibiotics. WHO also recommends the use of oxygen for children who are unable to feed or drink, or have cyanosis, respiratory rate of 70 or more, or severe chest wall in-drawing. Recent evidence shows that children with chest wall in-drawing who do not have any of the danger signs can be successfully treated with oral amoxicillin (Addo-Yobo et al. 2004). The safety and effectiveness of this approach is now being further evaluated. If confirmed, this could result in a substantially lower number of hospitalizations.

In HIV-positive children, who should be on oral co-trimoxazole prophylaxis, oral amoxicillin is recommended as the first-line treatment of non-severe pneumonia. Children older than 2 months who have severe pneumonia should receive therapy for *Pneumocystis jiroveci* in addition to the standard injectable antibiotics.

Malaria

Malaria kills more than a million people annually, 90 per cent of them in sub-Saharan Africa and the majority of whom are children under five. Chapter 9.15 on malaria describes malaria interventions in greater detail (Morrow & Moss 2008).

Prevention

Vector control remains the most generally effective measure to prevent malaria transmission in all ages. Insecticide-treated nets (ITNs) are a form of effective vector control and have been shown to be particularly effective in reducing mortality in young children (Lengeler 2004).

Case management

The two diagnostic approaches currently used are based on clinical diagnosis and detection of the causative parasite or its products. The IMCI strategy has practical algorithms for management of the sick child presenting with fever where there are no facilities for laboratory diagnosis. The additional use of parasitological diagnosis, either by light microscopy or by rapid diagnostic tests (RDTs), is becoming particularly important with the introduction of the more expensive artemisinin-based combinations in national malaria and IMCI treatment guidelines of many countries.

Once diagnosed as malaria, either on a clinical or parasitological basis, the child should be treated early with a safe and effective antimalarial medicine because a delay in treatment could result in progression to severe disease, which is associated with a high case-fatality rate. Malaria case management has been greatly affected by the emergence and spread of chloroquine and sulfadoxine-pyrimethamine (SP) resistance, which have been replaced by artemisinin-based combinations in many countries (World Health Organization 2006a). In areas with poor access to health facilities, early recognition and prompt and appropriate treatment of malaria in children requires treatment in the home or community.

HIV and AIDS

Currently, an estimated 2.3 million children under the age of 15 are living with HIV, and every day more than 1400 are newly infected. Without interventions, over half of the infected children die before their second birthday. Chapter 9.13 on HIV and AIDS describes HIV and AIDS interventions in greater detail (Karim et al. 2008).

Prevention

Over 90 per cent of HIV-infected children are infected through mother-to-child transmission (MTCT), which occurs during pregnancy, during birth, or through breastfeeding. Without any interventions, the risk of transmission is between 20 and 45 per cent, but this can be reduced to less than 2 per cent with a package of evidence-based interventions (World Health Organization 2004c).

Antiretroviral therapy (ART) for all pregnant women who are eligible for treatment is the most effective method of preventing MTCT. Pregnant women with HIV who do not yet require ART should be offered prophylactic regimens (World Health Organization 2004a).

The most effective way of eliminating the risk of HIV transmission through breastfeeding is by avoiding it altogether. However, exclusive breastfeeding for the first six months of life is the most effective preventive measure available for reducing child mortality in low- and middle-income countries. UN agencies have developed recommendations that recognize this dilemma and help in balancing the risks, considering the HIV-infected mother's individual circumstances and health services, counselling, and support available to her (World Health Organization 2006d):

◆ Exclusive breastfeeding is recommended for HIV-infected women for the first six months of life unless replacement feeding is acceptable, feasible, affordable, sustainable, and safe for them and their infants before that time; it has been shown that exclusive breastfeeding carries a lower risk of HIV transmission than mixed feeding (i.e. breastfeeding while also giving other fluids or foods).

◆ When replacement feeding is acceptable, feasible, affordable, sustainable, and safe, avoidance of all breastfeeding by HIV-infected women is recommended.

◆ Breastfeeding mothers of infants and young children who are known to be HIV-infected should be strongly encouraged to continue breastfeeding.

Management and care of HIV-exposed and HIV-infected children

All children born to HIV-infected mothers are considered to be HIV-exposed, whereas those in whom HIV has been transmitted from the mother are HIV-infected. Diagnosis of HIV-infection in children is based on demonstrating the presence of HIV (PCR-virological test) at age less than 18 months and on the presence of antibodies to HIV (ELISA) beyond this age. This is because maternal antibodies to HIV can pass through the placenta and will be present in HIV-exposed children until the age of 18 months.

HIV-exposed or HIV-infected children may acquire a serious life-threatening form of pneumonia caused by an organism called *Pneumocystis jirovecii* (previously *carinii*), which often occurs before their HIV status has been confirmed. Regular prophylaxis with trimethoprim-sulfamethoxazole (co-trimoxazole) provides a simple, inexpensive, and effective strategy to prevent this illness, and has been shown to reduce mortality of HIV-infected children by up to 40 per cent even in the absence of ART (Chintu *et al.* 2004).

HIV-exposed and HIV-infected children should receive all vaccines as early in life as possible, except BCG and yellow fever vaccines. In asymptomatic children, the decision to give late BCG should be based on the local risk of tuberculosis. Infants with symptomatic HIV infection should not receive yellow fever vaccines.

ART, which means antiretroviral drugs given in the correct way and with adherence, can substantially improve survival of HIV-infected children.

Malnutrition

Malnutrition contributes to more than half of all under-five deaths globally. Malnourished children, particularly those who are severely malnourished, have substantially higher risks of death from common childhood illness such as diarrhoea, pneumonia, and malaria.

Prevention

Interventions to prevent malnutrition include promotion of optimal feeding of infants and young children, prevention and treatment of illness, and amelioration of micronutrient deficiencies in the diet.

Early initiation of breastfeeding, ideally within the first hour after birth, has been shown to be associated with a reduced risk of neonatal mortality (Edmond *et al.* 2006). Exclusive breastfeeding during the first six months of life is associated with about a tenfold lower risk of death due to any cause than not breastfeeding at all, and a two- to threefold lower risk of death than partial breastfeeding (Bahl *et al.* 2003). Continued breastfeeding into the second year of life has also been shown to reduce the risk of child mortality and malnutrition (World Health Organization Collaborative Study team 2001). WHO, therefore, recommends early initiation of breastfeeding, exclusive breastfeeding up to six months of age, and continued breastfeeding along with complementary foods up to at least two years of age. Multiple approaches exist to promote breastfeeding through health facility and community programmes, including health education, professional support, lay support, and mass media campaigns.

Safe and appropriate complementary feeding started at six months of age can reduce the prevalence of malnutrition and contribute to reduced mortality. Promotion of safe and appropriate complementary feeding has been shown to improve weight-for-age and height-for-age gains by 0.24–0.87 SD in pilot studies (World Health Organization 1998). Effects of this magnitude if reproduced on a large scale could translate into tangible reductions in rates of malnutrition and the mortality attributable to it.

Prevention and prompt case management of common childhood illness, as discussed in the earlier subsections, can reduce the nutritional adverse effects of illness and, thereby, help break the vicious cycle of malnutrition–infections–malnutrition.

Common micronutrient deficiencies such as that of vitamin A, iron, iodine, and zinc, both at clinical and subclinical levels, contribute to illness and mortality in children. Approaches to prevent these deficiencies include supplementation, food fortification, and dietary diversification.

Case management of severe malnutrition

Children with severe malnutrition are usually identified by the weight-for-height criterion (< 70 per cent or < −3 SD of WHO reference median) and/or the presence of bilateral oedema. An additional independent criterion that can be used is mid-upper arm circumference (MUAC) of < 110 mm in children 6–59 months of age. For infants < 6 months of age, 'visible severe wasting' can be used to identify severe malnutrition in addition to the weight-for-height criteria (Prudhon *et al.* 2006).

Severely malnourished children without any complications can be managed in the community, whereas those with complications should be admitted to a hospital for treatment. These complications include anorexia, severe oedema, or both severe wasting and mild or moderate oedema.

In communities with limited access to proper local diets for nutritional rehabilitation, ready-to-use therapeutic foods (RUTFs) have been shown to be highly effective in the treatment of severe malnutrition in children 6–59 months of age without complications

(Collins *et al.* 2006). When families have access to nutrient-rich foods, children with severe malnutrition without complications can be managed in the community (without RUTFs) by carefully designed diets using low-cost family foods, provided appropriate minerals and vitamins are given. Children under six months, however, should not receive RUTFs or any solid family foods. They need milk-based diets and should be managed in a hospital, where their mothers can obtain support to re-establish breastfeeding.

Children with severe malnutrition who have complications should be admitted in a hospital. They need careful evaluation and treatment of infections, electrolyte imbalance, hypoglycaemia, and hypothermia. They should be fed carefully during the acute phase and should be given micronutrient supplements but no iron during the acute or stabilization phase. Subsequent rehabilitation, when appetite has returned and there is no severe oedema, can be done at home using RUTFs or nutrient-dense family foods, along with micronutrient supplements (World Health Organization 1999).

Integrated delivery of interventions

Despite the fact that effective interventions exist against all major conditions from which children die, the coverage of these interventions remains low in general. The key to achievement of substantial mortality reduction in children is universal coverage of the interventions described in the previous subsection.

Before the mid-90s, child health programmes in low- and middle-income countries focused on immunization, control of diarrhoeal diseases, ARIs, and nutrition. Their implementation led to reduction in under-five mortality in many countries, but this approach also encountered limitations. The narrow focus on single interventions has failed to consider the child in a holistic manner, leading to many missed opportunities for care in contacts with a health practitioner. Also, it was difficult to resolve upstream health-system constraints such as management or human resource policies by using this approach.

Solving these problems involves ensuring access to an integrated package of interventions that are organized around a 'continuum of care' from pregnancy, birth, neonatal period, infancy, childhood, and adolescence into adulthood. It also means that care should span across the home, community, health centre, and hospital. Trying to do so has profound consequences for the way programmes are organized. It requires realigning the scope of programme activities, specifying the packages, establishing benchmarks, and integrating delivery strategies. It also means adapting programme management procedures to reflect integration and to embed them within health-system development processes.

Packaging interventions for health-system delivery

The advantages of delivering interventions as packages include the following:

1. Many interventions go naturally together because they are delivered by the same person at the same time; for example, keeping the baby warm immediately after birth and initiation of breastfeeding within one hour.

2. Packaging is more cost-effective in terms of training, implementation, and supervision; for example, it is more efficient to run a course for IMCI than four separate courses on management of diarrhoea, pneumonia, malaria, and infant and young child feeding.

3. Packaging meets the needs of the individual caregiver and the child much better than isolated and uncoordinated single-intervention delivery, thus reinforcing the continuum of care.

Individual interventions should, therefore, be packaged and, if new interventions become available, they should be integrated within the existing packages and current strategies for their delivery. The delivery levels at which the programmes will focus for each of the packages should be decided, with the aim of achieving high and equitable coverage. The following is a suggested list of packages, which could be adapted to the country situation:

1. Care before pregnancy—reproductive health package, including family planning

2. Care during pregnancy—antenatal care package, including birth preparedness, syphilis screening, intermittent preventive treatment for malaria during pregnancy, HIV and AIDS counselling, nutrition counselling, and micronutrient supplementation

3. Care during labour, birth, and immediate 1–2 hours after birth—skilled birth attendant, basic and comprehensive emergency obstetric and neonatal care package (Basic and Comprehensive EmONC)

4. Care during postnatal period—postnatal or neonatal care package, including warmth, early initiation of exclusive breastfeeding, hygienic eye and cord care, and early recognition of and timely care seeking for signs of illness

5. Management of childhood illness—integrated management of newborn and childhood illnesses, based on assessment and classification of signs that are highly sensitive and specific, and that can be completed by a health practitioner with minimal equipment

6. Community-based promotion of optimal newborn and child care practices which have an impact on survival and health of infant and young children

Potential obstacles to packaging of interventions should also be considered. This may include those related to policy, programmes, and the organizational structure of ministries and health services. For example, managers responsible for single issue-focused programmes such as EPI, malaria, or HIV may feel that packaging their interventions with other maternal and child health services might make their delivery less efficient. Another concern about packaging interventions is that vulnerable groups may not get any of the interventions if enough attention is not given to equitable delivery of the package.

To overcome the gaps in access to care, which is a barrier to improved health in many countries with a high burden of newborn and child mortality, governments increasingly invest in strengthening provision and quality of care that can be provided by community health workers. For example, in Pakistan, a cadre of lady health workers now acts as the first line of contact in many villages. In India, the government is complementing the role of the village-based *anganwadi* worker with that of an *ayah*, both of whom are responsible for delivering health promotion, nutrition counselling, and basic medical care for the mother and child. The Government of Ethiopia has recently adapted a new policy that will put in place over 30 000 health extension workers. Where such effectors are undertaken, it remains critical to invest in strengthening other levels of care simultaneously in order to ensure functional referral pathways and care, as well as adequate supervision and other health-system supports.

Integrated management of childhood illness as a key strategy for improving child survival

IMCI was developed as an integrated primary health-care approach to child health based on the principles of primary health care as set out in the Alma Ata Declaration. This approach includes strengthening health workers' skills at the first level of the health system for appropriate treatment of common diseases, promotion of proper nutrition, and reduction of missed opportunities for immunization. Further, it includes strengthening the provision of essential drugs and supplies, supervision, and referral links. Finally, the promotion of key family and community practices contributes to the remaining components of PHC as related to children.

The IMCI approach to managing common childhood diseases is practical and scientifically sound. It focuses on the child as a whole, including his or her nutrition and immunization status, and not just a particular disease. IMCI addresses the major global causes of mortality and morbidity (malnutrition, newborn conditions, pneumonia, diarrhoea, malaria, measles, and HIV) (Bryce *et al.* 2005). It can be adapted to include or exclude conditions based on the national- and subnational-level epidemiological data. The key family and community practices to promote are also based on scientific evidence.

Where it has been implemented well, IMCI has been shown to improve health-worker performance (Gouws *et al.* 2004), drug availability, rational use of drugs, organization of work at health facilities, use of referral notes, and maintenance of records at district level, and to increase health facility utilization (Arifeen *et al.* 2004).

Strengthening of child health services

It will not be possible to scale-up child health interventions effectively without dealing with the challenges that affect health systems in many low-income countries. In order to translate knowledge of effective interventions into practical action, programme management is a key function at all levels of the health system (e.g. national, subnational, district, and community levels). Many countries have established a national programme that is responsible for child health, bringing together diarrhoea and ARI control programmes, in addition to a national immunization programme. However, considering the range of interventions that impact on the health of children, the inputs of other programmes are also required to ensure that a complete package is delivered with the desired level of coverage. In this context, programme management involves specific tasks of:

◆ Strategic planning—required periodically (every five years or so) to identify or reformulate the main strategic directions to improve child health, which is based on priority needs and resource availability, and with a view to building a continuum of care. This should promote harmonization of inputs across various programme areas (such as IMCI, nutrition, EPI, malaria, HIV and AIDS, maternal and newborn health) and among partners.

◆ Operational planning—required more frequently (often annually) to identify the concrete activities that will be implemented based on the strategic plan. Operational planning can involve activities in the areas of policies, guidelines, training, supervision, provision of drugs and supplies, health management information, monitoring, and evaluation.

◆ Implementation—the application of the operational plan in conducting activities. It requires programme managers to have skills of organization, facilitation, negotiation, and supportive supervision, among others.

Programme management for child health will also need to consider the broader context of health-systems development. In many countries, health-sector reforms that will affect the way child health programmes are planned and implemented are in progress. If covered by the definition of an essential health package, it is important that child health interventions are well reflected therein. Sector-wide approaches promote pooling of finances to address wider health-sector needs and are often accompanied by decentralization. It may not always be easy to harmonize the specific interests of child health programmes and the needs of the health sector as a whole; hence the need for programme managers who have a good understanding of health policy and planning. In this regard, human resources and health financing are two areas that are of specific relevance for scaling-up the implementation of interventions in order to achieve high population coverage (World Health Organization 2005b).

Economic hardship and financial crises have eroded the health sector in many countries over the past two decades. Many national health systems are in disarray, with a deteriorating infrastructure and a public health sector subject to the resource restrictions consequent to structural adjustment and macroeconomic ceilings. As a result, human resources working in the health sector have been destabilized and undermined. Low density of health workers, poor motivation, and drainage of the most qualified staff to urban centres and abroad have left rural population and even the urban population in some low-income countries deprived of the much needed human resources to provide adequate health care.

It is estimated that there is a global shortage of more than 4 million health professionals worldwide (World Health Organization 2006e). A global assessment of the shortfall has suggested that, on average, countries with fewer than 2.5 health workers per 1000 population failed to achieve 80 per cent coverage rates for deliveries by skilled attendants or for measles immunization. For child health services specifically as well to increase access among deprived populations, the deployment of an equivalent of 100 000 full-time multipurpose professionals backed up by many more community health workers is required. Governments in various countries are responding to this challenge by instituting a new cadre of community health workers or upgrading the skills of existing community resource persons, to deliver an essential package of health services that include child health interventions.

Ensuring universal access to child health services, however, is not merely a question of increasing the supply of services. Financial barriers to access have to be reduced or eliminated as well. In many countries, households spend considerable amounts on health care and out-of-pocket expenditures for health services can be between two and three times greater than the total health expenditure by governments and donors. User fees refer to the payment of out-of-pocket charges at the time of use of health care and constitute the largest share of out-of-pocket payments.

The higher the proportion of user payments in the total mix of financing for health, the greater is the relative share of the financing burden falling on poor people. The poorest population groups often forgo the care they need because it is unaffordable. When people do use available services, the costs incurred can force them to miss out on other necessities such as food, clothing, or children's education. Household expenditure surveys suggest that more than 150 million individuals globally face severe financial hardship each year because of health-care costs. Rather than relying on user fees and out-of-pocket payments, systems of prepayment can be used to promote fair access to health services.

Prepayment systems involve advance collection of funds through tax-based insurance or social health insurance schemes. Both provide financial risk protection and promote equity through prepayment of health-care costs and pooling of health risks. WHO recommends that out-of-pocket expenditures should be gradually converted into prepayment schemes, including community finance programmes. Unfortunately, to move from a situation of limited supply of health services, high out-of-pocket expenditures, and exclusion of the poor to a situation of universal access and financial protection can take many years.

Monitoring child health programmes

The phrase 'what gets measured gets done' summarizes the importance of monitoring and evaluation in programme planning and implementation.

Health status indicators

Health status of children is usually measured in terms of mortality, morbidity or disability, growth, and development. Changes in health status are influenced by social, economic, behavioural, and environmental determinants of health, as well as by the health system. Some examples of frequently used health status indicators relevant for child health programmes are:

- Under-five mortality rate
- Neonatal mortality rate
- Proportion of infants infected by HIV
- Proportion of wasted, stunted, or underweight children

The following methods are used to collect data on health status indicators:

- Large, nationally representative household surveys—large sample-size surveys are used to calculate health status indicators such as under-five, infant, and neonatal mortality rates.
- Vital registration—it is the best source of information related to the number and causes of death. However, many low- and middle-income countries have low coverage of vital registration.
- Qualitative research studies—research that uses focus groups, in-depth interviews, participatory approaches, and observations is conducted to get information on local beliefs, attitudes, terms, and cultural practices.
- Quantitative studies—these research studies are used to evaluate the effectiveness of different intervention delivery approaches.

Outcome indicators

Outcomes are the changes in the coverage of selected effective interventions produced as a result of programme activities. Improved coverage is expected to contribute to improved health status. Changes in outcome measures usually cannot occur unless programme outputs have changed. Some examples of outcome indicators used in child health programmes are:

- Proportion of children with diarrhoea who received oral rehydration treatment
- Proportion of children with pneumonia treated with antibiotics
- Proportion of HIV-exposed infants on co-trimoxazole prophylaxis
- Proportion of newborns who receive at least one postnatal care visit within 2 days of birth
- Proportion of infants less than 6 months who are exclusively breastfed
- Proportion of HIV-exposed infants less than 6 months who receive either replacement feeding or exclusive breastfeeding

Methods that can be used to collect data on outcome indicators are as follows:

- Large, nationally representative household surveys—commonly conducted large household surveys include the DHS and the UNICEF Multi Intercountry Cluster Survey (MICS).
- Small-sample household surveys, such as 30 cluster household surveys.

Reports from health facilities—routine reports from health facilities are sometimes used to estimate coverage of an intervention.

Inputs and output indicators

Inputs are the financial, material, and human resources that must be mobilized and made available to carry out programme activities. These include supportive laws and policies, human resources to carry out planned activities, health financing that supports universal access to health care, and efficient organization of services.

Some examples of input indicators are as follows:

- Countries or districts have a strategy and costed implementation plan for improving newborn and child survival.
- Countries or districts are implementing IMCI.
- Countries have adopted a policy promoting the new WHO/UNICEF recommendations on the management of diarrhoea.
- Countries have adopted a policy of community management of pneumonia for areas with low access to facilities.
- Countries have adopted a national policy on IYCF, including national targets.

Outputs are immediate results that are produced by a combination of making inputs available and conducting the planned activities. For example, the proportion of training courses or supervisory visits that have been completed as planned and according to an acceptable level of quality, and the proportion of trainees who had been trained and who are competent at the end of training. Some other examples of output indicators are:

- Proportion of first-level health facilities with at least 60 per cent of health workers who care for children trained in IMCI
- Proportion of first-level health facilities that have all the essential drugs for IMCI available
- Proportion of mothers who received early and exclusive breast-feeding advice during pregnancy or the first day of the infant's life

Methods which can be used to collect data on input and output indicators are listed as follows:

- Small-sample household surveys (output indicators)—these provide the best data related to knowledge and practices of caretakers for the prevention and treatment of illness in children and newborns.

◆ Health facility or provider surveys (output indicators)—these provide the best data on case-management practices and on the availability of facility supports.

◆ Reports from health facilities (output indicators)—almost all health facilities prepare and send routine reports to higher levels, usually the district health managers, providing information on patient treatment and availability of supplies.

◆ Supervisory visits (input and output indicators)—during supervisory visits, one can frequently also obtain information on human resources, and on material and drug supplies.

◆ Health facility auditing (input and output indicators)—the process of auditing allows comparison of the provision of a selected intervention or service with the standard set by the country.

◆ National or district programme records (input indicators)—details of availability of health workers, training activities, purchase of drugs and supplies and their distribution, and monitoring visits are usually available with programme managers.

International goals to accelerate progress in child survival

At the United Nations Millennium Summit in September 2000, 189 national leaders endorsed 'The Millennium Declaration' with an aim to promote the achievement of poverty elimination, which includes the development of education, promotion of and respect for human rights and equality, and improvement of the environment. As a roadmap to accomplish these aims, a commitment to attain eight specific goals by 2015 was made. Although all the Millennium Development Goals (MDGs) are relevant to child health, MDGs 1, 4, 5, and 6 are directly related to child survival (*see* Box 11.3.2). The fourth MDG has the explicit target of 'reducing by two-thirds, between 1990 and 2015, the under-five mortality rate'.

The global target (based on an U5MR of 94 per 1000 live births in 1990) is, therefore, to reach a mortality rate of 31 per 1000 live births by 2015. However, if recent trends (2000–2005) continue unchanged, the global U5MR is likely to be still more than twofold higher than the target for 2015. Even more worrisome are the facts that progress has been slowing down in recent years and it is not equally distributed across countries and regions (Fig. 11.3.6).

Box 11.3.2 The millennium development goals
Goal 1 Eradicate extreme poverty and hunger
Goal 2 Achieve universal primary education
Goal 3 Promote gender equality and empower women
Goal 4 Reduce child mortality
Goal 5 Improve maternal health
Goal 6 Combat HIV/AIDS, malaria and other diseases
Goal 7 Ensure environmental sustainability
Goal 8 Develop a global partnership for development

In May 2002, the UN Special Session on Children (UNGASS) adopted a declaration and plan of action set out in a document 'A World Fit for Children'. The document committed governments to a time-bound set of goals for children and young people, with particular focus on (a) promoting healthy lives; (b) providing quality education; (c) protecting children against abuse, exploitation, and violence; and (d) combating the HIV/AIDS epidemic. The UNGASS goals and targets provide an intermediate framework for assessing progress towards the MDGs, with many targets set for 2010, and a periodic review process agreed on as part of the UN General Assembly that takes places every year.

The Millennium Declaration and the Roadmap towards its implementation, as well as the UNGASS Declaration, stress the need for placing human rights at the centre of peace, security, and development programmes. As emphasized in the Roadmap, a rights-based approach to development should be the basis for equality and equity, both in the distribution of developmental gains and in the level of participation in the developmental process. From a child health perspective, therefore, integration of human rights norms and standards into country and United Nations system policies, programmes, and strategies is a crucial contribution towards achieving more equitable child health outcomes.

In this context, the United Nations Convention on the Rights of the Child (CRC) provides an important, holistic, legal, and normative framework for addressing child health, and for tackling the prevailing equity gaps within countries. It provides guidance for identifying and clarifying the legal obligations of governments and other actors to address and improve child health, and enhances accountability at the national and international levels. It requires a systematic and in-depth assessment of the possible impact that child health policies and programmes may have on the health and development of all children within a country.

Measuring progress towards MDGs

In 2005, the 'Countdown to 2015: Tracking progress in child survival' initiative was launched This initiative biennially measures and publishes the progress made in improving coverage of essential health interventions and in mortality reduction in the 60 countries that suffer the highest burden of child deaths. The second Countdown report 2008 showed that 16 countries were on track to achieving MDG 4, 26 were judged to have made insufficient progress in reducing child mortality, and 26 countries had made no progress at all (UNICEF, WHO, UNFPA and partners 2008).

The neonatal period stands out as one in which too few children are reached by effective care, and data on postnatal visits are yet to be systematically collected and reported. Given the important contribution of newborn mortality to under-five mortality, it is expected that in most countries, newborn mortality needs to be halved in order to achieve the MDG 4. To achieve MDG 4, efforts are also necessary to achieve MDGs 5 and 6, as they contribute to improved newborn survival and reduction in incidence and case fatality of malaria and HIV/AIDS, respectively.

Emphasis on children's early development is also needed given that two of the major United Nations 2000 MDGs are to reduce poverty and to ensure that all children complete primary schooling. These goals will not be achieved in countries where a large proportion of children live in poverty, suffer from poor nutrition and health, or lack psychosocial care.

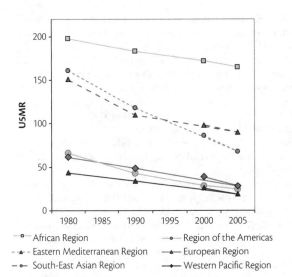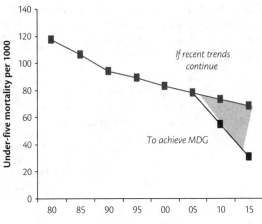

Fig. 11.3.6 Global and regional under-five mortality trend, 1980–2015.
Source: WHO mortality database. Data available on request from WHO-CAH Department.

Mobilizing resources for children

To achieve improved health outcomes for all children, development strategies and programmes need to increase the investments on building the capacity of families and communities in order to provide for and protect the physical, emotional, and cognitive development of children. It is important to ensure universal access to good-quality basic health, clean water, sanitation, and other social sector services such as education. This also includes creating the national legal, policy, and budget frameworks to promote the realization of children's rights to these services.

WHO and UNICEF support programmes to improve health and advocate protecting the rights of children across the world, along with other UN and external partners. The responsibility of success of child health programmes lies ultimately with governments. Only a fraction of resources for health in low- and middle-income countries originates in the international system, most of the resources being national. Scaling-up delivery of child health interventions will require additional investments in commodities, equipment, and human resources, as well as strengthening of the operational health system. This has cost implications. It has been estimated by WHO that universal coverage with known child health interventions will require an additional US$50 billion in the ten years from 2005 to 2015. At country level, financial needs for child survival will depend on the current situation as well as the targets set and the strategies employed for reaching those targets. Undertaking a cost assessment for child survival can help bring national programmes together to address priority needs, set joint targets, and plan complementary activities.

Once a multiyear budgeted child survival plan is available, it can be inserted into insurance plans, sector-wide approaches, poverty reduction strategy papers, and medium-term expenditure frameworks, allowing financing options to be discussed concretely with actors both inside and outside the health sector.

The additional financial resources will have to be mobilized by increasing both the national health budgets and the amount of official development assistance for health. In addition to these increased resources, greater efficiency and equity are required for their allocation and use.

Conclusion

Almost 10 million children under five die each year, 4 million of them dying in the neonatal period. Most neonatal deaths are due to three causes: Infections, prematurity, and birth asphyxia. ARIs, diarrhoea, malaria, measles, and HIV are the main causes of death in children aged 28 days to 5 years. Undernutrition is associated with over 35 per cent of these deaths. Child deaths are unequally distributed in the world. Three-quarters of child death occur in Africa and Southeast Asia; half of the child deaths take place in 6 countries. Within countries, child mortality tends to be higher in the rural areas and within the poorer and least educated families.

Key points

◆ Approximately two-thirds of under-five deaths could be prevented by universal coverage with a small set of existing interventions that do not require expensive technology. Among these interventions, the promotion of breastfeeding, management and prevention of diarrhoea, ARIs, malaria, and HIV infection, in addition to improved feeding practices to prevent malnutrition have the highest impact in reducing child mortality.

◆ Coverage with the earlier-mentioned interventions remains low. Integrating the interventions into packages of care that are organized along a continuum from pregnancy, birth, neonatal period, and childhood, and delivered at all levels—from the home and community through the first-level facility and hospital—would contribute to improved efficiency in intervention delivery and to the achievement of high coverage.

◆ Strengthening the health system will be key for increasing the coverage of health interventions. This requires improved programme management, with attention to strategic and implementation planning, implementation, monitoring, and evaluation.

◆ The development of an operational plan to which programmes can be held accountable, along with a good financing strategy, will yield long-term benefits for the child and the health system at large and is an essential element to follow the development of a child survival strategy.

◆ The achievement of the MDG of reducing child mortality by 2015—with a target of a two-thirds reduction from its 1990 level—will require significant acceleration in investments in child survival.

References

Addo-Yobo E., Chisaka N., Hassan M. *et al*. Oral amoxicillin *versus* injectable penicillin for severe pneumonia in children aged 3 to 59 months: a randomised multicentre equivalency study. *Lancet* 2004;**364**(9440):1141–8.

Arifeen S.E., Blum L.S., Hoque D.M.E. *et al*. Integrated management of childhood illness (IMCI) in Bangladesh: early findings from a cluster randomized study. *Lancet* 2004;**364**:1595–602.

Badan Pusat Statistik-Statistics Indonesia (BPS), ORC Macro. *Indonesia demographic and health survey 2002–3*. Calverton (MD): Badan Pusat Statistik-Statistics Indonesia, ORC Macro; 2003.

Bahl R., Frost C., Kirkwood B.R. *et al*. Infant feeding patterns and risks of death and hospitalization in the first half of infancy: multicentre cohort study. *Bulletin of the World Health Organization* 2003;**83**: 418–26.

Black R.E., Morris S.S., Bryce J. Where and why are 10 million children dying every year? *Lancet* 2003;**361**:2226–34.

Bryce J., Boschi-Pinto C., Shibuya K. *et al*. and the Child Health Epidemiology Reference Group. WHO estimates of the causes of death in children. *Lancet* 2005;**365**:1147–57.

Caulfield L.E., de Onis M., Blössner M. *et al*. Undernutrition as an underlying cause of child deaths associated with diarrhoea, pneumonia, malaria, and measles. *American Journal of Clinical Nutrition* 2004;**80**:193–8.

Chintu C., Bhat G.J., Walker A.S. *et al*. Co-trimoxazole as prophylaxis against opportunistic infections in HIV-infected Zambian children (CHAP): a double-blind randomized placebo-controlled trial. *Lancet* 2004;**364**:1865–71.

Collins S., Dent N., Binns P. *et al*. Management of severe acute malnutrition in children. *Lancet* 2006;**368**:1992–2000.

Collison D., Dey C., Hannah G. *et al*. Income inequality and child mortality in wealthy nations [e-pub ahead of print]. *Journal of Public Health* (*Oxford*) 2007 Mar 13.

DfID, UNICEF, USAID, WHO. The analytic review of the integrated management of childhood illness strategy. Geneva: World Health Organization; 2003.

Edmond K.M., Zandoh C., Quigley M.A. *et al*. Delayed breastfeeding initiation increases risk of neonatal mortality. *Paediatrics* 2006;**117**:380–6.

El-Zanaty F., Way A. *Egypt demographic and health survey 2005*. Cairo, Egypt: Ministry of Health and Population, National Population Council, El-Zanaty and Associates, ORC Macro; 2006.

Euro HIV. *HIV/AIDS surveillance in Europe: end-year report 2005*. Saint-Maurice, France: Institut de Veille Sanitaire; 2006. Number 73.

Fontaine O. Effect of zinc supplementation on clinical course of acute diarrhoea. Report of a meeting held in New Delhi, India; 2001 May 7–9. *Journal of Health, Population, and Nutrition* 2001;**19**:338–46.

Gouws E., Bryce J., Habicht J.P. *et al*. Improving antimicrobial use among health workers in first-level facilities: results from the multicountry evaluation of the integrated management of childhood illness strategy. *Bulletin of the World Health Organization* 2004;**82**:509–15.

Grantham-McGregor S., Cheung Y.B., Cueto S. *et al*. (on behalf of the International Child Development Steering Group). Developmental potential in the first 5 years for children in developing countries. *Lancet* 2007;**369**:60–70.

Hanh S.K., Jim Y.J., Garner P. Reduced-osmolarity oral rehydration solution for treating dehydration due to diarrhoea in children: a systematic review. *British Medical Journal* 2001;**323**:81–5.

Institut National de la Statistique du Rwanda (INSR), ORC Macro. *Rwanda demographic and health survey 2005*. Calverton (MD): Institut National de la Statistique du Rwanda, ORC Macro; 2006.

Jamison D.T., Breman J.G., Measham A.R. *et al*. editors. *Diseases control priorities in developing countries*. 2nd ed. Oxford: Oxford University Press; New York (NY): World Bank; 2006.

Jones G., Steketee R.W., Black R.E. *et al*. and the Bellagio Child Survival Study Group. How many child deaths can we prevent this year? *Lancet* 2003;**362**:65–71.

Karim S.S.A., Karim Q.A., Detels R. Acquired immunodeficiency syndrome. In: Detels R, Beaglehole R, Lansang MA, Gulliford M, editors. *Oxford Textbook of Public Health*. Oxford: Oxford University Press; 2008.

Kosek M., Bern C., Guerrant R.L. The global burden of diarrhoeal disease, as estimated from studies published between 1992 and 2000. *Bulletin of the World Health Organization* 2003;**81**:197–204.

Lengeler C. Insecticide-treated bed nets and curtains for preventing malaria. [Cochrane review]. Cochrane Database Syst. Review 2004;(2). CD000363.

Maroc Ministère de la Santé, ORC Macro, Ligue des États Arabes. *Enquête sur la population et la santé familiale (EPSF) 2003–4*. Calverton (MD): Ministère de la Santé, ORC Macro; 2005

Morrow R., Moss W. Malaria. In: Detels R., Beaglehole R., Lansang M.A., Gulliford M, editors. *Oxford Textbook of Public Health*. Oxford: Oxford University Press; 2008.

National Bureau of Statistics, ORC Macro. *Tanzania demographic and health survey 2004–5*. Dar es Salaam, Tanzania: National Bureau of Statistics, ORC Macro; 2005.

National Institute of Population Research and Training (NIPORT), Mitra and Associates, ORC Macro. *Bangladesh demographic and health survey 2004*. Dhaka, Bangladesh: National Institute of Population Research and Training; 2005.

National Institute of Public Health, National Institute of Statistics, ORC Macro. *Cambodia demographic and health survey 2005*. Phnom Penh, Cambodia, Calverton (MD): National Institute of Public Health, National Institute of Statistics, ORC Macro; 2006.

National Scientific and Applied Center for Preventive Medicine (NCPM), ORC Macro. *Moldova demographic and health survey 2005*. Calverton (MD): National Scientific and Applied Center for Preventive Medicine, Moldova Ministry of Health and Social Protection, ORC Macro; 2006.

National Statistical Service, Ministry of Health, ORC Macro. *Armenia demographic and health survey 2005*. Calverton (MD): National Statistical Service, Armenian Ministry of Health, ORC Macro; 2006.

National Statistics Office (NSO), ORC Macro. *National demographic and health survey 2003*. Calverton (MD): National Statistics Office (Philippines), ORC Macro; 2004.

Ndiaye S., Mohamed A. *Enquête Démographique et de Santé au Sénégal 2005*. Calverton (MD): Sénégal Centre de Recherche pour le Développement Humain, ORC Macro; 2006.

Prudhon C., Briend A., Weise Prinzo Z. *et al*. guest editors. WHO, UNICEF, and SCN informal consultation on community-based management of severe malnutrition in children. *Food and Nutrition Bulletin* [supplement] 2006;**27**. SCN Nutrition Policy Paper Number 21.

Qazi S. Short-course therapy for community-acquired pneumonia in paediatric patients. *Drugs* 2005;**65**:1179–92.

Rudan I., Tomaskovic L., Boschi-Pinto C. *et al*. and the WHO Child Health Epidemiology Reference Group. Global estimate of the incidence of clinical pneumonia among children under five years of age. *Bulletin of the World Health Organization* 2004;**82**:895–903.

Secretaría de Salud (SS), Instituto Nacional de Estadística (INE), Macro Internacional. *Encuesta nacional de salud y demografía 2005–6*. Tegucigalpa, Honduras, Calverton (MD): Secretaría de Salud, Instituto Nacional de Estadística, Macro International; 2006.

UNICEF, WHO, UNFPA and partners: Countdown to 2015: Tracking progress in maternal, newborn and child survival. The 2008 Report. New York: UNICEF, 2008. www.Countdown2015MNCH.org).

United Nations Children's Fund, World Health Organization. *Low birth weight: country, regional, and global estimates*. New York (NY): UNICEF; 2004.

United Nations Children's Fund. *Child poverty in rich countries*. Florence, Italy: UNICEF Innocenti Research Centre; 2005. Innocenti Report Card Number 6. Available from: http://www.unicef.org/brazil/repcard6e.pdf [Accessed 2007 Oct 1].

United Nations Children's Fund. The state of the world's children 2007. Women and children: the double dividend of gender equality. New York (NY): UNICEF; 2006.

Victora C.G., Kirkwood B.R., Ashworth A. *et al*. Potential interventions for the prevention of childhood pneumonia in developing countries: improving nutrition. *American Journal of Clinical Nutrition* 1999;**70**:309–20.

World Bank. *Data and statistics*. Washington (DC): World Bank; 2007. Available from: http://www.worldbank.org/ [Accessed 2007 May 14].

World Health Organization and United Nations Children's Fund. *Joint statement: clinical management of acute diarrhoea*. Geneva: World Health Organization; New York (NY): UNICEF; 2004.

World Health Organization Collaborative Study team on the Role of Breastfeeding on the Prevention of Infant Mortality. Effect of breastfeeding on infant and child mortality due to infectious diseases in less developed countries: a pooled analysis. *Lancet* 2001;**355**:451–5.

World Health Organization. Antiretroviral drugs for treating pregnant women and preventing HIV infection in infants: guidelines on care, treatment, and support for women living with HIV/AIDS and their children in resource-constrained settings. Geneva: World Health Organization; 2004a.

World Health Organization. Complementary feeding of young children in developing countries: a review of current scientific knowledge. Geneva: World Health Organization; 1998. WHO/NUT/98.1.

World Health Organization. Family and community practices that promote child survival, growth, development—a review of the evidence. Geneva: World Health Organization; 2004b.

World Health Organization. *Guidelines for the treatment of malaria*. Geneva: World Health Organization; 2006a.

World Health Organization. *HIV transmission through breastfeeding—a review of available evidence*. Geneva: World Health Organization; 2004c. WHO/UNICEF/UNFPA/UNAIDS

World Health Organization. Integrated management of childhood illness: complementary course on HIV/AIDS. Geneva: World Health Organization; 2006b.

World Health Organization. *Management of severe malnutrition: a manual for physicians and other senior health workers*. Geneva: World Health Organization; 1999. ISBN 92 4 154511 9 (NLM Classification: WD 101).

World Health Organization. Pregnancy, childbirth, postpartum, and newborn care: a guide for essential practice. 2nd ed. Geneva: World Health Organization; 2006c.

World Health Organization. *Strategic directions for improving the health and development of children and adolescents*. Geneva: World Health Organization; 2002. WHO/FCH/CAH/02.21 Available from: http://www.who.int/child-adolescent-health/publications/OVERVIEW/CAH_Strategy.htm [Accessed 2007 Oct 1].

World Health Organization. *Strategic framework for the prevention of HIV infection in infants in Europe*. Copenhagen, Denmark: Regional Office for Europe of the World Health Organization; 2004d. Available from: http://www.who.int/hiv/mtct/PMTCTEURO.pdf and http://www.unicef.org/ceecis/Strategic_framework_for_the_prevention_of_HIV.pdf [Accessed 2007 Oct 1].

World Health Organization. *The European health report 2005: public health action for healthier children and populations*. Copenhagen, Denmark: Regional Office for Europe of the World Health Organization; 2005a.

World Health Organization. *The world health report 2005: make every mother and child count*. Geneva: World Health Organization; 2005b.

World Health Organization. *WHO HIV and infant feeding technical consultation consensus statement*. Held on behalf of the interagency task team (IATT) on prevention of HIV infections in pregnant women, mothers, and their infants; 2006 Oct 25–7. Geneva: World Health Organization; 2006d. Available from: http://www.who.int/child-adolescent-health/publications/NUTRITION/consensus_statement.htm [Accessed 2007 Oct 1].

World Health Organization. WHO mortality database

World Health Organization. *World health report 2006: working together for health*. Geneva: World Health Organization; 2006e.

World Health Organization. *World health statistics 2007*. Geneva: World Health Organization; 2007. Available from: http://www.who.int/whosis/whostat2007.pdf [Accessed 2007 Oct 1].

11.4

Adolescent health

Pierre-André Michaud,
Venkatraman Chandra-Mouli,
and George C. Patton

Abstract

Around 30% of the world's population is aged 10–24 years, and close to 90% of these young people live in low- and middle-income countries. In recent decades, there have been marked shifts in the health problems affecting this age group. Infectious diseases, including HIV and TB, have become prominent and are major causes of death in Africa and South Asia. Accidents and injuries have also become common and are a greater cause of mortality and morbidity in this age group than others. Chronic illnesses, including mental and behavioural disorders, are the leading cause of disability in the age group. There are emerging problems with obesity in many parts of the world, but undernutrition also remains important in lower-income countries.

Various strategies are likely to be useful in responding to the health problems of young people. The health care system should offer 'youth-friendly' services that take into account the social context, developmental stage, and emerging autonomy of their young patients. The school setting can be used in many countries to implement and sustain broader health promotion initiatives in the age group. Ideally, young people, their parents, and the broader community in which young people live and work should be engaged in the implementation of preventive health programs.

At a broader level, policies that promote easy access to health care and contraception, traffic safety, limitation of access to licit and illicit drugs as well as weapons, and better access to health foods are likely to have a great effect on the health of this age group. Some of the most effective health interventions are likely to be around ongoing engagement in education and promoting a smooth transition into the workforce.

Adolescence and youth: A bio-psychosocial developmental concept

The WHO defines 'adolescence' as the age group of 10–19 years and 'youth' as the age group of 15–24 years. These two overlapping age groups are combined in the category of 'young people', covering the age range of 10–24 years. In this chapter, we will interchangeably use the words 'adolescents' and 'young people', as the categories are arbitrary and the health problems faced are similar. Indeed, adolescence is better viewed as a flexible life phase rather than a fixed time period.

In most cultures and in individuals, it begins with the appearance of puberty and ends with a transition to greater emotional and social autonomy. This stage of transition between childhood and adulthood is largely shaped by biological and socioeconomic factors.

There is considerable variation in the onset of adolescence. At an individual level, there is a 4–5 year variation in the age of onset of puberty among healthy individuals, which is a physiological peculiarity of man and is observed even where living conditions are similar for all members of a group. At a population level, there are variations in the timing of puberty across races and across time periods. In Western countries, since around 150 years, pubertal timing has decreased by 4–5 years: The mean age for menarche is now 12–13 years in most high-income countries, whereas it used to occur between 16 and 17 years some centuries ago (Ong et al. 2006).

This biological trend is accompanied by an increasing duration of education and training, with a later acquisition of professional capabilities that are the hallmarks of an adult status (Patton & Viner 2007). In pre-industrial societies, the adolescent transition from puberty to adult roles, as defined by the onset of sexual activity, marriage, and parenthood, ranged from around two years in girls to four years in boys. In today's developed economies, longer periods of education, increased affluence, and the availability of effective contraception mean that adolescence commonly persists for well over a decade. Current concepts of adolescence typically encompass a biological onset at puberty and highly variable social transitions that mark its completion. The biological processes initiated at puberty interact with the social context to affect an individual's emotional and social development.

A modern pattern for reproductive capacity, as well as sexual activity, to precede (by more than a decade) role transitions into parenthood and marriage has been accompanied by a rise in the number of sexual partners before marriage and higher rates of sexually transmitted diseases. Similarly, the delay in taking on mature social roles and responsibilities in marriage, parenthood, and employment, associated with earlier initiation of substance use, has been linked to rises in substance use and mental health problems among young people. This phenomenon was limited to high-income countries for many years, but is increasingly being observed in low- and middle-income countries (Lloyd 2005).

Recent neuroscience research has shown that many brain changes continue to take place until the end of the third decade of life. Some changes precede and initiate puberty; others continue well beyond puberty. The possibility that behavioural problems arise because of a mismatch between the emotional reactions and cognitive capacities of young adolescents has long interested clinicians. The importance of this biological gap might be accentuated for those adolescents who mature earlier than their counterparts. Indeed, it has been repeatedly shown that early maturers, both boys and girls, engage in health-compromising behaviours at a higher rate than normal or late maturers and as such may represent a subgroup of adolescents with special vulnerability (Michaud et al. 2006).

This gap between the biological maturation of the brain and the acquisition of an adult status within society has important implications, as it creates a period of psychosocial vulnerability: Young people are offered tools and opportunities that they cannot master in terms of their cognitive abilities (Steinberg 2004). For instance, the use of fast motorized vehicles requires anticipation skills that are not necessarily acquired in middle adolescence. Therefore, public health professionals, as we will review later in this chapter, should not expect too much from purely educational strategies and need to place as much emphasis as they can on developing safe environments for adolescents.

Adolescents are a heterogeneous group (Steinberg & Morris 2001). There are great differences between a 12-year-old girl struggling to come to terms with a new body and the emergence of her menstrual periods, and a 19-year-old young woman who is pregnant and engaged to be married. For these reasons, adolescence has been divided into three phases:

- Early adolescence is marked by puberty and a rapid physical growth, with a raised interest in one's self image.

- Middle adolescence is characterized by a period of experimentation with potentially risky behaviours such as unprotected sexual intercourse, and the use of legal and illegal psychoactive substances. Many health-risk behaviours are transitory, but some can have harmful long-term consequences, such as unsafe sex resulting in an HIV infection.

- Late adolescence is a period of progressive stabilization during which young people tend to form more stable relationships and acquire long-term perspectives, a developmental process that extends into early adulthood.

In low- and middle-income countries (mainly in Africa and South Asia), young people currently represent 1.3 billion individuals, a number that will continue to increase up to 1.5 billion by the middle of the century. This is largely due to the improved child survival initiatives implemented over the last three decades. However, in the rest of the world, the proportion of young people within the total population will slowly decrease over the next few decades; that is, the relative size of the youth population will fall. This is largely due to the growing number of people who remain alive at older ages. Another demographic factor that impacts on the health of young people is the increasing age of marriage. Postponing marriage allows young female adolescents to access better education. It also alleviates some of the harmful consequences of very early childbearing.

Also, over the last 20 years, a steadily growing number of low- and middle-income countries have placed emphasis on education (Lloyd 2005; United Nations 2005; World Bank 2007). Learning gives the individual the knowledge and skills needed to master daily tasks and make decisions, including those that relate to health. In the poorest countries, efforts have been directed at ensuring that all children receive primary school education, and in many middle-income countries, authorities have invested in the development of post-primary education. The rate of achievement still varies a great deal across countries: Whereas the retention rate in Thailand up to the ninth grade is around 80 per cent, it drops to 20–40 per cent in countries such as Nicaragua or Senegal, with a large discrepancy between pupils from low and high socioeconomic groups.

The level of education attained should be looked at as one of the main determinants of health. Health literacy is closely linked with the learning process: Adolescents from poor families who drop out of school do much worse than those from wealthier families who have greater access to education and employment (World Bank 2007). With the emergence of new electronic media, young people around the world have access to information that was not previously available. The Internet and other information and communications technologies have created new means of socialization in which young people can reach out without geographic limits. Media use can be considered as potentially harmful in some instances (e.g. depriving physical activity or promoting violent behaviour among vulnerable youngsters), but it should also be viewed as an effective way to disseminate information, especially information on health that could potentially have a positive influence on young people's behaviour.

Adolescence can be viewed as a period of great opportunity and also of vulnerability during which public health interventions can greatly affect current and future health. According to the WHO (World Health Organization 2002a), there are at least three reasons for investing in the health and development of adolescents:

1. Reduction in the burden of morbidity and mortality in later life, because healthy behaviours and practices adopted during adolescence tend to last a lifetime.

2. From an economic perspective, gains in national productivity when healthy and well-educated adolescents enter the workforce.

3. Lastly, adolescent health is a basic human right. The UN Convention on the Rights of the Child (CRC) declares that, 'children and adolescents have a right to life, development, and to benefit from the highest attainable standard of health'.

The health of adolescents and young people: An overview

The health of young people is determined by influences within and outside the health system. Epidemiological research has highlighted the role of these risk and protective factors in shaping the health of young people at an individual and collective level. Figure 11.4.1, adapted from a recent publication (Blum et al. 2002), summarizes some of the biological, psychological, and socioenvironmental determinants that have been found to affect adolescent health.

Preventive intervention should address these determinants in the environment, in addition to interventions that are addressed to young people directly. For example, in injury prevention, strategies aimed at improving the environment have been shown to be more effective in reducing injuries than those attempting to directly modify the behaviour of young people (Toroyan & Preden 2007).

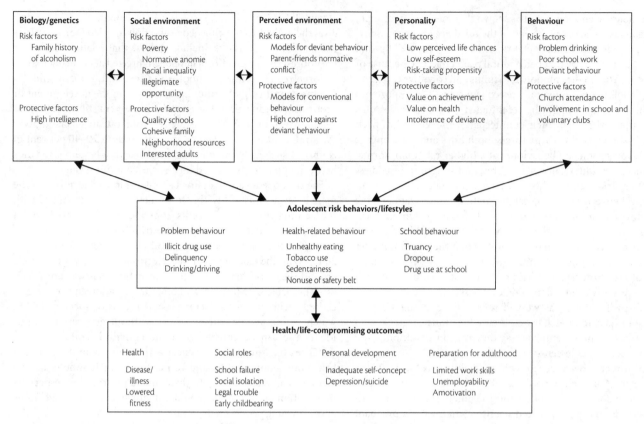

Fig. 11.4.1 Risk and protective factors that impact on the health of adolescents at the individual, family, community, and environmental levels. (Adapted from Blum RW, McNeely C, Nonnemaker J. Vulnerability, risk, and protection. *The Journal Adolescent Health* 2002;**31** Suppl 1:28–39.)

Although the scope and magnitude of health problems among youth vary greatly from one continent and country to another, the profile of problems and burdens found around the world is quite similar. The main current fatalities, diseases or burden of disease, and future threats to health can be observed in both rich and poor countries—such as malnutrition; self-inflicted violence and violence directed at others; HIV, sexually transmitted infections (STIs), and unplanned pregnancies; health problems resulting from substance use; mental health problems; and health and social problems arising from chronic conditions.

Overall, the health of young people has improved over the last decade. Between the 1970s and 1990s, life expectancy at birth increased in low- and middle-income countries more than in high-income countries (Lloyd 2005). This is largely due to the decline in infant mortality and a decrease in the rate of infectious diseases. A notable exception is the epidemic of HIV/AIDS in Africa, particularly in sub-Saharan Africa, where around 60 per cent of deaths among 15–29 year old individuals is attributed to the epidemic. The situation is far less dramatic in Middle East and Asia, but could deteriorate in the future.

In most countries, rich or poor, the overall mortality rate of young people is low in comparison with that of infants, adults, and older people, but the likelihood of premature death is much higher in poor countries. The average 15 year old boy has a 90 per cent chance of surviving to the age of 60 in Western Europe or North America, but only a 50 per cent chance in sub-Saharan Africa,

primarily because of communicable diseases such as AIDS. In most parts of the world, with the exception of sub-Saharan Africa and South America, the main cause of premature deaths among young people is injuries, as exemplified in Table 11.4.1.

The second highest cause of death is suicide, which represents but one consequence of the burden of mental health problems and disorders among young people. Homicides are a notable cause of deaths among young people: Although it is often the result of crimes due to a violent environment in some US suburbs and in South America, it should not be forgotten that in other parts of the world, notably in Africa, it is the result of war and armed conflict. In 2003, more than 70 countries were considered as 'unstable' (UNAIDS 2006), and UNICEF estimates that there are approximately 300 000 young people under the age of 18 enrolled as soldiers, many of them forcibly recruited (United Nations 2005). Finally, in Africa, Southeast Asia, and to some extent in Eastern Mediterranean countries, other infectious diseases constitute an important cause of mortality and morbidity (Blum 1991).

The data on the global burden of disease estimated by Lopez *et al.* (2006) represent another view of the top-priority health concerns among young people. Health habits and lifestyles acquired during adolescence will impact on the future state of health and the global burden of disease. Among the top ten conditions that affect the global burden of disease worldwide, at least five are directly linked with health behaviours largely developed during the adolescent period: Unsafe sex, legal and illegal use of psychoactive

Table 11.4.1 Five leading causes of mortality in 15–29-year-olds[a]

World regions	Leading causes of death[b]				
	Unintentional injuries	AIDS	Other infectious causes	Homicide/war/other intentional injuries	Suicide/self-inflicted injuries
All world regions	1 (531 000)	2 (326 000)	3 (229 000)	4 (227 000)	5 (124 000)
South America/Caribbean	2 (64 000)	5 (11 000)	4 (12 000)	1 (72 000)	3 (14 000)
Africa	4 (56 000)	1 (225 000)	2 (104 000)	3 (66 000)	5 (6 000)
Southeast Asia	1 (178 000)	3 (72 000)	2 (81 000)	5 (33 000)	4 (37 000)
Western Pacific	1 (119 000)	5 (8 000)	3 (19 000)	4 (17 000)	2 (32 000)
Eastern Mediterranean	1 (40 000)	4 (7 000)	2 (21 000)	3 (15 000)	5 (5 000)
Europe	1 (74 000)	5 (2 000)	4 (10 000)	3 (23 000)	2 (30 000)
North America[c]	1	6	5	3	2

[a] Between brackets: Number of deaths worldwide.
[b] Data on maternal mortality among 15–29-year-olds not available.
[c] In North America, cancer is the fourth leading cause of death in the adolescent/young adult years.
Source: Blum RW, Nelson-Mmari K. The health of young people in a global context. *The Journal of Adolescent Health* 2004:**35** 402–16.

substances and of tobacco, physical inactivity, and high body mass index (BMI).

Injuries and other forms of violence inflicted against and among adolescents

Injuries among young people are mainly due to traffic accidents, interpersonal violence, war, and suicide, and account for substantial mortality and morbidity. Apart from sub-Saharan Africa, where HIV accounts for a large proportion of deaths, in the rest of the world, violent deaths make up half of the mortality. A recent review run by the Department of Injuries and Violence Prevention of the WHO (World Health Organization 2002b) gives a good overview of the importance of injuries to the health of young people. In 2002, worldwide, among males aged 15–29 years, road traffic injuries accounted for approximately 285 000 deaths per year and for 12.4 billions disability-adjusted life years (DALYs), whereas the figures for females were 70 000 deaths and 2.7 billions DALYs. As motorized transportation grows, it is expected that the number of deaths linked with traffic accidents will also grow.

Overall, the profile of deaths by injuries varies greatly between males and females: Males experience more than twice the rate of fatalities than females do. Whereas road traffic injuries are the most common injuries among males, self-inflicted injuries (suicide) are the most common among females. Among males, interpersonal violence is the second most common cause of violent deaths: In some regions of the world (e.g. in South America), it is the most frequent cause of death as well as the leading cause of DALYs among both males and females. In Africa, the leading cause of death and of DALYs is war; in 2000, an estimated 53 856 young people aged 15–29 years lost their lives as a result of armed conflict. These deaths are not only those of young people enrolled in the army, but also of barbaric acts perpetrated among young people, especially among females.

The problem of violence affecting young people is not only reflected by high rates of mortality, but also of various injuries and handicaps. Severe traffic injuries often result in permanent brain or limb damage. The same applies to young people who are victims of anti-personnel mines. It is in the Americas that one observes the highest rates of homicide among young people. In many countries of this region, homicides account for one-third of the deaths among young people. Homicide is the second highest cause of death among young people in half of the South American countries and accounts for high rates of death in the United States as well (McAlister 2006).

Violence prevention needs to address risk factors at the individual, family, community, and societal levels (Dahlberg & Potter 2001; World Health Organization 2004c). Evidence shows that life-skills and social development programmes for children and adolescents aged 6–19 years are effective, as are mentoring programmes to develop attachments between at-risk youth and caring adults (Tremblay 2006). Visiting and supporting parents of young children at home and building their skills in problem solving and non-violent disciplining have also been shown to be effective in reducing parental violence. Preschool enrichment programmes (for children aged 3–5 years), and life-skills and social development programmes (for children and adolescents aged 6–19 years) have been shown to be effective in reducing violent behaviour later in life.

Several school-based violence prevention programmes have been implemented with a special focus on dating violence prevention and the promotion of healthy relationships. Those which have been proven effective have usually involved the surrounding community. A good example of such a programme is the Seattle Social Development Project, a theory-guided preventive intervention that strengthened teaching and parenting practices, and taught children interpersonal skills during the elementary grades, as well as showed wide-ranging beneficial effects on functioning in early adulthood, including better mental functioning and reduced crime and substance abuse (Hawkins *et al.* 2005).

Reducing the availability of alcohol and other legal substances, and decreasing the demand for and access to lethal weapons are effective ways of reducing violence. Actions to make health systems more responsive and to build the empathy and competence of health workers can help ensure that adolescents who experience violence, including sexual violence, get effective and sensitive care and treatment. Also, the provision of ongoing psychological and social support can help adolescents deal with the long-term psychological effects of violence, and reduce the likelihood of their becoming perpetuators of violence in the future. Finally, it should be stressed that reducing poverty, economic inequality, and social exclusion, which strongly impact on the occurrence of violence, is probably among the most effective strategies. However, outcome evaluation research to test all these strategies in low- and middle-income countries is urgently needed.

Road traffic accidents are increasing alarmingly in some low- and middle-income countries. This is due to the growth of motorized transport, a rise in the number of vehicles, and perhaps, a lack of education in driving skills. Four main types of strategies can be developed to address traffic injuries: Modifying the road environment, increasing the safeness of vehicles, providing guidance and support, and reducing the exposure of young people to traffic (Munro *et al.* 1995). Traffic calming measures and enforcing speed limits have proven particularly effective. Another environmental measure tested in high-income countries is preventing driving while under the influence of alcohol by providing alternative means of transportation for young people during late hours of the night. The use of seat belts and helmets is another very effective way to diminish the potential health impact of accidents.

Mental health

In nearly all countries, mental disorders account for an important, and often underestimated, part of the burden of disease. Five of the ten leading causes of DALYs in people aged 15–44 years are mental disorders: Unipolar depressive disorders, alcohol use disorders, self-inflicted injuries, schizophrenia, and bipolar affective disorders (Patel *et al.* 2007). One of the reasons for this is that several mental disorders start during adolescence (Michaud & Fombonne 2005). Mental health problems during adolescence constitute a heavy burden at the individual as well as the societal level, because they are not only a significant source of suffering for the adolescent and his or her family, but also often negatively influence the future of life course emotionally, socially, and professionally. Also, suicide, which frequently is a result of a mental disorder, represents one of the leading causes of deaths in many countries.

It is not easy to distinguish mental health problems from true disorders. Mental disorders are defined as situations characterized by lasting behavioural or psychological burden accompanied by a concomitant distress and/or a raised risk of death, or an important loss of freedom, involving an unexpected cultural response to any situation (Michaud & Fombonne 2005). Over the last few decades, it has been estimated that the rate of adolescents suffering from mental health problems and disorders is on the rise (Rutter & Smith 1995). In industrialized countries, the most prominent increase has been observed in the area of substance use, eating disorders, and conduct disorders (antisocial behaviour).

Many adolescents suffer from several mental health problems that tend to cluster. For example, psychoactive substance use disorder (PSUD) is often associated with depression and suicide attempts. The WHO estimates that this trend will continue and that there will be a 50 per cent increase in the percentage of young people suffering from mental disorders worldwide (World Health

Organization 2003). One important problem linked with mental health disorders is that adolescents are often reluctant to seek help or to express their mental health problem in a way that is readily identifiable by family members, teachers, peers, or even health practitioners.

Public health interventions must tackle both risk and protective factors for mental health. Promoting mental health, preventing mental health problems, and responding to them if and when they arise requires a continuum of responses ranging from the community level, through health services at the primary level, to specialist health and social services at the referral level (Patel *et al.* 2007). The fact that mental health problems are very often correlated with other health problems (e.g. substance abuse and violence) must be taken into account. By identifying and treating individuals with attention-deficit hyperactivity disorder, psychoses, mood disorders, and anxiety disorders, one may well decrease the number of adolescents who will engage in violent behaviour, delinquency, or substance abuse.

A growing body of evidence suggests that effective interventions could reduce risk factors and enhance protective factors at the level of the child or adolescent, the family, and the community. These interventions include enhancing social skills, problem-solving skills, and self-confidence, and can address all the children in a community (universal interventions) or those at particular risk (selective interventions). They have been shown to help prevent specific mental health problems such as conduct disorders, anxiety, depression, and eating disorders, as well as other risk behaviours, including those that relate to sexual behaviour, substance use behaviour, and violent behaviour (World Health Organization 2004b).

There is some evidence that broad school-based approaches can have a beneficial midterm effect on the behaviour and mental health of pupils (Patton *et al.* 2006), as will be discussed later. These measures are particularly effective for young people who are at risk of developing mental health problems because of their family or social environment. Another complementary approach is to integrate mental health interventions with other existing youth programmes. For example, mental health prevention can be coupled with programmes focusing on sexual and reproductive health or programmes directed at the reduction of violent behaviours.

Also, another important area of intervention is to provide adolescents with mental health problems and disorders with better access to adequate treatment. Health workers at the primary level need to have the competencies to relate to young people, to detect mental health problems early, and to provide appropriate treatment, which includes counselling, cognitive-behavioural therapy and, where appropriate, psychotropic medication. However, these workers should be backed by specialist services at the referral level (Patel *et al.* 2007).

Worldwide, it is estimated that between 100 000 and 200 000 young people commit suicide every year. In industrialized countries, it is the first or second most common cause of death among young people, and also accounts for a large proportion of deaths in other countries (Wasserman *et al.* 2005). In 26 countries for which data were available for the period 1965–99, a rising trend of suicide in young males was observed, which was marked in the years before 1980 and in countries outside Europe. The determinants of suicide are multiple and complex, and include both personal vulnerability factors as well as family and psychosocial characteristics (Beautrais *et al.* 2006). Dysfunctional social networks, such as being disconnected from community and family ties, seem to play a predominant role.

Several countries have engaged in large, population-based, effective suicide prevention programmes (Wilson 2004), which include a sensitization of the whole population as well as training of target groups of professionals such as health workers, clergymen, policemen, teachers, and educators. Some countries have implemented formal teaching sessions addressing the issue of suicidal behaviours within the school setting. Most workers point out that such universal approaches show no evidence of a beneficial effect on suicide attempts and suicide. Ploed *et al.* (1996) suggest that more broadly based comprehensive school health programmes should be developed, addressing the determinants of adolescent risk behaviour. A promising more selective approach is the identification by lay professionals, such as teachers and social workers, of potentially suicidal adolescents who can then be referred to their doctor or to mental health facilities (Hawton & James 2005).

Substance use, misuse, and abuse

Psychotropic substances ('drugs') include both legal and illegal drugs such as, among others, tobacco, alcohol, psychoactive medication, cannabis, synthetic substances, cocaine, and heroin. Tobacco currently represents a major cause of death among adults in the world (Lopez & Mathers 2006): Nearly 5 million persons die every year from tobacco-related illnesses, with disproportionately higher mortality occurring in low- and middle-income countries. For instance, chronic obstructive lung diseases cause almost as many deaths as HIV/AIDS (2.7 million). Among those people who smoke, nearly a quarter had smoked their first cigarette before they reached the age of ten.

The Global Youth Tobacco Survey (GYTS), initiated in 1999 by WHO, the Centers for Disease Control, and the Canadian Public Health Association, is a school-based survey that provides self-reported data on the prevalence of cigarette and other tobacco products use within each of the six WHO regions (Centers for Disease Control 2007). The GYTS data indicate that nearly 2 of every 10 students report currently using a tobacco product (smoking: 8.9 per cent; other tobacco use: 11.2 per cent). Use of any tobacco products is highest in the American and European regions (22.2 per cent and 19.8 per cent, respectively) and lowest in the Southeast Asian and Western Pacific regions (12.9 per cent and 11.4 per cent, respectively). Boys are significantly more likely than girls to use any tobacco products in the Eastern Mediterranean, Southeast Asian, and Western Pacific regions, and significantly more likely than girls to smoke cigarettes in the African, Southeast Asian, and Western Pacific regions. Deterring young people from starting tobacco use is one of the big public health challenges health policy makers currently face.

The use of alcohol is heavily linked with cultural and religious contexts, which explains why its use varies considerably across countries. Although no evidence exists of significant health benefits from moderate alcohol consumption for young adults, it is essentially the hazardous use of alcohol (also named 'alcohol misuse' or 'problematic alcohol use') that represents a serious problem during adolescence because of its short- and long-term consequences, such as violence, unprotected sex, and injuries while driving under the influence of alcohol, or developing alcohol dependence once

they enter adulthood (Bonomo *et al.* 2004). In Western countries, especially in Europe, the rate of adolescents reporting hazardous use of alcohol (on a more or less regular basis) has increased over the last two decades (Zaborskis *et al.* 2006). In Africa and South America, alcohol use and hazardous use are also on the rise, because of societal changes.

Besides alcohol, cannabis is the most frequently used illicit drug worldwide. The lifetime prevalence of cannabis use, however, differs greatly from one country to another. The available data suggest that lifetime prevalence rates of cannabis use, misuse (problematic use), and abuse are increasing in many countries. According to the Global Youth Network of the UN Commission on Narcotic Drugs (CND) (United Nations Economic and Social Council, Commission on Narcotic Drugs 1991), the percentage of young people having ever used cannabis varies between 1 per cent in poor countries such as Romania and 40–45 per cent in countries with high prevalence such as Canada, the United States, and Switzerland, with several countries such as those in Asia displaying intermediate figures (~5 per cent). A much lower but still substantial percentage of young people have access to other illicit drugs such as ecstasy, cocaine, and heroin, especially in high-income countries.

Young people initiate substance use for a range of reasons that may include curiosity and some peer pressure. Perceptions of prevailing norms on substance use are relevant to the extent that young people commonly conform to such norms in defining their identity (Hawkins *et al.* 1991). Influences on continuing and escalating use include vulnerability related to mental health, family difficulties, school failure, and unemployment, but the cultural, economic, and legal contexts in which adolescent development takes place also influence patterns of initiation and progression of substance use (Kodjo & Klein 2002). Several countries are currently debating whether the penalties for possessing small amounts of cannabis should be reduced: Reducing penalties for cannabis use does not necessarily lead to widespread use in the young. In the Netherlands, where cannabis use is not a criminal offence, the lifetime prevalence of cannabis use is lower than in the United States, which has some of the toughest cannabis laws in the Western world (Korf 2002).

Public health responses to adolescent substance use may take a variety of forms (Toumbourou *et al.* 2007). As mentioned before, regulatory interventions seek to limit the availability of substances through taxation and legislation. Legislation includes regulation of sales through age restrictions on purchase as well as regulation at points of sale, on hours of sale, and on quantities that can be sold. Regulation extends to limiting use in public spaces, a strategy that has been the cornerstone of tobacco control, although with less success in young people than in adults. Developmental interventions seek to reduce demand for substances by promoting healthy development and tackling risks that arise in the course of development.

Improving the social climate of secondary schools and/or implementing a life-skills approach among pupils could contribute to decreasing the likelihood of engagement in both licit and illicit substance use (Tobler 2000). Screening of young people and brief psychological interventions may be effective in reducing substance abuse (McCambridge & Strang 2004). Family interventions also appear very relevant and effective for the younger adolescent substance abuser (Kumpfer & Alvarado 2005). Finally, harm-reduction interventions are important in an overall public health response to substance abuse (Toumbourou *et al.* 2007). In those with harmful use, abuse, and dependence, these interventions seek to reduce the likelihood of negative outcomes without necessarily affecting the level of substance use. For example, needle and syringe exchange programmes have been shown to be effective in preventing HIV transmission without encouraging an increase in substance use through injection or other routes.

Nutritional problems and obesity

Chronic malnutrition in earlier years is responsible for widespread stunting and adverse health and social consequences throughout the life span. This is best prevented in childhood, but actions to improve access to food could benefit adolescents as well. Anaemia is one of the key nutritional problems in adolescent girls. Preventing too-early pregnancy and improving the nutritional status of girls before they enter pregnancy could reduce maternal and infant mortality, and contribute to breaking the cycle of intergenerational malnutrition. This will involve improving access to nutritious food and to micronutrient supplementation and, in many places, preventing infections as well. Adolescence is a timely period to shape healthy eating and exercise habits that can contribute to physical and psychological benefits during the adolescent period and to reducing the likelihood of nutrition-related chronic diseases in adulthood.

Over the past decade, WHO has recognized that overweight and obesity represent a major public health challenge, reaching pandemic proportions among adults as well as among children and adolescents. This pandemic was first observed and is still prominent in high-income countries such as the United States and those in Western Europe (Ogden *et al.* 2003), but has also occurred in Eastern Europe (Musaiger 2004), South America, and East Asia (Wang *et al.* 2002). The prevalence of overweight and obesity has increased markedly in the last two decades in most high- and middle-income countries (Wang *et al.* 2002). For instance, in the European Union, the number of overweight children is increasing by at least 400 000 every year, of which 85 000 are obese (Lobstein & Frelut 2003). This trend has arisen as a result of obesogenic environments, more sedentary time, diminished physical activity, and increasing calorie consumption. Urbanization encourages the use of automobiles and other motorized vehicles; in high-income countries, suburbs lack stores, entertainment, or other destinations within walking distance. Also, outside Northern European countries, infrastructure that supports walking and cycling has been neglected.

Linked with the area of obesity is an upward trend in the incidence of eating disorders in high- and middle-income countries. Anorexia nervosa is a condition that typically affects adolescents (0.5–1 per cent of the female population below 20 years), whereas bulimia nervosa tends to affect young adult females (3–5 per cent of this population). Increasingly, more girls (and even boys) suffer from typical and atypical eating disorders (so-called EDNOS for 'eating disorder not otherwise specified'), which are conditions only partially fulfilling the criteria for anorexia or bulimia, but are the source of much suffering, and often, of an overuse of health care (Chamay-Weber *et al.* 2005).

Most public health strategies addressing the area of overweight and obesity of young people have focused on the school setting. Several recent meta-analyses have reviewed the factors that contribute to the success of interventions in the field (Flodmark *et al.* 2006). In general, long-lasting programmes with a sound conceptual framework appear successful. Multifaceted interventions addressing intake as well as energy expenditure appear to be the most effective. An example of this approach is the CATCH intervention (Coordinated Approach to Child Health) run in 24 schools of the San Diego County in the United States, and directed at elementary and middle-school children. The intervention was designed to modify the pupils' environment by increasing the number and intensity of physical education sessions and modifying available food within the school. These principles apply to interventions targeting specifically obese adolescents as well.

Although encouraging youngsters to engage in physical activity has only a modest effect on their weight, it has a significant effect on health-compromising correlates of obesity such as glucose metabolism and cardiovascular fitness. The prevention of obesity should be progressively achieved through environmental measures set up in close collaboration with the food industry, such as political and economic measures, and large media campaigns. Physical and sports activities should be encouraged by increasing opportunities and facilities both within and outside the school. For instance, the European community set up the European Childhood Obesity Group, which has developed a comprehensive programme in cooperation with the food industry, advertisement agencies, and associations of consumers, and puts a strong emphasis on environmental measures (Widhalm & Fussenegger 2005).

Sexual and reproductive health

There is no area that has been more influenced by the biological and societal shifts reviewed at the beginning of this chapter as has the sexual and reproductive health of young people. Both societal transformation and behavioural patterns create a situation of unique vulnerabilities and expose young people to heightened risks for poor health outcomes, such as unplanned (early) pregnancy, STIs including HIV/AIDS, and sexual coercion and abuse (Bearinger *et al.* 2007). Biological as well as psychosocial factors contribute to this vulnerability: For example, young girls are at increased risk for acquiring an STI or facing difficulty in childbirth because of the immaturity of their reproductive and immune systems. The psychological vulnerability of adolescents, both girls and boys, also places them at greater risk of sexual exploitation, and in several countries, adolescents who are compelled to become sex workers are at heightened risk of STIs, pregnancy, and violence.

Sexual behaviour, contraception, and safe sex

Several surveys conducted among young people in high-income countries show that they tend to engage in premarital sexual activity in a progressive way; that is, from kissing to petting, and then, non-penetrative and penetrative intercourse (Brown *et al.* 2001), but this may not apply to some low-income countries where sexual activity starts with marriage, at least among women. Indeed, cultural and contextual factors do play an important role in the sequencing of these events. For instance, in the United States, which has promoted 'abstinence-only programmes', young people tend to replace penetrative vaginal intercourse with oral sex, which has raised a number of controversies in that country about the adequacy of this strategy (Brown *et al.* 2001).

The age at which young people tend to engage in sexual experiences varies, depending on contextual and cultural factors (Bearinger *et al.* 2007). In Africa, the percentage of young people aged 15–24 years reporting being sexually experienced varies between 30 and 60 per cent among males, and between 7 and 60 per cent among females. In Eastern Europe and Central Asia, the percentages among females and males are lower. In Latin America, they are between 40 and 60 per cent among males, and between 10 and 25 per cent among females ; whereas in high-income countries, the rates vary between 45 and 60 per cent, and are fairly similar among males and females.

In high-income as well as in many low- and middle-income countries, the gap between the first sexual intercourse and marriage is widening, which means that most early sexual experiences occur among unmarried young women and men. However, it has to be recognized that, in some places, many adolescent girls (an estimate of 100 million within the next 10 years) have their first sexual intercourse while married, with the consequence that they often do not use any contraception or protection and could be at high risk of acquiring STIs (Wellings *et al.* 2006).

The use of effective contraception and protection among young people has increased considerably over the last decades; around 1990, the reported rates were as low as 2–4 per cent in Africa and South America and between 10–30 per cent in the Middle East and Asia (Lloyd 2005). According to the most recent data available, in Africa and Latin America, it is around 20 per cent in the Middle East and around 50 per cent in Asia. As can be seen, the rates vary substantially from one region to another: In Western Europe, in the year 2000, 70–80 per cent of young people reported to have used effective contraception at first intercourse (Bajos & Guillaume 2003).

The most readily available contraceptive device is the condom, which also protects against STIs. It is thus very important to assess to what extent young people are informed on the issues of both contraception and infection protection, and are provided easy access to condoms. Many countries have embarked on information campaigns, resulting in increased condom usage among sexually active young people. Unfortunately, even in regions with high rates of HIV/AIDS, a substantial proportion of young people still do not use condoms: For example, the rates of males aged 15–24 years using condoms vary between 20 (e.g. in Mali, Haiti, and Malawi) and 40 per cent in many low-income countries.

Early childbearing and abortion

The average birth rate for young people varies considerably across regions (World Health Organization 2004a). In countries in sub-Saharan Africa, it ranges from 40–230 per 1000 adolescents; in North Africa, the Middle East, and Central and South Asia, the figures are lower (~7–120 per 1000). In Europe, the rates vary between a low of 5 per 1000 in Switzerland and a high of 40 per 1000 in Bulgaria. In South America, the figures vary roughly between 50 and 150 per 1000. The United States has a high rate of birth of around 40 per 1000, one of the highest among high-income countries, whereas Canada's rate is much lower at around 15 per 1000.

As a result of their biological immaturity and psychosocial vulnerability, adolescents who are pregnant face higher risks of medical complications and death. Indeed, maternal mortality and morbidity related to pregnancy constitute a significant threat to the health of many young women in low- and middle-income countries, especially among adolescents younger than 14 or 15 years of age. Worldwide, the death rates vary between around 6 per 100 000 in East Asia and 25 per 100 000 in North Africa and the Middle East (WHO 2001b). The gap between high-income countries and

low- and middle-income countries is impressive: The lifetime risk of dying from maternal causes is 1 in 2800 in wealthy countries whereas it reaches 1 in 61 in sub-Saharan African countries (Lloyd 2005). Besides death, childbearing at a younger age has a greater likelihood of complications such as infection, haemorrhage, eclampsia, obstructed labour, and vesicovaginal fistula. Many of these adverse consequences are linked with absence of services, poor access to adequate medical care, and lack of confidentiality, and may thus be addressed in the future by more adequate coverage of the specific needs of pregnant adolescents.

Faced with an unplanned pregnancy, girls may choose to have the baby or elect to have an abortion. Such decisions are not only dependent on personal and family factors, but are heavily linked to environmental and cultural factors as well. The number of abortions taking place outside the formal or legal health-care system or taking place in countries in which it is considered illegal is obviously difficult to estimate. Performed in adequate conditions, with up-to-date methods, abortion is safe and carries little health risks.

However, every year, about 19–20 million abortions are performed by individuals without adequate skills and in unsafe environments; 97 per cent of these are in low- and middle-income countries (Grimes *et al.* 2006). Young women aged 15–24 years account for about 25 per cent of these unsafe abortions in Africa, whereas the percentages are lower in Asia and Latin America. A recent comparison of birth and abortion rates among 46 countries showed that the adolescent birth rate has declined in the majority of industrialized countries over the past 25 years and that pregnancy rates in 12 of the 18 countries with accurate abortion reporting showed declines (Lloyd 2005).

Sexual coercion and violence, female genital mutilation

Sexual coercion can be defined as an act of forcing, or attempting to force, an individual to engage in sexual behaviour against his or her will, using violence, threats, verbal insistence, and deception. The consequences of such sexual violence both among females and males are important, including intense mental suffering, depression, post-traumatic stress disorder, and even suicide. Moreover, some young people may engage in casual and unsafe sex as a result of having experienced forced sex. Young female and young male adolescents with homosexual orientation are at high risk for such events because of their inexperience and because of the age gap with the perpetrator.

For social and cultural reasons, female genital mutilation (FGM) remains common in many countries, including African countries where over 136 million women have been 'multilated' despite persistent and consistent efforts by various governments (Magoha & Magoha 2000). Besides measures such as repression through legislation, which can be set up in these countries, proper education of young girls, and above all, sensitization of families and communities to change social norms in this area should be set up. Moreover, health professionals should be sensitized to this issue: Even Western high-income countries should consider the risk of FGM when caring for migrant adolescents from countries where these operations still take place.

STIs and HIV

The WHO (World Health Organization 2001a) estimated that there were 340 million new cases of syphilis, gonorrhoea, chlamydia, and trichomoniasis worldwide in 1999 in men and women aged 15–49 years, whereas in 1990, the figure was around 250 million new cases. Within and between countries, the prevalence and incidence of STIs vary greatly due to many factors such as differences between urban and rural environments, levels of knowledge, and availability of protection. STIs tend to occur at a younger age in females than in males, which may be explained by differences in patterns of sexual activity and in the relative rates of transmission from one sex to the other (World Health Organization 2001a). Data in this field must be interpreted with caution, because the surveillance of STI spread is a neglected field in many countries worldwide.

An estimated 38.6 million people worldwide were living with HIV in 2005. Every year, around 4.1 million become newly infected with HIV and around 2.8 million lose their lives to HIV-related illnesses. Globally, an estimated 10.3 million young people aged 15–24 years are living with HIV/AIDS, and half of all new infections—over 6000 daily—are occurring among young people. About two-thirds of young people aged 15–24 years with an HIV infection live in sub-Saharan African countries (Bearinger et al. 2007). Many young people are vulnerable to HIV because of unsafe sexual behaviour, substance use, and their lack of access to HIV information and prevention services.

Young people who are marginalized and homeless, injecting drugs, or working in the sex industry have the highest risks. The UN estimates that there are more than 150 million street children worldwide injecting drugs using non-sterile needles and syringes, accounting for an estimated 10 per cent of all new HIV infections. Intravenous drug use (IDU) is often initiated at a young age and, in some places, the injecting trend among young people is increasing. Moreover, it is estimated that only 16 per cent of HIV-positive youth know their serological status, which means that the vast majority of young people who are HIV-positive do not know that they are living with HIV. Moreover, few young people engaging in sex know the HIV status of their partners.

Primary prevention is the cornerstone of HIV/AIDS prevention and does actually also address the transmission of other STIs. A recent publication of the WHO (World Health Organization 2006) provides a comprehensive review of evidence-based strategies to reach this objective. A second important area of intervention is secondary prevention: Public health programmes should focus on offering HIV testing to young people to identify those who are already HIV-positive and to help them access the services that will keep them healthy and teach them the skills needed to protect their sex partners. Moreover, testing and identifying young people who are HIV-negative helps them to stay negative as long as they are provided counselling sessions along with the test itself.

Although the search for an effective vaccine against HIV is still on its way, the recent introduction of the human papilloma virus (HPV) vaccine gives a good example of future avenues to control the spread of some STIs. Worldwide, HPV infections are responsible for approximately 493 000 cervical cancer cases annually, about half of which result death each year (Bosch & de Sanjose 2003). It remains to be shown that, given the price of the vaccine and the logistics required to vaccinate young people, this vaccine will represent an effective means to prevent cervical cancer, especially in low- and middle-income countries.

Services, community health, and policies

The continuum–of–care approach is one that has been applied to maternal and child health and which is also applicable to adolescent health, in which interventions commonly aim to affect more than one health outcome (Mahler 1986). In this subsection, we describe approaches at three levels of care: Hospital care, ambulatory or primary-level care, and the scope for health promotion.

Youth-friendly health services

The WHO, in collaboration with UNICEF, developed the concept of adolescent- or youth-friendly health services (YFHS) (McInthyre 2003). This approach stressed the need for a holistic and developmental approach to ambulatory care for young people. Factors contributing to adolescent-friendly service delivery are outlined in Table 11.4.2. The principles of YFHS have initially been conceptualized and implemented in specialized ambulatory youth clinics. They are, however, relevant to other health-care settings such as inpatient hospital care.

There is growing evidence that younger patients experience better quality of care in adolescent wards compared to child or adult wards (Viner 2007), but this seems particularly relevant in high-income countries. A recent review concluded that: 'Enough is known to recommend that each country, state, and locality has a policy and support to encourage provision of innovative and well-assessed youth-friendly health services' (Tylee et al. 2007). The principles of adolescent-friendly health services are not only appropriate for creating specific youth clinics, but they also apply to existing school health centres, primary-care clinics, private practice, and outreach facilities.

Indeed, primary-care physicians play a role in promoting adolescent health through a strategy of providing health guidance

Table 11.4.2 Basic principles of youth-/adolescent-friendly services

Policies	◆ Fulfil the right of adolescents
	◆ Address the special needs of vulnerable adolescents
	◆ No stigmatization (ethnicity, social status, etc.)
	◆ Confidentiality guaranteed
	◆ Affordability of services
Procedures	◆ Easy access
	◆ Easy registration
	◆ Short waiting time
Healthcare providers	◆ Technically competent
	◆ Communication skills
	◆ Adequate time
	◆ Provide information and support
	◆ Evidence-based approach
Environment	◆ Convenient location
	◆ Convenient opening hours
	◆ Outreach activities
	◆ Link with the community
Youth participation	◆ Young people consulted/youth council
	◆ Young people's satisfaction surveyed
	◆ Young people disseminating information

Source: McInthyre P. Adolescent-friendly health services. Geneva: World Health Organization; 2003.

to adolescents and parents, screening, and encouraging immunizations; the rationale is that many aspects of lifestyle relevant to health are adopted in adolescence (Elster & Levenberg 1997). Goldenring and Rosen (Goldenring & Rosen 2004) proposed a simple mnemonic tool, HEEADSSS, to define the main areas to be covered in screening: Home, Education, Eating, Activities, Drugs, Sexuality, Suicide, and Security.

School-based preventive strategies

Adolescents, up to the age of 15–18 years, spend just under half their waking hours in school. Thus, schools remain one of the most important settings for health promotion and preventive interventions for young people, which include the following:

- Programmes aimed at increasing physical activity, often with a nutrition component: As in other instances, the available evidence suggests that programmes extending outside the school zone and involving the parents are more effective than those targeting the pupils only (Van Sluijs *et al.* 2007).

- Drug education, such as programmes promoting the adoption of life and social skills: Some evidence from efficacy trials shows that modest sustained effects in reducing uptake of licit and illicit drugs can take place with such programmes, but there are few models of effective, sustained, and system-wide implementation (Tobler 2000). Interventions involving parents and the community are more effective than those involving the students only (Kumpfer & Alvarado 2005).

- Sexuality education programmes: The issue of sexual education is a hotly debated one; carefully designed interventions such as those based on sound theoretical frameworks have had positive effects on the adoption of safe sex behaviours, without increasing the percentage of young people engaging in active sexual life (World Health Organization 2006).

The extension of health education to health promotion led the WHO to develop the concept of a health promoting school (HPS). The network of HPSs currently involves more than 35 countries. Schools commit to establishing a healthy physical and social environment. Youth participation such as setting up pupils' councils, or mediation sessions in case of conflict, and the use of life-skills interventions are encouraged. Some evidence supports key components of the HPS programme, namely that the programmes should be sustained, multifaceted, and have the commitment of the head of the school to provide appropriate training to the staff and to work in a holistic way (World Health Organization 2006). An excellent example of this approach was the Gatehouse project (Patton *et al.* 2006), a multilevel systemic programme focusing on promoting social inclusion of students with a view to promoting mental health and diminishing health-risk behaviours. Reductions in health-risk behaviours over a period of four years ranged from around 25 per cent for substance use and socially disruptive behaviours to around 50 per cent for levels of very early sexually activity. These are substantially greater than the effects obtained from health education alone and, given that they are largely based on changes in the schools' environment, offer a better prospect for sustainable system change.

Community health and policies

Other promising community strategies to promote the health of young people include media campaigns, the adoption of policies outside the health sector, and interventions within the community. In the field of smoking prevention, a recent review has shown some superiority of programmes involving the whole community over traditional approaches targeting young people only (Sowden *et al.* 2003). Community-based preventive interventions have shown an effect on youth substance use (Wu *et al.* 2002), suicide (Omar 2005), harmful drinking (Stafstrom *et al.* 2006), and rates of teen pregnancy (Cassell *et al.* 2005).

The International Policy Context around Adolescent Health and Development has received considerable attention in the past five years with a range of initiatives affecting the way in which health and other systems address young people and their development. Several of these initiatives have frameworks that extend beyond a health focus, a concept referred to as the 'new public health'. The World Bank Report on (Adolescent) Development and the Next Generation (World Bank 2007) dealt with the potential for interventions around young people to have a impact on the health and development of the next generation. The report took important steps in outlining a comprehensive framework for youth health and development. It focused on investments in five areas: Reducing health risks, promoting education, ensuring transition into employment, promoting citizenship, and family formation. The report stressed the value of a broad policy framework in that education and the transition to employment affect health risks.

Another broad initiative with a potential impact on the health of young people is the Millennium Development Goals (MDGs) which was adopted by the UN General Assembly in 2000. They have provided a framework for cooperation across the UN agencies. The MDGs grew out of an overall aim of reducing extreme poverty. As far as adolescent health is concerned, they focus on HIV prevention and the prevention of mortality in young mothers.

As already mentioned, all the available evidence accumulated in these reports show that, besides the quality of the health-care system and the preventive strategies set up, in most if not all countries, the level of education attained should be looked at as one of the main determinants of health. Adolescents from poor families who drop out of school do much worse than those from wealthier families who have greater access to education and employment (World Bank 2007). Thus, improving health literacy and the level of education of the adolescent population as well as providing young people with a perspective of their professional future and role in the society is probably one of the single most effective ways to improve their health and well-being.

Future directions

The advances in developing policy frameworks and recommendations outlined earlier raise questions about how to measure the progress made as well as the functioning of service systems. Several groups have proposed indicators ranging from health measures to sociodemographic determinants and health-system indicators (Harris *et al.* 2006). Currently, most agencies do not provide numbers by five-year strata, even for such basic data as mortality. Because indicators are essential for the monitoring of public health policies as well as for advocacy, it is important to achieve a fair consensus in this area in the future. Also, although we have more and more data showing evidence of what works (Evidence for Policy and Practice Information and Co-ordinating Centre 2002; Health Evidence Network, World Health Organization 2006), such information remains limited by the paucity of available evidence-based evaluations conducted outside high-income countries. Some of the approaches that have been validated in specific settings and ethnic backgrounds may not be as effective for young people and communities outside the cultural mainstream. Still another limitation is that most of the 'evidence-based' approaches that are available have emerged from randomized controlled trials (RCTs), which may limit their broad application in the public health context. Several authors have proposed more feasible and valid alternatives to RCTs, insisting on the importance of taking into account the context of the research and the interest of measuring trends over time (Victora *et al.* 2004).

Another more strategic issue is whether to put emphasis on the prevention of specific health problems or to use a more holistic health-promotion approach. Both strategies work, and may need to be used in judiciously in combination. 'New public health' has called for an approach to adolescent health that cuts across traditional fields such as social welfare, education, environment, and the health sectors. In many countries, basic public health engineering has been achieved, such as immunization, but new factors including psychological, social, and economic, and are becoming increasingly relevant as determinants of health and causes of illness, such as access to higher education and reduction of socioeconomic disparities.

Conceptual approaches targeting the whole population (and not only adolescents) may indeed positively impact on the health of young people. It requires better sensitization of politicians and policy makers to the health consequences of decisions and policies developed outside the field of health. An example of such a strategy comes from the Swedish Parliament, which in 2003 adopted a policy aimed to create social conditions that would ensure good health for the entire population, identifying the contribution of other sectors in creating safe environments and products, including the participation of the society (Hogstedt *et al.* 2004).

Conclusion

Young people aged 10–24 years represent a large part of the population, especially in low- and middle-income countries, where they will constitute about 1.5 billion people by 2050. Important epidemiological shifts have occurred and are still occurring in terms of the main health problems affecting young people. We have reviewed several types of strategies that can potentially address these important issues, which are as follows:

♦ The health-care system has to develop specific responses, taking into account the bio-psychosocial and developmental specificities of adolescents and their struggle for autonomy. Health-care settings and staff have to become more accessible and user-friendly to young people.

♦ We now have good evidence that the school setting can implement and sustain effective programmes to address specific problems as well as, more globally, the well-being of pupils. Implementing sound information provision and life skills building approaches as well as fostering a climate of confidence and trust among pupils and between pupils and teachers has a positive impact in terms of healthy habits as well as mental health.

♦ Young people as well as their parents and the community members should participate in the conceptualizing and implementing

of preventive programmes. Young people represent an enormous resource that has proven extremely useful when used appropriately by health professionals, educators, or even policy makers.

♦ At a global level, there is substantial evidence showing that legislative and environmental policies—such as easy access to health care and contraception, improvement of traffic conditions, limitation of access to legal drugs or to lethal weapons, control of the quality of foods served in school or provided in shopping areas, and better access to sports areas—impact positively on the health of young people.

♦ Improving the socioeconomic conditions in which deprived families live positively affects the health of young people as well as the other segments of the population.

♦ Above all, improving health literacy and the level of education of adolescents as well as providing them with a perspective of their role in society is probably one of the single most effective ways to improve their health and well-being.

References

Bajos N., Guillaume A.K.O., editors. *Reproductive health behaviour of young Europeans*. Strasbourg, France: Council of Europe; 2003.

Bearinger L.H., Sieving R.E., Ferguson J. *et al.* Global perspectives on the sexual and reproductive health of adolescents: patterns, prevention, and potential. *Lancet* 2007;**369**:1220–31.

Beautrais A.L., Wells J.E., McGee M.A. *et al.* Suicidal behaviour in Te Rau Hinengaro: the New Zealand Mental Health Survey. *The Australian and New Zealand Journal of Psychiatry* 2006;**40**:896–904.

Blum R. Global trends in adolescent health. *Journal of the American Medical Association* 1991;**265**:2711–9.

Blum R.W., McNeely C., Nonnemaker J. Vulnerability, risk, and protection. *The Journal Adolescent Health* 2002;**31** Suppl 1:28–39.

Blum R.W., Nelson-Mmari K. The health of young people in a global context. *The Journal of Adolescent Health* 2004;**35**:402–18.

Bonomo Y.A., Bowes G., Coffey C. *et al.* Teenage drinking and the onset of alcohol dependence: a cohort study over seven years. *Addiction* 2004;**99**:1520–8.

Bosch F.X., de Sanjose S. Human papilloma virus and cervical cancer – burden and assessment of causality. *Journal of the National Cancer Institute (Monographs)* 2003;**31**:3–13.

Brown A.D., Jejeebhoy S., Shah I. *et al.*, editors. Sexual relations among young people in developing countries: evidence from WHO case studies. Geneva: World Health Organization; 2001.

Cassell C., Santelli J., Gilbert B.C. *et al.* Mobilizing communities: an overview of the Community Coalition Partnership Programs for the Prevention of Teen Pregnancy. *The Journal of Adolescent Health* 2005; **37** Suppl 3:S3–10.

Centers for Disease Control. Use of cigarettes and other tobacco products among students aged 13–15 years worldwide, 1999–2005. *Morbidity and Mortality Weekly Report* 2007;**55**:553–6.

Chamay-Weber C., Narring F., Michaud P.A. Partial eating disorders among adolescents: a review. *The Journal of Adolescent Health* 2005;**37**:417–27.

Dahlberg L.L., Potter L.B. Youth violence. Developmental pathways and prevention challenges. *American Journal of Preventive Medicine* 2001; **20** Suppl 1:3–14.

Elster A.B., Levenberg P. Integrating comprehensive adolescent preventive services into routine medicine care. *Rationale and approaches. Pediatric Clinics of North America* 1997;**44**:1365–77.

Evidence for Policy and Practice Information and Co-ordinating (EPPI) Centre. Barriers to and facilitators of the health of young people: a systematic review of evidence on young people's views and on interventions in mental health, physical activity, and healthy eating.

London: Evidence for Policy and Practice Information and Co-ordinating Centre; 2002.

Flodmark C.E., Marcus C., Britton M. Interventions to prevent obesity in children and adolescents: a systematic literature review. *International Journal of Obesity (2005)* 2006;**30**:579–89.

Goldenring J., Rosen D. Getting into adolescent heads: an essential update. *Contemporary Pediatrics* 2004;**21**:64–90.

Grimes D.A., Benson J., Singh S. *et al*. Unsafe abortion: the preventable pandemic. *Lancet* 2006;**368**:1908–19.

Harris K.M., Gordon-Larsen P., Chantala K. *et al*. Longitudinal trends in race/ethnic disparities in leading health indicators from adolescence to young adulthood. *Archives of Pediatrics and Adolescent Medicine* 2006;**160**:74–81.

Hawkins J.D., Abbott R., Catalano R.F. *et al*. Assessing effectiveness of drug abuse prevention: implementation issues relevant to long-term effects and replication. *NIDA Research Monograph* 1991;**107**:195–212.

Hawkins J.D., Kosterman R., Catalano R.F. *et al*. Promoting positive adult functioning through social development intervention in childhood: long-term effects from the Seattle Social Development Project. *Archives of Pediatrics and Adolescent Medicine* 2005;**159**:25–31.

Hawton K., James A. Suicide and deliberate self-harm in young people. *British Medical Journal* 2005;**330**:891–4.

Health Evidence Network, World Health Organization. *What is the evidence on school health promotion in improving health or preventing disease?* Geneva: World Health Organization; 2006.

Hogstedt C., Lundgren B., Moberg H. *et al*. The Swedish public health policy and the National Institute of Public Health. *Scandinavian Journal of Public Health (Supplement)* 2004;**64**:6–64.

Kodjo C.M., Klein J.D. Prevention and risk of adolescent substance abuse. The role of adolescents, families, and communities. *Pediatric Clinics of North America* 2002;**49**:257–68.

Korf D.J. Dutch coffee shops and trends in cannabis use. *Addictive Behaviors* 2002;**27**:851–66.

Kumpfer K.L., Alvarado R. Family-strengthening approaches for the prevention of youth problem behaviors. *The American Psychologist* 2005;**58**:457–65.

Lloyd C. *Growing up global: the changing transitions to adulthood in developing countries*. Washington (DC): National Research Council and Institute of Medicine, National Academies Press; 2005.

Lobstein T., Frelut M.L. Prevalence of overweight among children in Europe. *Obesity Reviews* 2003;**4**:195–200.

Lopez A.D., Mathers C.D. Measuring the global burden of disease and epidemiological transitions: 2002(2030. *Annals of Tropical Medicine and Parasitology* 2006;**100**:481–99.

Magoha G.A., Magoha O.B. Current global status of female genital mutilation: a review. *East African Medical Journal* 2000;**77**:268–72.

Mahler H. International Conference on Health Promotion in industrialized countries; 1986 Nov 17–21; Ottawa, Canada. *Canadian Journal of Public Health* 1986;**77**:387–92.

McAlister A.L. Acceptance of killing and homicide rates in nineteen nations. *European Journal of Public Health* 2006;**16**:260–6.

McCambridge J., Strang J. The efficacy of single-session motivational interviewing in reducing drug consumption and perceptions of drug-related risk and harm among young people: results from a multi-site cluster randomized trial. *Addiction* 2004;**99**:39–52.

McInthyre P. *Adolescent-friendly health services*. Geneva: World Health Organization; 2003.

Michaud P.A., Fombonne E. Common mental health problems. *British Medical Journal* 2005;**330**:835–8.

Michaud P.A., Suris J.C., Deppen A. Gender-related psychological and behavioural correlates of pubertal timing in a national sample of Swiss adolescents. *Molecular and Cellular Endocrinology* 2006;**254–255**:172–8.

Munro J., Coleman P., Nicholl J. *et al*. Can we prevent accidental injury to adolescents?. *A systematic review of the evidence. Injury Prevention* 1995;**1**:249–55.

Musaiger A.O. Overweight and obesity in the Eastern Mediterranean region: can we control it?. *Eastern Mediterranean Health Journal* 2004;**10**:789–93.

Ogden C.L., Carroll M.D., Flegal K.M. Epidemiologic trends in overweight and obesity. *Endocrinology and Metabolism Clinics of North America* 2003;**32**(vii):741–60.

Omar H.A. A model program for youth suicide prevention. *International Journal of Adolescent Medicne and Health* 2005;**17**:275–8.

Ong K.K., Ahmed M.L., Dunger D.B. Lessons from large population studies on timing and tempo of puberty (secular trends and relation to body size): the European trend. *Molecular and Cellular Endocrinology* 2006; **254–255**:8–12.

Patel V., Flisher A.J., Hetrick S. *et al*. Mental health of young people: a global public-health challenge. *Lancet* 2007;**369**:1302–13.

Patton G.C., Bond L., Carlin J.B. *et al*. Promoting social inclusion in schools: a group-randomized trial of effects on student health risk behaviour and well-being. *American Journal of Public Health* 2006;**96**:1582–7.

Patton G.C., Viner R. Pubertal transitions in health. *Lancet* 2007;**369**:1130–9.

Ploeg J., Ciliska D., Dobbins M. *et al*. A systematic overview of adolescent suicide prevention programs. *Canadian Journal of Public Health* 1996;**87**:319–24.

Rutter M., Smith D. Psychosocial disorders in young people. Time trends and their causes. New York (NY): Wiley; 1995.

Santelli J., Ott M.A., Lyon M. *et al*. Abstinence and abstinence-only education: a review of U.S. *policies and programs. The Journal of Adolescent Health* 2006;**38**:72–81.

Sowden A., Arblaster L., Stead L. Community interventions for preventing smoking in young people. [Online]. *Cochrane Database of Systematic Reviews* 2003;(1):CD001291.

Stafstrom M., Ostergren P.O., Larsson S. *et al*. A community action programme for reducing harmful drinking behaviour among adolescents: the Trelleborg Project. *Addiction* 2006;**101**:813–23.

Steinberg L., Morris A.S. Adolescent development. *Annual Review of Psychology* 2001;**52**:83–110.

Steinberg L. Risk taking in adolescence: what changes, and why?. *Annals of the New York Academy of Sciences* 2004;**1021**:51–8.

Tobler N. School-based adolescent drug prevention programs: 1998 meta-analysis. *The Journal of Primary Prevention* 2000;**20**:275–336.

Toroyan T., Preden M. *Youth and road safety*. Geneva: World Health Organization; 2007.

Toumbourou J.W., Stockwell T., Neighbors C. *et al*. Interventions to reduce harm associated with adolescent substance use. *Lancet* 2007;**369**: 1391–401.

Tremblay R.E. Prevention of youth violence: why not start at the beginning?. *Journal of Abnormal Child Psychology* 2006;**34**:481–7.

Tylee A., Haller D.M., Graham T. *et al*. Youth-friendly primary-care services: how are we doing and what more needs to be done?. *Lancet* 2007;**369**:1565–73.

UNAIDS. AIDS epidemic update: December 2006. Geneva: UNAIDS; 2006.

United Nations Economic and Social Council, Commission on Narcotic Drugs. Youth and drugs: a global overview. Report of the 42nd session of the Secretariat; 1991 Mar 16–25; Vienna. Available from: http://www.unodc.org/pdf/document_1999-01-11_2.pdf [Accessed on 2008 Feb 4].

United Nations. Millennium development goals. Available from: http:// www.un.org/millenniumgoals/

United Nations. *World youth report*. New York (NY): United Nations; 2005. p. 148–60.

Van Sluijs E.M., McMinn A.M., Griffin S.J. Effectiveness of interventions to promote physical activity in children and adolescents: systematic review of controlled trials. *British Medical Journal* 2007;**335**:703.

Victora C., Habicht J., Bryce J. Evidence-based public health: moving beyond randomized trials. *American Journal of Public Health* 2004;**94**:400–5.

Viner R.M. Do adolescent inpatient wards make a difference? Findings from a national young patient survey. *Pediatrics* 2007;**120**:749–55.

Wang Y., Monteiro C., Popkin B.M. Trends of obesity and underweight in older children and adolescents in the United States, Brazil, China, and Russia. *The American Journal of Clinical Nutrition* 2002;**75**:971–7.

Wasserman D., Cheng Q., Jiang G.X. Global suicide rates among young people aged 15–19. *World Psychiatry* 2005;**4**:114–20.

Wellings K., Collumbien M., Slaymaker E. *et al.* Sexual behaviour in context: a global perspective. *Lancet* 2006;**368**:1706–28.

Widhalm K., Fussenegger D. Actions and programs of European countries to combat obesity in children and adolescents: a survey. *International Journal of Obesity (2005)* 2005;**29** Suppl 2:130–5.

Wilson J.F. Finland pioneers international suicide prevention. *Annals of Internal Medicine* 2004;**140**:853–6.

World Bank. World development report: development and the next generation. Washington (DC): World Bank; 2007.

World Health Organization. *Adolescent pregnancy: issues in adolescent health and development.* Geneva: World Health Organization; 2004a.

World Health Organization. *Caring for children and adolescents with mental disorders.* Geneva: World Health Organization; 2003.

World Health Organization. Global prevalence and incidence of selected curable sexually transmitted infections. Geneva: World Health Organization; 2001a.

World Health Organization. Growing in confidence: programming for adolescent health and development. Geneva: World Health Organization; 2002a.

World Health Organization. *Injury: a leading cause of the global burden of disease.* Geneva: World Health Organization; 2002b.

World Health Organization. Preventing HIV/AIDS in young people: a systematic review of the evidence from developing countries. Geneva: World Health Organization; 2006.

World Health Organization. Preventing violence: a guide to implementing the recommendations of the world report on violence and health. Geneva: World Health Organization; 2004c.

World Health Organization. *Prevention of mental disorders. Effective interventions and policy options.* A report of the WHO, Department of Mental Health and Substance Abuse in collaboration with the Prevention Research Unit of the Universities of Nijmegen and Maastricht. Geneva: World Health Organization; 2004b.

World Health Organization. *World health report. Mental health: new understanding, new hope.* Geneva: World Health Organization; 2001b.

Wu Z., Detels R., Zhang J. *et al.* Community-based trial to prevent drug use among youths in Yunnan, China. *American Journal of Public Health* 2002;**92**:1952–7.

Zaborskis A., Sumskas L., Maser M. *et al.* Trends in drinking habits among adolescents in the Baltic countries over the period of transition: HBSC survey results, 1993–2002. *BMC Public Health* 2006;**6**:67.

Ethnic minorities and indigenous peoples

Myfanwy Morgan, Martin Gulliford, and Ian Anderson

Abstract

This chapter considers the health of ethnic minorities and indigenous peoples. The term *ethnicity* is currently employed to refer to
groupings of people defined according to shared characteristics
including ancestral and geographical origins, cultural tradition,
language, and religion. Ethnicity is a fluid, multifaceted construct
whose characteristics are not fixed or easily measurable, with classification dependent on context. The concept of ethnicity has
superseded the largely discredited biological notion of racial differences that emerged in the first half of the nineteenth century as the
basis for differentiating groups in a population. The term *indigenous
peoples* refers to groups who are descendants of populations that
inhabited a country or geographical region at the time of conquest
or colonization and who retain some or all of their own social, economic, cultural, and political institutions. Ethnic-minority and
indigenous populations generally have younger age distributions
than the majority of the population, and often show some degree
of concentration into geographically distinct areas or communities.
Where data are available, ethnic minorities and indigenous peoples
may have increased mortality and diminished life expectancy compared with the majority, demonstrating an ethnic patterning of
cause-specific mortality and morbidity. Determinants of health
that are of particular relevance for explaining the ethnic patterning
of health outcomes include genetics, culture and lifestyles, consequences of migration and discrimination, lack of access to services,
and socioeconomic inequalities and poverty, all of which are inter-
related. The significance of these determinants may vary for different
health outcomes and in different contexts. More recent perspectives regard cultural beliefs and identities as flexible and shaped by
the structural conditions of people's lives and experiences. The
final section of the chapter considers policies at the societal level,
including the question of self-determination for indigenous peoples, the assumptions and ideology of multiculturalism, and the
critiques of this approach.

Introduction

This chapter analyses, from the standpoint of public health, the
health of ethnic minorities and indigenous peoples. The health
status of ethnic-minority groups and indigenous populations is
important for several reasons. From the perspective of the 'right to
the highest attainable level of health', the ethnic patterning of
health outcomes observed in many populations may indicate that
the right to health is not equally respected, protected, or fulfilled
for all groups. Ethnic inequalities in health are particularly likely
to be inequitable and unfair, stemming from wider social inequalities and the experience of deprivation across a range of social and
environmental domains. Ethnic variation in health status may also
be indicative of particular health needs that should be addressed
through appropriate policies and services. Research into ethnicity
and health may sometimes also provide insights into the causes of
disease.

The first section of the chapter explores the concepts of ethnicity,
race, and indigenous peoples. It also examines approaches to the
classification of ethnic groups. The next section presents empirical
data for several aspects of health status in relation to ethnic-minority
or indigenous status. This is followed by an analysis of traditional
approaches for explaining health risks and behaviour patterns of
ethnic minorities and indigenous people in terms of distinct determinants, including economic disadvantage and cultural beliefs and
behaviours. This is contrasted with more recent perspectives that
regard cultural beliefs and identities as flexible and shaped by the
structural conditions of people's lives and experiences, with examples of the significance of ethnicity and identity.

The concept of ethnicity

The concept of ethnicity is derived from the Greek word *ethnos*—
meaning a nation, people, or tribe—and is currently employed to
refer to groupings that people belong to, or are perceived to belong
to, based on certain shared characteristics. These characteristics
typically include ancestral and geographical origins, cultural tradition, language, and religion. Ethnicity is, thus, a multifaceted
construct whose characteristics are not fixed or easily measurable.
The concepts of ethnicity and ethnic groups have increasingly
replaced the biological notion of racial differences that emerged in
the first half of the nineteenth century as the basis for differentiating
groups in the population.

Concept of race: Use and misuse

The historical notion of racial groups assumed that humankind could be differentiated into distinct subgroups based on physical characteristics, such as skin colour, hair type, eye colour, shape of head and face, and specific features such as the nose and lips. Underpinning this interest in racial types were questions of whether these biological differences were associated with indicators of social worth, particularly intelligence, and thus with the superiority and inferiority of different peoples. This notion of racial differences reflected the belief in a natural biological hierarchy, and led to the development of various crude classifications. These were based on continental groupings and trace their origin to Linnaeus (1806), a biologist who devised a biological classification of all living things (cited in Bhopal 2007). Linnaeus' grouping of humans had four categories: *Homo afer* (later synonyms: Black, African origin, Negro, Negroid), *Homo europaeus* (later synonyms: white, European origin, Caucasian, Caucasoid), *Homo asiaticus* (later synonyms: Mongoloid, Asian), and *Homo americanus* (later synonyms: American Indian, North American Indian, Native American). Variants of such classifications also have a grouping for the Aborigines (Australia).

From the 1930s, the concept of race was increasingly criticized for its use in justifying the unequal treatment of racial groups, involving economic exploitation, segregation, and genocide. This criticism was fuelled by the Nazi's abuse of the concept of race during World War II. Attempts to distinguish racial types have been shown to lack biological foundation and scientific legitimacy. This view was supported by evidence that 90–95 per cent of the genetic variation occurs within rather than among allegedly different races. Furthermore, only small differences in genotype are identified as being responsible for differences in facial and skin colour characteristics that form supposedly essential markers of racial difference (Cooper *et al.* 2003). Another conceptual distinction can be made based on much of contemporary thinking in population genetics, that the distribution of many gene frequencies is graduated across populations. Whereas a biological concept of race assumes a particular genetic structure within a racially defined population this does not hold for the socially based concept of ethnicity. However, the concept of ethnicity does not discount the role of genetic factors in some health conditions.

Concerns regarding both the biological basis and social misuse of racial categorizations has led to a shift from crude biological notions of race to the recognition that the variable of race measures some combination of social class, culture, and genes (Jones 2001). The concept of race, particularly the distinction between black and white racial groups, continues to be identified as a key social division in many countries. However, there is also increasing use of the concept of ethnicity to distinguish migrant groups, with the term *indigenous peoples* being used to refer to non-migrant minority groups, notably the Maoris (New Zealand), Native Americans, and the Inuit (Canada).

There are currently differing views regarding the importance of racial categories in the health field. Goldberg (1993), recognizing the contribution of genetic factors to disease, has argued for retention of the concept of races, while acknowledging that the use of this concept in modernity differs from the notions of superiority and inferiority that marked earlier usage and now merely identifies difference. Jones (2001), from a US perspective, similarly recommends the analysis of race-observed differences in health in order

to eliminate them, with the important provisos that race is regarded as a social rather than a biological category, the diversity within racial groups is acknowledged, and the impacts of social class and racism are measured in explaining differences in health. A more critical view is to reject racial classifications altogether on the grounds that race-based research is inherently racist. Osborne and Feit (1992) take this approach, observing that explanations of differences between blacks and whites in stigmatized conditions such as sexually transmitted diseases and mental illness are frequently attributed to race rather than to socioeconomic status and other aspects of their conditions of life. This often reflects a general failure to move beyond associations between racial groups and disease, with the causal mechanisms such as poverty or lack of access to services remaining unknown and hidden from view.

Concept of ethnicity

Concerns about the misuse of racial categories has led to an increased emphasis on the concept of ethnicity in order to describe the social groupings that people identify based on common descent and shared culture or history. Sivanandan (1987) has argued that differentiating racial groups in terms of ethnicity can have the negative effect of dividing people who experience racism. He favoured expanding boundaries and using the political term 'black' as a social construct (as opposed to a biological construct) to signify the shared interests of peoples of African, African-Caribbean, and South Asian descent. However, as Modood (1994) noted, many members of minority groups reject inclusion in the political term 'black', as this does not acknowledge the substantial variations that exist in economic advantage with a consequent lack of shared class interests.

Classification of ethnicity

The development of acceptable and useful ethnic classifications has proved difficult and classifications currently vary between countries (see Bhopal 2007). This partly reflects the particular composition and characteristics of migrant groups arising from historical patterns of migration. For example, the group categorized as 'Asian' in the United States reflects particular patterns of migration to that country and comprises people of Chinese, Japanese, and Malayan descent, whereas in the United Kingdom the category of 'Asian' refers to people from the Indian subcontinent, reflecting the major migrations from India, Pakistan, and Bangladesh. Other differences are in the numbers of categories identified and variations in the marker of ethnicity employed (e.g. ethnic origin or self-identity).

The Canadian census uses one of the most detailed ethnic classifications and focuses on individuals' origins as the marker of ethnicity. The 2001 Canadian census identified 25 ethnic categories and sub-categories that included British Isles origins; Aboriginal origins; Caribbean origins; Latin American, Central American, and South American origins; African origins; Arab origins; West Indian origins; and South Asian origins. In the United States census, five major groups have been identified: black or African-American; white; Asian; native Hawaiian or other Pacific Islander; and American Indian or Alaska native. A distinction is also made between Hispanic and non-Hispanic ethnicity. In the United Kingdom, an ethnic classification that focused on self-perceived ethnicity as the marker was first introduced in the 1991 census, at a time when over half the black ethnic groups were born in the United Kingdom. Subsequently, a more comprehensive classification was included in the 2001 census. New features were to specifically identify Irish self-identity within the white population (although neglect of other white groups reflects the tendency to regard white ethnicity as invisible) and the introduction of categories that acknowledge the increasing numbers of people of mixed parentage and identity (14.6 per cent of the ethnic-minority population; Table 11.5.1).

Ethnic classifications lend themselves to subdivision, as with the distinction between black African and black Caribbean. White people may similarly perceive themselves as English, Turkish, Irish, Swedish, etc. However, individuals' self-perceived ethnicity may depend on context. For example, people who identify themselves as Nigerian in their country of origin may define themselves as black African or black British in the United Kingdom. Differences in self-perceived ethnicity also occur across generations. Migrants from the Caribbean to the United Kingdom in the 1950s and 1960s often identified themselves as coming from a particular island or from the West Indies, whereas today second- and third-generation migrants tend to perceive themselves as black British, black Caribbean, or African-Caribbean. Broad ethnic groupings also describe heterogeneous categories that may mask important variations by country of origin, religion, education, language, and diet. In the United Kingdom, people categorized as Asian were characterized by differences in language, religion, education, and place of origin,

with the Indian group including Hindu (45 per cent), Sikh (29 per cent), and Muslim (13 per cent). People classified as black African come from a number of African countries with different cultural traditions, religions, and languages and include disproportionate numbers in the professional classes, and unemployed and semi-skilled workers. Neglect of such substantial within-group variations leads to dangers of stereotyped assumptions.

Examples of ethnicity in different contexts

Table 11.5.1 provides data on the ethnic composition of three countries: Trinidad and Tobago, England and Wales, and the United States of America. In these countries, both the classification of ethnicity and the ethnic distributions of populations reflect the differing histories and cultures of the three countries.

In Trinidad and Tobago, before the first arrival of Europeans, there was an indigenous population of 30 000–40 000; however, this population declined rapidly after European colonization and is no longer distinguishable. The largest groups are now formed of well-established populations of African or Indian-subcontinent descent who migrated to the islands, under varying degrees of coercion, as agricultural workers mostly in the period between 1783 and 1919 (Brereton 1981). There is an increasing group of 'mixed ethnicity', as well as small but economically significant

Table 11.5.1 Distribution of population by ethnic group in three countries

Trinidad and Tobago (2000)		England and Wales (2001)		United States (2000)	
Ethnic group	Per cent population	Ethnic group	Per cent population	Ethnic group	Per cent population
African descent	37.5	White:		White	75.1
Indian descent	40.0	British	87.0	Black/African American	12.3
White	0.6	Irish	1.3	American Indian/Alaska native	0.9
Chinese	0.3	Other	2.7	Asian:	3.6
Mixed	20.5	Mixed:		Asian Indian	0.6
Other	0.3	White and black Caribbean	0.5	Chinese	0.9
Not stated	0.8	White and black African	0.2	Filipino	0.7
		White and Asian	0.4	Japanese	0.3
		Other	0.3	Korean	0.4
		Asian/Asian British:		Vietnamese	0.4
		Indian	2.1	Other Asian	0.5
		Pakistani	1.4	Native Hawaiian and Other	
		Bangladeshi	0.6	Pacific Islander	0.1
		Other Asian	0.5	Some other race	5.5
		Black/black British:		Two or more races	2.4
		Caribbean	1.1		
		African	1.0		
		Other	0.2		
		Chinese	0.4		
		Other	0.4		

Source: Trinidad and Tobago Central Statistical Office. *Statistical pocket digest*. Port of Spain: Central Statistical Office; 2004; Office for National Statistics. *Census 2001: ethnicity and religion in England and Wales*. London: Office for National Statistics; 2007; United States Census Bureau. *Overview of race and Hispanic origin*. Washington (DC): United States Census Bureau Population Division; 2007.

groups of Chinese, Portuguese, and Lebanese or Syrian origin. In Fenton's (1999) classification, Trinidad and Tobago provides an example of ethnic groups in a plural society.

In England, the white population remains the largest ethnic group, but there are significant populations of Indian-subcontinent and African descent who migrated to England in the period after 1945. The group of African descent can be separated into earlier migrants from the Caribbean islands and more recent arrivals from various African countries. The Indian-subcontinent-origin population in England includes groups that are diverse with respect to language, religion, culture, and national origin, including people from India, Pakistan, and Bangladesh, as well as migrants from Indian-origin communities in East Africa and elsewhere. There are a wide range of smaller ethnic groups, including significant numbers from Southern Europe, and a growing population of migrants from Eastern Europe. England exemplifies the typology of ethnic groups as urban minorities derived from migrant worker populations (Fenton 1999).

In the United States, indigenous populations now represent a small minority. The largest ethnic grouping is formed from the descendants of settler migrants who travelled from Western Europe between the seventeenth and twentieth centuries. However, there is a significant African-American population mostly descending from involuntary migrants from West African countries between the seventeenth and nineteenth centuries. There is also a significant 'Asian' grouping in the United States, but this is more diverse in origin than in the United Kingdom. In the United States, ethnic minorities represent three distinct typologies including an indigenous minority, a post-slavery minority, and an urban-migrant minority group (Fenton 1999).

These data from three countries in the Western hemisphere illustrate how the ethnic composition of contemporary populations is generally formed through the interaction between the indigenous population and migrant groups that have moved to a country at different times in history. Migration is driven by social, political, and economic forces that are, to a greater or lesser extent, unique to a given national context. These influences also determine the experience of immigrant populations. In the United States, the African-American population was for a long time the subject of systematic segregation, discrimination, and denial of civil rights. These problems have only begun to be addressed in recent decades. In Trinidad and Tobago, a somewhat similar state of affairs existed during the colonial era but, in contrast to the United States, this experience generally applied to each of the major population groups and was ended as the country became independent (Brereton 1981). In England, large-scale immigration is a more recent phenomenon and, although difficulties with discrimination exist, the civil rights of ethnic minorities as well as their access to services are officially protected and promoted. These formative influences have implications for the determinants of health experienced by ethnic groups and influence the comparative age distribution of different ethnic groupings, their socioeconomic position, and geographical concentration.

Age distribution

Table 11.5.2 shows the proportion of the population in different age groups for the three countries. In Trinidad and Tobago, the population has a young age distribution, consistent with its status as a middle-income country. However, the age distribution of the

Table 11.5.2 Age-distribution in relation to ethnicity in three countries

Country and ethnic group	Age group (years)	
	< 15	≥ 65
Trinidad and Tobago (1990)		
African descent	33	8
East Indian	31	4
Mixed	41	6
United Kingdom (2001)[a]		
White British	19	16
Indian	22	6
Pakistani	35	4
Bangladeshi	38	3
Other Asian	22	4
Black Caribbean	25	9
Black African	33	2
Mixed	55	2
United States (2000)		
White	19	14
African-American	26	8
Asian	20	8

Figures are percentages of the total.

[a] Data are for <16 years.

Source: Trinidad and Tobago Central Statistical Office. *Statistical pocket digest*. Port of Spain: Central Statistical Office; 2004; Office for National Statistics. *Annual local area labour force survey*. London: Office for National Statistics; 2002; United States Census Bureau. *Overview of race and Hispanic origin*. Washington (DC): United States Census Bureau Population Division; 2007.

population is similar in each ethnic group, which reflects the fact that the majority of the population have been established in the country over several generations. In the United Kingdom, in contrast, ethnic-minority populations are generally more youthful, with a higher proportion of children and a much smaller proportion of old people. This is a consistent finding across all the ethnic groups. There is also a different age distribution between older first-generation migrants and younger second-generation immigrants who were born in Britain. Data for the United States are between those obtained from the other two countries.

Geographical concentration and deprivation

Ethnic-minority groups are typically unevenly distributed geographically forming, to a greater or lesser extent, defined communities characterized by concentration according to ethnic group. In Trinidad at the 1990 census, African and Indian groups each contributed about 40 per cent of the total population, but people of Indian descent only comprised 11 per cent of the population of the capital Port of Spain; in contrast, in the town of Chaguanas in Central Trinidad, 65 per cent of the population were of Indian descent (Republic of Trinidad and Tobago, Central Statistical Office 1994). This distribution reflects local employment patterns; the immigrant Indian population was initially employed in agriculture and is still now more heavily concentrated in the former sugar-producing areas of the country.

In the United Kingdom, there is also significant spatial concentration of minority ethnic groups, in this case towards the inner cities. At the 1991 census, 35 per cent of the total UK population was located in nine metropolitan areas compared with 81.1 per cent for black Caribbeans, 86.5 per cent for black Africans, 67.8 per cent for Indians, 71.1 per cent for Pakistanis, and 77.6 per cent for Bangladeshis (Peach 1996). This concentration was still present at the 2001 census but there was evidence of ethnic minorities migrating out from these areas of concentration, leading to increasing diversity in other areas (Rees & Butt 2004). Data for the 2001 census in England have been analysed in relation to a small-area Index of Multiple Deprivation (IMD 2004), which summarizes measures of deprivation across seven domains (including income, employment, education, health and disability, housing, living environment, and crime). In the most deprived decile of areas, people of Bangladeshi and Pakistani origin made up a four-times higher proportion of the population than they did for England as a whole, whereas people of black Caribbean and black African descent represented a two and half times higher proportion of the population than they did for England as a whole. The distribution of the Indian-origin population varied in different regions. In London, Indians lived in areas with intermediate deprivation scores, whereas in the West Midlands they were more heavily concentrated in the most deprived areas.

In the United States, there is also a high degree of segregation of ethnic-minority groups by neighbourhood. Polednak (1997) used an index of residential dissimilarity to evaluate the segregation of African-Americans. The index gives an indication of the per cent of African-Americans that would have to move in order to achieve an even distribution. Across 38 metropolitan areas in 1990, the index gave values of 89 in Detroit, 87 in Chicago, 86 in Cleveland, and 84 in Milwaukee and Buffalo, with only two out of 38 metropolitan areas having values less than 50. Recently, African-American segregation has shown a modest decrease but segregation has increased for US 'Asians' and 'Hispanics' (Logan *et al.* 2004).

The geographical separation of minorities often provides a context in which the processes of social exclusion may be enacted (Peace 2001). The quality of housing, employment opportunities, and access to education and health services are characteristic of particular areas. The geographical context may therefore be associated with the social, economic, and health outcomes achieved by ethnic minorities. In the United States, for example, black:white mortality differentials at area level are strongly associated with indicators of segregation (Polednak 1997). These processes of social exclusion are particularly relevant to the experience of indigenous peoples.

The concept of indigenous peoples

On 13 September 2007, the United Nations General Assembly adopted a Declaration on the Rights of Indigenous Peoples (hereafter the Declaration). There had been over two decades of negotiations between representatives of indigenous peoples and governments within the United Nations system. The international political movement that led to this result provoked considerable—at times apparently intransigent—debate on the definition of indigenous peoples and the rights that were consequent to this. There was, for example, an ongoing dispute between indigenous delegates and states about whether the appropriate terminology should be indigenous peoples, indigenous people, or indigenous populations (Niezen 2003). Some governments resisted the use of the first

construct—on the basis that the other terms inferred that indigenous people had collective rights, such as self-determination (Niezen 2003; Feiring & Partners 2003). Others governments denied that there were indigenous peoples within their jurisdiction notwithstanding the contrary claims of representatives of those peoples.

In 1972, a United Nations study proposed the following 'working definition':

Indigenous communities, peoples, and nations are those having a historical continuity with pre-invasion and pre-colonial societies that developed on their territories, consider themselves distinct from other sectors of the societies now prevailing in those territories, or parts of them (Coates 2004: p. 6).

In 1989, The International Labour Organization (2007), an agency of the United Nations that deals with labour issues, defined indigenous peoples in its convention on Indigenous and Tribal Peoples as follows:

Peoples in independent countries who are regarded as indigenous on account of their descent from the populations which inhabited the country, or a geographical region to which the country belongs, at the time of conquest or colonization or the establishment of present State boundaries and who, irrespective of their legal status, retain some or all of their own social, economic, cultural, and political institutions (Office of the High Commission for Human Rights 2007).

These formulations continue to be influential within the United Nations system. However, the representatives of indigenous organizations who were involved in the negotiation of the Declaration rejected the idea of a formal definition of indigenous peoples that would be adopted by States. This view was supported by governmental delegations for whom it was 'neither desirable nor necessary to elaborate a universal definition of indigenous peoples (Department of Economic and Social Affairs 2004: p. 3). Indigenous delegates resisted the inclusion of formal definitions on the basis that they did not wish to exclude groups from participating in debates on the basis of a technicality. This also reflected the emphasis placed by many indigenous delegates on the right to self-definition, a view that was preserved in the final version of the Declaration in Article 33 clause 1, which states:

Indigenous peoples have the right to determine their own identity or membership in accordance with their customs and traditions. This does not impair the right of indigenous individuals to obtain citizenship of the States in which they live (United Nations General Assembly 2007).

Many contemporary commentators, when surveying the application of the concept of indigeniety internationally, have commented on the difficulty in developing definitions that satisfactorily embrace the full range of this diversity (Niezen 2003; Coates 2004; Barsch 1989; Stamatopoulou 1994; Kingsbury 1998; Stephens & Nettleton 2006). Indigenous identities are also contested within and between indigenous communities (Weaver 2001). These debates between indigenous peoples do have considerable social significance, but they are not unusual in their own right, as is attested to by many other similar disputes among people who belong to communities of religion, language, or ethnicity.

When the medical journal, *The Lancet*, put out a call for papers on indigenous health as part of a series that it intended to run on these issues (Stephens & Nettleton 2006), one anthropologist felt so troubled by the use of the term *indigenous* that he wrote to the journal arguing that the word 'is commonly used as a euphemism for primitive' when in fact those contemporary indigenous peoples who are hunters and who are seen as 'the contemporary heirs to the Upper Paleolithic way of life [when] the relation between contemporary and Upper Paleolithic hunting is very distant indeed' (Kuper 2006: p. 983). Kuper argues that peoples such as the Kalahari Bushmen (the San) and Central African pygmies have been interacting with African farming communities for centuries, whereas other hunting peoples such as the Inuit in Northern Canada have been integrated within a global trade network for a similar period of time. As a consequence of these definitional problems and the difficulties in identifying 'genuine' indigenous people, Kuper argues that:

> *The category of indigenous peoples is so problematic, it is unwise for The Lancet to devote a series of papers to their supposedly special health problems* (Kuper 2006: p. 983).

Despite the misgivings of Kuper and others, the concept persists and it has growing currency in global political processes. Further, given the entanglement with this idea and rights, there are compelling reasons to intellectually engage with this agenda. The various attempts to define indigenous peoples have resulted in two distinct, but related, definitional strategies: Culturist and political (Coates 2004).

The culturalist framework emphasizes the cultural characteristics of indigenous communities, placing particular emphasis on cultural difference relative to urban capitalist societies. Classically, the cultural and social organization of indigenous communities are characterized as small-scale societies which are generally a society of a few dozen to several thousand people who live by foraging wild foods, herding domesticated animals, or non-intensive horticulture on the village level. Such societies lack cities as well as complex economies and governments. Kinship relationships are usually highly important in comparison to the common pattern of large-scale societies (O'Neil 2007).

Indigenous communities that might be candidates in this regard include the Aborigines living in remote areas; the Yanomami of the Amazon River basin; and the San, who live a mobile lifestyle in the Kalahari Desert. However, this approach tends to fix indigenous peoples at a particular point in history, and ignores the impact of colonialism and globalization on even the most traditional of indigenous communities. Four-wheel-drive vehicles, Coca-Cola, and welfare payments are as characteristic of contemporary indigenous lifestyles in many remote regions of the globe as are classificatory kinship structure and hunting or foraging. Furthermore, during the twentieth century, many indigenous populations have became increasingly urbanized and integrated within capitalist economies—even though they many have continued to maintain traditional economic practices and occupy a relatively marginal position within the broader economy. Although many indigenous peoples were historically mobile peoples, the demography of indigenous peoples has changed within the context of colonial history.

However, not all pre-colonial societies were mobile; many, such as in Central America, had long histories of urbanization.

Although it is not possible to identify a cultural archetype for indigenous society, indigenous peoples may respond to social trends and cultural change in a way that is distinct from the dominant society. Some change may be resisted for a range of complex reasons, even though indigenous peoples may also embrace some forms of development. Although it is not possible to predict responses to mining or the incursion of other economic modes of production (such as agriculture) into indigenous territories, the fault lines for these conflicts do re-inscribe the social and political relations between indigenous communities and dominant societies. In that respect, many indigenous peoples retain the desire to maintain a distinct identity and cultural practices in the face of a history of dispossession and social marginalization; they continue to maintain an understanding and sense of connection to a pre-colonial past, often passed on through oral testimony, ceremonies, and cultural activities, which serve to preserve the understanding of history.

Political definitions of indigenous people emphasize the relationship between indigenous people and states in which ethnic settler majorities dominate. Indigenous peoples are commonly political minorities in nation states dominated by settler societies or other ethnic majorities. Their contemporary political circumstance has been historically shaped by colonization in which they have been dispossessed from their traditional lands and natural resources, and subsequently incorporated within the institutional and political structures of the settler state. The management of indigenous peoples by the settler state has often involved the development of administrative structures and programmes. The rights of indigenous peoples and those of the settler majority are frequently differentiated. This pattern of political disempowerment is reflected in other forms of social and cultural marginalization. Increasingly, and perhaps most significantly, indigenous peoples, in the face of ongoing social and political incorporation into the state-centric structures, have increasingly over the last forty years formed political alliances with other indigenous peoples. These alliances are a response to globalizing processes and in working through the United Nations system have attempted to transcend the local politics of exclusion and marginalization.

The development of a globally applicable terminology that is sufficiently flexible for all contexts is clearly a challenge. However, this problem may have greater significance for jurists and legal scholars than the public-health practitioner. The anthropologist Ronald Neizen (2003), who spent some time observing the political machinations of the United Nations processes in the negotiations that led to the Declaration on the Rights of Indigenous Peoples, took the view that the ongoing debate about definitions were valuable in that they continued to draw attention to the different social and political contexts in which this idea has currency. The concept of indigeniety provides a conceptual lens through which we can frame our understanding of the health and social status of distinct populations. It directs our analytical gaze towards the historically unfolding relationships of power within the context of colonial relationships and it also focuses our attention on the role of the state in the production of social inequalities. The diversity of indigenous experience and context should keep our analytical attention on the particular histories and social relations of the peoples in question.

Indigenous peoples in a global context

People who either describe themselves as indigenous or who are defined as such by others are found around the world in widely varying social, cultural, political, and geographical contexts. This includes those peoples who are descended from the 'aboriginal' populations of Australia, New Zealand, North America, and most of Latin America where the history of European colonialism has produced and maintained the social distinction between native peoples and European-settler colonial societies (Stephens *et al.* 2006). The Aborigines inhabited the continent of Australia and the island of Tasmania for up to 60 000 years. Most were hunter–gatherers and there were up to 500 distinct language groups at the time of British colonization in 1788 (Anderson *et al.* 2006). The Maoris of New Zealand are descendants of Pacific Polynesian peoples and share an older cultural and linguistic heritage with many indigenous peoples in the Pacific including Native Hawaiians (Anderson *et al.* 2006). Despite the much longer history of European colonization in the Caribbean and Latin America, indigeniety here is also 'most clearly defined as those who pre-dated European conquistadores' (Montenegro & Stephens 2006: p. 1859). There is considerable linguistic and cultural diversity between indigenous peoples across this region. This includes the present-day descendants of the pre-Columbian complex societies of Central America such as the Maya and the many diverse cultures of the Amazon basin. It is estimated that there are nearly 400 different indigenous languages across the region (Montenegro & Stephens 2006). Indigenous peoples in this region also vary considerably in the extent to which they constitute the population of various nation states—from 71 per cent of the population of Bolivia and 66 per cent of the population of Guatemala to 0.2 per cent of the population of Brazil and 0.03 per cent of the population of Uruguay (Montenegro & Stephens 2006). Although the link between indigenous identities and colonial histories might lend an appearance of definitional clarity for these particular contexts, in other regions of the world—such as in Asia, the Middle East, and Africa—the history of colonialism is more complex and layered. In these contexts, 'colonization took place between ethnic groups within and between countries, and in some case native populations were almost entirely eradicated' (Stephens *et al.* 2006).

A number of Asian minority groups were involved in the global political processes that led to the adoption of the Declaration. These include tribal peoples from India, Taiwanese aboriginal groups, the Ainu, West Papuans, the Hmong peoples from Southeast Asia, and indigenous groups from the Philippines and the Republic of South Mollucas. In India, social hierarchy such as the caste system has created social categories in which social position is established at birth with some groups recognized as indigenous or tribal on a sociocultural basis (Stephens *et al.* 2006). Here, there are about 532 scheduled tribes, speaking over 100 different languages, each with its own ethnic or cultural identity (FAO Investment Centre 2006). Historically, these communities were characterized on the basis of their distinct non-agrarian lifestyles. Their forest-based subsistence economy used a combination of cultivation, hunting, and foraging strategies. British colonial rule had a significant impact on these communities through both the appropriation of forests and the loss of access to their traditional modes of economic production (FAO Investment Centre 2006).

By contrast, the Ainu people of Japan are a small proportion of the total Japanese population, found mainly on the island of Hokkaido. In 1999, there were approximately 23 767 Ainu people living in Hokkadio and 5000 in the Kanto area (Cheung 2003). Over the last four centuries, they have retained a distinct cultural identity—although in the contemporary world very few speak the Ainu language or practice a traditional way of life. They have over this period of time been subject to different political and legislative interventions such as the 1899 Law for the Protection of Native Hokkaido Aborigines, which attempted to impose a policy of assimilation on the Ainu (Cheung 2003).

Benedict Kingsbury (1998) documented some of the political controversy that followed the recognition of some Asian peoples as indigenous peoples. One group of delegates petitioned a meeting of the United Nations Working Group on Indigenous Populations in 1991:

First and foremost, we want to bring to your attention the denial of some Asian governments of the existence of indigenous peoples in our part of the world. This denial presents a significant obstacle to the participation of many indigenous peoples from our region in the Working Group's deliberations. The denial also seeks to withhold the benefits of the Declaration from the indigenous, tribal, and aboriginal peoples of Asia. We hereby urgently request that peoples who are denied the rights to govern themselves, and are called tribal, and/or aboriginal in our region, be recognized, for the purpose of this Declaration, and in accordance with [International Labor Organization] practice, as equivalent to indigenous peoples (Kingsbury 1998: p. 417).

In 1995, the People's Republic of China put the following position to a working group of the UN Commission on Human Rights:

The Chinese Government believes that the question of indigenous peoples is the product of European countries' recent pursuit of colonial policies in other parts of the world. As in the majority of Asian countries, the various nationalities in China have all lived for aeons on Chinese territory. Although there is no indigenous peoples' question in China, the Chinese Government and people have every sympathy with indigenous peoples' historical woes and historical plight. China believes it absolutely essential to draft an international instrument to protect their rights and interests. The special historical misfortunes of indigenous peoples set them apart from minority nationalities and ethnic groups in the ordinary sense. For this reason, the draft declaration must clearly define what indigenous peoples are, in order to guarantee that the special rights it establishes are accurately targeted at genuine communities of indigenous people and are not distorted, arbitrarily extended, or muddled (Kingsbury 1998: p. 417–418).

Within Africa, the recognition of some minorities as indigenous is even more highly contested. Many of these critics would claim to the contrary that all Africans are indigenous in relation to European colonization (Stephens *et al.* 2006; Ohenjo & Willis 2006). According to Ohenjo *et al.* (2006), there are 14.2 million people in Africa who identify as indigenous; these people can be historically grouped into three major categories: Hunter–gatherers (such as the Pygmy peoples of Central Africa and the San of Southern Africa); fisher peoples; and pastoralists (such as the Masai of Kenya and Tanzania, pastoral communities in Ethiopia and Sudan, the Taureg of West and Northern Africa, and the Himba of Namibia). One of the problems in the African context is that within this longer history, which pre-dates European colonial expansion in the continent, the patterns of settlement and political relations between various groups are contested. This situation is rendered more complex in the political context of the era following European colonization, when negotiation of post-colonial borders disrupted many existing cultural and political alliances. Ohenjo *et al.* (2006) take the view that being indigenous is related to the relation between peoples and the state and its dominant and economic and political structures. To that end, they point out that the national identity movements that emerged in the twentieth century sought to disregard internal ethnic differences with numerically dominant populations such as the Twana in Botswana being established as culturally normative and politically dominant with respect to the indigenous populations, such as the San peoples, who were now spliced within and between the political boundaries of a post-colonial Africa.

Health and social outcomes for indigenous peoples

Health status of indigenous peoples

The social circumstance of indigenous peoples across the globe varies considerably; in part, this reflects their different histories and location in resource-poor or resource-rich nations. However, it is the social inequalities experienced by indigenous peoples that have provided the political momentum for the increasing focus on indigenous issues in the international arena. These inequalities are evident in the measurement of health and social outcomes. There are a few instances in which some health indicators match that of benchmark populations. Patterns of disease also reflect the broader social context of the indigenous people in question, with patterns of disease varying between those peoples who live in resource-rich and resource-poor nations.

Despite the increasing global attention on the question of indigenous health, specific and accurate information concerning their health status is fragmented and incomplete. This quality of health data varies considerably, and in part reflects the capacity or political will of various nations to develop health-information systems that enable the disaggregation of data according to indigenous status. In resource-poor countries, the capacity to develop health-information systems more generally impacts on the collection of indigenous health data. For example, the US-associated Micronesia, where indigenous peoples constitute a majority of the population, does not have the capacity to support a sophisticated health-information system (Anderson *et al.* 2006). Not all nations record indigenous status in health data collections. Even in those that do, the quality of the data collected and recorded is variable. In Australia, for example, good-quality mortality data are available for only 60 per cent of the indigenous population (Anderson *et al.* 2006). Factors that compound some of these difficulties include the extent to which health services can systematically record indigenous status, when indigenous people may be a relatively invisible minority. There are also different approaches to how indigenous status is defined. Some communities cross international and other jurisdictional boundaries—making it even more difficult to get an accurate picture of health and social status (Stephens & Porter 2006).

Life expectancy

In general, indigenous populations experience lower life expectancies relative to other benchmark populations. The life expectancy among the Maya of Guatemala is 17 years shorter than that for non-Indigenous (Feiring & Partners 2003). The life expectancy for indigenous Australians for the years 1996–2000 was 59.4 years for men (compared with 76.6 years for non-Aboriginal men) and 64.8 years for women (compared with 82 years for non-Aboriginal women) (Anderson *et al.* 2006). The Maoris, in 1996–1999, had a life expectancy of 66.3 years for men and 71 years for women compared with 75.7 years and 80.8 years, respectively, for the non-Maori, non-Pacific population (Anderson *et al.* 2006). For the peoples of the Federated States of Micronesia (FSM), life expectancy was 68 years for men and 71 years for women compared with US benchmarks (Anderson *et al.* 2006). In 2001, the differences between the Mexican indigenous population were 67.6 years for men (72.4 years in the total population) and 71.5 years for women (78.1 years for the total population) (Feiring & Partner 2006).

Infant mortality

Measures of infant mortality rates also provide a useful insight in the differences between health outcomes for indigenous and non-indigenous peoples. The infant mortality rate among indigenous peoples of Mexico is almost double that of its non-indigenous population. In Australia and the FSM, indigenous infant mortality rates are approximately three times that of their benchmark populations (Freemantle & Read 2006). In New Zealand, Maori infants had twice the mortality rate (Anderson *et al.* 2006). Native Hawaiians have a similar rate of infant mortality with the non-native population of Hawaii (Anderson *et al.* 2006). Tribal peoples in the Indian state of Bihar had approximately three times the infant mortality rate, with over half of the children of this group experiencing malnutrition (FAO Investment Centre 2006). There are also documented differences in the prevalence of low birth weight. In Australia, 12.9 per cent of the total indigenous births were under 2500 g (compared with 6.1 per cent for the total Australian population), and in New Zealand, 7.9 per cent of Maori births were low birth weight compared with 6.1 per cent of the non-Maori non-Pacific population. However, the figures for native Hawaiians and non-native Hawaiians were very similar in 2001 at 8 and 8.1 per cent, respectively (Anderson *et al.* 2007).

Morbidity

It is difficult to make global generalization with respect to patterns of morbidity. In part, this reflects differences in the global pattern of disease. Many indigenous populations have higher incidences of chronic diseases such as diabetes, mental disorders, and cancers. In wealthy countries, diseases that are now relatively rare, such as tuberculosis and rheumatic fever, are significantly over-represented in indigenous populations.

Disability is often more frequent; for instance, 31 per cent of First Nations people in Canada report some form of disability linked to high accident rates, poor housing, substance abuse, or chronic disease. Alaskan Natives report unintentional-injury death rates more than three times the national average (Beavon & Cooke 2003). The suicide rate among indigenous Hawaiians is more than 150 per cent greater than that of non-Indigenous Hawaiians.

Indigenous health inequalities are reflected in broader social inequalities (Anderson *et al.* 2006). For example, in Peru, the rate of poverty among indigenous populations is 150 per cent that of the non-indigenous (Feiring & Partners 2003). Ninety-one per cent of the indigenous people in Guatemala lived in extreme poverty in 1989, compared to 45 per cent of the non-indigenous. In Ecuador, 76 per cent of the indigenous children live in poverty. The impact of poverty is clear from figures found in Honduras where an estimated 95 per cent of indigenous children under the age of 14 are malnourished (Feiring & Partners 2003).

Social determinants of indigenous health

There are a range of different explanatory frameworks that have been used to account for the persistent health and social disparities experienced by indigenous peoples. These include racial or genetic models; health behaviours; socioeconomic models and approaches, which have drawn upon the social and historical analysis of colonialism and the social relations that this has produced. With the exception of the latter, there is in fact a considerable degree of overlap with some of the approaches taken to theoretical and research agenda in ethnic health disparities (e.g. Dressler *et al.* 2005).

In contemporary analysis, there is a growing interest in the application of thinking drawn from the work on the social determinants of health of indigenous populations (e.g. Anderson *et al.* 2007; Carson *et al.* 2007). The convergence of thinking in indigenous health with this broader agenda in public health recognizes that many of those social processes which have been demonstrated to play a role in the production of health outcomes in other populations—such as economic circumstances, access the health and social services, experiences of racism and other forms of discrimination—are likely to play a role in the production of health inequalities for indigenous peoples. Nonetheless, it is also possible that there are particular social processes, or more likely a particular sociohistorical configuration of social processes, that conceptually distinguishes indigenous social determinants of health. To date, most of this analysis in indigenous health has been at the more theoretical end of the spectrum—with a relatively smaller body of research that empirically investigates the relationship between social processes and health outcomes.

The World Health Organization's Commission on the Social Determinants of Health (CSDH) decided to establish a process at its meeting in Nairobi in June 2006 to inquire into the role of the social determinants in the health of indigenous peoples. As a consequence, an International Review of Social Determinants of Indigenous Health was established to synthesize existing knowledge and expertise in this field (Mowbray 2007). This review included a commissioned international situational analysis and an international call for case studies, both of which formed the background papers for an International Symposium on the Social Determinants of Indigenous Health, which was convened by the CSDH in Adelaide, Australia, in April 2007, and attended by seventy-four participants from Australia, Belize, Cambodia, Canada, Chile, China, Ecuador, Guatemala, New Zealand, the Philippines, and the United Kingdom. The workshop subsequently covered a number of themes that were consistent with the analysis emerging from the document review. They included issues such as the following:

- The politics of indigenous self-determination
- The health consequences of ecological and environmental change
- Economic factors such as poverty or prosperity, fairness, and equity
- The development of indigenous leadership and capacity building in indigenous communities

- The impact of racism, political dominance, and imperialism
- Healing the access to health services, systems, and structures
- Cultural sustainability, protection, stewardship
- Land tenure, territorial integrity, and human rights

These ideas and themes had remained remarkably consistent through the entire process, in both the written material and workshop process. Despite the differences in the social and political contexts of indigenous peoples worldwide, there was a high degree of concordance throughout this process in the collective understanding about the role played by social processes in the development of disparities in indigenous health. However, it was also clear, particularly through the more detailed local case studies, that these broad ideas need to be critically interpreted within particular historical and social environments. In this sense, local research is required to identify how these more broadly defined processes might impact on local lives and realities.

Another significant finding was the understanding that, although the influence of social determinants on health can be identified in all populations, there is a specific cluster of factors and relationships that can be identified in the indigenous context. The role of work and other economic relationships is likely to be different within the context of the Aborigines, where the realm of social life is distinctly organized relative to other Australians. The historical processes of colonialism, and the ongoing processes of social marginalization, have effects on the health of indigenous Australians that require the development of a particular approach to the analysis of social relationships critical to health outcomes. These challenges are pivotal to the future development of research in this field.

Health status of ethnic minorities

A sizeable literature has described differences in health status and health outcomes between ethnic groups at different stages in the life course that are comparable to those described for indigenous peoples. The description of such variations is dependent on the collection of data for ethnicity in systems for vital registration, as well as population censuses and special surveys. These types of data may not be available in some countries and less satisfactory measures, such as the country of birth, may sometimes be collected instead of ethnic group. Systems for classification may also differ for health events as numerators as compared with population data as denominators. Much attention has focused on relative differences between ethnic groups, but evaluation of absolute risks will also be relevant for developing appropriate policy responses. For example, people of African descent in Europe are characterized as having a high risk of stroke and a low risk of coronary heart disease compared with white Europeans, but the absolute risk of coronary heart disease in the African group is generally higher than for stroke, as it is in most populations.

Mortality and life expectancy

Differences in mortality in relation to ethnic group or race are well documented in the United States (Tables 11.5.3 and 11.5.4). Infant mortality is twice as high in African-Americans and is 50 per cent higher in Native Americans, when compared to whites. In the Hispanic and Latino group, overall infant mortality is similar to that in whites, but the rate for Puerto Ricans (8.3 per 1000) is close to that for Native Americans. All-cause mortality is increased in African-Americans; life expectancy at birth in 2004 was 73.1 years

Table 11.5.3 Infant mortality rate by ethnic group in the United States, 2001–2003

Ethnic group	Infant mortality per 1000 live births
White	5.7
African American	13.6
Hispanic/Latino	5.6
Asian/Pacific Islander	4.8
American Indian/Alaskan Native	8.9

Source: United States Department of Health and Human Services. Health United States, 2006. Washington (DC): US Department of Health and Human Services; 2006.

for African-Americans compared with 78.3 for whites. There is considerable variation in the relative increase for different causes of death. African-American mortality shows greatest relative increases for HIV, homicide, diabetes, and cerebrovascular disease with no increase observed for unintentional injuries, chronic liver disease and cirrhosis, and chronic lower respiratory disease (Table 11.5.4).

In the United Kingdom, mortality has been analysed according to country of birth since 1981 (Balarajan 1995; Wild & Mckeigue 1997; Harding *et al.* 2008). These analyses are derived from the collection of data for country of birth in the national census and in death certification. Increased mortality from coronary heart disease in Indian-subcontinent-origin populations is a consistent finding, especially at younger ages. In the population under 65 years, mortality from coronary heart disease in people born in the Indian subcontinent is 1.5–1.7 times higher than in people born in England and Wales, and mortality for stroke is 1.8–2.5 times higher. For people born in Africa or the Caribbean, relative mortality is higher for stroke and lower for coronary heart disease. For migrants born in Europe, the evidence is conflicting; migrants from Ireland have increased mortality from both coronary heart disease and stroke, whereas mortality for both outcomes is lower among those born in continental Europe. Recent analyses by Harding *et al.* (2008) have shown that this ethnic patterning of mortality has been consistent over the three decades from 1979 to 2003, but mortality relative to those born in England and Wales has increased as mortality rates declined more rapidly in the England-and Wales-born population. Elevated mortality from coronary heart disease has been observed in Indian-subcontinent-origin populations in a number of countries including Trinidad and Tobago (Miller *et al.* 1988).

Diabetes, hypertension, and metabolic syndrome

A number of studies have shown that ethnic patterning of mortality is associated with variation in risk-factor profiles. The prevalence of type 2 diabetes is generally higher among people of African or Indian-subcontinent descent when compared with white Europeans (Chaturvedi *et al.* 1994; Simmons *et al.* 1992). The prevalence of hypertension, and mean blood pressure levels, are also higher among people of African descent (Chaturvedi *et al.* 1993). There is also variation in lipid profiles and anthropometric measures, including the prevalence of obesity and abdominal fatness, among ethnic groups that are also patterned by gender (Chaturvedi *et al.* 1994).

These observations have been used to raise questions concerning whether anthropometric reference standards should be developed for different groups; most present reference data having been obtained from white European-origin populations. One illustration is provided by the ethnic-group-specific criteria suggested for the definition of metabolic syndrome, a clustering of risk factors that is associated with increased risk of diabetes and vascular

Table 11.5.4 Age-adjusted mortality rates by ethnic group and cause in the United States, 2004

Cause of death	Age-adjusted mortality rate per 100 000		Rate ratio
	White	African American	
All causes	786.3	1027.3	1.31
Ischaemic heart disease	149.2	179.8	1.21
Cerebrovascular disease	48.0	69.9	1.46
Lung cancer	53.6	59.8	1.12
Breast cancer	23.9	32.2	1.35
Chronic lower respiratory disease	43.2	28.2	0.65
Chronic liver disease and cirrhosis	9.2	7.9	0.86
Diabetes	22.3	48.0	2.15
HIV	2.3	20.4	8.87
Unintentional injuries	38.8	36.3	0.94
Homicide	3.6	20.1	5.58

Source: United States Department of Health and Human Services. Health United States, 2006. Washington (DC): US Department of Health and Human Services; 2006.

disease (Okosun *et al.* 2000; Alberti *et al.* 2005). Lower cut-points for the definition of abdominal obesity have been proposed for men of Indian subcontinent or Chinese origin because diabetes is generally more frequent at lower values for waist circumference in these groups (Alberti *et al.* 2005). However, the significance of this observation is unclear (see Chapter 9.5 on obesity for further discussion).

Results from multi-site international studies make it clear that environmental influences are important in conditioning health outcomes within groups. For example, the International Collaborative Study on Hypertension in Blacks included population surveys in rural and urban populations in West Africa, in several Caribbean islands, and in Maywood, Illinois (Kaufman *et al.* 1996). The prevalence of obesity ranged from 5 per cent in rural African men to 36 per cent in African-American women in the United States. The prevalence of hypertension, with blood pressure ≥ 140/90 mm Hg or treated, ranged from 12 per cent in rural African men to 35 per cent in African-American women (Kaufman *et al.* 1996). These results draw attention to the potential importance of environmental determinants on supposed 'ethnic differences' and raise questions concerning how these differences may be explained.

Determinants of health among ethnic groups

As for indigenous peoples, a number of determinants of health are considered to have particular relevance to the ethnic patterning of health outcomes. These include variations in gene frequencies between populations; culture and lifestyles; migration, including selection effects and the consequences of migration; discrimination; lack of access to services; and socioeconomic influences, including poverty and deprivation in terms of income, education, and housing. The significance of these explanations varies for different health outcomes and different contexts. As we shall see, these explanations are not separate but closely interconnected and dependent.

Gene frequencies

Single gene defects

Inherited disorders of haemoglobin, including sickle cell disease and thalassaemias, are the most frequent diseases associated with single gene defects, with up to 7 per cent of the world population being carriers and up to half a million severely affected births each year (Weatherall *et al.* 2007). Disorders of haemoglobin vary greatly in frequency between ethnic groups in high-income countries. This is because the genes associated with these conditions are only present at low frequency in Northern European populations but in other regions—including Africa, South Europe, the Middle East, and South and Southeast Asia—up to 40 per cent or more of the population may be carriers. As a result of migration, there are significant numbers of affected births among minority ethnic groups in countries whose populations are primarily of Northern European origin. There is important morbidity, including transfusion dependency in thalassaemia or painful crises and increased risk of stroke in children with sickle cell disease, leading to increased health-care utilization.

As a policy response, neonatal screening programmes have been introduced to facilitate earlier detection and treatment of affected infants together with antenatal screening to facilitate prenatal diagnosis, so as to provide parents with an opportunity for informed choice concerning reproductive outcomes. An important question in the implementation of these programmes concerns whether screening should be universal, covering all pregnancies and births, or whether a selective strategy should be introduced to target minority ethnic groups. In the United Kingdom, universal antinatal screening is implemented in high-prevalence areas whereas a selective strategy is employed in low-prevalence areas. In the selective strategy, a preliminary screening question is used to identify individuals who, because of their ethnicity or family origin, may be more likely to be carriers of inherited haemoglobin disorders. This screening question asks 'What are your family origins?', with responses classified by geographical region, and does not depend on self-assigned ethnicity (Aspinall *et al.* 2003; Dyson *et al.* 2006). Screening is thus performed according to the restricted criterion of parental family origin in a region of the world where the population has a high gene-carrier frequency, rather than according to the broader, self-assigned concept of ethnicity.

Complex traits

The genetic evaluation of complex traits and their associations with ethnicity has generally been intractable. Interest in the genetic determinants of ethnic variation in complex traits has been stimulated recently by the development of pharmacogenomics, the study of the effect of genetic variation on responses to drug therapy. This raises the commercially attractive possibility that drugs may be tailored to the expected responses of patients in different groups. For example, it has been proposed that selection of antihypertensive drug therapy should be guided by assessment of ethnicity (Brown 2006). Those interested in the genetic evaluation of ethnic variations in complex traits must be sensitive to the antecedent history of research into race and health (Bhopal 1997). One example of a research study is provided by a case–control study in Trinidad that evaluated genetic markers of West African ancestry as risk factors for systemic lupus erythematosus (SLE) (Molokhia *et al.* 2003). The authors proposed that their results were consistent with a genetic basis for the difference in risk of SLE between West Africans and Europeans.

Culture and lifestyle

The term *culture* has several different meanings. It was defined by the United Nations Educational, Scientific, and Cultural Organization (UNESCO 2007) as 'the set of distinctive spiritual, material, intellectual, and emotional features of society or a social group that encompasses, in addition to art and literature, lifestyles, ways of living together, value systems, traditions, and beliefs'. The contribution of culture to ethnic variation in health status may derive from the distinct traditions and beliefs of communities that contribute to different lifestyles and ways of living which are associated with risk of illness and disease. Differences between communities are graded. On the one hand, there is usually substantial within-group variation in the degree of conformity with cultural norms; on the other hand, differences between groups are non-specific. There is cultural regulation or modulation of the uptake of the main lifestyle risk factors for diseases. Different cultures also vary in their social construction of illness and appropriate responses in terms of help-seeking behaviour.

An example of a culturally specific behavioural norm is provided by the requirement for women in some Muslim communities to be covered by clothing when outdoors. There is a concern that this might contribute to low vitamin D production in the skin with potential risks to women's bone health and the potential for development of rickets in children who are breastfed. A study in Turkey found that women who were habitually veiled had substantially lower serum 25-hydroxy vitamin D concentrations than women who usually wore western clothes (Guzel *et al.* 2001). In England, early clinical reports of rickets, osteomalacia, and vitamin D deficiency in people of Indian-subcontinent-origin led to the introduction of local strategies for vitamin D supplementation (Dunnigan *et al.* 1981). Recently, there has been a re-emergence of vitamin D deficiency among second-generation immigrants, leading to renewed calls for vitamin D supplementation in pregnancy to prevent foetal and maternal vitamin D deficiency (Shaw & Pal 2002). However, the causes for this vitamin D deficiency are unclear. Both men and women of Indian origin have been found to have low serum vitamin D concentrations (Shaunak *et al.* 1985), and this deficiency is not confined to particular religious groups (Jonnalagadda & Diwan 2002). Low vitamin D levels have also been found among African-Americans in the United States and in other minority groups (Dawson-Hughes 2004). Dietary deficiency and lack of vitamin D supplementation appear to be the more important causes of this increased susceptibility to vitamin D deficiency (Dawson-Hughes 2004).

Analysis of data for other lifestyle determinants of health reveal important differences between groups (Sproston & Mindell 2006). Smoking cigarettes and drinking alcohol are generally less frequent among ethnic minorities than in the general population. In particular, Indian, Pakistani, Bangladeshi, and Chinese women in England generally do not smoke. Alcohol is generally not used by men and women from Pakistan and Bangladesh. The proportion of men and women of Indian-subcontinent origin achieving recommended levels of physical activity is considerably lower than in the general population, more so among women. Crude dietary indicators such as consumption of fruit and vegetables generally reveal less variation between groups, but these crude measures conceal substantial differences between groups in the types of foods consumed, with further differences between first- and second-generation immigrants (Landman & Cruickshank 2001).

Data such as these are important in contributing to the development of strategies to promote health and prevent disease. They inform, for example, strategies to promote physical activity in women of Indian subcontinent origin (Carroll *et al.* 2002). Culturally-appropriate interventions are required that address the needs of groups in the context of their particular cultural traditions, beliefs and norms.

Migration and discrimination

The experience of migration is generally key to the formation of ethnic-minority groups in the high-income countries; these countries have a need to attract skilled as well as less-skilled workers and may offer a destination for asylum-seekers and refugees. Migrants are often in better general health than the populations from which they are drawn, contributing to the 'healthy migrant effect'. However, migration may itself have significant negative consequences for health and this is well illustrated with respect to mental health problems (Bhugra & Minas 2007).

Much research has addressed the question of differing frequency of schizophrenia and other psychoses among ethnic groups.

In England, there is a well-documented excess of new diagnoses of schizophrenia in African-Caribbean populations. The AESOP study (Fearon *et al.* 2006) evaluated the incidence of schizophrenia and other psychoses among different ethnic groups in three areas of England with a combined population of just over 1 million. The results (Table 11.5.5) show a 6.7-fold increase in risk of new-onset psychosis in African-Caribbean men and women, a 4.1-fold excess risk in Africans, with more modest elevations in risk in other ethnic groups. This has led to suggestions that genetic predisposition or experiences of migration and racial discrimination may contribute to the increased risk of schizophrenia in people of African descent.

Studies in Trinidad (Bhugra *et al.* 1996), Jamaica (Hickling & Rodgers-Johnson 1995), and Barbados (Mahy *et al.* 1999) have evaluated the incidence of new-onset schizophrenia in Caribbean populations. These studies show that the incidence of schizophrenia in the Caribbean is similar to that observed in other regions, including the white British population in England, and much lower than those observed in Caribbean-origin populations in England. These studies provide strong evidence that environmental factors are responsible for the increased incidence of schizophrenia among ethnic minorities in England.

In the AESOP study (Fearon *et al.* 2006), the absence of a major elevation in risk in 'Asians' was viewed as diminishing a potential role for racial discrimination in the aetiology of schizophrenia, as the Asian group may be equally exposed to problems of racial discrimination as black Caribbean and Africans. A modest elevation in risk of psychosis among non-British whites was also regarded as important, as this group is exposed to the stresses of migration and acculturation. This is consistent with the findings of a systematic review, which found that both first- and second-generation migrants has an increased relative risk of schizophrenia compared with non-migrants in the same population (Cantor-Graae & Selten 2005).

Bhugra and Minas (2007) discuss four interrelated reasons why migration may represent a significant stressor with respect to mental health. First, migration generally occurs between communities with different cultural orientations. Immigrants are often derived from poor communities which have a collectivist or 'sociocentric' outlook, but the destination country will often be more affluent

Table 11.5.5 Age-adjusted incidence rate ratios (95 per cent confidence intervals) for all psychosis using the white British group as reference

Ethnic group	Relative risk of all psychosis (95 per cent confidence interval)
White British	1.0
African-Caribbean	6.7 (5.4–8.3)
Black African	4.1 (3.2–5.3)
Asian	1.5 (0.9–2.4)
Other	2.6 (1.7–3.9)
White other	1.6 (1.1–2.2)

Source: Fearon P, Kirkbride JB, Morgan C et al. AESOP Study Group. Incidence of schizophrenia and other psychoses in ethnic minority groups: results from the MRC AESOP Study. *Psychological Medicine* 2006; **36**: 1541–50.

and have a more individualistic or 'egocentric' culture. The resulting tensions may lead to mental distress (Bhugra & Minas 2007). Second, removing an individual from his or her familiar context including family and social support, together with the problems encountered in settling into a new environment, may increase the risk of mental illness. Third, experiences of racial discrimination may have significant impacts on mental well-being. These may result from individual-level interactions or from institutional racism, which may be more difficult to confront. Institutional racism is a term attributed to Stokely Carmichael and is defined as 'the collective failure of an organization to provide an appropriate and professional service to people because of their colour, culture, or ethnic origin' (Wikipedia 2007). Accusations of institutional racism have been specifically levelled at mental health services with the suggestion that methods for diagnosing and managing ethnic-minority patients with serious mental illness may be discriminatory (Singh & Burns 2006). However, these suggestions have not generally been supported by epidemiological studies in the United Kingdom (Singh & Burns 2006; Morgan et al. 2004). Fourth, the dominant majorities in countries that receive migrants may not embrace the prospect of increasing cultural pluralism and may not develop adequate responses to linguistic and ethnic diversity (Bhugra & Minas 2007). Questions of cultural sensitivity may be of most immediate concern in the delivery of health services used by ethnic-minority groups.

Access to services

The access that ethnic-minority groups have to health services is a significant source of concern, but the extent to which equity of access is achieved depends on the health-system context. In countries such as England and Trinidad and Tobago, which offer universal eligibility to health services, all groups may be said to have access to services, but there may be significant barriers to utilization that prevent particular groups from gaining access on an equitable basis. In other settings which, such as the United States, do not offer services with universal coverage, there are generally greater threats to achieving equity of access.

In Trinidad and Tobago, successive governments have adopted a strongly egalitarian approach to the provision of services. Findings from ad hoc surveys suggest that a fair degree of equity may be achieved in respect of ethnicity (Gulliford et al. 2002). In health-care services, the main threat to equity comes from the expanding private sector with access dependent on ability to pay, regardless of ethnic group.

In England, ethnic minorities are more concentrated in deprived areas that generally have less well-developed primary-care services consistent with the 'inverse-care law'. However, a number of studies have found that, after allowing for differences in needs, ethnic-minority groups are generally higher users of primary-care consultations then the white English population (Smaje & LeGrand 1997). Analysis of utilization of preventive medical care reveals a mixed picture. Local studies have shown increased uptake of immunization among ethnic minorities, especially those of Indian-subcontinent origin (Mixer et al. 2007; Deshpande 2004), but lower uptake of breast- and cervical-cancer screening (Webb et al. 2004; Atri et al. 1996). Some studies suggest that there is evidence of inequitable uptake of specialist services by people from ethnic minorities, especially with respect to the management of coronary heart disease (Feder et al. 2002), but this has not been confirmed in other studies

(Britton et al. 2004). Significantly, there do not appear to be important differences in health-care-seeking behaviour with respect to chest pain between different ethnic groups (Adamson et al. 2003). Although these studies suggest that a fair degree of equity of access is achieved overall, local studies show that difficulties may be encountered when services do not deliver services that are sufficiently tailored to the needs of specific groups. The concepts of 'linguistic competence' and 'cultural competence' have been developed to describe organizations' ability to communicate effectively with minority groups and deliver services that are sensitive to cultural concerns which may influence the acceptability, uptake, and outcomes of services (Szczepura 2004).

In the US health system, there is strong and consistent evidence of inequitable treatment of ethnic minorities, especially African-Americans. The evidence was summarized most authoritatively in the US Institute of Medicine (Institute of Medicine 2003) report 'Unequal Treatment'. This report found that, even when difficulties of accessing health care because of financial barriers or lack of insurance coverage were excluded, there were significant racial or ethnic inequalities in the delivery of care that were sufficient to impact negatively on health outcomes. The report identified persistence of racial and ethnic discrimination at the societal, health-service, and practitioner levels as significant causes of these inequalities. In particular, bias and prejudice on the part of health-care providers were identified as significant causes of the lower-quality care received by ethnic minorities (Institute of Medicine 2003; Betancourt & King 2003). One example of the impact of such inequalities in access and delivery of care is provided by an analysis of black:white mortality differentials from human immunodeficiency virus (HIV) in the United States before and after the introduction of highly active antiretroviral therapy (HAART) (Levine et al. 2007). In men aged 25–34 years, the black:white mortality rate ratio for HIV was 3.1 in the period 1990–1995, but this ratio increased to 6.36 in the period 1997–2002 after the introduction of HAART. In women of the same age, the mortality rate ratio was 8.25 in the pre-HAART period and 13.24 after the introduction of HAART (Levine et al. 2007).

Socioeconomic position and deprivation

Deprivation and poverty are key determinants of the health of ethnic minorities. In a plural society such as Trinidad and Tobago, the social stratifiers of education, income, and wealth generally have similar significance for all ethnic and cultural groups (Ryan 1991). In other settings, ethnic minorities—or significant portions of minority populations—may, to a greater or lesser extent, be at risk of marginalization or social exclusion with ethnicity contributing tacitly to social stratification.

The concept of social exclusion is hard to define but has found wide application to social policy in recent years (Peace 2001). In a narrow sense, social exclusion refers to income poverty, encompassing groups that are not included in the labour market or who are confined to low-paid work. In this sense, the concept of social exclusion is often applicable to urban minorities. In a wider sense, social exclusion refers to a combination of lack of resources and denial of social rights that contributes to deprivation across multiple domains, in turn leading to a breakdown in social ties and a loss of sense of purpose (Peace 2001).

Evaluation of individual measures of socioeconomic position in England reveals a complex picture (Sproston & Mindell 2006).

Whereas African-Caribbean, Pakistani, and Bangladeshi men are less likely to have educational qualifications, black African and Indian men are more likely than the general population to be educated to degree level. Pakistani and Bangladeshi women have particularly low educational qualifications, but Chinese and African women in England are better-educated than the general population. In terms of occupational social class, ethnic-minority groups are more likely to be classified into routine or semi-routine occupations, but people of Indian-subcontinent origin as well as the Chinese are more likely than the general population to be small employers or working on their own account. It is an oversimplification to characterize ethnic-minority groups as invariably associated with lower socioeconomic position and social exclusion. There is considerable diversity both within and between groups, the effect of gender varies between groups, with inconsistency among indicators of socioeconomic position. In spite of this complexity, there are recognizable vulnerable groups within ethnic-minority populations that are excluded through lack of access to education and employment or because of poor health.

Nazroo (2003) and Smith (2002) have analysed the complexity of the interrelationship between ethnicity and socioeconomic position. Analyses have usually focused on the average socioeconomic position of different ethnic groups, but within ethnic groups, there is gradation of socioeconomic circumstances with some households having more, or less, advantaged status leading to socioeconomic inequalities within groups. Thus, in England, poor self-rated health in Bangladeshis is observed among lower-income groups and not in the top-income tertile. The overall poor health of the Bangladeshi group may be 'explained' by poverty and not ethnicity (Nazroo 2003).

The significance of indicators of socioeconomic status may vary between groups as, for example, if the income achieved for a given level of occupational social class is not the same between groups (Nazroo 2003). This is a methodologically important point because in conventional multiple regression analyses, adjustment for indicators of socioeconomic position, such as occupational social class, may not fully account for socioeconomic differences between groups. Proposed ethnic differences may in reality be explained by residual confounding with socioeconomic position (Nazroo 2003; Smith 2002). The same social indicator may sometimes have different associations with health measures in different ethnic groups. For example, in white European families, children's height diminishes as the number of children in the family increases, but this association is generally less apparent in children of African or Indian-subcontinent descent (Gulliford et al. 1991), perhaps because of the differing cultural significance of family size across ethnic groups.

At the societal level, segregation and discrimination may be important in restricting social and economic freedoms, contributing to the lower socioeconomic status of minority ethnic groups (Nazroo 2003). This is particularly evident in the situation of African-Americans in the United States. Furthermore, in a system in which there are significant financial barriers to accessing health care, lack of access to good-quality care and effective treatment may compromise outcomes in treatable conditions such as HIV infection. The low socioeconomic status of poorly educated migrant workers is often associated with poverty and poor overall health status, as is evident in some migrant groups in England. However, although cigarette smoking is a significant contributor to social inequalities in health in the general population, a lower cultural acceptance of smoking makes this a less significant hazard in African- and Indian-origin ethnic-minority groups, in whom there is a relatively low incidence of lung cancer (Wild & Mckeigue 1997).

Ethnicity and identity

Whereas cultural factors have traditionally been viewed as major but fairly static influences on the beliefs and health-related practices of ethnic minorities, increasingly the cultural beliefs and identities of minority ethnic groups are viewed as flexible and shaped by the structural conditions of people's lives and experiences, including those of racism and disadvantage. As Bhopal et al. (1991: p. 244) observed:

> Far from being immutable categories, the labels to which ethnicity give rise vary in time and space, and according to social and political context.

Ethnicity has thus been described as a 'hybrid' identity that is influenced by internal and external factors, including a group's history, prevailing circumstances, and the responses of the wider society. For example, the finding that smoking rates are strongly related to age on migration to the United Kingdom, with those migrating at younger ages or born in the United Kingdom having higher rates of smoking, may reflect the differing circumstances and experiences of different age groups (Nazroo 2003). Similarly, differences may arise from an ethnic groups varying experience of the wider society in terms of acceptance or discrimination, and from the extent to which traditional beliefs and practices conform or differ from those of the dominant culture. Ethnic categories are, therefore, shaped by their particular experiences as members of a group, rather than global categories for whom findings can be generalized from one context or group to another. Ethnicity, although a key dimension of identity, is also only one aspect of individuals' identity that includes socioeconomic position, gender, and age, with differing aspects of identity varying in importance between different peoples and in different contexts. Where race and ethnicity tend to be the organizing principle of people's lives, this has been described as 'thick' identity, and is contrasted with 'thin' ethnic identity that occurs where there are less frequent and less dense ethnic interactions, and where other dimensions of social life (including class and occupation) tend to be more powerful shapers of daily life and experiences (Cornell & Hartman 1998).

Recent research has aimed to move beyond the mere identification of differences in patterns of behaviour between ethnic groups to explain these behaviours in terms of the meanings and significance of ethnic identity in people's lives. For example, there is concern about low levels of participation by some marginalized groups in local-community consultation exercises and activist networks, including those focusing on the provision of facilities for children, women's issues, health issues, neighbourhood safety, policing, and leisure and entertainment facilities, which limits their access to community resources. This has traditionally been explained in terms of lack of knowledge or awareness and motivation. However, in-depth interviews conducted with a sample of African-Caribbean residents in a deprived multi-ethnic area in the United Kingdom indicated that such non-participation partly arose from experiences of racism and exclusion at school and work, which led to feelings of being an 'outsider' (Campbell & McLean 2002).

In addition, African-Caribbean residents' collective identity as a group was identified as weak and thus failed to unite people at the local-community level beyond particular face-to-face networks. This lack of solidarity was attributed to a number of factors including the relatively low numbers of African-Caribbean residents in the area relative to other groups, their partial integration into mainstream culture, and life and decline of black consciousness, together with the divisions that existed within the African-Caribbean community associated with social class and their particular island identity as 'Jamaican', 'Trinidadian', etc.

The authors concluded that policy recommendations which simply advocate grassroots participation in community networks as a means of tackling health inequalities are likely to fail without acknowledging the obstacles to such participation that arise from a groups collective identity and experiences, and making recommendations for addressing these barriers. Similar barriers to participation among the African-Caribbean population in the United Kingdom were identified in a qualitative interview study to understand the reasons for their low-organ-donor registration (Morgan et al. 2008). This indicated that these respondents' low levels of trust in the medical profession and the process of organ donation reflected their feelings of a lack of 'belonging' to mainstream society and reported experiences of discrimination and exclusion in relation to major social institutions such as hospitals, the police, and schools. Respondents also placed considerable emphasis on their ideal of returning 'home' to the Caribbean for burial, thus reaffirming their ethnic identity at death, which was associated with a desire that their body should return home 'whole', or without organs removed. In contrast, studies with South Asian communities in the United Kingdom indicate that their major concerns about the body associated with a reluctance to donate arise from religious concerns. This includes requirements among Muslims for rapid burial and proper handling of the corpse (Alkhawar et al. 2005) and concerns among Sikh Asians about whether their body will be reincarnated if tampered with (Exeley et al. 1999). This identifies ways in which similar negative attitudes in terms of the survey responses of ethnic groups may reflect differing cultural and situational factors arising from collective and personal experiences as an ethnic minority (Morgan et al. 2006).

Policy responses

Indigenous peoples and self-determination

The Declaration on the Rights of Indigenous peoples was passed with an overwhelming majority of 143 votes in favour. Only four countries—Canada, Australia, New Zealand, and the United States—cast negative votes, and there were 11 abstentions (Morgan et al. 2006). The inclusion of the term self-determination in the declaration was the most significant cause of controversy in this debate. The idea of self-determination has a long genesis outside the indigenous arena and is generally seen as a universal right that protects all peoples from political tyranny. Those who are opposed to the idea of indigenous self-determination argue that this concept threatens the unity of nation states—even though there are relatively few examples, if any, of indigenous secessionists in recent global history. Niezen (2003) argues that indigenous peoples have not pursued a secessionist political strategy for a number of reasons which include the fact that this would discharge nation states from their treaty obligations and further result in the creation of

relatively poor nations. Indigenous peoples have preferred to develop global political alliances rather than internal secessionist movements.

The political idea of self-determination has been manifest in a number of ways. At one end of the spectrum, some indigenous peoples have sought forms of regional autonomy; at the other end, they have insisted that governments consult with them on issues that impact of the development of policy, services, and indigenous social and economic development.

However, although most indigenous peoples have some form of self-determination in health policy, the range of policy responses have been quite diverse. These have included strategies to improve access to health services (particular primary-care services), address the social determinants of health, improve health data, and develop strategies that address the broad range of health inequalities in indigenous populations.

Ethnicity and health policy

Policies and provision for ethnic minorities in the health field are shaped by wider assumptions and policies that accord with either multicultural or assimilationist perspectives. Multiculturalism (or cultural pluralism) is an ideology advocating that society should allow and include distinct cultural and religious groups with equitable status, and is generally supported by the view that cultural diversity is a positive force for society and justified in terms of civil rights to equality of cultures. In contrast, assimilationist policies and practices encourage forms of acculturation to the norms and language of the dominant culture to achieve a monoculture.

In the United States, the mass immigrations of the early nineteenth century were associated with what was termed as the 'melting pot' concept, which emphasized the assimilation of each group of immigrants into American society at their own pace, although Federal and state governments now support many multiculturalist policies in the United States. Multiculturalism as an official national policy is regarded to have started in Canada, which in 1971 became a bilingual and bicultural country, and was followed by Australia in 1973. Multiculturalism has since been adopted by most member states of the European Union as the official policy. In the healthcare field, this ideology has led to considerable emphasis on the provision of culturally sensitive services to respond to differences in language, religion, diet, and lifestyles through the provision of interpreter services, patient advocates and link workers, information provided in minority languages, and provision for women patients to be attended only by women staff where this is a cultural expectation (Kai 2003).

A number of governments have recently expressed concerns that multiculturalism is divisive, and several European countries have begun to reverse this policy and to emphasize the importance of acculturation, often accompanied by the provision of compulsory language and citizenship courses to achieve this goal. The emphasis on cultural sensitivity has also been criticized from an anti-racist perspective as focusing overwhelmingly on supposed 'problems' of ethnic-minority groups that are internally generated through inappropriate cultural, familial, and community traditions. This in turn leads to a benevolent model of health-service provision in which the solution to problems are essentially technical and professional rather than political, based on the assumption that services will be improved with greater knowledge of different cultures, with improved skills in cross-cultural communication, and through the creation of particular ethnic specialisms. In contrast, an anti-racist perspective takes racism rather than culture as the starting point, and views racism as a pervasive reality structuring interactions at the interpersonal, organisational or institutional, and the structural or societal levels (Stubbs 1993). Thus, rather than merely responding to differences in cultural beliefs and practices, key requirements are to address the relatively disadvantaged position occupied by many ethnic-minority groups that increases health risks and discourages participation, and in particular to achieve the goal of equity among ethnic groups in the provision of health services (Bhopal 2007).

References

Adamson J., Ben ShlomoY., Chaturvedi N. *et al.* (2003). Ethnicity, socio-economic position and gender—do they affect reported health-care-seeking behaviour?. *Social Science and Medicine*;57:895–904.

Alberti K.G.M., Zimmet P., Shaw J. (2005). The metabolic syndrome—a new worldwide definition. *Lancet*;366:1059–62.

Alkhawar F.S., Stimson G.V., Warrens A.N. (2005). Attitudes towards transplantation in UK Muslim Indo-Indians in West London. *American Journal of Transplantation*;5:1326–31.

Anderson I., Baum F. *et al.* (2007). *Beyond bandaids: exploring the underlying social determinants of Aboriginal health*. Papers from the Social Determinants of Aboriginal Health Workshop, Adelaide, 2004 Jul. Darwin, Australia: Cooperative Research Centre for Aboriginal Health.

Anderson I., Crengle S., Kamaka M.L. *et al.* (2006). Indigenous health Part 1: indigenous health in Australia, New Zealand and Pacific. *Lancet*;367:1775–6.

Aspinall P.J., Dyson S.M., Anionwu E.N. (2003). The feasibility of using ethnicity as a primary tool for antenatal selective screening for sickle cell disorders: pointers from the research evidence. *Social Science and Medicine*;56:285–97.

Atri J., Falshaw M., Livingstone A. *et al.* (1996). Fair shares in health care? Ethnic and socioeconomic influences on recording of preventive care in selected inner London general practices: Healthy Eastenders Project. *British Medical Journal*;312:614–7.

Balarajan R. (1995). Ethnicity and variations in the nation's health. *Health Trends*;27:114–9.

Barsch R.L. (1989). United Nations seminar on indigenous peoples and states. *American Journal of International Law*; 833:599–604.

Beavon D., Cooke M. (2003). An application of the United Nations human development index to registered Indians in Canada, 1996. In: White JP, Maxim PS, Beavon D, editors. *Aboriginal conditions: research as a foundation for public policy*. Vancouver, Canada: University of British Columbia Press.

Betancourt J.R., King R.K. (2003). Unequal treatment: the Institute of Medicine report and its public health implications. *Public Health Reports*;118:287–92.

Bhopal R. (1997). Is research into ethnicity and health racist, unsound, or important science? *British Medical Journal*;314:1751.

Bhopal R.S., Phillimore P., Kohli H.S. (1991). Inappropriate use of the term 'Asian': an obstacle to ethnicity and health research. *Journal of Public Health Medicine*;13:244–6.

Bhopal R.S. (2007). Ethnicity, race, and health in multicultural societies. Oxford: Oxford University Press.

Bhugra D., Hilwig M., Hossein B. *et al.* (1996). First-contact incidence rates of schizophrenia in Trinidad and one-year follow-up. *British Journal of Psychiatry*;169:587–92.

Bhugra D., Minas I.H. (2007). Mental health and global movement of people. *Lancet*;370:1109–11.

Brereton B. (1981). *A history of modern Trinidad 1783 to 1962*. Oxford: Heinemann International.

Britton A., Shipley M., Marmot M. *et al.* (2004). Does access to cardiac investigation and treatment contribute to social and ethnic differences in coronary heart disease? The Whitehall II prospective cohort study. *British Medical Journal*;329:318.

Brown M.J. (2006). Hypertension and ethnic group. *British Medical Journal*;332:833–6.

Campbell C., McLean C. (2002). Ethnic identities, social capital and health inequalities: factors shaping African-Caribbean participation in local community networks in the UK. *Social Science and Medicine*; 55:643–57.

Cantor-Graae E., Selten J.P. (2005). Schizophrenia and migration: a meta-analysis and review. *American Journal of Psychiatry*; 162:12–24.

Carroll R., Ali N., Azam N. (2002). Promoting physical activity in South Asian Muslim women through 'exercise on prescription'. *Health Technology Assessment*;6:1–101.

Carson B., Dunbar T. *et al.* (2007). *Social determinants of indigenous health*. Crows Nest, NSW: Allen and Unwin.

Chaturvedi N., McKeigue P.M., Marmot M.G. (1994). Relationship of glucose intolerance to coronary risk in Afro-Caribbeans compared with Europeans. *Diabetologia*;37:765–72.

Chaturvedi N., McKeigue P.M., Marmot M.G. (1993). Resting and ambulatory blood pressure differences in Afro-Caribbeans and Europeans. *Hypertension*;22:90–6.

Cheung S.C.H. (2003). Ainu culture in transition. *Futures*;35:951–9.

Coates K.S. (2004). A global history of indigenous peoples struggle and survival. New York (NY): Palgrave Macmillan.

Cooper R.S., Kaufman J.S., Ward R. (2003). Race and genomics. *New England Journal of Medicine*;348:1166–70.

Cornell S., Hartman D. (1998). Ethnicity and race: making identities in a changing world. London: Pine Forge Press.

Dawson-Hughes B. (2004). Racial/ethnic considerations in making recommendations for vitamin D for adult and elderly men and women. *American Journal of Clinical Nutrition*;80:S763–6.

Department of Economic and Social Affairs (2004). The concept of indigenous peoples: workshop on data collection and dissagregation for indigenous peoples. New York (NY): United Nations.

Deshpande S.A. (2004). Ethnic differences in the rates of BCG vaccination. *Archives of Disease in Childhood*;89:48–9.

Dressler W.W., Orths K.S. *et al.* (2005). Race and ethnicity in public health research: models to explain health disparities. *Annual Review of Anthropology*;34:231–52.

Dunnigan M.G., McIntosh W.B., Sutherland G.R. *et al.* (1981). Policy for prevention of Asian rickets in Britain: a preliminary assessment of the Glasgow rickets campaign. *British Medical Journal*;282:357–60.

Dyson S.M., Culley L., Gill C. *et al.* (2006). Ethnicity questions and antenatal screening for sickle cell/thalassaemia [EQUANS] in England: a randomised controlled trial of two questionnaires. *Ethnicity and Health*;11:169–89.

Exeley C., Sim J., Reid N. *et al.* (1999). Attitudes and beliefs within the Sikh community regarding organ donation: a pilot study. *Social Science and Medicine*;43:23–8.

FAO Investment Centre (2006). Overview of socio-economic situation of the tribal communities and livelihoods in Madhya Pradesh and Bihar. Rome: FAO Investment Centre.

Fearon P., Kirkbride J.B., Morgan C. *et al.* (2006). AESOP Study Group. Incidence of schizophrenia and other psychoses in ethnic minority groups: results from the MRC AESOP Study. *Psychological Medicine*;36:1541–50.

Feder G., Grook A.M., Magee P. *et al.* (2002). Ethnic differences in invasive management of coronary disease: prospective cohort study of patients undergoing angiography. *British Medical Journal*;324:511–6.

Feiring B., Partners M. (2003). Indigenous peoples and poverty: the cases of Bolivia, Guatemala, Honduras and Nicaragua. London: Minority Rights Group International.

Fenton S. (1999). *Ethnicity: racism, class and culture*. Basingstoke: Macmillan.

Freemantle C.J., Read A.W. et al. (2006). Patterns, trends, and increasing disparities in mortality for Aboriginal and non-Aboriginal infants born in Western Australia, 1980–2001: population database study. *Lancet*;367.

Goldberg D. (1993). Racist culture: philosophy and the politics of meaning. Oxford: Blackwell.

Gulliford M.C., Chinn S., Rona R.J. (1991). Social environment and height: England and Scotland 1987 and 1988. *Archives of Disease in Childhood*;**66**:235–40.

Gulliford M.C., Mahabir D., Rocke B.C. et al. (2002). Free school meals and children's social and nutritional status in Trinidad and Tobago. *Public Health Nutrition*;**5**:625–30.

Guzel R., Kozanoglu E., Guler-Uysal F. et al. (2001). Vitamin D status and bone mineral density of veiled and unveiled Turkish women. *Journal of Women's Health and Gender-Based Medicine*;**10**:765–70.

Harding S., Rosato M., Teyhan A. (2008). Trends for coronary heart disease and stroke mortality among migrants in England and Wales, 1979–2003: slow declines notable for some groups. *Heart* 94, 463–70.

Hickling F.W., Rodgers-Johnson P. (1995). The incidence of first-contact schizophrenia in Jamaica. *British Journal of Psychiatry*;**167**:193–6.

Institute of Medicine (2003). Unequal treatment: what healthcare providers need to know about racial and ethnic disparities in healthcare. Washington (DC): Institute of Medicine.

International Labour Organization (2007). International Labour Organization 1996–2007. [Online]. Available from: http://www.ilo.org/global/lang--en/index.htm [retrieved 2007 Nov 6]

International Work Group for Indigenous Affairs (2007). Declaration on the rights of indigenous peoples 2007. [Online]. Available from: http://www.iwgia.org/sw248.asp [retrieved 2007 Oct 19]

Jones C.P. (2001). Invited commentary: 'Race', racism and the practice of epidemiology. *American Journal of Epidemiology*;**154**:299–304.

Jonnalagadda S.S., Diwan S. (2002). Nutrient intake of first-generation Gujarati Asian Indian immigrants in the US. *Journal of the American College of Nutrition*;**21**:372–80.

Kai J., editor (2003). *Ethnicity, health, and primary care*. Oxford: Oxford University Press.

Kaufman J.S., Durazo-Arvizu R.A., Rotimi C.N. et al. (1996). Obesity and hypertension prevalence in populations of African origin. *Epidemiology*;**7**:398–405.

Kingsbury B. (1998). 'Indigenous peoples' in international law: a constructivist approach to the Asian controversy. *American Journal of International Law*;**92**:414–57.

Kuper A. (2006). Indigenous people: an unhealthy category. *Lancet*;**366**:983.

Landman J., Cruickshank J.K. (2001). A review of ethnicity, health and nutrition-related diseases in relation to migration in the United Kingdom. *Public Health Nutrition*;**4**:647–57.

Levine R.S., Brigs N.C., Kilbourne B.S. et al. (2007). Black–White mortality from HIV in the United States before and after introduction of highly active antiretroviral therapy in 1996. *American Journal of Public Health*;**97**:1884–92.

Linnaeus C. (1806). A general system of nature through the three grand kingdoms of animals, vegetables and minerals: Systems Naturae. London: Lackington Allen and Co.

Logan J.R., Stults B.J., Farley R. (2004). Segregation of minorities in the metropolis: two decades of change. *Demography*;**41**:1–22.

Mahy G.E., Mallett R., Leff J. et al. (1999). First-contact incidence rate of schizophrenia in Barbados. *British Journal of Psychiatry*;**175**:28–33.

Miller G.J., Kirkwood B.R., Beckles G.L. et al. (1988). Adult male all-cause, cardiovascular and cerebrovascular mortality in relation to ethnic group, systolic blood pressure and blood glucose concentration in Trinidad, West Indies. *International Journal of Epidemiology*;**17**:62–9.

Mixer R.E., Jamrozik K., Newsom D. (2007). Ethnicity as a correlate of the uptake of the first dose of mumps, measles and rubella vaccine. *Journal of Epidemiology and Community Health*;**61**:797–801.

Modood T. (1994). Political blackness and British Asians. *Sociology*; **28**:859–76.

Molokhia M., Hoggart C., Patrick A.L. et al. (2003). Relation of risk of systemic lupus erythematosus to West African admixture in a Caribbean population. *Human Genetics*;**112**:310–8.

Montenegro R.A., Stephens C. (2006). Indigenous health in Latin America and the Caribbean. *Lancet*;**367**:1859–69.

Morgan C., Mallett R., Hutchinson G. et al. (2004). Negative pathways to psychiatric care and ethnicity: the bridge between social science and psychiatry. *Social Science and Medicine*;**58**:739–52.

Morgan M., Hooper R., Mayblin M. et al. (2006). Attitudes to kidney donation and registering as a donor among ethnic groups in the UK. *Journal of Public Health*;**28**:226–34.

Morgan M., Mayblin M., Jones R. (2008). Ethnicity and registration as a kidney donor: the significance of identity and belonging. *Social Science and Medicine*;**66**:147–58.

Mowbray M. (2007). The social determinants of indigenous health. The international experience and its policy implications. Adelaide: Commission on Social Determinants of Health.

Nazroo J.Y. (2003). The structuring of ethnic inequalities in health: economic position, racial discrimination, and racism. *American Journal of Public Health*;**93**:277–284.

Niezen R. (2003). The origins of indigenism. Human rights and the politics of identity. Berkeley (CA): University of California Press.

O'Neil D. (2007). Social organisation: glossary of terms, 2005. [Online]. Available from: http://anthro.palomar.edu/status/glossary.htm [retrieved 2007 Oct 25]

Office for National Statistics (2007). *Annual local area labour force survey*. London: Office for National Statistics; 2002. Available from: http://www.statistics.gov.uk/StatBase/Expodata/Spreadsheets/D6300.xls [accessed 2007 Dec 3]

Office for National Statistics (2007). Census 2001: ethnicity and religion in England and Wales. London: Office for National Statistics; 2007. Available from: http://www.statistics.gov.uk/pdfdir/ethnicity0203.pdf [accessed 2007 Dec 3]

Office of the High Commission for Human Rights (2007). Convention concerning indigenous and tribal peoples in independent countries No.169 [Online].Available from: http://www.unhchr.ch/html/menu3/b/62.htm [retrieved 2007 Aug 10]

Ohenjo N.O., Willis R. et al. (2006). The health of indigenous people in Africa. *Lancet*;**367**:1937–46.

Okosun I.S., Rotimi C.N., Forester T.E. et al. (2000). Predictive value of abdominal obesity cut-off points for hypertension in Blacks from West African and Caribbean island nations. *International Journal of Obesity*;**24**:180–6.

Osborne N.G., Feit M.D. (1992). The use of race in medical research. *Journal of American Medical Association*;**267**:275–9.

Peace R. (2001). Social exclusion: a concept in need of definition? *Social Policy Journal of New Zealand*;**16**:1172–438.

Peach C. (1996). The ethnic minority populations of Great Britain. In: *Ethnicity in the 1991 census;* vol. 2. London: Office for National Statistics.

Polednak A.P. (1997). Segregation, poverty and mortality in urban African Americans. New York (NY): Oxford University Press.

Rees P., Butt F. (2004). Ethnic change and diversity in England 1981 to 2001. *Area*;**36**:174–86.

Republic of Trinidad and Tobago, Central Statistical Office (1994). Age structure, religion, ethnic group, education. In: *Population and housing census 1990;* vol. 2. Port of Spain: Office of the Prime Minister, Central Statistical Office.

Ryan S. (1991). *Social and occupational stratification in contemporary Trinidad and Tobago*. St Augustine: Institute of Social and Economic Research, University of the West Indies.

Shaunak S., Colston K., Ang L. *et al.* (1985). Vitamin D deficiency in adult British Hindu Asians: a family disorder. *British Medical Journal*;**291**:1166–8.

Shaw N.J., Pal B.R. (2002). Vitamin D deficiency in UK Asian families: activating a new concern. *Archives of Disease in Childhood*;**86**:147–9.

Simmons D., Williams D.R., Powell M.J. (1992). Prevalence of diabetes in different regional and religious South Asian communities in Coventry. *Diabetic Medicine*;**9**:428–31.

Singh S.P., Burns T. (2006). Race and mental health: there is more to race than racism. *British Medical Journal*;**333**:648–51.

Sivanandan A. (1987). RAT and the degradation of the black struggle. In: *Racism awareness training: a critique*. London: Strategic Policy Unit; p. 54–87.

Smaje C., Le Grand J. (1997). Ethnicity, equity and the use of health services in the British NHS. *Social Science and Medicine*;**45**:485–96.

Smith D.G. (2002). Learning to live with complexity: ethnicity, socioeconomic position, and health in Britain and the United States. *American Journal of Public Health*;**90**:1694–8.

Sproston K., Mindell J. (2006). *Health survey for England 2004*. The health of minority ethnic groups. Leeds: The Information Centre.

Stamatopoulou E. (1994). Indigenous peoples and the United Nations: human rights as a developing dynamic. *Human Rights Quarterly*;**16**(1):58–81.

Stephens C., Nettleton C. *et al.* (2006). Indigenous peoples' health—why are they behind everyone, everywhere? *Lancet*;**366**:10–13.

Stephens C., Porter J. *et al.* (2006). Disappearing, displaced, and undervalued: a call to action for indigenous health worldwide. *Lancet*; **367**:2019–28.

Stubbs P. (1993). 'Ethnically sensitive' or 'anti-racist'? Models for health research and service delivery. In: Ahmad W.I.U., editor. *'Race' and health in contemporary Britain*. Buckingham: Open University Press; p. 34–50.

Szczepura A. (2004). Access to health care for ethnic minority populations. *Postgraduate Medical Journal*;**81**:141–7.

Trinidad and Tobago Central Statistical Office (2007). *Statistical pocket digest*. Port of Spain: Central Statistical Office; 2004. Available from: http://cso.gov.tt/files/cms/Pocket%20Digest%202004.pdf [accessed 2007 Dec 3.

UNESCO (2007). Universal declaration on cultural diversity, 2001. [Online]. Available from: http://unesdoc.unesco.org/images/0012/001271/127160m.pdf [accessed 2007 Nov 29]

United Nations General Assembly (2007). United Nations declaration on the rights of indigenous peoples. United Nations General Assembly; A/RES/61/295.

United States Census Bureau (2007). Overview of race and Hispanic origin. Washington (DC): United States Census Bureau Population Division; 2007. Available from: http://www.census.gov/population/www/cen2000/briefs.html [accessed 2007 Dec 3].

United States Department of Health and Human Services (2006). Health United States, 2006. Washington (DC): US Department of Health and Human Services.

Weatherall D., Akinyanju O., Fucharoen S. *et al.* (2007). Inherited disorders of haemoglobin. In: Jamison D.T. *et al*, editors. *Disease control priorities in developing countries*. 2nd ed. Washington (DC): World Bank Publications; 2007. Available from: http://files.dcp2.org/pdf/DCP/DCP34.pdf [accessed 2007 Nov 29]

Weaver H.N. (2001). Indigenous identity: what is it, and who really has it. *American Indian Quarterly*;**25**:240–55.

Webb R., Richardson J., Esmail A. *et al.* (2004). Uptake for cervical screening by ethnicity and place-of-birth: a population-based cross-sectional study. *Journal of Public Health*;**26**:293–6.

Wikipedia (2007). Stokely Carmichael. [Online]. Available from: http://en.wikipedia.org/wiki/Stokely_Carmichael [accessed 2007 Nov 29]

Wild S., Mckeigue P. (1997). Cross-sectional analysis of mortality by country of birth in England and Wales, 1970–92. *British Medical Journal*;**314**:705.

11.6

People with disabilities

Donald Lollar

Abstract

Disability is traditionally associated with morbidity and mortality as the negative public health outcomes. Primary prevention activities addressing birth defects, developmental disabilities, injuries, and chronic illnesses associated with disabling conditions are seminal to public health. There are, however, always going to be people in the population who fall through the primary prevention net and live with disabling conditions. Public health is beginning to acknowledge the potential role it plays in promoting the health and well-being of this population. This chapter addresses the emerging field of public health and disability.

The essential public health functions of assessment, policy development, and assurance are outlined for this population across countries and age groups. The World Health Organization's *International Classification of Functioning, Disability and Health* provides the framework for the conceptual and scientific issues. Clarifying definitions of 'disability' for purposes of public health surveillance and epidemiology, as well as research, are major emphases, including child disability measurement and caregiving or carers. Policy development emerges from the national and international conventions and activities, including the recently adopted UN Convention on the Rights of People with Disabilities, and supports the notion that the public health and disability communities have mutual responsibility for improving the health and well-being of this population. Assurance begins by asserting the relationship between poverty and disability, and includes discussion on interventions such as clinical preventive services, along with community-based rehabilitation activities.

Finally, the chapter outlines directions for public health and disability to develop more fully. Recommendations are made for improving communication, cooperation, and coordination of activities between the public health and disability communities. Curricula are coming available for the education and training of public health professionals in disability. Use of these curricula is strongly encouraged so that people with disabilities are included in public health science, programmes, and policy activities.

Introduction

Disability has traditionally been placed alongside morbidity and mortality as the negative public health outcomes. Preventing disabilities, therefore, has been a goal of public health activities. The activities to prevent disabling conditions are, indeed, a crucial aspect of public health work in the areas of birth defects, injuries, chronic illnesses, and even aging. However, this primary prevention emphasis begs the question: 'What happens to those who become disabled in spite of our best primary prevention efforts?' Individuals who fall through the public health prevention net by experiencing disabling conditions have been regarded as best served by medical and rehabilitation systems and services, and thus are seemingly outside the purview of public health. Medical and rehabilitative services are, indeed, crucial to those living with disabilities, but in fact do not take the place of public health.

In recent years, public health practitioners have begun to rethink this traditional stance, acknowledging that people with disabilities as a population are at greater risk for additional health and health-related problems, and therefore, are worthy of appropriate public health intervention. The most basic premise of this chapter, however, is that people with disabilities can experience and should experience a health status comparable to their peers without disabling conditions. People with disabilities can live healthy lives.

Public health emphasizes prevention. In the public health field of disability, this would include preventing secondary conditions among those with existing disabling conditions, in addition to promoting health and well-being. In some countries, medical care and rehabilitation are equated with disability; however, these services are rarely identified with public health. This chapter will describe current issues surrounding the inclusion of disability as an evolving concept and people with disabilities as an emerging population in public health. The three core public health functions—assessment, policy development, and assurance—will be applied to this population (Institute of Medicine 1988). Dimensions of disability, crossing the lifespan, international comparisons, and the role of environmental factors, will be described as they interact with these three public health functions. This chapter is meant to redefine disability and its conceptual and scientific relationship to public health.

As a preface, however, recent history must be invoked to provide a context for how public health and disability are evolving towards each other. Public health, although concerned with the population as a whole, has become progressively more concerned about certain populations at greater risk for disease, injury, and other aetiologic agents. This trend has focused primarily on ethnic minorities and other excluded groups who are more susceptible to diseases by virtue of being poor and marginalized with less access to health care. Simultaneously, a civil rights movement has been emerging among people with disabilities over the past 25 years, culminating in the UN's adoption of a Convention on the Rights of Persons with Disabilities in 2006 (United Nations 2006a). Although public health has evolved naturally from a medical approach to disability conditions, the disability rights movement has focused on disability as a social construct. Although these two models have vastly different emphases, there is growing awareness among public health professionals that people with disabilities can be viewed as a large minority population who are more vulnerable to various co-morbid conditions or secondary conditions, those that are more probable due to a primary disabling condition. Table 11.6.1 provides an overview of basic differences between the perspectives. The World Health Organization (WHO) has developed a framework for viewing disability that accounts for both models, and is becoming both the conceptual and scientific framework for integrating public health and disability.

Over the past 40 years, several paradigms of disability have developed. Disability models are currently best represented by the WHO's *International Classification of Functioning, Disability and Health* (ICF) (World Health Organization 2001). The ICF was approved by the World Health Assembly in 2001, and it is becoming the global standard both conceptually and scientifically. The ICF combines the medical and social models into what is described as a bio-psychosocial model of disability. Figure 11.6.1 depicts the ICF model.

The WHO began work to revise a previous disability classification in the early 1990s. Over the course of almost a decade, over 800 individuals, including individuals living with disabling conditions, representing more than 60 countries participated in the revision process. The resultant product emerged as a member of the WHO family of international classifications, the most notable member being the *International Classification of Diseases* (ICD) (World Health Organization 1992). The ICF took a different conceptual approach, addressing components of health rather than consequences of disease—the focus of the earlier rendition. In addition, a most crucial conceptual and coding component was added to the ICF—environmental factors. The importance of the environment as it interacts with health and functioning is explicit in this system. Environmental elements for the ICF interact with every other component.

The ICF does not address causes or aetiologies, but rather addresses function and health. From the beginning, the emphasis

has been to provide a complement to the ICD. In addition, the purpose of the classification is to provide a foundation for the scientific study of function, health, and disability, as well as to provide a common language to be used across populations, sectors, ages, and users. The coding system outlined in the ICF allows public health professionals to collect data for population use, in addition to its use in clinical work to assess individual needs, plan interventions, and assess outcomes.

The components of the framework illustrated in Fig. 11.6.1 include functioning across all spheres—body structures and functions, personal activities, and societal participation. Body functions and structures refer to the physiological functions of body systems and the anatomical parts of the body, respectively. A problem with body functions or structures is referred to as *impairment*. A personal task or action undertaken by an individual is termed as an *activity*, and a difficulty in this area is called an *activity limitation*. Likewise, functioning in society in a life situation is termed as *participation*, with a problem in this functioning being called a *participation restriction*. Finally, an *environmental factor* includes any physical, social or attitudinal, and systemic element that affects the functioning of the individual, potentially in all components of body, person, and society (World Health Organization 2001). Figure 11.6.2 provides an outline of the one-level two-character codes for each of the components of the ICF. The full coding system allows coding up to six characters, permitting functional descriptions at both broad and specific levels. The functional codes can be used in both public health surveillance and in epidemiologic studies. Of particular importance for epidemiologic studies is the inclusion of qualifier codes that can be attached after the functional dimension. Qualifiers range from zero to four for severity and encompass a spectrum from 'no problem' to 'complete problem'. In addition, qualifiers can be used clinically to show changes in limitation and participation because of interventions and can be used to monitor change over time (World Health Organization 2001).

This framework provides the most plausible system for common understanding of disability concepts, definitions, and specific functional codes across countries, ages, and sectors, which are relevant for public health purposes related to assessment, policy development, and assurance.

Assessment

Public health assessment is defined as the regular, systematic collection and analysis of information on the health of a community or population. It should include data on health status, health needs of the population, and epidemiologic and other studies of health difficulties. Assessment begins with a most basic tenet—a definition of which health issue is to be assessed. Case definitions are crucial to appropriate identification and are the basis for surveillance, epidemiology, and potential intervention strategies.

Historically, definitions of disability and identification of those experiencing disability have varied greatly in those public health or other sector activities in which this population was included. Definitions for the purpose of identification of individuals with disabilities fall into one of several categories. Traditional approaches to defining disability for public health have focused on equating a particular diagnosis with disability: An individual with a diagnosis of cerebral palsy or blindness, for example, would be assumed to have a disability. A second approach has been to focus on the

Table 11.6.1 Differences between the medical and social model perspectives

Area of concern	Medical model	Social model
Locus of problem	Individual	Society
Focus of change	Individual behaviour	Societal attitudes/culture
Changes needed	Personal adjustment	Environmental changes
Intervention strategy	Individual treatment	Social action
Policy issues	Medical/health care	Human rights/access to care

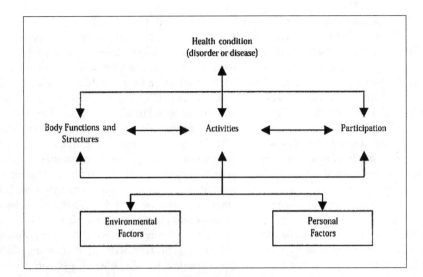

Fig. 11.6.1 Interactions among the *International Classification of Functioning, Disability and Health* components.
Source: Reprinted with permission of the World Health Organization.

impairment—that is, if someone cannot hear in one ear or has an intellectual or learning difficulty, he or she would be considered to have a disability. Third, limitations in particular activities, such as self-care or moving around, have been defined as disabilities. Another approach has been to identify those with problems in working or going to school because of a health problem as having a disability. Yet another approach is to identify those who need special programmes, such as special education or vocational rehabilitation, or special therapies such as physical, occupational, or speech therapy as having a disability. Further, another approach is to ask the individuals themselves if they or others would identify them as someone with a disability (self-identification).

Using these different definitions will produce different prevalence rates. For example, countries using a question such as 'Is anyone in the household deaf, blind, or mute?' as a disability identifier usually will find a prevalence of disability in the 1–2 per cent range. On the other hand, for an activity-oriented question or set of questions—such as, 'Does anyone in your household have difficulty seeing a friend across the street?' or 'Does anyone in your household have difficulty taking care of themselves in eating, drinking, toileting, or dressing?'—the prevalence of disability reaches double digits, and in some countries might approach 20 per cent (United Nations 1990). In more developed countries, several of the approaches to defining disability can be used according to the government agency

Body functions

b1 Mental functions
b2 Sensory functions and pain
b3 Voice and speech functions
b4 Cardiovascular, haematological, immunological, and respiratory
b5 Digestive, metabolic, and endocrine functions
b6 Genitourinary and reproductive functions
b7 Neuromusculoskeletal and movement-related functions
b8 Functions of the skin and related functions

Body structures

s1 The nervous system
s2 Eye, ear, and related structures
s3 Structures for voice and speech
s4 Cardiovascular, immunological, and respiratory structures
s5 Digestive, metabolic, and endocrine structures
s6 Genitourinary and reproductive structures
s7 Structures related to movement

s8 Skin and related structures

Activities and participation

d1 Learning and applying knowledge
d2 General tasks and demands

d3 Communication
d4 Mobility
d5 Self-care
d6 Domestic life
d7 Interpersonal interactions and relationships
d8 Major life areas
d9 Community, social, and civic life

Environmental factors

e1 Products and technology
e2 Natural environment and human-made changes to environment
e3 Support and relationships
e4 Attitudes
e5 Services, systems, and policies

Fig. 11.6.2 Outline of the one-level two-character codes for each of the *International Classification of Functioning, Disability and Health* components.

or purpose for the definition. For example, definitions to address civil rights issues for people with disabilities will be intended to be broad, whereas those providing compensation for disability related to work will be more stringent (Lollar & Crews 2003). Table 11.6.2 provides data on the prevalence of disability in selected countries by source, across low-, middle-, and high-income countries. These figures highlight the different rates outlined by the various definitions described—self-identification related to lower rates and functional approaches producing higher rates. In addition, this table highlights the trend towards higher rates of disability being found in surveys than in censuses. Censuses, however, need to be used for comparisons because low-income countries often have no other mechanism for data collection (Mont 2007a). Better approaches to question formation are needed for these countries.

The United Nations Statistics Division (UNSD) published the first compendium of disability statistics in 1990 (United Nations 1990), which included data from 55 countries and provided prevalence figures and differing case definitions. A major goal of the volume was to begin to develop international standards for disability statistics. Since that initial effort, the UNSD has published the *Guidelines and Principles for the Development of Disability Statistics* (United Nations 2001). This document provided clearer guidelines

Table 11.6.2 Prevalence of disability in selected countries, by source.*

Censuses			Surveys		
Country	Year	Per cent with disability	Country	Year	Per cent with disability
United States	2000	19.4	New Zealand	1996	20.0
Canada	2001	18.5	Australia	2000	20.0
Brazil	2000	14.5	Uruguay	1992	16.0
United Kingdom	1991	12.2	Spain	1986	15.0
Poland	1988	10.0	Austria	1986	14.4
Ethiopia	1984	3.8	Zambia	2006	13.1
Uganda	2001	3.5	Sweden	1988	12.1
Mali	1987	2.7	Ecuador	2005	12.1
Mexico	2000	2.3	Netherlands	1986	11.6
Botswana	1991	2.2	Nicaragua	2003	10.3
Chile	1992	2.2	Germany	1992	8.4
India	2001	2.1	China	1987	5.0
Colombia	1993	1.8	Italy	1994	5.0
Bangladesh	1982	0.8	Egypt	1996	4.4
Kenya	1987	0.7			

Note: Rates vary according to type of disability-identifier questions used, and are explained in the text.

* Statistics complied using data from UNSD, IBGR (Brazil), INEC (Nicaragua), INEC (Ecuador), INEGI (Mexico), Statistics New Zealand, INE (Spain), Census of India 2001, and SINTEF Health Research 2006 (Zambia).

Source: Reprinted with permission of the World Bank. SP Discussion Paper No. 0706 by Mont D; 2007 Mar.

on how national statistical offices could improve the questions used and data collection methods employed, as well as how they could approach the dissemination of data overall. The UN guidelines used the ICF framework to assist countries as they work towards harmonization and comparability in disability data.

In 2001, the UNSD convened a group of disability experts from around the world to address the need for more standardized disability measures. From this conference emerged the Washington City Group on Disability Measurement (city groups are a mechanism used by the UN to focus on specific topics and are named after the city in which they meet first.) This international group has developed a short set of questions that were field-tested in several countries. After intensive discussion and analysis of questions used in numerous countries, a set of six questions focusing on personal activities are being tested now. The questions currently cover difficulty seeing, hearing, walking or climbing stairs, remembering or concentrating, washing oneself, and communicating (Centers for Disease Control and Prevention 2006a). The conclusion has been that, in surveys and censuses, respondents can report person-level activities more reliably and validly than they can diagnoses or impairments. Therefore, across settings and countries, comparable data on disabilities can be generated. There is continuing discussion about how to ensure the inclusion of those with cognitive or mental health problems in short sets of disability questions.

As definitions are clarified, there are several kinds of questions that can be further asked by public health about a subpopulation, such as: 'What characterizes this group beyond its disability status?', 'Which conditions are most associated with disability?', and 'Are there disparities between this group and the general population?'

In a recent publication from the United States, data on chronic health conditions contributing to a limitation of activity (disability) indicated that arthritis and other musculoskeletal conditions were most frequently associated with limitations among working-age adults, aged 18–44 years. Mental illness was the second condition most associated with activity limitation, followed by fractures or joint injuries. With increasing age (45–64 years), arthritis was still the most frequently cited condition associated with activity limitation, but was followed by heart and circulatory conditions. Mental illness and diabetes were also mentioned often. The same conditions were associated with activity limitation in the 65–74 age group, but in the 75 years and over age group, senility and vision or hearing problems substantially increased. Throughout all age groups, however, arthritis and heart problems were most related to causing activity limitations (Centers for Disease Control and Prevention 2006b).

In Australia, data have indicated that 20 per cent of the people are living with a disability, also defined as limitation of activity but including impairments and participation restrictions. Among the population, 6.3 per cent have experienced a profound or severe core activity limitation, indicating a need for help with self-care, mobility, or communication. Australia uses a four-factor approach to the kind of disability reported—physical or diverse, sensory or speech, psychiatric, and intellectual or learning. Fifteen per cent of the population have reported physical or diverse category as the disability most affecting their everyday lives. Approximately 2 per cent of the population reported the psychiatric and sensory or speech categories, whereas the intellectual category contributed just less than 1 per cent. As with the United States, older age groups experience more disabling conditions, but the prevalence of severe disability is rather stable (Australian Institute of Health and Welfare 2006).

The Canadian Participation and Activity Limitation Survey from 2001 indicated that 12.4 per cent of individuals reported some degree of disability, defined as limitations in daily living due to a physical, psychological, or health condition. Among adults, the most common limitation was mobility, defined as having problems walking, climbing stairs, or moving from one room to another. Working-age adults reported that the next most common form of disability was from pain (69.5 per cent) (Statistics Canada 2002).

Data from the United Kingdom used 'limiting long-term illness' as the disability approach, and reported 16 per cent of the population in that category. Similar to the Canadian data, the most common limitation was mobility, followed by lifting, carrying, and dexterity. Musculoskeletal problems were most commonly reported as the cause of limitations, then heart and circulatory difficulties, followed by respiratory disorders (Department of Health 1991).

All of these high-income countries have the ability to collect disability data from several sources, such as censuses and varied surveys, and use several definitions of disability—from reported impairments, activity limitations, and participation restrictions. Population-based interventions can be better tailored to a particular group when the characteristics of the population are more clearly understood. Low-income countries, on the other hand, are usually able to collect disability data only during a decennial census and, thus, have substantially less information for the purpose of policy development or assurance of services.

An example of characterizing those identified as having a disability, regardless of the definition, is the data from the United States. The public health agenda for the country has been established every 10 years since the 1980s. The current *Healthy People 2010* includes 'disability status' as a demographic variable for many of the health objectives. For example, one objective is to reduce the number of adults with disabilities who feel sad, depressed, or unhappy; the disparity between those with and those without disabilities in the general population at baseline was 21 per cent (28 per cent adults with disabilities *versus* 7 per cent of the general population). Likewise, a 9 per cent disparity was reported on life satisfaction between adults with and those without disabilities (United States Department of Health and Human Services 2000). In the United States, people with disabilities report obesity at a rate of 31.2 per cent, whereas those without disability reported a 19.6 per cent rate. Physical inactivity was also twice as prevalent among people with disabilities as those without disabilities (22.4 per cent *versus* 11.9 per cent) (Centers for Disease Control and Prevention 2006c).

In a report from the Special Rapporteur on Disability of the UN Commission for Social Development in 2006, results of a UN survey were presented. The survey included questions related to national monitoring of disability. Of the 73 countries responding, about 50 per cent had adopted an official definition of disability and 48 per cent had worked on collecting disability data. In terms of the range of data, 43 per cent were collecting data on the prevalence of disability, and 55 per cent included the types of disabilities. Fifty-six percent reported using data to develop policy (United Nations 2006b).

Using the ICF framework, and given the importance of the environment on the health and well-being of individuals with disabilities, assessment of environmental factors is also emerging.

Satariano (1997) noted the importance of environment in the aging process and indicated that public health professionals need to understand and conceptualize the role of the physical environment so as to enhance the independence and mobility of this population. Altman *et al.* (2003), using data from the National Health Interview Survey in the United States, concluded that people with disabilities are more likely to report environmental barriers to their participation in everyday life. The type of functional or activity limitation appears to be related to which barriers are most reported, and respondents in this survey emphasized physical barriers rather than attitudinal or policy barriers. This element of assessment is continuing to develop.

Child disability measurement

Assessing children and youth can be just as or more difficult than assessing adults. First, a child or youth is not usually asked to respond to questions, rather a parent or other proxy. Second, if activity limitation is the approach used to assess disability, at early ages the inability to complete the tasks is developmentally appropriate—that is, the child is not supposed to be able to complete a task, such as dressing or toileting. Also, developmental stages make interpretation of limitations more problematic. Because of these differences, the WHO empowered a working group of international consultants in childhood disability to revise the ICF so that unique aspects of child and youth development and function would be captured (Lollar & Simeonsson 2005). The ICF-CY (Children and Youth) was approved by the WHO in 2006, and published in 2007 (World Health Organization 2007b).

In a 2006 report from the Australian Institute of Health and Welfare, 8.3 per cent of Australian children were reported to have a disability. The report indicated that the most prevalent disabling conditions related to intellectual or learning (4.3 per cent) and physical or diverse (4.2 per cent). Sensory or speech accounted for 3.4 per cent, and psychiatric conditions were reported for 1.2 per cent of the children and youth.

A 2003 study from the United States used the ICF as a framework and the National Health Interview Survey Disability Supplement from 1994–95 to show limitations in activities among children and youth (Fedeyko & Lollar 2003); a prevalence rate of 12 per cent was found using this approach. Learning limitations were more than twice as prevalent as the next highest contributors—communication and social or emotional difficulties. Sensory (vision and hearing) disability was a distant fourth. The *Chart Book on Trends in the Health of Americans* (Centers for Disease Control and Prevention 2006b) indicated that, according to age, different health conditions undermine function more often. Preschoolers have a higher prevalence of speech problems, breathing difficulties related to asthma, and learning or other developmental problems. Learning problems and attention-deficit hyperactivity disorder were the major contributors to activity limitations among school-age children. Older children added emotional and behavioural problems as important aetiologies. Stein and Silver (2002) compared four different definitions of chronic conditions and disabilities among children; the children and youth ranged in age from birth to 17 years. Using a common data set, the National Health Interview Survey from the United States, operational definitions identified between 13.7 and 17 per cent of the population of children with chronic conditions or disabilities. Differing definitions included those using specific diagnoses associated with developmental disabilities and those using consequences of conditions, such as limitations, need for therapies or medication, and the use of compensatory equipment or assistive technology. They concluded that there was significant overlap in the characteristics and prevalence rates, even using different conceptual definitions.

Durkin *et al.* (1995) employed an activity limitation approach to develop a screener of 10 questions for childhood disability. It has been used in several countries, including Bangladesh, Jamaica, and Pakistan where 15.6 per cent, 14.7 per cent, and 8.2 per cent, respectively, of children were identified as having disabilities (Durkin *et al.* 1994). The method used to identify the children was different, however, in that the studies are not usually population-based. The positive aspect is that children identified by the screener can be evaluated more thoroughly, if resources are available; intervention is then possible. The US National Survey of Children with Special Health Care Needs uses a similar activity-oriented approach, which more explicitly follows the ICF-CY model: It includes 13 questions, some of which are related to social and emotional limitations (Maternal and Child Health Bureau 2005). Analysis will allow a substantially greater understanding of both functioning and service use and satisfaction than has been previously possible.

Carers, caregivers, and personal assistance services (PAS)

Beyond obtaining the data to determine the prevalence of people with disabilities, public health should also address the health and well-being of those who provide assistance or care to individuals with disabilities. Most often, this involves family members but also includes paid caregivers or carers. Carers UK suggests that approximately 3 million carers work in the United Kingdom, and that 60 per cent of people will be a carer at some point in their life (ACE National Action for Carers and Employment 2007; Carers UK 2007). Australian data (Australian Institute of Health and Welfare 2006) indicates that 202 000 persons are the primary carers of individuals under 65 of age and live with the person for whom they care. These carers are primarily parents caring for a child or persons caring for a spouse or partner. It was reported that respite care was limited for these carers. Data from Canada indicate that parents of children with disabling conditions report substantial tension as a result of trying to coordinate work, family, and child-care duties, compromising the quality of life (Canadian Institute of Child Health 2000). In the United States, approximately 53 million people are caregivers, providing unpaid services estimated at US$257–389 billion (Arno *et al.* 1999). The persons providing the most intense level of care reported poor health more often than those providing moderate levels of care (Talley & Crews 2007). The numbers and economic impact of caregiving are substantial. Public health associations in high-income countries are only beginning to address this subject, and low-income countries are even less able to address this important health issue.

Measures of health and disability

As more data and sophisticated methods of data analysis are becoming available in many countries, attempts have been made to generate statistics that can better inform public health. Some statistics particularly focused on evaluating the relative effectiveness of public health interventions, among which are the years of healthy life (YHL), quality-adjusted life years (QALYs), and disability-adjusted life years (DALYs). The DALYs indicator was developed with support from the World Bank (Murray & Lopez 1996), and has been used in numerous reports to assess public health priorities and to set a future public health agenda. Because DALYs use the term disability, and because it is being employed so frequently to set public health priorities, it is important that public health professionals understand the relationship between DALYs and the 'current' definitions of disability.

DALYs are based on a definition of disability that correlates with individual disease states. This emphasis on disease assumes that all disease states translate into similar activity limitations and participation restrictions, and assumes no influence of, equal influence of, or only random influence of environmental factors. Over several years, public health professionals, economists, and the disability community have questioned several of the core terms, methods, and implications of the use of DALYs, including using the term disability to describe the statistics. Chamie (1995) suggested that DALYs misrepresent the concept of disability, and it would be better using a term such as *morbidity-adjusted* or *illness-adjusted*, given the method used to generate the measure.

The method requires health professionals to assess the burden of 22 disease-related conditions using preference weighting—the Person Trade-off (PTO) Method. Personal preferences, not population-based data, are used to characterize disability. The methodology used to generate DALYs, the lack of a functional definition of disability in most countries to identify people with disabilities, and the exclusion of people with disabilities in the development process makes the outcomes of this utility suspect (Grosse *et al.* 2009). Mont (2007b) suggested that DALYs were a poor indicator of how public health interventions affect or improve the lives of people with disabilities. He reported that the primary objective in the development of this indicator was to implement a metric that could help national policy makers in allocating resources to reduce poor health. Given the competing needs of people and the minimal resources available, governments have to make difficult decisions regarding public health improvement. Mont concluded that 'an indicator that does not properly embody the intended goals can build in systematic bias against achieving them' (Mont 2007b). The use of DALYs to inform public health policy is questionable, and methods incorporating increased levels of participation by people with disabilities compared to people without disabilities should be developed. Mont and Loeb (2008) have developed a protocol for addressing impact of activity limitations and impairments on participation using population-based data from Zambia. This approach provides a more scientific and generalizable approach to measuring the impact of disabling conditions on people with disabilities. In addition, it allows monitoring of changes in participation across the population and for comparisons across populations.

In summary, whatever the source (e.g. survey, census, or administrative data), public health data should be both periodic and predictable in timing. It is important that disability definitions be separated from outcomes so that analyses can compare groups with and without disabilities. When possible, environmental factors affecting outcomes should also be included in surveys, if not in censuses. Finally, if disability data are to be accepted for the purpose of policy development, people with disabilities should be included at each point in the development, collection, and analysis of data. The disability community dictum of 'nothing about us without us' is particularly important as public health assesses, characterizes, and compares this population with the general population.

Policy development

Data obtained about persons with disabilities alone do not make a difference in public health or in their own lives. Policy development addresses the need for public health policies to use scientific knowledge in decision making, as public health policy is best formulated on the foundation of strong data. Integral to the development of a more consistent approach to public health data collection on disability is the application of this data. Since 1982, when the World Programme of Action was adopted by the United Nations General Assembly, disability policy has been a global mandate (United Nations 1982). The Standard Rules on the Equalization of Opportunities for Persons with Disabilities (United Nations 1993) were developed by the UN to operationalize the Programme, and have been the basis for policy directions globally. Disability data allow countries to evaluate themselves, or have others evaluate them, as to how people with disabilities fare in relation with the general population.

The Standard Rules are divided into three groups—preconditions for equal participation (Rules 1–4), target areas for equal participation (Rules 5–12), and implementation measures (Rules 13–22). Figure 11.6.3 provides an outline of the rules. The end product of these rules is that people with disabilities have an opportunity to participate in society as equals to people without disabilities. It is a step beyond traditional public health and moves further than the emphasis on preventing disease, injury, and disability to embrace the higher-order outcome of participation. This move made when the WHO adopted as its mission 'to improve health and well-being' around the globe. This broader interpretation is the result of an ongoing interaction between public health professionals and the disability community.

It is noteworthy that Rules 2 and 3—medical care and rehabilitation—are the traditional roles acknowledged by public health. The emphasis in Rule 2 (medical care) is on early detection, assessment, and treatment of *impairment*, which can 'prevent, reduce, or eliminate disabling effects'. Also, states are encouraged to provide regular treatment and medication that is needed for people with disabilities to maintain or improve functioning. Rule 3 recommends that national rehabilitation programmes for all people with disabilities be developed. Programmes should focus on the daily needs of these individuals with the goal of full participation and equality. Recommendations are that individuals be involved in their own rehabilitation, that services be available in the local community, and that advocacy groups be included in national programme planning.

Implementation measures are, in fact, the processes that must be in place for the preconditions and target areas to be addressed. Most of the target areas are really the specific outcome areas in which opportunities should arise—for example, education, employment, recreation and sports, culture, and religion. Throughout the Document, the term *health* is rarely found. The concept of health promotion is also absent, and can only be found by an extensive reading of the early detection, assessment, and treatment of impairment or the provision of health care and related services to all people in order to reduce or prevent the 'disability effects of impairment' (United Nations 1993). An emerging area for public health intervention focuses specifically on promoting health and preventing secondary conditions often associated with primary disabilities—such as decubitus ulcers or skin sores among persons with spinal injuries. Physical activity and nutrition, smoking, and alcohol abuse, for example, are clear areas for public health policy and assurance in many countries. However, people with disabilities are often not seen as a vulnerable population for public health messages. Formulation of policy addressing not only rehabilitation and medical services but also health promotion and secondary condition prevention are important areas to be addressed among people with disabilities.

South Africa has provided arguably the most complete national strategy interpreting the UN Standard Rules (Office of the Deputy President 1997). The White Paper on an Integrated National Disability Strategy comprises policy guidelines for the major areas

---

Major areas

Preconditions	Target areas
Rule 1 Awareness raising	Rule 5 Accessibility
Rule 2 Medical care	Rule 6 Education
Rule 3 Rehabilitation	Rule 7 Employment
Rule 4 Support services	Rule 8 Income maintenance/social security
	Rule 9 Family life and personal integrity
	Rule 10 Culture
	Rule 11 Recreation and sports
	Rule 12 Religion

Implementation measures

Rule 13 Information and research	Rule 18 Organizations of persons with disabilities
Rule 14 Policy making and planning	Rule 19 Personnel training
Rule 15 Legislation	Rule 20 National monitoring/evaluation of disability programmes
Rule 16 Economic policies	Rule 21 Technical and economic cooperation
Rule 17 Coordination of work	Rule 22 International cooperation

Fig. 11.6.3 Adapted from outline of the standard rules on the equalization of opportunities for persons with disabilities.
Source: United Nations. *Standard rules on equalization of opportunities for disabled persons*. New York [NY]: United Nations; 1993.

of the Standard Rules, including prevention, health care, and rehabilitation. Secondary prevention is included and suggests that the targets might be the prevention of complications, such as contractures for those with cerebral palsy. Inclusion of secondary prevention is a critical element in health policy related to disability. A national data base is being developed to provide an array of medical- and disability-related services, as well as to collect information on health-related needs and incidence of impairments. The policy objectives for data and research focus on the gaps between physical and mental conditions and their causes, including the environmental factors influencing them.

In 2007, countries began to sign the first UN convention of the new century—a convention establishing the rights of people with disabilities. This convention provides a roadmap to end discrimination and marginalization of people with physical or mental conditions and has a goal to eliminate exploitation and abuse. Its premise is that people with disabilities have an inherent right to life equal to that of people without disabilities and should receive equal protection and rights, including control of their own financial affairs and the right to privacy. Health is addressed in Article 25, and addresses access to health care, financing, and health professionals' training. Provision of population-based health programmes equivalent to the general population is included—for the first time. Implicit, though not explicitly stated, is the notion that people with disabilities can live healthily.

Although public health professionals can be faulted for not including people with disabilities in health messages for the population, and not recognizing their unique characteristics of vulnerability (for example, the difficulty of balancing nutrition and exercise among those using wheelchairs), the disability community must also recognize its complicity in this omission. In many policy debates surrounding the rights of people with disabilities, there has been an ambivalence to include health. For many people living with disabilities, health is equated with medical intervention and contact. At times, if not often, both medical care and rehabilitation are a source of (1) painful physical experiences, even for treatment; (2) difficulty accessing services; and (3) negative attitudes from medical staff. Therefore, when issues such as civil rights emerge, there is emphasis on employment, education, accessibility to public accommodations, transportation, and so forth, but little acknowledgment of the importance of health as one of the foundations for use of these other rights.

Countries have begun formulating public health policy by setting national health goals. *The Health of the Nation* was published by the Department of Health in the United Kingdom in 1991 (Department of Health 1991). Key areas were selected for attention, which included causes of substantial mortality such as cancer, causes of substantial ill health such as diabetes and mental health, factors contributing to mortality and morbidity such as smoking and diet, areas having potential for great harm (e.g. HIV/AIDS), and areas in which there was clear scope for improvement. This final area included rehabilitation services for people with a physical disability. Emphasis is placed on raising the awareness of medical professionals about care of individuals with chronic physical conditions by raising expectations for people with disabilities. Employing doctors with training in rehabilitation is seen as a step towards better service and higher expectation for function. The assumption is that better rehabilitation services will reduce pressure sores, contractures, and incontinence. Tailored health messages for wheelchair users or relating smoking to elevated skin breakdown associated with decubitus ulcers, however, are not considered as a possible broader public health awareness approach.

Healthy People 2010 (HP 2010) is the national public health agenda for the United States. The inclusion of a chapter in this volume that focuses on improving the health and well-being of people with disabilities is a major step forwards for public health policy in the United States. Addressing four basic misconceptions is at the core of the HP2010 chapter on disability and secondary conditions. First, there is a misconception that people with disabilities are, by definition, in poor health by virtue of living with a disabling condition; it follows, then, that people living with disabilities cannot be healthy. Second, public health has no responsibility for promoting the health of people with disabilities and is responsible only for preventing disabling conditions. Third, there is no need, therefore, to create or develop a case definition for 'people with disabilities'. Fourth, there is a misconception that the environment is unrelated to disability and that any disabling condition lies within the person. The 13 HP 2010 objectives address these misconceptions most clearly by setting targets that match those for the general population. For example, Objective 6-3 has the goal of reducing the proportion of adults with disabilities who are depressed to a level that has parity with all adults aged 18 years and older without disabilities in the United States. Objective 6-13 addresses the goal of having data and programmes for people with disabilities and caregivers in all 50 states by 2010. Figure 11.6.4 outlines the HP2010 objectives for Chapter 6: Disability and Secondary Conditions (United States Department of Health and Human Services 2000).

Regional reports from countries selected in Asia and the Americas have been completed by the International Disability Rights Monitor (Center for International Rehabilitation 2003; Center for International Rehabilitation 2004; Center for International Rehabilitation 2005). These reports include information from 33 countries and reflect policy data on disability measures, as well as on health, rehabilitation, and medical issues.

Child disability policy

As with public health assessment, policy issues are different for children with disabling conditions. The 1989 UN Convention on the Rights of the Child specifically addresses children with disabilities in Article 23 (United Nations 1989). It is committed to the view that these children should enjoy a full life under conditions that allow them to live with dignity, self-determination, and participation in the life of their community. It indicates the right to special care and assistance for them and their families or caregivers. Finally, any such help should come without cost and should include education, training, health care, rehabilitation, and services with the goal of individual development and social integration. This convention has been signed by virtually all countries in the world, and provides the foundation for national policies addressing the needs of children with disabilities. As noted, health care and rehabilitation are included in those rights.

Assessment can identify the magnitude of problem and the population to be targeted. Policies that provide special attention to those needing it can be developed. The final core function of public health, however, is most crucial to those individuals living with a disability—assurance.

Goal: Promote the health of people with disabilities, prevent secondary conditions, and eliminate disparities between people with and without disabilities in the US population.

Number	Objective short title
6-1	Standard definition of people with disabilities in data sets
6-2	Feelings and depression among children with disabilities
6-3	Feelings and depression interfering with activities among adults with disabilities
6-4	Social participation among adults with disabilities
6-5	Sufficient emotional support among adults with disabilities
6-6	Satisfaction with life among adults with disabilities
6-7	Congregate care of children and adults with disabilities
6-8	Employment parity
6-9	Inclusion of children and youth with disabilities in regular education programmes
6-10	Accessibility of health and wellness programmes
6-11	Assistive devices and technology
6-12	Environmental barriers affecting participation in activities
6-13	Surveillance and health-promotion programmes

Fig. 11.6.4 Outline of the *Healthy People 2010* objectives for Chapter 6: Disability and Secondary Conditions. *Source:* United States Department of Health and Human Service, 2000.

Assurance

Assurance focuses on the certitude that needed services will be provided to individuals and communities so that health goals can be reached. Assurance also suggests that services must not only be present but also maintained so that goals can be met. Implicit in these assertions is the notion that there are challenges or barriers to the provision and use of services that must be addressed. Assurance advises that the use of authority may be required to ensure that services will be provided and will not be too costly to access (IOM 1988).

Assurance of services includes not only the presence of services but also the access to those services. Access includes physical proximity or reasonable transport to travel to the services, physical accessibility to the services, policies and systems that allow financial access, and attitudes that encourage participation in the services. The services include clinical preventive services usually set as a baseline for everyone in any particular country, health promotion activities, and prevention of secondary conditions, in addition to basic medical care and rehabilitation.

A basic barrier to assurance of public health services and attention is poverty. Poverty not only contributes to disability but the presence of a disability contributes to poverty, particularly in low-income countries. This applies to any country or group, and it is applicable to people with disabilities because employment rates among them are substantially lower (in the United States, 75 per cent *versus* 37 per cent for individuals with and without disabilities, respectively) (United States Department of Health and Human Services 2000).

In public health, primary prevention programmes are extremely important across the life span. However, even with intense efforts to prevent birth defects, developmental disabilities, injuries, and chronic illnesses, for the foreseeable future, children and adults will continue to live with disabling conditions. They will be affected by poor nutrition, prenatal exposures and events, poorly controlled diseases, conflicts, and environmental factors. A recent Canadian report reflects that 'among those experiencing the worst income inequity are children with disabilities or children with parents who have disabilities' (Canadian Institute of Child Health 2000).

The relationship between poverty and disability has long been established, alongside the general relationship between health status and poverty (Fujiura & Kiyoshi 2000; United Kingdom Public Health Association 2007; Park *et al.* 2002). Yeo and Moore (2003), in discussing the relationship between poverty and disability, concluded that people with disabilities are among the poorest of the poor and are not represented in international development organizations and activities.

Often, people with disabilities, for reasons such as stigma, few resources, or transport, are unable to access appropriate health, medical, or rehabilitation services. In many countries, public health activities are difficult to implement for any of the general population. It is important, however, to remember that societies are judged by the way they relate to the most vulnerable of their citizens. In 2004, the World Bank held a conference on development and disability. James D. Wolfensohn, the World Bank Group President at that time, reported that the Millennium Development Goals set by the UN and the World Bank could not be achieved without the inclusion of people with disabilities (Wolfensohn 2004). Increasing development and improving economic standards cannot be successful without all populations being included.

Public health services

Primary prevention messages can be of equal importance for all segments of a population, including persons with disabilities. For example, people with disabilities might be just as vulnerable, or more so, to heart problems as the general population. Public health messages are often not tailored to ensure that those living with disabilities feel included. Sometimes, people with disabilities are even shown in messages to demonstrate the outcome of inappropriate behaviour, such as showing someone in a wheelchair in a message to promote safe driving. It is important, therefore, that prevention messages be developed so as to acknowledge that people with disabilities can be affected by the same images as the general population. At times, messages should be customized to reach individuals with disabilities. For example, people who have limited mobility are at greater risk for weight gain than the general population because of reduced physical activity (United States Department of

Health and Human Services 2006). However, some in the disability community might interpret primary prevention activities related to injuries or screening for birth defects as inimical to their being alive, and thus, might be suspicious, if not angry, about such activities. Communication between public health professionals and the disability community is critical so that important public health education can be delivered with appropriate input from people having disabilities, but without losing the impact of poignant messages.

Perhaps, the most important public health message for individuals with disabilities is consistent with that for the general population. Encouraging children, youth, and adults to be responsible for their own health is a powerful message that is particularly cogent for people with disabilities. For anyone who experiences multiple medical interventions, a sense of losing control over one's body can develop, which can further be equated with a loss of control over one's health as well. Both at the individual and population level, self-efficacy—a belief in one's ability to have control over one's life and health—is an important mediating factor for positive health outcomes.

Beyond public health education are the clinical services that all countries, whether well-developed or less-developed, attempt to provide for their citizens (US Preventive Services Task Force 1996). These services include immunizations, cancer screenings for both men and women, health guidance regarding nutrition and physical activity, sexuality and pregnancy education, drug use education including alcohol and smoking, and other important health information. In more-developed countries, medical care and rehabilitation are emphasized, whereas clinical preventive services are not. Often, rehabilitation becomes equated with medical rehabilitation and providers focus on the disabling condition and its medical complications. Primary care is not emphasized, with the assumption that medical-care generalists will provide the immunizations, health screenings, education, and other primary-care activities. Also, specialists might not be familiar with or sensitive to the need for these services in this population. Many individuals with disabilities, if they have specialized care, do not use primary care, and therefore, might not receive appropriate services. Jones and Kerr (1997) reported that individuals with cognitive impairments did not receive annual health screenings. Austin (2003) found that people with disabilities, in the US state of Oregon, using services funded through public mechanisms are at greater risk of developing smoking-related cancers, are more likely to be diagnosed at a later stage of cancer, and therefore, not receive timely screening for it. In addition, treatment was more often delayed among this population. A public health responsibility is to ensure that people with disabilities are not lost to the provision of clinical preventive services.

Secondary conditions prevention

The term *secondary conditions* is new and is evolving in the vocabulary and objectives of public health. Introduced in the early 1990s into public health in the United States, the term has come to denote those conditions that are preventable but are present because of a pre-established primary disabling condition. A secondary condition is one to which an individual is more susceptible by virtue of living with a disability. 'Secondary' does not reflect the level of importance but rather means that it comes after the primary condition (Lollar 1999). 'Conditions' was chosen to indicate that this

secondary problem could have characteristics beyond the medical or even physical ones. Thus, depression could be a primary disabling condition, but could also be a secondary condition associated with a physical impairment. Social isolation is another common secondary condition not physical in nature, but certainly related to the presence of and vulnerability associated with a disabling condition. Of course, more common examples are physical fatigue from the exertion of moving a wheelchair or urinary tract infections associated with but not a required co-morbid diagnosis of spinal cord injury or spina bifida.

To reiterate, an important characteristic of a secondary condition is that it can be prevented. Thus, medical, rehabilitative, and public health professionals are involved with activities to prevent secondary conditions at the individual and the population level. Given that Disabled Persons International has affiliates in more than 120 countries (Disabled Persons International 2007), it is clear that people live with disabilities around the globe. The health of people with disabilities, however, should not be assumed to be poor by virtue of having a disabling condition. Health is also a right for people with disabilities.

Ravesloot *et al.* (1997) completed a study on adults with disabilities across several diagnostic categories. They indicated that the results were surprising because they had assumed that each diagnostic group would report different secondary conditions. Instead, the results indicated common secondary conditions across all diagnoses. Traci *et al.* (2002) used a survey of common secondary conditions in a study on individuals with developmental disabilities. Physical fitness and conditioning problems were the most prevalent (590/1000), followed by communication and mobility difficulties (573/1000 and 509/1000, respectively). Low frustration tolerance and weight problems were next in prevalence. They concluded that these difficulties included major behavioural and lifestyle limitations, whereas more medically oriented conditions, such as bowel problems or respiratory difficulties, were substantially less reported.

This topic is not complete without a mention of the 'secondary benefits'. Disabling conditions usually challenge the individual and family's functioning and participation, and often lead to secondary conditions. There are, however, benefits that may come as a result of living with a disability or being a family member of such an individual. Benefits often include openness to and acceptance of differences in other human beings and seeing the humanity beyond the difference. Creative problem solving is also frequently required in adapting to a world that is often not accommodating. Strength of will is more developed due to increased physical and emotional energy required to complete tasks (Lollar 2006). Friendships based on the shared experience of disability provide both social and emotional support, and the identifications created are often long lasting. These benefits may become protective factors in future adjustment and participation for both children and adults, and should be included in public health evaluation, policy, and assurance. Prevention of secondary conditions should be an integral part of any nation's public health agenda for people with disabilities, regardless of the health-care financing system.

Public health interventions

Interventions must be provided at both an individual and a population level. Using a self-efficacy conceptual model, several programmes have been developed to improve the health and well-being of people with disabilities. Seekins *et al.* (1991) developed an eight-session workshop, Living Well with a Disability, co-led by people with disabilities and a professional who helps participants learn to set health goals and find ways to meet them. This approach has reduced secondary conditions and medical visits among the participants. Fifteen US states have implemented the programme. In addition, state programmes that educate health-care providers about how to make their physical office space and medical staff attitudes more accessible to those with disabilities have also been instituted (North Carolina Office on Disability and Health 1999).

Many low-resource countries have medical and rehabilitation services—usually proportionate to their overall level of resources. These services, however, are not equivalent to public health. This translation of medicine and rehabilitation into public health is a necessary, but not sufficient, approach to improving the health and well-being of people with disabilities. Medical care is important, even critical, for all citizens regardless of disability status. Rehabilitation services, whether medical, educational, vocational, or social, are specific services focused on outcomes related to the designated area—for example, work or school. The experiences of individuals with disabilities are much broader than just medicine or rehabilitation, even defined broadly. Public health must encompass these services, but must also include those services discussed in previous subsections—health education, preventive services, prevention of secondary conditions, and environmental facilitators of health and well-being.

Towards this end, community-based rehabilitation (CBR) activities have been developed in more than 90 countries and strive to provide comprehensive strategies to include people with disabilities in the life of their communities (World Health Organization 2007a). This emphasis, sponsored by the WHO, focuses on providing equal access to medical and rehabilitation services, but also to education, employment, and numerous other community activities. Public health professionals, in conjunction with CBR staff, can collaborate to provide the expertise from both public health and the disability community to improve the health of people with disabilities.

Major directions

Communication, cooperation, coordination

The most pressing need is for public health and disability communities to acknowledge their respective perspectives of the other. Public health professionals do not easily acknowledge that people with disabilities are a legitimate population—a minority population, even—who deserve public health attention. The disability community must accept that health is a core issue for all, and particularly, for themselves because they are often more vulnerable to additional health problems. The public health community can be a strong partner towards improving health and well-being among people with disabilities. Likewise, the disability community can assist the public health community in achieving these goals.

There is a growing interaction between public health professionals and members of the disability community. A prime example of this cooperation was a leader from Disabled Persons International (DPI) co-chairing the WHO Environmental Task Force to complete the ICF. On the DPI website, there is support for use of the ICF to conceptualize disability and to collect data using ICF definitions. In the United Kingdom, a report on The Life Chances of Disabled People has been completed by disability researchers and

addresses inclusion of people with disabilities. The Office on Disability Issues has created an advisory body of 23 people with disabilities called Equality 2025, whose responsibility is to advise the Government on disability issues, including health and well-being. Likewise, in 2006, the UN Department of Social and Economic Affairs commissioned an audit to evaluate the accessibility of the Internet for people with disabilities (Nomensa 2006). Five sectors from the Convention on the Rights of Persons with Disabilities were selected for assessment—travel, finance, media, politics, and retail. Interestingly, health was again not included. The evaluation concluded that only 3 sites, among the 100 audited from 20 countries, achieved appropriate accessibility ratings and that there was a failure around the world to provide basic levels of Internet accessibility for those living with disabilities.

In 2001 and 2002, the UN sponsored two workshops on measuring disability. The groups were composed equally of disability advocates and national statistical office representatives from the same countries. Representatives of English-speaking countries from Eastern Africa met in Kampala, Uganda in 2001 and those from the ESCWAR region, including Arab-speaking countries and Israel, met in Cairo, Egypt in 2002 (United Nations Statistics Division 2001, 2002). During each of the 2 weeks, the groups interacted to come to a better understanding of how disability statistics and disability policy were connected; the advocates and statisticians developed pilot questions to be used in censuses or surveys in their countries. These activities have not, until now, been the norm, but should become part of every nation's public health efforts to achieve valid disability data and pragmatic disability policy.

Disability framework and measurement

The WHO disability framework approved in 2001 along with the children's version approved in 2006 provide the foundation for public health functions to be achieved. The ICF is finding more traction in countries around the world. Clinical use of ICF codes can be found, in Germany, in the work of Stucki et al. (2002a, 2002b) Physicians throughout Italy are being trained to use ICF coding alongside ICD codes in clinical work (Disability Italian Network 2005). The Measuring Health and Disability in Europe (MHADIE) project of the European Union is implementing an ICF approach in addressing a standardized method to data collection on disability in its 25 member states (Measuring Health and Disability in Europe 2005).

Surveys have been incorporating the ICF framework in Qatar (Simeonsson RJ, Evaluation of children with activity limitations in Qatar schools, personal communication; 2007) and in the United States (Maternal and Child Health Bureau 2005). The Washington Group on Disability Measurement included 75 countries in its early efforts to develop a short set of ICF-based functional questions in order to identify people living with some of the most prevalent activity limitations associated with disability (Centers for Disease Control and Prevention 2006a). There is still the challenge of identifying individuals with mental health problems or with cognitive impairments, but the process has begun. Because the process for revision of both the ICD and the ICF are under the auspices of the Committee on Family of International Classifications (WHO-FIC), there will be growing congruence in the use of these complementary classifications in both clinical and public health settings.

Public health education and training

Public health education is expanding around the world. A study by Tanehaus *et al.* (2000) indicated that schools of public health in the United States are beginning to include disability-related course work. They recommend the inclusion of dedicated courses addressing disability issues, as well as integration of disability issues into courses across the public health curricula. As an outgrowth of this study, two products have been developed. A course dedicated to disability and public health has been developed by the Oregon Office on Disability and Health (Drum *et al.* 2004). In addition, a handbook of disability and public health has been completed. This volume encompasses all major public health core areas—epidemiology, health services, global health, environmental health, and ethics. Public health experts in these fields have contributed chapters that provide a link between public health and disability in their particular specialty and provide references and case studies for each area. Using this approach, any discipline within public health could integrate disability into its courses (Allen & Garberson 2009).

Conclusions

People living with disabilities have traditionally not been included in public health activities. As more people with disabilities live longer because of better nutrition, medical interventions, and public health interventions such as immunizations, there is a greater need for this population to be included in public health interventions, to be a target for specific public health messages, and to be acknowledged as a population worthy of attention when public health planning is being instituted. This 'epidemic of survival' provides an opportunity for public health to address a minority population around the world.

People with disabilities need to be encouraged to take responsibility for their health behaviours, but also to challenge the systems that undermine progress towards health and well-being. Both groups can address environmental barriers to health, including non-health issues such as access to health care and education, societal attitudes towards those with disabling conditions, and policies and systems. Training of public health professionals in disability issues is emerging, and this education of young people can lead to long-term changes in public health perceptions and practice.

References

ACE National Action for Carers and Employment. Work and Families Act 2006 [Online]. 2007. Available from: www.acecarers.org.uk

Allen D., Garberson W., editors. *One in Five: Public Health Perspectives on Disability.* 2009. New York: Springer Publishing Co.

Altman B., Lollar D.J., Rasche E. The experience of environmental barriers among persons with disabilities. Presentation to the American Sociological Association; 2003.

Arnesen T., Nord E. The value of DALY life: problems with ethics and validity of disability-adjusted life years. *British Journal of Medicine* 1999;**319**:1423–5.

Arno P.S., Levine C., Memmott M.M. The economic value of informal caregiving. *Health Affairs* 1999;**18**(2):182–8.

Austin D. Disabilities are risk factors for late stage or poor prognosis cancers. Paper presentation on Changing Concepts of Health and Disability at the Science and Policy Conference. Portland (OR): Oregon Health and Science University; 2003.

Australian Institute of Health and Welfare. Disability and disability services in Australia. Canberra: Australian Institute of Health and Welfare; 2006.

Canadian Institute of Child Health. *The health of Canada's children.* Ottawa: Canadian Institute of Child Health; 2000.

Carers UK. The voice of carers [Online]. 2007. Available from: www.carersuk.org

Center for International Rehabilitation. *International disability rights compendium.* Washington (DC): Center for International Rehabilitation; 2003.

Center for International Rehabilitation. *International disability rights monitor: regional report of the Americas 2004.* Chicago (IL): International Disability Network; 2004.

Center for International Rehabilitation. *International disability rights monitor: regional report of Asia 2005.* Chicago (IL): International Disability Network; 2005.

Centers for Disease Control and Prevention. *Chart book on trends in the health of Americans.* Washington (DC): Centers for Disease Control and Prevention; 2006b.

Centers for Disease Control and Prevention. *Disability and health state chart book.* Atlanta (GA): Centers for Disease Control and Prevention; 2006c.

Centers for Disease Control and Prevention. Washington City group report on disability measurement. Washington (DC): Centers for Disease Control and Prevention; 2006a.

Chamie M. What does morbidity have to do with disability? *Disability and Rehabilitation* 1995;**17**(7):323–7.

Department of Health. *The health of the nation.* London: Her Majesty's Stationery Office; 1991.

Disability Italian Network. *ICF: basic and advanced course.* Gardolo, Italy: Disability Italian Network; 2005.

Disabled Persons International [Online]. Available from: http://v1.dpi.org/lang-en/index

Drum C.E., Krahn G.L., Ritacco B.A. *et al.*, editors. *Disability and public health curriculum outline.* Portland (OR): Oregon Office on Disability and Health; 2004.

Durkin M.S., Islam S., Hasan Z.M. *et al.* Measures of socioeconomic status for child health research: comparative results from Bangladesh and Pakistan. *Social Science and Medicine* 1994;**38**(9):1289–97.

Durkin M.S., Wang W., Shrout P.E. *et al.* Evaluating a ten-questions screen for childhood disability: reliability and internal structure in different cultures. *Journal of Clinical Epidemiology* 1995;**48**(5):657–66.

Fedeyko H.J., Lollar D.J. Classifying disability data. In: Barnarrt S, Altman B, Hendershot G *et al.*, editors. *Using survey data to study disability: results from the national health interview survey on disability.* Research in Social Science and Disability. Vol. 3. Oxford: Elsevier; 2003. p. 55–72.

Fujiura G.T., Kiyoshi Y. Trends in demography of childhood poverty and disability. *Exceptional Children* 2000;**66**(2):187–99.

Grosse S., Lollar D.J., Campbell V.A., and Chamie M. (2009) Disability and disability-adjusted life years (DALYs): not the same. *Public Health Reports,* accepted for publication.

Institute of Medicine. *The future of public health.* Washington (DC): National Academy Press; 1988.

Jones R.G., Kerr M.P. A randomized control trial of an opportunistic health screening tool in primary care for people with intellectual disability. *Journal of Intellectual Disability Research* 1997;**41**:409–15.

Lollar D.J., Crews J.E. Redefining the role of public health in disability. *Annual Review of Public Health* 2003;**24**:195–208.

Lollar D.J., Simeonsson R.J. Diagnosis to function: classification for children and youths. *Developmental and Behavioral Pediatrics* 2005;**26**(4): 323–30.

Lollar D.J. Clinical dimensions of secondary conditions. In: Simeonsson RJ, McDevitt LN, editors. *Issues in disability and health: the role of secondary conditions and quality of life.* Chapel Hill (NC): University of North Carolina; 1999. p. 41–50.

Lollar D.J. Preventing secondary conditions and promoting health. In: Rubin IL, Crocker AC, editors. *Medical care for children and adults with developmental disabilities.* Baltimore (MD): Paul H Brookes Publishing; 2006. p. 33–42.

Maternal and Child Health Bureau. Survey of children with special health care needs. Washington (DC): Maternal and Child Health Bureau; 2005.

Measuring Health and Disability in Europe. MHADIE Press Release 2005 [Online]. Available from: http://www.mhadie.it/aboutus.aspx

Mont D. and Loeb M. (2008). *Beyond DALYs: Developing Indicators to Assess the Impact of Public Health Interventions on the Lives of People with Disabilities.* SP 0185. World Bank: Washington, DC.

Mont D. Measuring disability prevalence. *Social protection discussion paper.* New York (NY): World Bank; 2007a.

Mont D. Measuring health and disability. *Lancet* 2007b;**369**:1658–63.

Murray C.J.L., Lopez A.D., editors. The global burden of disease: a comprehensive assessment of mortality and disability from diseases, injuries and risk factors in 1990 and projected to 2000. Cambridge (MA): Harvard University Press; 1996.

Nomensa. United Nations global audit of web accessibility [Online]. 2006. Available from: http://www.nomensa.com/resources/research/united-nations-global-audit-of-accessibility.html

North Carolina Office on Disability and Health. Removing barriers: tips and strategies to promote accessibility. Chapel Hill (NC): North Carolina Office on Disability and Health; 1999.

Office of the Deputy President. Integrated national disability strategy: a white paper. Ndabeni, South Africa: Office of the Deputy President; 1997.

Park J., Turnbull A.P., Turnbull H.R. Impacts of poverty on quality of life in families of children with disabilities. *Exceptional Children* 2002;**68**(2):151–70.

Ravesloot C., Seekins T., Walsh J. A structural analysis of secondary conditions experienced by people with physical disabilities. *Rehabilitation Psychology* 1997;**42**(1):3–16.

Satariano W.E. The disabilities of aging—looking to the physical environment. *American Journal of Public Health* 1997;**87**(3):331–2.

Seekins T., Clay J., Kirchmyer S. *et al.* Developing and implementing a program for preventing and managing secondary conditions experienced by adults with physical disabilities. Missoula (MT): Research and Training Center on Rural Rehabilitation; 1991.

Statistics Canada. Participation and activity limitation survey: a profile of disability in Canada. Ottawa: Statistics Canada; 2002.

Stein R.E.K., Silver E.J. Comparing different definitions of chronic conditions in a national data set. *Ambulatory Pediatrics* 2002;**2**:63–70.

Stucki G., Cieza A., Ewert T. *et al.* Application of the international classification of functioning, disability and health in clinical practice. *Disability and Rehabilitation* 2002a;**24**:281–2.

Stucki G., Ewert T., Cieza A. Value and application of the ICF in rehabilitation medicine. *Disability and Rehabilitation* 2002b;**24**:932–8.

Talley R.C., Crews J.E. Framing the public health of caregiving. *American Journal of Public Health* 2007;**97**(2):224–8.

Tanehaus R.H., Meyers A.R., Harbsion L.A. Disability and the curriculum in US graduate schools of public health. *American Journal of Public Health* 2000;**90**:1315.

Tracy M.I., Seekins T., Szalda-Petree A. *et al.* Assessing secondary conditions among adults with developmental disabilities: a preliminary study. *Mental Retardation* 2002;**40**(2):119–31.

United Kingdom Public Health Association. The state of Britain's health: poverty and inequality [Online]. Available from: http://www.ukpha.org.uk/default.asp?action=article&ID=71&KeyWords=poverty%2Cand%2Cinequality

United Nations Statistics Division. *Workshop report on disability statistics for Africa.* 2001 Sept 10–14; Kampala, Uganda.

United Nations Statistics Division. *Workshop report on disability measurement for ESCWA countries.* 2002 Jun 1–5; Cairo, Egypt.

United Nations. Convention on the Rights of Persons with Disabilities; 2006 Aug 25. New York (NY): United Nations; 2006a.

United Nations. *Convention on the rights of the child.* New York: United Nations; 1989.

United Nations. *Disability statistics compendium.* New York (NY): United Nations; 1990.

United Nations. Global survey on government action on the implementation of the standard rules on the equalization of opportunities for persons with disabilities. New York (NY): United Nations; 2006b.

United Nations. Guidelines and principles for the development of disability statistics. New York (NY): United Nations; 2001. Series Y, No. 10.

United Nations. Standard rules on equalization of opportunities for disabled persons. New York (NY): United Nations; 1993.

United Nations. *World programme of action.* New York (NY): United Nations; 1982. Resolution 37/52.

United States Department of Health and Human Services. Disability and secondary conditions. In: *Healthy people 2010.* Washington (DC): Department of Health and Human Services; 2000.

United States Department of Health and Human Services. *Midcourse review on healthy people 2010: disability and secondary conditions.* Washington (DC): Department of Health and Human Services; 2006.

US Preventive Services Task Force. *Guide to clinical preventive services.* 2nd ed. Alexandria (VA): International Medical Publishing; 1996.

Wolfensohn J.D. Disability and inclusive development. Keynote presentation at the World Bank Conference; 2004 Dec 1; Washington (DC).

World Health Organization. Disability and rehabilitation team [Online]. 2007a. Available from: www.who.int/disabilities/cbr/en.

World Health Organization. *International classification of diseases.* 10th revision. Geneva: World Health Organization; 1992.

World Health Organization. *International classification of functioning, disability and health.* Geneva: World Health Organization; 2001. pp. 29–30.

World Health Organization. International classification of functioning, disability and health—children and youth. Geneva: World Health Organization; 2007b.

Yeo R., Moore K. Including disabled people in poverty reduction work: 'nothing about us without us'. *World Development* 2003 Mar;**31**(3):571–90.

Health of older people

Shah Ebrahim and Julie E. Byles

Abstract

Declines in death rates and fertility have resulted in population ageing and associated epidemiologic transition from infectious to chronic diseases. Dramatic improvements in life expectancy have occurred, although these have not been equally distributed among socioeconomic groups or seen in politically or economically unstable countries. Ageing is associated with increased health- and social-care needs, not only due to increased risk of chronic diseases but also due to multiple pathologies, and ironically, greater risk of iatrogenic problems associated with polypharmacy. Measures of functioning and disability provide a comprehensive and pragmatic means of assessing older people's needs and evaluating the effects of interventions. Older people are capable of benefiting from a wide range of preventive interventions that reduce mortality and morbidity in middle age—such as cardiovascular disease (CVD) risk factor reduction, increased physical activity, and a healthy diet. Specific preventive interventions—such as falls-prevention schemes and screening or anticipatory care—are probably of less value than was thought, which may reflect the increased access and acceptability of high-quality health services for older people in many high-income countries. These include disease-specific services—such as stroke units, orthogeriatric units, and psychogeriatric units—and general services such as assessment and rehabilitation units, day hospitals, and long-term care. Many countries, particularly low- and middle–income ones, have yet to establish these essential requirements for meeting older people's needs. Informal family support remains the backbone of care for older people in all countries, and without these contributions, statutory formal health- and social-care sectors would be inundated. The costs of care are wrongly considered to increase with age; in reality, costs are more strongly concentrated in the short period before death. Long-term care in institutions is expensive, and reducing the need for such care by increasing home care and avoiding the use of acute-sector institutions are both important measures for reducing costs. Considerable debate is required in order to develop new policies on societal and individual responsibilities for meeting the costs of long-term care. Public health has responsibilities for monitoring trends and transition in risk factors, disease, and disability in ageing populations. In addition, it has roles in encouraging effective health-promotion practices and in setting policy for the equitable and efficient use of health-care resources for the growing population of older people.

Introduction

This chapter considers the phenomenon of population ageing and the public health implications. The case for considering older people as a special-needs group is discussed, together with the health problems they face. The available evidence on the efficacy of preventive intervention, primary care and hospital services, and long-term care and social support is reviewed.

Concepts of ageing vary across societies and settings, over time, and from person to person. Even the definition of 'old age' is imprecise, and varies with the situation and purpose. In the past, the United Nations and other international agencies defined 'the elderly' as 60 years and over, but more recently, there is a growing consensus that it be defined as 65 years and over. However, people over this age are not one homogenous group. Indeed, older people are a very heterogeneous group comprising those who are actively pursuing careers in industry or politics, enjoying healthy retirement, or caring for frail and dependent relatives or friends, and others who are themselves very frail and dependent. Such diverse people are frequently grouped together as 'the elderly', as if they have similar needs and would respond uniformly to interventions. It is essential to recognize this heterogeneity when defining needs, assessing effects and relevance of intervention, and planning for the future.

It is common to categorize older people as the 'young old'—aged 60–69 years, the 'old old'—aged 70–79 years, and the 'oldest old'—aged 80 years and over. Further, as more and more people reach older ages, there is increasing interest in studying the needs and characteristics of centenarians and 'super-centenarians' (110 years and over). However, ageing is a biological and social process that affects individuals at different rates and which is related to but not synonymous with chronological age. Characteristics, apart from age, also contributing to the differences between older people include gender, geographic location, and socioeconomic and ethnic background. At any age, there is great variance in experience, capacity, and health status between individuals. The process of ageing is universal but not uniform.

Demographics and projections

Over the last century, the world has undergone an extraordinary demographic transition. The proportion of people aged 65 years is expected to increase from around 1 per cent of the world's population 100 years ago to an estimated 20 per cent by the middle of the twenty-first century (United Nations 2002). Currently, the world population is around 6.5 billion, of whom an estimated 485 million (7.4 per cent) were aged 65 and over in 2006 (United States Census Bureau 2007). The relative size of the population aged 65 years and over is expected to increase to more than 9 per cent in 2020 and to almost 17 per cent by 2050.

Figure 11.7.1 shows the age and sex structure of the world's population in 2000 and the projected structure in 2050. Figure 11.7.2 shows the proportions of people aged 65 years and over in various world regions in 2002.

More affluent countries tend to have older average population ages than lower-income regions. In affluent countries, ageing involves a large cohort of people born out of post-World War II prosperity. A majority of these people are health conscious, educated, and resourceful, and have access to a wide range of technologies. They also have relatively low levels of disability and have the health capacity to remain productive well into their old age. However, the majority of the world's older people live in low-income countries. In low-income countries, ageing is occurring rapidly against a background of prevailing poverty, immense social and cultural change, changes in family structure, vast urban–rural differences, the existing endemic diseases (e.g. malaria), and newer epidemic diseases (e.g. AIDS and obesity).

Moreover, the pace of population ageing in many low-income countries is more rapid than in high-income countries (see Fig. 11.7.3). In low-income countries, the annual population growth of people aged 65 years and over is almost 3 per cent per year, whereas in high-income countries, the growth has fallen to less than 2 per cent per year (Kinsella 1996). Belgium took over 100 years to double the

proportion of its 60-plus population from 9 to 18 per cent. China will take 34 years to undergo the same transition, and Singapore will take only 20 years.

In high-income countries, the proportion of the 'oldest old' is growing more rapidly than any other age group. In the United States, the proportion of persons aged 85 years and over increased by 274 per cent from 1960 to 1994, compared with 100 per cent for persons aged 65 years and 45 per cent for the total population (United States Census Bureau 2007). It is these oldest old who tend to present major challenges for health and social services in these regions. Figure 11.7.4 illustrates the numbers of people aged 80 years or over projected to 2050.

Projections of population ageing are important for planning services, but are subject to error. These are particularly sensitive to assumptions about mortality rates at older ages and tend to underestimate the true numbers of older people. Population projections are also sensitive to phenomena such as changes in fertility rates, mass migrations, wars, and pandemics. The AIDS pandemic has had a major impact on the age and sex structure of many countries (most particularly those in sub-Saharan Africa), and the full effects are yet to be seen. The other population phenomenon of current interest is the post-war 'baby boom', which has created a bulge in the mid-aged populations of many high-income countries. Maintenance of the health and productivity of these people as they age is of particular importance for the sustainability of health services and welfare systems.

Determinants of population ageing

Population ageing is not only due to greater numbers of people living longer, but also due to lower fertility rates resulting in fewer

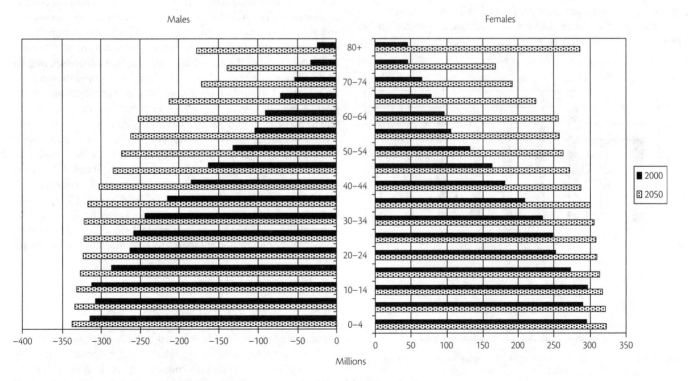

Fig. 11.7.1 World population pyramids, showing age and sex structure, in 2000 and the 2050 projection.
Source: United States Census Bureau (Online). Available from: http://www.census.gov/

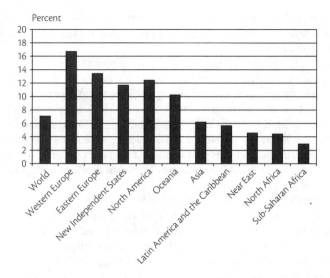

Fig. 11.7.2 Population aged 65 years and over in 2002 represented as a percentage of the total population, by region.
Source: United States Census Bureau. Global population profile 2002 (Online). Available from: http://www.census.gov/

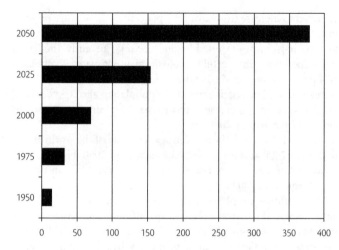

Fig. 11.7.4 World population aged 80 years or over, 1950–2050.
Source: Adapted from Department of Economic and Social Affairs. New York (NY): Population Division, United Nations; 2001. Available from: www.un.org.au

young people entering the population. Therefore, although improvements in medical care have contributed to population ageing, the major drivers are declines in fertility and childhood mortality. In the United Kingdom, the drop in infant and childhood mortality began in the nineteenth century, pre-dating the era of modern effective medical care by many decades. In the twentieth century, population ageing was accelerated by lower infant and child mortality, initially because of improved living conditions and sanitation, and then as a result of better nutrition, immunization, antitoxins, immune sera, and antibiotics. From the mid-twentieth century, reductions in deaths from heart disease and strokes further extended life expectancy at older ages (Charlton & Murphy 1997).

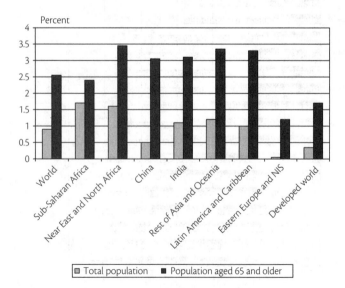

Fig. 11.7.3 Percentage annual change in population aged 65 years and over compared with the total population, by region, 2002–2025.
Source: Adapted from United States Census Bureau (Online). Available from: http://www.census.gov/

However, even recently in the United Kingdom, mortality declines have only been experienced by the better-off, demonstrating the continuing influence of social and economic factors (Drever & Whitehead 1997). In low-income countries, the successful infant and child health programmes (such as growth-chart monitoring, oral rehydration for diarrhoea, breastfeeding, and immunization for common infections) are probably responsible for the rapid rates of mortality decline at younger ages.

Declines in fertility are attributed to urbanization, industrialization, and social mobility, which have all had an influence on family structures. In addition, the emancipation of women, their greater chances for education, later age at marriage, and access to contraception have all played a part. It seems likely that education of women and access to contraception explain the rapid rates of population ageing in the countries of Latin America and Southeast Asia. China's implementation of the one-child policy has had a dramatic impact on fertility and has contributed to its rate of population ageing (Riley 2004). Currently, it is estimated that at least 50 per cent of the world's people live in a region where fertility rates are below replacement level (Office of National Statistics 2007). In high-income countries with low mortality rates, the replacement rate is based on an average of 2.1 children per woman in the population. In 2003, fertility rates were 2.07 in the United States, 1.71 in the United Kingdom, and 2.91 in Japan. At present, the country with the highest fertility rate is Niger (7.46) and lowest is Hong Kong (0.95) (Central Intelligence Agency 2006). Lower fertility rates not only affect population ageing, but, in the longer term, also have an impact on population size (assuming that mortality rates remain fairly constant).

Demographic and epidemiological transitions

Population ageing is accompanied by a change in the patterns of prevalent and incident diseases. To some extent, this change is due to the same factors that contributed to declines in mortality and fertility. In populations with high fertility, infections affecting infants and children were very common. As environmental conditions contributing to risk of infections improved, and as nutritional patterns changed from periods of famine to a more plentiful food supply throughout the year, so were the seeds of chronic and degenerative diseases sown. These epidemiological transitions have been defined as the age of pestilence and famine, the age of receding pandemics, and the age of degenerative and man-made diseases (Omran 1971). However, rapidly ageing low-income countries are experiencing high levels of infectious diseases that take their toll on infants and children, and also, emerging burdens of smoking- and diet-related diseases, particularly cardiovascular diseases, cancers, and diabetes mellitus. An additional 'age' has been defined to accommodate the populations experiencing reversals in longevity due to economic and political instability (Yusuf *et al.* 2001).

Mortality rates and life expectancy

Mortality rates tend to increase at older ages; however, in recent decades, the rate of death has slowed at all ages. Also, at advanced ages (after age 70 or 80), 'old-age mortality deceleration' takes place. The mortality rates of a population can be summarized in a 'life table', which can be used to calculate life expectancy of people at different ages. Table 11.7.1 shows the life expectancy at birth and at age 65 years for men and women in England and Wales. Note that for people who achieve 'old age', their life expectancy is greater than life expectancy at birth. A male born in 1841 could be expected to survive to 40.2 years, but another male who had already survived childhood and reached 65 years could expect to live a further 10.9 years. The difference between the situation in 1841 and now is that far fewer people actually survived the hazards of early life then.

Over recent decades, there has been a substantial increase in life expectancy at birth. Global life expectancy was around 46 years in 1950 and increased to 66 years in 1998. Even in the two decades since 1978, life expectancy increased by 5 years for men (reaching 65 years in 1998) and by 6 years for women (reaching 69 years in 1998) (World Health Organization 1999). Gains in life expectancy have been most pronounced at younger ages, but even at older ages increases have occurred due to falling death rates. Life expectancy gains have mainly benefited the better-off.

Life expectancy shows great variation between countries and even within countries. The country with the highest life expectancy at birth is Andorra, where a child born in 2006 can be expected to live 83.5 years. The lowest life expectancy is found in Swaziland, where the life expectancy at birth is only 32.6 years. Even among the most developed countries, there is substantial variation, with Australia at 80.5, Canada at 80.2, Great Britain at 78.5, and the United States at 77.8 years (Central Intelligence Agency 2006). Many of the countries with the lowest life expectancies have very high rates of HIV infection or AIDS. In sub-Saharan Africa, life expectancy in several countries has been reduced by 15–20 years following increases in the prevalence of HIV, and is now as low as 30 years (Mathers *et al.* 2001).

Other factors can also have a dramatic influence on life expectancy. Life expectancy for men in the former Soviet Union and Eastern European countries has declined following political reforms (Chenet *et al.* 1998; Leon *et al.* 1997). The reason for this trend is unclear, but sudden deaths due to binge alcohol drinking, increased risks of violent death, and suicide play a part (Chenet *et al.* 1996; Shkolnikov *et al.* 2001). The reunification of the former East Germany with West Germany shows a different picture; in the decade since the removal of the Berlin Wall in 1989, mortality rates in the East have fallen towards those in the West among women but not men (Haussler *et al.* 1995) These 'natural experiments' of the effects of social and economic engineering provide examples of how public health is influenced by political change. It also reinforces the importance of social and economic factors as major forces in determining life expectancy.

Differences in life expectancy between groups within countries have been long recognized. William Farr calculated average life expectancies in 1841 for Liverpool, Surrey, and London, which were 26, 45, and 37, respectively. By 1992, although the rank order by place of residence was much the same, life expectancy over the age of 65 years showed even greater variation than it did in 1841. Similarly, life expectancy shows a marked social-class gradient. As shown in Fig. 11.7.5, the difference in life expectancy for men in England and Wales at age 65 years between social class I (professional) and V (unskilled manual) has increased from 3.4 years in 1972–76 to 5 years in 1997–2001: Similar gradients exist for women. Analysis of health inequalities indicate that the cause of these gradients is more complex than simply poverty, but that relative deprivation is also important (Marmot 2001).

Table 11.7.1 Life expectancy at different ages in England and Wales, 1841–2005.

Year	Birth		65 years	
	Male	Female	Male	Female
1841	40.2	42.2	10.9	11.5
1901–10	48.5	52.4	10.8	12.0
1930–32	58.7	62.9	11.3	13.1
1960–62	68.1	74.0	12.0	15.3
1990–92	73.4	79.0	14.3	18.1
1993–95	74.1	79.3	14.6	18.2
1998–2000	75.3	80.1	15.5	18.8
2003–05	76.9	81.2	16.8	19.6

Source: Charlton J, Murphy M. *The health of adult Britain 1841-1994*. London: Her Majesty's Stationery Office; 1997.
Office of National Statistics [Online]. Available from: www.statistics.gov.uk

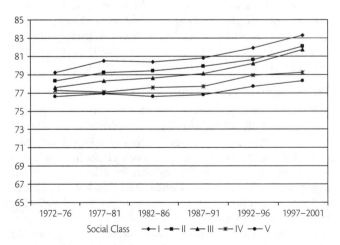

Fig. 11.7.5 Life expectancy for men at age 65, by social class, in England and Wales. *Source*: Office of National Statistics (Online). Available from: www.statistics.gov.uk/downloads~Life_Expect_Social_Class_1972-2001.pdf (accessed 9 February 2007).

Within the United States, African-American men have a life expectancy at birth of up to 20 years less than white men (Murray *et al.* 1998), and the difference in life expectancy is increasing. Levine *et al.* (2001) reported a 29-year lag in age-adjusted all-cause mortality, with the value for African-Americans in 1998 (6.9 per 100 000) equalling the value for white people in 1969. The age-adjusted all-cause mortality rate for African-Americans in 1965 showed a lag of 27 years compared with the rate for white persons (Levine *et al.* 2001). Interestingly, beyond the age of 80 years, African-Americans have better life expectancy than white populations—perhaps suggesting survival of the fittest (Manton 1980).

Similar differences in life expectancy exist between indigenous and non-indigenous populations in many countries, including New Zealand, Australia, Canada, and the United States. Within these developed, 'rich' countries, indigenous people regularly suffer from poorer levels of general health, and have an excess of early mortality and lower life expectancy when compared with the non-indigenous population. A study by Bramley *et al.* (2004) found that indigenous male life expectancy was highest in New Zealand (69 years) and indigenous female life expectancy was highest in Canada (76.6 years). The lowest life expectancy for indigenous people, males (56 years) and females (63 years), was in Australia. According to the Australian Bureau of Statistics (2000), 53 per cent of Aboriginal male deaths occur at ages less than 50 years.

Life expectancy is different from the maximum lifespan, which is the longest an individual member of a species or group has survived. Animals in the wild seldom achieve their maximum lifespan; in captivity, they are capable of reaching much older ages because major risks of predation, starvation, and accidents have largely been eliminated (Kirkwood 1999). Although the maximum lifespan that humans can achieve is widely debated, it is unlikely that we have reached it yet.

Other measures of ageing and health

Health-adjusted life expectancy provides an index of the equivalent years of full health that a person can expect to live at any given age, taking account of prevalent health states in the population and the value placed on ill health.

Figure 11.7.6 presents the inequalities in life expectancy (LE) and health-adjusted life expectancy (HALE) at birth across regions. The best HALE is seen in low-mortality countries such as Japan, where healthy life expectancy is estimated to be 75 years at birth (Mathers *et al.* 2001). Low-income countries have lower healthy life expectancy; furthermore, people in these countries can expect to spend a greater proportion of their life in ill health.

Compression of morbidity

With increases in life expectancy, there has been debate on whether added years of life will be spent in good health or in disability. If healthy life expectancy increases relative to life expectancy, then people will spend a greater proportion of their life in good health and 'compression of morbidity' will operate (Fries 1980, 1989). If people live longer due to reduction in fatal illness but with disability due to chronic disease, then 'expansion of morbidity' will occur. A third scenario, 'dynamic equilibrium', could occur if the prevalence of some chronic diseases increases with ageing, but the progression of some degenerative diseases reduces. In this scenario, people might suffer chronic illness for a longer period, but with less serious effects (Andrews 2001). This steady state could also be

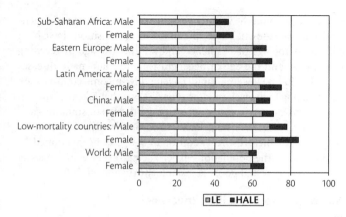

Fig. 11.7.6 Inequalities in years of life expectancy (LE) and healthy life expectancy (HALE) at birth, by gender and region, in 2002.
Source: Adapted from Mathers CD, Iburg KM, Salomon JA *et al.* Global patterns of healthy life expectancy in the year 2002. *BMC Public Health* 2004;**4**:66.

achieved if there are parallel declines in both disease incidence and total mortality (Manton 1982).

Fries (2005) argues that compression of morbidity may be prevailing in some populations. However, data to test this hypothesis are difficult to find and hard to interpret. Very few countries are capable of making reliable assessments over time, between geographic regions, or between socioeconomic groups. Investment in research infrastructure is required to ensure that regular health and disability surveys using comparable methodology are established. The US Health and Retirement Study has found that successive cohorts of people aged 51–56 years are in relatively poorer health, reporting more difficulty with daily tasks, more pain, more chronic conditions, more psychiatric problems, and higher use of alcohol (Soldo *et al.* 2006). Similar findings have also been reported for people in the United Kingdom (Banks *et al.* 2006).

Evidence of compression of morbidity is mostly seen among higher socioeconomic status people, particularly those with low levels of risk factors for chronic disease. In the United States, not only are disability rates higher among African-Americans than white people, but also the trends between 1990 and 1996 show that white people have enjoyed a reduction in disability whereas African-Americans people have suffered an increase (National Center for Health Statistics 1999). Among university alumni followed prospectively, those with high-risk health behaviours (i.e. smoking, high body mass index [BMI], and lack of physical exercise) suffered twice the cumulative incidence of disability, with the onset of disability postponed by an average of 5 years in those with low-risk health behaviours (Vita *et al.* 1998). If compression of morbidity is to occur at a population level, greater health-promotion and risk-reduction activities will be needed for disadvantaged groups who have high levels of health risks. Moreover, even if preventive activities were highly successful in reducing or postponing disability, increasing numbers of people living to very old ages mean that there will also be greater numbers of people with disabling conditions. At a population level, even if compression of morbidity dominates, there will be increasing needs for health and other care as the population ages.

Ageing in specific populations

Ageing in rural areas

The experience of ageing, need for care, and service availability vary greatly between people living in large cities and those living in rural and remote areas. Living in rural areas is also generally associated with economic hardship and poorer quality housing. Not only are incomes lower in rural areas, but prices of commodities such as fuel and food are higher as well.

The special circumstances of ageing in rural communities have not received much attention. However, the majority of the world's elderly live in rural and remote areas. Even in highly urbanized countries, a significant minority of the elderly live in rural and remote parts. Moreover, as younger people leave rural areas to work in cities, the proportion of older people in the rural population increases; so, rural and remote populations are ageing at a faster rate than urban populations. This effect is magnified when rural communities become popular places to live in retirement. Migration of young adults away from rural areas diminishes opportunities for family support, which is particularly important in rural areas, where societies tend to be more traditional and there is greater reliance on family structures.

The UN Madrid International Plan of Action on Aging considers the need to improve living conditions and infrastructure in rural areas, and to alleviate the marginalization of rural-dwelling older persons, particularly in low-income countries. Environmental factors, including lack of safe drinking water and poor sanitation, inadequate housing and absence of electricity, and poor roads and transport make life increasingly difficult for elderly people in rural areas. Further, in times of stress, such as during drought or other natural disasters (or war), rural elderly are likely to be particularly vulnerable (Mitka 2000).

Ethnic minority elders

Immigrations associated with trade, the colonial past, wars, and famine have produced complex multicultural societies in many countries. Different countries will have experienced immigration at different times and the contexts that will affect how ethnic minorities are viewed, their place in society, and their absolute and relative numbers will differ. Australia, for instance, has had a long history of immigration, from the early settlers and convicts, to the wave of immigrants from Europe following the Second World War, to more recent immigrants from Southeast Asia and other countries. The population is drawn from 200 countries, and 23 per cent of the population were born overseas (Australian Bureau of Statistics 2001). Ethnic minority populations that emigrated from other countries are now ageing rapidly and are often at a disadvantage due to poor health, poor economic circumstances and reliance on public services, as well as cultural and racial discrimination (Villa & Wallace 2007).

Data from United States indicate that immigrants such as Latinos and Asians, as well as African-American elders, are more likely to live in poverty and have lower median incomes than the general population. Further, many of these people are in poor health. African-Americans, for instance, have higher rates of disease and disability as compared to the rest of the population, and also appear to be more vulnerable to the impacts of disease (Villa & Wallace 2007).

Census information from the United Kingdom also shows older people from major ethnic minority groups, with the exception of the Chinese, to have more long-standing disability than the Anglo-Saxon majority. Explanations for excess morbidity may be found in poverty, poor housing and diet, and limited physical activity, all of which are likely to contribute to higher rates of CVD, diabetes, and other chronic health problems. The aetiology of ethnic minority health problems may be classified as 'home' country influences, influences of the new adopted country, selection of who migrates, and processes of adaptation and adjustment to migration (Marmot et al. 1984). However, once people from ethnic minorities reach old age, the selective 'healthy migrant' factors attenuate and they become prey to the common causes of chronic ill health in the wider population. Moreover, relocation and adaptation to a new country is a major lifetime stress that may have negative effects on health at later ages (Noh & Kaspar 2003). People who emigrate at older ages are particularly vulnerable; not only do they have poor health associated with ageing and disadvantage, but they also have more difficulty adjusting to a new culture and language than younger people, and they may also be less likely to use health care than others with similar needs.

Subtle barriers to referral, investigation, and treatment may also affect the care received by ethnic minority elders (Ebrahim 1996). People from ethnic minorities are less likely to receive social-support services, although given their need, they should be represented in greater proportion. In Australia, older people from non-English speaking backgrounds comprise around 25 per cent of the population aged 65 years and over, but only represent 16 per cent of the home-care clients and 7 per cent of the residential aged-care clients (Australian Institute of Health and Welfare 2002). Much more work is required to develop and evaluate appropriate services for ethnic minority elders.

Age and gender

Although the main conditions that affect people at older ages are similar among men and women (except for breast cancer and reproductive cancers), there are differences in the incidence of these conditions and the peak age of onset. For instance, men experience peak incidence of coronary artery disease earlier than women do. Lung cancer is more common among men who have had higher rates of smoking, although lung cancer is now the second most common cancer among women, reflecting their increasing smoking habits. There are also gender differences in terms of social roles and human rights, and these will have significant effects on the experience of ageing. Although there are few differences in self-rated health and long-standing illness, older women have higher rates of functional disability than men. Women also tend to live longer than men do, and so are more likely to experience disease and disability associated with advanced age.

Women's longevity also means that they are more likely to experience the death of their spouse and to spend a proportion of their older age widowed. Single older men, however, are more likely to be admitted to residential care than single older women, and married men are more likely to remain living in the community than married women (Arber & Cooper 1999).

Older women are especially vulnerable in the event of crises such as war, natural disaster, and famine, partly because they generally control fewer economic resources than older men do and because much of the care of children and other vulnerable people falls to older women.

Gender differentials in health and ageing have been poorly studied, but are important because of the gender imbalance in the population at older age due to women's longer life expectancy. In 2002 healthy life expectancy at the global level was 57.8 years for women, 2 years higher than that for men at 55.8 years. In Russia, healthy life expectancy was 66.4 years for women, 3 years below the European average, but just 56.1 years for men, 7 years below the European average (Mathers *et al.* 2004).

Health needs of older people

As people age, they have increased risk of disease and disability, and often, increasing health needs. Many conditions become more common at older ages, partly because of physiological changes associated with ageing, accumulated exposure to adverse health behaviours and risk factors across the life course, toxins and injury, and simple 'wear and tear'. Older people also tend to experience more than one health problem at any given time, and these problems are frequently under-reported and under-treated. In many cases, social circumstances add to the difficulties that people face as they age, making it harder for them to manage their health problems, and requiring a given broad and special consideration for the health needs of older people.

Physiological and functional changes

Physiological changes that occur with ageing affect all body systems. These normal changes limit bodily reserves, reduce the ability to maintain homeostasis, and increase the potential for illness. Obvious external signs of ageing appear on the skin, but along with these cosmetic changes skin also loses some of its function with age. The dermis becomes thinner and more fragile, and there are fewer and slower dividing keratinocytes—which means slower healing and less efficient production of vitamin D. Other changes in skin function include increased vulnerability to extremes of temperature and reduced sensitivity to touch. Muscle and bone mass decline with age, tendons become shorter, and cartilages become stiffer. Diseases such as osteoporosis and osteoarthritis exacerbate these losses and effects.

Changes to the cardiovascular system include stiffening of arteries (even among those with normal blood pressure), slowed electrical activity, postural hypotension, and reduced right ventricular function. The lungs become stiffer, alveoli enlarge, bronchioles collapse, and the chest muscles weaken, reducing respiratory capacity. Also, the cough reflex is reduced, leading to increased susceptibility to infection. The digestive system becomes less efficient at absorbing nutrients (especially vitamins), leaving older people vulnerable to nutritional deficiencies, particularly folate-deficiency anaemia. Changes in smooth muscle function can predispose to constipation. The liver reduces in size and becomes less efficient at synthesizing proteins and metabolizing toxins (increasing the risk of drug toxicity). Likewise, there is a decrease in kidney mass and renal function. Older people find it harder to maintain fluid and electrolyte balance, and are vulnerable to dehydration. Bladder capacity is reduced and bladder muscles may become weak and unstable (increasing the risk of incontinence), and in men, the prostate enlarges (increasing the risk of obstruction).

Physiological changes in body function are not due to disease (just as menopause is the loss of reproductive function but is not a disease). However, certain diseases and states can accelerate the onset of disability and shorten life. A number of longitudinal studies have been conducted in an attempt to disentangle the effects of

ageing and disease on health and well-being (see United States National Institute of Ageing 2007). For example, the MacArthur Study of Successful Aging followed 1189 relatively healthy people aged between 70 and 79 years, for a period of seven years, to investigate factors that influence physical and cognitive functioning. They found that 'successful ageing' was associated with exercise, social engagement, and a positive mental attitude, including feelings of being useful to others (Seeman & Chen 2002; Gruenewald *et al.* 2007).

Common conditions affecting older people

Causes of death and disability

Some conditions are particularly strongly associated with age. These include conditions that are rapidly fatal (such as lung cancer) and which contribute greatly to years of life lost (YLL), and those that are chronic and associated with years of life lost to disability (YLD).

The most common recorded causes of death among people aged 60 years and over are diseases of the circulatory system, diseases of the respiratory system, and malignant neoplasms (see Box 11.7.1).

Worldwide, ischaemic heart disease and cerebrovascular disease are the leading causes of disability and death among people aged 60 years and over, measured by disability-adjusted life years (DALYs), (see Box 11.7.2).

Other major causes of DALYs include chronic obstructive lung disease, dementias, and cataract (and other vision disorders). Older people are also particularly susceptible to respiratory infections such as pneumonia. In regions where TB is endemic, older people are particularly vulnerable.

Musculoskeletal conditions (such as osteoarthritis and osteoporosis) are also common among older people, although they tend to contribute to disability more than death. In high-income countries, more than one in four women will have sustained at least one osteoporotic fracture by the age of 70. In 1990, a worldwide estimate of 1.7 million hip fractures occurred as a result of

Box 11.7.1 Mortality—adults aged 60 years and over		
Rank	**Cause**	**Deaths (1000)**
1	Ischaemic heart disease	5825
2	Cerebrovascular disease	4689
3	Chronic obstructive pulmonary disease	2399
4	Lower respiratory infections	1396
5	Trachea, bronchus, lung cancers	928
6	Diabetes mellitus	754
7	Hypertensive heart disease	735
8	Stomach cancer	605
9	Tuberculosis	495
10	Colon and rectum cancers	477

Source: World Health Organization. *World health report 2003: shaping the future*. Geneva: World Health Organization; 2003.

Box 11.7.2 Disease burden—adults aged 60 years and over

Rank	Cause	DALYs (1000)
1	Ischaemic heart disease	31 481
2	Cerebrovascular disease	29 595
3	Chronic obstructive pulmonary disease	14 380
4	Alzheimer and other dementias	8569
5	Cataracts	7384
6	Lower respiratory infections	6597
7	Hearing loss, adult onset	6548
8	Trachea, bronchus, lung cancers	5952
9	Diabetes mellitus	5882
10	Vision disorders, age-related, and other	4766

Source: World Health Organization. *World health report 2003: shaping the future*. Geneva: World Health Organization; 2003.

osteoporosis; this number is expected to exceed 6 million by 2050 (World Health Organization 2001).

These common conditions are associated with a range of functional limitations such as cognitive impairment, mobility restrictions, and urinary incontinence. Urinary incontinence affects 10–30 per cent of older people, and women are affected twice as often as men (Chiarelli *et al.* 2005). Under-nutrition is another problem that commonly underlies and exacerbates many conditions affecting older people, even in countries where food supplies are generally reliable and plentiful.

Multiple pathology

Most older adults have a range of active health problems that interact with one another and complicate approaches to treatments. Figures vary from study to study, but at least 80 per cent of the people older than 65 years have one chronic condition or more, and 65 per cent have multiple chronic conditions (Wolff *et al.* 2002). For example, in one Australian study of men and women aged 70 years and over, the median number of conditions per person was 7 (Byles *et al.* 2005). This state (called multi-morbidity or co-morbidity) is important because it is associated with many important health outcomes such as quality of life, activities of daily living, health-service utilization, and mortality (Byles *et al.* 2005).

Population statistics often do not recognize the prevalence of co-morbidity among older people. For instance, deaths are enumerated according to the underlying cause and contributing causes are often not counted. However, although the recorded cause of death may be quite specific, the reality is that a number of co-morbid conditions could have caused or contributed to the person's death. In other cases, deaths among older people are attributed to 'senility' or to 'ill-known and undefined causes'. These cases represent the notion of multiple system failure, which accompanies old age, but again they do not provide information on those conditions that contribute most to morbidity and mortality.

Iatrogenic disease

Iatrogenic disease is common in older people, particularly in those taking multiple medications. Although medications can be beneficial in the management of multiple health problems of older people, they also have the potential to cause serious adverse effects. Older people have a reduced volume of distribution for drugs, and slower rates of drug metabolism and elimination, and so are vulnerable to overdose. Reduced physiological reserve renders older people more susceptible to drug toxicity. Also, multiple medications increase the risk of drug–drug interaction. Multiple medicines also increase medication complexity, which can increase risk of medication error and reduce adherence. In high-income countries, an estimated 60–90 per cent of community dwelling people aged 65 years and over take medications. Over 50 per cent use at least one drug on a regular basis, with the average number of medications used ranging from two to five (Byles *et al.* 2003). Adverse reactions are estimated to account for up to 22 per cent of hospital admissions, 35 per cent of unplanned readmissions, and almost half of nursing home admissions (Schmader *et al.* 1997). It is estimated that up to half of these adverse reactions could be prevented (Simonson & Feinberg 2005).

Functioning, disability, and health

The International Classification of Functioning, Disability and Health (known as the ICF) recognizes that functioning and disability occur in personal, environmental, and social contexts (World Health Organization 2007). This new classification scheme replaces the original International Classification of Impairment, Disability and Handicap.

The ICF has two parts: Part 1—Functioning and Disability (Body Functions and Structures, and Activities and Participation) and Part 2—Contextual Factors (Environmental Factors and Personal Factors). Any significant problem in body function or structure is classified as 'impairment'. Depending on the amount of impairment and on personal and environmental factors, impairments can result in activity limitations and restrictions on an individual's involvement in everyday life. A person can have impairment without having any limitation (e.g. disfigurement), but a person may also have activity limitations without obvious impairment (e.g. incontinence). The interaction with environmental and personal factors means that a person may have capacity limitations without assistance, but no performance restrictions when provided with a supportive social and physical environment.

People who work in aged care and in rehabilitation use the terms *activities of daily living* (ADL) and *instrumental activities of daily living* (IADL) to describe the functional limitations of many of the people they care for and to evaluate the effects of rehabilitation. ADLs are the basic functions of being able to walk, wash, dress, eat, groom, and go to the toilet. IADLs are higher-order activities that are needed to function independently in modern life, including using the telephone, going shopping, cooking meals and housekeeping, doing the laundry, using transport, using medications, and managing finances.

Frailty and geriatric syndromes

Although *frailty* is a term that is commonly used to describe older people, it is poorly defined and not well understood. Fried *et al.* (2001) have developed an operational definition of frailty that includes decreased resiliency and reserve, cycles of decline across multiple systems, negative energy balance, sarcopenia, and decreased strength and exercise tolerance. The symptoms and signs include exhaustion, weight loss, weak grip strength, slow walking pace, and low energy expenditure.

The common coexistence of disease in older people has led some to describe certain combinations of conditions as 'geriatric syndrome'. As with frailty, this term is not well defined and various usages are made. Common combinations associated with this term include falls, dementia, and incontinence.

Health-related quality of life

With longer lifespans, importance is placed not only on the quantity of life but also the quality of life. Quality of life is a subjective element that relates to the adequacy of people's circumstances and to their feelings about these circumstances. In terms of health, relevant aspects of the quality of life range from negatively valued aspects such as pain and disability to more positively valued aspects such as role function or happiness. Recently, there has been great attention given to quantification of quality of life as a measure of general health status, and for comparing outcomes of different treatments.

Health-related quality of life in older age is affected not only by disease but also by symptoms, which may not be associated with specific pathology, and by social circumstances. Common symptoms include joint stiffness, constipation, incontinence, and memory complaints. However, despite the presence of symptoms, medical conditions, and disability, older people often report their health as good or better and record high quality of life scores. This is a 'disability paradox' (Albrecht & Devlieger 1999), and was explored quantitatively in a national sample of British women, where it was found that one-fifth reported 'fairly' to 'very severe' levels of difficulty with daily living activities, but 62 per cent of these women rated their quality of life as 'good' or better. Multivariable analysis indicated that worse-perceived health, chronic diseases, and sociopsychological resources, including perceived control over life, distinguished between those who perceived their quality of life to be good in the face of functional difficulties (Bowling et al. 2007).

Trajectories of ageing and functional decline

The Established Populations for Epidemiologic Studies of the Elderly (EPESE) analysed four classical trajectories of functional decline by comparing activity of daily living scores for 4190 people who died in the first six years of follow-up (Lunney et al. 2003). Of the people studied, 15 per cent experienced sudden death, 21 per cent had a primary diagnosis of cancer and demonstrated a rapid decline to death, 20 per cent had congestive heart failure or chronic lung disease and exhibited a fluctuating level of function due to organ failure, and 20 per cent with none of these diseases had been in a nursing home in the year before death and had a prolonged steady decline in function, probably attributable to a dementia syndrome. The remaining 24 per cent were classified as 'other', and died outside of a nursing home. The different modes of death were associated with age (people dying of cancer were generally younger, people dying in nursing homes were generally older), gender (those dying of following a steady decline were more likely to be women), and race (those experiencing sudden death were more likely to be non-white). Importantly, only deaths from cancer had a predictable terminal period, which is important information for elderly people, their relatives, and those planning and funding palliative aged care.

Health and social care for older people

Health-care policy makers and planners are often challenged by concerns about the rising costs of health care in the face of an ageing population. The argument is that increasing numbers of older people will result in an explosion of costs and an unsustainable demand on services. People aged 65 years and over tend to have more admissions to hospital than younger people, and they have longer lengths of hospital stay. They also have more visits to doctors and use more medications. However, people aged 65 years and older contribute only modestly to time trends in per-capita costs of health care compared with the rest of the population. It has also been noted that the proportion of health-care expenditure that is allocated to older people is actually decreasing as the population ages. Rather, it is terminal illness that is expensive, not age as such, and the costs of health care increase with proximity to death (Normand 1998; Dixon et al. 2004). Also, very old people have lower health-care costs than young people with the same survival prospects (Himsworth & Goldacre 1999). The notion that we should restrict expensive acute- and tertiary-level services for older people overlooks the important benefits that even very old people can gain from both acute and technologically innovative health care.

Health promotion for old age

Three stages in promoting healthy old age have been described (see Fig 11.7.7). The first is increasing capacity for health in early life, which includes good maternal nutrition, and optimizing the development of vital organs such as brain, muscle, bone and blood vessels during childhood and early adulthood to build resources that may affect later capacity (such as increasing peak bone density to protect against osteoporosis). The second stage occurs in adult life and involves strategies to reduce damage (such as avoiding smoking), to protect against damage (a balanced fruit- and vegetable-focused diet), or to prevent loss through lack of use (such as physical activity). The third stage is in late life and involves minimizing the progression of disease and disability, protecting against increased environmental demands or stresses, and compensating for lost capacity. Examples of these approaches to health promotion include secondary prevention of stroke, rehabilitation, exercise and strength training, social support, correction of deficits in vision and hearing, and modifications to domestic and outdoor environments.

Several key health behaviours are associated with diseases that are common in older age. These associations would suggest that primary-prevention approaches are likely to be effective in reducing the incidence of disease at older ages. However, randomized

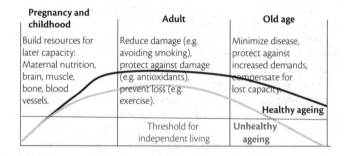

Fig. 11.7.7 Health promotion for old age.
Source: Adapted from Alexandre Kalache World Health Organization, personal communication 2008.

controlled trials have frequently failed to show that behavioural interventions addressing these risk factors are effective. For example, large-scale randomized controlled trials of dietary advice, smoking cessation advice, and exercise did not demonstrate a reduction in disease incidence (Ebrahim & Davey Smith 1997). This does not mean that reducing these risk factors is not important, rather that standard approaches to health promotion are not sufficiently effective. Strategies that take a more holistic approach, that involve the whole community (not just individuals), and that address environmental and cultural determinants of ill health are more important.

Social inequity is one of the major determinants of ill health at all ages (Marmot 2005). Poor circumstances have their first impact during pregnancy, when deficiencies in nutrition, maternal stress, smoking, and misuse of drugs and alcohol, insufficient exercise, and inadequate prenatal care can inhibit optimal foetal development. As seen in the life-course approach to health promotion, poor foetal development is a risk for health in later life. The impact of disadvantage continues throughout childhood and adult life, and is manifest in terms of psychosocial stress (which can have both physical and mental health impacts), poor education, poor nutrition, social exclusion, underemployment and poor job security, and work-related stress and injury. Smoking, alcohol, and drug use are higher among people in disadvantaged circumstances. Disadvantaged people also tend to live in poorer neighbourhoods with high rates of violence and crime, in overcrowded circumstances, and in areas with high levels of environmental hazards. Thus, although it is useful to highlight behaviours of individuals as risk factors for ill health at later ages, addressing these problems requires that the social circumstances that underpin these behaviours are also understood and improved where possible.

Smoking is a risk factor for CVD, stroke, respiratory disease, and many cancers, and smoking prevention is important in reducing the incidence of these conditions, even at older ages. The British Doctor's Study shows that over seven years of life expectancy are gained by avoiding smoking after the age of 35 years (Doll et al. 2004). Quitting smoking is also important in reducing up to 36 per cent of future coronary events. Systematic reviews of many trials show that brief advice and nicotine supplements do help people to stop smoking (Lancaster & Stead 2005a, 2005b).

Physical activity is strongly associated with lower rates of CVD, depression, and osteoporosis in many observational studies, and some small trials have demonstrated short-term health benefits among older participants. However, older people may find it difficult to maintain high levels of exercise, and the encouragement of exercise requires attention to physical environments as well as education of the individual. Neighbourhood factors such as the availability of transport, housing density, pedestrian-oriented urban design, and diversity of land use can increase physical activity (Handy et al. 2002; Saelens et al. 2003).

Observational studies suggest a clear association between nutrition and health at older ages. For example, the Baltimore Study of Ageing found that men who consumed at least five servings of fruits and vegetables per day and who obtained 12 per cent energy or less from saturated fat had 31 per cent lower all-cause mortality ($P < 0.05$), and were 76 per cent less likely to die from coronary heart disease (CHD; $P < 0.001$) than other men in the study (Tucker et al. 2005). However, dietary intervention studies and studies of vitamin supplementation have not demonstrated significant health benefits (Bengmark 2006; Davey Smith & Ebrahim 2005).

Obesity and overweight are increasing in prevalence and are associated with increased risk of stroke, coronary artery disease (CAD), diabetes, arthritis, and some cancers (World Health Organization 2000). There is currently little evidence from well-designed randomized controlled trials of the effectiveness of weight reduction on reducing longer-term morbidity.

A number of studies have demonstrated an association between social support and improved survival, reduced disability and health-care use, and improved quality of life (Berkman & Syme 1979; Bowling & Browne 1991; Steinbach 1992; Mendes de Leon et al. 1999). It is thought that these health effects are mediated through the influence of social support on health behaviour, improved access to care, and possibly through physiological pathways. A systematic review of 30 studies of social-support interventions for older people identified some evidence that educational- and social-activity group interventions that target specific groups can alleviate social isolation and loneliness among older people (Cattan et al. 2005). However the methods and generalizability of the reported studies varied, and more work is required to develop both theoretically sound social-support interventions and better methods for evaluating the outcomes of these approaches.

Prevention of specific conditions affecting older people

CVDs and diabetes

Many clinical trials provide evidence in support of the effectiveness of drug therapy in primary and secondary prevention of CVDs. It has been estimated that six preventative drugs in combination (three low-dose anti-hypertensives, a statin to lower cholesterol, aspirin, and folic acid) could prevent up to 88 per cent of CHDs and 80 per cent of strokes (Wald & Law 2003). This therapy has been proposed for all people over the age of 55 years regardless of CVD risk, but may be more beneficial among older people and people with pre-existing disease among whom the risk–benefit ratio is greater. However, there are many cost and safety issues to consider before universal multi-chemoprophylaxis becomes common practice. Furthermore, recent randomized trials of folate supplementation have not demonstrated the anticipated reductions in CVD risk, suggesting that this component of any combination treatment will not be useful.

Hormone replacement therapy (HRT) was thought to be cardioprotective (Stampfer & Colditz 1991), but large trials have demonstrated an increase in CHD among women on long-term HRT (Lawlor et al. 2004). However, a recent re-analysis of the Women's Health Initiative trials has shown that among women started on HRT shortly after the menopause, there was no evidence of an increased risk of CHD, a finding that has rekindled the HRT debate (Rossouw et al. 2007).

When treating diabetes in elderly patients, one must consider not only the importance of glucose control, but also other health risks and priorities as well as patient preferences. Life expectancy should also be considered. Control of other risk factors such as lipids and hypertension, as well as glucose control, is also important and may have considerable short-term advantages. For people with shorter life expectancy, long-term control of hyperglycaemia may be less important than for younger patients (Durso 2006). As with many conditions affecting older people, randomized controlled trial evidence is lacking. Observational evidence suggests that intensive control of diabetes mellitus can have favourable effects on microangiopathy (Katakura et al. 2007). Trials among people with impaired glucose tolerance have revealed that physical activity reduces the likelihood of developing diabetes (Toumilehto & Lindstrom 2003; Bethel & Califf 2007).

Mental health

Depression is the most common psychiatric disorder in the elderly, and is commonly under-diagnosed and under-treated. Once detected, however, it responds well to pharmacotherapy and/or psychotherapy (Wilson *et al.* 2001).

Dementia is a major cause of years of life lost to disability (Mathers *et al.* 2000). At this stage, there is no evidence that any treatment will prevent or slow the progression of dementia. However, many dementias appear to be partially attributable to CVD risk factors such as hypertension and control of these risk factors may reduce the incidence of dementia.

Falls and fractures

Numerous modifiable risk factors for falls and osteoporosis have been identified. However, reduction of fall-related injury at a population level requires that preventive activities become embedded within everyday social functions and physical structures (McClure *et al.* 2005). A number of interventions have been shown to reduce the risk of falls, including health and environment risk factor screening or intervention programmes, muscle strengthening and balance retraining, and home hazard assessment and modification (Gillespie *et al.* 2003). Multifactorial fall-prevention programmes have been shown to be effective in reducing falls among community-dwelling older people, OR 0.73 (0.63 to 0.86), and for older people with a history of falling, OR 0.79 (0.67 to 0.94) (Tinetti *et al.* 1994). Increased calcium and vitamin D as well as physical activity may also protect against osteoporosis (Boonen *et al.* 2006), although recent large-scale randomized trials of calcium and vitamin D supplementation in community-dwelling people did not demonstrate reductions in the risk of fracture (Porthouse *et al.* 2005; Jackson *et al.* 2006; The RECORD Trial Group 2005). A recent Cochrane review concluded that vitamin D has a significant effect in preventing fractures (including hip fracture) among people living in institutional care (Avenell *et al.* 2001). Evidence shows that bisphosphonates improve bone density and reduce osteoporotic fractures (Cranney *et al.* 2002). HRT may also reduce fractures; however, recent studies show increased risk of CVD and breast cancer, so HRT is not currently recommended for fracture prevention (Writing Group for the Women's Health Initiative Investigators 2002).

Osteoarthritis

Little attention has been paid to the prevention of osteoarthritis. Weight loss and prevention of obesity may have a role in prevention, and in the relief of symptoms and maintenance of activities of daily living for those with established disease (Bliddal & Christensen 2006). Established arthritis may also respond to exercise, orthotics, pharmacological therapies, and joint replacement.

Gains in healthy life expectancy due to the elimination of disease

The elimination of some diseases (such as CVD and cancer in men) would result in an increase in life expectancy, but with expansion of morbidity. Compression of morbidity is predicted with the elimination of musculoskeletal disorders and mental conditions; endocrine, nutritional, and metabolic disorders; respiratory and digestive disorders in men; and neoplasms in women (Mathers 1999). Population effects of preventing a condition such as arthritis would be considerable, as so many individuals are affected. Also, in addition to the direct effects of pain and stiffness, arthritis has indirect effects by limiting physical activity and thereby increasing risk of other conditions.

Preventive activities in primary care

Immunization

Vaccination of community-dwelling older people may be a cost-effective way to prevent hospitalization for influenza or pneumonia and to prevent deaths. However, much of the evidence on vaccination in the elderly comes from observational studies and may reflect other differences between vaccinated and non-vaccinated groups (Rivetti *et al.* 2006). In the United States, the Centers for Disease Control are aiming to achieve influenza vaccination coverage of 90 per cent for persons aged 65 years and over by 2010. Influenza vaccination levels have increased from 33 per cent in 1989 to 66 per cent in 1999 for people in this age group. However, vaccination rates are lower among certain groups (such as African-Americans and Hispanics) and among people in residential care, who are at greater risk and for whom there is also greater benefit (Centers for Disease Control 2006).

Medication review

Some studies have shown medication review to be beneficial for older people living in the community (e.g. Zermansky *et al.* 2002), but other studies did not find any effect of medication review on the use of medicines (e.g. Allard *et al.* 2001; Sellors *et al.* 2003). One large Australian randomized controlled trial demonstrated a positive effect on medication use and a reduced incidence of falls 12 months after the medication review (Pit *et al.* 2007).

Health assessments, case finding, and screening

Multiple problems: Reviews of the evidence on prevention-based assessment programmes for older people have come to varying conclusions: That the assessments have positive effects (Stuck *et al.* 2002), no effect (Cole 1998), or small mixed effects (Van Haastregt *et al.* 2000; Byles 2000; Elkan *et al.* 2001). These reviews also found differences between studies in content and duration of assessments and the length of follow-up. The effectiveness of assessments may depend on multiple follow-ups, and benefits may be most pronounced for the 'young old' (under 78 years) and for those with a low risk of death (Stuck *et al.* 2002). Further randomized controlled trials of health assessments have been published in the last four years (Byles *et al.* 2004; Fletcher *et al.* 2004), which demonstrated only limited health benefits associated with health assessments.

Cancer screening: Many cancer screening programmes for younger people are not promoted for older people; for instance, breast cancer screening is encouraged for women aged 40–70 years (United States Preventive Services Task Force 2006). Evidence for ceasing screening after age 70 is not clear because few mammography screening controlled trials enrolled women older than 69 years and no trials enrolled women older than 74 years. The incidence of breast cancer increases with age, but the benefits of screening may be outweighed by competing morbidities among older women. Screening for cervical cancer is not recommended for women over the age of 70 years if they have had three normal

Pap smears in the past ten years (United States Preventive Services Task Force 2006): The incidence of cervical cancer decreases at older ages, and so screening older women has low yield. Also, in Western countries, many women have had a hysterectomy and do not require cervical screening. Screening for colorectal cancer is recommended for adults over the age of 50 years and up to the age of 80 years depending on the person's health and co-morbidities (United States Preventive Services Task Force 2006). As for breast cancer, few trials enrolled older patients. Although there is limited evidence of the benefit of screening for oral cancer, assessment of the mouth, teeth, and gums is helpful for older people with cognitive impairment and who may have conditions that limit chewing, swallowing, and communication (Research Dissemination Core 2002). Box 11.7.3 lists some recommended screening procedures for older adults.

Cardiovascular diseases: Treatment of high blood pressure as a means for preventing stroke among relatively fit people up to the age of 80 years is supported by strong evidence from randomized controlled trials (Insua *et al.* 1994; Mulrow *et al.* 1994). Treatment of people over the age of 80 years has been examined in a subgroup analysis of seven randomized controlled trials of drug treatments. Reductions in non-fatal cardiovascular events were found with no overall reduction in total mortality (Gueyffier *et al.* 1999). However, increased efforts to screen for high blood pressure, either by case finding or screening, have not shown improvements in population coverage,

adherence to treatment, or blood pressure control (Ebrahim 1998). Screening for lipid disorders is not considered to be important for older people because lipid levels are less likely to increase after age 65 years (United States Preventive Services Task Force 2006).

Osteoporosis: Although there is no direct evidence that screening for osteoporosis prevents fractures, the prevalence of osteoporosis and fractures increase with age, and the short-term risk of fracture can be estimated by bone measurement tests and risk-factor assessment. Treatment may reduce fracture risk among women with low bone density (Nelson *et al.* 2002).

Vision and hearing: Annual screening for vision and hearing problems is recommended for adults after the age of 65 years (Mouton & Espino 1999). However, screening for visual problems has not been associated with improvements in visual impairment (Smeeth & Iliffe 2003).

Mental health: Screening for depression may improve the recognition and treatment of this condition as well as quality of life or mood. A meta-analysis of screening for depression among adults showed screening to be associated with a 13 per cent reduction in relative risk and a nine-percentage-point absolute reduction in the proportion of patients with persistent depression (Pignone *et al.* 2002). Available evidence is insufficient to recommend for or against routine screening for dementia in older adults (United States Preventive Services Task Force 2006).

Box 11.7.3 Screening procedures for older adults

	US Preventive Services Task Force	UK National Screening Committee
Breast cancer (women)	• Up to age 70 years	• Age 50–70 years
Cervical cancer (women)	• Up to age 70 years	• Age 25–64 years
Colorectal cancer	• Up to age 80 years (depending on co-morbidities)	• Age 50–75 years
Blood pressure	• No age limit	• All adults
Lipids	• Up to age 65	• Relatives of people with familial hypercholesterolaemia
Diabetes	• Screening recommended for adults with hypertension or hyperlipidaemia	• General population screening not recommended
Osteoporosis	• Women aged 65 years and older, women 60 years and older with increased risk for osteoporotic fractures	• Screening not recommended
Dementia	• Insufficient evidence to recommend for or against	
Depression	• Recommended if appropriate systems for follow-up	• Screening not recommended
Smoking	• Screening and advice to quit recommended for all adults	
Glaucoma	• Insufficient evidence	• Screening not recommended
Elder abuse	• Insufficient evidence	

Sources: United States Preventive Services task Force. *The guide to clinical preventive services, 2006.* Rockville (MD): Agency for Healthcare Research and Quality; 2006. UK National Screening Committee. Policy positions. 2006 Jul. Available from: http://www.nsc.nhs.uk/pdfs/policy position chart july06%5B1%5D.pdf. Last accessed 2007, Feb 09.

Elder abuse: There is little evidence to make recommendations about screening for elder abuse (United States Preventive Services Task Force 2006). Elder abuse, however, is common and health workers should remain alert. Factors associated with the abuse of older adults include increasing age, low-income status, functional impairment, cognitive disability, substance use, poor emotional state, low self-esteem, cohabitation, and lack of social support.

In summary, efforts to improve disability and to prevent disease through health assessments and systematic case finding are not well supported by currently available evidence. It is likely that the failure to achieve benefits is due to inadequately specified actions to be taken in the light of problems detected by case finding. Further work in this area needs to ensure that interventions are better planned and should evaluate how well the processes of care operate, in addition to examining outcomes. Also, the trials of preventive approaches are subject to many methodological problems; of these problems, small sample sizes and loss to follow-up are the most common. Reliance on trials performed in diverse health-care systems is unwise owing to the very different barriers to care, expectations of people, and differences in need. More data are required to guide policy on the application of trial evidence for the prevention of morbidity and disability among elderly people.

Systems of care

There are many strategies that enable people to successfully manage existing specific conditions and live a normal life. Quality care for chronic diseases to prevent complications and to compensate for functional impairment is essential in order to optimize health and quality of life for older people.

Primary care

Primary care is considered to be of great importance in reducing health-care inequalities and in improving the quality and outcomes of health care among older people. However, training in health care for older people is not a high priority in undergraduate curricula in many medical and health schools. It is essential that the needs of the growing numbers of older people are reflected in health-care education. The first step is to examine the common health problems among older people seen in primary care and to match training to meeting these needs. Without appropriate training, it is likely that older people will simply receive an increasing number of pills for each of their symptoms, running the risk of iatrogenesis, and potentially diagnosable and treatable problems will be missed.

Hospital services

People are more likely to use hospital services as they age and occupy hospital beds for longer (McCallum *et al.* 2003). It is, therefore, expected that older people will consume an increasing proportion of the available hospital resources in the future. Older people presenting to hospital tend to be sicker, with more urgent conditions, and have more co-morbid diseases and medications than young people (Bridges *et al.* 2005). Cardiopulmonary disorders are among the most common medical reasons for presentation, and fall-related injury is the most common surgical emergency among older people presenting to emergency departments. Adverse drug-related events (unfavourable medical events related to medication use or misuse) account for around 10 per cent of emergency department visits, the most frequently implicated medications being non-steroidal anti-inflammatory drugs (NSAIDs), antibiotics, anticoagulants, diuretics,

hypoglycaemics, β-blockers, calcium-channel blockers, and chemotherapeutic agents.

Older patients tend to have complex health problems, with longer length of stay; the discipline of geriatric medicine has evolved to meet these needs, and specialist geriatric units now exist within major hospitals. A systematic review shows positive effects of hospital geriatric evaluation and management units on mortality, place of discharge, and change in functional status (Stuck *et al.* 1993). Although these results support current working methods, there is a possibility that these results are affected by publication bias. Also, better characterization of the process of care in trials of complex interventions is essential for the interpretation and implementation of findings.

Disease-specific services

Specialist services for patients suffering strokes have been evaluated in several small randomized controlled trials and appear to reduce mortality, disability, and institutionalization by about 20 per cent at 12 months. A meta-analysis of these studies concluded that the outcome appeared to be better in stroke units based in a discrete ward (Stroke Unit Trialists' Collaboration 2001). Similar models have also been applied for the management of diabetes, respiratory disease, and CVD (Gentles & Potter 2001). Specialist services for fractured neck-of-femur patients (orthogeriatric services) have also been examined in systematic reviews of small randomized controlled trials; pooled effects show a non-significant trend towards improved survival and less dependence. However, the trials are very heterogeneous in terms of the interventions used and do not provide secure evidence for or against such services (Cameron *et al.* 2001).

Health services for elderly people suffering from functional mental illnesses (largely, depressive illness) and organic brain syndromes (largely, dementia) have followed the general trend of moving out of psychiatric hospitals and into the community. The specialty of geriatric psychiatry has developed to meet the needs of an ageing population with an increased burden of dementia (Arie & Jolley 1998). As with hospital services for physically ill people, convincing evidence to support particular styles of psychogeriatric practice in terms of costs and outcomes is not available.

Hospital-at-home and day services, rehabilitation, and transitional care

Various 'hospital-at-home' and early-discharge schemes have been promoted in efforts to reduce demand on acute hospital services. A review of 22 trials evaluating early-discharge and hospital-at-home schemes found little evidence of benefits or costs savings. However, early-discharge schemes for older patients may reduce the pressure on acute hospital beds (Shepperd & Iliffe 2001).

There is an increasing demand for rehabilitation for older people. Traditionally, this process has occurred in hospital or other institutional settings, but more recently community-based rehabilitation options have been explored. In countries lacking investment in hospital services for elderly people, community-based rehabilitation offers an alternative model, but requires evaluation. Many studies have been undertaken to evaluate this approach to rehabilitation, but these studies have not been considered adequate to provide evidence of its effectiveness (Ward *et al.* 2003).

Specific issues that need further study are the role of families in the process of rehabilitation, local low-cost production of disability aids and appliances, and education and training in rehabilitation for primary-care teams.

Long-term care

A common approach to population ageing has been to establish institutional care, despite its costs and very limited accessibility for a majority of elderly people. In Egypt, for example, the number of aged-care institutions has more than doubled over the past 20 years (Boggatz & Dassen 2005).

At any one time, the majority of older people will not live in institutions, but many will require some form of long-term care during the course of their life. In high-income countries, there is a trend towards care being increasingly provided in community settings. Care in the community is now the preferred and most common care arrangement, and there has been a reduction in the numbers of people in institutional care, despite the ageing of the population.

Future need for long-term care will be determined by demographic trends, the strong relationship between age and disability, the extent to which community care permits people to stay at home, and the willingness of relatives to provide continued unpaid help. Most of these factors will tend to result in more rather than less need for long-term institutional care. In many countries, current levels of provision will be inadequate to meet future needs. Ignoring the problem is likely to have predictable consequences for waiting lists and admission of acutely ill elderly people as beds become 'blocked' with people waiting for some alternative to an acute hospital bed.

Informal care and social support, community and social care

In the United Kingdom, almost three million people provide care for someone over the age of 75 years, and informal care is recognized as an essential component of aged care and support (Department of Health 1999). Many people providing care for older people are themselves old.

The move to community care relies on the availability of informal carers, and there is increasing concern about who will care for older people in need. Not only will there be more people in need of care, but also the demands of modern society reduce people's ability to provide adequate care for their friends and families. For example, the increased emphasis on community care has come at the same time as a massive increase in the numbers of women who work in paid jobs.

Although both caregivers and care recipients generally regard home-based care as preferable to institutionalization, there is a lot of evidence that care giving can be physically and emotionally taxing (e.g. Schulz & Martire 2004; Lee 2001). Lee and Porteous (2002) found that mid-age women who have never had a role in providing care were more likely to be in full-time employment, and had better physical and mental health as well as lower levels of stress than carers. They were more likely to be within a healthy weight range, were less likely to use medications for sleeping difficulty or depression, and had higher life satisfaction scores and lower depression scores. When women gave up their caring roles, they reported fewer general-practice visits and less use of medications for nerves than current caregivers. In many cases, people who took on caring were already in poor health themselves. The demands of being in or taking on caring roles are frequently overlooked by health professionals, who may actually trade on the emotional ties between daughters and parents to achieve community care for very dependent patients.

The tradition of family support for older people is changing in many countries as a result of economic and political conditions, and where diseases such as AIDS have affected mid-aged adults leaving older people and children without support. In China, where filial piety is a traditional value, family responsibility for older people is made explicit in policy and is incorporated into the marriage contract (Zavoretti 2006). Even so, economic development, urbanization, and demographic transition are having an impact on intergenerational support.

Costs of care

There is much concern about costs associated with an ageing population. However, many analysts predict that the cost implications will be small in relation to the overall economies of most high-income countries. Across countries belonging to the Organization for Economic Cooperation and Development (OECD), population ageing is not associated with health expenditure as a proportion of gross domestic product (GDP). For example, 17.3 per cent of the Swedish population were aged 65 years or older in 2001, and 8.6 per cent of the Swedish GDP was spent on health. In contrast, around 12.7 per cent of the Australian population were aged 65 years and over, but 9.3 per cent of the GDP was spent on health (Coory 2004). Other analyses suggest that the greatest proportion of lifetime health-care costs are incurred in the last two years of life, and are more closely associated with the proximity to death than with chronological age (Dixon et al. 2004).

The major increases in costs associated with ageing occur in association with community and residential aged care. Nursing home costs in the United States have grown at a far faster rate since the 1960s than other sectors of health-care spending (National Center for Health Statistics 1999). British long-term care costs also dominate the overall projections over a period of decades, far outstripping primary-care and hospital-sector costs (Laing et al. 1991). Hotel 'board and lodging' costs make up a high proportion of long-term care costs and individual payment for these costs is generally acceptable (Royal Commission on Long-Term Care 1999; Fitzgerald 2000).

A number of studies have compared the relative costs of residential and community care. A study in British Columbia found that, although people receiving community care spent more days in hospital than people in residential care, the overall costs of community care were half to three-quarters the cost of residential care. However, much of this cost difference is contributed by families (Chappell et al. 2004). Variation in costs of care depend on levels of dependency, the number of residents and number of short-stay admissions, qualified nursing staff and supervisory staff, and building standards (Fitzgerald 2000). However, although the relationship between severity of dependency and cost of care is relatively flat for institutional care, costs for care at home increase exponentially with increasing dependency (Evans 1993). Anyone can be looked after at home if sufficient resources are available.

The issue of who pays for long-term care is important, as 'protection' of health- and social-services budgets coming from different sources may not result in the optimal use of resources or good standards of care. A move towards private funding also raises concerns regarding equity of access to care, especially for people with the greatest need. Older people who would benefit from specific interventions (e.g. coronary revascularization) are less likely to receive them (Bowling 1991). Ironically, acute hospital beds are used by older patients waiting for transfer to a social-care sector, either their own homes or institutional accommodation.

Increasing the barriers to gaining entry into secondary care for older people is an obvious but misplaced response because it exacerbates inequity for some. Ensuring that both health- and social-care costs are considered in economic appraisals, rather than just the costs of one or other system, should guarantee that the balance of care is of net benefit to society and not simply to one payer. The role of family and community in reducing costs of care need to be recognized as being of fundamental importance.

Unfortunately, much of urban planning has ignored the needs of older people, is designed inappropriately (e.g. high-rise public housing), and is suited to small nuclear families rather than larger extended families. Also, although promoting care at home is a desirable policy, the practice may be unaffordable for poor families.

Rationing of care

Rationing of care for older people may result from paternalistic ageism or from (often incorrect) assumptions and value judgments that older people are less likely to benefit from treatments than younger people. In many circumstances, the old, who have the greatest need for care and the greatest potential to benefit, are least likely to receive care. Moreover, there is often a dearth of evidence on which to base decisions about what care is most appropriate and effective for older people.

How much should be spent on care for older people can only be determined by reference to ethical principles. If no value is placed on life once economic productivity ceases, then an argument to not waste resources on health services for elderly people will prevail. But if quality of life in older age is seen to have its own value, then there is an argument for providing care. The amount that one generation should spend on supporting earlier generations remains to be decided. The 'fair innings' argument—after so many years, old people should not expect any more—is used by health economists to argue for transfers from old to young rather than vice versa (Williams & Evans 1997). An obvious flaw in such arguments is the notion that we only get sick and in need of health and social care when we get old ; the 'fair innings' does not relate to health status or to the ability to benefit from health care, only to years lived.

An alternative economic argument can also be made, that older people have contributed to society for their whole lives and are denied the support of society at the point in their lives when they need it most. Of importance in this debate is a consideration that most health care for older people is not about prolonging life but about ensuring that their old age is as comfortable and humane as possible. For the most part, it is not health care at older age that contributes to longevity, but rather survival from health risks at younger ages. Furthermore, provision of timely and appropriate health care for older people may potentially offset other costs.

The ethics of state provision of a health service is based on utilitarianism—the greatest good for the greatest number. Healthcare policy generally aims at targeting resources to where they will do the most good, rather than issue them in response to the distribution of disease. This approach appears appropriate at one level, but may have unintended consequences if the ability to gain health benefits are not distributed equitably across the population in need (Aldrich et al. 2003). Targeting also requires relevant information on service inputs and health outcomes. In the face of inadequate information on costs and benefits, it seems inevitable that doing the best for the patient regardless of cost should gain hold over utilitarianism. With stronger evidence on the effects of pharmacological interventions, it is also inevitable that conflicts between groups holding different ethical precepts (and with different financial incentives) will emerge. Older people will stand to lose on two counts: First, evidence is weakest and hardest to obtain for complex non-pharmacological interventions from which they may benefit, and second, the inherent ageism of society will ensure that elderly people will lose in an individual or collectivist fight for resources. Without better and wider evidence on the benefits of innovative patterns of care for elderly people, more resources will not necessarily mean better care.

Public health implications of population ageing

As seen in this chapter, population ageing is a global phenomenon that will have a major impact on disease and disability patterns, and on health-service use. A coordinated and appropriate public health response is essential if this phenomenon is to translate into an opportunity for longevity and healthy ageing, rather than a threat to global health and resources. Public health is important in monitoring trends and transitions in risk factors, disease, and disability, in encouraging effective health-promotion practices, and in setting policy for equitable and efficient use of health-care resources for this growing population. Health promotion for older age begins in early life and continues throughout life to the oldest age. Much more knowledge is needed as to how we can optimize the conditions and experiences of ageing. The recognition of contributions made by older people themselves to their families and communities as well as to national wealth is also of fundamental importance in meeting the challenges of an ageing population and in meeting the health needs of increasing numbers of older people.

Key points

- Ageing is occurring at far greater rates in low- and middle-income countries than it does in high-income countries, which will place considerable strain on the health- and social-care sectors.

- Increased longevity has not been experienced uniformly across socioeconomic groups or in different countries.

- Severe disability is becoming less common in successive cohorts of elderly people, indicating that a compression of morbidity and disability is occurring.

- Health services for older people have had dramatic effects in improving survival and reducing disability associated with the inevitable increases in chronic diseases at older ages.

- In all countries, families provide a major part of the care needed by older people, but require the knowledge and support of formal health and social services.

- Public health has major roles in surveillance, prevention, and development of services for older people.

References

Albrecht G.L., Devlieger P.J. The disability paradox: high quality of life against all odds. *Social Science and Medicine* 1999;**48**:977–88.

Aldrich R., Kemp L., Williams J.S. *et al.* Using socio-economic evidence in clinical practice guidelines. *British Medical Journal* 2003;**327**(7426):1283–5.

Allard J., Hebert R., Rioux M. *et al.* Efficacy of a clinical medication review on the number of potentially inappropriate prescriptions prescribed for community-dwelling elderly people. *Canadian Medical Association Journal* 2001;**164**(9):1291–6.

Andrews G.R. Care of older people: promoting health and function in an ageing population. *British Medical Journal* 2001;**322**:728–9.

Arber S., Cooper H. Gender differences in health in later life: the new paradox. *Social Science and Medicine* 1999;**48**:61–76.

Arie T., Jolley D. Psychogeriatric services. In: Tallis R.C., Fillit H.M., Brocklehurst J.C., editors. *Brocklehurst's textbook of geriatric medicine and gerontology.* 5th ed. Edinburgh: Churchill Livingstone; 1998.

Australian Bureau of Statistics. Australia demographic statistics. Canberra: Australian Bureau of Statistics; 2001. Cat. No. 3101.

Australian Bureau of Statistics. Mortality of Aboriginal and Torres Strait islanders. Canberra: Australian Bureau of Statistics; 2000. Occasional paper 3315.0.

Australian Institute of Health and Welfare. Australia's health 2002. Canberra: Australian Institute of Health and Welfare; 2002.

Avenell A., Gillespie W.J., Gillespie L.D. *et al.* Vitamin D and vitamin D analogues for preventing fractures associated with involutional and post-menopausal osteoporosis. [Online]. Cochrane Database Systematic Reviews 2001;1:CD000227.

Banks J., Marmot M., Oldfield Z. *et al.* Disease and disadvantage in the United States and in England. *Journal of the American Medical Association* 2006;**295**(17):2037–45.

Bengmark S. Impact of nutrition on ageing and disease. *Current Opinion in Clinical Nutrition and Metabolic Care* 2006;**9**(1):2–7.

Berkman L.F., Syme S.L. Social networks, host resistance and mortality: A nine year follow-up study of Alameda County residents. *American Journal of Epidemiology* 1979;**109**:186–204.

Bethel M.A., Califf R.M. Role of lifestyle and oral anti-diabetic agents to prevent type 2 diabetes mellitus and cardiovascular disease. *American Journal of Cardiology* 2007;**99**:726–31.

Bliddal H., Christensen R. The management of osteoarthritis in the obese patient: practical considerations and guidelines for therapy. *Obesity Reviews* 2006;**7**(4):323–31.

Boggatz T., Dassen T. Ageing, care dependency, and care for older people in Egypt: a review of the literature. *International Journal of Older People Nursing* 2005;**14**:56–63.

Boonen S., Vanderschueren D., Haentjens P. *et al.* Calcium and vitamin D in the prevention and treatment of osteoporosis—a clinical update. *Journal of Internal Medicine* 2006;**259**(6):539–52.

Bowling A., Browne P.D. Social networks, health, and emotional well-being among the oldest old in London. *Journal of Gerontology* 1991;**46**(1): S20–32.

Bowling A., Seetai S., Morris R. *et al.* Quality of life among older people with poor functioning. *The influence of perceived control over life. Age and Ageing Advance Access* 2007;**36**(3):310–5.

Bowling A. Ageism in cardiology. *British Medical Journal* 1991;**319**: 1353–5.

Bramley D., Hebert P., Jackson R. *et al.* Indigenous disparities in disease-specific mortality, a cross-country comparison: New Zealand, Australia, Canada, and the United States. *New Zealand Medical Journal* 2004;**117**:1207.

Bridges J., Meyer J., Dethic L. *et al.* Older people in accident and emergency: implications for UK policy and practice. *Reviews in Clinical Gerontology* 2005;**14**:15–24.

Byles J., Heinze R., Nair K. *et al.* Medication use among older Australian veterans and war widows. *Internal Medicine Journal* 2003;**33**:388–91.

Byles J.E., D'Este K., O'Connel R. *et al.* Single index of multi-morbidity did not predict multiple outcomes. *Journal of Clinical Epidemiology* 2005;**58**(10):997–1005.

Byles J.E., Tavener M., Nair K. *et al.* A randomized controlled trial of health assessments for older Australian veterans and war widows. *Medical Journal of Australia* 2004;**181**:186–90.

Byles J.E. A thorough going over: evidence for health assessments for older persons. *Australian and New Zealand Journal of Public Health* 2000;**24**:117–23.

Cameron I.D., Handoll H.H.G., Finnegan T.P. *et al.* Co-ordinated multidisciplinary approaches for inpatient rehabilitation of older patients with proximal femoral fractures. [Online]. Cochrane Database of Systematic Reviews 2001;(3):CD000106.

Cattan M., White M., Bond J. *et al.* Preventing social isolation and loneliness among older people: a systematic review of health promotion interventions. *Ageing and Society* 2005;**25**:41–67.

Centers for Disease Control. Prevention and control of influenza: recommendations of the Advisory Committee on Immunization Practices. *Morbidity and Mortality Weekly Report* 2006;**55**:1–42.

Central Intelligence Agency [Online]. 2006. Available from: www.cia.gov [accessed 2007 Feb 9].

Chappell N.L., Haven B., Hollander M.J. *et al.* Comparative costs of home care and residential care. *Gerontologist* 2004;**44**:389–400.

Charlton J., Murphy M. The health of adult Britain 1841–1994. London: Her Majesty's Stationery Office; 1997.

Chenet L., Mckee M., Fulop N. *et al.* Changing life expectancy in central Europe: is there a single reason? Journal of Public Health Medicine 1996;**18**:329–36.

Chenet L., McKee M., Leon D. *et al.* Alcohol and cardiovascular mortality in Moscow; new evidence of a causal association. *Journal of Epidemiology and Community Health* 1998;**52**:772–4.

Chiarelli P., Bower W., Wilson A. *et al.* Estimating the prevalence of urinary and faecal incontinence in Australia: systematic review. *Australasian Journal on Ageing* 2005;**24**(1):19–27.

Cole M.G. Impact of geriatric home screening services on mental state: a systematic review. *International Psychogeriatrics* 1998; **10**:97–102.

Coory M.D. Ageing and healthcare costs in Australia: a case of policy-based evidence? Medical Journal of Australia 2004;**180**:581–3.

Cranney A., Guyatt G., Griffith L. *et al.* the Osteoporosis Methodology Group, the Osteoporosis Research Advisory Group. Meta-analyses of therapies for postmenopausal osteoporosis. IX: *Summary of meta-analyses of therapies for postmenopausal osteoporosis. Endocrine Reviews* 2002;**23**(4):570–8.

Davey Smith G., Ebrahim S. Folate supplementation and cardiovascular disease. *Lancet* 2005;**366**:1679–81.

Department of Health. Caring about carers: a national strategy for carers. London: Her Majesty's Stationery Office; 1999.

Dixon T., Shaw M., Frankel S. *et al.* Hospital admissions, age and death— 'the cost of ageing' or 'the cost of dying'? A retrospective cohort study. *British Medical Journal* 2004;**328**:1288.

Doll R., Peto R., Boreham J. *et al.* Mortality in relation to smoking: 50 years observations on male British doctors. *British Medical Journal* 2004;**328**:1519.

Drever F., Whitehead M. Health inequalities. London: Office for National Statistics, Her Majesty's Stationery Office; 1997. DS No. 15.

Durso S. Using clinical guidelines designed for older adults with diabetes mellitus and complex health status. *Journal of the American Medical Association* 2006;**295**:1935–40.

Ebrahim S., Davey Smith G. Systematic review of randomized controlled trials of multiple risk factor interventions for preventing coronary heart disease and stroke. *British Medical Journal* 1997;**319**:1358–60.

Ebrahim S. Detection, adherence and control of hypertension for the prevention of stroke: a systematic review. *Health Technology Assessment* 1998;**2**:1–78.

Ebrahim S. Ethnic elders. *British Medical Journal* 1996;**313**:610–3.

Elkan R., Kendrick D., Dewey M. *et al.* Effectiveness of home based support for older people: systematic review and meta-analysis. *British Medical Journal* 2001;**323**:719.

Evans J.G. Institutional care and elderly people. *British Medical Journal* 1993;**306**:806–7.

Fitzgerald V. Financial implications of caring for the aged. Melbourne: Myer Foundation; 2000.

Fletcher A., Price G., Ng E. *et al*. Population-based multidimensional assessment of older people in UK general practice: a cluster-randomized factorial trial. *Lancet* 2004;**364**(9446):1667–77.

Fried L.P., Tangen C.M., Walston J. *et al*. Frailty in older adults: evidence for a phenotype. *The Journal of Gerontology Series A: Biological Sciences and Medical Sciences* 2001;**56**:146–57.

Fries J.F. Aging, natural death, and the compression morbidity. *New England Journal of Medicine* 1980;**303**:130–5.

Fries J.F. Frailty, heart disease, and stroke: the compression of morbidity paradigm. American Journal of Preventive Medicine 2005;**29** (5 Suppl 1):164–8.

Fries J.F. The compression of morbidity: near or far? The Milbank Quarterly 1989;67:208–32.

Gentles H., Potter J. Alternatives to acute hospital care. *Reviews in Clinical Gerontology* 2001;**11**(4):373–8.

Gillespie L.D., Gillespie W.J., Robertson M.C. *et al*. Interventions for preventing falls in elderly people. [Online]. Cochrane Database Systematic Review 2003;(4):CD000340.

Gruenewald T.L., Karlamangla A.S., Greendale G.A. *et al*. Feelings of usefulness to others, disability, and mortality in older adults: the MacArthur Study of Successful Aging. *Journals of Gerontology Series B: Psychological Sciences and Social Sciences* 2007;**62**:28–37.

Gueyffier F., Bulpitt C.J., Boissel J.P. *et al*. the INDIANA Group. Antihypertensive drugs in very old people: a sub-group meta-analysis of randomized controlled trials. *Lancet* 1999;**353**:793–6.

Handy S.L., Boarnet M.G., Ewing R. *et al*. How the built environment affects physical activity: views from urban planning. *American Journal of Preventive Medicine* 2002;**23**:64–73.

Haussler B., Hempel E., Reschke P. Changes in life expectancy and mortality in East Germany after reunification (1989–1992). *Gesundheitswesen* 1995;**57**:365–72.

Himsworth R.L., Goldacre M.J. Does time spent in hospital in the final 15 years of life increase with age at death? A population based study. *British Medical Journal* 1999;**319**:1338–9.

Insua J.T., Sacks H.S., Lau T.S. *et al*. Drug treatment of hypertension in the elderly: a meta-analysis. *Annals of Internal Medicine* 1994;**121**:355–62.

Jackson R.D., LaCroix A.Z., Gass M. *et al*. Calcium plus vitamin D supplementation and the risk of fractures. *New England Journal of Medicine* 2006;**354**:669–83.

Katakura M., Naka M., Kondo T. *et al*. Development, worsening, and improvement of diabetic microangiopathy in older people: six-year prospective study of patients under intensive diabetes control. *Journal of the American Geriatrics Society* 2007;**55**:541–7.

Kinsella K. Demographic aspects. In: Ebrahim S, Kalache A, editors. Epidemiology in old age. London: BMJ Publishing; 1996. p. 32–40.

Kirkwood T. The time of our lives: the science of human ageing. London: Weidenfield and Nicolson; 1999.

Laing W., Hall M., Lumley P. Agenda for health. The challenges of ageing. London: Association of the British Pharmaceutical Industry; 1991.

Lancaster T., Stead L.F. Individual behavioural counselling for smoking cessation. [Update of Cochrane Database Syst Rev. 2002;(3):CD001292; PMID:12137623]. Cochrane Database of Systematic Reviews 2005b;(2): CD001292.

Lancaster T., Stead L.F. Self-help interventions for smoking cessation. [Update of Cochrane Database Syst Rev. 2002;(3):CD001118; PMID:12137618]. Cochrane Database of Systematic Reviews 2005a;(3): CD001118.

Lawlor D.A., Davey Smith G., Ebrahim S. Commentary: The hormone replacement–coronary heart disease conundrum: is this the death of observational epidemiology?. *International Journal of Epidemiology* 2004;**33**:464–7.

Lee C., Porteous J. Experiences of family caregiving among middle-aged Australian women. *Feminism and Psychology* 2002;**12**(1):79–96.

Lee C. Experiences of family caregiving among older Australian women. *Journal of Health Psychology* 2001;**6**:393–404.

Leon D.A., Chenet L., Shkolnikov V.M. *et al*. Huge variation in Russian mortality rates 1984–94: artefact, alcohol or what? Lancet 1997;**350**:383–8.

Levine R.S., Foster J.E., Fullilove R.E. *et al*. Black–white inequalities in mortality and life expectancy, 1933–1999: implications for healthy people 2010. *Public Health Reports* 2001;**116**:474–83.

Lunney J.R., Lynn J., Foley D.J. *et al*. Patterns of functional decline at end of life. *Journal of the American Medical Association* 2003;**289**(18): 2387–92.

Manton K.G. Changing concepts of morbidity and mortality in the elderly population. *Milbank Memorial Fund Quarterly – Health and Society* 1982;**60**:183–244.

Manton K.G. Sex and race specific mortality differentials in multiple causes of death data. *Gerontologist* 1980;**20**:480–93.

Marmot M., Adelstein A.M., Bulusu L. Lessons from the study of immigrant mortality. Lancet 1984;**1**(8392):1455–7.

Marmot M. Inequalities in health. *New England Journal of Medicine* 2001;**345**(2):134–6.

Marmot M. Social determinants of health inequalities. *Lancet* 2005;**365**(9464):1099–104.

Mathers C. Health differentials among older Australians. Canberra: AGPS ; 1999. Health Monitoring Series No. 2.

Mathers C.D., Iburg K.M., Salomon J.A. *et al*. Global patterns of healthy life expectancy in the year 2002. *BMC Public Health* 2004;**4**:66.

Mathers C.D., Sadana R., Salomon J.A. *et al*. Healthy life expectancy in 191 countries, 1999. *Lancet* 2001;**357**(9269):1685–91.

Mathers C.D., Vos E.T., Stevenson C.E. *et al*. The Australian Burden of Disease Study: measuring the loss of health from diseases, injuries and risk factors. *Medical Journal of Australia* 2000;**172**:592–6.

McCallum J., Simons L., Simons J. The Dubbo Study of the Health of the Elderly 1988–2002. Sydney: University of Sydney; 2003.

McClure R., Turner C., Peel N. *et al*. Population-based interventions for the prevention of fall-related injuries in older people. [Online]. Cochrane Database Systematic Review 2005;(1):CD004441.

Mendes de Leon C.P., Glass T.A., Beckett L.A. *et al*. Social networks and disability transitions across eight intervals of yearly data in the New Haven EPESE. *Journal of Gerontology SeriesB: Psychological Sciences and Social Sciences* 1999;**54**:S62–72.

Mitka M. International conference considers health needs of the rural elderly. *Journal of the American Medical Association* 2000;**284**(4): 423–34.

Mouton C.P., Espino D.V. Problem-oriented diagnosis: health screening in older women. *American Family Physician* 1999;**59**(7):1835–42.

Mulrow C.D., Cornell J.A., Herrera C.R. *et al*. Hypertension in the elderly. Implications and generalizability of randomized trials. *Journal of the American Medical Association* 1994;**272**:1932–8.

Murray C.J.L., Michaud C.M., McKenna M.T. *et al*. US patterns of mortality by county and race: 1965–1994. Cambridge (MA): Harvard School of Public Health; Atlanta (GA): Centers for Disease Control and Prevention; 1998.

National Center for Health Statistics. Health, United States 1999. Hyattsville (MD): National Center for Health Statistics; 1999.

Nelson H.D., Helfand M., Woolf S.H. *et al*. Screening for postmenopausal osteoporosis: a review of the evidence for the US Preventive Services Task Force. *Annals of Internal Medicine* 2002;**137**:529–41.

Noh S., Kaspar V. Perceived discrimination and depression: moderating effects of coping acculturation, and ethnic support. *American Journal of Public Health* 2003;**93**(30):232–8.

Normand C. Ten popular health economic fallacies. *Journal of Public Health Medicine* 1998;**20**:129–32.

Office of National Statistics. Population trends 119 [Online]. Spring 2005. Available from: http://www.statistics.gov.uk/downloads/theme_population/PT119v2.pdf [accessed 2007 Feb 9].

Omran A.R. The epidemiologic transition: a theory of the epidemiology of population change. *Milbank Memorial Fund Quarterly* 1971;**49**(4): 509–38.

Pignone M.P., Gaynes B.N., Rushton J.K. *et al.* Screening for depression in adults: a summary of the evidence for the US Preventive Services Task Force. *Annals of Internal Medicine* 2002;**136**:765–76.

Pit S.W., Byles J.E., Henry D.A., Holt L., Hansen V., Bowman D.A. A Quality Use of Medicines program for general practitioners and older people: a cluster randomised controlled trial *Medical Journal of Australia* 2007; **187**(1):23–30.

Porthouse J., Cockayne S., King C. *et al.* Randomized controlled trial of calcium and supplementation with cholecalciferol (vitamin D3) for prevention of fractures in primary care. *British Medical Journal* 2005;**330**:1003–8.

Research Dissemination Core. Oral hygiene care for functionally dependent and cognitively impaired older adults. Iowa City (IA): University of Iowa Gerontological Nursing Interventions Research Center; 2002.

Riley N.E. China's population: new trends and challenges. *Population Bulletin* 2004;**59**:3–35.

Rivetti D., Jefferson T., Thomas R. *et al.* Vaccines for preventing influenza in the elderly. [Online]. Cochrane Database of Systematic Reviews 2006;(2):CD004876.

Rossouw J.E., Prentice R.L., Manson J.E. *et al.* Postmenopausal hormone therapy and risk of cardiovascular disease by age and years since menopause. *Journal of the American Medical Association* 2007;**297**:1465–77.

Royal Commission on Long-Term Care. With respect to old age: long-term care— rights and responsibilities. London: Her Majesty's Stationery Office; 1999.

Saelens B.E., Sallis J.F., Frank L.D. Environmental correlates of walking and cycling: findings from the transportation, urban design, and planning literatures. *Annals of Behavioral Medicine* 2003;**25**:80–91.

Schmader K.E., Hanlon J.T., Landsman P.B. *et al.* Inappropriate prescribing and health outcomes in elderly veteran outpatients. *Annals of Pharmacotherapy* 1997;**31**(5):529–33.

Schulz R., Martire L. Family caregiving of persons with dementia: prevalence, health effects, and support. *American Journal of Geriatric Psychiatry* 2004;**12**:240–9.

Seeman T., Chen X. Risk and protective factors for physical functioning in older adults with and without chronic conditions: MacArthur Studies of Successful Aging. *Journals of Gerontology Series B: Psychological Sciences and Social Sciences* 2002;**57**:S135–44.

Sellors J., Kaczorowski J., Sellors C. *et al.* A randomized controlled trial of a pharmacist consultation program for family physicians and their elderly patients. *Canadian Medical Association Journal* 2003;**169**(1):17–22.

Shepperd S., Iliffe S. Hospital at home versus in-patient hospital care. [Online].Cochrane Database of Systematic Reviews 2001;(3): CD000356 [last update 2005 May].

Shkolnikov V., McKee M., Leon D.A. Changes in life expectancy in Russia in the mid-1990s. *Lancet* 2001;**357**:917–21.

Simonson W., Feinberg J.L. Medication-related problems in the elderly: defining the issues and identifying solutions. *Drugs Aging* 2005;**22**(7):559–69.

Smeeth L., Iliffe S. Community screening for visual impairment in the elderly. [Online]. Cochrane Database Systematic Reviews 2003;(4): CD001054.

Soldo B.J., Mitchell O.S., Tfaily R. *et al. Cross-cohort differences in health on the verge of retirement.* Cambridge (MA): National Bureau of Economic Research; 2006. Working paper 12762.

Stampfer M.J., Colditz G.A. Estrogen replacement therapy and coronary heart disease: a quantitative assessment of the epidemiologic evidence. *Preventative Medicine* 1991;**20**:47–63.

Steinbach U. Social networks, institutionalization, and mortality among elderly people in the United States. *Journal of Gerontology* 1992; **47**:S183–90.

Stroke Unit Trialists' Collaboration. Organized inpatient (stroke unit) care for stroke. In: The Cochrane Library. Issue 3. [Online]. Oxford: Update Software; 2001.

Stuck A.E., Siu A.L., Wieland G.D. *et al.* Comprehensive geriatric assessment: a meta-analysis of controlled trials. *Lancet* 1993;**342**(8878): 1032–6.

Stuck A.Q., Egger M., Hammer A. *et al.* Home visits to prevent nursing home admission and functional decline in elderly people. *Journal of the American Medical Association* 2002;**287**:1022–8.

The RECORD Trial Group. Oral vitamin D3 and calcium for secondary prevention of low-trauma fractures in elderly people (Randomized Evaluation of Calcium Or vitamin D, RECORD): a randomized placebo-controlled trial. *Lancet* 2005;**365**:1621–8.

Tinetti M., Baker C., McAvay G. *et al.* A multifactorial intervention to reduce the risk of falling among elderly people living in the community. *New England Journal of Medicine* 1994;**331**:821–7.

Toumilehto J., Lindstrom J. The major diabetes prevention trials. *Current Diabetes Report* 2003;**3**:115–22.

Tucker K.L., Hallfrisch J., Qiao N. *et al.* The combination of high fruit and vegetable and low saturated fat intakes is more protective against mortality in aging men than is either alone: the Baltimore Longitudinal Study of Aging. *Journal of Nutrition* 2005;**135**:556–61.

United Nations. World Population Ageing 1950–2050. New York (NY): Population Division, United Nations; 2002. Available from: http://www.un.org/esa/population/publications/worldageing19502050/[accessed 2007 May 8].

United States Census Bureau [Online]. Available from: http://www.census.gov/[accessed 2007 Feb 6].

United States National Institute of Ageing [Online]. Available from: http://www.nia.nih.gov/[accessed 2007 May 8].

United States Preventive Services Task Force. The guide to clinical preventive services, 2006. Rockville (MD): Agency for Healthcare Research and Quality; 2006.

Van Haastregt J.C.M., Diederiks J.P.M., van Rossum E. *et al.* Effects of preventive home visits to elderly people living in the community: systematic review. *British Medical Journal* 2000;**320**:754–8.

Villa V.M., Wallace S.P. Diversity and ageing: implications for aging policy. In: Carmel S., Morse C.A., Torres-Gil F.M., editors. Lessons of ageing from three nations. Volume I: The art of ageing well. New York (NY): Baywood Publishing Company Inc; 2007.

Vita A.J., Terry R.B., Hubert H.B. *et al.* Aging, health risks and cumulative disability. *New England Journal of Medicine* 1998;**338**:1035–41.

Wald N.J., Law M.R. A strategy to reduce cardiovascular disease by more than 80%. *British Medical Journal* 2003;**326**:1419–24.

Ward D., Severs M., Dean T. *et al.* Care home versus hospital and own home environments for rehabilitation of older people. In: The Cochrane Library. Issue 2. [Online]. Oxford: Update Software; 2003.

Williams A., Evans J.G. The rationing debate. *Rationing health care by age. British Medical Journal* 1997;**314**:820–5.

Wilson K., Mottram P., Sivanranthan A. *et al.* Antidepressants versus placebo for the depressed elderly. [Online]. Cochrane Database Systematic Review 2001:CD000561.

Wolff J.L., Starfield B., Anderson G. Prevalence, expenditures, and complications of multiple chronic conditions in the elderly. *Archives of Internal Medicine* 2002;**162**:2269–76.

World Health Organization. International Classification of Functioning, Disability and Health. Geneva: World Health Organization. Available from: www.who.int/icf [accessed 2007 May 8].

World Health Organization. Obesity: preventing and managing the global epidemic. Report of a WHO consultation. Geneva: World Health Organization; 2000. Technical Report Series 894.

World Health Organization. The bone and joint decade. Geneva: World Health Organization; 2001.

World Health Organization. World health report 1999: making a difference. Geneva: World Health Organization; 1999.

Writing Group for the Women's Health Initiative Investigators. Risks and benefits of estrogen plus progestin in healthy postmenopausal women: principal results from the Women's Health Initiative Randomized Control Trial. *Journal of the American Medical Association* 2002;**288**:321–33.

Yusuf S., Reddy S., Ounpuu S. *et al.* Global burden of cardiovascular diseases—Part II: variations in cardiovascular disease by specific ethnic groups and geographic regions and prevention strategies. *Circulation* 2001;**104**(23):2855–64.

Zavoretti R. Family-based care for China's ageing population. *Asia Europe Journal* 2006;**4**:211–8.

Zermansky A.G., Petty D.R., Raynor D.K. *et al.* Clinical medication review by a pharmacist of patients on repeat prescriptions in general practice: a randomized controlled trial. *Health Technology Assessment* 2002;**6**(20):1–86.

Forced migrants and other displaced populations

Catherine R. Bateman and Anthony B. Zwi

Abstract

This chapter provides an overview of the global health dimensions of forced migration and the associated public health challenges. The chapter begins by identifying different categories of forced migrants including refugees, internally displaced persons, asylum seekers, trafficked or smuggled persons, as well as environment and development displacees. The causes must be viewed in global context in which globalization is simultaneously a force for greater integration while at the same time contributing to forced migration. Global influences include economic inequalities, armed conflicts, human rights abuses, environmental degradation, and natural disasters among others. The problem of forced migration is difficult to quantify, and statistics are contested. In 2006, the United Nations High Commissioner for Refugees (UNHCR) recognized 32.9 million 'persons of concern' including 9.9 million refugees and 12.8 million internally displaced persons. Legal frameworks, including the 1951 UN Convention on Refugees and its successors, identify formal protections to which refugees and other groups of forced migrants are entitled. Nevertheless, the public health situation of forced migrants are varied and often poor. They may form distinct populations or be dispersed amongst host populations; they may be displaced within their own country, to a nearby country, or to a more distant country of asylum; and they may dwell in a developing country experiencing conflict, a more peaceful but poverty-stricken developing country, or a wealthy developed nation. The health of each forced migrant population will be shaped by these contextual factors, but also by prior health and social conditions, the journeys they have had to take, the social structures within which they now live, including access to services, and the stability of these new structures. The role of public health professionals in developing a comprehensive understanding of these dynamics, advocating for forced migrant health, and enabling forced migrants to speak and be heard, aiding them in transforming their own health outcome is discussed.

Introduction

This chapter provides a global overview of forced migration and the public health challenges facing populations forced to move from their usual homes. It begins by presenting a brief history of forced migration and the legal definition of 'refugee'. We describe the emergence of categories of forced migrants that do not meet the legal definition of 'refugee', describe how these groups are treated by states, and the implications for peoples' lives and health. The chapter then explores the social and political factors that have influenced the treatment of refugees by states. We lay out some of the major health issues that refugees face in both developing and developed countries. The wide variety of actors involved in both protecting forced migrants and providing health services is presented, along with a discussion of the contextual conditions that have an impact, often detrimental, on the health of forced migrants. As well as describing the structural factors that create and limit health outcomes, this analysis seeks to highlight the agency and voice of forced migrants, exploring the importance of understanding and projecting these, and of appreciating the rationales for how forced migrants may act in the often chaotic situations in which they find themselves. We consider how interactions with other actors, within the complex social, political, and legal context of forced migration, may lead to seemingly unhealthy choices, and at times, barriers to engaging with services. Yet, forced migrants make choices, when possible, seeking to protect their well-being and fight for better, and healthier, outcomes.

Categories of forced migrants

Definitions of forced migration have been debated for more than 50 years, dating back to the first UN Convention on Refugees in 1951. The legal framework that emerged under the Convention centred on 'refugees' as a specially defined group and is based upon the 1951 Convention and a subsequent 1967 protocol. According to these, a refugee is a person who:

owing to a well-founded fear of being persecuted for reasons of race, religion, nationality, membership of a particular social group, or political opinion, is outside the country of his nationality, and is unable to or, owing to such fear, is unwilling to avail himself of the protection of that country (UNHCR 2007).

This definition has been modified by regional instruments in Africa and Latin America, as described in a later section.

The International Association for the Study of Forced Migration (IASFM), however, defines forced migration much more widely as:

a general term that refers to the movements of refugees and internally displaced people (those displaced by conflicts) as well as people displaced by natural or environmental disasters, chemical or nuclear disasters, famine, or development projects (FMO 2008).

This definition encompasses a wide range of forced migrants, and these can be distinguished into several distinct groups (Box 11.8.1).

The definitions of other forced migrant groups, and their sources, are outlined below. They highlight the increased attention devoted to both describing, and defining, the many forms of forced migration that exist. The discourse and narratives presented have a marked impact on how people see, and respond, to those forced to leave their usual homes and livelihoods.

Internally displaced persons (IDPs)

Unlike refugees, there is no legal definition of an IDP. It is generally accepted that if a person meets the definition of a refugee, but their displacement does not take them across an international border, then they are internally displaced. The Secretary General of the United Nations has appointed a representative to deal with IDPs and the Office of the United Nations High Commissioner for Human Rights (OHCHR) has produced a set of Guiding Principles to address the specific needs of IDPs who are described as:

persons or groups of persons who have been forced or obliged to flee or to leave their homes or places of habitual residence, in

particular as a result of, or in order to, avoid the effects of armed conflict, situations of generalized violence, violations of human rights or natural or human-made disasters, and who have not crossed an internationally recognized State border (Deng 1998).

Asylum seekers

Asylum seekers are those who are fleeing persecution and are seeking refugee status in another country. According to UNHCR, an asylum seeker:

is a person who has left their country of origin, has applied for recognition as a refugee in another country, and is awaiting a decision on their application (UNHCR 2007).

The application referred to relates to being recognized under the 1951 Convention as a refugee and therefore entitled to the protection and support stipulated by the Convention. They may or may not arrive in a country with authorization, nevertheless, they have a legal right to claim asylum and are therefore not 'illegal'.

Trafficked persons

The 2003 Protocol to Prevent, Suppress and Punish Trafficking in Persons, especially Women and Children, describes trafficking as:

recruitment, transportation, transfer, harbouring, or receipt of persons, by means of the threat or use of force or other forms of coercion, of abduction, of fraud, of deception, of the abuse or power or of a position of vulnerability or of the giving or receiving

Box 11.8.1 **Categories of forced migrants**	
Refugee	A person who 'owing to a well-founded fear of being persecuted for reasons of race, religion, nationality, membership of a particular social group, or political opinion, is outside the country of his nationality, and is unable to or, owing to such fear, is unwilling to avail himself of the protection of that country' (UNHCR 2008).
Internally displaced persons	'Persons or groups of persons who have been forced or obliged to flee or to leave their homes or places of habitual residence, in particular as a result of, or in order to, avoid the effects of armed conflict, situations of generalized violence, violations of human rights or natural or human-made disasters, and who have not crossed an internationally recognized State border' (Deng 1998).
Asylum seeker	'A person who has left their country of origin, has applied for recognition as a refugee in another country, and is awaiting a decision on their application' (UNHCR 2007).
Trafficking in persons	'Recruitment, transportation, transfer, harbouring or receipt of persons, by means of the threat or use of force or other forms of coercion, of abduction, of fraud, of deception, of the abuse for power or of a position of vulnerability or of the giving or receiving of payments or benefits to achieve the consent of a person having control over another person, for the purpose of exploitation' (United Nations 2003).
Smuggling in persons	'The procurement, in order to obtain, directly or indirectly, a financial or other material benefit, of illegal entry of a person into a state, party of which the person is not a national or permanent resident' (United Nations 2000) [Article 3 (a)].
Environmentally displaced person	'A person displaced owing to environmental causes, notably land loss and degradation, and natural disaster' (United Nations 1997).
Development displacees	"People who are compelled to move as a result of policies and projects implemented to supposedly enhance 'development'" (Forced Migration Online 2008).

of payments or benefits to achieve the consent of a person having control over another person, for the purpose of exploitation. Exploitation shall include, at a minimum, the exploitation of the prostitution of others or other forms of sexual exploitation, forced labour or services, slavery or practices similar to slavery, servitude or the removal of organs (United Nations 2003).

Smuggled persons

Smuggling of aliens or 'illegal migrant smuggling' is defined by the UN 2000 Protocol Against Smuggling of Migrants by Land, Sea and Air, which supplemented the UN Convention Against Transnational Organized Crime, to mean:

the procurement, in order to obtain, directly or indirectly, a financial or other material benefit, of illegal entry of a person into a state, party of which the person is not a national or permanent resident (United Nations 2000) [Article 3 (a)].

Environmentally displaced persons

The OECD glossary of statistical terms 2001 describes an environmental refugee as 'a person displaced owing to environmental causes, notably land loss and degradation, and natural disaster' (United Nations 1997). However, the term was first described by Essam El-Hinnawi (1985), a researcher from United Nations Environment Program (UNEP) in 1985, who defined environmental refugees as:

those people who have been forced to leave their traditional habitat, temporarily or permanently, because of a marked environmental disruption (natural and/or triggered by people) that jeopardized their existence and/or seriously affected the quality of their life.

'Environmental disruption' in this definition is taken to mean any physical, chemical, and/or biological changes in the ecosystem (or resource base) that render it, temporarily or permanently, unsuitable to support human life. The validity of the term 'environmental refugees' has been debated greatly since that time. Actors emerge from a realm of perspectives including environmentalists, economists, and refugee advocates, each with a different interpretation of the term. Some prefer to use the term 'environmental migrant' or 'environmental displacee'; different terms establish different implications for both the individuals and states involved.

Development displacees

There is no legal definition for development displaces; however, Forced Migration Online (http://www.forcedmigration.org) suggests they are:

people who are compelled to move as a result of policies and projects implemented to supposedly enhance 'development'. These include large-scale infrastructure projects such as dams, roads, ports, airports; urban clearance initiatives; mining and deforestation; and the introduction of conservation parks/reserves and biosphere projects. Affected people usually remain within the borders of their country. People displaced in this way are sometimes also referred to as 'oustees', 'involuntarily displaced' or 'involuntarily resettled' (Forced_Migration_Online 2008).

Interestingly, large-scale agricultural projects do not seem to be specifically mentioned.

Causes of displacement

The global context

Forced migration cannot be fully understood without considering the global context and the shifting global forces that shape the form and patterns of migration. Globalization and its role in shaping the dynamics of forced migration need to be considered. Although globalization is a contested concept with disputed definitions, most people accept it as a global process of integration which affects sociocultural, economic, and political domains (see Chapter 2.1).

There is a polarized debate over the affects of globalization on health. Some commentators argue, like Feachem (2001), that the forces of economic globalization can be beneficial to the poor, increasing wealth and therefore health; while others (Baum 2001; MacDonald 2007) highlight the poor health situation in many developing countries and the vast inequities present, and suggest that globalization plays a part in generating these conditions. The latter argue that globalization cannot be separated from economic policies that serve the interests of the wealthy, reinforcing or exacerbating inequalities, fuelling conflicts and contributing to public health crises in developing countries. This analysis suggests that the only way to improve health is to seriously restructure the dominant international financial institutions. Taking the middle ground, Lee (2004) suggests that rigorous, ongoing analysis is required to assess the positive and negative impacts on health within the overall conceptual domain of globalization. Zwi and Alvarez-Castillo (2003) argue that globalization has often led to poor health outcomes for vast populations and that this in turn is responsible for fuelling forced migration. Regardless of our standpoint on globalization, what it is, how it impacts on health, and its influence, what is clear is that global health inequities exist and are dramatic, producing some of the major contributors to forced migration, whether or not associated with violence.

Castles' (2004) analysis suggests that the global context should be carefully examined when considering forced migration dynamics. He argues that the current perception of a global 'asylum crisis' should be seen more as a crisis of North–South relationships, within which 'asylum' is but one aspect. The current picture of forced migration, he argues, is a result of disparities between North and South. While these disparities exist and people search for a better life, or simply for survival, forced migration will continue. The disparity is also reflected in how the effects of forced migration are absorbed globally, further deepening the crisis in North–South relations. He shows that while there has repeatedly been a perception of impending asylum crises ever since the 1800s, which largely do not fully emerge as feared, there are some new features. He cites the increase in endemic violence and human rights violations as a feature that has increased the volume of forced migration in recent times. Castles (2004) shows, however, that for the North, there is no significant economic or social crisis resulting from forced migration and contrary to popular belief, the North has not had to absorb large influxes of people. The situation is nonetheless construed by those in the North as a crisis because it highlights the 'erosion of nation-state sovereignty'. The South, however, has absorbed the vast majority of forced migrants from neighbouring countries (Allotey & Reidpath 2003). This combined with increasingly restrictive policies of wealthy countries that seek to limit refugee absorption from the South, leads to a tension in North–South relations, and opens space for people smuggling and trafficking, further threatening the sense of control over borders that the North is seeking to maintain, and therefore deepening the sense of crisis perceived by the North. Hence the burden has been left largely with the South, while in the North, incomplete pictures of fear that exclude vulnerable people have been painted and promoted (Grove & Zwi 2006). In their review of globalization, forced migration, and health, Zwi and Alvarez Castillo (2003) suggest that public health professionals have a responsibility to examine the context and whole picture, and in so doing, to advocate for a more humane globalization that has a chance of decreasing forced migration and the associated poor health outcomes.

Immediate causes of displacement

There is general agreement on the range of factors that contribute to displacement and forced migration. However, the importance of particular factors, and the linkages between them, varies in different contexts. Identification of specific causes has implications for both the states involved and the migrants themselves, given that the perceived cause of displacement has an impact on the international response, the level of funding support provided and the attitudes of host populations to those seeking protection. The health consequences of forced migration will be shaped by not only the causes of displacement, but by the perceptions of all actors regarding these causes and their relationship to them. In this respect, the terms and context within which forced migrants are described and 'presented' greatly affects the societal response and opportunities, or constraints, operating.

Forced migration has traditionally been associated with war and violence. The conception of a refugee as defined by the UN Convention, fleeing from persecution to a place of safety in another country, was clear-cut and well understood. As Moore and Shellman (2004) describe, the central model was one of:

Violence in = Forced migration out

However, whilst the main causes of involuntary displacement remain armed conflict, repression and war, other factors such as natural disaster and development projects are also important, as are the more complex set of economic, social, and political circumstances that may lead to trafficking and people smuggling.

Martin (2002) focuses attention on natural and man-made disasters and border changes leading to statelessness, as factors which lead to forced migration, alongside the well recognized factors related to persecution, human rights violations, repression, and conflict. Environmental factors, such as rising sea levels and extreme weather conditions, are also increasingly recognized as important. Some argue that these causes may, over time, supercede conflict as a primary cause of forced migration (Myers & Kent 1995). Resource constraints, including depleted access to land and water, and conflict over precious minerals, are likely to become increasingly important, especially as the global population increases from around six billion people at present to nearly nine billion by 2050.

While all these factors are important, quantifying their effects is difficult. Data are available regarding numbers of 'Convention' refugees and also, more recently, regarding IDPs. These data may give some indication of the level of displacement produced by conflicts and violence, alongside immediate natural disasters such as tsunami and earthquakes. However, more insidious environmental and economic effects are far harder to quantify.

The increased complexity of recent times in describing and understanding factors that cause displacement rise new concerns that go beyond the simple 'violence = migration' model therefore calls for new approaches. Major challenges include an increased focus on economic migrants and those who are forced to move as a result of environmental and climate changes; there is also a rise in 'mixed migration', a term which recognizes that many migrants fall somewhere on the spectrum between forced and voluntary migration and are hard to categorize as one or the other.

Particularly important is a call for a shift in policies of protection for host countries to developing policies which address the root causes within countries from which people are forced to migrate; and a growing understanding that understanding causes may allow predictions of impending displacement as well as the identification of the means to avert large-scale displacement.

Some analyses continue to support the primacy of violent conflict, or threat of conflict as the major predictor of populations leaving their homes. Moore and Shellman (2004) analysed a global sample of 40 countries and using a model that incorporated a wide range of indicators (government threat, dissident threat, government-dissent interaction, ethnic or non-ethnic civil wars, war on territory, income opportunity, political freedom and the rule of law, and cultural and family ties), they found that the first three were the primary determinants of forced migration flows. These were more important than other factors such as size of economy or type of political institution. Apodaca (1998) analysed a variety of models developed to predict forced migration and concluded that human rights violations are one of the most important predictors.

Economic migration has often been portrayed in the media as freely chosen migration that should not confer a responsibility to protect on accepting states. However, analysts such as Castles (2003) argue that forced migration is linked to economic migration and that the two are 'closely related (and indeed often indistinguishable) forms of expression of global inequalities and societal crises'. These inequities have intensified since the end of the Cold War. He argues that studies of the causes of forced migration have neglected the over-arching economic and social structures which should be seen in relation to 'US political and military domination, economic globalization, North–South inequality and transnationalism'.

Debates regarding causes of displacement have particular salience in relation to the protection offered to forced migrants. As subsequent sections of the chapter describe, the nature and extent of protection is often determined by perceived cause. Therefore, understanding these debates is crucial as they may have effects on what and how protection, if any, is offered to forced migrant populations.

Forced migration statistics

Assessing the volume of global flows of forced migrants is valuable in identifying trends, and the patterns of distribution with respect to where the burden for providing assistance and care lies. In specific countries and contexts, where people are forced to migrate from their place of origin, the first step in addressing public health and other more general concerns is often to define the size of the population at risk. Donors, governments, aid agencies, and community organizations require basic demographic and related data to inform planning and service delivery. The collection of data is complicated and surrounded by controversy, having the potential to immediately reframe what looks like a technical issue into a political one.

The two main sources of statistics on forced migrants are the United Nations High Commissioner for Refugees (UNHCR) and the US Committee for Refugees and Immigrants (USCRI). These organizations produce differing estimates for different types of forced migrants in different geographical contexts. The logistic difficulties of collecting reliable data from shifting forced migrant populations leaves space for political interests to enter, and seek to shape, the field. This is compounded by disagreement over definitions of forced migrants and which groups to include in which categories, as mentioned earlier, with significant implications for the rights and entitlements of such groups, as well as for who bears the responsibilities for addressing their needs. Despite contested data, available sources provide valuable information on trends and distribution.

UNHCR provides data based on 'persons of concern', an increasingly wide-ranging term. 'Persons of concern' includes refugees (as defined by the 1951 Convention or the 1969 Organisation of African Unity (OAU) Convention); persons granted complementary protection (alternative forms of protection for those that fall outside of the terms of the 1951 Convention) and those with forms of temporary protection; asylum seekers who in the year of data collection are still pending a final decision on an application for protection; stateless persons; refugees who returned to their country of origin in the year of data collection; and IDPs. For the purposes of UNHCR the latter are limited to conflict-generated IDPs to whom UNHCR protection or assistance is extended, but does not include all IDPs.

The changes seen between 2005 and 2006 in the UNHCR estimates (Tables 11.8.1 and 11.8.2) illustrate how dramatically statistics may fluctuate due to real, methodological, and political influences on data.

The number of 'persons of concern' to UNHCR increased substantially in 2006. Although 2006 saw a real increase in refugee numbers as a result of 1.2 million Iraqis seeking refuge in Syria and Jordan, there were other factors that led to the increased numbers (Tables 11.8.1 and 11.8.2). The UNHCR became involved at this point as a player in the cluster approach, through which UN agencies have been seeking to enhance their efficiency, and consequently extended its activities to include a larger number of IDPs. Methodological changes in collecting data also contributed to the increase partly as a result of moves to better reflect individual refugee registration in UNHCR operations, but also due to a review of the caseload of countries such as the United States.

It is important to note that 4.3 million Palestinian refugees falling under the mandate of the United Nations Relief and Works Agency for Palestinian Refugees in the Near East (UNRWA) are not included in these UNHCR figures. The Palestinian community has been one of the largest groups of refugees that has remained without being fully resettled or absorbed into host-nations; a reflection of how community members on the ground suffer while local, national, regional, and global powers resolve, or fail to resolve, higher-level strategic and political issues.

Given the importance of these numbers, they are invariably contested and debated; with key actors seeking to shape what data are collected and presented, who are counted, and what the implications are for future activities. Indeed each 'player' in the system, whether they be a UN or non-governmental agency, a recipient or state of origin, a local community or professional group, and many others, has their own rationale for inflating or deflating the numbers of people whether they be refugees or IDPs, in or outside of camps, dependant or free of other major influences.

Legal framework

Refugees

The 1951 Convention, which forms the basis of all international refugee law, was drafted in the aftermath of World War II in response to the large numbers of displaced people caused by the war. The Convention included restrictions on who would be classified as a 'refugee' based on geographical and temporal factors that were specific to the European context. As a result, the 1967 Protocol relating to the Status of Refugees was adopted which removed these restrictions and allowed for more general application of the Convention. The Convention and Protocol laid out not only the definition of a refugee but also the scope of protection to which refugees were entitled. The most fundamental of these is *non-refoulement*, the right to remain rather than be returned to a place where their lives or freedoms would be at risk. Debate has raged over the continuing relevance of the Convention definition, given that it excludes large numbers of people in need of international protection, notably internally displaced persons and those that have migrated as a result of generalized (as opposed to individualized) violence, civil war, and widespread human rights abuses.

Africa and Latin America responded to the limitations of the Convention and Protocol by adopting their own regional laws and standards. The Organisation of African Unity (now known as the African Union) adopted the 1967 Convention Governing the Specific Aspects of Refugee Problems in Africa (Barnett 2002).

Table 11.8.2 World Refugee Survey (USCRI 2006, 2007)

	2005[a]	2006[b]
Refugees and asylum seekers	12 million	13.9 million
New refugees and asylum seekers	1.04 million	1.1 million
IDPs	21 million	–
New IDPs	2.1 million	–

[a] World Refugee Survey (2006) reports data from 2005.
[b] IDP data not available in World Refugee Survey (2007).

Table 11.8.1 'Persons of concern' to United Nations High Commissioner of Refugees (UNHCR, April 2007, December 2007)

	2005	2006
Refugees	8.7 million	9.9 million
Asylum seekers	773 500	744 000
IDPs	6.6 million	12.8 million
Stateless	2.4 million	5.8 million
Returnees	1.6 million	2.6 million
Resettlement	80 000	71 700
Others of concern	960 400	1 million
Total	20.8 million	32.9 million

This is the only legally binding regional instrument and has a refugee definition similar to that of the convention but includes those who flee due to 'external aggression, occupation, foreign domination or events seriously disturbing public order in either part or the whole of his country of origin or nationality' (OAU 1969).

In Latin America, the Cartagena Declaration, adopted in 1984, included a definition of refugee similar to that of the OAU Convention but which also included reference to 'massive violation of human rights' (Cartagena Declaration 1984). The latter is not legally binding but has been adopted by many states and incorporated into some national legislation in the region.

Persons who have participated in war crimes and violations of humanitarian and human rights law, including the crime of terrorism are specifically excluded from the convention and cannot be recognized as refugees.

The UNHCR has been given a mandate to provide international protection to refugees and seek permanent solutions to their problems through its Statute, adopted by the UN General Assembly (UNGA) in December 1950. Over the years, the UNGA has allowed UNHCR to extend its responsibilities and is increasingly focused not only on refugee protection but also on managing refugees in the field.

IDPs

Whilst IDPs do not have the same legal framework of protection, they have become included in UNHCRs 'people of concern' and are therefore often covered by its mandate. The United Nations Office for Coordination of Humanitarian Affairs (OCHA) has produced a set of Guiding Principles to address the specific needs of internally displaced persons (OCHA 1998). The guidelines identify rights and guarantees that should be afforded to IDPs although they are not legally binding.

Asylum seekers

The Declaration of Territorial Asylum (DTA) adopted by the UN General Assembly in 1967 is based on article 14 of the Universal Declaration of Human Rights, which declares that 'everyone has the right to seek and to enjoy in other countries asylum from persecution'. The principles of the DTA are that all States recognize asylum granted by one State, that States themselves evaluate the grounds for asylum, and that no one seeking asylum should be rejected at borders or if already within a country should not be compulsorily returned to any State in which they may be subject to persecution. Exceptions can only be made in situations of national security or for asylum seekers that have committed a crime against humanity, against peace or a war crime.

Asylum may be granted by States on the basis of the 1951 Refugee Convention, in which an individual has been deemed a 'refugee' as defined by the Convention. However, given the restrictions of this definition and the increasing numbers of people who are seeking protection but do not fit the Convention definition, alternative forms of protection have developed. Often termed 'complementary' or 'subsidiary' protection, McAdam (2006) describes the plethora of alternative forms of protection for 'non-Convention refugees' that previously had been treated much the same as Convention refugees by states.

'Non-Convention' refugees, such as those fleeing widespread violence rather than targeted individual persecution, have to look to instruments of human rights law, rather than refugee law, for protection. However, human rights instruments do not attach the same clear rights and standards as the Refugee Convention and it has also been argued that human rights law can be weak on implementation (McAdam 2006). This has led many to argue that complementary protection is a lesser form of protection, and there is a danger of States using these forms of protection to decrease the numbers of Convention refugees and therefore their level of commitment. Debate continues as to whether expanding the current Convention definition, or expanding systems of complementary protection, will weaken or broaden protection to those seeking asylum.

Trafficking and smuggled persons

Although the reasons for a person to be trafficked or smuggled are very similar, international agreements and national laws treat them quite differently. Unlike trafficking, which may occur internally in a country, smuggling always involves the illegal crossing of an international boundary. Smuggling is seen as a crime against a *state* whereas trafficking is a crime against an *individual*. Consequently persons that are trafficked or smuggled are likely to be treated quite differently. The UN Convention on Trafficking mandates states to consider granting victims permanent or temporary resident status, whereas the Smuggling of Migrants Protocol calls on states to facilitate the return of smuggled persons to the country from which they came.

Environmental and developmental displacees

The concept of environmental refugees or displacees is particularly contentious and the subject of much current debate. There is little agreement on the whether environmental factors can be seen as primary causes of displacement and equally no consensus on a definition for those displaced from their homes by these factors. As a result the legal protection available is marginal. The current legal regime has no specific mandate to protect environmental displaces, if they are displaced across international borders, however, 'natural or human-made disasters' are covered by the Guiding Principles on Internal Displacement. These place the primary duty for protection with the national authority, however, no duty is placed on other states to recognize the need for protection. A growing body of opinion has begun calling for a system of global governance that recognizes environmental factors as a cause of displacement and for the displacees to be protected under international law (Courtland Robinson 2003; Biermann & Boas 2007).

Similarly developmental displacees do not have frameworks of protection of their own but are covered by the Guiding Principles on Internal Displacement. There is a need to recognize the needs of this group and for research on displacement not to fall into a dichotomy that separates conflict-related displacement from development-related displacement (Cernea 2007).

Evolving rights of protection

Protection based on a definition of refugees fleeing from the effects of violent conflict has been the prevailing paradigm, and whilst the centrality of conflict-related displacement has been debated, conflict and violence clearly remain significant causes of forced migration and suffering. Analysis reflecting the increasingly complex drivers of forced migration, including economic and environmental concerns, whilst vital, should be careful not to compromise existing rights of protection. These rights of protection, based on conflict as the central tenet, should not be further eroded by the recognition that there are other causes of forced migration that need to be seriously considered.

Political interests and control

Harrell-Bond (1992), the doyen of analysts examining forced migration, along with other key commentators such as Crisp (1999), and Bakewell (2008), demonstrate how resources to deal with forced migration are structured by broader ideological, political, and economic decisions. Harrell-Bond (1992) argues that refugee camps and many of the structures and organizations set up are part of a system of control of those in need. She argues that the allocation of resources (whether aid, political or military resources), is a 'central component in an ideology of control'. The granting of aid often legitimizes a group and their struggles; politics influences the status and visibility accorded to different groups. Even where humanitarian and development assistance are well targeted at forced migrants in need, the impact of services, systems, and funds, may be both positive and negative. While the forced migrants in great need may be able to access resources, these are not distributed equitably, and local populations, which often bear the brunt of providing for such community members, frequently are marginalized and unable to access new resources or services.

A valuable compilation of insights (Essed *et al.* 2004) highlights how forced migrants interact with agencies and the implications for ethics, policies, and politics. A case study by Turner (2004) in the same volume, for example, demonstrates how UNHCR effectively displaces older men as providers in their families and in so doing creates new dependencies. UNHCR becomes 'a better husband'—at the same time undermining and transforming traditional household and family relationships.

Public health situation of forced migrants

Forced migrants live in a range of different social, political, and geographical conditions. They may form distinct populations or be dispersed amongst host populations; they may be displaced within their own country, to a nearby or distant country of asylum; and may dwell anywhere from a developing country experiencing conflict, to a more peaceful but poverty-stricken developing country, to a wealthy developed nation. The health of each forced migrant population, and each individual within the group, will be shaped by these factors, as well as their prior health and social condition, the journeys they have had to take, the stability and security present in their new environments, the social structures within which they live, and the access they have to services and social support.

Gushulak and MacPherson (2000) describe migration health in terms of 'three distinct but interdependent undertakings: The pre-departure phase, the migratory journey itself, and the arrival at destination', each of which influences health. Factors such as social networks, assets, language, knowledge, information or access to services, food security issues, poor shelter, sanitation, and availability of safe water will influence health outcomes.

In this section we describe the major health challenges facing forced migrant populations. This is followed by an overview of the public health responses and an indication of where more detailed technical advice may be found.

Refugees in developing countries

Developing countries continue to absorb the vast majority of forced migrants, in particular as developed nations have become more restrictive. Within developing countries, people who are forcibly displaced either within or across borders may find themselves in a variety of possible contexts, settling short or long term either in a camp situation or dispersed within a host population. Each presents threats and opportunities.

The type of settlement formed has implications for health and well-being. The typical refugee camp setting has presented a range of problems, although improvements in public health knowledge and experience, and informing policy and practice with evidence, have led to better outcomes.

The impact of forced migration falls heavily on developing nations, and within these countries, on host populations. This is particularly so where forced migrants reside in non-camp situations.

Camps and non-camp settlements

Camps, whilst constructed with the intention of providing protection, safety and access to services, may also pose risks. Poorly planned refugee settlements may have inadequate infrastructure, may pose risks to safety, or set up new inequalities. The combination of overcrowding, poor hygiene and sanitation, lack of water, poor nutrition, and inadequate shelter provides conditions for spread of many diseases, particularly communicable disease. Refugees may arrive in a poor condition, suffering from malnutrition, and with poor immunity, reflecting limited access to immunization services. Disrupted social structures decrease the capacity to deal with sickness. Communicable disease spreads quickly and may be particularly severe. Psychological distress is also a major issue due to the insecure, restricted environment and lack of resources.

Debates over the utility of camps are highlighted by Harrell-Bond (2000) who argues that as a concept they have failed. Originally based on modernization theory, the premise was that camp settlements would become new agricultural centres and eventually be integrated with host populations to the benefit of all. However, this was abandoned as the theory became discredited and was replaced by a view that refugees should be seen as temporary. Harrell-Bond suggests that those in camps are in 'prison-like' settlements with poor conditions, increased vulnerability to disease and often poor nutrition. She also argues that camps do not help host populations, as large sums of money are diverted to camps which may be demolished if refugees do move on, as well as diverting scarce human and material resources from the host population. She suggests that it would be far more appropriate and cheaper to help integrate refugees into host populations and invest in the country and strengthening existing social structures, as a whole.

In many situations of forced migration, for example, when the Kosovar Albanians fled from Kosovo over the border into Albania, integration with host populations there was the norm. Following political instability and violence in Timor-Leste in 2006, 4 years after independence, makeshift camps were established within Dili, the capital city, for IDPs, while many also fled and were integrated with host communities in the districts. The latter necessarily absorbed a portion of the social and economic costs associated with accommodating those who fled.

However, Salama *et al.* (2004) show that, despite the problems associated with camps, there are also benefits. The increased knowledge base and co-ordination of humanitarian interventions have led to improvements in health, with better nutrition, sanitation, and health services. The burden of ill-health may shift from displaced populations who are relatively well serviced, especially if they cross international borders and become refugees, relative to host populations and IDPs whose needs may be greater and who have less access to assistance.

Mortality

Crude mortality rates are often used as an indicator of the immediate impact of complex emergencies. Toole and Waldman (1990) proposed a definition of the acute phase of a complex emergency as greater than one death per 10 000 people per day, based on a doubling of the baseline mortality rate in sub-Saharan African countries. Surveillance systems to monitor the impact of emergencies have been established in the past 15 years based on this definition. In recent decades, it has not been unusual to see CMRs in refugee populations of 30 times the baseline in the country of origin (Toole & Waldman 1997); some of the highest recorded were amongst Rwandan refugees who flooded into North Kivu in 1994 where average crude mortality rates were 20–35 deaths per 10 000 (Salama *et al.* 2004). In refugee camps, CMRs of 2 per 10 000 are now rarely seen, however, the situation in non-camp situations has deteriorated (Salama *et al.* 2004). Refugees are usually at greatest risk in early days of displacement, with mortality rates subsequently diminishing. The highest risk group is young children with most deaths occurring in the under-5 age group, demonstrated dramatically in one Somali camp in which 70 per cent of children under 5 appear to have died over an 8-month period (Moore *et al.* 1993; cited in Toole & Waldman 1997).

Causes of death

The main causes of death in developing country refugee situations are similar to those of developing country populations in general. The most common causes of death in Africa are diarrhoeal disease, measles, acute respiratory infections, and malaria (where endemic), exacerbated by a high prevalence of acute malnutrition (Toole & Waldman 1997). These diseases typically account for the vast majority of reported deaths in refugee populations, at times up to 95 per cent thereof. This is in contrast to European countries affected by war, where the most common causes of death are injuries, as well as communicable diseases, neonatal problems, and nutritional deficiencies. Recent analyses suggest that chronic diseases require attention, given the ageing population, and violence, instability, and forced migration in populations in which communicable diseases have been relatively well controlled and chronic diseases have emerged as problems (Chan & Sondorp 2007).

The conditions affecting refugees may have been brought with them from the country of origin, may be acquired in the host country (with refugees susceptible due to lack of sufficient immunity), or may result from the camp conditions themselves.

Diarrhoeal disease

Possibly the greatest threat to life amongst refugees is diarrhoeal disease. The main pathogens of concern are usually cholera and shigella. In some refugee camps, more than 40 per cent of deaths in the acute phase of an emergency can be attributed to diarrhoeal disease, and over 80 per cent of these deaths are in children under the age of 2 years (Salama *et al.* 2004). Outbreaks are exacerbated by factors such as the sharing and contamination of water sources and food, the scarcity of soap, and inadequate sanitation.

Amongst Rwandan refugees in camps in North Kivu, 85 per cent of the 50 000 deaths amongst the 800 000 people that flooded into the area early July 1994 were caused by diarrhoea, with 40 per cent

from shigella dysentery and 60 per cent from cholera (Salama *et al.* 2004). The primary drinking source, which was lake water, became rapidly contaminated, and as water was also scarce, infection spread swiftly through the refugees. Deaths in Goma were associated with a number of preventable causes (Siddique *et al.* 1995). Among Kurdish refugees, 70 per cent of deaths were a result of diarrhoea (Toole & Waldman 1997). In the elderly and young children, dysentery case-fatality rates can be as high as 10 per cent. Important public health interventions include the need to supply sufficient water, control excreta and hygiene, and increase public awareness of basic rules of hygiene. Evidence-informed case management is necessary to avoid unnecessary deaths.

Measles

Another of the most feared diseases in camps is measles—a particularly large problem in refugee situations in the 1970s and 1980s until it was recognized that vaccination should be accorded priority. The risk of death from measles is exacerbated in the presence of malnutrition, a common occurrence amongst refugee populations, as are secondary complications. Globally, measles kills approximately 450 000 people each year. While it is less of a problem in previously well-vaccinated populations, in developing countries, measles death rates can range from 1–5 per cent, and in refugee settings among malnourished children, the death rate may reach 10–30 per cent.

In 1985, 53 and 42 per cent of refugee deaths in eastern Sudan and Somalia, respectively, were caused by measles (Salama *et al.* 2004). The situation has improved in refugee camps due to mass vaccination, but IDPs still suffer as they have less access to vaccinations and, since 1990, it is more common to find high rates of measles in IDPs than in refugees. Measles is included in the Expanded Program on Immunisation but there is often low coverage in young children especially where human resources for health are limited or conflict affects normal service delivery. Increasing attention is being devoted to ensuring that services can continue to be supplied in fragile states.

Malaria

In areas where malaria is endemic, it can cause high rates of mortality and morbidity amongst refugees. This is particularly the case when people are displaced from an area of low endemicity to one of high endemicity. Drug resistance also plays a large part with chloroquine resistance and more recent resistance to fansidar reported in Rwandan refugees in Zaire. Local communities in low endemic areas may be placed at risk by refugees arriving from high endemic areas, especially if local conditions favour the mosquito. In Africa, 30 per cent of annual malarial deaths occur in complex emergency settings. This is because in complex emergencies (CEs) overcrowding increases the frequency of bites and also delays intervention thereby increasing the time that the parasite is in the blood (Salama *et al.* 2004). An example is Burundi which had a major epidemic in 2000–2001 when the population of 7 million reported 2.8 million cases of malaria, the war in 1993 caused control efforts to break down, populations were moving and there was widespread resistance to chloroquine.

Acute respiratory infections (ARIs)

Refugee camp conditions facilitate the spread of ARIs and rank amongst the leading causes of death in displaced populations. The lack of shelter, overcrowding with poor ventilation, and exposure that characterize the refugee existence contribute to the susceptibility to ARIs with poor outcomes. Young children are particularly affected. In Kabul, in 1993, 30 per cent under-five deaths and 23 per cent of deaths in displaced persons were a result of ARIs (Salama *et al.* 2004). Vaccinations against malaria, diphtheria, and pertussis have led to decreased mortality from ARIs. It is not just that these pathogens cause ARIs but they also render hosts less able to defend themselves from bacterial infection.

Tuberculosis (TB)

Tuberculosis is becoming increasingly important in complex emergencies and situations of forced migration—in part as a result of disrupted therapy (Connolly *et al.* 2004). TB can become a major problem, leading to a large numbers of deaths. Poor nutrition and over-crowding exacerbate the risk of TB, as may underlying HIV in some populations. A recent study of instability and internal displacement in Timor-Leste revealed a number of problems in maintaining continuity of treatment for those with TB. As a result many may have incomplete or inadequate treatment.

Meningococcal meningitis

Meningococcal meningitis is a potentially major problem for refugees when they are in overcrowded settlements in an endemic area, such as the 'meningitis belt' of sub-Saharan Africa that stretches from Senegal to Ethiopia. In Africa, a threshold incidence of 15 cases per 100 000 population per week is used to define the presence of an 'epidemic'. In CEs, large epidemics have also been reported outside the traditional malaria belt. Democratic Republic of the Congo had six epidemics in 6 months in 2002 and epidemics have also occurred in Uganda, Rwanda, Tanzania (Salama *et al.* 2004). Immunization has proved to be an effective control measure but is only effective in epidemics, routine immunization is not effective as the current vaccines only produce immunity for 3–5 years and may not be used in children under two. Therefore, WHO only recommends mass immunization in areas where epidemic proportions have been reached, and they estimate that this can reduce deaths by up to 70 per cent.

Hepatitis

Outbreaks of hepatitis E have occurred in African refugee camps. It is transmitted by the entero-faecal route, and therefore water supplies are often involved. Case-fatality rates vary from 1–4 per cent but there have been particularly high attack rates and case-fatality rates (up to 20 per cent) reported amongst pregnant women. The high level of previous exposure to hepatitis A and B in developing countries makes it likely that any hepatitis epidemic with high attack rates in adults is likely to be caused by hepatitis E.

HIV/AIDS and other sexually transmitted diseases (STIs)

The pattern of HIV/AIDS and STIs amongst refugee populations in developing countries will depend on many factors, including the level of infection prior to displacement (Dualeh & Shears 2002). Spiegel (2004), working at the UNHCR, has highlighted the key preventive and other responses to HIV/AIDS. Conflict situations and camp conditions have often been thought to exacerbate the spread of sexually transmitted infections, due to breakdown of social structures, behavioural change, sexual violence, and lack of access to services and testing (Zwi & Cabral 1991). However, Spiegel (2004) describes other factors inherent in refugee situations that may retard the spread of these diseases, such as decreased mobility,

and the possibility of a host country having increased services in comparison to the country from which people have fled. He argues that each situation should be examined independently and that the spread of sexually transmitted infections are most likely to be determined by the complex interactions between a number of groups: Refugees and their hosts, the original conflict-affected population, IDP populations in the country of origin and host communities in country of origin. He argues for public health responses to be broad and focus not only on camps but the entire situation, including host populations.

Other communicable diseases

Outbreaks of other less common communicable diseases have been reported in some refugee camps, as highlighted by Dualeh and Shears (2002). Typhoid fever is endemic in many tropical areas and may occur sporadically in refugee situations. Leishmaniasis and Trypanosomiasis have also been reported in epidemic proportions amongst displaced populations in Uganda and Sudan. Viral haemorrhagic fevers occur in selected areas and may place refugee communities at risk. Rift valley fever has been documented among Somali refugees in Kenya, Yellow fever occurred amongst displaced populations from Ethiopia to Sudan, and Dengue affect refugees in endemic areas of Southeast Asia.

Connolly *et al.* (2004) provide an excellent overview of the literature on communicable diseases and complex emergencies.

Malnutrition—protein energy deficiencies

Moderate to severe acute malnutrition is a common occurrence in refugee settings. Children are particularly affected, with some deteriorating in terms of nutritional status after arrival in camps, due to inadequate nutrition or diarrhoeal disease. Surveys undertaken between 1988–1995 documented a range of 11–81 per cent of children under 5 years suffering acute malnutrition in conflict affected populations (Toole & Waldman 1990). Acute malnutrition can be both the cause and effect of other illnesses, and contributes to mortality both directly and indirectly. Malnutrition and measles are particularly linked with malnutrition exacerbating measles, and measles itself contributing to high malnutrition rates in those that survive it (Toole & Waldman 1990). This 'synergistic relationship' that malnutrition has with communicable disease requires an integrated response aimed at improving nutrition combined with efforts to improve public health services.

Micronutrient deficiencies

As a result of inadequate food rations micronutrient deficiencies occur frequently in refugee populations. The most common diseases seen are iron and vitamin A deficiencies but other diseases include scurvy (vitamin C deficiency), pellagra (niacin and/or trytophan deficiency), and beriberi (thiamine deficiency). As Prinzo and Benoist (2002) discuss, the solutions are not simple and each setting may require a different approach, including providing fortified blended cereal and finding ways to exchange rations for locally produced fresh fruit and vegetables.

Food and nutritional interventions need to be responsive to cultural as well as economic issues.

Reproductive health

The reproductive health needs of refugees have gained recognition since the mid-1990s. The burden is undeniably greater for women as a result of insecurity in their social situations and gender-based violence.

Women lack basic necessities such as sanitary napkins and condoms, and pregnancy itself can be a serious health threat in settings in which services are lacking or overwhelmed (Krause *et al.* 2000). Referral services are often non-existent and birthing or abortion may be undertaken in unsafe situations. Women may have no, or limited, access or means to carry out family planning, rape and sexual coercion are typically increased, and pressures on women to rebuild the population. Female genital mutilation may occur and sexually transmitted infections, including HIV, may be relatively common (Krause *et al.* 2000). A particularly important set of risks relate to sexual and other forms of gender-based violence, common in all societies and increased where societal norms are less able to be enforced or reinforced, and in which men with guns can demand whatever they like in return for precious resources such as safety, food, and onward passage. Intense efforts have focused on improving all aspects of reproductive health for women affected by complex emergencies and forced migration—and a Minimum Initial Services Package has been produced to address these needs. A study by Hynes *et al.* (2002) showed that due to the strength of the response there have actually now been better reproductive health outcomes in refugee camps than in host population or origin countries. However, the lessons learned require expansion across settings.

Mental health and psychosocial needs

Mental health problems are recognized as an important source of morbidity globally (Prince *et al.* 2007) and are likely to be even greater amongst displaced populations. Epidemiological assessments have documented high rates of mental illness in these populations. Studies have tended to focus on trauma-related conditions, although low prevalence conditions such as psychosis have also proven significant in post-conflict and refugee setting. There is much debate about the validity of western-derived measurement and about the trauma focus, with further development of relevant culturally valid ways to measure psychiatric morbidity still required. Despite the measurement debate, there is clearly a substantial burden of mental distress in these settings, and support for vulnerable people is vital in situations of social breakdown, especially where usual systems of social support and healing are disrupted (Silove *et al.* 2000). It may be of value to identify and respond to the needs of three different groups of people who experience psychosocial and mental distress in these situations: Those who are mentally ill, who need treatment; those who have had particularly horrific experiences and need care and support in order to recover; and the vast majority who need a more stable social and political environment in which they can resume their normal day-to-day activities necessary to promote mental health.

IDPs

While IDPs in developing countries have very similar health problems to refugees, they also have particular vulnerabilities. Some of these result from falling through gaps in a system geared to protect a particular group of forced migrants (i.e. 'Convention refugees'). Particularly in developing countries, but also in more developed states, the limited data available suggest higher morbidity and mortality in IDPs compared with refugees (Salama *et al.* 2001). With limited protection granted by the international community, the responsibility for protection and assistance often lies with their own governments. Yet, it is these governments themselves that have often contributed to the displacement experienced.

Governments may not even officially recognize the existence of IDPs for fear of international scrutiny or interference. A growing number of countries have developed laws and policies to govern responses to IDP populations but not all make concerted attempts to implement these policies, and even when there is political will the states involved are often the poorest countries of the world limiting their ability to respond. There is no mandated international body although UNHCR may include them amongst their persons of concern and they are increasingly supported by agencies which follow the UN's Guiding Principles on Internal Displacement.

IDP populations rarely experience access to health services at the same standard as offered to other citizens and are likely to be markedly poorer than those available to refugees. Recent efforts to improve quality and responsiveness of interventions in humanitarian crises and complex emergencies have contributed to better health outcomes. IDPs, however, have poor access to these improved systems of protection and assistance.

Collection of data is more difficult amongst IDP populations and relatively few studies focus specifically on IDPs. However, the IDP-specific health data that are available suggest that access to health care for IDPs is often extremely limited. Salama *et al.* (2001) show how some of highest mortality rates in humanitarian emergencies have been found in IDP populations; Sudan and Somali, for example, reached 8 per 10 000/day and 17 per 10 000/day (Salama *et al.*, quoting Toole & Waldman 1993). In Ethiopia and DRC, delays in vaccinations led to measles outbreaks. In Ajiep (southern Sudan), severe acute malnutrition amongst IDPS reached 36 per cent during a famine in 1998.

Although international humanitarian law applies to all civilians affected by armed conflict and therefore IDPs should be afforded the same protection and assistance as the un-displaced host population, they may be multiple reasons why IDPs face discrimination and therefore do not receive the help they need.

Even in developed countries IDPs may have poor health outcomes. They are often subject to the discrimination and exclusion experienced by their developing country counterparts. The Internal Displacement Monitoring Centre (IDMC) describe the situation for a number of IDP groups in developed nations; 'While IDPs in the Balkans generally have satisfactory access to water, sanitation and health care, they are more likely than the local population to suffer from trauma-related problems. Roma IDPs usually live in informal settlements with very poor sanitary conditions. IDPs in Azerbaijan and the Russian Federation access health care less easily than the local population in some areas, due to administrative inconsistencies, lack of health care facilities and the demand for informal payments for medical treatment' (Internal Displacement Monitoring Centre 2008).

IDPs, whether in developing or developed countries, are clearly living with a higher burden of illness and mortality than many other forced migrant groups. Initiatives are emerging that aim to support this extremely vulnerable population, but they are yet to be supported by any legal framework.

Refugees and asylum seekers in developed countries

Refugees and asylum seekers often reach destinations in developed countries after long, precarious journeys. Prior to the journey, they will have faced many of the routine health problems that present themselves in disrupted developing country settings. The journey itself will have produced health challenges; people may have been detained at points along the way or experienced significant anxiety and distress through difficult and dangerous journeys and experiences. On arrival, the range of situations they find themselves in will further shape their health condition. Those who have applied for refugee status prior to arrival may have undergone health checks already in the country of origin, as is the practice of many developed countries; therefore, certain health conditions may have been picked up. Depending on the country they arrive in, they will then have a different range of options available to address their health problems. However, those applying for refugee status on arrival have an even more complicated journey; they may be detained for short or long periods, they may have extensive periods on temporary visas or they may find themselves living illegally without authorization from the host country. Typically asylum seekers are often isolated with difficulty in communication, in a situation of poverty, discrimination and a lack of social structure, causing many to suffer from trauma-related problems and many general health problems, exacerbated by poor provision of health information and barriers to accessing to services.

Biggs and Skull (2003) discuss the specific medical conditions that may be present amongst refugees in developed countries. These include communicable disease such as TB, HIV, STIs, hepatitis B and C, and parasitic diseases, all compounded by incomplete immunization. In addition, nutritional deficiencies (vitamin D in particular), mental health problems, and other non-communicable diseases such as diabetes and reproductive health issues are common.

Screening for health problems among newly 'arrived' refugees, or prior to arrival for those applying for refugee status overseas, is common practice. Biggs and Skull (2003) point out that there is little evidence demonstrating that screening has proved effective as many people have limited contact with services and many are lost to follow up. Refugees seeking asylum in the United States are screened before arrival to identify 'inadmissible conditions' such as HIV, TB, and leprosy. They may also be screened for diseases that are known to be prevalent and targets of public health intervention. For example, Somali refugees were mass treated for malaria and intestinal parasites. The types of health problems sought and treated in newly arrived immigrants also reflect particular areas of concern for asylum seekers, including infectious disease, gynaecological health (rape, genital surgery, STIs), and mental health (torture, trauma) (Adams *et al.* 2007).

Burnett and Peel (2001) evaluated the health needs of asylum seekers and refugees in Britain. They point out that these groups are subject to 'poverty, dependence, and lack of cohesive social support' as well as racial discrimination. They consider a range of studies examining the health status of refugees and found, for example, that 21 per cent of migrants to Spain from sub-Saharan Africa were chronic carriers of hepatitis B, and 3.4 per cent of refugees arriving in the United States in 1988 had tuberculosis. They highlight the lack of screening programmes available and how the focus has tended to be on protecting hosts rather than a responsibility to provide health care to all.

One specific refugee and asylum health condition that has been investigated somewhat more extensively than other health issues is mental health (see Chapter 9.7). Gerritsen *et al.* (2004) describe how early research focused on those who used services, or victims of trauma, followed by early population-based studies in Western settings which have tended to focus on psychiatric disorders such as post traumatic stress disorder (PTSD), anxiety, and depression. In a review of the literature, Fazel *et al.* (2005) show documented

rates of PTSD from 4–70 per cent, depression 3–88 per cent, and anxiety 2–80 per cent. Their meta-analysis suggests that 1 in 10 refugees in Western countries have PTSD, 1 in 20 has major depression, 1 in 25 has a generalized anxiety disorder. Although lower than some estimates, this is still 10 times higher than rates of PTSD in the general population in the United States. Data for asylum seekers alone is sparse but there are reasons to believe even they have even higher rates due to their vulnerability because of disruption, separation from family members, increased levels of torture and trauma, lack of language skills and the often hostile reception from host population fuelled by media perceptions. The current trend towards detention, and temporary rather than permanent protection have added extra stress, as evidenced by studies of asylum seekers in detention centres and on temporary protection visas showing very high rates of mental illness (Silove *et al.* 2000, 2007).

Problems that asylum seekers in particular face, rather than refugees, relate to issues of having a temporary and often contested legal status, and in some cases actually being considered illegal, with implications (real or perceived) for access to health services. Many countries such as the United Kingdom and Australia have fluctuating policies with regards to what asylum seekers, of differing categories, may be entitled to in terms of health care. This can act as a barrier to health for many asylum seekers. The increased use of detention for asylum seekers, whilst claims are processed, has been challenged heavily by health professionals as a result of evidence that it is detrimental to health. The other popular policy of extending only temporary protection to some asylum seekers, therefore also causing confusion with regards to health entitlements, and long-term insecurity with associated health risks, has also caused concern to health professionals (Silove *et al.* 2000). Health care for asylum seekers may be difficult to access on many levels; policies of active deterrent of asylum seekers may mean they are not entitled to care, or there may be lack of prioritizing refugees, health professionals often misunderstand what the policies are and may refuse to register asylum seekers, they also fear the burden of vulnerable groups, those that do offer treatment may lack of understanding of the refugee health situation, temporary registration with GPs may be offered rather than permanent (limiting access to immunizations and screening), language problems are also a great barrier, with many practitioners having inadequate access to interpreting services.

Harris and Telfer (2001) estimated that in 1999–2000 there were over 10 000 asylum seekers living in the community in Australia. Many had to survive for many months or years with no right to work and no medical cover through the national Medicare scheme, resulting in untreated medical conditions. A study in Sydney suggested that most presenting to a Asylum Seeker Centre (ASC) providing health services had fairly serious psychological or physical symptoms. Some related to trauma and torture, others were infectious diseases, musculoskeletal complaints, and gynaecological problems. Up to 40 per cent of the asylum seekers were denied Medicare. A few are picked up by Asylum Seeker Assistance Scheme (ASAS) and the Red Cross assists others. Hospital fees are particularly high and case studies have shown that some are denied hospital treatment until assurance of payment is provided.

Trafficked and smuggled people

People that are trafficked or smuggled are not an entirely distinct group from other types of forced migrants already described.

Trafficked people have been coerced or tricked into allowing another person to organize their passage to another country; also smuggled across borders are those who 'voluntarily' migrate for a vast range of reasons but feel unable to do so through legal channels. Although these groups may appear distinct from refugee populations they may include convention refugees and others whose circumstances are very close to those of refugees. Resorting to illegal and clandestine methods of migrating to another country, either through being coerced and misled or through having such limited choices as to choose this route, is often a result of many of the factors behind the forced migration of refugees and internally displaced people.

Gushulak and MacPherson (2000) describe some of the reasons why people may fall into a trafficking situation. Poverty, exposure to violence, restrictive barriers—e.g. screening for certain diseases or security barriers, slow processing of routine immigration application which may cause delay to family reunification—all may encourage people to take alternative routes—especially when traffickers may offer what appear to be attractive possibilities. They state that the reasons why someone is more likely to migrate through these illegal methods are also reasons that place a person at higher risk of having poor health prior to migration. The journeys faced by trafficked and smuggled people are often extremely precarious, with high levels of morbidity and mortality attached as a result. Un-seaworthy and over crowded boats on long journeys, stowed in containers, attached to carriers, attempts to cross inhospitable land with extremes of temperature, drowning from swimming attempts, violence from traffickers, illegal activities such as smuggling drugs with people. On arrival people are then subject to many of the difficulties already outlined that face asylum seekers. Some trafficked and smuggled people may seek asylum and depending on the policies of the countries may incur some health benefits, however, many will be forced into illegal employment and be either too scared or prevented from approaching health services. Disease prevention and control in this population will be extremely poor—leading to increased prevalence of disease in the trafficked community as a whole.

Busza et al. (2004) examine the need for careful understanding of trafficking situations and to unravel the local dynamics. They state that even when intermediaries are involved, and even when they are taking people into exploitative arenas such as sex work, these situations remain a complex mixture of voluntary and forced migration. Whilst economic disadvantage may fuel the choice, there is still a choice being made in some contexts and organizations seeking to stem the flow or break up these systems may compromise the health or the individuals involved more than it helps. Attempts to 'save' people may make them even more vulnerable—e.g. the raiding of brothels and other such moves can force vulnerable people to go underground making engagement with health services difficult.

The health of trafficked and smuggled people is affected by fact they cannot easily be separated out from each other or from other types of 'voluntary' migration that are not truly voluntary but have strong forces pushing people on. The policies developed by states towards any of these groups are likely to impact on the capacity of other groups to access health care. Displaced people are more vulnerable to trafficking and may in desperation turn to smugglers. This should be kept in mind by health professionals to avoid vulnerable people missing out on essential services and support.

Public health solutions and interventions

Forced migration, as described above, clearly has major impacts on public health. Specific solutions and interventions need to be sensitive to culture and context.

Key actors and organizations in refugee health

There is an extensive range of organizations involved in addressing forced migration. The United Nations has designated the United Nations High Commissioner for Refugees as the key multilateral agency for identifying and dealing with refugee issues. More recently, the mandate of UNHCR, as described earlier, has been extended to include other 'people of concern' including IDPs and asylum seekers. Other agencies with a specific mandate for dealing with forced migrants include the International Organisation on Migration, the International Centre for Migration and Health, the American Refugee Committee International, the US Committee on Refugees, and the Global IDP Project.

A wide range of multilateral agencies including the World Health Organization (WHO), UN Population Fund (UNFPA), UNICEF, International Committee of the Red Cross (ICRC), International Federation of Red Cross and Red Crescent Societies (IFRC), and UNAIDS have some concern with forced migrants. Key non-governmental organizations (NGOs) include Merlin, Medicines sans Frontieres (MSF), International Medical Corps (IMC), International Rescue Committee (IRC), OXFAM, Save the Children Fund, CARE, Caritas, CONCERN, and the Norwegian Refugee Council. Academic bodies include the Oxford University Refugee Studies Program, the Centers for Disease Control (CDC), and the Refugee Studies Program in Cairo. A number of important journals, notably the *Journal of Refugee Studies, Disasters, Conflict and Health*, and *Forced Migration Online*, provide avenues for academic debate.

Developing countries and complex emergency settings

The principles of public health and epidemiology only began to be systematically applied to complex emergency situations from the early 1970s (Salama et al. 2004). Since then, new academic and practitioner fields have developed, including emergency public health and public health nutrition. With the introduction of an indicator to measure the impact of a complex emergency through crude mortality rates (CMRs), alongside the development of simplified measurements of malnutrition, and threshold rates for epidemics, it has become increasingly possible to draw meaningful inferences from data collected.

An understanding of the dynamics of disease and related mortality in CEs has grown, and practice improved on the basis of experience and research evidence. Guidelines and technical manuals have been produced and efforts enhanced to promote organizational learning and enhanced service delivery, building on a growing evidence-base. The call for evidence with which to inform policy and practice (Banatvala & Zwi 2000) reinforced what was already happening in the field where practitioners and academics were drawing lessons from experiences and enhancing the quality of their responses.

Mortality rates are now much lower than previously seen, malnutrition declining in many settings, and measles, a major killer in the past, less catastrophic following efforts to ensure early immunization of children. Enhanced understanding of risks of communicable diseases has decreased risks, although failures to apply evidence, such as in Goma following the Rwandan genocide, still lead to tens of thousands of preventable deaths. Epidemics of some communicable diseases are better controlled and may be less serious and last for shorter periods given improved surveillance and earlier detection of outbreaks. The pattern seen is often similar to the baseline in developing countries, in terms of the major killers. However, the shift has been to seeing many of the highest mortality rates outside of camps, where the public health response has not been as well developed.

Toole and Waldman (1997) describe the need for primary, secondary, and tertiary prevention. In primary prevention, they argue that political and diplomatic mechanisms should be developed to prevent conflicts evolving to the point of mass displacement, and that epidemiology may be able to add value in studying some of the dynamics that indicate conflict developing on a large scale. Secondary prevention comprises early detection of population movements, contingency planning so that relevant actors are prepared for the scale and nature of likely public health crises, having well trained personnel with knowledge and experience in dealing with the health problems associated with refugee situations and able to rapidly assess and intervene in partnership with local organizations, along with the capacity to monitor and evaluate programmes swiftly and effectively. Tertiary prevention involves channelling resources into combating the sources of morbidity and mortality already outlined. This involves providing shelter and protection, adequate food rations, adequate clean water and sanitation facilities, programmes for preventing specific communicable diseases, preparing for epidemics, specific programmes such as maternal and child health or mental health, managing diarrhoeal disease, and setting up health information systems.

The social, cultural, and political challenges of instituting these levels of prevention, alongside the practical implications of working in such settings, are substantial. Salama *et al.* (2004) describe how the field has been growing over 30 years, with increasing attention by humanitarian actors since the 1990s to codify technical guidelines. In the early 1990s, there was a growing disappointment and recognition amongst the actors attempting to engage with these complexities, and provide emergency assistance to refugees, that the field was uncoordinated and lacking in technical direction. Research, adverse publicity, and heightened calls for accountability around standards of service delivery and to the supposed beneficiaries of humanitarian interventions, all pointed to the need for significant improvements.

Initiatives were beginning to emerge that were investigating ways to address these issues, but the field was ultimately galvanized by events in 1994 in Goma, Zaire. The unprecedented rapid influx of refugees and the resulting massive cholera epidemic, producing one of the highest mortality rates recorded, led to a serious reappraisal of humanitarian work in these settings. The Joint Evaluation of Emergency Assistance to Rwanda was an impressive, multi-agency, multi-donor-funded initiative, paving the way to a deep review of the humanitarian and relief field and the standards of care and conduct.

In terms of future public health directions, Salama *et al.* (2004) describe the need to move beyond the current refugee and IDP paradigms, as non-camp populations affected by conflict are now often greater in number and burden, and mechanisms to deliver services to such populations are less clear. There is a need for enhanced coverage in all settings of known effective public health interventions, and for the more upstream causes of CEs to be addressed. The technical needs identified include the development of more context-specific methods for assessing mortality rates as an indicator based on surrounding baseline CMRs, and considering which other indicators may point to a deteriorating situation such as fluctuations in disease incidence, levels of displacement, and decreasing food security. They suggest that implementation of control measures should be early, not when mortality and malnutrition are already high, and that whilst communicable disease control should continue to be prioritized along with nutrition and food security, that enhanced efforts at addressing mental health, reproductive health, and neonatal health should also be incorporated. Important policy issues include better means of determining direction and co-ordination of public health interventions, early identification of a lead agency, and greater effort to support fledgling governments to take the lead with the support of a coherent international system. They suggest that the skills of relief workers should be strengthened and broadened to include knowledge of assessment and prevention of disease, monitoring and evaluation, and international systems, policies, and regulatory bodies.

Ensuring equity in the response and equity in access to services and resources made available remains a considerable and under-emphasized challenge.

Developed countries

In developed countries, the complex political arena and the increasingly restrictive views of host populations towards asylum seekers and refugees complicates the task of addressing the public health of forced migrants. Whilst an array of motivated and effective actors plays a number of different roles in this field, there are few central bodies charged with overseeing the public health of forced migrants as a whole. The policies of the host nations themselves are likely to shape the public health landscape and in situations where these policies seem to be detrimental to the health of this population, public health professionals may find themselves having to take increasingly political roles to fulfil their public health duties.

Advocacy groups and health professional organizations have set up refugee and asylum seeker health networks and centres through which to provide services and support and advocate for more inclusive social and health policies.

The Health of London Project established a health centre in 1999 to provide access to good-quality primary care for forced migrants. The service aims to provide a thorough initial health assessment, along with effective responses to issues such as mental health problems and communicable diseases. In Europe, Medecins du Monde, an NGO, has stepped in to provide care for groups with restricted access to healthcare, particularly failed asylum seekers.

The best way in which to organize health care for resettled refugees, and for asylum seekers, remains contentious. A key issue point of debate is whether they should be integrated within mainstream services, or offered separately through distinct services for these marginalized groups (Finney Lamb & Cunningham 2003). Such centres are often voluntarily run and unable to cover the full extent of need. Hull and Boomla (2006) discuss the implications of such NGO provision, including some of the unanticipated negative aspects.

Another potential theoretical divide that can emerge with health approaches to asylum seekers and refugees is that between public health and human rights frameworks. Governments are more responsive to public health arguments whereby health problems of forced migrant populations may be addressed for the benefit of the wider population, often highlighting the risk brought with incoming refugees and forced migrants of communicable diseases. However, these approaches focus more on protecting the host than the forced migrants' right to receive health care (Burnett & Peel 2001) and may reinforce discrimination and marginalization of the migrants who are seen as posing a risk to the general community and demanding excessive use of public services (Grove & Zwi 2006). Tarantola *et al.* (2008) argue for much closer links between public health, human rights and development—all equally relevant to forced migration.

Hull and Boola (2006) describe recent UK government proposals to deny GPs the discretion of registering overseas visitors including failed asylum seekers, and to provide care to them. They highlight the possibility that such a policy will inadvertently increase costs through more emergency admissions, and they stress that such a policy is a breach of human rights, ethically unsupportable, and may place clinicians in conflict with their professional duties.

Ashcroft (2005) describes the language of the UK and Australian governments as 'Orwellian' in an overview of their approaches to asylum seekers and health. In discussing the UK government's move to make failed asylum seekers pay for all non-emergency care, despite not having the right to work, he states that the treatment of asylum seekers is an ethical issue and that denial of medical treatment should not be used as a lever to exclude people or get them to leave the country. In some cases, the presence of HIV seropositivity has been used to exclude refugees from the opportunity to resettle in a third country; this is of particular concern given the heightened risk of violence and infection that may characterize the lives of many refugees. Using this against such vulnerable community members is a double victimization.

As Silove et al. (2000) stated 'the medical profession has a legitimate role in commenting on the general and mental health risks of imposing restrictive and discriminatory measures on asylum seekers, especially when some of these administrative procedures threaten one of the fundamental principles underpinning the practice of medicine: primum non nocere' (do no harm).

Further study to document the patterns of disease, the links to the asylum experience and impact of policies, not only on forced migrant health but also the implications for host populations are required. Given the more restrictive policy environment, health professionals require a strong evidence base from which to lobby for improved access to services as a first step in improving the health of refugees and asylum seekers in developed countries.

Emerging issues for public health professionals

Many of the issues raised above have a technical focus, even if their links with broader sociopolitical issues have been acknowledged. In this concluding section of the chapter, we highlight some of the many issues which challenge professionals and societies, not only on a technical level, but in terms of the values underpinning how we, individually and collectively, whether as citizens or professionals, see and respond to others, especially those who have been forced to flee.

This section seeks to highlight, briefly, a number of key themes: Globalization and poverty, quality and accountability, ethics and researching with forced migrants, voice, visibility, and agency. They are central to understanding the context within which forced migration arises and health needs should be understood and addressed.

Globalization and poverty

There is increasing evidence of widening gaps in income and basic needs between the well-off and the impoverished in many settings. Labonte and Schrecker (2005) identify the key links between current patterns of globalization and the influence these have on the social determinants of health. The challenges are evident in the failure to address the Millennium Development Goal (MDG) targets, while extreme wealth continues to be generated and monopolized by small fractions of the world's population. Resource constraints are likely to increase; countries engaging actively with global economic and political opportunities may do well but not all their citizens will necessarily benefit.

Evidence of gaps are widespread; and it is apparent that the MDGs, a major driving force at present in international development, do not adequately address issues of equity (Attaran 2005). Such concerns are likely to be amplified in relation to especially vulnerable and socially excluded communities such as forced migrants, data on whom may be unavailable and systems of response to which will be fragmented, uncoordinated, and inadequately monitored. Colson (2007) argues cogently that much greater emphasis should be placed on understanding the 'factors that provide the impetus to leave' and not focusing only on the aftermath of such forced migrations.

Quality and accountability

A key challenge in engaging with situations of violence, social exclusion, and disempowerment is in ensuring that work undertaken to assist those affected does no harm, or at least strives to limit the potential harm and maximize the potential value. The international community, through the United Nations, other multilateral and bilateral agencies, international NGOs, all ostensibly seek to assist those forced to flee or migrate.

One way in which evidence improvements are underway is in relation to enhancing and seeking to assure the quality of humanitarian and relief work. Major Quality and Accountability initiatives such as SPHERE, the Humanitarian Code of Conduct, the Humanitarian Accountability Partnership, and many others contribute to enhanced practice. There remains a need to facilitate self-reflection and open review, transparency of difficulties limitations and failures, and promotion and funding for the search to do better.

The vast majority of incentives currently in place, however, encourage the hiding, rather than the declaration, of weaknesses, so as to elicit the next tranche of funding. This is counter-productive when seeking to reflect and improve services and their responsiveness to need. New thinking is required: How do we develop systems of trust and collegiality, mutual support between affected communities, services providers, and agencies, to ensure that all incentives operate to maximize the gain for those at greatest risk?

New initiatives in the humanitarian and relief areas of activity seek to enhance practice and open out debate and public scrutiny. In so doing, weaknesses are identified, guidelines and lessons for better practice formulated, and processes which seek to engage and creatively respond to problems, developed. Taking forward such action requires promoting an ability to report and record limitations and inadequacies, and to carefully and systematically document strengths and limitations, weaknesses and potentials, to address real problems. Services are never ideal and always have constraints and limits; it is crucial to establish ways of examining them such that opportunities to change, to experiment, to creatively engage with solving problems are established.

New and enhanced knowledge management systems would be most valuable if they assisted in finding innovative means of conceptualizing problems, sharing information and insights of what works in different contexts, and develop systems to ensure accountability to the intended beneficiaries, the forced migrants themselves.

Ethics and researching with forced migrants

Ethical issues require considerable attention especially given the power imbalances present and in relation to research. Forced migrants may be especially vulnerable and risk being abused, either through their stories and survival strategies being exposed and used by their opponents to undermine them; the very practice of talking with an outsider or sharing information may heighten risk, vulnerability, and the attention of those seeking further to undermine and disempower. Real risks may result from security lapses, confidentiality lapses, exposure of coping strategies and adaptations; as well as stigma and reinforcement of difference and of 'otherness'.

A major challenge in research with refugees and other forced migrants is to assist them in documenting their experiences of forced migration (Mackenzie et al. 2007). In so doing, the locus of power in the research relationship has the potential to shift from the researcher him or herself, to the communities being researched. The project may shift from research *on* refugees to research *with* refugees and research *by* refugees for action and change.

While this may be conceptually and morally attractive, the practicalities of achieving this are impeded at multiple levels, not least of which is establishing a trusting relationship between the researcher and the communities with whom they research. Engaging with forced migrants is itself a major challenge: Such communities are often highly dependent on others, and may be reliant on outside agencies with expertise and resources and/or on local power-brokers in control of the basic necessities of life and survival—food, water, shelter, and security.

Zwi et al. (2006) have highlighted the importance of reconceptualizing such research to consider the potential to ensure benefit and reciprocity for the subjects of research and to shift the locus of decision-making in their direction. They offer a model to describe this process, while Mackenzie et al. (2007) present a case study of applying many of these considerations to work with forced migrants on the Thai–Burmese border. Of note is the transfer of power to community organizations, with women's groups from the Thai–Burmese border having control over the stories and narratives collected from them and academics being required to obtain permission from them to publish and distribute and write up such material.

Innovative approaches to research are emerging and warrant support. Youth-focused research highlights the importance of young people in exploring and documenting their own lives and experiences. Young people play a central role in refining and redefining the issues, identifying the challenges and the potential approaches to solving them through new models of participatory action research. Such collaboration needs to build skills, resilience, and opportunities to shape the future.

Voice, visibility, and agency

There is increasing recognition of the importance of hearing from those most affected by any public health condition and ensuring that their voices are heard; empowering them to help shape the proposed solutions. Black (2003) emphasizes the importance of advocacy as a central component of work with marginalized and disempowered groups and reinforces the centrality of ensuring that the voices of those affected, and of the range of stakeholders engaged, is heard.

The voices of forced migrants may be silenced while those of powerful agencies and governments are privileged in shaping our understanding both of the problems and of the solutions which surround forced migration (Harrell-Bond & Voutira 2007). Power imbalances, vulnerability, and cultural and linguistic differences are among the many barriers to creating an environment in which refugees and IDPs are able to take an active part in shaping solutions. As with the youth, truly participatory models of action and research require sensitivity to the challenges of the context and understanding of the conditions that usually deny refugees a voice.

It is crucial that we hear the voices of those most affected by forced migration if we are to recognize the range of experiences, and the positive and negative change and transformation which results. As Eastmond (2007) states eloquently: 'while transformation and change are part of the refugee experience, not all change is perceived as loss or defined as problematic or unwelcome by all individuals involved. Nor are refugees necessarily helpless victims, but rather likely to be people with agency and voice'. Learning and recognizing how agency, transformation, resilience, adaptation and change are shaped, notably, but not only, in relation to gender and power, would not be possible without hearing from and learning with, those most affected.

Concluding remarks

Forced migrant populations frequently suffer vast health challenges. Their experiences need to be understood within the context of accelerating globalization, with its positive and negative features transforming the lives of millions of people.

The role of public health professionals in working alongside forced migrants to bring about improvements in their health is demanding and complex. A comprehensive understanding of the dynamics of forced migration and sensitivity to the constraints placed on individuals and populations is vital to gain trust and provide opportunities for transforming health outcomes. Particularly, given the increasingly restrictive environments that forced migrants find themselves in, public health professionals can have a crucial role in advocating for forced migrant health, enabling forced migrants to speak and be heard, and to bring about improvements in their own health.

Improving knowledge and understanding is central to affirming the rights and the agency of those affected. Public health can play an important role, and indeed has done so, in improving technical quality of service delivery. Key gaps remain, however, in understanding, appreciating, and responding to the varied ways in which those forced to move seek to shape, transform, and better their own lives and experiences.

Further reading

The following manuals give technical advice in managing public health aspects of forced migration.

Médecins Sans Frontières (MSF)(1997) *Refugee health: an approach to emergency situations*. London: Macmillan. Available at http://www.refbooks.msf.org/msf_docs/en/Refugee_Health/RH1.pdf accessed 28th May 2008.

World Health Organization (2006). Communicable disease control in emergencies. A field manual. Available at http://www.who.int/infectious-disease-news/IDdocs/whocds200527/whocds200527chapters/ accessed 28th May 2008.

Relevant websites

Forced Migration Online—http://www.forcedmigration.org/

The Humanitarian Accountability Partnership—http://www.hapinternational.org/

SPHERE—www.sphereproject.org

ALNAP—'learning, accountability, performance in humanitarian action' www.alnap.org

United Nations High Commission for Refugees—www.unhcr.org

References

Adams, K., Gardiner, L., and Assefi, N. (2007). Healthcare challenges from the developing world: post-immigration refugee medicine. *British Medical Journal*, **328**, 1548–52.

Allotey, P.A. and Reidpath, D.D. (2003). Refugee intake: reflections on inequality. *Australian and New Zealand Journal of Public Health*, **27**, 12–6.

Apodaca, C. (1998). Human rights abuses: precursor to refugee flight? *Journal of Refugee Studies*, **11**, 80–93.

Ashcroft, R. (2005). Standing up for the medical rights of asylum seekers. *Journal of Medical Ethics*, **31**, 125–6.

Attaran, A. (2005). An immeasurable crisis? a criticism of the millennium development goals and why they cannot be measured. *PLoS Medicine*, **2**(10): e318 doi:10.1371/journal.pmed.0020318.

Bakewell, O. (2008). Can we ever rely on refugee statistics? Radical statistics. Available at http://www.radstats.org.uk/no072/article1.htm accessed 25th May 2008.

Banatvala, N. and Zwi, A.B. (2000). Public health and humanitarian interventions: developing the evidence base. *British Medical Journal*, **321**, 101–5.

Barnett, L. (2002) Global governance and the evolution of the international refugee regime. *International Journal Refugee Law*, **14**, 238–262.

Baum, F. (2001). Health equity justice and globalisation: some lessons from the People's Health Assembly. *Journal of Epidemiology and Community Health*, **55**, 613–6.

Biermann, F. and Boas, I. (2008). Preparing for a warmer world – towards a global governance system to protect climate refugees. Available at http://www.glogov.org/images/doc/WP33.pdf accessed 27th May 2008.

Biggs, B. and Skull, S. (2003). Refugee health: clinical issues. In *The health of refugees: public health perspectives from crisis to settlement* (ed. P. Allotey), pp. 54–67. Oxford University Press, Melbourne.

Black, R. (2003). Ethical codes in humanitarian emergencies: from practice to research? *Disasters*, **27**(2), 95–108.

Burnett, A. and Peel, M. (2001). Asylum seekers and refugees in Britain: health needs of asylum seekers and refugees. *British Medical Journal*, **322**, 544–7.

Busza, J., Castle, S. and Diarra, A. (2004). Trafficking and health. *British Medical Journal*, **328**, 1369–71.

Cartagena Declaration on Refugees. (1984). Colloquium on the International Protection of Refugees in Central America, Mexico and Panama. Available at http://www.unhcr.org/cgi-bin/texis/vtx/research/opendoc.htm?tbl=RSDLEGAL&id=3ae6b36ec accessed 27th May 2008.

Castles, S. (2003). Toward a sociology of Forced Migration and Social Transformation. *Sociology*, **37**, 13–34.

Castles, S. (2004). Confronting the realities of forced migration. Available at http://www.migrationinformation.org/Feature/print.cfm?ID=222 accessed 27th May 2008.

Cernea, M. (2007). Development-induced and conflict-induced IDPs: bridging the research divide. *Forced Migration Review*, March, 25–7.

Chan, E.Y. and Sondorp, E. (2007). Medical interventions following natural disasters: missing out on chronic medical needs. *Asia Pacific Journal of Public Health*, **19**(Special Issue), 45–51.

Colson, E. (2007). Linkage methodology: no man is an island. *Journal of Refugee Studies*, **20**, 321–33.

Connolly, M.A., Gayer, M., Ryan, M.J. *et al.* (2004). Communicable diseases in complex emergencies: impact and challenges. *The Lancet*, **364**, 1974–83.

Crisp, J. (1999). *'Who has counted the refugees?' UNHCR and the politics of numbers*. UNHCR, Geneva.

Courtland Robinson, W. (2003). Risks and rights: the causes, consequences, and challenges of development-induced displacement: The Brookings Institution-SAIS Project on Internal Displacement. Available at http://www.brookings.edu/~/media/Files/rc/reports/2003/05humanrights_robinson/didreport.pdf accessed 27th May 2008.

Deng, F. (1998). The guiding principles on internal displacement. United Nations, New York, February 11.

Dualeh, M. and Shears, P. (2002). *Refugees and other displaced populations*. In *Oxford Textbook of Public Health* (eds. R. Detels, J. McEwen, R. Beaglehole, H. Tanaka). Oxford University Press, Oxford.

Eastmond, M. (2007). Stories as lived experience: narratives in forced migration research. *Journal of Refugee Studies*, **20**, 248–64.

El-Hinnawi, E. (1985). *Environmental refugees*. United Nations Environment Programme, Nairobi.

Essed, P., Frerks, G. and Schrijvers, J. (eds.) (2004). *Refugees and the transformation of societies. Agency, policies, ethics and politics*. Berghahn Books, New York and Oxford.

Fazel, M., Wheeler, J. and Danesh, J. (2005). Prevalence of serious mental disorder in 7000 refugees resettled in western countries: a systematic review. *Lancet*, **365**, 1309–14.

Feachem, R. (2001). Globalisation is good for your health, mostly. *British Medical Journal*, **323**, 504–6.

Finney Lamb, C., Cunningham, M. (2003). Dichotomy or decision-making: specialization and mainstreaming in health service design for refugees. In: Allotey P, ed. *The Health of Refugees. Public Health Perspectives from Crisis to Settlement*. Melbourne: Oxford University Press. pp. 156–168.

Forced_Migration Online. (2008). *What is Forced Migration?* Available at http://www.forcedmigration.org/whatisfm.htm accessed 25th May 2008.

Gerritsen, A., Bramsen, I., Deville, W., van Willigen, L., Hovens, J. and van derPloeg, H. (2004). Health and health care utilisation among asylum seekers and refugees in the Netherlands: design of a study. *BMC Public Health*, **4**, 1–10.

Grove, N. and Zwi, A.B. (2006). Our health and theirs: forced migration,othering and public health. *Social Science and Medicine*, **62**, 1931–42.

Gushulak, B. and MacPherson, D. (2000). Health issues associated with the smuggling and trafficking of migrants. *Journal of Immigrant Health*, **2**, 67–78.

Harrell-Bond, B. (2000). 'Are refugee camps good for children?' UNHCR, Geneva. Available at http://www.jha.ac/articles/u029.htm accessed 28th May 2008.

Harrell-Bond, B. and Voutira, E. (2007). In search of 'invisible actors': barriers to access in refugee research. *Journal of Refugee Studies*, **20**, 282–98.

Harrell-Bond, B., Voutira, E., and Leopold, M. (1992). Counting the refugees: gifts, givers, patrons and clients. *Journal of Refugee Studies*, **5**, 205–25.

Harris, M.F. and Telfer, B.L. (2001). The health needs of asylum seekers living in the community. *Medical Journal of Australia*, **175**, 589–92.

Hull, S. and Boomla, K. (2006). Primary care for refugees and asylum seekers. *British Medical Journal*, **332**, 62–3.

Hynes, M., Sheik, M., Wilson, H.G. and Spiegel, P. (2002). Reproductive health indicators and outcomes among refugee and internally displaced persons in postemergency phase camps. *Journal of the American Medical Association*, **288**, 595–603.

Internal Displacement Monitoring Centre (2008). Health and IDPs. Accessed 27th May 2008. http://www.internal-displacement.org/8025708F004D404D/(httpPages)/61944755DF644EE1C12570C9005BAC3A?OpenDocument

Krause, S.K., Jones, R.K., and Purdin, S.J. (2000). Programmatic Responses to Refugees' Reproductive Health Needs. *International Family Planning Perspectives*, **26**, 181–7.

Labonte, R. and Schrecker, T. (2005). Globalization and social determinants of health: promoting health equity in global governance (part 3 of 3). *Globalization and Health*, **3**, 7.

Lee, K. (2004). Globalisation: what is it and how does it affect health? *Medical Journal of Australia*, **180**, 156–8.

MacDonald, T.H. (2007). *The Global Human Right to Health – dream or possibility?* Radcliffe Publishing, Oxford, New York.

Mackenzie, C., McDowell, C., and Pittaway, E. (2007). Beyond 'Do No Harm': The Challenge of Constructing Ethical Relationships in Refugee Research. *Journal of Refugee Studies*, **20**, 299–319.

Martin, S. (2002). Averting forced migration in countries in transition. *International Migration*, **40**, 25–40.

McAdam, J. (2006). The Refugee Convention as a rights blueprint for persons in need of international protection. UNHCR, Geneva.

Moore, W. and Shellman, S. (2004). Fear of persecution: forced migration 1952–1995. *Journal of Conflict Resolution*, **48**, 723–45.

Moore, P.S., Marfin, A.A., Quenemoen, L.E., Gessner, B.D., Ayub, Y.S. and Sullivan, K.M. (1993). Mortality rates in displaced and resident populations of Central Somalia during the famine of 1992. *Lancet*, **341**, 935–8.

Myers, N. (1993). Environmental refugees in a globally warmed world. *BioScience*, **43**, 752–61.

Myers, N. and Kent, J. (1995). *Environmental Exodus: An Emergent Crisis in the Global Arena*. Climate Institute, Washington DC.

Organisation of African Unity (1969). *OAU Convention Governing the Specific Aspects of the Refugee Problems in Africa*. Addis-Ababa. Available at http://www.unhcr.org/basics/BASICS/45dc1a682.pdf accessed 28th May 2008.

Office for the Coordination of Humanitarian Affairs (1998). *Guiding Principles on Internal Displacement*. Available at http://www.reliefweb.int/ocha_ol/pub/idp_gp/idp.html accessed 28th May 2008.

Prince, M., Patel, V., Saxena, S. *et al.* (2007). No health without mental health. *Lancet*, **370**, 859–77.

Prinzo, W.Z. and Benoist, B. (2002). Meeting the challenges of micronutrient deficiencies in emergency affected populations. *Proceedings of the Nutrition Society*, **61**, 251–7.

Salama, P., Spiegel, P., and Brennan, R. (2001). No less vulnerable: the internally displaced in humanitarian emergencies. *Lancet*, **357**, 1430–2.

Salama, P., Spiegel, P., Talley, L., and Waldman, R. (2004). Lessons learned from complex emergencies over past decade. *Lancet*, **364**, 1801–13.

Siddique, A.K., Salam, A., Islam, M.S., Akram, K., Majumdar, R.N., Zaman, K., Fronczak, N., and Laston, S. (1995). Why treatment centres failed to prevent cholera deaths among Rwandan refugees in Goma, Zaire. *The Lancet*, **345**, 359(3).

Silove, D., Steel, Z., and Watters, C. (2000). Policies of deterrence and the mental health of asylum seekers. *Journal of the American Medical Association*, **284**, 604–11.

Silove D., Ekblad S., Mollica R. (2000). The rights of the severely mentally ill in post-conflict societies. *Lancet*. Vol 355, issue 9214, 1548–1549.

Silove, D., Austin, P., and Steel, Z. (2007). No refuge from terror: The impact of detention on the mental health of trauma-affected refugees seeking asylum in Australia. *Transcultural Psychiatry*, **44**, 359–93.

Spiegel, P. (2004). HIV/AIDS among conflict-affected and displaced populations: dispelling myths and taking action. *Disasters*, **28**, 322–39.

Stanley, J. (2008). *Development induced displacement and resettlement – global overview*. Forced Migration Online. Available at http://www.forcedmigration.org/guides/fmo022/ accessed 28th May 2008.

Tarantola D., Byrnes A., Johnson M., Kemp L., Zwi A.B., Gruskin S. (2008). Human rights, health and development. *Australian Journal of Human Rights*, **13**, 2.

Toole, M. and Waldman, R. (1990). Preventing excess mortality in refugee and displaced populations in developing countries. *Journal of the American Medical Association*, **263**, 3296–302.

Toole, M. and Waldman, R. (1997). The public health aspects of complex emergencies and refugee situations. *Annual Review of Public Health*, **18**, 283–312.

Turner, S. (2004). New opportunities: angry young men in a Tanzanian refugee camp. In *Refugees and the transformation of societies. Agency, policies, ethics and politics* (eds. P. Essed, G. Frerks and J. Schrijvers) pp. 94–105. Berghahn Books, New York and Oxford.

United Nations General Assembly (2003). *Protocol to Prevent, Suppress and Punish Trafficking in Persons, Especially Women and Children, Supplementing the United Nations Convention Against Transnational Organized Crime*, G.A. Res. 25, Annex II, U.N. GAOR, 55th Sess. UN; 2003. p. Supp. No. 49, at 60.

United Nations (2000). *Protocol against the smuggling of migrants by land, sea and air*. United Nations, New York.

United Nations (1997). *Glossary of environment statistics, studies in methods*. United Nations, New York. Available at http://stats.oecd.org/glossary/detail.asp?ID=839 accessed 28th May 2008.

United Nations High Commissioner for Refugees (2005). *Statistical Yearbook 2005 – trends in displacement, protection and solutions*. UNHCR, Geneva. Available at http://www.unhcr.org/cgi-bin/texis/vtx/home/opendoc.pdf?id=464049e80&tbl=STATISTICS accessed 28th May 2008.

United Nations High Commissioner for Refugees (2006). *Statistical Yearbook 2006 – trends in displacement, protection and solutions*. UNHCR, Geneva. Available at http://www.unhcr.org/cgi-bin/texis/vtx/home/opendoc.pdf?id=478ce2e62&tbl=STATISTICS accessed 28th May 2008.

United Nations High Commissioner for Refugees (2007). *Definitions and obligations*. Available at http://www.unhcr.org.au/basicdef.shtml accessed 28th May 2008.

US Commitee for Refugees and Immigrants (2006). *World Refugee Survey 2006*. Available at http://www.refugees.org/article.aspx?id=1565&subm=19&ssm=29&area=Investigate& accessed 28th May 2008.

US Commitee for Refugees and Immigrants (2007). *World Refugee Survey 2007*. Available at http://www.refugees.org/article.aspx?id=1941&subm=19&ssm=29&area=Investigate accessed 28th May 2008.

Zwi, A.B. and Cabral, A.J. (1991). Identifying "high risk situations" for preventing AIDS. *British Medical Journal*, **303**, 1527–9.

Zwi, A.B. and Alvarez-Castillo, F. (2003). *Forced migration globalization and public health: getting the big picture into focus*. In *The health of refugees* (ed. P. Allotey), pp. 14–34. Oxford University Press, Melbourne.

ZWI, A.B. *et al.* (2006) Placing ethics in the centre: Negotiating new spaces for ethical research in conflict situations. *Global Public Health*, **1**(3): 264–277.

SECTION 12

Public health functions

12.1

Need: What is it and how do we measure it?

Di McIntyre, Gavin Mooney, and Stephen Jan

Abstract

The concept of need is interpreted in different ways. The principle adopted in this chapter is that need is defined by the notion of 'capacity of benefit'. This means that need derives its meaning from the various pathways in which it can contribute to the achievement of a particular objective, i.e. it is 'instrumental'. Here we focus on need in relation to healthcare; a need for healthcare can be seen to be instrumental to the achievement of the objective of health. As a consequence, the type of healthcare that is needed in any given circumstance is a function of factors such as the level of prevailing resources, the availability and effectiveness of healthcare, and the perspective and values of whomsoever is making the assessment.

Need is a critical concept in the pursuit of efficient healthcare, in terms of maximizing health benefits, given the limited resources. There are a number of tools such as programme budgeting and marginal analysis and quality-adjusted life years (QALY) league tables which enable decision makers to systematically allocate resources efficiently according to need. Recent policy initiatives such as the Oregon Health Plan, the World Bank's essential package concept, and the Commission for Macroeconomics and Health have also incorporated cost-effectiveness as a basis for determining need to ensure best use of limited resources.

Need is also useful in planning for the equitable allocation of resources as it provides a measure by which policy makers may pursue objectives such as 'equal access for equal need' or 'equal use for equal need'. The application of these principles in practice can be seen most readily in health needs assessment exercises such as those carried out in the United Kingdom in the 1990s and the various needs-based resource allocation formulae that have been employed over recent decades in the United Kingdom, Australia, and recently in a number of low- and middle-income countries. One of the challenges in implementing these policies is in ensuring that any measure of need takes into account social values, absorptive capacity constraints, and is sensitive to variations in mortality and morbidity. These are issues that provide a focus for future research on this topic.

There is a beguiling simplicity about the proposition that healthcare services should be designed to meet the needs of the community. Indeed, the healthcare policies of a great many countries have as a key goal meeting the needs of the population. Faced with the obvious appetite for healthcare exhibited by virtually all communities exposed to it, it is traditional to distinguish between wants and needs: Wants, by implication, being less rational, possibly even related to greed. Needs, by contrast, are seen as objective states, things that can be measured and agreed upon by rational people often on behalf of those who have them, as deserving attention.

The purpose of this chapter is first to explore the concept of need and its relevance within a public health framework. The purposes for which need might be measured—for action in the clinical and population settings and for planning—are then reviewed. Some currently available measures of need are then examined and some conclusions are drawn. Given the elusive nature of the concept of need, a glossary of relevant terms used in this chapter is provided in Box 12.1.1 as a reference point for readers.

The concept of need within the context of public health

Need as an instrumental concept

The starting point for exploring the concept of need is to address the question of the need for what? If we are focusing on the health sector, there is general agreement that we are concerned with the need for healthcare—it is this need for healthcare that is the focus of this chapter. However, the need is not for healthcare as an end in itself; instead, healthcare is instrumental to achieving improved health, which is the ultimate objective. It is evident that there are instruments other than healthcare that are able to promote health, such as good housing and sanitation services, but we restrict ourselves mainly to health sector services in this chapter, even though many interventions outside the health sector are of relevance from the public health perspective (Culyer 1991; Culyer & Wagstaff 1993).

There is often a tendency to refer to healthcare needs in very general terms, usually with an implication that all needs ought to be addressed. However it is important to recognize that any given form of healthcare can be one of a number of instruments to achieving health benefit. For example, it would be helpful to indicate that a particular person with arthritis needs a hip-replacement *in order that* they are able to walk more easily and suffer less pain. This allows for critical assessment of whether a hip-replacement is

Box 12.1.1 Glossary of terms	
Capacity to benefit	The notion that health care need is measured by the extent to which individuals or populations are able to benefit from care. One implication of using this criterion is that need is directly associated with the effectiveness and cost-effectiveness of health care.
Need as an instrumental concept	Health care is seen to have no intrinsic value; it is valued only insofar as it contributes to health or health related benefits such as information and autonomy. Therefore the need for health care is seen as instrumental in achieving these outcomes.
Need as a subjective concept	Need is seen to be a function of individual and community perception and therefore may vary across individuals and communities.
Equal health as a health care objective	The view that the objective of health care systems is the achievement of equal health across individuals
Equal access for equal need	The view that the objective of health care systems is the achievement of equal access to health services for individuals with the same level of need. It says nothing about how individuals with different needs should be treated relative to one another.
Equal use for equal need	The view that the objective of health care systems is the achievement of equal use of health services for individuals with the same level of need. The difference between this objective and the previous one is that 'equal access' implies a tolerance for inequalities in the use of services based on differing preferences, i.e. some individuals may choose not to use services whilst others in the same position do use them.
Absorptive capacity	This relates to the ability of a community or organization to utilize fully the resources which it has been allocated. It is a problem with resource allocation formulae, particularly in low income settings, where the policy of shifting resources to poorer regions is undermined by the inability of those regions to transform such investment into additional services.

really necessary, based on whether this intervention is appropriate for achieving the specified health improvement goal and whether or not there are other interventions that may be more effective and more cost-effective in achieving that goal. These sorts of critical assessments assist in deciding which needs should be addressed and to what extent, given that there is a scarcity of resources.

The instrumental nature of healthcare highlights firstly that effectiveness is closely associated with need; a need can only exist for effective healthcare. Thus, it is necessary to ask whether specific health services will actually prolong life, improve quality of life (e.g. improved mobility, relief of pain) or at least prevent further deterioration in quality of life. Secondly, it also underlines that need has a forward-looking perspective. Need is not equivalent to a person's or a group's existing health or illness status but focuses on how healthcare could lead to improved health.

Need as capacity to benefit

A useful concept that encapsulates this perspective is that of capacity to benefit from healthcare, in that there should be the potential for health to be improved relative to what it would be in the absence of the healthcare intervention. Culyer and Wagstaff (1993) define need as 'the minimum resources required to exhaust an individual's capacity to benefit from healthcare'. Defining need in this way not only points to the instrumental nature of healthcare but also places a limit on the amount of healthcare needed.

Whose perspective?

While the above ideas seem to provide quite clear guidance on the issue of need, they are quite difficult to implement in practice.

They also fail to recognize that need can be viewed from different perspectives. A community experiencing high levels of infant mortality due to tetanus might be seen by a preventivist as one in need of the development of an effective maternal education programme focusing on hygiene at the time of cutting the umbilical cord, and maternal immunization. Conversely, an intensive care physician may see the same phenomena and compute them in terms of needs for neonatal intensive care beds to effect rescue of the young victims. The individuals involved—the parents of the children affected—may have a third interpretation of what they need, which may have little to do with healthcare.

These constructs of need—which is what they are, melding essentially the same 'facts' into different shapes—each have their legitimacy. Unless health is to be seen as something occupying a quiet biological space, independent of culture and society, then these different constructs should be accepted. Each derives from the fact that any relevant concept of need is subjective. Definitions of need vary depending on whose perception, interpretation and values are in play. As it is most unlikely that some universally valid construct of need can be adopted that will be apposite in all circumstances, the question arises of whose values ought to come into play and in which circumstances. Thus, another key issue is who should determine that a need exists and what the value is of meeting it in part or full.

Need is most frequently seen as being formed or perceived in the eyes of another, a third party. Thus, Liss (1990) wrote 'A need for healthcare exists when an assessor believes that healthcare ought to be provided'. With this conceptualization of need it is not the patient who is doing the assessing but someone else, an agent (often a medical doctor), on behalf of the patient. (While it would be possible to deduce from the quote from Liss (1990) that need might be self-assessed, it is clear elsewhere in his and in much other literature in this area that is not what he intends).

Such third-party assessment requires, for the assessment to have legitimacy, that wider concerns are at play. If a doctor, for example, assesses a patient's needs, this is only of interest if that assessment leads to rights for the patient or clarification or quantification of rights which then provide the patient with access to services which might be of assistance in addressing the problems identified by the doctor. It is not the assessment by the doctor that provides the needs with their rights base, with their element of 'social legitimacy'. That can only come from the concept of a social contract. When it is claimed that individuals have a right to certain basic necessities, that is the language of a social contract. As Loewy (1990) stated 'Social contract consists of those things which "go without saying" and which we consider to be the legitimate expectations we have of others and of our community'.

Tension arises with respect to what sort of community it is in which we are trying to assess needs. As Loewy (1990) reminded us, according to the Aristotelian dictum 'justice consists of giving everyone their due'. He continues, however:

What is and what is not someone's due . . . is another matter. Minimalist communities which . . . accept freedom as an absolute condition of the moral life will see what is due quite differently than will more generously based communities. What is due in minimalist communities is doing to each other no harm; what is due in broader-based communities is a far more difficult matter and one which will ultimately be determined by an ongoing dialectic between communal values and individual interests.

Needs and wants

It immediately follows that the separation of wants and needs, which for some seems so simple, in practice is far from simple. There is an astonishing lack of research into individuals or communities as to what they actually want from their healthcare services and so the pejorative view of wants as little more than expressions of greed by the ignorant is particularly unfortunate. Paternalistic professionalism has blocked progress in understanding how the community views health and healthcare and where they place them in the context of other things that they also want for their lives.

Distinctions between needs and wants are made still more difficult by the fact that different disciplines also use different definitions. A potentially useful set of constructs is provided by the discipline of economics. Wants are the preferences of individuals on behalf of themselves but do not have to be expressed through taking action to have the wants 'fulfilled'. 'Demands' are based on wants, that is on an individual's own preferences, by some action on the part of the individual in seeking to have the wants addressed. Thus, a want for better health can be expressed as a demand for healthcare if the individual visits a general practitioner. A need for healthcare would arise if the general practitioner were to agree that some relevant and effective action could be taken by the healthcare services on behalf of the patient. It is clear that need could exist without want or demand, demand could exist without need but not without want, and want could exist without demand or need.

This distinction between need on the one side and wants and demands on the other emphasizes still further the value-laden nature of these phenomena. Such emphasis is merited. While wants and demands are normally readily recognized as being subjective in this way, this is less commonly the case with the conceptualization of need.

Need over time

Need is also likely to be dynamic over time. The need for care today, for example, is very different from the need for care 20 years ago. Partly, it is that the incidence and prevalence of diseases have changed. Also, expectations and values of both the population and the health professional have changed. Technological change and changing availability of services have also altered the extent and pattern of needs. Similarly, needs are likely to vary in moving from one culture or one society to another.

Need within the paradigms of public health

Policy and research in public health have not often adopted a multidisciplinary approach to the understanding of either wants or needs for healthcare. A great deal of ignorance thus lies undisturbed and the strengths and limits of the various public health sciences and discourses are thrown into relief when each comes to examine the nature of need. Epidemiology, with its reductionist roots, can provide a count of cases, deaths, and denominators, and can also provide insights into some of the causal pathways that manifest as these health states that we declare as needs. The social sciences can provide an interpretation of needs in terms of how society views departures from health—ranging from their perception as religious events through to secular phenomena that require government intervention that reinforces social values such as equity and efficiency. As indicated above, health economists can contribute to the understanding of healthcare needs by setting them within the context of what demands individuals and society place upon the resources available to them, in terms of their individual and corporate happiness and satisfaction. For example, where do healthcare needs fit in the total spectrum of needs, alongside the basic ones in the lower orders of the Maslow hierarchy (food, shelter, etc.) and in relation to the more sophisticated ones for education, justice, and freedom of speech (Maslow 1943)?

Any simple interpretation of need must therefore be suspect. The reductionist quality of measures of need should be understood if we are to avoid making useless extrapolations from them. Nevertheless, reductionist measures of need share with much reductionist science a remarkable capacity to get the job done, things improved, wars won, and health status elevated. The major issue confronting those involved in public health, therefore, is not so much to search endlessly for an all-embracing definition of need, but to be willing to live with pared-down versions of need that may be useful within a particular context, whilst recognizing their limitations. The debate about measuring need therefore shares much with the debate about measuring the quality of life.

What is not to be applauded, however, are those interpretations of need which are driven by data availability rather than the purpose for which the need measure is required. There are too many examples in the literature of needs estimation based on inappropriate grasping at available numbers without due consideration as to whether in ordinal or cardinal terms the interpretation of the numbers does reflect the construct of need which is claimed implicitly or explicitly.

The purpose of measuring need

If we accept that the generic notion of need is complex and elusive, we can proceed to identify different settings in which different measures of need, each with their limitations, may prove useful.

Need in the clinical setting

Within clinical practice, the measurement of need is an integral part of the daily routine. While it is a necessary and accepted part of such practice, it is not always judged explicitly.

The relevance of need and its usefulness in clinical decision-making are obvious and seemingly unchallenged and unchallengeable. Yet a challenge does arise from the extent to which there are substantial variations in clinical practice for similar or even identical health conditions. At this level, seemingly similar problems—identified perhaps with respect to reduced health status—are interpreted quite differently by different clinicians in terms of what is needed to deal with them. Manifestations of such apparent variations in interpretation can be a function not only of a diversity in respect of need but also of availability of resources to treat particular problems.

However, variations in the rates of performing various surgical procedures exist to a very great extent, even after allowing for or controlling for variations in the supply of resources and the characteristics of the populations being served. There is little doubt that this is a function of differences in perception and/or interpretation of needs at a clinical level across different clinicians.

In the face of a value-laden concept of need, the 'medical model'—if A, then B—can appear somewhat mechanistic. Neither A (the diagnosis) nor B (the choice of therapy) is devoid of value judgements on the part of the clinician. Yet historically it was possible to read into the concept of need in clinical medicine something that appeared concrete, objective, and largely value free. At the very heart of clinical medicine lies an increasing recognition of the extent to which medicine is about values, including the assessment and interpretation of needs.

At a clinical level there will be variations in interpretation of need across similar conditions but in different contexts. This can very clearly be influenced by the nature and structure of incentive systems (and not just financial incentives), which emphasizes still more the subjective nature of need. It is not possible to interpret the results of various studies on changes in remuneration systems in any other way. Need at a clinical level is a function, among other things, of how doctors are paid. As a consequence, care is sometimes provided that may not be 'needed' as viewed by a third party.

To point this out is not to criticize or to express regret about such a phenomenon. More importantly it is to recognize that there is potentially a useful tool for influencing clinical practice, in terms of not only the effectiveness of that practice but also its efficiency and its contribution to concerns for equity. Given the central place of need in clinical decision making, the fact that need can be perceived differently within different remuneration systems (Krasnik *et al.* 1990) has to be an important consideration for policy-makers. Yet the potential for using the remuneration system for policy purposes has been underexploited to date although recent initiatives in the United States and United Kingdom highlight growing interest in this area (Institute of Medicine 2001; Berwick *et al.* 2003; Mason *et al.* 2005).

Need at the level of the population

Although need may be considered in absolute terms, it is principally in relative terms that it finds its place in contemporary health service development and appraisal. Thus, 'standardized mortality ratios', that is mortality rates standardized to some common population, are compared from one region or country to another and implications are drawn about need. A community that has a 10 per cent higher mortality rate from ischaemic heart disease than the national average is seen, in particular by the popular press, as being 'in need'—of more coronary care beds, or more preventive programmes, or more ambulances fitted with defibrillators, etc.

Need is defined in these settings as some correlate of mortality, in no small part because mortality statistics despite all their weaknesses are, like democracy, pretty good compared with anything else. However, there is a particular problem in low- and middle-income countries in that many deaths are unreported and, hence, mortality statistics are very unreliable. What is of particular concern is that death reporting is especially poor in rural areas and, although residents of these areas in reality often bear the greatest burden of ill-health, this is not reflected in official mortality data. This is to some extent being addressed by the practice in a great many low- and middle-income countries of regularly conducting Demographic and Health Surveys (DHS), which provide data on infant, child and maternal mortality that are more reliable than official statistics.

Where there is a problem with mortality measures is with respect to answering the question: 'need for what?' Other things being equal, a higher level of mortality implies a higher level of need in some general rather unspecific sense—but greater need for what? It might be for health services but perhaps also for many other goods, services or activities. We believe that in the continuing tension between, on the one hand, treatment services for meeting health-care needs and, on the other hand, public health services, one of the reasons why the latter may 'lose out' in resource allocation is the failure to specify needs adequately in terms of instrumentation. Instruments or interventions in treatment services tend to be of a much more specific and identifiable nature than is the case with public health measures. The former are also drawn from a defined set of healthcare services whereas public health interventions can be present in very many areas of the economy—transport, housing, the environment, food policy, etc.

Doctors working in the acute hospital sector always have seductively simple and clear instruments at hand. In the battle for meeting needs at that level as opposed to the public health level, they have the imperative of current sickness to provide still more weight to their claims over a still greater share of society's scarce resources. The latter is difficult to push aside and there are arguments that in the context of rescue, there is no reason to push them aside. It is important, however, to decide the extent of influence since it cannot be the case that treating current sickness can be seen as an absolute, or at least ought not to be. An important issue to draw into such considerations is that of effectiveness of alternative interventions, in that even though current sickness exists, there may not be the 'capacity to benefit' from currently available interventions.

Need from a planning perspective

The discussion in this section is framed largely within the context of tax funded health systems. However, many of the same issues apply to planning in health systems that are funded primarily through social or national health insurance. There are two places where need impacts upon planning. The first is in relation to what economists refer to as 'allocative efficiency'. This involves first an acceptance that resources are scarce, and second that the over-riding goal is to maximize benefits with the available resources. In terms of needs, this translates as maximizing the needs met or the value of the needs met with the resources available.

The second place where need and planning converge is in the pursuit of equity. In relation to equity, issues of distribution are often set in terms of 'equal use for equal need' or 'equal access for equal need'.

Allocative efficiency issues

For allocative efficiency, the health service planner approaches needs as but one ingredient in a complex equation which he or she is expected to solve. In this context, the planner may identify 'need' as being those margins of existing programmes for which additional resources might achieve more than similar sized investments in other programmes. An implication of this is that there may be situations for which resources might be withdrawn and devoted elsewhere with greater well-being than is currently derived from the system.

The following statement might be made: The returns to health of monies spent here, on this programme, in this location, on this group of patients, on this effort on prevention, are not high enough—the money would be better spent over there on that other programme, on that other group of patients. If it is possible to take US$100 000 from the treatment of cancer patients and do still more good in treating the elderly for, perhaps, chronic arthritis, then it should be done. If the reverse is true then the direction of the resource shift should be reversed.

It is not enough to be able to say that resources which are scarce are being well spent; the issue is rather, could they be better spent? Are there more needs or more highly valued needs that resources could be used to address?

The idea of shifting resources to where they can meet the greatest need (or more correctly where they will do most good)—what economists call marginal analysis—is not difficult to grasp. If more good can be done than is being done, if more needs can be met with the same resources, then the argument is that that is what should be done.

It is here that the necessity for measurement of need becomes paramount, as judgements have to be made about where resources will meet the greatest need. If, with the same amount of resources, pain, suffering and death can be reduced still more, then let us do so. That is the simple notion of economic efficiency.

The concept of need incorporated into this planning framework is that of capacity to benefit (Culyer 1991), outlined earlier. This concept is a somewhat different type of need as compared with that which is used frequently at the population level, which is interpreted in terms simply of the extent of illness and death in a population (as described above). Even if a health problem exists, if there is no capacity to benefit, such as where no effective treatment exists for that particular health problem, under this definition there is no need.

Programme budgeting and marginal analysis

This planning framework stands to benefit if we can obtain a picture of how resources are currently being spent and linked in an appropriate way to what the objectives and priorities are. This picture is what is known as a set of 'programme budgets'.

Most commonly in healthcare, expenditure data are available categorized by inputs, for example, expenditure on doctors, nurses, pharmaceuticals, and linen. In programme budgeting the interest is in categorization of sets of needs that we seek to alleviate or meet—the needs of the elderly, children, cancer patients, etc. The link is thus between expenditure and health objectives for relevant social or disease groupings.

Therefore, prior to proceeding with the marginal analysis or shifting resources, it is relevant to find out what is being spent on these groupings or 'programmes'. The two keys to designating programmes are first that the programmes together are comprehensive in that, first, all the health services—hospital, general practitioner, and community—are included, and second, the programmes are output or outcome orientated and not input orientated as is the case with most forms of budgeting.

This approach—programme budgeting plus marginal analysis—is what economists recommend for use in pursuing the meeting of needs at a planning level (*Health Policy* 1995). With respect to the marginal analysis part of the approach, trying to form a judgement about whether US$1 million is better spent on maternity care rather than on care of the elderly is difficult. There are major measurement problems here and greater effort needs to be invested in developing appropriate measures to enable these comparisons to be made.

A recent example of the use of programme budgeting and marginal analysis (PBMA) is that undertaken by two of the regional health authorities in New Zealand to inform their purchasing of health services (Bohmer *et al.* 2001). This PBMA initiative focused on identifying the optimal allocation of resources between existing and potential respiratory disease interventions. Respiratory diseases are seen as important given that they account for up to 16 per cent of deaths in these two regions. The establishment of an advisory group for the PBMA process allowed for the inputs of all concerned groups, including community representatives. As a result of the PBMA, both regions prioritized additional or new investment in smoking cessation programmes and educating health professionals and communities in respiratory disease issues including appropriate antibiotic use, amongst others, and prioritized disinvestment in lung transplants and relatively ineffective treatments such as the use of cough syrups and bronchodilators. Although decision-makers viewed the process as having been of considerable value and the results were being implemented, it was noted that PBMA can be very data and resource intensive (Bohmer *et al.* 2001).

Quality-adjusted life years (QALYs) league tables

QALY league tables may be seen as a form of marginal analysis. Such tables allow comparisons to be made between conditions according to the impact they have on the quantity and quality of life of sufferers. As discussed in more detail below, the QALY, which weights chronological survival according to the quality of life, has also been used as an output currency to compare what is attainable for investment in various healthcare procedures. Thus, for US$10 000 spent on treatment for one condition one may purchase 300 QALYs, compared with 700 QALYs for the same price if one is treating a different condition. Yet QALY league tables have limited applicability in resource allocation contexts for several reasons (Gerard & Mooney 1993). For example, different studies will often be based on different comparators for the intervention being assessed. There are difficulties in making meaningful QALY league tables if the comparators do not reflect current standard practice.

Recent initiatives

The moves in, for example, the United States (through the Patient Outcome Research Team programme etc.), the United Kingdom (through health needs assessment—see later section), New Zealand, and New South Wales in Australia, to plan health services with the focus on health outcomes or health gain, place emphasis on efficiency and equity in the context of needs. Such an emphasis demands that objectives be more precisely and explicitly stated and needs identified more carefully and then quantified. It is to the quantification of needs that we will turn shortly.

Attempts to reallocate limited Medicaid dollars to a wider pool of recipients in Oregon attracted great attention, in no small part because need, effective therapy and cost were subject to public scrutiny in determining a pattern of resource expenditure for healthcare (Dixon & Welch 1991; Kitzhaber 1993). In 1991, after extensive consultation, a proposal was put forward that Medicaid coverage for the poor in Oregon should cease to cover everything possible for the poorest 200 000 recipients of aid and instead provide for 709 disease categories and paired treatments for an additional 100 000 recipients. The plan was approved by President Clinton on 19 March 1993.

Teng (1996) argues that compromises which led to the development of the list of services to be covered meant that the original objective of cost-effectiveness was largely undermined. Regardless of how the list was devised, however, it is doubtful whether cost-effectiveness is compatible, in general, with an approach to funding that partitions services above and below a fixed line. Its main limitation is that it takes no account of differences across individuals in terms of their capacity to benefit from the same treatment.

Despite this, the Oregon Health Plan was successful in one of its major objectives; increasing healthcare coverage across the state (Oregon Health Plan 1997; Jacobs et al. 1999). Conversely, it has been less successful in reducing overall healthcare expenditure and has relied to a large extent on funding from increases in tobacco taxes (Jacobs et al. 1999).

On the basis of the success of the Oregon Health Plan, which achieved its goal of providing cover to an additional 100 000 people, in 2002 the State decided to pursue a further extension to an additional 46 000 low income Oregon residents. The proposal was to move the cut-off point on the service priority list up, i.e. reduce the services covered in order to reallocate funds to cover new enrolees. As expressed by a senior Oregon health department official: 'It comes down to an old issue. Is it better for everybody to have something than for some to have a lot and others to have nothing?' (Oberlander 2007). Co-payments, both for premiums and at the point of service use, were also introduced. These changes were introduced in early 2003, with unexpectedly negative consequences. While there were 104 000 'additional' enrollees from the original Oregon Health Plan by January 2003, this had declined to 49 000 by December 2003 and even further to 24 000 by 2006. Instead of achieving a 50 per cent increase in enrolment for the Oregon Health Plan, the changes resulted in a 75 per cent decrease in enrolment. This decline has been attributed largely to the introduction of cost-sharing. In thinking about how to resuscitate the Oregon Health Plan, policy makers wanted to reorder the list of priorities, emphasizing chronic care and preventive services, with an emphasis on reducing costs of the services covered (Oberlander 2007).

Another initiative to prioritize among interventions which has received considerable attention is the World Bank's efforts to promote the development of 'essential packages' in low- and middle-income countries. The essential package concept was linked to the 1993 World Development Report, in which it was argued that governments should only finance those public health services which have *substantial* externalities and a defined package of essential clinical services (World Bank 1993). It was recommended that the essential package should include the most cost-effective health services which address the major health problems within that country (determined in terms of the 'burden of disease' measured as disability-adjusted life years or DALYs—discussed in more detail in 'DALYs'). A key component of this reform measure was the creation of an enabling environment for the private health sector to grow and to finance and provide all services outside of this essential package. Another World Bank (1994) publication that followed shortly thereafter, designed an 'essential package' that was seen to be appropriate for a wide range of low- and middle-income countries. Countries could determine which elements of the package to include based on their major diseases and available funds. Although the World Development Report suggested that each country should undertake its own burden of disease study and cost per DALY calculations in order to develop a country-specific essential package, the package defined in a wide range of African countries is almost identical to the package proposed in the World Bank's 'Better Health in Africa' report (World Bank 1994). The fact that the relative cost-effectiveness of specific interventions may vary considerably in different country contexts was not acknowledged by the World Bank.

The Commission on Macroeconomics and Health recommended an almost identical approach stating that low- and middle-income countries should identify essential interventions that are the most cost-effective and address the main contributors to the burden of disease (World Health Organization 2001). The main differences are that the Commission recommended that 'the needs of the poor should be stressed', estimated that the essential package would cost about US$35 per person per year, compared to the World Bank's previous estimate of US$13 per person per year and called for greater national and international investment in health. A veritable 'industry' has arisen around these suggestions, with each African country being encouraged to set up a National Commission on Macroeconomics and Health (see, for example, http://www.afro.who.int/cmh/index.html). The practice of identifying need in relation to measures such as DALYs and defining limited service packages in relation to these 'needs', is firmly entrenched in many African countries as well as some other low- and middle-income countries.

The dilemma of deciding which health services can be provided to meet the needs of the population best is not unique to tax funded health systems. Indeed, this challenge is even more evident in insurance funded systems; while tax funded systems often avoid making explicit decisions about service rationing and effectively leave these decisions to clinicians, health insurance schemes (whether voluntary private or mandatory social health insurance) have to specify the benefit package to which their members will be entitled.

Equity issues

The second consideration that planners will be interested in concerns equity. One of the most problematical aspects of this is that there is so much confusion in healthcare policy circles as to what this word means. The chief contenders are 'equal health', 'equal use for equal need', and 'equal access for equal need'. Clearly the last two of these incorporate some view of need within them. Here our concern is restricted to the relationship between equity and need and, within that, the issue of resource allocation formulas.

The international industry of needs-based (or weighted capitation) resource allocation formulas began with the Resource Allocation Working Party (RAWP) in England whose report was published in 1976 (DHSS 1976). The approach has been used in several other places since (e.g. New South Wales in Australia, New Zealand, Portugal, as well as several African and Latin American countries such as Ghana, Tanzania, Zambia, Brazil, Chile, Colombia and Mexico).

What the original RAWP sought was a formula for allocating resources fairly to the 14 geographical regions of England based on the principle of equal access for equal need (although in practice it did not go beyond equal expenditure for equal need). The RAWP formula (and the various versions it has spawned) emphasized horizontal equity, i.e. equity that ensures that individuals with similar characteristics are treated equally. Vertical equity—the unequal, yet equitable, treatment of unequals—is not included directly in the formulation except in so far as different needs are weighted by the cost of dealing with each.

In the last decade, some attention has been devoted to Mooney's (1998) argument that there may be a case for developing the notion of 'communitarian claims' to replace needs or at least to complement them. It is normally the case that need is conceptualized in terms of purely health and that in meeting need, all nominally equal health gains (such as QALYs) be weighted equally. Communitarian claims, it is suggested, allow for other considerations (e.g. information or respect for patient dignity) to enter and for health gains to some recipients (e.g. those in particularly poor health) to be weighted more highly than others. A further claimed advantage is that it is the community who determine first what constitutes a claim, and second the differential strengths of different claims. These would determine what healthcare resources were to be made available to different groups in society. These claims are communitarian not only in the sense that the responsibility to arbitrate over them lies with the community but also that it is beneficial to the community that they do so. For example, in Australia the overall community may feel better as a result of knowing that it has contributed to the betterment of the health of its Indigenous peoples.

Measuring need—available instruments and their application

Needs-based formulas

In several countries measures of need have been constructed to guide the allocation of healthcare resources. The methods vary from allocating resources to geographical areas on the basis of prevailing patterns of mortality and social class, through to case-mix payment to hospitals on the basis of the need (in terms of diagnosis and severity) of patients admitted to their care.

The approach adopted in the RAWP formula (see above) aimed at measuring relative (and not absolute) need for healthcare in different regions. Such healthcare was divided into seven categories: Non-psychiatric inpatient services, all day-patient and outpatient services, mental illness inpatient services, mental handicap inpatient services, community services, ambulance services, and administration of general practitioner services but not these services *per se*.

The relative need for each of these services in each region was calculated on the basis of a formula which weighted the population according to a number of factors. For example, the factors relevant to non-psychiatric inpatient services were size of population, age/sex composition, morbidity (although in practice this was actually the standardized mortality rate), cost, patient cross-boundary flows, medical education and capital investment. Relative need was calculated for each of the services listed and then weighted according to the national proportion of the total spending on that service. These were then summed to give an overall regional weight. Thus, if a region with a population of, say, 5 million was above average in terms of need, for example to the extent of 10 per cent, then it would receive funding which assumed a weighted population of 5.5 million. In a later revision of the RAWP formula (DHSS 1986), the regional population was also weighted by a deprivation index (i.e. a composite index of socioeconomic indicators). This was in response to criticisms that standardized mortality rates do not account for regional variations in the need for health services arising from differences in socioeconomic conditions. Subjective indicators of health, in the form of self-rated health in household surveys, have also been used in the United Kingdom, although concerns exist about their validity given their high variability and low statistical association with mortality (O'Reilly 2005).

As indicated earlier, the idea of needs-based formulas to guide resource allocation has been taken up by a wide range of high-, middle- and even low-income countries. This is probably due to the success that RAWP had in effecting a relative redistribution of healthcare resources between regions in England. The difference in expenditure per capita (of weighted population) between the poorest and wealthiest regions was approximately 30 per cent when the RAWP report was published; this gap had virtually been eliminated one and a half decades later.

Box 12.1.2 provides an overview of the indicators of 'need' included in resource allocation formulas in a range of low- and middle-income countries. These countries face particular challenges in that there is limited access to data on many indicators. While all formulas have a common starting point, namely population size, and many adjust for the age and sex composition of the population, low- and middle-income countries tend to use infant or child mortality instead of standardized mortality ratios. Many also include some measure of socioeconomic status (poverty or a broader deprivation index) and adjust for the differential cost of providing services (particularly in rural or low-density areas). A factor that was not relevant in the English context, but is critical in many low- and middle-income countries is that of funds that may accrue at district or regional level other than central government tax funding. Given that different areas have different abilities to attract donor funding or to generate their own revenue (e.g. through local government rates and taxes or user fees charged at health facilities), it is necessary to take such revenue into account in order to promote equity in the overall funding envelope but at the same time, avoid undermining incentives to raise revenue locally.

What these formulas assume is that the total relative need in a region and across regions is a meaningful entity. That is open to challenge, however, if total need for healthcare is seen as in part a function of supply. Thus total relative need cannot be defined in the absence of some budget constraint which makes the argument for using total relative need as a measure for allocating a budget between different regions somewhat circular. It further assumes that the relative total need can be measured sufficiently accurately by just a few factors. Thirdly, it assumes that using standardized mortality rates (or infant or child mortality) as a measure of relative morbidity is a valid measure (again a doubtful assumption).

Box 12.1.2 Examples of low- and middle-income countries using a needs-based resource allocation formula

Africa

Ghana

Since 2004, Ghana has been allocating its tax funded and donor pooled fund health budget between regions using a formula which includes the regional population size, weighted for deprivation (measured as the population below the poverty line) and under 5 mortality.

Tanzania

The Tanzanian formula for the allocation of 'basket' (donor-pooled) funds to districts includes population size, under-five mortality as a proxy for disease burden, poverty level and adjusts for the differential cost of providing health services in rural and low population density areas.

Uganda

The primary health care budget is allocated between districts using a formula based on population size, the inverse of the Human Development Index (HDI), the inverse of per capita donor and NGO spending and a supplement for districts with a difficult security situation and those with no district hospital. In this formula, the HDI component includes measures of both socio-economic status and ill-health. Taking account of donor and NGO funding ensures that the full resource envelope for each district is taken into account when determining the allocation of government funds.

Zambia

Initially, a simple per capita formula was used in Zambia because of the scarcity of accurate data on other needs-based indicators. However, weightings for remoteness and disease patterns have been recently included in the formula.

Latin America

Chile

Resources for primary health care are allocated from central government to municipalities on the basis of population size, with an adjustment for rurality and municipal poverty level.

Colombia

Central government in Colombia allocates general funds to municipalities on the basis of a formula that includes the size of the municipal population, adjusted for poverty level, unmet basic needs, quality of life indicators and locally-generated revenue. A portion of these funds is explicitly earmarked for health services. Thus, they use a needs-based formula to determine an overall allocation for all municipal services but limit municipal autonomy in deciding on the distribution of these funds between types of services by protecting part of the grant for health (and similarly for education). This approach has dramatically promoted equity in the distribution of health care resources between municipalities.

Mexico

The Mexican Ministry of Health quite recently introduced a resource allocation formula which includes population size, child mortality rate and a 'marginalization index'. The last is a composite index of socio-economic status which includes educational status, access to potable water and to sanitation and overcrowding.

Source: Bossert *et al.* (2003); Pearson (2002); Rocha *et al.* (2004)

Finally, it assumes that differences in need are proportional to the resources required to address them. For example, if a particular region is judged to have needs that are on average 10 per cent greater than the national average, they are allocated 10 per cent more resources than they would have received based purely on their population size. In effect, this procedure for allocating resources is not consistent with the concept of allocating resources according to capacity to benefit *at the margin*.

We would not want to appear overcritical of this process, as these formulas have been instrumental in breaking historical inertia in resource allocation patterns and contributing to considerable resource redistribution in some countries. What we would emphasize is the desirability in many instances of trying to fund health services on an equitable basis and that using some concept of need is the way to follow. It remains the case, however, that the assumptions typically used in needs-based formulas and the problems of measurement are

such that we are less than convinced that this is the best way to proceed. In particular, we would submit that not weighting different needs according to social values remains problematical.

Weighting need to reflect social values

In order to weight needs on the basis of social values, some form of survey needs to be carried out to determine such weights. Various methods have been posited in the literature including both surveys and citizen jury-based approaches—typically entailing scenario-based allocations across hypothetical populations differing with respect to various characteristics such as socioeconomic status, age and sex. For examples of such approaches, see Mooney *et al.* (1995), Nord *et al.* (1995), Wiseman *et al.* (2003), and Mooney and Blackwell (2004).

Similar efforts to elicit social views on the relative weights that should be accorded to different needs have been undertaken in low- and middle-income countries such as Zambia and Namibia. In Namibia, 101 people were interviewed, with two-thirds being elected representatives at national, regional or local level (MHSS & WHO 2005). The vast majority were in favour of adopting a vertical equity approach and weighting the needs of certain groups more highly than others (e.g. rural residents and the poor).

Absorptive capacity issues

When efforts are made to reallocate resources to promote equity in meeting the needs of the population, it is important to ensure that communities benefiting from additional allocations are able to 'absorb' and benefit from these resources. There are too many examples of substantial budgetary resource redistribution occurring where historically under-funded areas are unable to utilize all the funds allocated to them while historically well-resourced areas struggle to cope with budget cuts. This was experienced in South Africa, for example, shortly after its first democratic elections, where an overly ambitious initiative to achieve equal per capita spending in each province within 5 years (the term of government) encountered major absorptive capacity problems (Gilson et al. 1999). In this instance, this was clearly a problem of too rapid a pace of change, which the original RAWP had avoided by setting explicit 'floors and ceilings' which limited the annual percentage decrease or increase in any region's budget. There are, however, other issues that are important to take into account in relation to absorptive capacity, and it may be necessary to explicitly invest in developing such capacity.

It has been proposed that this be done through the building of 'MESH' infrastructure (where MESH is management, economic, social and human) (Mooney & Houston 2004). The idea is simple. The capacity to benefit from any set of resources allocated to improving health will in practice be realized only to the extent that there is an adequate infrastructure available to use the resources in an efficient way. If in some jurisdiction there is a lack of leadership and other skills to operate programs successfully to the benefit of their communities, then the capacity to benefit will not be realized as fully as it otherwise might be. The policy response should then be to build MESH. This governance issue is one that internationally is increasingly recognized as important in Indigenous affairs (Cornell et al. 2004) but the ideas are applicable in any population. (see, for example, Thomas, Mooney and Mbatsha 2007 in relation to South Africa).

Thus, different jurisdictions and communities may differ in terms of their capacities to produce benefits for the people they serve. This can be for three reasons: (i) some populations already have relatively good health, so the capacity to benefit further is limited compared with others; (ii) even where the health levels of two populations are similar, one population's health problems can be more amenable to health service interventions, i.e. its capacity to benefit from healthcare interventions is greater; and (iii) even where both the health levels and the health problems are similar, one health service may be better placed or better equipped to deliver benefit to its population than the other. In the case of (iii), the capacity to benefit is inhibited because the service lacks the necessary MESH infrastructure to deliver health benefits to its population.

The basis of the approach to resource allocation outlined here takes as its starting point the issue of governance. If progress is to be made in improving the health of any population, it must be through the preferences and the wishes of the people concerned.

Insofar as there are variations in the abilities of different communities and health services with respect to MESH infrastructure, this can result in uneven implementation of health service interventions and consequent inequities and inefficiencies for the relevant populations.

It is thus necessary to address this problem of variation through providing support to those jurisdictions that are deficient in these abilities. The building of MESH infrastructure can be seen as a major plank in any equity strategy, as it may well be those jurisdictions with the greatest healthcare need that are most often lacking in MESH. The lack of MESH in these communities will then exacerbate the inequities in healthcare need between communities.

Needs-based formulas in insurance-funded systems

While the needs-based resource allocation formulas discussed above refer largely to the allocation of nationally collected general tax funds to provinces, regions, districts or similar geographical localities, a similar approach is also used in the case of what is termed 'risk-equalization' between different health insurance schemes (van Vliet & van de Ven 1992; Beck et al. 2003). 'Risk' in actuarial terms has a similar meaning to need as discussed in this chapter. Risk-equalization has both equity and efficiency objectives. It particularly aims to respond to 'cream-skimming' (or risk selection) by competing health insurance schemes, whereby they seek to attract young, healthy members leaving other schemes with a large share of older and less healthy members. The risk profile of individual schemes is assessed, particularly using demographic variables such as age and gender but may also include the number of members with particular chronic diseases. Schemes with a high proportion of low-risk members are required to pay into a 'risk-equalization fund' while those with a high proportion of high-risk members will receive payments from the fund. This applies pressure on schemes to operate efficiently and promotes risk cross-subsidies (the healthy subsidising the costs of the ill), which are seen as a key component of promoting equity in health service benefits, between schemes. This risk equalization process thus seeks to promote equal expenditure for equal need.

Risk-equalization or risk-adjustment between competing health insurance schemes exists in many high-income countries with a mandatory requirement for the population to purchase health insurance cover, such as the Netherlands, Switzerland, and Ireland. However, in many cases, the risk-equalization is based purely on demographic variables (age and gender), with these variables only being able to predict a small proportion of the variance in health expenditure, thus allowing for schemes to continue to 'cream-skim' (van Vliet & van de Ven 1992; Beck et al. 2003). Interestingly, it is a middle-income country, South Africa, that has developed one of the more comprehensive risk-equalization methodologies. This includes age, a maternity or delivery indicator, the number of people with any of the 25 most prevalent chronic conditions, the number of people with multiple chronic conditions and the number of people with HIV on antiretroviral therapy (McLeod 2004). At the time of writing (March 2007), the risk-equalization methodology has been finalized, all health insurance schemes have submitted information of these variables and the process will be fully implemented within the next year or two.

Health needs assessment

Health needs assessment (HNA) has been described as 'a systematic method for reviewing the health issues facing a population, leading to agreed priorities and resource allocation that will improve health and reduce inequalities' (Cavanagh & Chadwick 2005). The HNA approach was developed to assist in the 'commissioning' of services in the United Kingdom after the separation of purchaser and provider functions within the National Health Service in the early 1990s. Its growing importance as a planning instrument has been promoted by the trend towards evidence-informed decision making in the health sector. In recent years, considerable emphasis has been placed on HNA as a mechanism for ensuring that community views are taken into account in the planning process.

HNA is described as a five-step planning process:

1. Preliminary activities, including: The identification of the population to be considered (particularly from an equity perspective such as a group or area which suffers from multiple deprivation); and establishing clear objectives

2. Identifying health priorities, including: Gathering general information on the target population; identifying how the population perceives its own needs; identifying the health conditions and underlying factors that have a significant impact (in terms of size and severity) on health status in this population (using a broad health determinants framework) and whose health is most at risk from these priority conditions; which priority conditions or factors influencing these conditions can effectively be improved; and shortlisting priorities for action

3. Assessing a health priority for action, including: Identifying effective interventions for the health priority; defining the specific target population; identifying the changes required; confirming that the proposed changes will help reduce health inequalities; identifying the most acceptable interventions; and assessing the resource feasibility of the interventions including a marginal analysis of whether resources can be shifted from their current use to more cost effective interventions

4. Planning for change which focuses on detailed programming of the necessary actions and tasks to implement the identified interventions

5. Monitoring and review, particularly to assess if the planned impact is being achieved and ways of improving impact

There are a number of ways in which HNA is an advance on previous efforts to measure needs within a planning context. Firstly, it recognizes the instrumental nature of need for healthcare, as the explicit goal is the improvement of health, and it focuses on areas where effective interventions exist. Throughout the HNA process, decision-makers are required to consider two criteria in the selection of priorities: 'impact' and 'changeability' (Cavanagh & Chadwick 2005). In terms of 'impact', one is required to evaluate whether the specific health problem being considered has a significant impact on the health functioning of the population, both in relation to severity and size of the impact. The criterion of 'changeability' requires explicit assessment of the extent to which the health problem can be addressed *effectively* within the local context and by the groups involved.

Secondly, HNA also ensures that resource scarcity is explicitly taken into consideration and is designed as a marginal analysis. In the third step of the HNA process, decision-makers have to estimate the resources required to implement a priority intervention and to address questions such as: 'Can existing resources be used differently?'; 'What resources might be released if existing ineffective interventions are stopped?'; and 'Which actions will achieve the greatest impact on health for the resources used?' (Cavanagh & Chadwick 2005). In effect, a marginal analysis is required to identify existing interventions that are less cost-effective and should be de-prioritized.

Third, equity is an explicit objective and a vertical equity approach is used in that there is an emphasis on identifying particularly deprived populations and assessing whether interventions identified as priorities will achieve a reduction in health inequalities. In the first step, the population to be prioritized is identified on the basis of answering the questions 'Does this population have significantly worse health than others locally' and do they suffer from 'significant health inequalities'? (Cavanagh & Chadwick 2005). In addition, groups that suffer not only worse health status but also social and material deprivation are given priority. There is also explicit consideration of whether an intervention will reduce inequalities, before it is included on the priority list.

Finally, the community is extensively involved in identifying priority interventions. Community involvement is required at various stages of the HNA, including to contribute to identifying the key health issues affecting that community, the interventions regarded as most acceptable, and prioritizing the target population, health conditions and potential interventions. Particular emphasis is placed on ensuring that marginalized communities are reached and that their perspectives and preferences are taken into account (Cavanagh & Chadwick 2005).

Measuring instruments

Measuring needs, as indicated above, is likely to be problematical for the various reasons already stated. Whatever process is adopted, it involves establishing a measure of some shortfall in health status from some ideal, some norm, from some achievable health status, or some measure of 'capacity to benefit'.

There are many ways of trying to measure needs which are severely deficient and reflect more the availability of data than any real attempt to grapple seriously with the conceptualization of needs as spelt out so far in this chapter. Various activity measures—number of admissions, visits to general practitioners, vaccinations carried out, etc.—are sometimes used to measure need. Yet, it is readily apparent that such indicators reflect not only need (although visits to general practitioners may perhaps be designated a measure of consumer demand, in particular first visits during a specific episode) but also supply-side considerations such as availability and appropriateness of services.

Certainly, there are a number of vehicles that can be adopted to allow measurement of need to take place. Most common here would be epidemiological and social surveys. The question then is how to measure needs within any such survey. The emphasis around the world is on identifying measures of need that combine indicators of length of life (mortality) and quality of life or health (morbidity). We first consider some of these aggregate quantity and quality of life measures and then consider in more detail specific instruments frequently used to measure health-related quality of life.

QALYs

The QALY, and its later 'stable mate' the healthy year equivalent (HYE), have been developed largely by economists (Williams 1985;

Torrance 1986; Mehrez & Gafni 1989) to allow health status to be measured in various circumstances. Both are based on the concept of health-related utility which recognizes that health, as an output of health services and of other activities that promote health, is a function of both quantity of health and quality of health—or mortality and morbidity.

The QALY allows individuals, groups, or societies to 'trade-off' quantity of life against quality of life arguing, for example, that according to people's preferences, 10 years living with a chronic condition which results in the individual being confined to his or her own home is equivalent to 8 years of full health. The implication is that the 'quality adjustment' for the chronic condition is 0.8. Furthermore, it is implied that intervening to cure the chronic condition would result in an improvement in quality of life of 0.2 per annum which over 10 years means 2 QALYs.

While there are various criticisms that can be made of QALYs (Loomes & McKenzie 1989), they do have considerable merit over the more conventional measures of health status and of need such as mortality rates or standardized mortality rates in that they do endeavour to combine both quantity of life and quality of health. The development of QALYs has helped to gain greater acceptance for the point that health status, and in turn need, have large subjective elements (Sculpher 2006). In practice, to date QALYs have been used to measure need, essentially marginal-met need, in the context of priority setting through QALY league tables, as discussed above.

DALYs

The DALY is a variant of the QALY. DALYs were first introduced by the World Bank in the early 1990s (World Bank 1993) as a means of calculating the burden of different diseases. The approach involves the measurement of health status (strictly lost health status) into a universal index of mortality and morbidity.

Specifically, the DALYs for a given condition or disease are the sum of years of life lost due to premature mortality and the number of years of life lived with disability, adjusted for the severity of the disability (Murray & Lopez 1997). In terms of the disability severity weights, these were originally based on the opinions of experts in international health and fell into six classes of severity ranging from 0 (for perfect health) to 1 (for death) but, more recently, social values have been incorporated in DALYs (Murray & Lopez 1997a).

DALYs and their use as an aggregate measure of health status in the monitoring of population health, in the establishment of priorities between interventions, and as a guide to research priorities have been criticized by a number of authors (Ugalde & Jackson 1995; Anand & Hanson 1997; Paalman et al. 1998). One of the most controversial aspects of the DALY calculation is the differential age weighting applied to life years lost (Barendregt et al. 1996). Murray (1994), a key designer of DALYs, argues that it is valid to weight life years lost for working age adults more highly than for young children and the elderly, given that 'because of social roles the social value of that time may be greater' and that it is purely 'an attempt to capture different social roles at different ages'. Anand and Hanson (1997) highlight the extent of age discrimination by noting that 'in the construction of a DALY, a year lived at age 2 counts for only 20 per cent of a year lived at age 25 where the age-weighting function is at a maximum, while that lived at age 70 counts for 46 per cent of the maximum'. The effect of this age weighting is that

if two people have the same illness and can be treated effectively for the same cost, preference would be given to treating a young adult rather than an older person or a child. A number of authors have argued that the age weights should be considered 'inequitable in principle' (Paalman et al. 1998; Anand & Hanson 1997). Others have commented that DALYs inadequately reflect social preferences for health, that the assumed or posited goals of healthcare systems are not validated, that such goals are assumed to be constant across all societies, and that using DALYs, as is advocated, to measure the burden of disease to assist with priority setting is at best a misuse of analytical resources and at worst potentially misleading (Mooney & Creese 1993; Sayers & Fliedner 1997; Wiseman & Mooney 1998; Williams 1999).

More recently, Murray and colleagues have developed variations of DALYs, namely disability-free life expectancy (DFLE) and disability-adjusted life expectancy (DALE) (Murray & Lopez 1997b). For these measures, they developed seven categories of disability and associated weights ranging from 0 (for minimal disability) to 1 (for very severe disability). The weights were based on preferences for different health states according to nine groups of people from 25 countries. A single set of disability weights was developed, which the authors regard as applicable across the world.

This reflects one of the key challenges with measures such as QALYs, HYEs, DALYs, and DALEs. It is unlikely that a single set of social values can be developed that is universally applicable, or that a set of values developed in one country would be applicable or reflect social values in a very different country. Values of health, trade-offs between quantity and quality of life, and the influence of spirituality on health are all likely to vary from culture to culture. Even the very construct of health can be culturally specific. For example, the construct of Australian Aboriginal health is holistic in a way not recognized in Western biomedical definitions. It also includes elements of reciprocity, mutuality, and obligation (Houston 2004).

It is of concern that little work has been undertaken in low- and middle-income countries to develop quality of life or disability weights that are relevant within specific country contexts, although more work has been undertaken in this regard in recent years. Low- and middle-income countries most frequently take an existing instrument for measuring health-related quality of life, which usually has been developed in the United States or in a European context, translate it into the local language and collect data to estimate locally relevant valuation of different health states (Bowden & Fox-Rushby 2003). Nevertheless, the emphasis appears to be placed more on ensuring that the quality of life measures are equivalent to that in other countries than on ensuring that the measures are appropriate for assessing need within the individual country contexts. The preoccupation with being able to perform cross-country comparisons appears to take precedence over appropriately informing local decision-making.

Measuring quality of life

What are some of these generic health-related quality of life instruments that are used around the world? The two most widely used instruments are 'SF-36' (or Short Form 36) and EuroQol (European Quality of Life) EQ-5D. The SF-36 was developed by the RAND Corporation in the United States for use in the Health Insurance Study Experiment/ Medical Outcomes Study (Ware et al. 1993). It is a concise 36-item health status questionnaire and has become one of the most widely used measures of subjective health status (Ware *et al.* 1993; Jenkinson *et al.* 1996).

The SF-36 contains 36 items which measure eight dimensions: Physical functioning (ten items), role limitations due to physical problems (four items), role limitations due to emotional problems (three items), mental health (five items), energy/vitality (four items), social functioning (two items), pain (two items), and general health perception (five items). There is also a single item about perceptions of health changes over the past 12 months.

The validity and reliability of the SF-36 in patient populations has been confirmed in the United States (McHorney *et al.* 1992, 1993). For example, patients with chronic heart failure reporting oedema, orthopnoea, or dyspnoea on exertion were classified as having a serious medical condition. The SF-36 could detect difference in health status among these patient groups across all eight scales. Garratt *et al.* (1993) claim on the basis of their own empirical work in the United Kingdom that the SF-36 seems 'acceptable to patients, internally consistent, and a valid measure of the health status of a wide range of patients'.

However, not all studies have been favourable to the SF-36. For instance, it has been criticized for failing to detect low levels of morbidity in some patient groups (Bowling 1997). Kurtin *et al.* (1992) reported 'floor' effects in the role of functioning scales in severely ill patients, where 25 to 50 per cent of patients obtained the lowest score possible, the implication being that deterioration in condition will not be detected by the scale. Other studies have revealed that it has little discriminatory power among women receiving different treatments for stage II breast cancer (Levine *et al.* 1988; Guyatt *et al.* 1989). Detailed reviews of the instrument are given by Anderson *et al.* (1993) and Bowling (1997).

More recently, an abbreviated version of the SF-36, the SF-12, has been developed (Ware *et al.* 1996). The SF-12 health survey generates the physical and mental component summary scores of the SF-36 'with considerable accuracy, while imposing less burden on the respondents' (Jenkinson & Layte 1997). However, there do appear to be trade-offs in terms of reliability. For example, Jenkinson and Layte (1997) warn that 'the questionnaire contains a number of areas of health tapped with only a single item ... consequently the SF-36 will provide a more reliable profile of scores across the eight domains than could be gained using the SF-12'.

Both the SF-36 and SF-12 can now be used to estimate QALYs through the SF-6D algorithm. This provides a single summary measure of quality of life based on preference-based weights (Brazier *et al.* 2002; Brazier & Roberts 2004). Likewise, the EQ-5D, provides a simple summary measure of quality of life based on five questions (The EuroQol Group 1990).

Recently there has also been the development of the World Health Organization's Quality of Life Measure (WHOQOL) which seeks to assess inter alia the relevance of spirituality, religion and personal beliefs to health (WHOQOL SRPB Group 2006). These factors are likely to vary, sometimes markedly, from one culture to another, as will their influence on health. This measure is thus particularly important in acknowledging the diversity of cultures and the fact that the construct of health is a cultural phenomenon.

The measurement of both need and health status is thus constantly undergoing improvement and development. That will undoubtedly continue in the future.

Which measure is to be preferred in measuring need is not only a function of why need is being assessed but also the context or environment in which it is being assessed. Many normative factors influence health perceptions including the health of others in the individual's community or group, the nature and severity of the illness, demographic characteristics, and social class (Festinger 1954; Sen 1987; Crawford 1994; Olsen & Dahl 2007). While many measurement efforts are mathematically sophisticated and some are reliable in the sense that they can reproduce the same results from one application to another, they tend to be of questionable validity in so far as they fail to recognize the importance of these normative factors. Currently, most health status indices do not take account of the variation in criteria that individuals or groups use to make judgements about their own health status.

The consistent underperception of ill health observed in many disadvantaged and marginalized groups has 'obvious implications for the design and implementation of public health programs particularly if these programs aim to bring treatment to those most in need of such help' (Wiseman 1999). Secondly, resource allocation decision-making which relies on potentially different subjective measures of health may provide a misleading picture of the resource requirements of some groups in society. This will have implications for estimating healthcare priorities and the funding and planning of health services. There is a need to learn more about the criteria of health which are relevant in judging the well being of these groups and to investigate alternative elicitation procedures which would allow for a more accurate reflection of the preferences of such groups.

Conclusion

The concept of need is elusive but useful. In confronting the notion of need, we acknowledge the value-laden quality of the community's expectation of health services, whether these be for the relief and treatment of illness or the preservation and maintenance of good health. Need derives its meaning from the instrumental pathways we can follow in meeting it and inevitably involves third parties in its definition. Key issues identified in this chapter include:

◆ The focus of the need for healthcare is on the outcome of such care, namely improved health. This implies that there must be a capacity to benefit from healthcare and that a need can only exist for effective healthcare.

◆ In determining how to meet need in a setting of limited resources, the allocation of resources must take account of the likely health gain and the cost of that achievement. Moving resources at the margins of our principal programmes of care and health development, according to estimates or measurement of the cost and outcome, offers ways in which we can move in the direction of the wisest use of those resources in meeting need.

◆ Needs-based formulas have been important in pursuing equitable resource allocation in many countries, generally in relation to promoting equal expenditure for equal need. More emphasis should be placed on incorporating social values in this process, to identify whose needs should be given relatively greater weight in the allocation of limited resources.

◆ Measuring needs involves assessing the shortfall in health status from some achievable norm, generally using a measure that combines indicators of length of life (mortality) and quality of life (morbidity). There are a few instruments, developed in the United States and Europe, for measuring health-related quality of life that are regarded as valid and reliable. However, further work is required to assess the appropriateness of these instruments in different cultural contexts and how to account for normative factors that influence health perceptions in need measures.

◆ Despite the considerable outstanding agenda of work in refining concepts and measures of need, disappointingly little published work has been forthcoming over the past few years. If we are to progress in addressing health sector efficiency and equity, this trend should be reversed.

Acknowledgement

We are grateful to Steve Leeder and Virginia Wiseman for allowing us to use materials contained in previous versions of this chapter, which they co-authored with Gavin Mooney, and the latter also with Stephen Jan.

References

Anand S. and Hanson K. (1997). Disability-adjusted life years: a critical review. *Journal of Health Economics*, **16**, 685–702.

Anderson R., Aaronson N., and Wilkin D. (1993). Critical review of the international assessments if health-related quality of life. *Quality of Life Research*, **2**, 369–95.

Barendregt J.J., Bonneux L., and Van der Maas P.J. (1996). DALYs: the age-weights on balance. *Bulletin of the World Health Organization*, **74**(4), 439–46.

Beck K., Spycher S., Holly A. *et al.* (2003). Risk adjustment in Switzerland. *Health Policy*, **65**, 63–74.

Berwick D.M., DeParle N.A., Eddy D.M. *et al.* (2003). Paying for performance: Medicare should lead. *Health Affairs (Millwood)*, **22**, 8–10.

Bohmer P., Pain C., Watt A. *et al.* (2001). Maximising health gain within available resources in the New Zealand public health system. *Health Policy*, **55**, 37–50.

Bossert T., Larranaga S., Giedion U. *et al.* (2003). Decentralization and equity of resource allocation: evidence from Colombia and Chile. *Bulletin of the World Health Organization*, **81**, 95–100.

Bowden A. and Fox-Rushby J.A. (2003). A systematic and critical review of the process of translation and adaptation of generic health related quality of life measures in Africa, Asia, Eastern Europe, the Middle East, South America. *Social Science and Medicine*, **57**, 1289–306.

Bowling A. (1997). *Measuring health. A review of quality of life measurement scales* (2nd edn). Open University Press, Milton Keynes.

Brazier J.E. and Roberts J. (2004). Estimating a preference-based index from the SF-12. *Medical Care*, **42**(9), 851–9.

Brazier J.E., Roberts J., and Deverill M (2002). The estimation of a preference-based measure of health from the SF-36. *Journal of Health Economics*, **21**, 271–92.

Cavanagh S. and Chadwick K. (2005). *Health needs assessment: A practical guide.* Health Development Agency (now National Institute for Health and Clinical Excellence), London.

Cornell S., Curtis C. and Jorgensen M. (2004). *Joint Occasional Paper on Native Affairs No 2004–02: The concept of governance and is implications for First Nations.* The Harvard Project on American Indian Economic Development, Boston.mhttp://www.jopna.net/pubs/jopna_2004-02_Governance.pdf

Crawford R. (1994). The boundaries of the self and the unhealthy other: reflections on health, culture and AIDS. *Social Science and Medicine*, **38**, 1347–65.

Culyer A.J. (1991). *Equity in health care policy.* Paper presented to the Ontario Premier's Council on Health, Well-Being and Social Justice. University of Toronto, Toronto.

Culyer A.J. and Wagstaff A. (1993). Equity and equality in health and health care. *Journal of Health Economics.* **12**, 431–57.

DHSS (Department of Health and Social Security) (1976). *Report of the Resource Allocation Working Party (RAWP).* HMSO, London.

DHSS (Department of Health and Social Security) (1986). *Review of the Resource Allocation Working Party Formula.* Report by the NHS Management Board. DHSS, London.

Dixon J. and Welch H.G. (1991). Priority setting: Lessons from Oregon. *Lancet*, **337**, 912–6.

The EuroQol Group (1990). EuroQol: A new facility for the measurement of health-related quality of life. *Health Policy*, **16**, 199–208.

Festinger L. (1954). A theory of social comparison processes. *Human Relations*, **7**, 117–40.

Garratt A., Ruta D., Abdalla M. *et al.* (1993). The SF36 Health survey Questionnaire: an outcome measure suitable for routine use within the NHS? *British Medical Journal*, **306**, 1440–4.

Gerard K. and Mooney G. (1993). QALY league tables: handle with care. *Health Economics*, **2**, 59–64.

Gilson L., Doherty J., McIntyre D. *et al.* (1999). *The Dynamics of Policy Change: Health Care Financing in South Africa 1994–99. Monograph No. 66.* Centre for Health Policy and Health Economics Unit, Johannesburg.

Guyatt G., Nogradi S., Halcrow S. *et al.* (1989). Development and testing of a new measure of health status for clinical trials in health failure. *Journal of General Internal Medicine*, **4**, 101–7.

Health Policy (1995). Special issue on programme budgeting and marginal analysis. *Health Policy*, **33**.

Houston S. (2004). *Aboriginal Health Policy: The Past, the Present, the Future.* PhD Thesis. Curtin University, Perth.

Institute of Medicine (2001). *Crossing the quality chasm: a new health system for the 21st century.* National Academy Press, Washington, D.C.

Jacobs L., Marmor T., and Oberlander J. (1999). The Oregon Health Plan and the political paradox of rationing: what advocates and critics have claimed and what Oregon did. *Journal of Health Politics, Policy and Law*, **24**, 161–80.

Jenkinson C. and Layte R. (1997). Development and testing of the UK SF-12. *Journal of Health Services Research and Policy*, **2**, 14–8.

Jenkinson C., Layte R., Wright L. *et al.* (1996). *The UK SF-36: an analysis and interpretation manual.* Health Services Research Unit, Oxford.

Kitzhaber J.A. (1993). Prioritizing health services in an era of limits: the Oregon experiment. *British Medical Journal*, **307**, 373–7.

Krasnik A., Groenewegen P., Pedersen P.A. *et al.* (1990). Changing remuneration systems: effects on activity in general practice. *British Medical Journal*, **300**, 1698–701.

Kurtin P., Davies A., Meyer K. *et al.* (1992). Patient-based health status measurements in outpatient dialysis: early experiences in developing an outcomes assessment program. *Medical Care*, **30** (Supplement 5), MS136–49.

Levine M., Guyatt G., Gent M. *et al.* (1988). Quality of life in stage II breast cancer: an instrument for clinical trials. *Journal of Clinical Oncology*, **6**, 1798–810.

Liss P.E. (1990). *Health care need: meaning and measurement.* Linkoping University, Linkoping.

Loewy E.H. (1990). Commodities, needs and health care: a communal perspective. In: *Changing values in medical and health care decision making* (ed. J.J. Jensen and G. Mooney), pp. 17–31. Wiley, Chichester.

Loomes G. and McKenzie I. (1989). The scope and limitations of QALY measures. *Social Science and Medicine*, **28**, 299–308.

McLeod H. (2004). *Social Health Insurance: An introduction for practitioners.* University of Pretoria, Pretoria.

McHorney C., Ware J., Rogers W. *et al.* (1992). The validity and relative precision of MOS short- and long-form health status scales and Dartmouth COOP charts: results from the medical outcomes study. *Medical Care*, **30** (Supplement 5), MS253–65.

McHorney C., Ware J., and Raczek A. (1993). The MOS 36-item short form health survey. II: Psychometric and clinical tests of validity in measuring physical and mental health constructs. *Medical Care*, **31**, 247–63.

Maslow A.H. (1943). A theory of human motivation. *Psychological Review*, **50**, 370–396

Mason A.R., Drummond M.F., Hunter J.A. *et al.* (2005). Prescribing incentive schemes: a useful approach? *Applied Health Economics and Health Policy*, **4**(2), 111–117

Mehrez A. and Gafni A. (1989). Quality adjusted life years, utility theory and healthy year equivalents. *Medical Decision Making*, **9**, 142–9.

MHSS (Ministry of Health and Social Services) and WHO (World Health Organization), Namibia (2005). *Equity in health care in Namibia: Towards needs-based allocation formula.* Regional Network for Equity in Health in Southern Africa (EQUINET), Harare. (http://www.equinetafrica.org/bibl/docs/DIS26finNamibia.pdf)

Mooney G. (1998). 'Communitarian claims' as an ethical basis for allocating health care resources. *Social Science and Medicine*, **47**, 1171–80.

Mooney G.H. and Blackwell S.H. (2004) Whose health service is it anyway? Community values in healthcare. *Medical Journal of Australia*, **180**, 76–8.

Mooney G. and Creese A. (1993). Priority setting for health service efficiency: the role of measurement of burden of illness. In *Disease control priorities in developing countries* (ed. D. Jamison, W. Mosely, A. Measham and J. Bobadilla). Oxford University Press, New York.

Mooney G. and Houston S. (2004). An alternative approach to resource allocation: weighted capacity to benefit plus MESH infrastructure. *Applied Health Economics and Health Policy*, **3**(1), 29–33.

Mooney G., Jan S., and Wiseman V. (1995). Examining preferences for allocating health gains. *Health Care Analysis*, **3**, 261–5.

Murray C.J.L. (1994). Quantifying the burden of disease: the technical basis for disability-adjusted life years. *Bulletin of the World Health Organization*, **72**(3), 429–45.

Murray C. and Lopez A. (1997a). The utility of DALYs for public health policy and research: a reply. *Bulletin of the World Health Organization*, **75**, 377–81.

Murray C.J.L. and Lopez A.D. (1997b). Regional patterns of disability-free life expectancy and disability-adjusted life expectancy: Global Burden of Disease Study. *The Lancet*, **349**, 1347–52.

Nord E., Richardson J., Street A. *et al.* (1995). Maximising health benefits versus egalitarianism: an Australian survey of health issues. *Social Science and Medicine*, **41**(10),1429–37.

Oberlander J. (2007). Health reform interrupted: The unravelling of the Oregon Health Plan. *Health Affairs*, **26**(1), 96–105.

Olsen K.M. and Dahl S.A. (2007). Health differences between European countries. *Social Science and Medicine* (in press).

Oregon Health Plan (1997). *The uninsured in Oregon 1977.* Office for Oregon Health Plan Research, Salem.

O'Reilly D., Rosato M., and Patterson C. (2005) Self reported health and mortality: ecological analysis based on electoral wards across the United Kingdom. *British Medical Journal*, **331**(7522), 938–939.

Paalman M., Bekedam H., Hawken L. *et al.* (1998). A critical review of priority setting in the health sector: the methodology of the 1993 World Development Report. *Health Policy and Planning*, **13**(1), 13–31.

Pearson M. (2002). *Allocating Public Resources for Health: Developing Pro-poor Approaches.* DFID Health Systems Resource Centre, London.

Rocha G., Martinez A., Rios E. *et al.* (2004) Resource allocation equity in northeastern Mexico. *Health Policy*, **70**, 271–9.

Sayers B.M. and Fliedner T.M. (1997). The critique of DALYs: a counter-reply. *Bulletin of the World Health Organization*, **75**, 383–4.

Sculpher M. (2006) The use of quality-adjusted life-years in cost-effectiveness studies. *Allergy*, **61**(5), 527–30.

Sen A. (1987). *On ethics and economics.* Basil Blackwell, Oxford.

Teng T.O. (1996). An evaluation of Oregon's Medicaid rationing algorithms. *Health Economics*, **5**, 171–81.

Thomas S., Mooney G., and Mbatsha S. (2007). The MESH approach: strengthening public health systems for the MDGs. *Health Policy*, **83**(2-3), 180–5.

Torrance G.W. (1986). Measurement of health state utilities for economic appraisal. *Journal of Health Economics*, **5**, 1–30.

Ugalde A. and Jackson J.T. (1995). The World Bank and international health policy: A critical review. *Journal of International Development*, **7**(3), 525–41.

van Vliet R.C.J.A. and van de Ven P.M.M. (1992). Towards a capitation formula for competing health insurers: An empirical analysis. *Social Science and Medicine*, **34**(9), 1035–48.

Ware J., Kosinski M., and Keller S. (1996). A 12-item short-form health survey: construction of scales and preliminary tests of reliability and validity. *Medical Care*, **34**, 220–33.

Ware J., Snow K., Kosinski M. *et al.* (1993). *SF-36 survey manual and interpretation guide.* Health Institute, New England Medical Center, Boston, MA.

WHOQOL SRPB Group (2006). A cross cultural study of spirituality, religion, and personal beliefs as components of quality of life. *Social Science and Medicine*, **62**(6), 1486–97.

Williams A. (1985). Economic of coronary artery bypass grafting. *British Medical Journal*, **49**, 825–31.

Williams A. (1999). Calculating the global burden of disease: time for a strategic reappraisal? *Health Economics*, **8**, 1–8.

Wiseman V. (1999). Culture, self-rated health and resource allocation decision-making. *Health Care Analysis*, **7**, 207–23.

Wiseman V. and Mooney G. (1998). Burden of illness estimates for priority setting: a debate revisited. *Health Policy*, **43**, 243–51.

Wiseman V., Mooney G., Berry G. *et al.* (2003). Involving the general public in priority setting: experiences from Australia. *Social Science and Medicine*, **56**, 1001–12.

World Bank (1993). *World Development Report 1993: Investing in Health.* Oxford University Press for The World Bank, New York.

World Bank (1994). *Better Health in Africa: Experience and Lessons Learned.* The World Bank, Washington, D.C.

World Health Organization (2001). *Macroeonomics and Health: Investing in Health for Economic Development. Report of the Commission on Macroeconomics and Health.* World Health Organization, Geneva.

Needs assessment:
A practical approach

Aileen Clarke, John Powell, and
Mary Ann Lansang[1]

Abstract

Needs assessment is an essential part of planning for health care and public health. This chapter describes a practical approach to needs assessment, building on the previous chapter on need and its measurement (McIntyre *et al.* 2009). Needs assessment aims to ensure a population-based, epidemiological, and public health approach to the planning of health interventions. It is of particular importance in publicly funded systems but is also of value in other systems. A needs assessment should provide a specific plan for meeting the needs of a specific population, with a specified health condition or set of conditions, taking questions of effectiveness, affordability, allocative efficiency, equity, and access into account and independent of competing clinical or commercial interests. A conventional needs assessment includes epidemiological, comparative, and corporate components although this chapter also considers rapid needs assessment and participatory community appraisal techniques. In the past, needs assessment has been seen as failing to contribute expected benefits; however, needs assessment has great potential to contribute valuable practical public health inputs to any health organization's activities.

Introduction

Need for needs assessment

In any health system, decisions must be made about the introduction of new services, the closure of old services, and the re-organization of others. How should such decision be taken? While there is often an underlying emphasis on financial considerations, health and health improvement have to be key considerations.

Health planning often follows an incremental approach, with a varying ability of planners and managers to respond rationally to changes in demography, the epidemiology of disease or the availability of new pharmaceuticals or technologies (Buse *et al.* 2007). Needs assessment can provide a rational, systematic, and analytical approach to planning health care as part of a cycle of planning, execution, or implementation of change, management, and review (Fig. 12.2.1).

Definitions and issues of definition in needs assessment

Needs assessment is the process of identifying need for health interventions and its distribution in a population. Need has been defined as 'the capacity to benefit' (McIntyre *et al.* 2009), but it is important to consider definitions of both 'capacity' and 'benefit'. Capacity is defined here as the ability to make use of a needed intervention. Benefit is defined as a reduction in disease or disability or an improvement in health. However, need is a value-laden and contested concept as McIntyre, Mooney, and Jan demonstrate (McIntyre *et al.* 2009). This raises questions concerning whose view of capacity should be taken into account? And whose estimate of the extent of a reduction in disease or disability should be considered as representing a legitimate benefit?

It is also important to distinguish 'need' from 'demand or want' and from 'utilization' or 'supply' (Fig. 12.2.2). Need has sometimes

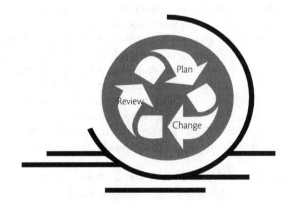

Fig. 12.2.1 Forward rolling cycle of management planning, implementing change, and review.

---

[1] M. A. Lansang, chapter co-author, currently works at The Global Fund to Fight AIDS, Tuberculosis and Malaria. The views expressed in this chapter are those of the named authors and do not necessarily reflect the decisions or stated policy of The Global Fund.

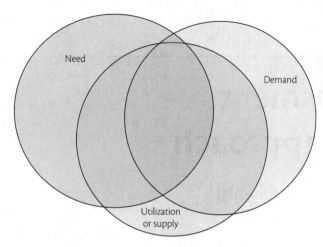

Fig. 12.2.2 Overlapping circles of need, demand, and utilization. (For most conditions there is little empirical evidence for the extent to which these circles overlap.)

been defined as the professional view of capacity to benefit; if the clinical professional view is that those with a certain level of severity of a condition will benefit from a specific intervention, then they are considered to have a 'need'. If a person believes that they have a capacity to benefit from an intervention that is considered a 'want'. The want can be translated into a demand by a request for that intervention. Need and demand can of course co-exist or exist separately. When professionally-defined need is not addressed by services, there is said to be 'unmet need'.

Utilization (or use or supply) of health services can exist in the absence of need. As an example, some would say that high rates of upper gastrointestinal endoscopy may represent utilization without need (NICE 2007). It is much rarer for utilization to occur without demand. Usually if a person takes up a service or intervention, it can be assumed that it is demanded (although compulsory psychiatric intervention could be seen as utilization without demand).

It is also important to be aware that supplier-induced demand can occur, as for example, where suppliers (health care organizations or clinicians) increase intervention levels to rates which are higher than expected, given levels of need. Supplier-induced demand is often found where financial incentives encourage intervention. This has been demonstrated in many health systems in relation to fee-for-service payments, for example, in dentistry, or where excessively high Caesarean section rates occur. The phenomenon of supplier-induced demand is recorded in many clinical areas and in different parts of the world (Murray 2000; Delattre & Dormont 2003).

Rates of utilization of services are the end result of a complex interplay of population demography, need, and demand. They are related to the extent of unmet need, supplier-induced demand, and the availability of services, as well as a population's ability to access them (McKee & Clarke 1995). In some rare urgent and emergency cases, for example severe head injury due to road accidents (Williams *et al.* 1997), utilization rates may come close to reflecting the actual level of need within a population, but in most cases, utilization rates used in this way will not give an accurate estimate of need.

Levels of needs assessment

It is important to be aware that needs assessment as defined may be undertaken at a number of different levels. Needs assessment can be undertaken for:

a) A whole population

b) A subgroup of the population (McNeil *et al.* 2006; Wright & Tomkins 2006)

c) A subgroup of the population suffering from a specific condition, e.g. stroke (Mant *et al.* 2004) or drug misuse (Marsden *et al.* 2004) or for specific interventions, e.g. hip replacement (Dawson *et al.* 2004), carotid endarterectomy (Ferris *et al.* 1998), or emergency obstetric care (Orinda *et al.* 2005)

d) For a population using a particular service, e.g. psychology and counselling services, rural primary care services, accident and emergency services (Williams *et al.* 1997); and prison health service (Cresswell *et al.* 2005)

e) For an individual person or family. Need for healthcare, housing, food, sanitation, safety, etc., can be gauged for individuals and a service or treatment plan put in action

This chapter will focus mainly on needs assessment at levels c and d in the above classification (subgroups of the population either suffering from a specific condition or in need of a specific intervention, and assessment of need for a particular health service). Level e will not be considered further because in this chapter concentrates on needs assessment at the population level. The principles of needs assessment for levels a and b are similar to those for c and d, although this sort of needs assessment can sometimes be important (McNeil *et al.* 2006). The process of starting from a zero base to work out the whole health care needs of a population is rarely undertaken except in emergency situations (McNeil *et al.* 2006). Thinking further about levels c and d, it is also possible to undertake needs assessment either for a service, e.g. blood transfusion services or smoking prevention services or for a recognized disease or problem, e.g. alcohol misuse (Cook 2004). Needs assessment can be undertaken for different types of health intervention, e.g. for health protection and infectious disease control; for health education, health promotion and disease prevention; for screening and immunization; for diagnostics; for acute treatments and ongoing treatment for chronic disease, for rehabilitation, and for terminal and palliative care. A public health approach would normally include health education, health promotion, and disease prevention as part of the range of interventions for any condition.

Timing of needs assessment

When should a needs assessment be undertaken? Ideally, a needs assessment should be undertaken whenever a major change in a health services or programme is anticipated or occurs. Of course, a needs assessment should be undertaken in advance of a planned change in order to inform that change. A needs assessment should not be undertaken simply to provide a post hoc justification for a change that has already been agreed.

When does a needs assessment end? This is not a spurious question since many models of needs assessment discuss the process of implementing change. This chapter will cover the process of needs assessment until a recommended, evidence-based, and costed plan for change has been produced, but many would suggest that the needs assessment does not end here and that the management processes for implementing change are also part of the needs assessment.

The definitions and distinctions outlined in this section are important because they impact on methods for undertaking needs assessments. Often in needs assessments, normative judgements of need are used, demands are not always included or viewed as legitimate, unmet need is considered too difficult to measure, and utilization rates are used as a proxy for need. However, needs assessment should distinguish between demand and need and evaluate met and unmet needs taking into account the contextual and value-laden nature of the definition of need. This may be of particular importance if either the health care intervention under consideration or proposed changes are controversial. Community participatory techniques and rapid assessment procedures (RAP), which are discussed later in the chapter, both tackle some of these issues directly.

Undertaking a needs assessment

The aim of needs assessment is to deliver practical information to change public health and health services. One useful definition is; 'to maximize the appropriate delivery of effective health interventions or care and to minimize both the provision of ineffective health intervention or care and the existence of unmet need for healthcare in an evidence-based way', and to 'maximize equity' (Powell 2006). This definition gives the overall aim of a needs assessment and in the following section we will break down the practicalities of needs assessment into a series of steps. In practice these will require adaptation to local circumstances.

A needs assessment is highly dependent on data. Variations occur in the availability, extent, reliability, and validity of data sources both for the evidence of effectiveness and for the underlying demography of the population of interest. One of the recurring themes in needs assessment is to what extent can, or should, new data be gathered? We would suggest that for a practical needs assessment to be of value in usual health management timescales, new data collection should be kept to an absolute minimum, but that pragmatism should prevail. In some low- and middle-income countries, there are often no alternatives to the collection of new data as many routine health statistics are incomplete, unreliable, and inaccurate. In emergency situations, *ad hoc* data collection is the rule. Rapid Appraisal Procedures are of particular value in this context.

A number of models for undertaking a needs assessment have been proposed including those of Cavanagh and Chadwick (2005) and Stevens and Raftery (2004), and we draw on both of these in the following sections. In particular, we will draw on an 'epidemiological, corporate and comparative' model (Stevens & Raftery 2004) in the following plan of action for a needs assessment.

Problem definition

As with any project, planning is required in the early stages to clarify aims and objectives and the reasons for undertaking a needs assessment. It is important to clarify who the 'customer' or commissioner of the needs assessment is, what they hope to achieve from the needs assessment, how much resource they can offer for the needs assessment to be undertaken, their role within the health or public health system and their relationships with other stakeholders. Needs assessments can present those managing health services with hard choices and difficult decisions, and it is important that those undertaking a needs assessment are aware of this

---

Box 12.2.1 Seven questions to be asked before undertaking a needs assessment

1. Why is this needs assessment needed now?

2. Who will be affected?

3. What would be the consequences of doing nothing?

4. How much time is available? There may be pivotal decision points within the organization for which the results of the needs assessment will be needed.

5. How can the results and recommendations of the needs assessment be produced and presented to facilitate informed action?

6. Are sufficient resources available? This includes managerial support at the appropriate level for implementation

7. How will the needs assessment itself be assessed and evaluated?

---

from the outset. Certain questions should be asked, and answered, at this stage before a needs assessment can proceed, and these are shown in Box 12.2.1.

Stakeholder advisory group

A number of stakeholders will need to give their view on the definition of the problem and the issues which will need to be included. Ideally at the earliest stage, a stakeholder advisory group should be set up. The group should include the commissioner of the needs assessment, and other key stakeholders. These would usually include clinical or health experts in the field (current providers of services either may or may not be included); and may also include methodological experts; members of local communities, users of services and their representatives; voluntary sector, religious and charity representatives, and representatives of other concerned organizations (e.g. local councils or local or district authorities) or individuals. While it is very important to be clear about the advisory nature of these stakeholders' roles, is also important to be inclusive at this stage, in order to offer the needs assessment the optimal chance of legitimacy and implementation. Community participatory needs assessments tend to afford greater emphasis to engagement of members of the community at this stage. Box 12.2.2 shows an example of stakeholder involvement.

Project plan

The next phase of the needs assessment is to develop a formal costed project plan. The work should be broken down into manageable steps. For each step, an estimate of how long it will take, and how much it will cost should be made, and tasks should be allocated so that is clear who will undertake the work and how dependencies in timings between different project components will be managed. Production of a project plan may seem either a luxury or a nuisance; however, this planning stage is invaluable in developing a proper understanding of the work. The project plan can be used to monitor progress and can be amplified and modified as a working document which can be built on to produce the report of the work.

Box 12.2.2　Stakeholders in a needs assessment for male circumcision for HIV/AIDS prevention and control

Recent evidence from three randomized controlled trials in Africa shows reduction of HIV/AIDS by more than half among males who were circumcised (see detailed discussion of the evidence in Chapter 6.11, this volume). Male circumcision has been hailed by many international health organizations as an important intervention for HIV/AIDS prevention, particularly in high-burden areas like sub-Saharan Africa, India, and China.

But Sawires *et al.* (2007) have identified at least 13 issues that need to be considered for effective implementation, for example, acceptability among men and women, and among different ethnic and religious groups; perceptions of benefits and risks; timing of circumcision; safety and complications; and health system requirements.

For a needs assessment for services to increase the use of male circumcision for HIV/AIDS prevention, stakeholders will include:

- Experts: HIV/AIDS, epidemiology, behavioural sciences, mathematical modelling, health economics, communications, bioethics
- Policy makers: Local, regional, and national
- Health service payers and providers
- NGOs
- Religious and rights-based groups
- Community representatives especially for young people, and people living with AIDS

Box 12.2.3　Stages of a needs assessment

A. *Epidemiological needs assessment*—which answers the questions: How many people 'need' care for this condition in the local population and what effective interventions should be available for them?

B. *Comparative needs assessment*—which answers the question: How do others provide services for this condition?

C. *Corporate or local needs assessment*—which answers a series of questions. How are services currently provided locally? How does this compare with expected provision given evidence on incidence and prevalence? How do current treatments and interventions compare with the evidence of effectiveness? How do local services compare with those in other places? How do local treatments and services compare with what others consider should be done? (e.g. patient groups, government departments insurers, payers, etc.). What are the gaps? What are the options for improvement? What changes are required and how much will they cost?

Models of needs assessment

Drawing on Stevens and Raftery (2004) we are going to describe a detailed plan for how to undertake a needs assessment using epidemiological, corporate, and comparative approaches. Box 12.2.3 shows these stages of the Stevens and Raftery model. After describing this approach we will describe Rapid Assessment Procedures which are useful to provide information where data sources are limited and/or when the needs assessment is required urgently.

Epidemiological needs assessment: The population of interest

How many people 'need' care for this condition in the local population and what effective interventions are available for them?

The first phase of the actual work is to begin to understand the underlying characteristics of the population of interest from whom the population of those with a need for the service/s under consideration is drawn. As mentioned in the introductory section, the local population may be defined geographically, or by a particular insurance plan, or as a particular subgroup of a community. The demography of the local population, including age and sex structure and mortality, needs to be understood, along with any information available on broader health, welfare, and public health issues, health status, inequalities, and socioeconomic status, demand for health care, and underlying relevant risk factors.

Gathering data on the local or denominator population will be important for two reasons. First, it is important to be able to locate a needs assessment properly within an understanding of competing priorities for both the organization and for the population itself. This can only be done by developing an understanding of the population of interest. Secondly, much of the available epidemiological evidence for particular conditions is available, using age- and sex-standardized rates per hundred thousand population. In order to derive local estimates and to understand need (absolute numbers of those requiring interventions), the age and sex structure and characteristics of the local population need to be understood.

Many organizations publish demographic data which are relatively easily accessible for geographic areas and for appropriate reference populations. In many countries, routine data collection and manipulation, including censuses, death certification statistics and population projections, and estimates together allow for a picture of the structure of a population to be built up (National Statistics 2007). Insurance companies keep their own enrollees' demographic data (Young *et al.* 1991). Exceptions exist in poor countries or countries where breakdown in civil structures has occurred, during war, for example, where censuses are non-existent or unreliable, where special surveys may have to be undertaken to provide estimates of the relevant population structure. For some countries, where national information systems are weak, there have been efforts over the past 30 years to establish health and demographic surveillance systems to provide longitudinal, population-based data on important health and vital events for specific geographic areas or sentinel sites (Adazu *et al.* 2005). The INDEPTH Network (an International Network of field sites with continuous Demographic Evaluation of Populations and Their Health in developing countries) has 37 demographic surveillance sites in 19 countries. Problems can also arise in attempting to undertake a needs assessment for a subgroup of a community where no reliable population data exist and the issue of whether such data should be collected *de novo* arises.

Information on the structure of the local population may be relatively easy to access in many countries, but information on broader health and welfare, inequalities, socioeconomic status, and health status and demand for health care, and underlying relevant risk factors, may be much more difficult to obtain. In many countries, data on mortality by cause are collected which have been used as a measure of demand for health care, although there are drawbacks to this use of mortality data in needs assessments, as McIntyre, Mooney, and Jan point out (McIntyre *et al.* 2009). In the United Kingdom, the Health Survey for England (DH Health Survey 2007) provides data on levels of smoking or obesity, or health status but these rates are derived from relatively small samples of the overall UK population and are not always valid for smaller population groups. However, many local public health organizations undertake local health surveys, which document demography, health determinants (e.g. health risks and health behaviours), and health status, and these can be extremely valuable. Community participation can also be valuable here, where communities themselves can participate in local data collection. This is discussed again later in this chapter.

Epidemiological needs assessment: Conditions and levels of severity

The next step is to consider the conditions or diseases for which the needs assessment is being undertaken and, in particular, to consider known levels of severity, since need for intervention will vary with levels of severity. The main sources of information include published research literature, grey literature, policy documents, guidelines, and textbooks, but in some countries there will be morbidity surveys, or disease registries, for example, cancer registry data, which can be used. It may also be the case that others have already undertaken a needs assessment in the area and already listed relevant categories of severity. Literature searching techniques are not covered in detail in this chapter, but for this stage of a practical needs assessment, literature searching in order to understand categories of severity does not have to be exhaustive and governed by the same strict rules as for systematic reviews. It does, however, need to be systematic in its coverage of the important information and reasonably up-to-date since methods of categorizing diseases change.

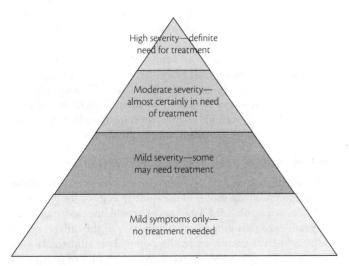

High severity—definite need for treatment

Moderate severity—almost certainly in need of treatment

Mild severity—some may need treatment

Mild symptoms only—no treatment needed

Fig. 12.2.3 Subcategories and levels of need in a population.

For some conditions and diseases, reliable and valid methods for measuring grades of severity are well documented. Examples include the American Urologists Association (AUA) categorization for prostatic hypertrophy (Barry *et al.* 1992), the international TNM (tumour, node, metastasis) systems for the classification of cancers (UICC and TNM 2007), the Oxford hip score (Dawson *et al.* 2001), and many more. Figure 12.2.3 gives a diagrammatic representation of the information to be collected on levels of severity.

A common scenario is that it is only possible to obtain estimates of incidence and prevalence for those in the most severe category of illness. However, a 'public health' approach, means that all those in each relevant category including those in the general population eligible for screening or primary prevention should also be estimated.

Epidemiological needs assessment: Risk factors

While it is very important to know the likely numbers of people in each grade of severity, it is also important to understand these differential risk subgroups in the population of interest who may experience a different rate of the disease under consideration. They may be either unequally exposed to an important determinant or unequally susceptible to the exposure and the likelihood of disease. There may be specific risk factors for the condition under consideration which need taking into account. One example would be in needs for diabetes services where the levels of people in any particular severity category are related to characteristics of the underlying population, e.g. levels of diet and physical activity (Chowdhury *et al.* 2005). For example, in hepatic cirrhosis, levels of alcohol consumption in the population will need to be measured or estimated.

Epidemiological needs assessment: Numbers affected by conditions and levels of severity within the reference population

Information on the population of interest and information on the diseases or conditions under consideration should be combined to estimate the absolute numbers of people suffering from the condition both overall and within each category of severity. It is important at this stage to be clear about absolute numbers in each level of severity and not to confuse absolute and relative measures of risk. Ideally, it would be possible to obtain incidence and prevalence values directly for the local population itself, but the possibilities either of data being available or for them to be collected within the time available for a needs assessment are low. There are often gaps in the evidence, and it is almost always necessary to extrapolate from other populations from epidemiological surveys or from health needs assessments elsewhere.

Given this extrapolation it is important for assumptions made to be made explicit. For example, one might assume that epidemiology of cataracts of the eye might be comparable between different cities in the same country (Wadud *et al.* 2006), or that rates of severe ankle sprain in children and young people apply equally in two different European cities. These are testable assumptions and contestable if clearly stated in the needs assessment. Figure 12.2.4 gives an example of an epidemiological study where information might be used in a needs assessment. Figure 12.2.4 shows World Health Organization (WHO) estimated numbers of new TB cases in different countries in the world in 2005. This map illustrates variations in numbers, and the complete lack of data from some countries. Of course, for a local or regional needs assessment it is very important to have more detailed data on absolute numbers of

Estimated numbers of new TB cases, 2005

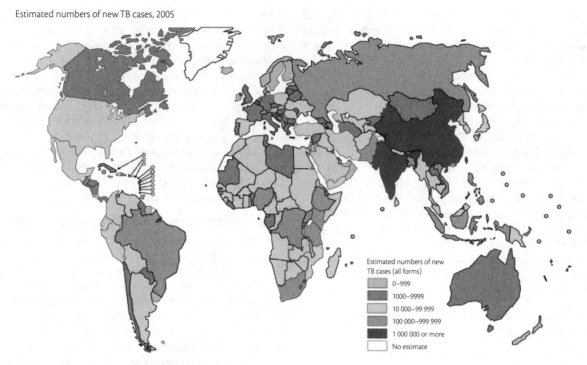

Fig. 12.2.4 Estimated numbers of new cases of TB by country in 2005.
Source: WHO Report 2007. Global Tuberculosis Control. Surveillance, Planning and Financing http://www.who.int/tb/publications/global_report/2007/pdf/full.pdf

those affected. An ideal approach is to have estimates of both incidence and prevalence. Need for services varies with stages in the trajectory of illness, but service use is often highly concentrated around the time of diagnosis, and assessment of needs is enhanced if absolute numbers of both incident cases per year and prevalent cases can be estimated. A significant problem in this part of a needs assessment is that often there is very little evidence relating to the natural history of disease. Little is known about what happens in the absence of treatment. However, natural history is important when 'unmet need' is being considered. Evidence may be sparse or lacking in this area, and discussion with clinicians may provide the most fruitful information. Another problem is attempting to understand factors affecting demand. This may not be an easy task although there is some literature which is published on this topic for different disease areas (e.g. reluctance to attend for screening appointments (Chan *et al.* 2002), but the relationship between need and demand is under-researched, and there may be little evidence to find.

Epidemiological needs assessment: The evidence on effectiveness and costs

The next stage of the needs assessment is to find and appraise evidence of the clinical and cost-effectiveness of interventions for the condition and for its different subcategories. This part of the needs assessment again requires searching of the research literature, grey literature, and policy documents to find the range of interventions available and estimates of their effectiveness. Interventions can act at a number of different levels and may include methods for screening or prevention as well as pharmaceutical or surgical interventions, rehabilitation services, etc. It is customary to take as much account of the hierarchy of evidence as possible in deriving the evidence base in a needs assessment. Therefore, for example, evidence consisting of systematic reviews of large number of large

randomized controlled trials (RCTs) should clearly be given more weight than single RCTs which should themselves be given more weight than observational designs and other evidence further down the hierarchy. However, it is often hard to find evidence to support the use of a particular well-known intervention which is believed to be beneficial. It is important to document these evidence gaps, and many needs assessments include recommendations for further research, recognizing a need for more and better evidence for common interventions. It is important at this stage not to be constrained by an awareness of the health services that are already currently provided to the population for the conditions under consideration but to approach the evidence in a spirit of inquiry. Sometimes radically different combinations of treatments or specific interventions can be shown to be more beneficial than those which are currently provided. Cost-effectiveness (e.g. expressed as cost per unit health benefit) or cost-utility (e.g. expressed as cost/QALY) evidence are equally as important as evidence of clinical benefit at this stage. The Disease Control Priorities Project, has developed cost-effectiveness estimates for some public health problems, especially those affecting low- and middle-income countries (The Disease Control Priorities Project 2006). However, evidence may often be lacking, and estimates of relative costs and benefits will sometimes be required in order for decisions to be made between different options.

Epidemiological needs assessment: Synthesis

At this stage, it should be possible to synthesize the information gathered to produce a model of the epidemiology of the condition in the local population. The model would include incidence and prevalence (absolute numbers) of each of the different subcategories of the condition in the population, adjusted (up or down) for underlying relevant risk factors; with a list of treatments and interventions ranked according to evidence of effectiveness and evidence relating to costs effectiveness and estimated actual likely costs where available. Often, the information estimated will be incomplete and imprecise, but this summary is the basis on which the next stages can be built.

Comparative needs assessment

How do others provide services for this condition?

Armed with the evidence of clinical and cost-effectiveness and an understanding of the local populations' needs, the aim of this phase of the needs assessment is to investigate how others approach meeting need and organizing services for the condition under consideration.

Comparative needs assessment: Models of care in practice

The research and grey literatures may be helpful in investigating others' approaches to organizing services and care pathways and patterns. It will be important to identify similar populations, systems, and services to the one under study and to meet those providing those services, to investigate what they do and the problems and issues that they face. This phase does not have to be restricted by country, and other countries may offer useful insights into how to provide care for particular conditions.

This phase may also simply be about opening a dialogue with other health service or health care providers to find out how they plan and offer services for this condition. It may help to be reasonably systematic about data gathering especially if a number of providers are being consulted at this stage, in order to ensure that all important items are covered. This part of the needs assessment should result in a list of models of care including patient care patterns and pathways and their relative strengths in practice.

Comparative needs assessment: The existence of variation

The existence of variation in intervention rates presents a problem for comparative needs assessment. Internationally, substantial variation in health care provision and utilization has been described, much of it not explained by known factors such as the apparent level of morbidity or 'need' within a population (Weinstein 2004). Therefore, it should be recognized that chosen comparators may be outliers, either under- or over-providing services for patients with a particular condition. Figure 12.2.5 illustrates this graphically. Women living in different districts in England had a varying likelihood of undergoing hysterectomy within the NHS between 1999 and 2003. Age-standardized rates can be seen to vary dramatically (Goldacre *et al.* 2005). Although the best comparators from a population point of view should be chosen, the possibility should also be considered that these chosen comparators may not be representative.

These figures show that quantitative, comparative needs assessment can be useful for highlighting variation and raising questions about that variation. However, comparative needs assessment may be most useful for providing a list of organizational models and patterns of care.

Corporate needs assessment

How are services currently provided locally? How does this compare with expected provision given evidence on incidence

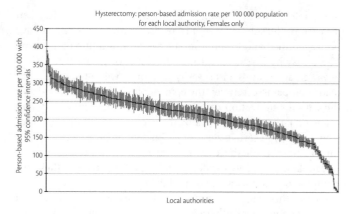

Fig. 12.2.5 Standardized admission rates (SARs) for hysterectomy per 100 000 women for a 3-year period (1998–1999 to 2002–2003), by local authority area with 95% confidence intervals.

Source: Unit for Health care Epidemiology, University of Oxford. (Each dot shows the rate for women in a single local authority and the border shows 95% confidence intervals.)

and prevalence? How do current treatments and interventions compare with the evidence of effectiveness? How do local services compare with those in other places? How do local treatments and services compare with what others consider should be done (e.g. patient groups, government departments insurers, payers, etc.)? What are the gaps? What are the options for improvement? What changes are required, and how much will they cost?

Corporate needs assessment: Current model of care

The corporate needs assessment is the stage where ongoing input from the stakeholder group will be most useful. For the first task of the corporate needs assessment, it is necessary to understand current service provision and utilization statistics. The best approach to this phase is a thorough and systematic data gathering process where all providers, and all relevant service users and members of the public are identified. Utilization data should be collected for all aspects of the care pathway, to organize data into a current working model of care used in practice. Routine data should, if possible, be gathered from primary or first contact care, from secondary and tertiary care, and from community and local government providers. There will be a problem in many regions and countries of missing, incomplete, or out-of-date data. Some commercial providers are unwilling to release data on patient flows through specific care pathways, and in some countries such data are not collected at all and often best estimates of current provision need to be made. At this stage, it is important to attempt to gather information in the same subcategories of disease that were developed earlier. However, information is not always collected in this way and again a pragmatic approach may be needed.

Corporate needs assessment: Comparison of current model of care with epidemiological needs assessment

Next a comparison needs to be made between the current model of care, 'the observed model', and the 'expected model' based on evidence derived from the epidemiological needs assessment. Is the pattern and level of provision equivalent to expected levels, given the known epidemiology, the evidence base, and the local demography of the reference population? This process needs to be undertaken for each of the subcategories of the disease or condition that have been identified and for appropriate age-groups in the population. These may be 5-year age-groups, to allow for greatest precision, however, age-groups and severity categories will often need to be made comparable between the epidemiological data collected and the data for utilization or actual provision. This is not easy and again may require assumptions to be made, for example, about epidemiology in certain age groups. Epidemiological evidence may, for example, omit the over 85-year-olds or the under-5s, and extrapolation of likely incidence and prevalence rates in these age groups and need for care may need to be made.

Also at this stage, it is important to consider inequalities and equity. The needs of otherwise underserved groups need special consideration. People such as the very elderly, those with social or language barriers to accessing services (the homeless, refugees, etc.), and those who are very poor, will almost certainly need special consideration. There may or may not be relevant evidence to cover the needs of these groups, but best efforts should be made to ensure that the model being constructed of care pathways is inclusive of the relevant social and care groups.

However, the idea here is not to build up the perfect definitive picture of expected provision versus observed utilization—but to derive practical working estimates of the discrepancies between the two, whilst acknowledging assumptions which have had to be made on the way.

At this stage, the issue of 'use-for-need' needs consideration. Although observed and expected levels of treatment for a particular condition may be consistent, it is possible that both unmet and over-met needs exist. Figure 12.2.6 illustrates this point.

This model, referred to previously in Fig. 12.2.3, can also be used to consider the problem of unmet need. There is a small group at the top of the pyramid who have a clear and definite need for the intervention(s) under consideration. At lower levels, there are more people in each layer but their need for intervention is less. If we assume that everybody above line B 'needs' intervention but that most services are provided along line C, then some people who need services do not receive it, whilst others who do not need it receive it. Needs assessment should be able to help make line B more horizontal, reducing 'unmet' and also 'over-met' needs. This diagram can also be used to consider equity and inequalities.

Perhaps some of those inappropriately above line C are more vociferous and demanding, and some of those who are below the line do not come forward even though they 'need' services. It is important to consider how current treatments and interventions compare with the evidence of effectiveness that has been compiled. Which interventions are commonly used for our population under consideration, and what is the evidence in favour of them? As we mentioned previously, for some areas of care there is very little good evidence. But if relevant evidence is already being used in providing care it is important to understand this.

Corporate needs assessment: Consultation with stakeholders

This is the stage where the input of the different pressure groups and interest group views can formally be taken into account. Systematic qualitative data collection should be undertaken to understand the views of the stakeholders and interest groups about what should be changed and why. It is valuable at this stage to include patient groups and providers as well as those involved in strategic planning for the service. Stakeholders will include patient and community groups, professional bodies, government departments, insurers, and payers, clinicians, auditors, and managers and others. Information on stakeholders' views of what currently works badly and what works well will also help with planning for change. At this stage, it is important to remember that some 'corporate' contributors may have their own strong agenda to bring to the table, and it will be important to consider the best strategy for dealing with these stakeholders, especially where there may be vested interests. There may also be national governmental or regional or local imperatives related to legislation or guidance. In many countries 'evidence-based' clinical practice guidelines or treatment guidelines have been adopted by national disease control programmes, which should be taken into account.

Community participation in needs assessment

Community participation can be included at many different stages of a needs assessment. Community participation might be thought of as part of the 'corporate' phase of a needs assessment where

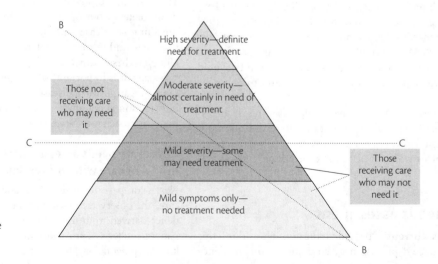

Fig. 12.2.6 Levels of need in a population. Line B represents the 'line of treatment or utilization'. Line C represents the 'line of need'.

stakeholders are consulted, but communities can play an important role in many different stages of a needs assessment in data collection; in understanding and making informed choices; in determining collective needs and priorities; and in reconciling these priorities to externally driven programme objectives. Through community participation, a sense of empowerment and ownership can be engendered among local stakeholders, increasing the chances of success of programme implementation and optimizing the use of local resources. This is in contrast to more superficial models of 'participation', which can range from passive participation, participation in information giving, participation in consultation and participation for material incentives.

Box 12.2.4 gives some examples of community participation.

Rapid assessment procedures (RAP)

Rapid assessment procedures cover a shorter period of systematic data collection than in the usual needs assessment, to provide information on health needs and status of a given community for planning and programming purposes. RAP has also been labelled as rapid ethnographic studies (RES) or rapid ethnographic procedures (REP). A related approach that allows clients and the community some control over some needs assessment tools has been labelled participatory rural appraisal (PRA). Uses include:

◆ Where health statistics and information are very limited or unreliable: For example, to assess needs among highly mobile such as urban slum dwellers (Rifkin et al. 1992) or refugees.

Box 12.2.4 Some examples of community participation in needs assessment

A. *Epidemiological needs assessment:* This was a health needs assessment using a thirty-cluster survey method in three urban areas in Dublin where there were inadequate health information systems, weak planning data and a history of inadequate recipient involvement in health service planning. Local community members, local general practitioners and other healthcare providers were trained and participated as data collectors in the surveys while the local health boards and NGOs were involved in the planning that ensured from the needs assessment (Smith *et al.* 2005)

B. *Epidemiological and 'corporate' needs assessment:* In Bangladesh communities with arsenic contamination of the water supply, a public participatory geographical information system and focus groups resulted in the development of community priorities for spatial planning of deep tubewell water for reducing arsenic contamination (Hassan 2005).

C. *Epidemiological and 'corporate' needs assessment:* Community members and local leaders in an area affected by conflict were involved in data collection and in in-depth discussions on their values and priorities for a reproductive health care needs assessment in southern Sudan. Findings revealed clear needs in reproductive health; a mismatch between the views of service providers and the community; variation in perception of need according to age, sex and whether the community was settled or displaced; lack of supplies and other barriers to accessing services (Palmer 1991).

◆ During disease outbreaks, health emergencies, and disasters where health statistics and information may have broken down, to determine needs and plan interventions rapidly (McNeil *et al.* 2006).

The steps of RAP basically follow the general methodology of health needs assessment, as described earlier in this chapter. RAP, as its name suggests, is quick and generally uses less resources and RAP studies often have small samples of key informants or other respondents. As a result RAP is often the less rigorous option—although it may be the only option available in some cases.

Methods of RAP are both quantitative and qualitative. RAP is often more participatory, partly as a pragmatic necessity. The range of qualitative research methods used in RAP and PRA are varied. They include: In-depth interviews, formal and informal observation, participant observation, focus group discussions, community mapping, case studies, community assemblies and discussions, and other cognitive or ethnographic techniques. A detailed description of some of the most commonly used ethnographic methods are provided in Chapter 7.1 of this Textbook (Morgan *et al.* 2009). Quantitative methods such as quick surveys are used in RAP to supplement or validate qualitative findings.

Synthesis and constructing the case for change

All the information gathered must be synthesized to construct the 'case for change'. It is important to be aware of how the many possible models now available—(what is *currently* in place—'the observed model'; what the evidence and epidemiology tell us *ought* to be done—'the expected model'; what the stakeholders and community *believe* should be done or *want* done—the 'hoped for' model) compare with each other. Gaps in treatments and services need to be identified, along with options for improvement, the likely changes required and the costs of such changes. Sometimes the gaps will be relatively minimal or require reorganization and changed patient care pathways within a service, but occasionally whole services will need providing. It is also important at this stage to continue to bear in mind inequalities, equity, and access to services.

Costed options are essential to allow for decision makers to understand the overall strengths and weaknesses of possible courses of action and to select between them. It is at this stage also that questions of allocative efficiency come in. How does investment in the area covered by the needs assessment compare with investment in other areas? How can the efficiency of the organization of the whole be maximized? Formal decision-making tools may be employed at this stage in order to make explicit the values, assumptions, and evidence that are being taken into consideration.

Discussion: Value and potential contribution of needs assessment

Value of needs assessments

Two evaluations of needs assessment have been undertaken (Hensher & Fulop 1999; Jordan *et al.* 2002) in the United Kingdom, and a critique has also been produced by the Department of Health in England and Wales (South Eastern Public Health Observatory 2007). Critiques suggest a lack of focus by needs assessments on population health and health outcomes, rather than on health care services; a lack of focus on prevention rather than treatment; a failure of some needs assessment to involve patients and the public; and the lack of actual use of needs assessments to change services in the 'real world'. Although important health-related costs and benefits have been identified in needs assessments, these have not necessarily been used in decision-making in the same way as purely financial considerations. It is unfortunate that evaluations paint a somewhat negative picture, and this research may need further investigation. The redesignation in 2006–2007 by the Department of Health for England and Wales as 'strategic' needs assessment suggests that needs assessments should be better tied into the needs and values of the organizations they are designed to help (South Eastern Public Health Observatory 2007).

However, it is always worth being reflective in public health practice. What went well? What went badly? What are the important research needs? Table 12.2.1 shows some of the strengths and weaknesses of the different elements of needs assessments. Later, for evaluation and audit, questions such as whether and how the needs assessment was valuable should be asked.

Boxes 12.2.5 and 12.2.6 show examples of successful needs assessments in different countries. The stages are not necessarily ordered in the same way as in this chapter but are nevertheless identifiable.

Needs assessment can be thought of as essential 'public health action' designed to tailor health programmes not to demand, or to unthinking cost restrictions, but to objectively assessed need. It has huge potential to allow for a rational approach to changing health care. As such it should be recognized as a key component of any health organization's planning framework.

The aim of needs assessment is to deliver practically useful information to change health services; to maximize the appropriate delivery of effective healthcare and to minimize the provision of ineffective care and the existence of unmet need for healthcare in an evidence-based way; and to maximize equity (Powell 2006). In this chapter, we have seen how many of the basic skills of public health, including epidemiology, statistics, and ethnographic skills, provide useful information for a needs assessment. The main steps of a needs assessment were shown to be: Understanding the rationale for the needs assessment; developing a good project plan; involving stakeholders; constructing a model of the problem in the population using the best evidence and information available (epidemiological needs assessment); comparing the model with practice in other areas (comparative needs assessment); understanding current practice and consulting widely on the problem and possible plans for change within the organization (corporate needs

Table 12.2.1 Some of the strengths and weaknesses of the different elements of needs assessments

Needs assessment	Strengths	Weaknesses
Epidemiological	◆ Rigorous ◆ Valid ◆ Reliable ◆ Uses best available evidence ◆ Gives absolute numbers ◆ Potentially less biased ◆ Potentially allows for clear understanding of 'the ideal model'	◆ Statistical expertise required ◆ Time-consuming ◆ More costly ◆ May require primary data collection ◆ Adaptation for local factors ◆ Data may not be available
Comparative	◆ Face validity ◆ Improved communications with colleagues, other stakeholders ◆ Can use routine data if available ◆ Provides comparators and benchmarks ◆ Good for identifying models used in practice	◆ Variation in service provision and organization and in health systems may make comparisons problematic ◆ Other may not be acting on the best evidence ◆ Requires adaptation for local factors
Corporate or local	◆ Essential basis on which to plan change ◆ Can use routine data if available ◆ Improved communications with decision makers and other stakeholders—allows for understanding of 'the hoped-for model' ◆ Potentially allows for clear understanding of 'what we do now—the observed model'	◆ May be swayed by local stakeholders with strong vested interests
Rapid assessment procedures	◆ Good use of limited resources ◆ Useful in an emergency situation ◆ Potentially allows for strengthened community involvement and partnerships ◆ Possibility of deeper understanding of community health needs and resources ◆ Potential for development of working hypotheses for future research or explanatory models for quantitative findings	◆ May require primary data collection ◆ Restricted generalizability of findings beyond the community studied ◆ Potential for 'bias' owing to small numbers of participants or respondents ◆ Potential for subjectivity in interpretation of qualitative data and of cultural differences in perceptions of different respondents

Box 12.2.5 Example of needs assessment for severe (morbid) obesity

The need

A local health board serving a population of 450 000 adults identified an increasing number of referrals of patients to specialist centres for the treatment of severe (morbid) obesity. There was no systematic approach to these referrals, and patients were sent to a variety of centres for a range of treatments such as various bariatric surgery procedures, with or without other interventions such as psychological assessment, and modifications to diet or physical activity The health board needed a consistent strategy for the future management of this population who have high health needs due to the associated morbidity.

Epidemiological approach

An epidemiological approach was used to estimate the numbers of adults in the local population likely to fit the clinical criteria for severe (morbid) obesity. This approach combined local population statistics with results from a health and lifestyle survey undertaken in the same region. This gave a prevalence figure for severe obesity (BMI > $40kg/m^2$) of 0.80 per cent (95% confidence interval 0.61–0.99%), implying a local population prevalence of 3 600 adults with severe obesity (95% confidence interval 2 750 to 4 460). Secondly, a systematic review was undertaken to determine the effectiveness and cost-effectiveness of the five main interventions for severe (morbid) obesity, namely diet, physical activity, psychological treatments, drug therapy, and surgery.

Corporate approach

A variety of local and national stakeholders were interviewed to capture their views on future service provision. Interviews were held with user representatives (including a voluntary organization for people with severe obesity), local clinical managers, local commissioners, local finance managers, national policymakers, and national experts on obesity treatment. A search was undertaken for relevant local or national guidelines. Finally routine activity data were examined to determine the current level of service provision. This showed that very few people with severe obesity were receiving effective interventions from the health service.

Comparative approach

Local health boards with similar populations were contacted to compare current policies and levels of service provision. Routine data collected nationally were also used to compare local provision with national averages. This data showed that the local level of need, and the local level of provision, was very similar to neighbouring areas.

Problems faced

Some of the problems faced in this needs assessment included:

- Difficulty ensuring involvement of a representative range of stakeholders
- Difficulty finding the evidence and in ensuring adequate time and skill available to synthesize it
- Difficulty with not having direct population statistics and therefore relying on extrapolation

- difficulty in incorporating new treatments (especially drugs) as they are being developed and introduced all the time with insufficient (cost)effectiveness data.

The conclusion

Nevertheless, through using the three approaches it was possible to identify and quantify significant unmet treatment needs for the local population with severe (morbid) obesity. Recommendations were made regarding future service provision, based on epidemiology, evidence of effectiveness and cost-effectiveness, expert opinion, and practice in neighbouring areas. These included increasing local provision of psychological assessment, dietary and physical activity advice. In addition local guidelines for the prescribing of obesity drugs and for the referral of patients for bariatric surgery were drawn up, to provide consistency in the future management of individuals. The prior involvement of stakeholders in the corporate element was important in ensuring implementation of the recommendations.

Source: Personal communication

Box 12.2.6 Example of needs assessment for services for mobile populations at high risk for HIV/AIDS along selected border towns in southern Africa

The need

The 'Corridors of Hope' Initiative, focused on mobile populations at high risk for HIV/AIDS along selected border towns in southern Africa. Overall, the plan was to develop 'a standard participatory methodology for evaluating HIV risk, identifying prevention opportunities and designing grounded, coordinated regional prevention initiatives'. To achieve this, a needs assessment was done from July to November 1999 in four border towns in 3 southern African countries, namely: Messina in northern South Africa, Beitbridge in southern Zimbabwe, Chirundu in northern Zimbabwe and Chirundu in southern Zambia. Specific objectives relating to these border towns were: (1) to identify STI/HIV risk factors and STI/HIV prevention opportunities at the Beitbridge–Messina and Chirundu highway and borders; and (2) to develop an implementation plan for priority STI/HIV prevention initiatives at these sites.

Epidemiological approach

Literature searches and reviews were undertaken, focusing on: Socioeconomic and health status, and morbidity and mortality data on STI and HIV/AIDS.

Corporate and comparative approaches

Policy documents and programme reports relating to STI/HIV/AIDS were reviewed.

As part of the stakeholder consultations on policy and programme priorities, the seven-member needs assessment team interviewed regional, national and provincial policymakers in the three southern African countries, including donor representatives, health employees, AIDS programme staff, NGO staff, and experts in various aspects of STI/HIV/AIDS health service delivery and education/communication.

Box 12.2.6 Example of needs assessment for services for mobile populations at high risk for HIV/AIDS along selected border towns in southern Africa (continued)

Rapid appraisal procedures approach

The field research in the selected sites employed a wide range of community participatory approaches, e.g. site inventories, mapping, behavioural surveys of sex workers, in-depth interviews, focus group discussions, ethnographic observations, and participatory learning appraisals. The field research focused on migrant men and women, including truckers, informal traders, and sex workers, but additional information on educational institutions and health services for STI.

Conclusions

The needs assessment found 'exceptional HIV vulnerability' at each border post, particularly among truckers and traders. While there were some interventions directed at sex workers, there was a notable lack of interventions for truckers as well as members of the permanent border communities who had migrant sexual partners. The needs assessment team recommended the following to the sponsoring agency and its government partners:

♦ A comprehensive prevention programme, with the following core services: Strengthened STI services, targeted interventions to protect truckers and their partners, workplace interventions; youth interventions; condom social marketing and targeted communication interventions for behavior change.

♦ Improved STI care for both sex workers and clients, including innovative strategies to reach truckers who may not avail of public health services, and regular screening for sex workers.

♦ Establishment of simple but effective project evaluation and quality assurance systems.

Acknowledgement: This regional assessment is part of the 'Corridors for Hope' Initiative funded by the United States Agency for International Development, in partnership with southern African governments and organizations. It was conducted under the auspices of Family Health International, which manages the Implementing AIDS Prevention and Care (IMPACT) Project, USAID's flagship effort for addressing the global HIV/AIDS pandemic (http://www.fhi.org/en/HIVAIDS/Projects/res_IMPACT±main±page.htm).

Source: Implementing AIDS Prevention and Care (IMPACT) Project (2007). Corridors of hope in southern Africa: HIV prevention needs and opportunities in four border towns. Family Health International and the United States Agency for International Development. Also available at: http://www.fhi.org/en/HIVAIDS/pub/guide/corrhope/correg.htm Last accessed on 5 May 2007

assessment); and developing a realistic, evidence-based, costed plan for change. We have described different methods of needs assessment including rapid appraisal techniques and their strengths and weaknesses and the special role of stakeholder, particularly community, involvement and participation. We have seen how important data are for needs assessment but how data systems and availability are likely to vary.

The next step is to act on the health needs assessment. At the beginning of the chapter we described the importance of locating a needs assessment within the planning and management cycles of the responsible organization (Box 12.2.1). We described a series of questions that should be asked before a needs assessment is undertaken. They relate to the timing of the needs assessment and its role. Perhaps the most important question of all to ask at the beginning is 'How can the results and recommendations of the needs assessment be produced and presented to best inform action?' If the needs assessment has been undertaken with care, using the best data available, and this question has been properly answered, then the likelihood of the needs assessment informing action is high.

References

Barry M.J., Fowler F.J. Jr., O'Leary M.P. *et al.* (1992). The American Urological Association symptom index for benign prostatic hyperplasia. *Journal of Urology*, **148**:1549–57.

Buse K., Walt G., Mays N. (2005) *Making Health Policy*. Open University Press, Maidenhead. England.

Busse J.W., Mills E., Dennis R. *et al.* (2009). Clinical epidemiology. In: Detels R., Beaglehole R., Lansang M.A., Gulliford M., eds. *Oxford Textbook of Public Health, 5th ed.* Oxford University Press, Oxford.

Cavanagh S., Chadwick K. (2005) *Health needs assessment: A practical guide.* UK National Institute for Health and Clinical Excellence (NICE). Available at http://www.nice.org.uk.

Chan C., Ho S.C., Chan S.G. *et al.* (2002) Factors affecting uptake of cervical and breast cancer screening among perimenopausal women in Hong Kong. *Hong Kong Medical Journal*, **8**(5):334–41.

Chowdhury P.P., Balluz L., Murphy W. *et al.* (2007) Centers for Disease Control and Prevention (CDC) (2007). Surveillance of certain health behaviours among states and selected local areas—United States, 2005. *MMWR Surveillance Summaries*, **56**(4):1–160.

Cook C. (2004) *Alcohol Misuse needs assessment*. Health Care Needs Assessment. First Series. Second Edition. Volume 1 Radcliffe Medical Press, Oxford.

Cresswell P., Learmonth A., Chappel D. (2005) *The Health Needs of Prisoners*. North East Public Health Observatory. Occasional Paper 16. Available at http://www.nepho.org.uk.

Dawson J., Fitzpatrick R., Frost S., *et al.* (2001) Evidence for the validity of a patient-based instrument for assessment of outcome after revision hip replacement. *Journal of Bone and Joint Surgery (British Volume)*, **83**(8):1125–9.

Dawson J., Fitzpatrick R., Fletcher J. *et al.* (2004) *Osteoarthritis affecting the hip and knee. Health Care Needs Assessment. First Series. Second Edition.* Volume 1 Radcliffe Medical Press, Oxford.

DH Health Survey for England (2007). Available at http://www.dh.gov.uk/en/Publicationsandstatistics/PublishedSurvey/HealthSurveyForEngland. Accessed 21 June, 2007.

Delattre E., Dormont B. (2003) Fixed fees and physician-induced demand: A panel data study on French physicians *Health Economics*, **12**(9):741–754.

Disease Control Priorities Project: Cost-Effective Interventions (2006). Available at http://www.dcp2.org.

Ferris G., Roderick P., Smithies A. *et al.* (1998) An epidemiological needs assessment of carotid endarterectomy in an English health region. Is the need being met? *British Medical Journal*, **317**:447–451.

Goldacre M., Yeates D., Gill L., *et al.* (2005) *A geographical profile of hospital admissions*. Published by Unit of Health-Care Epidemiology, Oxford University, and South East England Public Health Observatory.

Hassan M.M. (2005). Arsenic poisoning in Bangladesh: spatial mitigation planning with GIS and public participation. *Health Policy*, **74**, 247–60.

Hensher M., Fulop N. (1999) The influence of health needs assessment on health care decision-making in London health authorities. *Journal of Health Services Research & Policy*, **4**(2):90–5.

INDEPTH Network (2005) INDEPTH Demographic Surveillance Sites. Available at http://www.indepth-network.org/dss_site_profiles/dss_sites.htm.

International Union against Cancer (UICC) TNM (Tumour Node Metastasis) system. Available at http://www.uicc.org/index.php?id=508. Accessed 21 June 2007.

Jordan J., Wright J., Ayres P. *et al.* (2002) Health needs assessment and needs-led health service change: a survey of projects involving public health doctors. *Journal of Health Services Research & Policy*, **7**: 71–80.

Marsden J., Strang J. *et al.* (2004) Drug misuse needs assessment. *Health Care Needs Assessment. First Series. Second Edition*. Volume 2 Radcliffe Medical Press, Oxford.

Mant J., Wade D., Winner S. (2004) Stroke needs assessment. *Health Care Needs Assessment. First Series. Second Edition*. Volume 1 Radcliffe Medical Press, Oxford.

McIntyre D., Mooney G., Jan S. (2009) Need: What is it and how do we measure it? In: Detels R., Beaglehole R., Lansang M.A., Gulliford M., eds. *Oxford Textbook of Public Health, 5th ed*. Oxford University Press, Oxford.

McKee M., Clarke A. (1995) Guidelines, enthusiasms, uncertainty and the limits to purchasing. *British Medical Journal*, **310**;101–4.

McNeil M., Goddard J. *et al.* (2006) Rapid Community Needs Assessment After Hurricane Katrina—Hancock County, Mississippi. Centers for Disease Control (CDC) *MMWR*, **55**(09);234–236.

Morgan M., Reid M., Ogden J. (2009). Sociology and psychology in public health. In: Detels R., Beaglehole R., Lansang M.A., Gulliford M., eds. *Oxford Textbook of Public Health, 5th ed*. Oxford University Press, Oxford.

Murray S. (2000) Relation between private health insurance and high rates of Caesarean section in Chile: qualitative and quantitative study. *British Medical Journal*, **321**:1501–1505.

National Statistics. Available at http://www.statistics.gov.uk/StatBase/Product.asp. Accessed 21 June 2007.

Mortality Statistics: Cause (Series DH2).

National Institute for Clinical Excellence (2007) Determining local service levels for upper GI endoscopy: Assumptions used in estimating a population benchmark. Available at http://www.nice.org.uk. Accessed 13 June 2007.

Orinda V., Kakande H., Kabarangira J. *et al.* (2005) A sector wide approach to emergency obstetric care in Uganda. *International Journal of Genecology and Obstetrics*, **91**(3):285–291.

Palmer C.A. (1999). Rapid appraisal of needs in reproductive health care in southern Sudan: Qualitative study. *British Medical Journal*, **319**, 743–8.

Powell J. (2006) Health Needs Assessment: A systematic approach. National Library for Health; Health Management Specialist Library. Available at http://www.library.nhs.uk/healthmanagement/ViewResource.aspx?resID=29549.

Rifkin S., Annett H., Tabibzadeh I. (1992). Rapid appraisal to assess community health needs: A focus on the urban poor. In: Scrimshaw N.S. and Gleason G.R. (eds.). *Rapid assessment procedures: Qualitative methodologies for planning and evaluation of health related programs*, pp. 357–63. International Nutrition Foundation for Developing Countries, Boston, MA, USA.

Smith S.M., Long J., Deady J. *et al.* (2005). Adapting developing country epidemiological assessment techniques to improve the quality of health needs assessments in developed countries. *BMC Health Services Research* 5, 1472-6963-5-32. Available at http://www.biomedcentral.com/1472-6963/5/32.

South Eastern Public Health Observatory (SEPHO) 2007 Joint Strategic needs assessment. Available at http://www.sepho.org.uk/ViewResource.aspx?id=10769.

Stevens A., Raftery J. (2004) Health Care Needs Assessment. First Series. Second Edition. Volume 1 Radcliffe Medical Press, Oxford.

Young T.K., Roos N.P., Hammerstrand K.M. (1991) Estimated burden of diabetes mellitus in Manitoba according to health insurance claims: A pilot study. *Canadian Medical Association Journal*, **144**(3): 318–324.

Wadud Z., Kuper H., Polack S. *et al.* (2006) Rapid assessment of avoidable blindness and needs assessment of cataract surgical services in Satkhira District, Bangladesh. *British Journal of Ophthalmology*, **90**(10):1225–9.

Weinstein J.N., Bronner K.K., Morgan T.S. *et al.* (2004) Trends and geographic variations in major surgery for degenerative diseases of the hip, knee, and spine. *Health Affairs*, Suppl Web Exclusives:VAR81–9.

Williams B. Nicholl J. Brazier J. (1997) Accident and emergency departments. *Health Care Needs Assessment. Second Series*. Radcliffe Medical Press, Oxford.

Wright N., Tomkins C. (2006) How can health services effectively meet the health needs of homeless people? *British Journal of General Practice*, **56**(525):286–293.

12.3

Socioeconomic inequalities in health in high-income countries: The facts and the options

Johan P. Mackenbach

Abstract

Socioeconomic inequalities in health have been studied extensively in past decades. In all high-income countries with available data, mortality and morbidity rates are higher among those in less advantaged socioeconomic positions, and as a result differences in health expectancy between socioeconomic groups typically amount to 10 years or more. Good progress has been made in unravelling the determinants of health inequalities, and a number of specific determinants (particularly material, psychosocial and lifestyle factors) have been identified which probably contribute to explaining health inequalities in many high-income countries. Although further research is necessary, our understanding of what causes health inequalities has progressed to a stage when rational approaches to reduce health inequalities are becoming feasible. Although different countries are in widely different phases of awareness of, and willingness to take action on, health inequalities, several European countries have endeavoured to develop comprehensive policy programmes to tackle health inequalities.

Introduction

Socioeconomic inequalities in health have been studied extensively around the world in past decades. Inequalities in health have been documented from the United States (Davey Smith *et al.* 1996) to Russia (Shkolnikov *et al.* 2006), from Sweden (Ljung *et al.* 2005) and the Netherlands (Mackenbach & Stronks 2002) to Japan (Fukuda *et al.* 2007) and Korea (Khang *et al.* 2004), and from New Zealand (Shaw *et al.* 2005) to Canada (Lasser *et al.* 2006). At the start of the twenty-first century, all high-income countries are faced with substantial inequalities in health within their populations. People with a lower level of education, a lower occupational class, or a lower level of income tend to die at a younger age, and to have, within their shorter lives, a higher prevalence of all kinds of health problems. This leads to truly tremendous differences between socioeconomic groups in the number of years that people can expect to live in good health ('health expectancy'). In countries with available data, differences in health expectancy typically amount to 10 years or more, counted from birth. According to widely accepted principles, such differences in health are unjust (Whitehead 1990) and represent one of the greatest challenges for public health in these countries.

Historical notes

Historical evidence suggests that socioeconomic inequalities in health is not a recent phenomenon. However, it was only during the nineteenth century that socioeconomic inequalities in health were 'discovered'. Before that time, health inequalities simply went unrecognized due to lack of information. In the nineteenth century great figures in public health, such as Villermé in France, Chadwick in England, and Virchow in Germany, devoted a large part of their scientific work to this issue (Ackerknecht 1953; Coleman 1982; Chave 1984). This was facilitated by national population statistics, which permitted the calculation of mortality rates by occupation or by city district. Louis René Villermé (1782–1863), for example, analysed inequalities in mortality between 'arrondissements' in Paris in 1817–21. He showed that districts with a lower socioeconomic level, as indicated by the proportion of houses for which no tax was levied over the rents, tended to have systematically higher mortality rates than more well-to-do neighbourhoods. He concluded that life and death are not primarily biological phenomena, but are closely linked to social circumstances (Coleman 1982). Rudolf Virchow (1821–1902) went even further in his famous statement that 'medicine is a social science, and politics nothing but medicine at a larger scale' (Ackerknecht 1953).

Since the nineteenth century, the magnitude of socioeconomic inequalities in health has probably declined in absolute terms in developed countries. There has been a marked decline in the average mortality rate in the population, leading to a doubling of life expectancy at birth. This was largely due to improvements in living standards and public health. As a result, the absolute difference in mortality rates and in life expectancy at birth between people with a high and a low socioeconomic position has probably become smaller, as suggested by the limited historical evidence which has been uncovered in a few European countries (Pamuk 1985). It is less clear, however, whether inequalities in mortality have also declined in relative terms, i.e. in terms of the percentage excess death rates in lower as compared to higher socioeconomic groups. In the long run, the relative risks of dying for those with a low as compared to those with a high socioeconomic position seem to have remained very stable, and have even unexpectedly increased during the last decades of the twentieth century in many developed countries (Pamuk 1985; Mackenbach *et al.* 2003a). Particularly in Western Europe, with its high levels of prosperity and highly developed social security, public health, and health care systems, this was a disturbing finding. These developments have contributed to a heightened awareness of health inequalities, and of the challenge they pose to public health policy, around the world.

The start of the resurgence of an active interest in health inequalities in Europe can be linked to the publication of the Black Report in England in 1980 (Townsend & Davidson 1992), which first highlighted the widening of health inequalities despite the rise of the welfare state in the decades after World War II. The Black Report contributed to heightened awareness of health inequalities all around Europe as well as in developed countries in other parts of the world. As a result, an enormous amount of descriptive data has been collected and analysed in many countries, testifying to the existence of substantial inequalities in health in all countries with good data.

While all these descriptive studies were going on, the emphasis of academic research in this area has shifted from description to explanation, not only to satisfy scientific curiosities but also to find entry-points for policies and interventions to reduce health inequalities (Marmot & Wilkinson 2006; Mackenbach & Bakker 2002). This was greatly facilitated by increased research funding, both from national research programmes (e.g. in England, the Netherlands, and Finland), and by international agencies (e.g. the European Commission and the European Science Foundation) (Siegrist & Marmot 2006). As a result, our understanding of the causes of socioeconomic inequalities in health has expanded tremendously, and has allowed interested policy makers to start searching for strategies to reduce these inequalities. Countries are in widely different stages of policy development in this area, but in some countries (e.g. England) political windows of opportunity have arisen which have led to large-scale implementation of policies to tackle health inequalities.

The purpose of this chapter

This chapter aims to review the available evidence on the description and explanation of socioeconomic inequalities in health in high-income countries, and to present the current (2007) state of the art with regard to the available options for reducing health inequalities.

For the purpose of this chapter, socioeconomic inequalities in health will be defined as systematic differences in morbidity or mortality rates between people of higher and lower socioeconomic status, as indicated by, e.g. level of education, occupational class, or income level. Where possible, we will draw upon international overviews, such as comparative studies, in order to avoid biases related to the selective experiences of single countries. We will,

however, mainly draw upon the European experience, which has become very well documented in the past two decades.

The facts: Description

Mortality

Although no individual can escape death, important differences in mortality *rates* are typically found between men and women, city dwellers and inhabitants of rural areas, native people and immigrants, and population groups classified according to many other characteristics. Some of the largest inequalities are found when individuals are classified according to their socioeconomic position. In all high-income countries with available data, mortality rates are higher among those in less advantaged socioeconomic positions, regardless of whether socioeconomic position is indicated by educational level, occupational class, or income level (Mackenbach 2006).

Levels and trends

Table 12.3.1 summarizes these inequalities for a wide range of European countries. The overall picture is extremely clear: The mortality rates are consistently higher in lower, than in higher socioeconomic groups. Many of the figures given in Table 12.3.1 apply to middle-aged adults, and this implies that differences in mortality rates can be interpreted as differences in the risks of dying prematurely. From studies that have included women, it has become clear that inequalities in mortality exist among women as they do among men, but that inequalities are smaller among women than among men (Mackenbach *et al.* 1999).

Not only is the size of these inequalities often substantial, in the order of an excess relative risk of dying in the lowest socioeconomic groups of 25–50 per cent. But inequalities in mortality have also risen substantially in the past decades, without much evidence that the widening of the mortality gap will stop in the near future. To the surprise of many, mortality differences between socioeconomic groups have widened in many Western European countries during the last three decades of the twentieth century. This has continued into the 1990s, and has led to considerable increases of the relative excess risk of dying in the lowest socioeconomic groups (Fig. 12.3.1) (Mackenbach *et al.* 2003a).

The explanation of this disturbing phenomenon is only partly known. One aspect which should certainly be taken into account, however, is that this widening of the relative gap in death rates is generally the result of a difference between socioeconomic groups in the speed of mortality *decline*. While mortality declined in all socioeconomic groups, the decline has been proportionally faster in the higher socioeconomic groups than in the lower. The faster mortality declines in higher socioeconomic groups were in their turn mostly due to faster mortality declines for cardiovascular diseases (Mackenbach *et al.* 2003a). In many developed countries, the 1980s and 1990s have been decades with substantial improvements in cardiovascular disease mortality. These have been due to improvements in health-related behaviours (less smoking, modest improvements in diet, more physical exercise, etc.), and to the introduction of effective health care interventions (hypertension detection and treatment, surgical interventions, thrombolytic therapy, etc.). Apparently, while these improvements have to some extent been taken up by all socioeconomic groups, the higher socioeconomic groups have tended to benefit more.

Table 12.3.1 Inequalities in mortality by socioeconomic position in 21 European countries[a]

Country	Indicator of socioeconomic position	Period	Age-group	Rate ratio[b]		Source
				Men	Women	
Austria	Education	1991–1992	45+	1.43*	1.32*	National census-linked mortality follow-up
Belgium	Education	1991–1995	45+	1.34*	1.29*	National census-linked mortality follow-up
	Housing tenure	1991–1995	60–69	1.44*	1.43*	
Czech Republic	Education	End 1990s	20–64	1.66*	1.09*	Unlinked cross-sectional study
Denmark	Education	1991–1995	60–69	1.28*	1.26*	National census-linked mortality follow-up
	Housing tenure	1991–1995	60–69	1.64*	1.47*	
	Occupation	1981–1990	45–59	1.33*	n.a.	National census-linked mortality follow-up
England/Wales	Education	1991–1996	45+	1.35*	1.22*	National census-linked mortality follow-up
	Housing tenure	1991–1996	60–69	1.65*	1.58*	
	Occupation	1981–1989	45–59	1.61*	n.a.	National census-linked mortality follow-up; representative sample
Estonia	Education	2000	20+	2.38*	2.23*	National cross-sectional study
	Education	1988	20–74	1.50*	1.31*	National cross-sectional study
Finland	Education	1991–1995	45+	1.33*	1.24*	National census-linked mortality follow-up
	Housing tenure	1991–1995	60–69	1.90*	1.73*	
France	Education	1990–1994	60–69	1.31*	1.14	National census-linked mortality follow-up
	Housing tenure	1990–1994	60–69	1.27*	1.25*	
	Occupation	1980–1989	45–59	2.15*	n.a.	National census-linked mortality follow-up; representative sample
	Occupation	1984–1985	45–64	1.61	1.33	National cross-sectional study
Ireland	Occupation	1980–1982	45–59	1.38*		National cross-sectional study
Italy	Education	1991–1996	45+	1.22*	1.20*	Urban census-linked mortality follow-up (Turin)
	Housing tenure	1991–1996	60–69	1.37*	1.33*	
	Education	1981–1982	18–54	1.85*	n.a.	National census-linked mortality follow-up
	Occupation	1981–1982	45–59	1.35*	n.a.	National census-linked mortality follow-up
Latvia	Education	1988–1989		1.50	1.20	National cross-sectional study
Lithuania	Education	2001	25+	2.40*	2.90*	Unlinked cross-sectional analysis
Netherlands	Education	1991–1997	25–74	1.92*	1.28	GLOBE Longitudinal study (Eindhoven)
Norway	Education	1990–1995	45+	1.36*	1.27*	National census-linked mortality follow-up
	Housing tenure	1990–1995	60–69	1.44*	1.36*	
	Occupation	1980–1990	45–59	1.47*		National census-linked mortality follow-up
Poland	Education	1988–1989	50–64	2.24	1.78	National cross-sectional study
Portugal	Occupation	1980–1982	45–59	1.36*	n.a.	National cross-sectional study
Slovenia	Education	1991 & 2002	25–64	2.44	2.66	Unlinked cross-sectional study
Spain	Education	1992–1996	45+	1.24*	1.27*	Urban and regional census-linked mortality follow-up (Barcelona & Madrid)
	Occupation	1980–1982	45–59	1.37*	n.a.	National cross-sectional study
Sweden	Occupation	1980–1986	45–59	1.59*		National census-linked mortality follow-up
Switzerland	Education	1991–1995	45+	1.33*	1.27*	National census-linked mortality follow-up
	Occupation	1979–1982	45–59	1.37*		National cross-sectional study

[a] Because of differences in data collection and classification, the magnitude of inequalities in health cannot always directly be compared between countries.

[b] Rate ratio: Ratio of mortality rate in lower socioeconomic groups as compared to that in higher socioeconomic groups. Asterisk(*) indicates that difference in mortality between socioeconomic groups is statistically significant. n.a. indicates 'not available'.

Source: Mackenbach 2006.

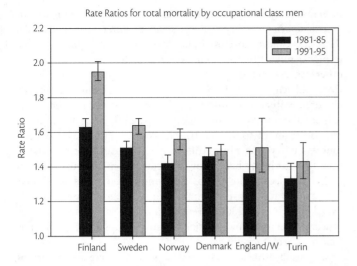

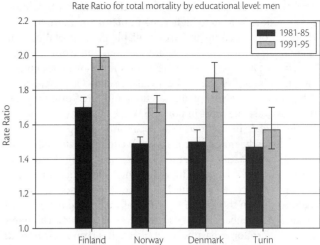

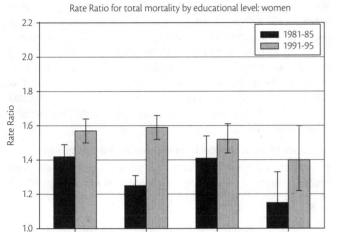

Fig. 12.3.1 Inequalities in mortality by educational level and occupational class, 1981–1985 and 1991–1995. Finland, Sweden, Norway, Denmark, England/Wales, Turin.
Source: Mackenbach *et al.* (2003).

Differences between countries

Some comparative studies have tried to assess whether the magnitude of inequalities in mortality differs systematically between countries. The most extensive of these studies have been performed in Europe (Mackenbach *et al.* 1997; Kunst *et al.* 1998, 1999; Huisman *et al.* 2004, 2005a) and have found that the range of between-country variation in relative inequalities is rather small within Western Europe. Due to the fact that countries differ substantially in average mortality rates for the population as a whole, absolute differences in mortality between socioeconomic groups usually do show clear between-country variations, in contrast to relative inequalities which tend to be more similar. For example, because of its low average death rates, Sweden has rather small absolute differences in mortality between socioeconomic groups, although relative differences are not clearly smaller than elsewhere (Mackenbach *et al.* 1997).

This is not to say that systematic differences between countries in the magnitude of relative inequalities in mortality do not exist: Relative inequalities in mortality are larger than elsewhere in some Eastern European countries, perhaps as a result of the economic and social developments following the political changes around 1990 (Mackenbach 2006). Since these transitions, mortality rates have changed dramatically in many countries in Eastern Europe, sometimes to the better (e.g. in the Czech Republic) but often to the worse, at least temporarily (e.g. in Hungary and Estonia), particularly among men. This is probably due to a combination of (interlinked) factors: A rise in economic insecurity and poverty; a breakdown of protective social, public health, and health care institutions; and a rise in excessive drinking and other risk factors for premature mortality. The available evidence clearly shows that these changes in mortality have not been equally shared between socioeconomic groups: In the countries with available data, mortality rates have generally improved less, or deteriorated more, in the lower socioeconomic groups. Apparently, people with higher levels of education have been able to protect themselves better against increased health risks, and/or have been able to benefit more from new opportunities for health gains. Evidence from several Eastern European countries (Estonia, Hungary, Russia) suggests a substantial widening of the gap in death rates (Leinsalu *et al.* 2003; Shkolnikov *et al.* 2006).

Cause-specific mortality

Variations in patterns of cause of death between socioeconomic groups provide valuable clues for the explanation of disparities in mortality, because they point to the mechanisms that link lower socioeconomic position to higher risk of premature mortality.

In all European countries with available data, mortality from cardiovascular disease is higher among men and women with a lower socioeconomic position. This does not, however, apply to all specific diseases of the cardiovascular system. Of these, ischaemic heart disease (myocardial infarction) and cerebrovascular disease (stroke) are the most important. While mortality from stroke is always higher in the lower socioeconomic groups, this is not the case for ischaemic heart disease (Avendano et al. 2004). For ischaemic heart disease, a north–south gradient within Europe has been found, with relative and absolute inequalities being larger in the north of Europe (e.g. the Nordic countries and the United Kingdom) than in the south (e.g. Portugal, Spain, and Italy) (Kunst et al. 1999; Mackenbach et al. 2000; Avendano et al. 2004). This international pattern for ischaemic heart disease has been interpreted as an expression of differences between countries in how the epidemiology of this disease has developed. In many countries, particularly in the north of Europe, mortality from ischaemic heart disease increased substantially after the World War II, probably as a result of changes in health-related behaviours, such as smoking, diet, and physical exercise. During the 1970s, however, a decline set in, and is still continuing. During this epidemiological development, important changes occurred in the association between socioeconomic position and ischaemic heart disease mortality. In the north of Europe, during the 1950s and 1960s ischaemic heart disease mortality was higher in the higher socioeconomic groups, leading to the notion of ischaemic heart disease being a 'manager's disease'. It was only during the 1970s, coinciding with the start of the decline of ischaemic heart disease mortality in the population as a whole, that a reversal occurred, and the current association emerged (Marmot & McDowell 1986). This is due to differences between socioeconomic groups in both the timing and the speed of decline of ischaemic heart disease mortality. As we have seen above, the widening of the gap in ischaemic heart disease mortality was still continuing in the 1990s. In the south of Europe, a similar 'epidemic' of ischaemic heart disease mortality has not occurred, and inequalities in ischaemic heart disease mortality have not undergone such clear-cut changes as in the north of Europe. It is possible that the lack of clear inequalities in ischaemic heart disease mortality in some southern European populations represents an earlier stage of epidemiological development, and will turn out to be a temporary phenomenon, because the protection of southern European populations against ischaemic heart disease which their traditional living habits offered, is gradually eroding.

Inequalities in cancer mortality tend to be smaller than those for cardiovascular disease mortality (Mackenbach et al. 1999; Huisman et al. 2005a). Among women, inequalities in mortality from all cancers combined are even negligible in magnitude in many countries. Among men, however, the usual pattern of higher mortality in lower socioeconomic groups applies to cancer as it does to most other diseases. These patterns for all cancers combined are the net result of strongly diverging patterns for specific forms of cancer. For some cancers, 'reverse' patterns (with higher death rates in the upper socioeconomic groups) are seen in some countries. Examples include prostate cancer among men, and breast and lung cancer in women. For colorectal cancer, another important cause of death, inequalities in mortality tend to be small everywhere. The 'reverse' or absent gradients *and* large contributions to cancer mortality

of breast, lung, and colorectal cancer in women explain the lack of excess cancer mortality in lower socioeconomic groups. In men, the excess cancer mortality in lower socioeconomic groups is due to higher mortality from lung cancer, as well as from a number of other cancers including stomach cancer and oesophagus cancers (Mackenbach et al. 1999; Huisman et al. 2005). Unfortunately, the favourable situation in women, with small or absent socioeconomic inequalities in total cancer mortality, is likely to be a temporary phenomenon. In some countries in Western Europe, it has been found that in younger birth cohorts rates of breast cancer mortality now tend to be higher in lower socioeconomic groups than in higher socioeconomic groups. For lung cancer, there are similar indications for a future change in gradient among women (Mackenbach et al. 2004). Prevention of the emergence of excess cancer mortality in lower socioeconomic groups among women is a clear priority for public health.

As a result of these cause-specific patterns, there are important differences between countries in the share of specific causes of death in the excess mortality in lower socioeconomic groups (Huisman et al. 2005). The most important difference is for ischaemic heart disease: Due to the north–south gradient in ischaemic heart disease inequalities mentioned above, ischaemic heart disease is a major contributor to inequalities in mortality in the north of Europe, and much less important (sometimes even 'protecting' lower socioeconomic groups against larger inequalities in mortality) in the south (Fig. 12.3.2).

Life expectancy is shorter in lower socioeconomic groups

As a result of these differences in the risk of dying at various ages, people from lower socioeconomic groups tend to live considerably

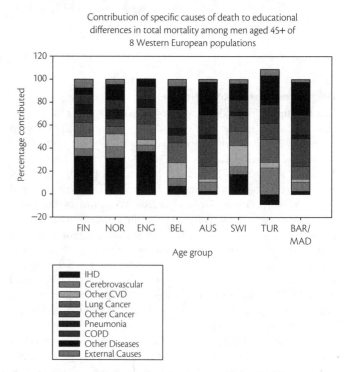

Fig. 12.3.2 Contribution (%) of specific causes of death to difference between low and high educational groups in total mortality in eight European populations, men and women aged 45 years and over, 1990s.
Source: Huisman et al. (2005).

shorter lives than those with more advantaged social positions. Differences in life expectancy at birth between the lowest and highest socioeconomic groups (e.g. manual versus professional occupations, or primary school versus postsecondary education) are typically in the order of 4–6 years among men, and 2–4 years among women, but sometimes larger differences have been observed (Mackenbach 2006). In England and Wales, for example, inequalities in life expectancy at birth among men have increased from 5.4 years in the 1970s to more than 8 years in the 1990s (Department of health 2004). A similarly strong increase has been observed in Finland (Martikainen et al. 2001).

Morbidity

Many countries have nationally representative surveys with questions on both socioeconomic status and self-reported morbidity (e.g. self-assessed health, chronic conditions, disability). Inequalities in the latter are substantial everywhere, and practically always in the same direction: Persons with a lower socioeconomic status have higher morbidity rates.

Inequalities in generic health indicators

For one indicator, self-assessed health (measured with a single question on an individual's perception of his or her own health), the availability of these data is almost as great as that for inequalities in mortality (Table 12.3.2). The overall pattern is clear again: Prevalence rates of less-than-'good' self-assessed health are higher in lower socioeconomic groups. No clear patterns have emerged in the magnitude of socioeconomic inequalities in self-assessed health between European countries (Mackenbach 2006).

These inequalities in self-reported morbidity persist into old-age. Beyond early adulthood, socioeconomic differences in self-reported morbidity have been found in all European countries where this has been examined (Cavelaars et al. 1998; Dalstra et al. 2005). For children and adolescents, however, the picture is more mixed. Some studies have suggested that in adolescence, the period between childhood and adulthood, there is a genuine narrowing of health inequalities, perhaps as a result of the transition between socioeconomic position of family of origin and own socioeconomic position. Among children the picture is more consistent: Many studies find that parents in lower socioeconomic groups report more ill-health for their children than parents in higher socioeconomic groups (Haldorsson et al. 2000).

Respondents to health interview surveys are unlikely to be perfect reporters of their health problems, and there may also be differences between socioeconomic groups in the accuracy of reporting health problems. Where more objective data have been available for comparison, however, similar pictures of higher incidence and prevalence of health problems have been obtained. Although height is partly genetically determined, it is also strongly influenced by childhood living conditions, such as nutrition, occurrence of disease, psychosocial stress, and housing conditions. It is often used as a summary indicator of health during childhood and adolescence, and shows consistent differences between socioeconomic groups. In all countries there are clear differences in average adult height between socioeconomic groups: The higher educated are 1–3 cm taller (Table 12.3.3) (Cavelaars et al. 2000a).

Inequalities in diseases and disabilities

Socioeconomic inequalities have not only been found for general health indicators, which are usually measured on the basis of self-reports, but can also be found for many specific indicators, including objective measurements of the incidence or prevalence of diseases and disabilities. In the large majority of these studies, higher incidences or prevalences of health problems have been found in the lower socioeconomic groups (Huisman et al. 2003; Dalstra et al. 2005).

No socioeconomic inequalities in the prevalence of cancer are usually found, while many epidemiological studies have found an increased incidence of many cancers in lower socio-economic groups. Among men, lung, larynx, oropharyngeal, oesophageal, and stomach cancers are among those with usually higher incidences in lower socioeconomic groups. Among women, this applies to oesophageal, stomach, and cervical cancer. Interestingly, some cancers have a higher incidence in higher socioeconomic groups: Colon and brain cancer and skin melanoma in men, and colon, breast, and ovary cancer and skin melanoma in women. We already saw similar patterns on the basis of cancer mortality (see 'Mortality') (Dalstra et al. 2005).

The fact that cancer prevalence is not higher in lower socio-economic groups can perhaps be explained by differences in cancer survival. Put simply, incident ('new') cases of cancer can either die or stay alive, and only those who stay alive contribute to the number of prevalent ('current') cases. There is extensive evidence for socioeconomic inequalities in cancer survival: Most studies show a survival advantage for patients with a higher socioeconomic position. The lower survival rates of cancer patients in lower socioeconomic groups may to some extent numerically 'compensate' the higher incidence rates, and contribute to the lack of an excess prevalence of cancer in lower socioeconomic groups. These data for cancer are illustrative for many other potentially fatal conditions: Patients from higher socio-economic groups are usually likely to have better survival, because of more favourable prognostic factors (e.g. less comorbidity, better psychosocial profiles, etc.), because of better treatment (better access, higher quality treatments, better compliance, etc.), or both. Although inequalities in health care utilization are not among the most important contributors to the explanation of socioeconomic inequalities in health, at least not in Western Europe, these data suggest that improvements in the health care system could still be of some help in tackling health inequalities.

Mortality data by cause of death show that suicide tends to occur more frequently in lower socioeconomic groups, particularly among men (Lorant et al. 2005). One of the underlying risk factors, mental ill-health, also tends to be more prevalent in lower socioeconomic groups. The higher prevalence of mental illness in lower socioeconomic groups is likely to have a complex explanation. In psychiatric epidemiology, there is a long tradition of looking at the possible effects of mental health problems on downward social mobility. This 'drift hypothesis' has indeed found some support, for example in the case of schizophrenia, whose onset usually occurs in adolescence and young adulthood, and which may consequently interfere with school and early work careers. On the other hand, incidence studies have also found higher rates of many mental health problems among those who are currently in a lower socioeconomic position. It seems likely that this at least partly reflects a causal effect, perhaps through a higher exposure to psychosocial stressors and/or a lack of coping resources.

As a result of the higher frequency of physical and mental health problems in lower socioeconomic groups, the prevalence of limitations in functioning and various forms of disability also tends to

Table 12.3.2 Inequalities in self-assessed health by socioeconomic position in 18 countries[a]

Country	Indicator of socioeconomic position	Period	Age	Odds ratio[b]		Source
				Men	Women	
Austria	Education	1991	25–69	3.22*	2.67*	Mikrozensus Fragen zur Gesundheit
Belgium	Education	1997	25–74	2.55*	2.36	Belgium Health Interview Survey
Bulgaria	Education	1997	18+	2.19*	2.84*	National representative survey of the population of Bulgaria
	Income			1.86	1.50	
Denmark	Education	1994	25–69	2.16*	3.00*	Danish Health and Morbidity Survey
	Occupation	1986–1987	25–69	2.19*	n.a.	Danish Health and Morbidity Survey
Estonia	Education	1996	25–79	3.11*	3.59*	Estonian Health Interview Survey
	Income			2.37*	1.66*	
Finland	Education	1994	25–69	2.99*	3.29*	Finnish Survey on Living Conditions
	Income			3.09*	2.43*	
France	Occupation	1991–1992	25–69	2.24*		Enquête sur la Santé et les Soins Médicaux
Germany (West)	Education	1990–1991	25–69	1.76*	1.91*	National Health Survey
	Income			2.05*	2.40*	
	Occupation			1.63*		
Great Britain	Income	1996	25–69	3.88*	3.92*	British General Household Survey
	Occupation	1991	25–69	2.32*	n.a.	General Household Survey
England	Education	1995	25–69	3.08*	2.66*	Health Survey for England
Italy	Education	1994	25–69	2.94*	2.55*	Health Interview Survey
Latvia	Education	1999	25–70	2.21*	2.48*	Norbalt-II Living Conditions Survey
	Income			5.10*	3.26*	
The Netherlands	Education	1997–1999	25–69	2.81*	2.12*	Permanent Survey on Living Conditions
	Income			4.50*	3.01*	
	Occupation	1991–1992	25–69	2.40*		Health Survey
Norway	Education	1995	25–69	2.30*	2.84*	Health Survey
Poland	Education	1993	35–64	1.27	1.72	Household Survey Pol-MONICA survey (Warsaw)
Poland	Education	1993	35–64	2.08	0.93	Household Survey Pol-MONICA survey (Tarnobrzeg)
Spain	Education	1997	25–69	2.58*	3.10*	Spanish Health Survey
Sweden	Education	1997	25–69	2.37*	3.06*	Swedish Survey on Living Conditions
	Income			4.11*	2.80*	
	Occupation	1991	25–69	2.79*	n.a.	Swedish Level of Living Survey
Switzerland	Occupation	1992–1993	25–69	2.12*	n.a.	

[a] Because of differences in data collection and classification, the magnitude of inequalities in health cannot always directly be compared between countries.

[b] Odds ratio: Ratio of odds (a measure of risk) of less-than-'good' self-assessed health in lower socioeconomic groups as compared to that in higher socioeconomic groups. Asterisk (*) indicates that difference in mortality between socioeconomic groups is statistically significant. n.a. indicates 'not available'.

Source: Mackenbach (2006).

Table 12.3.3 Differences in average height (cm) between higher and lower educational groups in 10 European countries, around 1990

	Men differences (95% CI)	Women differences (95% CI)
Norway	1.8 (0.7–3.0)	1.2 (0.1–2.2)
Sweden	2.5 (1.8–3.1)	1.5 (0.9–2.0)
Finland	1.6 (1.0–2.2)	1.5 (0.9–2.0)
Denmark	2.8 (2.0–3.7)	1.8 (1.0–2.6)
Netherlands	2.5 (2.1–3.0)	1.6 (1.2–1.9)
Germany	2.2 (1.7–2.6)	2.2 (1.8–2.6)
Switzerland	2.9 (2.4–3.4)	2.2 (1.8–2.6)
France	2.6 (2.2–3.0)	1.6 (1.2–2.0)
Italy	2.5 (2.2–2.7)	1.3 (1.1–1.5)
Spain	3.0 (2.7–3.3)	1.3 (1.0–1.7)

This table shows people with higher educational level to be 1–3 cm taller.
Source: Cavelaars *et al.* (2000).

be higher. This applies to many aspects of functioning (mobility, sensory functioning, grip strength, walking speed, etc.) and is particularly evident among the elderly (Avendano *et al.* 2005). These inequalities in functioning translate into inequalities in limitations with activities of daily living such as dressing and bathing (ADL), and limitations with instrumental activities of daily living such as preparing hot meals and making telephone calls (IADL). This illustrates the high burden of physical limitations among those with a lower socioeconomic position, and is likely to contribute to substantially higher professional care needs, including institutionalized care (e.g. nursing homes). As suggested by the results for objective measures of grip strength and walking speed, inequalities in self-reported disability are real, and not a matter of reporting bias.

'Healthy life expectancy' is shorter in lower socioeconomic groups

We have seen above that the higher mortality rates in lower socioeconomic groups lead to substantial inequalities in life expectancy: People in lower socioeconomic groups tend to live between 2 and 8 years less than people in higher socioeconomic groups. The fact that morbidity rates (among those who are still alive) are higher too, contributes to even larger inequalities in 'healthy life expectancy' (the number of years which people can expect to live in good health). Inequalities in the number of years lived in good health are often seen of more than 10 years (Sihvonen *et al.* 1998; Mackenbach 2006).

The facts: Explanation

'Selection' versus 'causation'

During the past decade, great progress has been made in unravelling the determinants of health inequalities, and although further research is certainly necessary, our understanding of what causes health inequalities has progressed to a stage when rational approaches to reduce health inequalities are becoming feasible.

Early debates about the explanation of socioeconomic inequalities in health focused on the question whether 'causation' or 'selection' was the more important mechanism (Townsend & Davidson 1992; Macintyre 1997). Social selection explanations imply that health determines socioeconomic position, instead of socioeconomic position determining health. The term 'selection' here refers to the process of social mobility (changes in socioeconomic position), during which a selection occurs on health or health-related characteristics.

The occurrence of health-related selection as such is undisputed: During social mobility, some degree of selection on (ill-)health does indeed occur, with people who are in poor health being more likely to move 'downward' (e.g. get a lower status job, or lose income) and less likely to move 'upward' (e.g. finish a high-level education, or obtain a highly paid job), than people who are in good health. It is less clear, however, what the contribution of health-related selection to the explanation of socioeconomic inequalities in health is. The few studies which have investigated this, have concluded that this contribution is likely to be small (Bartley & Plewis 1997; Van de Mheen *et al.* 1999).

Furthermore, longitudinal studies in which socioeconomic status has been measured before health problems are present, and in which the incidence of health problems has been measured during follow-up, show clearly higher risks of developing health problems in the lower socioeconomic groups. These studies have demonstrated clearly that 'causation' instead of 'selection' is the main explanation for socioeconomic inequalities in health (Marmot *et al.* 1991; Marmot & Wilkinson 2006).

The unspoken assumption in debates about the role of selection versus causation often was that social selection is less of a problem for public policy than social causation. This assumption was incorrect, however, because limiting the social consequences of health problems is one of the classical objectives of social security and public health policies in many developed countries.

Specific determinants

The 'causal' effect of socioeconomic status on health is likely to be largely indirect: Through a number of more specific health determinants which are differentially distributed across socioeconomic groups (Fig. 12.3.3). Many risk factors for morbidity and mortality are more prevalent in lower socioeconomic groups, and it is these inequalities in exposure to specific health determinants which should be seen as the main explanation of health inequalities.

There is no doubt that 'material' factors, i.e. exposure to low income and to health risks in the physical environment, are part of

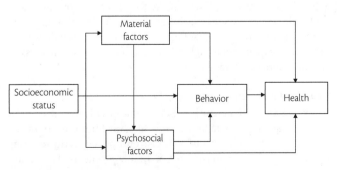

Fig. 12.3.3 Simple explanatory diagram: Factors which have been shown to 'mediate' between low socioeconomic position and risk of ill-health.

the explanation. All European countries have large inequalities in income. According to Eurostat, the 20 per cent of the population with the highest income in the European Union (EU-25) received 4.5 times more than the 20 per cent of the population with the lowest income in 2001. The proportion of the population who is at risk of poverty (defined as having an income less than 60 per cent of the national average) was 15 per cent in the EU as a whole. Although income inequality and poverty rates differ between countries, partly as a result of differences in income taxation and social security benefit schemes, it is quite likely that inequalities in financial disadvantage play an important role in the explanation of health inequalities in all developed countries. Financial disadvantage may affect health through various mechanisms: Psychosocial stress and subsequent risk-taking behaviours (smoking, excessive alcohol consumption, etc.), reduced access to health-promoting facilities and products (fruits and vegetables, sports, preventive health care services), etc. Occupational health risks (exposure to chemicals, accident risks, physically strenuous work, etc.) and health risks related to housing (crowding, dampness, accident risks, etc.) are other examples of 'material' factors which have been shown to make important contributions to the explanation of some health inequalities (Marmot & Wilkinson 2006; Siegrist & Marmot 2006).

The second group of specific determinants which contribute to the explanation of health inequalities are psychosocial factors. Those who are in a low socioeconomic position on average experience more psychosocial stress, in the form of negative life events (loss of beloved ones, financial difficulties, etc.), daily hassles, 'effort-reward imbalance' (high levels of effort without appropriate material and immaterial rewards), and a combination of high demands and low control. These forms of psychosocial stress can in their turn lead to ill-health, either through biological pathways (e.g. by affecting the endocrine or immune systems) or through behavioural pathways (e.g. by inducing risk-taking behaviours). Psychosocial factors related to work organization, such as job strain, have been shown to play an important role in the explanation of socioeconomic inequalities in cardiovascular health (Marmot & Wilkinson 2006; Siegrist & Marmot 2006).

The third group of contributory factors are health-related behaviours, such as smoking, inadequate diet, excessive alcohol consumption, and lack of physical exercise. In many developed countries, one or more of these 'lifestyle' factors are more prevalent in the lower socioeconomic groups, as will be discussed in the next section of this report. As we have seen above, many of the disease-specific patterns of health inequalities also suggest a substantial contribution of health-related behaviours to inequalities in mortality.

It is important to be aware of the fact that the three groups of explanatory factors are interlinked: For example, the higher frequency of material disadvantage in lower socioeconomic groups may partly explain their higher frequency of psychosocial stress or lack of leisure time physical exercise.

Health-related behaviours

By far the most widely available data on a specific determinant of health inequalities relate to smoking. In many European countries, particularly in the north of Western Europe, cigarette smoking is the number one determinant of health problems. This is not only because of its role in lung cancer and some other specific diseases, for which smoking is the main cause, but also because of its

role in (premature) mortality in general, less-than-'good' self-assessed health and disability, for which smoking is an important contributory factor. The prevalence of smoking differs strongly between socioeconomic groups in many European countries, so one can safely assume that it plays an important role in generating health inequalities (Cavelaars et al. 2000b; Huisman et al. 2005).

In general, the prevalence of smoking is higher in the lower socioeconomic groups, but there are important differences between countries in the magnitude, and sometimes even the direction, of these inequalities. A number of comparative studies within Europe have demonstrated a north–south gradient, with larger inequalities in current smoking in the north of Europe and smaller (sometimes even 'reverse') gradients in the south (Fig. 12.3.4) (Cavelaars et al. 2000b; Huismand et al. 2005). This is particularly clear in the case of women: Higher educated women smoke less in the north of Europe (represented by the Nordic countries, Great Britain, the Netherlands, Belgium, etc.), but they smoke more than lower educated women in the south of Europe (represented by Italy, Spain, Greece, Portugal, etc.). Current rates of smoking are the result of trends which have played out over the past decades: The habit of cigarette smoking started early in the twentieth century with the advent of industrially produced cigarettes, and in many European countries it was only after the World War II that smoking became highly prevalent, first among men

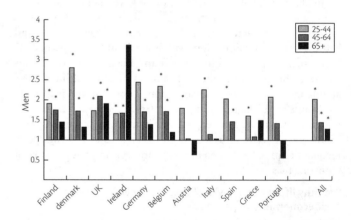

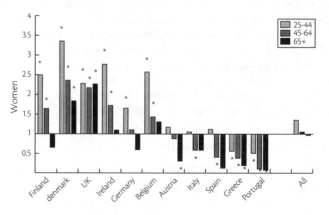

Fig. 12.3.4 Inequalities in current daily smoking by level of education in 11 European countries, 1998.
Source: Huisman, Kunst, and Mackenbach (2005).

(with rates of up to 90% smokers), then among women. In many countries, smoking prevalence has declined over the past decades, at least among men, as a result of health education efforts and other anti-tobacco measures such as raising excise taxes and bans on smoking in public places. This decline in smoking is still continuing, but there have been, and still are, clear socio-economic differences in this decline.

While smoking is clearly bad for health, alcohol is a more complex risk factor: Both abstinence and excessive alcohol consumption are bad for health (as compared to moderate drinking). Abstinence usually is more common in the lower socioeconomic groups, both among men and among women, but the pattern for excessive alcohol consumption is more variable. Many studies report a higher prevalence in lower socioeconomic groups, particularly among men, but the results for women are far from consistent (Droomers *et al.* 1999). These inconsistencies may well be due to real differences between countries in the social patterning of excessive alcohol consumption. In some countries, such as the Nordic countries (e.g. Finland) and several Eastern European countries, 'binge drinking' (drinking more than, say, 8 units on a single occasion) is a more serious source of health problems than regular overconsumption of alcohol. In these countries, binge drinking tends to be more common in lower socioeconomic groups, and is likely to contribute to the explanation of health inequalities, e.g. through a higher rate of ischaemic heart disease, stroke, and injury mortality (Makela *et al.* 1997).

Comparable data on dietary behaviour by socioeconomic status are even more difficult to obtain. The measurement of diet is notoriously difficult, and collecting nationally representative data on diet by socioeconomic position from a range of countries a costly exercise. Only a few comparative studies have been conducted, and these show that men and women in lower socioeconomic groups tend to eat fresh vegetables less frequently, particularly in the north of Europe. Differences in fresh vegetable consumption are smallest in the south of Europe, perhaps because of the larger availability and affordability of fruits and vegetables in Mediterranean countries. A similar north–south gradient has been found for the consumption of fruits (Cavelaars *et al.* 1997). Literature reviews have shown that it is likely that many other aspects of diet, such as consumption of meat, dairy products, and various fats and oils, also are socially patterned in many European countries, and that these social patterns differ between countries (Lopez-Azpiazu *et al.* 2003).

Lack of leisure-time physical activity tends to be more common in the lower socioeconomic groups, and so do overweight and obesity. Interestingly, this is one of the very few health aspects where patterns of social variation are clearer for women than for men. Among women, overweight and obesity are more prevalent in lower socioeconomic groups in all countries with available data, whereas the patterns are more variable among men (Fig. 12.3.5) (Sobal & Stunkard 1989; Cavelaars *et al.* 1997).

Additional perspectives

During the 1990s, substantial progress has been made in understanding the mechanisms and factors involved in generating these variations in health. What has emerged from recent research efforts is a rather complex picture of how individuals in the lower socioeconomic strata are exposed over their lifetime to a wide variety of unfavourable and interacting material, cultural and psychological

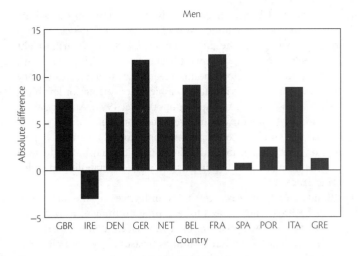

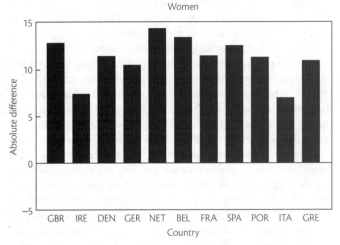

Fig. 12.3.5 Educational differences in overweight (% of individuals with body mass index higher than or equal to 25 kg/m²) in 10 European countries, men and women aged 20–74 years, ca. 1990.
Source: Cavelaars *et al.* (1997).

conditions, and how these exposures lead to ill-health—either directly, or indirectly through unhealthy behaviours or psychosocial stress. This research has opened a number of new perspectives which we review here: Life-course perspectives (dealing with the clustering of advantage and disadvantage over an individual's lifetime), and macrosocial perspectives (dealing with the effect of the wider social, economic, and political environment).

Life-course perspective

One of the interesting new perspectives on health inequalities has come from developmental research. The life-course perspective postulates that inequalities in the structure of society shape individuals' 'life chances'. Advantages and disadvantages not only cluster cross-sectionally, but also longitudinally (Davey Smith *et al.* 1997; Power & Matthews 1997). Interestingly, a life-course perspective also resolves the 'selection' versus 'causation' debate, because a material disadvantage in one stage of the life-course may translate into a health disadvantage in the next, which may then in turn lead to a material disadvantage 5 years later (Davey Smith *et al.* 1994).

The basis of health inequalities is evident even in the womb, because low socioeconomic status of the mother is associated with lower birth weight of the child (Stern *et al.* 1987). Low birth weight is not only associated with infant health, but surprisingly also with adult health, and socioeconomic inequalities in adult health may therefore partly be attributable to a higher prevalence of low birth weight in lower socioeconomic groups (Barker 1994). An association with low birth weight was first reported for adult coronary heart disease, but similar associations have been found for stroke, hypertension, and diabetes mellitus. The association may be due to 'fetal programming' of growth patterns and related metabolic and endocrine processes.

Quite clearly, however, early life influences on inequalities in adult health are not limited to fetal programming of growth patterns. There is now convincing evidence that childhood experiences leave their mark on adult health, as measured by both all-cause mortality and specific mortality rates for conditions varying from coronary heart disease to stomach cancer (Barker *et al.* 1990). For example, children's growth speeds decrease in response to a number of environmental hazards, such as poor housing, inadequate nutrition, and psychosocial stressors (Berney *et al.* 2001). Shorter adult height is associated with a range of health conditions, and the fact that adults with lower socioeconomic status are smaller on average thus suggests a role of adverse childhood living conditions in the generation of health inequalities. There is also growing evidence that socioeconomic circumstances literally shape the child and hence the adult in a process that has graphically been called 'neural sculpting' (Spencer 1996). The child's circumstances and experiences—in terms of psychosocial stress, cognitive stimuli, etc.—seem to be embodied in the adult through neuropsychological development and its impact on other biological systems that lead to potentially enduring differences in coping, competence, and health (Keating & Hertzman 1999). Circumstances in early life also set up a pattern of social learning, which may generate a sense of powerlessness reinforced by others in the social network who have been similarly disadvantaged and socially excluded, sometimes over generations (Keating & Hertzman 1999). The consequence of all this would be that observed socioeconomic differences in health in older people can plausibly be seen as the biological correlates of socially structured, differential exposure to health hazards over an entire lifetime (Berney *et al.* 2001). This view implies cumulative effects of adverse childhood living conditions, instead of latent effects.

Macrosocial perspectives

At the other end of the scale from biological factors is the macrosocial environment. Recent evidence suggests that factors such as 'social capital' and neighbourhood deprivation are independent determinants of health and may also play a part in generating health inequalities.

Partly spurred by studies suggesting that areas with more unequal income distribution have higher mortality rates, and that this may be due to less investments for the public good (Kaplan *et al.* 1996), there has been increased attention to the possible role of a lack of 'social capital' in generating health inequalities. Social capital can be depleted by high residential mobility, fear of strangers and by street crime that possibly inhibits people going to meetings and supporting their neighbours. There is some evidence that low social capital has an effect on overall levels of health, at ward

and state levels in the United States and elsewhere (Kawachi *et al.* 1999; Subramanian *et al.* 2001). While social capital is usually defined as the voluntary organizations that can bridge different social groups and whose activities can benefit members as well as those outside the membership, the concept remains contentious and has been employed quite differently by different schools of researchers.

In many countries, indices have been developed of socioeconomic deprivation of neighbourhoods and other geographical areas. These indices combine various factors known to be disadvantageous to health, such as being unemployed, part of a sole-parent household, or on a welfare benefit, and having no car or renting rather than owning a home. In recent years, a number of studies have consistently shown that even after taking account of individual circumstances, living in a deprived area is associated with ill-health both in subjective and objective terms (Diez-Roux *et al.* 2001). Pathways are likely to involve lack of access to amenities that are necessary to maintain or restore good health (such as sports facilities, stores with affordable fresh fruit and vegetables, health care), psychosocial effects (such as psychosocial stress, feelings of hopelessness, experiences of being disrespected by others), as well as depletion of social capital (Lynch *et al.* 2000; Marmot & Wilkinson 2001).

The options: How to build a strategy to reduce inequalities in health?

Policy developments vis-à-vis health inequalities

Different countries are in widely different phases of awareness of, and willingness to take action on, socioeconomic inequalities in health. Figure 12.3.6 illustrates these differences for nine countries from various parts of Europe (Mackenbach *et al.* 2003b). Four common

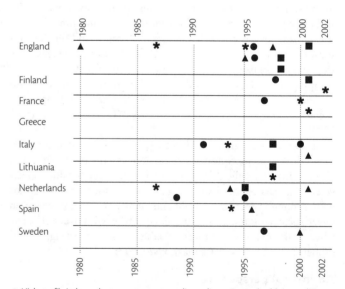

★ High-profile independent report recommending policy action on health inequalities
● Start of national research program on health inequalities
▲ Report of government advisory commission focusing on health inequalities reduction
■ Government policy document focusing on health inequalities reduction

Fig. 12.3.6 Time-lines representing concurrent policy development in nine European countries.
Source: Mackenbach and Bakker (2003).

milestones in policy development have been distinguished: High-profile independent reports recommending research or policy on health inequalities; national research programmes on health inequalities; government advisory committees recommending policies to reduce health inequalities; and coordinated government action to reduce health inequalities.

The first event included that is shown in Fig. 12.3.6 is the publication of the Black Report in 1980 in Britain (Townsend & Davidson 1992)—which has spurred research in Britain and increased awareness of health inequalities in the rest of Europe. It took more than a decade before further action was taken in Britain, first in the form of national research programmes and important government and non-government reports, then culminating in the Independent Inquiry published in 1998 (Acheson 1998). National governments in several other countries responded earlier, probably because of differences in political climate. In the Netherlands (late 1980s) and Italy (early 1990s), heightened awareness of health inequalities, partly generated by the Black Report, led to government-sponsored research programmes in this field. In Finland (mid-1980s) and Sweden (early 1990s), inequalities in health were addressed in major government policy documents on public health generally (not shown in Fig. 12.3.6) (Mackenbach et al. 2003b).

Whitehead has proposed a schematic 'action spectrum' to characterize the stage of diffusion of ideas on socioeconomic inequalities in health (Whitehead 1998). Starting with a primordial stage in which socioeconomic inequalities in health are not even measured, the spectrum covers the stages of 'measurement', 'recognition', 'awareness', 'denial/indifference', 'concern', 'will to take action', 'isolated initiatives', 'more structured developments', and 'comprehensive coordinated policy'. Among the countries included in the analysis shown in Fig. 12.3.6, which was carried out in 2002, Greece is the only one that found itself still in a pre-measurement stage. Data on socioeconomic inequalities in health were almost completely lacking, and awareness of the issue was limited to a small number of academics who do not have structural research funding for studies in this area. Spain, after a period with heightened awareness due to the publication of a Spanish 'Black Report', found itself in a 'denial/indifference' stage, largely because of a change in political colour of the national government. France and Italy both were in a 'concern' stage: Important reports on socioeconomic inequalities in health had been published, and policy-makers were increasingly paying attention to the issue. Lithuania, after the fall of the Soviet empire, has rapidly reached a 'will to take action' stage, as evidenced by parliamentary resolutions and reports from government advisory councils. The Netherlands and Sweden were in a 'more structured developments' stage, with national research programmes as well as high-level advisory committees that have recently issued comprehensive policy advice on how to reduce socioeconomic inequalities in health (see 'Blueprints for comprehensive strategies') (Mackenbach et al. 2003b).

The international comparison suggests that Britain, after a period of lagging behind other European countries, now is ahead of continental Europe in developing and implementing policies to reduce socioeconomic inequalities in health. It is the only country where policy advice has led to a significant number of new government initiatives specifically addressing health inequalities. Since the introduction of devolution in 1999, there have been a growing number of differences in health and other public policies between different parts of the United Kingdom, and it has therefore become difficult to make general statements. England seems to have entered a 'comprehensive coordinated policy' stage. Many recommendations from the Independent Inquiry have been accepted by the government in major policy documents (Department of Health 1999, 2001, 2004), and a series of new policies have been implemented ranging from neighbourhood renewal programmes to a fuel poverty strategy and from a national school fruit scheme to a child tax credit. Although from a European perspective some of these policies could be seen as a form of 'catching up' (similar programmes have been adopted long ago in other countries), the level of official government commitment was certainly unique at this point in time.

Innovative approaches

A number of innovative approaches to reduce health inequalities have been developed, some of which have been listed in Box 12.3.1.

Box 12.3.1 Innovative approaches for tackling socioeconomic inequalities in health developed during the 1990s in various European countries

Policy steering mechanisms
  Quantitative policy targets
    Reduction of inequalities in 11 intermediate outcomes (poverty, smoking, working conditions, etc.)—the Netherlands
  Health inequalities impact assessment
    Qualitative assessment of impact on health inequalities of EC agricultural policy—Sweden
Labour market and working conditions
  Universal approaches
    Strong employment protection and active labour market policies for chronically ill citizens—Sweden
    Occupational health services offering annual check-ups and preventive interventions to all employees—France
  Targeted approaches
    Reduction in retirement age for manual workers—Italy
    Job rotation among dustmen—the Netherlands
Health-related behaviours
  Universal approaches
    Serve low-fat food products through mass catering in schools and workplaces—Finland
  Targeted approaches
    Multi-method intervention to reduce smoking among low-income women—Britain
Health care
  Improving quality of care
    Nurse practitioners to support GPs working in deprived areas—the Netherlands
  Working with other agencies
    Community strategies led by local government agencies, but integrating care across all the local public sector services, including health—England
Territorial approaches
  Comprehensive health strategies for deprived areas
    Health Action Zones—England
    Municipal health policy towards Ciutat Vella, Barcelona—Spain

Source: Mackenbach and Bakker (2003).

For each of the innovations (with the exception of policy steering mechanisms), there is at least some empirical evidence suggesting that they can help to reduce health inequalities (Mackenbach & Bakker 2002). Here, we will only highlight a few examples in the areas of 'labour market and working conditions', 'health-related behaviour', and 'health care'.

Health inequalities are partly due to labour market and working conditions. Swedish labour market policies enforce strong employment protection and active promotion of labour market participation for citizens with chronic illness. A comparison with England suggests that these policies have been effective in protecting vulnerable groups from labour market exclusion during the recession of the 1990s (Burström *et al.* 2000). In France, occupational health services are mandatory and include an annual health check for every employee. This provides a good setting for introducing preventive activities for those who otherwise have few medical contacts, particularly those in manual occupations. Randomized controlled trials within this setting have shown that interventions aimed at detection and treatment of hypertension and smoking cessation were successful (Lang *et al.* 1995, 2000). In Italy, a financial crisis in the early 1990s led to a reform of the pension scheme and a postponement of retirement age. Trade unions called attention to socioeconomic inequalities in life expectancy, and negotiated a 1-year reduction in retirement age for manual workers (Costa *et al.* 2002). Improvements of working conditions have made important contributions to reducing health inequalities in the past, but a lot remains to be done. In the Netherlands, a recent intervention study suggests that task rotation among garbage collectors reduces sickness absenteeism. Rotation of tasks (truck driving and mini-container loading) reduces physical load and possibly also increases job control (Kuijer *et al.* 1999).

Health-related behaviours like food consumption, smoking, and physical exercise also contribute to socioeconomic inequalities in health. Finnish nutrition policies have followed the Nordic welfare ideology where universalism has been the general principle. School children, students, and employees in Finland receive free or subsidized meals at school or workplace, and special dietary guidelines have been implemented ensuring the use of low-fat food products. This has probably contributed to the favourable trend of narrowing socioeconomic inequalities in use of butter and high-fat milk in Finland (Prättälä *et al.* 1992). In many countries, smoking is increasingly concentrated in lower socioeconomic groups, and reviews show that a variety of policies and interventions is effective in reducing smoking in these groups. While the price weapon (raising excise taxes) is very effective, its regressive impact on the poorest smokers who cannot stop should be counteracted by active promotion of the use of nicotine replacement therapy and other cessation support. Low-income women are a group where it is particularly difficult to change smoking behaviour, and a promising Scottish initiative therefore combined various approaches (community development, drama and poetry, fitness, cessation services, social support) (Gaunt-Richardson *et al.* 1999).

Universal access to effective health care, regardless of income or other forms of social disadvantage, is another important factor. Unequal access to health care services (according to need) may aggravate socioeconomic inequalities in health or even cause them. In addition, health care can contribute to reducing health inequalities by offering dedicated services to lower socioeconomic groups and by taking the lead in working with other agencies. In England,

recent health service reforms gave local health authorities the lead responsibility for working with other agencies to improve health and reduce inequalities. The key integrating device is the production of a 3-year rolling plan for health, which feeds into a wider community strategy, committing all the local public sector services to a programme to improve the economic, social and environmental well-being of each area (Department of Health 2001).

Blueprints for comprehensive strategies

As it is unlikely that any single policy or intervention will significantly reduce socioeconomic inequalities in health, 'packages' of policies and interventions of a more comprehensive nature have been devised by government advisory committees in Great Britain, Sweden, and the Netherlands (Box 12.3.2).

Box 12.3.2 Comparison of three blueprints for comprehensive packages of policies and interventions to reduce inequalities in health

British Independent Inquiry into inequalities in health (1998)

39 main recommendations (123 with sub-clauses)

Seven overarching policy areas reviewed, corresponding to the major departments of state:

◆ Taxation and social security

◆ Education

◆ Employment

◆ Housing and environment

◆ Mobility, transport, and pollution

◆ Nutrition and the common agricultural policy

◆ National Health Service

Demographic factors over the life course considered, including:

◆ Mothers, children, and families

◆ Young people and adults of working age

◆ Older people

◆ Ethnicity

◆ Gender

Three priority areas are emphasized as crucial to addressing inequalities:

1. Health inequalities impact assessment

2. A high priority for the health of families with children

3. Reduction in income inequalities and improvement of living standards of poor households

The Dutch program committee on socioeconomic inequalities in health (2001)

26 recommendations

Four specific strategies:

1. Reduction of inequalities in education, income and other socioeconomic factors, e.g. no increase in income inequalities; anti-poverty measures; benefits to counter health effects of poverty

2. Reduction of the negative effects of health problems on socio-economic position, e.g. decent benefits for work-incapacity; improved labour market participation of chronically ill

3. Reduction of the negative effects of socioeconomic position on health, e.g. reduction of smoking, overweight, physical and psychosocial work load in lower socioeconomic groups

4. Improve access and quality of healthcare for lower socioeconomic groups, e.g. preserve equal access; strengthen primary care in deprived neighbourhoods

Eleven quantitative targets relating to intermediate outcomes.

In general, strong emphasis on continuation of research, development, monitoring, and evaluation.

Swedish National Public Health Commission (2000)

18 health policy objectives
Six overarching themes:

1. Strengthening social capital, e.g. reduce poverty; reduce segregation in housing; reduced isolation and loneliness

2 Growing up in a satisfactory environment, e.g. secure parent-child bond; schools that strengthen pupils' self-confidence

3. Improving conditions at work, e.g. low unemployment; adapt physical and mental work demands; reduced overtime

4. Creating a satisfactory physical environment, e.g. green areas and playgrounds; high standards of building; safe traffic environment

5. Stimulating health-promoting life habits, e.g. more physical exercise; reduce overweight; reduce unwanted pregnancies

6. Developing a satisfactory infrastructure for health, e.g. strengthening prevention; coordination of public health efforts; intensified research

Development of 'indicators for achievement' recommended.

Source: Mackenbach and Bakker (2003).

Great Britain

The Black Report, mentioned above, contained the first example of such a comprehensive strategy (Townsend & Davidson 1992), but was received coolly and largely ignored by the Conservative government that was in power when it was issued in 1980. Further high-profile reports, such as The Health Divide (Whitehead 1992), stimulated widespread debate in the late 1980s, but were rejected by the government of the day. By the mid-1990s, however, the political climate had softened, and the King's Fund revisited the area and made a systematic attempt to review the scientific evidence for effective policies and interventions to reduce socioeconomic inequalities in health (Benzeval *et al.* 1995). The King's Fund report paved the way for the Independent Inquiry into Inequalities in Health, held by the Acheson Committee. The committee came up with 39 recommendations (123 in total, counting sub-clauses) (Acheson 1998). Without a doubt, this is the most comprehensive set of recommendations ever prepared. It has consequently been criticized for its lack of clear priorities, although three areas were singled out as priorities in the report, as detailed in Box 12.3.2. There is a certain

emphasis on addressing 'upstream' factors like income, education, and employment, while recommendations on 'downstream' factors, like health-related behaviour, are presented as part of more general strategies directed towards groups defined in terms of age, gender, and ethnicity. The role of the National Health Service in reducing health inequalities is presented under a separate heading, probably to emphasize that even though deficiencies in health services are not a major cause of inequalities in health status, the health sector has an important part to play in any strategy to address observed health inequalities. Since the publication of the report, important progress has been made in implementing a number if its recommendations (Department of Health 1999, 2001, 2004).

The Netherlands and Sweden

Two recent reports from the Netherlands and Sweden provide an interesting contrast. In the Netherlands, a national 'Program Committee on Socioeconomic Inequalities in Health' has issued a set of 26 specific recommendations (Mackenbach & Stronks 2002). The committee is commonly called after its chairman, Albeda, a former Christian-Democrat Minister of Social Affairs. The committee had an equal representation of scientists and policy-makers, the latter representing different political parties. The recommendations were partly based on a series of intervention studies in which 12 different interventions addressing inequalities in health were subjected to, mostly quasi-experimental, process or outcome evaluations. A consultation exercise involving policy-makers and practitioners in various fields was part of the exercise (Stronks & Hulshof 2001). The recommendations were grouped in four strategies to address four different entry-points: Reduction of inequalities in socioeconomic factors; reduction of the negative effect of health on socioeconomic position; reduction of the negative effect of socioeconomic disadvantage on health (through reduced exposure to specific risk factors); and improved access and quality of health care. These entry points were derived from a simple and pragmatic model that was devised to help policy-makers understand how socioeconomic inequalities in health are generated. Examples of recommendations include 'no further increase in income inequality', 'no cuts in disability benefits', 'increase labour participation of the chronically ill', 'reduce physically demanding work', 'increase tobacco taxation', 'implement school health policies', and 'strengthen primary care in deprived areas' (Mackenbach & Stronks 2002). Due to recent political instabilities in the Netherlands, the national government has only recently started to implement some of the recommendations of the Albeda committee. At the local and regional level, however, many new initiatives have been taken to tackle health inequalities (Mackenbach & Stronks 2004).

In Sweden, the National Public Health Commission, a committee consisting of representatives of all political parties, scientific experts and advisers from governmental and non-governmental organizations, has recently developed a new national health policy with a strong focus on reducing health inequalities. The commission used a conceptual model resembling the Dutch model, but with contextual factors and the social consequences of disease added. Although the exercise involved a review of scientific evidence, like in the Independent Inquiry this review focused on explanations of inequalities in health, not on the evaluation of policies and interventions. It further involved extensive consultation of numerous organizations, and the proposal itself includes action by a wide range of actors in society. The commission formulated

18 health policy objectives grouped in six large areas: Strengthening social capital; growing up in a satisfactory environment; improving conditions at work; creating a satisfactory physical environment; stimulating health-promoting life habits; and developing a satisfactory infrastructure for health. Specific factors addressed by the strategy range from contextual factors such as social cohesion and housing segregation (with effects on children's educational opportunities) to work organization (with effects on job strain) and tobacco and alcohol consumption. The commission recommended to develop quantitative targets related to each of these policy objectives, but although specific targets were presented in draft versions of the strategy, these were withdrawn as the process progressed (Ministry of Health and Social Affairs, Stockholm 2000).

Towards evidence-based policy-making to tackle socioeconomic inequalities in health

The role of evidence

Within high-income countries, there is considerable diversity in the way scientific evidence has been used to underpin policies to reduce health inequalities. This is illustrated by the way the three comprehensive blueprints mentioned above were developed. The Acheson Committee commissioned 18 reviews of the evidence covering seven overarching policy areas, together with major socio-demographic factors over the life-course. Much of the evidence in the commissioned reviews related to the contribution of specific factors to the explanation of health inequalities, not to the effectiveness of policies and interventions tackling them (Macintyre *et al.* 2001). In contrast, the Dutch strategy was developed at the end of a 6-year research programme in which 12 studies were carried out to assess the effectiveness of various intervention options. The results of these studies were then discussed with experts and policy-makers, to see how these fitted into the existing evidence-base and in current policy (Stronks & Hulshof 2001). Although the approach proved only partly successful, because some entry-points for policy were not covered by evaluation studies, and some evaluation studies failed while others had design weaknesses, in the end a sizable fraction of policy recommendations was related to specific results of the programme (Mackenbach & Stronks 2002). In the Swedish case, the emphasis again was strongly on evidence relating to the explanation of health inequalities. The process was one of consultation with practitioners and policy-makers that ensured their commitment with the final recommendations. Evidence demonstrating that the strategies will actually work in terms of reducing health inequalities was not provided (Ministry of Health and Social Affairs, Stockholm 2000).

This diversity is also seen in the opinions of different researchers on what type of evidence is needed to underpin policies and interventions in this field. There are those who argue that in view of the urgency of starting to tackle health inequalities ('doing nothing is not an option') (Petticrew *et al.* 2004), one should be prepared to start intervening on the basis of plausibility. Political 'windows of opportunity' are usually short, e.g. 4 years at most, and they may be closed before careful evaluation studies have been conducted (Whitehead *et al.* 2004). A parallel has been drawn with nineteenth-century public health interventions for which controlled intervention studies have never been done, but which were implemented on the basis of plausibility and have proven to be highly successful (Davey Smith *et al.* 2001). Under the pressure of politicians wanting

to see rapid results, the best that can be achieved in terms of scientific evaluation may then be large-scale implementation accompanied by a 'real time' evaluation study of the intervention, concurrent with its implementation, using some quasi-experimental design (before-after study, interrupted time-series study, etc.) (Macintyre 2003).

On the other hand, there are those who argue that this is a strategy with serious risks. Like in other areas of social and health policy, the actual results of policies and interventions to reduce health inequalities could easily be counterintuitive. There are many historical examples of 'plausible' interventions and policies that did not work, or actually had adverse effects (Macintyre *et al.* 2001). The fact that there are no systematic differences between countries in the magnitude of health inequalities, despite large differences in health, social and economic policies, should also warn us against optimism about the effects of policies and interventions that seem plausible. Shouldn't one expect the magnitude of health inequalities in the Nordic countries, with their long histories of egalitarian economic, social, and health care policies, to be smaller than in other Western European countries? The fact that this is not the case, suggests that policies which could plausibly be seen as conducive to reducing health inequalities, may actually not be of much help, or at the very least far from sufficient. Several explanations have been suggested, including that the generous 'welfare state regimes' in the Nordic countries may actually have enabled people in lower socioeconomic groups to participate in an affluent life-style, including smoking, lack of physical exercise, overeating, and excessive alcohol consumption (Dahl *et al.* 2006). In addition to that, one could argue that any investment in reducing health inequalities should be justified on the basis of a comparison of its cost-effectiveness with that of other possible investments in health and well-being, and that producing credible evidence is therefore essential (Oliver 2001). A plea could therefore be made for more systematically collecting evidence on the (cost-)effectiveness of interventions and policies to reduce health inequalities (Macintyre *et al.* 2001).

What types and levels of evidence are needed?

Despite the disagreements on what types and levels of evidence are needed before policies and interventions to reduce health inequalities, there is a general consensus that collection of such evidence is needed. The next question then is what types and levels of evidence should be collected. Schematically, the evidence-base underpinning decisions to implement a policy or intervention to tackle health inequalities could be built up in the following sequence:

◆ Creating a theoretical rationale for the intervention or policy: Identifying factors which make a substantial, independent contribution to the explanation of health inequalities.

◆ Developing an intervention or policy which could target these factors: Adapting existing, or creating new, interventions or policies which are likely to do more good than harm, which will differentially benefit lower socioeconomic groups, and which can be implemented on a sufficiently large scale to have an impact on health inequalities at the population level.

◆ Demonstrating the (cost-)effectiveness of this intervention or policy: Showing empirically that the policy or intervention reduces health inequalities in settings similar to that in which it will be implemented, taking into account any harmful side-effects, and to an extent that justifies its cost.

For the first step, one must rely on evidence from carefully designed observational studies, such as longitudinal (or prospective cohort) studies in which exposure to low socioeconomic status and specific health determinants has been measured at base-line, and health outcomes are measured during follow-up. A number of such longitudinal studies have been set up over the past decades in some Western European countries, and have contributed importantly to the evidence-base (Marmot *et al*. 1991; Mackenbach *et al*. 1994). A variety of factors has been shown to make important contributions to the explanation of health inequalities, particularly inequalities in mortality or incidence of cardiovascular disease. Evidence on other outcomes is much more scarce. Because of the complexity of the explanation of health inequalities, in which chains of interconnected factors are thought to be operating over the life-course, one must be careful in interpreting the results of these studies. It is not necessarily the case that factors which have been identified by conventionally designed cohort studies, indeed make an 'independent' contribution to the explanation of health inequalities, in the sense that if this particular factor would be removed, the magnitude of health inequalities can be assumed to be reduced by its contribution as measured in multivariate analyses. It is important to be aware of the fact that the explanation of health inequalities, in terms of specific 'downstream' factors, is likely to be substantially different between Western European countries, and that theoretical rationales constructed for one country may have limited generalizability to other countries. This was illustrated above with the example of smoking.

Generally speaking, it is unlikely that suitable policies or interventions which effectively target factors identified in the first step are already available. Many of the factors known to be involved in the explanation of health inequalities, such as working and housing conditions, health-related behaviours, or psychosocial stressors, have been known to be health determinants for a long time, and many of them have been addressed by health or intersectoral policies. The fact that they still make important contributions to the explanation of health inequalities implies that current policies to address these factors are insufficiently effective in lower socioeconomic groups. More powerful and/or tailored approaches will therefore have to be developed, and carefully assessed, e.g. with regard to the balance between benefits and harms. In this stage of development, powerful evaluation designs are usually not necessary, just as in the case of drugs development where so-called phase I and II studies are usually small and uncontrolled (Thomson *et al*. 2004). Because of the scale of the problem of health inequalities, which requires changing the 'gradient' of health problems in whole populations, it is crucial that policies and interventions are developed which can effectively reach large sections of the population.

After the development stage, 'promising' new approaches will need to be evaluated for their effectiveness under 'real-life' circumstances. Clearly, randomized controlled trials will not always be feasible, particularly for the evaluation of policies and interventions that are applied on a population-wide scale. Sometimes, Community Intervention Trials, in which groups of people (school classes, neighbourhoods, etc.) instead of individuals are allocated to the intervention and control condition, will then be a good alternative. But in many circumstances one will have to rely on quasi-experimental or even observational designs to inform policy-makers on the effectiveness of new approaches. Controlled before-after studies or interrupted time-series designs could then be used, or observational studies of 'natural experiments', e.g. by making comparisons between countries (Thomson *et al*. 2004). A complicating factor in evaluating the effectiveness of policies and interventions to reduce health inequalities is that this effectiveness should be measured in terms of favourably changing the distribution of health problems in the population, not of reducing the rate of health problems in a particular group. A 'full' study-design therefore requires the measurement, in one or more experimental populations and one or more control populations, of changes over time in the magnitude of health inequalities. Any other design, such as an experimental study of changes over time in the rate of health problems in lower socioeconomic groups only, requires rather strong assumptions to be made, in this case on the absence of health effects in higher socioeconomic groups (Mackenbach & Gunning-Schepers 1997). Fulfilling this requirement is rather difficult in experimental study designs, which is an additional argument for accepting quasi-experimental and observational evidence in this area.

Conclusions

Whether it will actually be possible to substantially reduce socioeconomic inequalities in health remains an open question. Western European trends in inequalities in mortality during the last decades of the twentieth century have generally shown a widening of the gap in relative terms, and at best a stable situation in absolute terms (Mackenbach *et al*. 2003a). This was despite the WHO equity target for the period 1985–2000 (WHO 1985), but as previous analyses have shown, despite good intentions in some countries, scale and intensity of efforts aiming to reduce health inequalities have been very modest, at least until 1998 (Mackenbach *et al*. 2003b). It was only towards the end of the 1990s that a few countries reached a stage of policy development in which serious efforts can be, and sometimes are, considered.

There is a lot of good news too, however. First, in Western Europe, during the 1990s, there has been enormous progress in explanatory research, and this has identified a large number of targets for policies and interventions to tackle health inequalities. Second, there has also been a beginning of research and development for effective interventions and policies to tackle health inequalities. While this is still a modest beginning, it does put us in a better position to reduce socioeconomic inequalities in health in the coming decades. A number of innovative approaches have been developed for which there is at least some evidence of effectiveness. Blueprints of comprehensive packages have been developed in several countries that have a sound theoretical basis and clear inspirational value, and that have been taken or are being taken seriously by policy-makers. Progress in research and increased awareness among policy-makers have created an enormous 'window of opportunity' that should be used for moving policy forward.

Developing effective strategies to reduce health inequalities is a daunting task. No single country has the capacity to contribute more than a fraction of the necessary knowledge. This is a matter not only of restricted manpower or financial resources for research, but also of restricted opportunities for implementing and evaluating policies and interventions. Some policies can be implemented and evaluated in some countries and not in others, either because they have already been implemented or because they are politically infeasible. International exchange is therefore necessary to increase learning speed. Such international exchange should be supported strongly by international agencies such as the World Health Organization, the European Union, and the Cochrane and Campbell Collaborations.

References

Acheson, D. (1998) *Independent Inquiry into Inequalities in Health Report*. London: The Stationery Office.

Ackerknecht, E.H. (1953) Rudolf Virchow. Doctor, statesman, anthropologist. University of Wisconsin Press, Madison, WI.

Avendano, M., Kunst, A.E., Huisman, M. *et al.* (2004) Educational level and stroke mortality: a comparison of 10 European populations during the 1990s. *Stroke*, **35**, 432–7.

Avendano, M., Aro, A.R., Mackenbach, J.P. (2005). Socio-economic disparities in physical health in 10 European countries. In *Health, ageing and retirement in Europe. First results from the survey of health, ageing and retirement in Europe* (eds. A. Börsch-Supan, A. Brugiavini, H. Jürges, J.P. Mackenbach, J. Siegrist, G. Weber). Strauss GmbH, Morlenbach, pp. 89–94.

Barker, D.J.P. (1994) *Mothers, babies and health in later life*, 2nd ed. Churchill, Livingstone, Edinburgh.

Barker, D.J.P., Coggon, D., Osmond, C., Wickham, C. (1990) Poor housing in childhood and high rates of stomach cancer in England and Wales. *British Journal of Cancer*, **61**, 575–8.

Bartley, M., Plewis, I. (1997) Does health-selective mobility account for socioeconomic differences in health? Evidence from Engeland and Wales, 1971 to 1991. *Journal of Health Social Behaviour*, **38**, 376–86.

Benzeval, M., Judge, K., Whitehead, M. (1995) Tackling inequalities in health: An agenda for action. King's Fund, London.

Berney, L., Blane, D., Davey Smith, G. *et al.* (2001) Lifecourse influences on health in early old age.
In *Understanding health inequalities* (ed. H. Graham), pp. 79–95. Open Univ. Press, Buckingham.

Burström, B., Whitehead, M., Lindholm, C. *et al.* (2000) Inequality in the social consequences of illness: how well do people with long-term illness fare in the British and Swedish labor markets? *International Journal of Health Services*, **30**, 435–51.

Cavelaars, A.E.J.M., Kunst, A.E., Mackenbach, J.P. (1997) Socio-economic differences in risk-factors for morbidity and mortality in the European Community. An international comparison. *Journal of Health Psychology*, **2**, 353–72.

Cavelaars, A.E.J.M., Kunst, A.E., Geurts, J.J.M. *et al.* (1998) Morbidity differences by occupational class among men in seven European countries: an application of the Erikson Goldthorpe social class scheme. *International Journal of Epidemiology*, **27**, 222–30.

Cavelaars, A.E.J.M., Kunst, A.E., Geurts, J.J.M. *et al.* (2000b) Educational differences in smoking: international comparison. *British Medical Journal*, **320**, 1102–7.

Cavelaars, A.E.J.M., Kunst, A.E., Geurts, J.J.M. *et al.* (2000a) Persistent variations in average height between countries and between socio-economic groups: an overview of 10 European countries. *Annals of Human Biology*, **27**, 407–21.

Chave, S.P.W. (1984) The origins and development of public health. In *Oxford Textbook of Public Health* (ed. W.W. Holland, R. Detels, G. Knox). Oxford University Press, Oxford.

Coleman, W. (1982). Death is a social disease; public health and political economy in early industrial France. University of Wisconsin, Madison, WI.

Dalstra, J.A.A., Kunst, A.E., Borrell, C. *et al.* (2005) Socio-economic differences in the prevalence of common chronic diseases: an overview of eight European countries. *International Journal of Epidemiology*, **34**, 316–26.

Davey Smith, G., Neaton, J.D., Wentworth, D. *et al.* (1996). Socioeconomic differentials in mortality risk among men screened in the Multiple Risk Factor Intervention Trial: I: White men. *American Journal of Public Health*, **86**, 486–96.

Davey Smith, G., Blane, D., Bartley, M. (1994) Explanations for socioeconomic differentials in mortality. Evidence from Britain and elsewhere. *European Journal of Public Health*, **4**, 131–44.

Davey Smith, G., Hart, C., Blane, D. *et al.* (1997). Lifetime socio-economic position and mortality: Prospective observational study. *British Medical Journal*, **314**, 547–52.

Davey Smith, G., Ebrahim, S., Frankel, S. (2001) How policy informs the evidence. *British Medical Journal*, **322**, 184–5.

Department of Health (1999) *Reducing health inequalities: an action report*. Stationery Office, London.

Department of Health (2001) *From vision to reality. Stationery Office*, London.

Department of Health (2004) *Choosing health: making healthy choices easier*. Stationery Office, London.

Diez Roux, A.V., Merking, S.S., Arnett, D. *et al.* (2001) Neighborhood of residence and incidence of coronary heart disease. *New England Journal of Medicine*, **345**, 99–106.

Dahl, E., Fritzell, J., Lahelma, E. *et al.* (2006) Welfare state regimes and health inequalities. In *Health inequalities in Europe* (eds. J. Siegrist and M. Marmot). Oxford University Press, Oxford.

Dromers, M., Schrijvers, C.T., Stronks, K. *et al.* (1999) Educational differences in excessive alcohol consumption: the role of psychosocial and material stressors. *Preventive Medicine*, **29**, 1–10.

Fukuda, Y., Nakamura, K., Takano, T. (2007) Higher mortality in areas of lower socioeconomic position measured by a single index of deprivation in Japan. *Public Health*, **121**, 163–73.

Gaunt-Richardson, P., Amos, A., Howie, G. *et al.* (1999) Women, low income and smoking – breaking down the barriers. ASH Scotland/ Health Education Board for Scotland, Edinburgh.

Halldórsson, M., Kunst, A.E., Köhler, L. *et al.* (2000) Socioeconomic inequalities in the health of children and adolescents. A comparative study of the five Nordic countries. *European Journal of Public Health*, **10**, 281–8.

Huisman, M., Kunst, A.E., Andersen, O. *et al.* (2004) Socioeconomic inequalities in mortality among elderly people in 11 European populations. *Journal of Epidemiology and Community Health*, **58**, 468–75.

Huisman, M., Kunst, A.E., Bopp, M. *et al.* (2005a) Educational inequalities in cause-specific mortality in middle-aged and older men and women in eight Western European populations. *The Lancet*, **365**, 493–500.

Huisman, M., Kunst, A.E., Mackenbach, J.P. (2005) Educational inequalities in smoking among men and women aged 16 years and older in 11 European countries. *Tobacco Control*, **14**, 106–13.

Kaplan, G.A., Pamuk, E.R., Lynch, J.W. *et al.* (1996). Inequality in income and mortality in the United States: Analysis of mortality and potential pathways. *British Medical Journal*, **312**, 999–1003. Published erratum appears in *British Medical Journal*, **312**, 1253.

Kawachi, I.B.P., Kennedy, Glass, R. (1999) Social capital and self-rated health: A contextual analysis. *American Journal of Public Health*, **89**, 1187–93.

Keating, D.P., Hertzman, C. eds. (1999). *Developmental health and the wealth of nations: Social, biological and educational dynamics*. Guilford, New York.

Khang, Y.H., Lynch, J.W., Yun, S. *et al.* (2004) Trends in socioeconomic health inequalities in Korea: use of mortality and morbidity measures. *Journal of Epidemiology and Community Health*, **58**, 308–14.

Kuijer, P.P., Visser, B., Kemper, H.C. (1999) Job rotation as a factor in reducing physical workload at a refuse collecting department. *Ergonomics*, **42**, 1167–78.

Kunst, A.E., Groenhof, F., Mackenbach, J.P. and the EU Working Group on Socioeconomic Inequalities in Health (1998). Occupational class and cause-specific mortality in middle aged men in 11 European countries: a comparison of population based studies. *British Medical Journal*, **316**, 1636–41.

Kunst, A.E., Groenhof, F., Andersen, O. *et al.* (1999) Occupational class and ischemic heart disease mortality in the United States and 11 European countries. *American Journal of Public Health*, **89**, 47–53.

Lasser, K.E., Himmelstein, D.U., Woolhandler, S. (2006) Access to care, health status, and health disparities in the United States and Canada: results of a cross-national population-based survey. *American Journal of Public Health*, **96**, 1300–7.

Lang, T., Nicaud, V., Darne, B. *et al.* (1995) Improving hypertension control among excessive alcohol drinkers: a randomised controlled trial in France. The WALPA Group. *Journal of Epidemiology and Community Health*, **49**, 610–16.

Lang, T., Nicaud, V., Slama, K. *et al.* (2000) Smoking cessation at the workplace. Results of a randomised controlled intervention study. Worksite physicians from the AIREL group. *Journal of Epidemiology and Community Health*, **54**, 349–54.

Leinsalu, M., Vagero, D., Kunst, A.E. (2003) Estonia 1989-2000: enormous increase in mortality differences by education. *International Journal of Epidemiology*, **32**, 1081–7.

Ljung, R., Peterson, S., Hallqvist, J. *et al.* (2005) Socioeconomic differences in the burden of disease in Sweden. *Bulletin of the World Health Organisation*, **83**, 92–9.

López-Azpiazu, I., Sánchez-Villegas, A., Johansson, L. *et al.* (2003) FAIR-97-3096 Project. *Journal of Human Nutrition and Dietics*, **16**, 349–64.

Lorant, V., Kunst, A.E., Huisman, M. *et al.* (2005) Socio-economic inequalities in suicide: an European comparative study. *British Journal of Psychiatry*, **187**, 49–54.

Lynch, J.W., Davey Smith, G., Kaplan, G.A. *et al.* (2000) Income inequality and mortality: importance to health of individual income, psychosocial environment, or material conditions. *British Medical Journal*, **320**, 1200–4.

Macintyre, S. (1997) The Black Report and beyond: what are the issues? *Social Science and Medicine*, **44**, 723–45.

MacIntyre, S., Chalmers, I., Horton, R. *et al.* (2001) *Using evidence to inform health policy: case study. British Medical Journal*, **322**, 222–5.

Macintyre, S. (2003) Evidence based policy making. *British Medical Journal*, **326**, 5–6.

Mackenbach, J.P. (1994) Socioeconomic inequalities in health in the Netherlands: impact of a five year research programme. *British Medical Journal*, **309**, 1487–91.

Mackenbach, J.P., van de Mheen, H., Stronks, K. (1994) A prospective cohort study investigating the explanation of socioeconomic inequalities in health in The Netherlands. *Social Science of Medicine*, **38**, 299–308.

Mackenbach, J.P., Gunning-Schepers, L.J. (1997) How should interventions to reduce inequalities in health be evaluated? *Journal of Epidemiology and Community Health*, **51**, 359–64.

Mackenbach, J.P., Kunst, A.E., Cavelaars, A.E.J.M. *et al.* and the EU Working Group on Socioeconomic Inequalities in Health (1997) Socioeconomic inequalities in morbidity and mortality in Western Europe. *Lancet*, **349**, 1655–9.

Mackenbach, J.P., Kunst, A.E., Groenhof, F. *et al.* (1999) Socioeconomic inequalities in mortality among women and among men: an international study. *American Journal of Public Health*, **89**, 1800–6.

Mackenbach, J.P., Cavelaars, A.E.J.M., Kunst, A.E. *et al.* and the EU Working Group on Socioeconomic Inequalities in Health (2000) Socioeconomic inequalities in cardiovascular disease mortality: an international study. *European Heart Journal*, **21**, 1141–51.

Mackenbach, J.P., Bakker, M.J. (eds.) (2002) *Reducing inequalities in health: a European perspective*. Routledge, London.

Mackenbach, J.P., Stronks, K. (2002) A strategy for tackling health inequalities in the Netherlands. *British Medical Journal*, **325**, 1029–32.

Mackenbach, J.P., Bakker, M.J. and the European Network on Interventions and Policies to Reduce Inequalities in Health (2003b) Tackling socioeconomic inequalities in health: an analysis of recent European experiences. *Lancet*, **362**, 1409–14.

Mackenbach, J.P., Bos, V., Andersen, O. *et al.* (2003a) Widening socioeconomic inequalities in mortality in six Western European countries. *International Journal of Epidemiology*, **32**, 830–7.

Mackenbach, J.P., Stronks, K. (2004) The development of a strategy for tackling health inequalities in the Netherlands. *International Journal for Equity in Health*, **3**, 11.

Mackenbach, J.P., Huisman, M., Andersen, O. *et al.* (2004) Inequalities in lung cancer mortality by the educational level in 10 European populations. *European Journal of Cancer*, **40**, 126–35.

Mackenbach, J.P. (2006) *Health inequalities: Europe in profile*. Presidency of the EU, London, UK.

Mäkelä, P., Valkonen, T., Martelin, T. (1997) Contribution of deaths related to alcohol use of socioeconomic variation in mortality: register based follow up study. *British Medical Journal*, **315**, 211–6.

Marmot, M.G., McDowall, M.E. (1986). Mortality decline and widening social inequalities. *Lancet*, **2**, 274–76.

Marmot, M.G. *et al.* (1991) Health inequalities among British civil servants: The Whitehall II study. *Lancet*, **337**, 1387–93.

Marmot, M.G., Wilkinson, R.G. (2001). Psychosocial and material pathways in the relation between income and health. *British Medical Journal*, **322**, 1233–36.

Marmot, M., Wilkinson, R.G. (2006) *Social determinants of health*. Second Edition. Oxford University Press, Oxford.

Martikainen, P., Valkonen, T., Martelin, T. (2001) Change in male and female life expectancy by social class: decomposition by age and cause of death in Finland 1971-95. *Journal of Epidemiology and Community Health*, **55**, 494–9.

Mheen, H. van de, Stronks, K., Schrijvers, C.T.M. *et al.* (1999) The influence of adult ill health on occupational class mobility and mobility out of and into employment in The Netherlands. Results from a longitudinal study. *Social Science of Medicine*, **49**, 509–18.

Ministry of Health and Social Affairs. Hälsa på lika villkor – nationella mål för folkhälsan. Slutbetänkande av nationella folkhälsokommittén (Health on equal terms – final proposal on national targets for public health). (2000) Ministry of Health and Social Affairs, Stockholm (SOU 2000:91).

Oliver, A. (2001) Health inequalities policy: do we need evidence on effectiveness? [letter to the editor]. (rapid responses to: Davey Smith G, Ebrahim S, Frankel S. How policy informs the evidence.) *British Medical Journal*, **322**, 184–5.

Pamuk, E. (1985) Social class inequality in mortality from 1921 to 1972 in England and Wales. *Population Studies*, **39**, 17–31.

Petticrew, M., Whitehead, M., Macintyre, S.J. *et al.* (2004) Evidence for public health policy on inequalities I: The reality according to policymakers. *Journal of Epidemiology and Community Health*, **58**, 811–6.

Power, C., Mathews, S. (1997). Origins of health inequalities in a national population sample. *Lancet*, **350**, 1584–9.

Prättälä, R., Berg, M.A., Puska, P. (1992) Diminishing or increasing contrasts? Social class variation in Finnish food consumption patterns 1979-1990. *European Journal of Clinical Nutrition*, **42**(suppl), 16–20.

Shaw, C., Blakely, T., Crampton, P. *et al.* (2005) The contribution of causes of death to socioeconomic inequalities in child mortality: New Zealand 1981-1999. *New Zealand Medical Journal*, **16**, 118.

Shkolnikov, V., Andreev, E.M., Jasilionis, D. *et al.* (2006) The changing relation between education and life expectancy in central and Eastern Europe in the 1990s. *Journal of Epidemiology and Community Health*, **60**, 875–81.

Siegrist, J., Marmot, M. (eds.) (2006) *Health inequalities in Europe*. Oxford University Press, Oxford.

Sihvonen, A.-P., Kunst, A.E., Lahelma, E. *et al.* (1998) Socioeconomic inequalities in health expectancy in Finland and Norway in the late 1980s. *Social Science of Medicine*, **47**, 303–15.

Stern A. *et al.* (1987). Social adversity, low birth weight, and pre-term delivery. *British Medical Journal*, **295**, 291–3.

Stronks, K., Hulshof, J. (red.). (2001) *De kloof verkleinen*. Assen: Van Gorcum.

Subramanian, S.V., Kawachi, I., Kennedy, B.P. (2001). Does the state you live in make a difference? Multilevel analysis of self-rated health in the US. *Social Science and Medicine*, **53**, 9–19.

Thomson, H., Hoskins, R., Petticrew, M. *et al.* (2004) Evaluating the health effects of social interventions. *British Medical Journal*, **328**, 282–5.

Townsend, P., Davidson, N. (1992) The Black Report 1982. In *Inequalities in health: The Black Report and the health divide* (eds. Townsend, P., Whitehead, M., Davidson, N.), pp. 29–213. Penguin Books, London.

Whitehead, M. (1990) *The concepts and principles of equity and health.* World Health Organization, Copenhagen.

Whitehead, M. (1992) The Health Divide. In *Inequalities in health: The Black Report and the health divide* (eds. Townsend, P., Whitehead, M., Davidson, N.), pp. 215–450. Penguin Books, London.

Whitehead, M. (1998) Diffusion of ideas on social inequalities in health: a European perspective. *Millbank Quarterly*, **76**, 469–92.

Whitehead, M., Petticrew, M., Graham, H. *et al.* (2004) Evidence for public health policy on inequalities II: Assembling the evidence jigsaw. *Journal of Epidemiology and Community Health*, **58**, 817–21.

World Health Organization (1985) *Targets Health for All.* WHO, Copenhagen.

12.4

Reducing health inequalities in developing countries

Davidson R. Gwatkin

Abstract

This chapter provides a review of current thinking about health inequalities in developing countries and how to reduce them. The chapter initially discusses the relationship between three related indicators that describe distributional aspects of health status: The health of the poor, health inequality and health inequity. A concern for the health of poor flows from a broader concern for disadvantaged population groups. The definition of poverty may concern 'absolute poverty', with poverty defined in terms of a given level of income or consumption which is equally relevant for people wherever they may be. The concept of 'relative poverty' is more country-specific and attempts to define the poverty line in terms of relevance for a specific society. An alternative approach is to focus more on reducing inequalities, both in general and with respect to health in particular. Such a focus has traditionally occupied a particularly important place in thinking about international health issues and it is rare for a prominent international health statement not to give significant weight to inequality reduction. Poverty and inequality are both primarily empirical concepts. Equity, by contrast, is a normative concept, closely associated with the concept of social justice. One of the most widely cited definitions of health inequity is that it 'refers to differences in health which . . . are considered unfair and unjust'. At present, the greatest amount of attention in the overall economic development field is being paid to reducing absolute poverty, rather than to lessening relative poverty or decreasing inequality or inequity. This orientation is reflected most prominently in Millennium Development Goals (MDGs), a set of objectives that currently guide the strategy of most international and bilateral donor agencies. The second section of the chapter summarizes what is known about the dimensions and magnitude of health inequalities. The discussion focuses first on differences in life-expectancy and under-5 mortality between countries, and then describes variations in the distribution of health status and health service use within countries. The third section of the chapter presents a summary of current thought about how best to reduce inequalities and improve the health of the poor. This focuses on two, complementary issues. One is on reducing the social and economic inequalities that underlie the health inequalities described. The second is on reaching the poor more effectively with health and related services that are relevant to the principal health conditions from which they suffer. The chapter closes with a brief conclusion.

This is a review of current thinking about health inequalities in developing countries and how to reduce them. It is in three parts. The first is a discussion of the concept of health inequalities, and of the similarities and differences between other distributional concepts in current use. The second summarizes what is known about the dimensions and magnitude of health inequalities. The third presents a comparable summary of current thought about how best to reduce inequalities and improve the health of the poor. The review closes with a brief conclusion.

Concepts: The health of the poor, health inequality, health inequity

While the title of this chapter refers to health inequalities, it is important to recognize that such inequalities constitute only one of the several related indicators of interest to those dealing with the distributional aspects of health status and service use. Two others are health equity and the health of the poor.

These three indicators or concepts are similar in some ways, different in others. Those concerned with different ones of them all share a recognition that in health, as in many other fields, societal averages typically disguise as much as they reveal. Their interest is thus not in health conditions that prevail in society as a whole, but in the condition of different socioeconomic groups within society—especially in that of the lowest or most disadvantaged groups.

But within this shared concern lie a number of distinctions. Those interested with the health of the poor are typically concerned primarily with improving the health of that group alone, rather than with reducing differences between poor and rich. For those oriented towards equality, the principal objective is the reduction of poor–rich health differences. Those concerned with health inequities are concerned with righting the injustice represented by inequalities or poor health conditions among the disadvantaged.

These similarities and differences can most easily be understood by considering each the three indicators and concepts in turn, and then reviewing the practical implications of thinking in terms of one or the other:

The health of the poor

A concern for the health of poor flows from a broader concern of disadvantaged population groups that has occupied a central role in established thinking about overall socioeconomic development for over two decades. This concern emerged in the late 1960s and early 1970s in reaction to the then-dominant emphasis on countries' overall *per capita* income growth rates. At the time, a concern for distribution was thought likely to detract from the overall economic growth that was considered a necessary condition for the long-term alleviation of poverty. Concentrate first on overall growth, was the prevailing view. The result might be a rise in inequality over the short term. But, eventually, the benefits would trickle down to the poor and, over the long run, the poor would end up better off than under a development strategy oriented towards their immediate needs.

The 'trickle-up' and 'basic human needs' schools of thought, which emerged to counter the view just presented, advocated dealing directly with the poor as the best means of producing sustainable growth. The many discussions about how best to define the poor population groups of concern produced two approaches:

◆ *Absolute poverty*. The first, based on what is often called 'absolute poverty', takes a universal perspective and defines poverty in terms of a given level of income or consumption which is equally relevant for people wherever they may be. This is usually done by defining a 'poverty line' as the lowest amount of money sufficient to purchase the amount of food necessary for a minimally adequate diet (and still have enough left over to buy other essentials).

◆ *Relative poverty*. The second approach, more country-specific, deals with what is frequently referred to as 'relative poverty'. The practice here is to define the poverty line in terms of relevance for a specific society. This is typically done in one of three ways. One way, analogous to the international approach just described, is to determine how much income one needs to live decently according to some locally established definition of decency. The second approach is simply to define the national poverty line as some proportion—often arbitrarily determined—of a society's average per capita income or expenditure. The third is to define a certain percentage of a society's population, again usually arbitrarily established, as being poor.

Traditionally, advocates of absolute or relative approaches have both defined poverty in primarily in economic terms, with the poor seen as those suffering from inadequate incomes or purchasing power. However, the strictly materialistic view of this outlook has recently been increasingly challenged. Leading the charge has been the Nobel Laureate economist Amartya Sen, who has gained many adherents to his 'capabilities' approach, which defines poverty as a limited capability of an individual to realize his or her life aspiration (Sen 1999). Defined in this way, poverty becomes a much broader concept, since economic constraints constitute but one of the many obstacles that the poor must overcome. Other important ones include inadequate education, characteristics like race or religion that attract prejudice—and, of special interest for present purposes—poor health.

As of this writing, there is general agreement among those concerned with the health of the poor, and also with health inequalities as discussed in the next section, that poverty is a multi-dimensional phenomenon involving far more than economic status. There is less agreement on just which of poverty's many non-economic dimensions deserve highest priority, but many have been attracted to the dimensions included on what might be called 'the progress list'. In this case, 'progress' is an acronym, with each letter referring to a

dimension of poverty thought to be important: Place of residence, religion, occupation, gender, religion, education, socio-economic status, and social capital (Evans & Brown 2002). Yet another approach might be called 'pure' health inequality—that is, the ordering of people on the basis of their health status, from most to least healthy regardless of income or any other attribute, for the purpose of measuring health diversity in a society (Gakidou *et al.* 2000).

Health inequality

An alternative approach is to focus more on reducing inequalities, both in general and with respect to health in particular. Such a focus has traditionally occupied a particularly important place in thinking about international health issues. To be sure, it is possible to cite expressions of concern for poverty in prominent international health documents from at least the time of the 1978 Declaration of Alma-Ata onwards. But it is rare for a prominent international health statement not to give at least equal, if not more, weight to inequality reduction. For example, at the same time as the Declaration of Alma-Ata professed its concern for the unacceptable health conditions found among the hundreds of millions among the world's poor, it also advocated primary health care because of its potential 'to close the gap between the "haves" and the "have-nots"', i.e. to lessen health inequalities (World Health Organization 1978). Similarly, health inequalities have played a central role in a long European tradition of concern. Thus, for instance, well-known 1980 Black Report in the United Kingdom was titled *Inequalities in health* (Department of Health and Social Security 1980), as was the exercise that produced its successor, the 1998 Acheson Report (Independent Inquiry 1998). In the same vein, the 1984 targets of the WHO Regional Office for Europe (EURO) were expressed in terms of reducing poor–rich disparities. 'By the year 2000', said the WHO document in which these targets were presented, 'the actual differences in health status between countries and between groups within countries should be reduced by at least 25 per cent, by improving the health of disadvantaged nations and groups' (Whitehead 1990).

However, just as there are different approaches to poverty alleviation, so too are there various views about the most appropriate strategies for the reduction of inequalities. One, referred to in the previous section, concerns which dimension of health inequalities—economic, gender, ethnic, health status or some other—deserve highest priority. Other issues include:

◆ *How inequality is to be measured*. There are almost as many statistical definitions of inequality as there are statisticians; and the different definitions can produce very different interpretations of the same situation or trend. This is particularly true of measures of relative and of absolute inequality (e.g. a relative measure like the ratio of some death rate in the highest group under review relative to the rate in the lowest rate, or an absolute measure like the difference between the two rates). The measure that is currently in widest use is a relative one known as the concentration index. As in the case of the Gini coefficient for income distribution from which it is derived, the value of the concentration index can range from −1.0 (if all infant or under-5 deaths, for instance, occur in the poorest population group to +1.0 (if all deaths are in the richest group) (Wagstaff *et al.* 1991).

◆ *What aspects of inequality are most important*. Some would argue for considering inequality in health status as the outcome that counts, especially when poor health is seen as an important limitation to an individual's capability to realize his or her lifetime aspirations. Others favour focusing on health services, of any of several reasons. One is that health status can be determined by many factors, like diet and exercise practices, which are volitional; and thus, from a libertarian perspective, lie outside the realm of appropriate public policy. Another, more pragmatic reason for a health services focus is that health service access and coverage are the determinants of health status which health professionals can most easily influence.

Within each of these two streams of thought are further distinctions. Health status, for example, can be determined either through a physical examination or through self-assessment. (The two approaches can produce quite different results, in that people found to be relatively unhealthy through a physical examination do not always consider themselves to be less healthy than people whose health was determined by examination to be considerably better.) With respect to health services, there are distinctions between inequalities in service use and financing; among public, private non-profit and private for-profit services; and between preventive and curative services. People who come out ahead in one of these dimensions may lag from another perspective.

◆ *Whether the focus should be local or global.* A great deal of media and policy attention has been given to global inequalities, especially between wealthy regions like Western Europe and North America and particularly poor ones like sub-Saharan Africa, As will be discussed further below, this global outlook has recently been supplemented by the concern for inequalities among groups within countries that constitutes the principal focus of this review.

Health equity

Poverty and inequality, as described above, are both primarily empirical concepts. Equity, by contrast, is a normative one—a question of values, and closely associated with the concept of social justice. When applied to health, equity has traditionally been most often linked to the reduction of inequalities. Thus, one of the most widely cited definitions of health inequity is that it 'refers to differences in health which . . . are considered unfair and unjust'. In a similar vein, the above-cited WHO/EURO document on health equity indicated that 'equity requires reducing unfair disparities . . .' and that 'pursuing equity in health and health care development means trying to reduce unfair and unnecessary social gaps in health and health care . . .' (Whitehead 1990).

However, equity need not be exclusively a matter of reducing inequalities. It can also be associated with poverty, since one could argue that it is unjust to allow people to continue living in poverty when adequate resources are available within the society at large to lift them out of it. A particularly well-known example of poverty-oriented general thought about equity is the 'maximin' principle of distributive justice posited by John Rawls. That principle and others like it call for resources to be distributed in a way that the worst-off people in society (i.e. those occupying the 'minimum' position) get the maximum possible amount of gain. What happens to the better-off through such a pattern of resource distribution is extraneous to the maximin principle (Rawls 1971).

While not many equality-oriented advocates of health equity seem prepared to go this far, almost all incorporate at least traces of such a poverty-oriented equity definition in their statements.

The traces are to be seen most clearly in the tendency of equality-oriented discussions to disavow interest in one of the arguably more effective potential ways of reducing poor–rich health inequalities: Elimination of the rich. Rather, the focus of all known inequality-oriented health equity proposals is on lessening poor–rich differences through special efforts to improve the health of the poor.

However, regardless of whether one considers health equity to be related more to equality or poverty, the introduction of normative or social justice considerations also raises questions. For example:

◆ *When is an inequality unfair?* Not always, certainly. It is quite possible to imagine a situation marked by health inequalities that are not necessarily inequitable. One example is an inequality that is irremediable (Whitehead 1990). Another might be two population groups with similar incomes but marked differences in life expectancy attributable to different lifestyles. If the less healthy group adopts its lifestyle in full awareness of the risks involved, the resulting differences in life expectancy might be said to be simply a reflection of differences in the social preferences of the two groups, rather than any fundamental inequity. Or, to illustrate the same point by a more general example: If two individuals are in fact unequal in capacity, equal treatment would be unfair to the more capable of the two. In such a case, equity might well call for unequal treatment. In other words, equity and equality are by no means synonymous and need to be carefully distinguished from one another.

◆ *On what basis can one decide when the resources in a society are adequate to alleviate poverty?* 'Adequacy' is not a binary concept, such that there is one level of resource availability above which availability is totally adequate, and below which it is completely inadequate. Rather, there is a spectrum running from a total lack to infinite availability of resources, often with no obvious cut-off point along the way. Also, perceptions can differ: Resources that seem adequate to one person may not be so to another.

The policy and programme implications of the poverty-inequality-equity distinction

At present, the greatest amount of attention in the overall economic development field is being paid to reducing absolute poverty, rather than to lessening relative poverty or decreasing inequality or inequity. This orientation is reflected most prominently in MDGs, a set of objectives that currently guides the strategy of most, possibly all, international and bilateral donor agencies. The MDGs, which are contained in a declaration adopted unanimously in September 2000 by members of the United Nations drew together and enlarged a set of development objectives that had been agreed to during a set of global conferences over the preceding decade. As subsequently published (http://www.un.org/millenniumgoals/; http://www.undp.org/mdg/basics.shtml), they consist of eight specific aims. The overall tone of the MDGs is set by the by the first and most prominent of the eight is 'to eradicate extreme poverty and hunger'. This goal is accompanied by two targets that are unambiguously stated in terms of absolute poverty reduction. They are to halve, by 2015, the proportion of people with daily incomes of less that US$1.00, and suffering from hunger in 1990.

The three of the eight goals devoted explicitly with health are rather more ambiguously framed, in that all refer to improvements in national averages, without reference to how these improvements are to be distributed across groups within the nations concerned.

Goal four, on reducing child mortality, calls for reducing the under-5 mortality rate by two-thirds; goal five, to improve maternal mortality, sets a target of a three-quarters decline in the maternal mortality ration; goal six, on combating HIV/AIDS, malaria, and other diseases, says simply that the spread and incidence of these diseases should be halted and reversed.

While the ambiguity of these health goals leaves room for different interpretations, their association with goal one's unambiguous focus on the alleviation of absolute poverty implies at least to some degree that they, too, share this orientation. To the extent this is the case, they display less concern for lessening relative poverty, intergroup inequalities, or inequity than for improving the health of the people below the US$1.00 per day, who numbered just under one billion in 2004, representing around 18 per cent of the developing world's population in that year (World Bank 2007).

Whether the (apparent) adoption of this absolute poverty approach rather than some other has significant programme or policy approaches is a matter of debate. On the one hand, as has been noted, even those who seem furthest apart—those giving highest priority to reductions in poor–rich health inequalities in the name of equity, and those concerned with improving the health of the absolute poor—end up sounding rather similar once one realizes that the approach preferred by advocates of inequality reduction looks primarily to improvements in the health of the disadvantaged.

This is the approach taken in this article: Namely, that the most legitimate approach to reducing health inequalities is through improving the health of the poor, making the three terms close to synonymous In practice. However, it should be noted that there are at least some circumstances where an interest in improving the health of the poor can imply a different approach from that resulting from a concern for inequality reduction. An example concerns inter-regional resource allocations by international agencies:

◆ *An absolute poverty approach.* According to the World Bank figures cited earlier, nearly 80 per cent of the world's people living below the poverty line are in Asia and Africa (World Bank 2007). This being the case, an international agency guided by an absolute poverty objective would wish to put virtually all of its health resources into those regions. There would be much less justification for working in Latin America; and practically none at all for health activity in the Middle East or in Eastern Europe, where hardly anyone is so poor as to lie below the international poverty line.

◆ *A relative poverty approach.* Relative poverty exists in every country. From this perspective, there could thus be as strong a justification for supporting pro-poor health activities in one region of the world as in any other.

◆ *An equality approach.* Assuming that most of the existing health inequalities observed in the developing world are also inequitable and that inequality reduction interventions are equally effective, an equity approach would imply a particularly high priority to countries where health inequalities are greatest. Recent research points to the existence of large country-to-country differences in the degree of health inequality, which in turn suggests that some countries deserve much more attention than others from an equity perspective. According to the data presented in one recent review (Gwatkin *et al.* 2007a), intra-country economic inequalities in health (with regard to under-5 mortality) are highest in East Asia and the Pacific, and in Latin America so that these regions would deserve highest priority according to an

equality criterion. Countries in sub-Saharan Africa, where intra-country economic inequalities in health are lower, would receive less attention.

Evidence: The dimensions of the problem

Since space limitations prevent adequate coverage of the full range of health inequalities that might be considered, the discussion deals primarily, albeit not exclusively, on inequalities by economic status. It first covers global inequalities: Inequalities among regions and countries. It then turns to inequalities within countries.

A global perspective

To begin with what is perhaps obvious, the health of people in low-income regions is quite poor, much worse than in better-off countries. The situation is particularly deficient in sub-Saharan Africa.

Table 12.4.1 presents summary figures, drawn from the World Bank's *World Development Indicators*. In 2005, the latest year for which data are available:

◆ Life expectancy at birth in the low-income countries was around 59 years, 20 years or 25 per cent lower than the 79 years recorded in high-income countries. The worst conditions were in sub-Saharan Africa, where life expectance was only 47 years, more than ten years (20 per cent) below the low-income country average, more than thirty years (40 per cent) under the high-income country average.

◆ Under-5 mortality rates show the same pattern. In the low-income countries, 114 of all children born could be expected to die during the first 5 years of her or his life. This is nearly 100 (over 15 times) more than the seven who would die in the high-income countries. In sub-Saharan Africa, the 163 deaths would be almost 50 (30 per cent) higher than in the typical low-income country, over 150 (more than 23 times) above the average high-income one.

A comparison between the Table 12.4.1 figures for 2005 and 1980 provides an idea of how much the situation has changed in the past quarter-century. In brief:

◆ Life expectancy has improved significantly in almost all areas, rich and poor. But there are two exceptions: Eastern Europe, where the increase has been only one year, and in sub-Saharan Africa, where there has been a 1-year decline.

◆ Under-5 mortality has decreased in every region with available data, but the size of the increase has varied widely. Measured in absolute terms, the decrease has been largest in South Asia (97 deaths per thousand live births), lowest in the high-income countries (eight deaths per thousand live births). The percentage changes show quite a different picture, with under-5 mortality declining on the order of 50–60 per cent in all areas except sub-Saharan Africa, where a reduction of less than 15 per cent was recorded.

Any effort to summarize these trends is difficult, since the outcome varies widely with the trend and mortality measure used. All in all, however, it seems reasonable to conclude that overall conditions have improved significantly in most areas of the world, especially the middle-income countries. The major exceptions have been sub-Saharan Africa, which as clearly lagged behind the other regions; and Eastern Europe and Central Asia, where conditions appear to be improving only slowly at best.

Table 12.4.1 Global disparities in life expectancy at birth and in under-5 mortality, 1980 and 2005

Region	Life expectancy at birth (years)				Under-5 mortality (per 1000)			
	Levels in 1980, 2005		1980–2005 change		Levels in 1980, 2005		1980–2005 change	
	1980	2005	Absolute	Percentage	1980	2005	Absolute	Percentage
Low-income countries	53	59	+6	+11.3	177	114	−63	−35.6
Mid-income countries	60	70	+10	+16.7	79	37	−42	−53.2
High-income countries	74	79	+5	+6.8	15	7	−8	−53.3
East Asia, Pacific	65	71	+6	+9.2	82	33	−49	−59.8
East Europe, Central Asia	68	69	+1	+1.5	NA	32	NA	NA
Latin America, Caribbean	65	72	+7	+10.8	80	31	−49	−61.3
Middle East, North Africa	59	70	+11	+18.6	136	53	−83	−61.0
South Asia	54	63	+9	+16.7	180	83	−97	−53.9
Sub-Saharan Africa	48	47	−1	−2.1	189	163	−26	−13.8
High-income countries	74	79	+5	+6.8	15	7	−8	−53.3
World	63	68	+5	+7.9	123	75	−48	−39.0

Source: World Bank 2001, 2007

A country perspective

A concern for conditions among disadvantaged groups within developing countries is more recent than the attention given to the global situation outlined in the preceding section. To at least some degree, this resulted from the absence of standardized, comparable data that lent itself to easy review. However, this situation has changed greatly over the past few years, as international organizations have begun to provide increasing amounts of distributional information in the reports issued from comparable, multi-country household survey programmes that they have sponsored. The most readily available of these tables appear in programmes sponsored by the Demographic and Health Survey (DHS) Program, the World Bank in cooperation with the DHS Program, UNICEF, and the World Health Organization. Each has its strengths and limitations. To describe each briefly for the benefit of readers wishing to explore health equity issues more fully than is possible on the basis of information here:

◆ The DHS Program has conducted similar household surveys, focused on fertility and maternal/child health, in some 75 poor and middle-income countries. In many countries, there have been multiple surveys at different points in time. Many of the core tables in each country survey report (available at www. measuredhs.com/countries) have included data disaggregated according to such dimensions of poverty or inequality as gender, place of residence, and educational level. Since 2003, many tables have also provided information according to economic status.

◆ The World Bank, in cooperation with the DHS Program secretariat, has recently prepared a set of 56 country health and poverty reports based on information from 95 DHS surveys undertaken between 1990 and 2005. (Gwatkin *et al.* 2007a). While the reports contain information disaggregated by gender and place of residence, the principal focus is on economic disparities.

◆ UNICEF has sponsored a set of Multiple-Indicator Cluster (household) Surveys (MICS), which are generally similar to the DHS programme but cover a somewhat different set of countries and indicators. (Available at: www.childinfo.org/mics.) Like the DHS reports, those produced by MICS include data disaggregated by several dimensions of poverty.

◆ In 2002, the World Health Organization organized a World Health Survey, a set of comparable household surveys undertaken in some seventy developed and developing countries. (Available at www.who.int/healthinfo/survey/en/index.html.) These cover a considerably broader range of indicators than the mother/child-focused DHS and MICS: Self-assessed adult health status, for example; interventions against adult chronic diseases; household health expenditures; etc.

A flavour of what the massive amount of data available from these sources show can be gained from the contents of Table 12.4.2, based on DHS data. The figures presented there refer to the unweighted country averages for each of nine illustrative indicators, from as many of the 56 countries as had data available (ranging in number from 49 to 56). The average date of the surveys producing the data was around 2000. Among other things, they suggest that, overall:

◆ Economically disadvantaged groups are notably worse off with respect to almost all indicators of health status and health service use, and also with respect to almost underlying factors. For instance under-5 mortality and fertility in the lowest 20 per cent of the population is nearly twice as high as in the highest 20 per cent (135.4 vs. 73.5 for infant/child mortality, 5.7 vs. 3.0 for fertility); almost three times as high for severe malnutrition (18.0 per cent vs. 6.2 per cent). Coverage of basic health services is 50–200 per cent higher among the population's top 20 per cent as in its lowest 20 per cent, with attended deliveries being particularly skewed

Table 12.4.2 Distribution of health status, health service use in 56 low-and middle-income countries, ca. 2000

	Economic		Place of residence		Gender	
	Lowest 20%	**Highest 20%**	**Rural**	**Urban**	**Females**	**Males**
Health status						
Infant/child mortality	135.4	73.5	125.9	89.3	109.8	120.5
Severe malnutrition	18.0	6.2	15.0	8.6	12.6	13.5
Fertility	5.7	3.0	5.1	3.5	NA	NA
Health service use						
Immunization	40.7	64.0	46.6	59.3	50.9	50.7
Attended delivery	35.8	85.0	44.6	78.1	NA	NA
Contraceptive use	17.6	36.4	23.8	35.7	28.7	23.5
Underlying factors						
Breastfeeding	38.4	32.9	37.2	35.2	NA	NA
School completion	37.8	8.15	49.2	74.2	53.7	64.6
HIV/AIDS knowledge	64.3	88.2	69.9	83.3	69.7	83.9

Source: Gwatkin et al. 2007a. *Definitions:* Under-5 mortality for infant/child mortality (per 1000); third-degree stunting for severe malnutrition (%); total fertility rate for fertility (births/woman); full basic coverage for immunization (%); attendance by any medically trained person for attended deliveries (%); use of any modern contraceptive method for contraceptive use (%); exclusive breastfeeding up to six months for Breastfeeding (%); completion of five or more years of education for school completion (%); knowledge that HIV/AIDS is sexually transmitted for HIV/AIDS knowledge (%).

Note: Figures are unweighted averages for 49–56 low- and middle-income countries according to the indicator presented.

toward the best off. The only exception is breastfeeding, generally considered an important health-promoting behaviour, which tends to be somewhat higher in low economic groups.

◆ Rural-urban differences tend to parallel economic differences, presumably because of the fairly close relationship between place of residence and prevalence of economic poverty.

◆ Gender differences are quite mixed. For some indicators, there appears to be little difference among females and males, albeit with possibly higher rates among males. Examples include infant/child mortality (109.8 females, 120.5 males), severe malnutrition (12.6 per cent females, 13.5 per cent males), and immunization (50.9 per cent females, 50.7 per cent males). In some other respects, however, women seem clearly worse-off than males. School completion (53.7 per cent females, 64.7 per cent males) and HIV/AIDS knowledge (69.7 per cent females, 83.9 per cent males) are illustrations. There are yet other indicators where women seem to do better than men—as in contraceptive use (28.7 per cent female, 23.5 per cent male).

Averages, however, tell only part of the story, since there are large variations among regions and countries with respect to inequalities. A noteworthy example concerns female–male disparities with respect to infant/child mortality. Male infant/child mortality is higher than female in 50 of the countries covered; but it is lower is six. One of those six is India, which has one of the largest disparities in favour of males (female, 105.1; male 97.8). Since India is by far the most populous of the countries covered, an average figure weighted for population size—rather than unweighted as shown in Table 12.4.2—would probably show female mortality to be higher than male.

Further information on health services indicate clearly that government services, while less regressive on average that private

services, almost always deliver more benefits to the better-off than to the poor. This can be seen from Table 12.4.3, which indicates the amount of subsidy from government health expenditures accruing to the lowest and highest 20 per cent of the population in 21 countries (or large areas within countries). The highest 20 per cent of the population gained on average over 25 per cent of total financial subsidies provided through government health expenditures, compared with just over 15 per cent in the lowest 20 per cent of the population. Only four of these countries—all in Latin America—show a progressive pattern of subsidies through government services. But, in that region, government-provided services are usually accompanied by a large, highly regressive, government-sponsored social security system that provides services to formal sector employees and their families.

Benefits from government primary care expenditures seem much less inequitably distributed than those from total government health expenditures, with only about 20 per cent of primary care benefits going to the highest 20 per cent of the population, compared with 19 per cent of benefits going to the population's lowest 20 per cent. This is line with data for attended deliveries from the World Bank–DHS data exercise referred to above (but not presented here), strongly suggesting that coverage of lower-level services tends to notably less inequitable than that of higher-level ones.

The record with regards to trends in this pattern of intra-country inequalities has been limited largely to changes in economic disparities with regard to under-5 mortality. A notable exception has been the study of gender inequalities of infant and child mortality in Bangladesh, which shows a sharp decline in differences between boys and girls, which had disappeared by 2004 (Gwatkin *et al.* 2007b). The two known studies of this issue suggest that the picture has been mixed at best. This is the general conclusion from

Table 12.4.3 Subsidies from government health services accruing to top and bottom 20 per cent of a country/region's population

Subsidy from	Percentage of total subsidy to		Number of countries/regions where subsidy to bottom 20% of population is		
	Bottom 20% of population	Top 20% of population	Less than subsidy to top 20%	Same as subsidy to top 20%	More than subsidy to top 20%
All health expenditures	15.9%	26.4%	15	2	4
Primary health care expenditures only	18.8%	19.7%	12	0	9

Source: Filmer (2004).

a review, based on DHS data from the World Bank–DHS exercise. It found that among the 13 countries with a trend of decline in overall mortality, relative disparities had declined in only four, and had increased in five (Moser *et al.* 2005). The other study, by UNICEF researchers, relied on separate tabulations of DHS data. In the 24 countries covered, differentials were reduced in two, remained constant in a few others, but worsened in the majority (Minujin & Delamonica 2003).

The significance of these intra-country inequalities can be seen by considering the degree to which the total global health gap, in terms of potentially avoidable mortality, can be reduced by alleviating them. Around the year 2000, the global gap in child mortality stood at around 5 000 000 deaths, in the sense this is the number of deaths among infants and children under 5 years in the 56 countries covered by the World Bank–DHS exercise that would be eliminated by reducing mortality in those countries to the levels currently enjoyed in high-income societies. If instead, mortality levels in all economic groups within those 56 countries were reduced to the levels then experienced by the economically top 10 per cent in those same countries, slightly over 3 000 000 child deaths—representing about 60 per cent of the total global gap—would be averted. The crude nature of such estimates argues against drawing too firm a conclusion from them, but they are sufficient to suggest that intra-country disparities contribute at least as much to global health inequality as do differences among countries (Gwatkin 2007).

Evidence: Ways of remedying the problem

Current thought about how to reduce the inequalities discussed in the preceding sections focuses on two, complementary issues. One is on reducing the social and economic inequalities that underlie the health inequalities just described. The second is on reaching the poor more effectively with health and related services that are relevant to the principal health conditions from which they suffer.

Social and economic approaches

The rationale behind focusing on social and economic approaches is two-fold. The first is that social and economic improvement is in itself an important end—arguably the most important end—of development. From this perspective, while reducing health disparities between, say, economic groups is well worth doing, if one leaves the pre-existing economic inequalities unchanged, then the accomplishment is far smaller than achieving the broader goal of reducing both health and economic disparities. The second element of

the rationale is based on the argument that social and economic inequalities are the principal causes of health disparities, and only by tackling those underlying inequalities can one make significant progress toward reducing disparities in health.

Current efforts to reduce health inequalities through social and economic approaches can best be illustrated with reference to two active initiatives. One is the drive to achieve the MDGs, referred to earlier. The second is the work of a WHO Commission on the Social Determinants of Health (CSDH).

As noted previously, the MDGs consist of a set of development objectives adopted by the United Nations in 2000 that deal with a wide range issues related to human well-being: Income, hunger, education, health and others. While some of the indicators for progress toward the health MDGs refer to the coverage of health services (such as measles immunizations for reducing infant mortality and attended deliveries for improving maternal health), the goals themselves are stated in terms of health outcomes like mortality and disease prevalence levels that are influenced by far more than health services alone. Furthermore, the MDG health components are but one part of a broad, multi-pronged approach to development that focuses primarily on many other dimensions of economic and social improvement that affect health conditions.

The CSDH is a group of prominent international health professionals that began its 3-year programme of work in March 2005. The vision guiding this programme, as stated in the Commission's recent interim statement, is that 'strengthening health equity . . . means going beyond contemporary concentration on the immediate causes of disease . . . [and focusing on] the "causes of the causes"— the fundamental structures of socially determined conditions these structures crate in which people grow, live, and age—the social determinants of health'. (http://www.who.int/social_determinants/resources/ interim_statement/en/index.html) The Commission's principal aim is 'to set solid foundations for its vision: The societal relations and factors that influence health and health systems will be visible, understood and recognized as important . . . Success will be achieved if institutions working in health . . . will be using this knowledge to set and implement relevant public policy affecting health' (Marmot 2005).

At the heart of this work is the idea of a 'social gradient' in health, whereby health outcomes become worse as one descends the socioeconomic ladder. This means that not only do the poor have worse health than the rich, but the middle classes have worse health than the rich as well. While this is itself far from startling, the idea incorporates two other points that are much less intuitively obvious and that greatly increase its significance. One is the finding that these gradients exist not just in poor countries, but also in better-off ones where living conditions among even the lowest groups studied are far above any meaningful absolute poverty line. From this, it is pretty clear that there are causes of ill health that lie well outside the nexus of poor nutrition, inadequate education, unfavourable environmental surroundings, and the like that is normally blamed for particularly high rates of illness and death among the poor. The second is the identification of psychological factors—degree of control over one's work environment, for example—that appear to be responsible for these high rates, and the delineation of the biological channels through which such psychological and other factors work.

Such findings lead toward an emphasis on social and economic policies, more than on health services, as the most promising approaches to the reduction of socioeconomic health inequalities. One of the several examples that could be cited involves unemployment, which has been shown to affect health not only through loss of income, but also through the anxiety that it causes. Government moves to smooth the business cycle, and to ensure reasonable unemployment benefits illustrate ways of countering ill health and the other effects of this factor. Another illustration concerns transport, where government policies focusing on cycling, walking and the use of public transport can promote health by providing exercise, reducing fatal accidents, increasing social contact, and reducing air pollution (Wilkinson & Marmot 2003).

Thus far, most work on the social gradients of health has dealt with Northern, developed countries, particularly in Europe. If the Commission is successful, the same approach will be applied increasingly to health equity research and policy development in middle and lower income countries over the years ahead.

Health service approaches

For some, the case for reforming health services in order to reduce disparities rests on the view that the equal availability of social services is a desirable equity end in itself, regardless of how important or unimportant those services may be for reaching some other desired objective like improved health services. Recently, however, this rationale is becoming less common, and is being replaced by three others. All three acknowledge that improved health status is the desired end; that health service coverage constitutes only one of the many means to that end; and that its contribution to improved health status improvement may well be considerably less than that of broader social and economic progress. The first of the three rationales is that while health service coverage may well be a relatively minor contributor to better health, it is easier to influence than overall social and economic development. This is not to argue that even health service coverage and universal access are easy to achieve, just that it is not so difficult as the truly Herculean efforts require to increase, say, the incomes of poor people. Thus, when judged from a cost-benefit perspective, expanding health service coverage among the poor might compare quite favourably with other, social or economic approaches that might be considered. The second, closely related rationale is that with nearly US$400 billion being spent each year on health services in low- and middle-income countries, the sector is large and important enough to justify an effort to ensure that funds allocated to it are equitably spent as one component of an overall drive to improve health equity. The third rationale, also closely related to the other two, is that health

professionals have a far greater expertise in the health sector than in the other sectors related to social and economic development. Thus, while they no doubt have a potentially valuable supporting role to play in advocating and initiating change in these other sectors, the most direct contribution they can make is with respect to the health services whose provision they dominate. Some would add a moral dimension to this rationale, arguing that the first responsibility of health professionals to get their own house in order, before they try telling people in other sectors what they should be doing.

Among those working to improve health service coverage among the poor, there are two schools of thought about how to proceed. One would emphasize focusing on a few services of particular importance of health for the poor—basic immunization and attended deliveries, for example—and working to achieve universal coverage with respect to them. That is, the objective is to achieve 100 per cent coverage among all groups, better-off as well as poor. The other school prefers more targeted approaches—approaches that seek to identify the poor through one of the many methods described below—and focus on delivering services to them.

In cases where achievement of universal coverage can be realistically expected within an acceptably short period of time, the universal coverage approach would probably be generally accepted as the one of choice. When universal coverage is achieved, it provides 100 per cent coverage for the poor; and it is inherently egalitarian, in that the poor receive the same type and quality of the services concerned as do the better-off. This avoids the potential stigma, as well as the possibility of lower-quality services, that are present when special programmes are developed for disadvantaged groups. It also has the advantage of simplicity, in that it obviates the need for often-difficult and expensive mechanisms required to identify the poor and ensure that they are the ones who receive services. Also, when starting from a base of high initial overall coverage, a universal coverage approach is inherently targeted, in the sense that those not already covered are likely to be concentrated in disadvantaged groups.

There are a number of cases where universal care strategies can be shown to have largely achieved their objectives. Examples include the poor republics of the former Soviet Union, which have achieved high immunization coverage rates that are close to equal across economic classes, and even higher and well-distributed delivery attendance. Even here, however, there are notable class differences by type of delivery attendance with most deliveries in lower income groups handled by nurses or midwives, and most upper-income deliveries attended by doctors (Gwatkin *et al.* 2007a). Several Asian countries/areas with universal care strategies—Hong Kong, Malaysia, Sri Lanka, Thailand—have achieved government health service expenditure patterns that provides larger subsidies to the lowest than to the highest economic groups (O'Donnell *et al.* 2005).

The advantages of universal care strategies become considerably less obvious in settings where initial overall coverage is low, and where the prospects for achieving universal service availability in the foreseeable future are limited. Here, large numbers of people at all levels remain unserved. In such a situation is possible and tempting to increase national average rates by serving first the better-off uncovered groups, which are often the easiest to reach, and deferring expansion of coverage to the poor until some later stage of programme development. In the least unfavourable scenario, coverage of the poor can be delayed for an extended period marked by increased inequality as coverage rises among the better-off. In cases where the drive for coverage expansion slows or stalls before the achievement of universality, then this situation of heightened inequality could be extended indefinitely.

In these and other settings, an alternative is to use some 'targeted' approach. The expression 'targeting' refers to a set of techniques used to increase the percentage of benefits from a particular intervention that flow to the poor. There are many different targeting techniques available, and many ways of categorizing them. One of the more common categorization approaches features a distinction between 'individual', 'direct', or 'narrow' targeting on the one hand; and 'indicator/characteristic', 'indirect', or 'broad' targeting on the other.

The former type refers to efforts to identify poor individuals and see that as much of the service concerned reaches as many of them as possible. The objective is come as close as possible to the goal of 100 per cent coverage with 0 per cent leakage—that is, the goal of seeing that all of the poor are served and that all of those served are poor. The latter type of targeting deals with attributes rather than individuals. Rather than trying to identify individuals who are poor, for instance, it might feature the provision of services in slum areas in anticipation that the great majority of recipients will be poor. In doing so, it recognizes that it will not be able to reach all of the poor (some of whom live outside slums), and that at least some of those receiving services will not be poor (since not everyone living in a poor area is her/himself poor). But it accepts these limitations as prices worth paying in order to attain two important advantages. One is administrative practicality or efficiency, through avoidance of the considerable effort typically required to distinguish between poor and non-poor individuals with even a modest degree of precision. The second is political: The belief that poverty-oriented service programmes are much more likely to gain the political support needed for survival if members of the middle and upper classes gain enough from them to have an incentive to defend their continuation.

There are many specific targeting techniques available, each with unique features, strengths, and weakness. Three can serve to illustrate the different options. The three are individual targeting, and two forms of categorical targeting: Geographic and disease/age:

- *Individual targeting.* Recently, a great deal of attention has been given to the identification of poor individuals in order to exempt them from users' fees introduced in developing country government health facilities during health sector reforms. This is done with varying degrees of formality. At one end of the spectrum is the highly statistical 'proxy means test'. Under this approach, household possessions are taken as a proxy for income or consumption, the preferred measures of economic status; households are surveyed to determine what their residents possess; the results are amalgamated into a single index, using various statistical techniques to weight the different possessions; households are scored on the basis of this index; and those receiving below some specified score are deemed eligible for benefits. At the spectrum's other, least formal end are participatory approaches that leave it largely to village residents to determine what household characteristics best characterize poverty, and which households are poorest in terms of those characteristics.

- *Geographic targeting.* The idea behind geographic targeting is straightforward: The poorer the area to which resources are

allocated, the greater the likelihood that the individuals who benefit from those resources will be poor. Geographic targeting can be applied with widely varying degrees of precision. Perhaps the simplest, least precise form of geographic targeting is the emphasis often placed on rural areas, where the available information about suggests that poverty is in general considerably more prevalent than it is in the cities. Other, more precise forms of targeting involve a focus on poor states or provinces, or subdivisions within each. Typically, these are identified on the basis of data for per capita income or output produced by government statistical offices. Several countries, particularly in Latin America, have sought to be even more precise by using census data on things like house construction and educational levels to identify villages or other small communities that are especially poor. Recently, there has been experimentation with techniques to for identifying small areas on the basis of measures more obviously and directly related to consumption, traditionally the indicator preferred by economists concerned with poverty. The techniques concerned involve combining data from in-depth sample surveys, which ask many questions from a relatively small number of households, and from national censuses, which ask a few questions about all the households in a country. The basic idea is to identify those questions on the household survey instruments that: (1) are also included in the national census; and (2) best predict the consumption levels of the households covered. Then, average values for the questions thus identified can be calculated for individual villages covered by the census data in order to predict the average consumption levels prevailing in those villages; and the poorest villages can be selected on this basis. The amount of improved accuracy resulting from such increases in precision will depend upon the spatial distribution of poverty in the society concerned.

- *Targeting by disease and age.* While the poor generally suffer more at all ages and from all diseases than the better-off, the gaps tend to be considerably larger among young people suffering from communicable diseases. Also, because fertility is much higher among the poor, children tend to cluster in lower-income groups. For reasons like these, poverty-oriented health service programmes often focus on them through agencies like UNICEF and drives to deal with malaria, diarrhoea, immunization-preventable diseases, and acute respiratory infections. (However, as seen in the immunization figures of Table 12.4.2, many of the programmes that employ disease/age targeting end up achieving much lower coverage among the poor than among the better-off, indicating that this type of targeting alone is not necessarily sufficient to reach the poor children who suffer from the communicable diseases in question.)

These different targeting methods are not mutually exclusive and are often used in combination. Nor are they specific to health: They are also widely employed in determining the provision of other social services and benefits, and in public works programmes. There is no known instance of their achieving or even approaching perfection, when perfection is defined is full coverage of the poor, and all programme benefits flowing to them. However, there is considerable evidence that they often significantly increase the percentage of programme benefits flowing to disadvantaged groups.

A recent review of over 120 projects dealing with a wide range of development issues in nearly 50 low- and middle-income countries

(Coady *et al.* 2004) found that, on average, targeted programmes transferred around 25 per cent more to poor beneficiaries than they would have received under universal allocation. However, the range of experiences was wide, with a quarter of the interventions delivering more to the better-off. Some methods—proxy means testing and geographic means testing—seemed to work better than others. But the range of outcomes within each of the particular targeting approaches covered was very wide, suggesting that implementation effectiveness was more important in achieving success than was the targeting method selected.

Further evidence, specific to health, comes from a recent World Bank effort to identify programmes with reliable evidence concerning their record in reaching economically poor population groups (World Bank 2005). Of the 27 programmes it found, two-thirds delivered more than 20 per cent of their benefits to the population's poorest 20 per cent; in nearly a quarter of these cases, more than 40 per cent of the programme benefits went to the poorest quintile. Over half of these programmes also achieved coverage rates of over 50 per cent in the areas where they operated.

Illustrations of these programmes include:

◆ *Mexico's 'Progresa/Opportunidades' initiative* that pays rather than charges poor families for clinic and school attendance. The programme serves of 20 million people, and provides 20 per cent of the income to participating families. Almost 60 per cent of the people reached belong to the poorest 20 per cent of Mexico's population; 80 per cent of beneficiaries are in the poorest 40 per cent.

◆ *Colombia's use of a refined individual targeting technique* to provide subsidized health insurance to the disadvantaged. This raised insurance coverage in the poorest quintile of the population from well under 10 per cent in the early 1990s to nearly 50 per cent four years later. 35 per cent of the total programme subsidy went to the poorest 20 per cent of the population; 65 per cent to the poorest 40 per cent.

◆ *Cambodia's experiment in contracting with non-governmental organizations* to operate governmental rural primary health services, under contracts calling for attainment of specified coverage levels among the poor. During a 4-year experiment, the coverage among the poorest 20 per cent of the population of eight basic services rose from an average of below 15 per cent to over 40 per cent in two experimental districts with a total population of around 200 000. This increase was nearly two and one-half times as large as that experienced in two control districts that continued to receive standard government services.

◆ *Distribution of insecticide-treated bednets through measles immunization campaigns in Ghana and Zambia.* In Ghana, the Red Cross and the Government Health Service raised, from 3 per cent to nearly 60 per cent, the rate of treated bednet use among children in the poorest 20 per cent of people in a Northern district with a population of around 90 000. A similar programme in Zambia produced comparable results: An increase in ITN coverage from 18 per cent to 82 per cent in the poorest 20 per cent of the population in five rural districts with a total population of 450 000.

◆ *Marketing of insecticide-treated bednets in Tanzania.* In two southern districts, with a total population of about 60 000, the Ifakara Health Research and Development Centre developed and implemented a social marketing programme that raised the

ownership of bednets in the poorest 20 per cent of households from 20 per cent to 73 per cent. As in Ghana and Zambia, the increase in bednet use/ownership was higher among the poor than among the better-off.

As can be seen, the range of techniques featured in the apparently successful projects and programmes was wide (and included techniques that are believed not to have worked very well in other settings). Among the techniques were: Improved means of identifying poor individuals (Colombia, Mexico), cash payments for use of services (Mexico); services provided by NGOs working under contracts with carefully specified pro-poor performance indicators (Cambodia); mass campaigns (Ghana, Zambia); and social marketing (Tanzania). This is in line with the Coady-Grosh-Hoddinot finding reported above that differences in the effectiveness with which targeted programmes are administered, and in the care with which programme designs are fitted to the settings where they operate, are more important than the type of targeting approach used in determining success.

Conclusion

The conventional way to end a review of this kind is with a statement that further research is needed. Such a conclusion would no doubt be as valid with respect to health inequalities as with any of the other topics covered in this volume. Yet in the case of health inequalities, it would be difficult to argue that the need for further research is the highest priority. For, while much remains to be determined, a great deal is already understood, both about the magnitude and principal features of the problem that inequalities represent, and about approaches that can be taken to reduce them. As a result, much more is known than is being acted upon, and the principal constraints to progress are the many factors that prevent the translation of research findings into effective actions. Principal among these factors are the political ones that explain how societies determine which issues deserve their greatest attention. In other words: Political will.

References

Coady, D., Grosh, M., and Hoddinot, J. (2004). *Targeting of transfers in developing countries: review of lessons and experience.* World Bank: Washington.

Evans, T. and Brown, H. (2002). *Opportunities for action: applying an equity lens to global health initiatives.* Presentation at the National Press Club, Washington.

Evans, T. and Brown, H. (2002). *Applying an equity lens to the safe motherhood initiative.* Presentation to the Safe Motherhood Interagency Group, London.

Filmer, D. (2004). *The incidence of public expenditures in health and education.* Available at http://econ.worldbank.org/wdr/wdr2004/library/doc?id=29478.

Gakidou, E., Murray, C., and Frenk, J. (2000). Defining and measuring health inequality: an approach based on the distribution of health expectancy. *Bulletin of the World Health Organization,* **78**, 42–54.

Gwatkin, D., Rutstein, S., Johnson K. *et al.*(2007a). *Socio-economic differences in health, nutrition, and population within developing countries.* World Bank, Washington.

Gwatkin, D., Rutstein, S., Johnson K. *et al.* (2007b). *Socio-economic differences in health, nutrition, and population within in Bangladesh.* World Bank, Washington.

Gwatkin, D. (2007). *Health coverage for the poor*. Presentation at the Johns Hopkins University Bloomberg School of Public Health, Baltimore.

Marmot, M. (2005). Social determinants of health inequalities. *The Lancet*, **365**, 1099.

Minujin, A. and Delamonica, E. (2003) Mind the gap! widening child mortality disparities. *Journal of Human Development*, **4**, 397–418.

Moser, K., Leon, D., and Gwatkin, D. (2005) How does progress toward the child mortality millennium development goal affect inequalities between the poorest and least poor? Analysis of Demographic and Health Survey data. *British Medical Journal*, **331**, 2280–2.

O'Donnell, O. *et al.* (2005). *Who benefits from public spending on healthcare in Asia?* Equitap Working Paper No. 3. Institute for Health Policy, Colombo.

Sen, A. (1999). *Development as freedom*. Oxford University Press, Oxford.

Wagstaff, A., Paci, P., and van Doorslaer, E. (1991). On the measurement of inequalities in health. *Social Science and Medicine*, **33**, 545–s57.

Whitehead, M. (1990), *The concepts and principles of equity and health*. Document EUR/ICP/RPD/414. World Health Regional Office for Europe, Copenhagen.

Wilkinson, R. and Marmot, M. eds. (2003*). Social determinants of health: the solid facts*, 2nd ed., Healthy Cities 21st Century, and the International Centre for Health and Society. World Health Organization Regional Office for Europe, Copenhagen.

World Bank (2001). *2001 world development indicators*. World Bank, Washington.

World Bank (2005). *Reaching the poor with health, nutrition, and population services: what works, what doesn't and why*. Available at http://siteresources.worldbank.org/INTPAH/ Resources/Reaching-the-Poor/summary.pdf

World Bank (2007). *2007 world development indicators*. World Bank, Washington.

12.5

Prevention and control of chronic, non-communicable diseases[1]

Jørn Olsen, Virasakdi Chongsuvivatwong, and Robert Beaglehole

Abstract

Chronic, non-communicable diseases have reached epidemic proportions worldwide. These diseases include cardiovascular diseases, mainly heart disease and stroke; several important cancers; chronic respiratory conditions; and type-2 diabetes. They affect people of all ages, nationalities, and classes. Over the coming decades, the burden of chronic diseases is projected to rise particularly fast in low- and middle-income countries. Unfortunately, the prevention of disability and death from chronic diseases gets little attention worldwide. Fortunately, the main causes of these conditions are known and are similar in all regions of the world. Various strategies and interventions are available to prevent and control chronic diseases at relatively modest costs. Urgent action is required by multiple agencies to ensure that this knowledge is translated into action.

Introduction

Chronic, non-communicable diseases have reached epidemic proportions worldwide (WHO 2005). These diseases include cardiovascular diseases, mainly heart disease and stroke; several important cancers; chronic respiratory conditions; and type-2 diabetes; they affect people of all ages, nationalities, and classes. Over the coming decades the burden of chronic diseases is projected to rise particularly fast in low- and middle-income countries. Unfortunately, the prevention of disability and death from chronic diseases gets little attention worldwide, at least in part because of the persistence of myths and half-truths about them (WHO 2005). In poor sub-Saharan African countries, it is understandable that governments, donors, and research funding agencies have channelled most resources into infectious diseases. In most other richer countries, the focus of biomedical research on chronic diseases has been on treatment rather than prevention (Daar *et al.* 2007).

In response to the rising burden of chronic diseases, the World Health Assembly has adopted many resolutions—the first in 1956—calling for increased action to be taken to prevent and control the growing burden of chronic diseases. Most recently, the World Health Assembly has adopted a series of related resolutions which amplify WHO's mandate in the area of chronic diseases: Resolution WHA56.1 on the WHO framework convention on tobacco control; resolution WHA57.16 on health promotion and healthy lifestyles; resolution WHA57.17 on the global strategy on diet, physical activity and health; resolution WHA58.22 on cancer prevention and control; resolution WHA58.26 on public-health problems caused by harmful use of alcohol; and WHA 60.23 on prevention and control of non-communicable diseases: Implementation of the global strategy.

This chapter reviews the current and projected health and economic impacts of chronic diseases and strategies for their prevention and control with emphasis on low- and middle-income countries. Other chapters review the specifics of the major chronic diseases including mental disorders and their common risk factors.

The global burden of chronic diseases

Approximately 58 million deaths occurred in 2005. Around 17 million deaths, approximately 30 per cent, were due to infectious diseases (including HIV/AIDS, tuberculosis, and malaria), maternal and perinatal conditions, and nutritional deficiencies combined. An additional 5 million deaths, 9 per cent of the total, resulted from violence and injuries (WHO 2005; Abegunde *et al.* 2007).

Chronic diseases cause 60 per cent of all deaths. Cardiovascular diseases (mainly heart disease and stroke) are the leading cause of death, responsible for 30 per cent of all deaths (Fig. 12.5.1). Cancer and chronic respiratory diseases are the other leading causes of chronic disease deaths. The contribution of diabetes is underestimated because, although people may live for years with diabetes, their deaths are usually recorded as being caused by heart disease or kidney failure. About 80 per cent of all chronic disease deaths occur in low- and middle-income countries.

---

[1] The term 'chronic diseases' is preferred to 'noncommunicable diseases'.

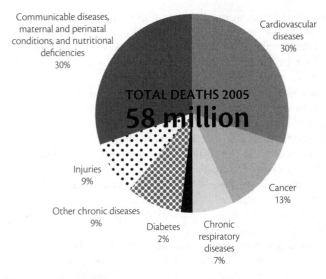

Fig. 12.5.1 Projected main causes of death, worldwide, all ages, 2005.

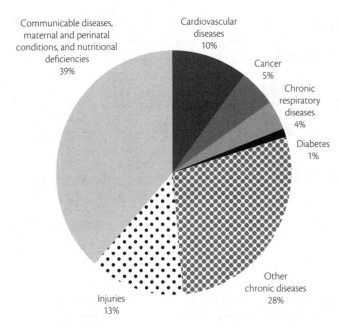

Fig. 12.5.2 Projected main causes of global burden of disease (DALYS), worldwide, all ages, 2005.

The number of deaths is similar in males and females. It is often assumed that chronic disease deaths are restricted to older people, but this is not the case. Moreover, chronic disease deaths occur at earlier ages in low- and middle-income countries than in high-income countries. The death rates for all chronic diseases rise with increasing age, but almost 45 per cent of chronic disease deaths occur under the age of 70 years.

Along with a high death toll, chronic diseases also cause disability, often for decades of a person's life. The most widely used summary measure of the burden of disease is the disability-adjusted life year (or DALY), which combines the number of years of healthy life lost to premature death with time spent in less than full health. One DALY can be thought of, under a number of conditions, as one lost healthy year of life (Murray & Lopez 1996). It focuses upon the health aspect of quality of life, and is based upon a number of assumptions; it is a concept that is population and time specific.

The projected global burden of disease for all ages, as measured by DALYs, is shown in Fig. 12.5.2, along with the burden of the leading chronic diseases. Approximately half of the burden of disease is caused by chronic diseases, 13 per cent by injuries, and 39 per cent by communicable diseases, maternal and perinatal conditions, and nutritional deficiencies combined. Cardiovascular diseases are the leading contributor, among the chronic diseases, to the global burden of disease. The number of DALYs caused by chronic disease is greatest in adults aged 30–59 years, and the rates increase with age. Overall, the burden of disease is similar in men and women. Approximately 86 per cent of the burden of chronic disease occurs in people under the age of 70 years.

Chronic disease is the leading cause of death in males and females in all WHO regions except Africa, as shown in Fig. 12.5.3 for males.

Chronic diseases are the leading cause of the burden of disease in all regions except Africa; HIV/AIDS is a major contributor in Africa (Fig. 12.5.4).

The challenges of prevention

Although, in principle it is known how to prevent many of the most important chronic diseases, it is not often known how best to

implement this knowledge. The common major risk factors for chronic diseases are the same for men and women in all regions of the world: Unhealthy diet, physical inactivity, and tobacco and excessive alcohol use. These risks, which are expressed through raised blood pressure, raised glucose concentrations in blood, abnormal concentrations of lipids in blood, overweight, obesity, and consequences of harmful use of tobacco and alcohol, are mainly driven by underlying social, economic, and environmental determinants of health (see Chapter 2.2). About 80 per cent of premature heart disease and stroke, 80 per cent of type-2 diabetes, and 40 per cent of cancers are probably preventable (WHO 2005).

Prevention aims to avoid diseases at a premature stage, not necessarily to prevent the diseases from occurring at the later stages of life. In fact, the occurrence of chronic diseases will increase with

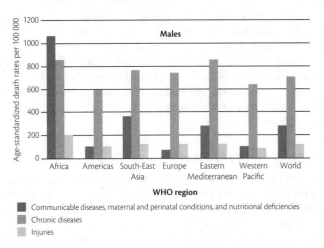

Fig. 12.5.3 Projected main causes of death by WHO region all ages, 2005—males.

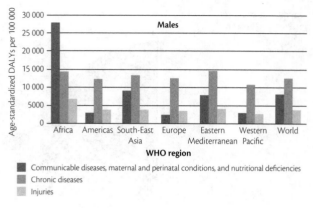

Fig. 12.5.4 Projected main causes of the burden of disease (DALYs) by WHO region, all ages, 2005, males.

the ageing of populations, in part as other risks for disease are controlled, and with the adoption of unhealthy behaviours. Basic health care will also lead to good-quality treatment of infections, and implementation of vaccination programmes will increase life expectancy; therefore, the lifelong occurrence of many chronic diseases will increase. The shift from communicable to chronic diseases in many low- and middle-income countries is in some respects a positive achievement. The challenges lie in reducing the avoidable deaths and disabilities related to chronic diseases at the same time as maintaining a focus on the remaining infectious diseases.

Although wealthy countries spend 90 per cent of world health resources on 10 per cent of world health problems, history clearly shows that expenditure of health resources on treatment alone has not been a very efficient way of reducing the number of non-communicable diseases. However, an increasing number of effective and cost-effective interventions are now available, including for chronic diseases (Jamison *et al.* 2006; Gaziano *et al.* 2007).

Social changes that make it easier to promote healthy habits will most likely have a large effect on life expectancy. For example, making it easy, safe, and pleasant to use the bicycle as a common means of transportation increases the number of people who take physical exercise every day, reduces air pollution, and saves fuel for more useful purposes. Accepting non-smokers' right to avoid passive smoke will reduce tobacco use and role models will have less influence when smoking is not performed in public places. Subsidizing healthy food or taxation on alcohol, tobacco, fat, and sugar may also facilitate a change towards a more prudent diet.

It is not possible to cover all options for preventing these diseases in a single chapter. Therefore, only certain aspects of prevention and health promotion will be discussed. Further details are to be found in the chapters dealing with the major chronic diseases and the main risk factors.

Types of prevention

Prevention is usually classified as primary, secondary, or tertiary (Rose 1992). Primary prevention aims at lowering the occurrence rate of the event, i.e. the incidence rate of the disease. Primary prevention includes programmes directed towards the whole population and high-risk groups. Secondary prevention aims at lowering the occurrence of later and more severe stages of the disease,

often by identifying diseases at a curable stage as in screening, thus reducing the prevalence of the disease through treatment. Tertiary prevention aims at reducing the consequences of the disease.

In many cases, the distinction between primary, secondary, and tertiary prevention is not clear, because the disease has no clear onset in time or a precise transmission time from one stage to another but is a result of processes which may be lifelong (Kuh & Ben-Shlomo 1997). The distinction between disease and non-disease is not as clear as many believe, not even for many cancers, and certainly not for cardiovascular diseases or mental disorders. Without a clear demarcation, it is difficult to base the taxonomy of prevention on the onset of certain stages of a disease, which may be unknown. For convenience, we often use the time when the clinician makes the diagnosis as a surrogate measure for the onset of disease.

For example, although smoking cessation may be seen as a primary prevention of lung cancer, it could also be viewed as secondary prevention if lung cancer is seen as a disease that starts with a first-stage transformation in a multistage carcinogenic process. A screening programme would aim at diagnosing lung cancer at a stage where treatment is possible and thereby removing the patient from the pool of prevalent cases (most attempts to do this have not been promising), but spiral CT screening may be an option (The International Early Lung Cancer Action Program Investigators 2006). Tertiary prevention would aim at securing work and income as long as possible and then to provide aid to reduce the losses following the disease, or to rehabilitate the patient to make it possible for him or her to work at a reduced physical or mental capacity.

The periconceptual intake of folic acid to prevent neural tube defects is primary prevention (Berry *et al.* 1999). Prenatal screening for neural tube defects by ultrasound examination is secondary prevention if a finding leads to an induced abortion, which removes the child from the pool of prevalent cases at birth. High-quality surgical treatment followed by extensive physical and social training is tertiary prevention, aimed at reducing the social consequences for the affected child and the family. Fortification of bread or flour with folic acid is primary prevention on a large scale and requires further knowledge about its consequences other than just its effects on the unborn child. Recent findings indicate that this vitamin (as well as other vitamins given in excess) may have unwanted side effects (Cole *et al.* 2007).

Screening

Screening is usually considered to be secondary prevention as it aims at identifying those with diseases at a time when they will still benefit from early detection and treatment (see Chapter 12.7). Thus, those with diseases are identified before reaching the critical point where only palliative treatment is available. Screening consists of a programme, not just the application of a screening test, and it must be evaluated as a programme. Even in situations where a well-accepted screening test is available, a health benefit is expected, and the necessary health-care facilities are available, a screening programme must be carefully evaluated before it is implemented; the screening programme takes up resources that could be spent in other areas, and also a screening activity often has severe side-effects for some of the participants. When a screening test is applied to people without symptoms, it aims at identifying the diseased before the disease has reached a non-reversible stage.

Table 12.5.1 Illustration of the outcome of a screening test

Test result	Diseased	Not diseased
Positive	True positive	False positive
Negative	False negative	True negative

An illustration of the simplest possible outcome after using a screening test on a population without symptoms shows how participants fall into four groups (Table 12.5.1).

The *true positives* benefit from the screening if they are diagnosed at a curable stage. Those who are diagnosed late may be harmed by the screening in some cases. The *true negatives* often benefit as they do not have the disease and are reassured by the testing. The false negatives may have the normal diagnostic routines delayed as the test was negative, and the false positives may have to go through unpleasant and perhaps even risky diagnostic routines due to the screening result. Therefore, the validity of the screening test is a key parameter for the success of a screening programme. It is usually measured as sensitivity, i.e. the probability of being tested positive given that you have the disease, and as specificity, i.e. the probability of being tested negative given that you do not have the disease. Screening tests often have a sensitivity ranging from 30 to 95 per cent and a specificity ranging from 80 to 95 per cent. When such a test is applied to a population with a low prevalence of the disease to be screened, many false-positive results are obtained, and not all with the disease are identified. Screening for a rare disease with a test that has low specificity will produce an unfavourable ratio between true and false positives (low predictive value; the number of true positives divided by all positives).

Randomized control trials have shown a reduction in cause-specific mortality after screening for breast cancer and colorectal cancer (Weitz *et al.* 2005). It is also generally believed that screening for cervical cancer is useful in affluent societies (WHO 2006). Identification of the subtypes of HPV that causes cervical cancer and the development of appropriate vaccines is one of the major success stories in preventive medicine and primary prevention may replace screening for cervical cancer in two to three generations (Muñoz *et al.* 2003, 2004). It is expected that more useful screening programmes will be available in cancer prevention in the future, but it would be dangerous to rely upon screening only in the fight against cancer.

Causation

The search for the causes of chronic diseases usually addresses proximal determinants of a disease because the cause must make a difference for at least some of the exposed. For example, tobacco smoking, asbestos, and some other exposures cause lung cancer, and by using counterfactual reasoning it is assumed that if these causes are removed some of the expected cases will not occur. Very few of the proximal determinants are in themselves sufficient or necessary causes. Most of the necessary causes are made necessary by including the cause in the definition of the disease (Olsen 1993). However, the component causal model presents a framework for causal thinking that matches actual evidence (Rothman & Greenland 1998). In many situations, prevention may, however, fail

if it is not taken into consideration that causes also have causes and more proximal causes may be more efficient. Poverty is probably a cause of many risk factors, and without eliminating poverty many preventive programmes will fail, especially in the most disadvantaged population groups.

WHO (2002) estimated that the five most important risk factors worldwide are malnutrition (underweight), unsafe sex, elevated blood pressure, tobacco, and alcohol misuse (in that order), with variations by level of development. Prevention should, if possible, aim at these proximal determinants directly, but in practice we may be more successful if we try to modify the determinants of, say, malnutrition or smoking. The first of these risk factors is to a large extent associated with poverty, and the tobacco, for example, is to some extent associated with ignorance and powerful marketing in some countries. Although it is known that specific subtypes of human papilloma virus are necessary causes of cervical cancer, dealing with more distal risk factors, such as reducing the number of sexual partners or encouraging condom use, may be the only way of preventing cervical cancers while we wait for an affordable vaccine to be available for the public in poor countries. Whether we should move upstream or downstream in the search for public health determinants remains an important topic for discussion.

Health promotion

Health promotion (see Chapter 7.3) includes activities that aim at improving health rather than preventing specific diseases. A prudent diet, physical exercise, better social networks, and a stimulating work environment will improve well-being and lower the risk of several diseases (see other chapters for details). Preventing chronic diseases will, with our present technology, rest upon encouraging healthy habits such as non-smoking, more physical exercise, a better diet low in fat and rich in fruit and vegetables, and better stress control by, for example, improving social networks. However, poverty-related problems such as homelessness, drug and alcohol abuse, and physical violence have not yet been eliminated, even in the most affluent societies. Basic needs concerning housing and food for all have not yet been secured, which makes health promotion meaningless for many people. A reduction in environmental exposures from pesticides, heavy metals, radon exposure, and other chemical and physical exposures are important, but at present these risk factors have a much smaller role than unhealthy lifestyle factors (WHO 2002). As many chronic diseases develop over the entire lifespan, prevention may be seen as a lifelong investment (Galobardes *et al.* 2006). The importance of taking a life course approach to disease prevention is perhaps best illustrated for obesity. Different growth curves at different age intervals correlate strongly with long-term obesity in a way we do not fully understand (Drake *et al.* 2007).

Changing behavioural risk factors is more difficult and perhaps also more expensive than changing environmental factors. Not all are willing to accept responsibility for their own health. Many people prefer, reasonably, to blame their bad health on some external factor—the environment in general, work conditions, or lack of social or personal support. Or they like to believe that medical treatment will solve all the problems that they may have in the future, perhaps not with the present technology but when they become patients in 10–20 years. The health-care industry has in many ways promised more than it could deliver. How much influence these promises have on health promotion and disease prevention is not known, but the detrimental effect could be substantial and it will continue since the health industry thrives on hope.

It is possible to change behaviour, and many private enterprises achieve this through repeated advertising. Usually large budgets are required as it is often necessary to create a perceived need and then to maintain it. Some health-related changes may benefit from being linked to profit-making enterprises. Commercial interest in selling smoking cessation tools may also be more efficient in reducing smoking habits than traditional anti-smoking campaigns. Recognition of the effectiveness of commercial methods has led to the development and application of the concept of 'social marketing', which aims to use marketing techniques to promote behaviour change for social good rather than commercial benefit.

Setting up systems that provided safe drinking water needed financial resources and political leadership in Europe in the nineteenth century (Holland & Stewart 1998). The same is true for organizing a well-functioning health-care system with a strong emphasis on health promotion. Strong political leadership is necessary to improve health behaviour. Health insurance companies, public health activities, private and public health care, pharmaceutical companies, strong medical professions, etc., do not have the same interests or goals, and they are powerful players in the health field and difficult to co-ordinate. Countries with a publicly funded health care system are often willing to provide the health care that is supported by evidence but rarely evidence-based prevention.

Building on the Ottawa Charter, the Bangkok Charter for Health Promotion (Tang *et al.* 2006) adds value to health promotion practice worldwide. Four new commitments were identified: To make the promotion of health central to the global development agenda, a core responsibility for all of government, a key focus of communities and civil society and a requirement for good corporate practices.

Prevention and healthcare

Usually only a small fraction of the overall budget for healthcare is spent on prevention, and most of the money is spent on screening and regular health examinations. Most experts agree that only changes in the most important lifestyle factors will succeed in substantially improving global health indicators in developed countries, and improving social conditions, reducing family size and providing safe water in developing countries. Still, it is difficult to see how the balance between treatment and prevention could change. Treatment deals with named patients in need. Prevention is about anonymous individuals who are at present healthy and who, in general, will not know whether or not they will benefit from the preventive action.

Convincing circumstantial evidence indicates that changing the sleeping position in early childhood from a prone to a supine position has saved thousands of children from sudden infant death syndrome (Gilbert *et al.* 2005), but there are no grateful parents who donate money to research or tell their member of parliament that prevention is an important activity to support. Prevention may be better than cure. Still, prevention will never be able to compete with cure on resources for many reasons, some of which are reasonable. A utilitarian approach to health care would allocate more resources to disease prevention, but a strictly utilitarian approach is not acceptable for ethical reasons and will be in conflict with the aim of equity in treatment (Jensen & Mooney 1990). In like manner it will not be acceptable to shift resources from necessary and efficient treatments to prevention. On the other hand, many treatments have little or no scientific justification and in these situations money is much better spent on evidence-based prevention. However, it may often be more difficult to obtain high-level evidence for preventive strategies than for clinical interventions.

A healthcare system needs to be organized towards well-defined health goals to make any difference in the priority setting. This message was probably the most important result of the WHO Health for All policy. Still, day-to-day problem solving and short-term goals, where the media's treatment of case stories plays an important part, drives most healthcare policy systems. WHO has proposed a global goal, additional to the Millennium Development Goals, which aims to reduce chronic disease death rates by an additional 2 per cent per year over current trends. The goal, if reached, would avert approximately 36 million chronic disease deaths by 2015 and would result in substantial economic savings (Abegunde *et al.* 2007). This goal is achievable even at our present level of knowledge. A small number of interventions directed towards the whole population and high-risk people will readily achieve the goal in 23 low- and middle-income countries at a relatively modest cost (Asaria *et al.* 2007; Lim *et al.* 2007).

Although prevention may be better than cure, few people act according to this precept. It is unlikely that this will change substantially in the near future, which is why every opportunity should be taken to discuss and change unhealthy habits. One such opportunity is illness. Stopping smoking after a myocardial infarction is late—too late in some cases, but not in all. Involving all healthcare workers in prevention carries an important potential for lowering the disease burden. In most countries, this potential resource has not been used to any large extent.

Social determinants of health

It is expected that disease and death would be closely correlated to poverty. It is disappointing that social inequalities in health are strong even in welfare states that have eradicated poverty in a materialistic sense for almost everyone in their societies and provided access to health care for all (see Chapter 2.2). It is perhaps difficult to avoid the fact that chronic disease can lead to unemployment and loss of income, but it should be within our reach to limit the inequalities in health that follow differences in social status. This has been one of the key targets in the WHO plan for Health for All by the Year 2000. However, in many countries, the trend has been the opposite. Reasons for social inequalities could be genetic, due to differences in access to health care, or due to differences in exposures to health hazards in the working environment or in personal life. Poor social conditions may also lead to greater exposure to stress and more changes in social conditions and other life events. In some of the East European states, there has been a substantial decline in life expectancy in males over the past 15–20 years (Eberstadt 2006).

Changes in the social classification system may explain some of the changes in social inequalities over time. If the population is classified into, say, quintiles according to a given social indicator, selection bias hardly explains changes in social inequalities. However, if the social classification system is based on educational levels, those who remain in the lower social groups need not be comparable with those from the same level in the past. This type of selection bias is expected to be present in many societies where social grouping is based on, for example, educational levels or the skill required to hold certain jobs (Cavelaars *et al.* 1998).

Social indicators are usually developed within social research. Although there are many possible ways that social factors may impair health (Marmot 2007), further knowledge is required on how best to classify social conditions in relation to health. Income, housing and working conditions, health behaviour, and access to health care may be related to health through very different mechanisms that may change over time and be different in different societies. How all these factors should be included in a social classification system that relates to health issues is not well understood.

It is likely that mandatory public health programmes, or programmes offered to all, such as vaccination programmes, free school meals, or control of work exposures help to reduce social inequalities in health. Health campaigns and voluntary screening programmes may, on the other hand, be better accepted by the best educated. Health-care workers have an important task in providing information to be used in primary or secondary prevention in a way that is understood by all. This potential for health improvements in patients with lifestyle-related diseases has not been widely used in most countries.

Genetic and molecular epidemiology

The mapping of the human genome provides new tools and new challenges in epidemiology. For most of the chronic diseases, the genetic risk factors will probably be complex and their individual contributions may be small. Stratifying the participants on genetic factors will sometimes make it easier to identify environmental and preventable causes of diseases, as has been shown for the Leiden V mutation and oral contraception (Appleby & Olds 1997). However, other gene–environment interactions may be much more difficult to detect. Important genetic determinants of breast cancer, colorectal cancer, cardiovascular diseases, obesity, and many other diseases have been identified (Frayling *et al.* 2007), but the importance of these findings in primary prevention is still not clear. The use of new genetic technologies has been most successful in identifying better treatment options by providing a better understanding of the causal pathways in disease progression. Although research may show that obesity to a large extent is a genetic disease this will not explain why obesity has an epidemic development in many countries. Even lung cancer would appear to be a predominantly genetic disorder in a population where all smoked 20 cigarettes per day. Epidemiology has had a strong link to public health. New research methods incorporating molecular biology have the potential to enhance the ability of epidemiologists to study disease processes; however, it is important for those epidemiologists using these new molecular tools to use them to help elucidate public health issues (Olsen *et al.* 1999). The development of diseases over time cannot be understood outside a social context. Diseases have causes and many of these causes are man-made and, therefore, often avoidable. Although these causes interact with genetic factors to produce their effect, it seems more appropriate to target or prevent these causes rather than change susceptibility, which may have unknown side-effects.

Environmental risk factors

Since Ramazzini published his book *De Morbis Artificium* about occupational diseases in the eighteenth century, many diseases have been accepted as having an occupational or environmental aetiology. Percival Pott was the first to identify an occupational cancer in 1775 when he recognized soot from chimney sweeping as the cause of scrotal cancer. Much later the culprit was identified as one of the polycyclic hydrocarbons. Now it is known that 4-aminophenyl, arsenic, asbestos, benzene, benzidine, chromium, polychlorinated biphenyls, vinyl chloride, and other compounds cause cancer but the fraction of cancers attributable to specific occupations is probably small in most affluent countries. Most countries have been successful in finding substitutes for some of the carcinogens or in reducing exposure levels to very low levels, but heavy metals and pesticides with very long biological half-lives are of concern, especially if they accumulate in human food chains. Asbestos exposure and exposure to radon daughter elements are still widespread and constitute important public health problems.

Environmental diseases have to be identified and their determinants located. Some diseases are so closely related to their causes that the task may be easy, such as cancer of the nose in furniture workers or liver cell angiosarcoma in people exposed to vinyl chloride. Most other diseases have environmental as well as non-environmental causes and thus are more difficult to detect despite the fact that they are much more frequent. Weak associations between exposure to high levels of electromagnetic fields and childhood leukaemia (UK Childhood Cancer Study Investigators 1999) or cell phone use and brain cancer have been difficult to interpret, as weak associations indicate that other causes of the disease are not included in the statistical model used.

In countries with very poor occupational standards, education may be the most cost-effective way of reducing exposures. Reducing environmental exposures need not be very expensive if the exposure levels are high. Exposure to, say, organic solvents may often be greatly reduced by minor rearrangements at the work site. Knowing what to do is often the first step to getting it done, but many newly industrialized countries lack the knowledge or the infrastructure to implement the knowledge.

A life-course approach to disease prevention

A growing body of evidence indicates that there may be new avenues of disease prevention in the future. The early phase of life from conception into early childhood may 'program' disease susceptibility, even for disease with an onset much later in life. As the field of life-course epidemiology evolves, it may lead to research results that can be translated into prevention (Gluckman & Hanson 2006).

It is well known that, for example, neurotoxic exposures in early life may permanently impair brain functioning, as is the case in fetal alcohol syndrome (Abel 1998). Infections may also cause damage that is not detected clinically within a short follow-up period, but could cause chronic disease in adulthood. Cardiovascular diseases, type-2 diabetes, and cancer have been seen as diseases that were the result of high-fat intake, smoking, and lack of physical exercise in adult life for genetically susceptible people. This susceptibility need not only be a function of genetic factors, but also a result of exposures that took place early in life (Gluckman & Hanson 2006). It is known from animal experiments that the functioning of some organs may be permanently altered if the diet is poor in nutritional components such as proteins, and this alteration is called 'programming'. The first human evidence came from

Forsdahl's (1977) studies in Norway showing that middle-aged males who were born in regions of high infant mortality at the time of their birth had a high mortality 50 years later, mainly due to cardiovascular diseases. Men born in regions with low infant mortality had a low risk of dying from cardiovascular diseases in middle age. A similar ecological correlation was found to be present for serum cholesterol (Bakketeig et al. 1991). Barker (1995) and Barker et al. (2005) followed up these ideas and established a link between birth weight and chronic diseases at the individual level. The mechanisms could operate via epigenetic changes where the fetus tries to adapt to the intrauterine environment. If this adoption does not match environmental conditions later it may have negative health consequences.

It is also believed that some cancers have a fetal aetiology, especially childhood cancers and cancer of the testis, but also breast cancers, ovarian cancers, and perhaps cancer of the prostate (Adami et al. 1998; Ekbom 1998). The intrauterine hormonal level may be of importance for these cancers, especially oestrogen or the balance between oestrogen and progesterone. Stress and nutrition are prenatal exposures with possible long-term effects (Ozanne & Hales 2004; St Clair et al. 2005).

The number of Sertoli cells at birth partly determines sperm production, and male fecundity may similarly be affected by external or internal disrupters of the hormonal balance acting during the time period of organogenesis (Sharpe & Skakkebæk 1993). New data indicates prenatal smoking may even be more important (Ramlau-Hansen et al. 2007). It is not known whether some types of medication have a programming effect or not but more than half of all pregnant women use medication during pregnancy.

However, whether or not these hypotheses are true is not crucial to the life-course approach in preventing chronic diseases. Arteriosclerosis is a process that starts very early in life, and dietary habits and the tendency to abuse alcohol, tobacco, or drugs depend on social and psychological factors in early life. Obesity in childhood is strongly associated with obesity in adult life. Given these conditions, health promotion as well as disease management must focus on the longitudinal track of a given disease process on the health status of individuals as well as populations. Antenatal care is only the first process in a lifelong health promotion and disease prevention endeavour and needs to take into consideration not only diseases that surface to clinical detection shortly after the onset of the programme but also health in the long run. A healthcare system strongly specialized within certain time periods of the lifespan or certain organ systems will not be well suited to meet the challenges raised by life-course research. Health promotion and diseases prevention must start early in life and should be an ongoing process like what is seen for many dental health plans.

Integrated prevention and control

Taking action

Creative solutions are necessary to address the escalating demands of reducing the frequency of chronic diseases and their common risk factors in countries with limited or stressed health systems where annual health expenditures are very low. With this limited funding, many countries must contend with a high prevalence of chronic malnutrition of children, relatively high maternal and neonatal mortality, an unfinished agenda around infectious diseases, and a steady increase in cardiovascular diseases, cancer, and

other chronic diseases. Within contexts such as these, ministries of health are faced with a seemingly daunting task: To rally support for chronic disease prevention and control; to provide a unifying vision and action plan to ensure that intersectoral action is emphasized at all stages of policy formulation and implementation; and to make certain that actions at all levels and by all sectors are mutually supportive. Additionally, actions need to be prioritized in keeping with the specific population needs for chronic disease prevention and control, range of possible interventions, and availability of human and financial resources to implement them.

Stepwise framework for preventing chronic diseases

The WHO stepwise framework offers a flexible and practical approach to assist ministries of health in balancing diverse needs and priorities while implementing evidence-based interventions (Epping-Jordan et al. 2005). The framework is guided by a set of principles based on a public health approach to chronic disease prevention and control:

- The national level of government provides the unifying framework for chronic disease prevention and control, so that actions at all levels and by all stakeholders are mutually supportive.

- Intersectoral action is necessary at all stages of policy formulation and implementation because major determinants of the chronic disease burden lie outside the health sector.

- Policies and plans focus on the common risk factors and cut across specific diseases.

- As part of comprehensive public-health action, population-wide and individual interventions are combined.

- In recognition that most countries will not have the resources to immediately do everything implied by the overall policy, activities that are immediately feasible and likely to have the greatest impact for the investment are selected first for implementation. This principle is the heart of the stepwise approach.

- Locally relevant and explicit milestones are set for each step and at each level of intervention with a particular focus on reducing health inequalities.

Figure 12.5.5 outlines the framework, which includes three main planning steps and three main implementation steps. The first planning step is to assess the current risk factor profile and burden of chronic diseases of a country or subpopulation. The distribution of risk factors among the population is the key information required by countries in their planning of prevention and control programmes, and can be assessed using WHO's stepwise surveillance approach (WHO 2003). This information must then be synthesized and disseminated in a way that successfully argues the case for the adoption of relevant policies. This is a key aspect of making the case for action.

The second planning step is to formulate and adopt a chronic disease policy that sets out the vision for prevention and control of the major chronic diseases and provides the basis for action in the next 5–10 years. In all countries, a national policy is essential to give chronic diseases appropriate priority and to organize resources efficiently. For example, China's Ministry of Health, with the support of WHO and the cooperation of relevant sectors, has been developing a national plan for chronic disease prevention and control that focuses on cardiovascular diseases, stroke, cancer, chronic

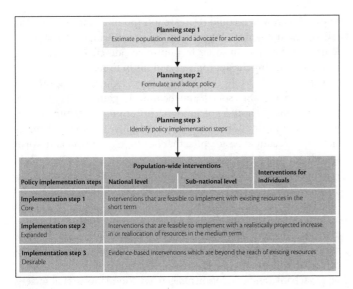

| Planning step 1 |
| Estimate population need and advocate for action |

| Planning step 2 |
| Formulate and adopt policy |

| Planning step 3 |
| Identify policy implementation steps |

| Policy implementation steps | Population-wide interventions | | Interventions for individuals |
	National level	Sub-national level	
Implementation step 1 Core	Interventions that are feasible to implement with existing resources in the short term		
Implementation step 2 Expanded	Interventions that are feasible to implement with a realistically projected increase in or reallocation of resources in the medium term		
Implementation step 3 Desirable	Evidence-based interventions which are beyond the reach of existing resources		

Fig. 12.5.5 Stepwise framework for prevention.

obstructive pulmonary disease, and diabetes. It will include an action plan for 3–5 years (Wang *et al.* 2005). Depending on the configuration of each country's governance, complementary policies can also be developed at the state, province, district, or municipal levels. In these cases, it is vital that subnational policies are fully integrated and aligned with national policies.

The third planning step is to identify the most effective means of implementing the adopted policies. The comprehensive approach requires a range of interventions to be implemented in a stepwise manner, depending on their feasibility and likely impact in the local conditions, and taking into account potential constraints and barriers to action. Some of the selected interventions might be primarily under the control of the health ministry, such as realigning health systems for chronic disease prevention and control. Others might be primarily the responsibility of other government sectors or the legislative branch, such as health financing, laws, and regulations, and improving the built environment. In these cases, the ministry of health must ensure coordination and cooperation with all government partners, civil society, and the private sector.

Planning is followed by a series of implementation steps: Core, expanded, and desirable. The chosen combination of interventions for core implementation forms the starting point and the foundation for further action. Each country must consider a range of factors in deciding the package of interventions that constitute the first, core implementation step, including capacity for implementation, likely impact, acceptability, and political support. Selecting a smaller number of activities and doing them well is likely to have more effect than tackling a large number haphazardly (Asaria *et al.* 2007; Lim *et al.* 2007). Countries should also try to ensure that any new activities complement those already underway locally, provincially or nationally.

Putting the framework into action

A number of countries, such as Vietnam and Tonga, have successfully used the stepwise framework for policy formulation and implementation (WHO 2005). They show how the stepwise approach has general applicability to solving chronic disease problems without sacrificing specificity for any given country.

Across these and other countries, the following factors have been associated with successful implementation:

◆ A high-level political mandate to develop a national policy framework

◆ A committed group of advocates who are often involved with estimating need, advocating for action, and developing the national policy and plan

◆ International collaboration providing political and technical support

◆ Wide consultation in the process of drafting, consulting, reviewing and re-drafting the policy until endorsement is achieved

◆ Development and implementation of a consistent and compelling communication strategy for all stages of the process

◆ Clarity of vision on a small set of outcome-oriented objectives

Involvement of civil society and the private sector

Any single organization or group is unlikely to have enough resources to address the complex public health issues related to the prevention and management of chronic diseases. The stepwise framework initiated by governments allows all health and non-health sectors to see how their role is an integral part of an overall framework. It becomes quickly apparent that it can be best implemented by working with the private sector, civil society, and international organizations. In the Philippines, for example, the Department of Health has assumed a coordination and advocacy role in the development of a response to chronic disease, marshalling the multiple inputs of local governments, non-governmental associations, and the Philippine Health Insurance Corporation. Using the stepwise framework as a basis for planning, a Philippine Coalition for the Prevention of Noncommunicable Diseases has been formed and a Memorandum of Understanding for action between these parties was signed in 2004 (Philippine Coalition for the Prevention of Noncommunicable Disease. Memorandum of understanding. April 14, 2004). The relations between government, civil society, and the private sector also apply at the international level, where WHO collaborates with a range of partners on chronic disease prevention and control.

The future of chronic diseases

'It is difficult to make predictions, especially for the future' was a statement made by the Danish writer Storm P., with which most people will agree. On the other hand, all preventive activities try to change undesirable expected future events and therefore are, or should be, based on predictions for the future. Not even the obesity epidemic was well predicted, although most of the risk factors were well known and monitored over time.

Most preventive activities address elimination or reduction of known risk factors, but often without giving much consideration to other consequences of behavioural or environmental changes. Most of the present predictions are based on what we know about the long-term consequences of present risk factors or long-term trends in, for example, life expectancy. Based on information of this type, we expect most populations to age in developed as well as in many developing countries and we expect chronic disease morbidity to increase from 28 million deaths worldwide in 1990 to 50 million in 2020. In 2020, the five leading causes of DALYs worldwide are expected to be ischaemic heart diseases, unipolar major depression, road traffic accidents, cerebrovascular diseases, and chronic obstructive pulmonary diseases (Murray & Lopez 1997). Although it is known how some of these diseases may be prevented, it is not in general known how to implement this knowledge. Predicting future trends rests upon many assumptions, guesses, and intuition that call for the use of many different sources of information coming from experts as well as non-experts. These methods include Delphi techniques, brainstorming, and simulation games, as well as quantitative approaches in time-series analyses, use of Markov chains, and many other related techniques (Garrett 1999; Kirchhoff et al. 1999).

The future will partly reflect the past (be predictable) but also partly reflect unpredictable opportunities and problems. Changes in climate, living conditions, wars, and behaviours will generate new diseases and provide new opportunities in new areas for existing diseases. Global warming may not only lead to mass migration from areas that will be flooded but will also lead to migration of diseases like malaria into areas where they do not exist at present. New infectious diseases may also emerge when conditions are right. Huge investments are being made in the hope that new technology may produce better predictions of pandemics and shorten the time for preventive measures like vaccines to be available.

A better understanding of diseases at the genetic and molecular level will change clinical medicine. It is less obvious it will change public health practice to the same extent but it has impact on public health research and large-scale studies are beginning to find results on genetic risk factors that are replicable in other studies as a better understanding of molecular pathways to diseases may reveal new hypotheses on gene–environment interaction which may advance a research area that focuses upon the avoidable causes of diseases.

Future research is a risky matter, as time will show if the prediction were accurate. It is necessary because it emphasizes the need to imagine what will happen with or without the preventive activity we want to implement. It is important to try to capture all consequences of preventive activities by focusing upon the larger picture rather than just single outcomes. For example, it is a noble aim to reduce childhood accidents in day-care centres, but as accidents are an unavoidable part of the way in which children explore and learn about the environment, they should not be reduced at all costs. Eradication of serious disease is extremely important for diseases such as smallpox, even though this makes the smallpox virus a frightening biological weapon. Elimination of measles will also be valuable if the virus is not replaced with other more harmful infectious agents, or if the disease or vaccination against it has no beneficial effect on the immune system in general.

Screening programmes may replace primary prevention if it is believed that the health problem can be solved by early treatment. However, if a screening programme is followed by increased risk behaviour at work or in personal life, the net benefit may be less than expected and could even be negative. If priorities were set entirely upon how much health a unit of cost would produce, the healthcare system would look very different from what we have at present. Few people would welcome such a radical approach as many other aspects have to be taken into consideration.

Setting higher standards for automobile safety equipment leads to more expensive cars and may make it impossible for poor people to own a car, which could decrease job mobility and increase the risk of unemployment. Futures studies aim at bringing these problems into the open in order to minimize side-effects as much as possible by taking the appropriate actions in time.

Although it is likely that lasting improvements in health can secure considerable social and economic gains (WHO 2001), priority setting should not be done on economic grounds only. Nor should prevention be implemented only if it saves resources elsewhere. It should be accepted that health in itself is an aim worth spending money on.

Chronic diseases will increase in numbers when life expectancy is prolonged due to better social conditions, better treatment of acute infections and active immunization. However, if the global health community gets serious about the prevention and control of chronic diseases, the onset of chronic diseases will be delayed and the time period of active life prolonged in all high-risk populations. Achieving this goal will require urgent action by WHO, the World Bank, regional banks and development agencies, foundations, civil society, non-governmental organizations, the private sector including the pharmaceutical industry, and academics (Beaglehole et al. 2007).

Key points

◆ Chronic diseases, principally cardiovascular diseases, cancer, chronic respiratory diseases, and diabetes, are leading causes of death and disability but grossly neglected on the global health agenda.

◆ Achievement of the global goal for chronic disease prevention and control would avert 36 million deaths by 2015 and would have major economic benefits.

◆ An integrated and stepwise approach to the prevention and control of chronic diseases will be the most efficient approach.

◆ Urgent action is required by WHO, the World Bank, regional banks and development agencies, foundations, civil society, non-governmental organizations, the private sector including the pharmaceutical industry, and academics.

References

Abegunde, D.O., Mathers, C.D., Adam, T. et al. (2007) The burden and costs of chronic diseases in low-income and middle-income countries. Lancet, 370, 1929–38.

Abel, E.L. (1998) Prevention of alcohol abuse-related birth effects. II: Targeting and pricing. Alcohol and Alcoholism, 33, 417–20.

Adami, H.O., Signorello, L.B., and Trichopoulos, D. (1998). Towards an understanding of breast cancer etiology. Seminars in Cancer Biology, 8, 255–62.

Appleby, R.D. and Olds, R.J. (1997). The inherited basis of venous thrombosis. Pathology, 29, 341–7.

Asaria, P., Chisholm, D., Mathers, C. et al. (2007) Chronic disease prevention: health effects and financial costs of strategies to reduce salt intake an control tobacco use. Lancet, 370, 2044–53.

Bakketeig, L.S., Magnus, P., and Sundet, J.M. (1991). In Problems and methods in longitudinal research (ed. D. Magnusson, L.R. Bergman, G. Rudinger, et al.). Cambridge University Press, Cambridge.

Barker, D.J. (1995). Fetal origins of coronary heart disease. British Medical Journal, 311, 171–4.

Barker, D.J., Osmond, C., Forsén, T.J. et al. (2005). Trajectories of growth among children who have coronary events as adults. New England Journal of Medicine, 353, 1802–9.

Beaglehole, R., Ebrahim, S., Voute, J. et al. (2007) Prevention of chronic disease: a call to action. Lancet, 370, 2152–7.

Berry, R.J., Li, Z., Erickson, J.D. et al. (1999). Prevention of neural-tube defects with folic acid in China. New England Journal of Medicine, 341, 1485–90.

Cavelaars, A.E.J.M., Kunst, A.E., Geurts, J.J. et al. (1998). Differences in self reported morbidity by educational level: a comparison of 11 Western European countries. Journal of Epidemiology and Community Health, 52, 219–27.

Cole, B.F., Baron, J.A., Sandler, R.S. et al (2007). Folic acid for the prevention of colorectal adenomas. JAMA, 297, 2351–9.

Daar, A.S., Singer, P.A., Persad, D.L. et al. (2007). Grand challenges in chronic noncommunicable diseases. Nature, 450, 494–6.

Drake, A.J., Tang, J.I., Nyirenda, M.J. (2007). Mechanisms underlying the role of glucocorticoids in the early life programming of adult disease. Clinical Science, 113, 219–32.

Eberstadt, N. (2006). Commentary: reflections on "The Health Crisis in the USSR". International Journal of Epidemiology, 35, 1394–7.

Ekbom, A. (1998). Growing evidence that several human cancers may originate in utero. Seminars in Cancer Biology, 8, 237–44.

Epping-Jordan, J.E., Galea, G., Tukuitonga, C. et al. (2005). Preventing chronic diseases: taking stepwise action. Lancet, 366, 1667–71.

Forsdahl, A. (1977). Are poor living conditions in childhood and adolescence an important risk factor for arteriosclerotic heart disease? British Journal of Preventive and Social Medicine, 31, 91–5.

Frayling, T.M., Timpson, N.J., Weedon, M.N. et al. (2007). A common variant in the FTO gene is associated with body mass index and predisposes to childhood and adult obesity. Science, 316, 889–94.

Garrett, M.J. (1999). Health Futures. WHO, Geneva.

Galobardes, B., Smith, G.D., Lynch, J.W. (2006). Systematic review of the influence of childhood socioeconomic circumstances on risk for cardiovascular disease in adult childhood. Annals of Epidemiology, 16, 91–104.

Gaziano, T.A., Galea, G., Reddy, K.S. (2007) Scaling up interventions for chronic disease prevention: the evidence. Lancet, 370, 1939–46.

Gilbert, R., Salanti, G., Hareden, M. et al. (2005). Infants sleeping position and the sudden infant death syndrome: systematic review of observational studies and historical review of recommendations from 1940 to 2002. International Journal of Epidemiology, 34, 874–87.

Gluckman, P. and Hanson, M. (2006). Developmental origins of health and disease. Cambridge University Press.

Gotzsche, P.C. and Olsen, O. (2000). Is screening for breast cancer with mammography justifiable? Lancet, 355, 129–34.

Holland, W.W. and Stewart, S. (1998). Public health. The vision and the challenge. Nuffield Trust, London.

Jamison, D., Breman, J., Measham, A. et al. (eds) (2006). Disease control priorities in developing countries. 2nd ed. New York, NY—Washington, DC: Oxford University Press; World Bank.

Jensen, U.J. and Mooney, G. (1990). Changing values in medical and health care decision making. Wiley, Chichester.

Kirchhoff, M., Davidsen, M., Bronnun-Hansen, H. et al. (1999). Incidence of myocardial infarction in the Danish MONICA population 1982–1991. International Journal of Epidemiology, 28, 211–18.

Kuh, D. and Ben-Shlomo, B. (eds) (1997). A life course approach to chronic disease epidemiology. Tracing the origins of ill-health from early to adult life. Oxford University Press, Oxford.

Lim, S.S., Gaziano, T.A., Gakidou, E. et al. (2007) Prevention of cardiovascular disease in high-risk individuals in low-income and middle-income countries: health effects and costs. Lancet, 370, 2054–62.

Marmot, M. (2007) Achieving health equity: from root causes to fair outcomes. Lancet, 370, 1153–63.

Muñoz, N., Bosch, F.X., de Sanjosé, S. et al. International Agency for Research on Cancer Multicenter Cervical Cancer Study Group. (2003) Epidemiologic classification of human papillomavirus types associated with cervical cancer. New England Journal of Medicine, 348, 518–27.

Muñoz, N., Bosch, F.X., Castellagué, X. et al. (2004) Against which human papillomavirus types shall we vaccinate and screen? The international perspective. International Journal of Cancer, 111, 278–85.

Murray, C.J.L. and Lopez, A.D. (1996). The global burden of disease: A comprehensive assessment of mortality and disability from diseases, injuries, and risk factors in 1990 and projected to 2020. Cambridge: Harvard University Press.

Murray, C.J.L. and Lopez, A.D. (1997). Global mortality, disability, and the contribution of risk factors: Global Burden of Disease Study. Lancet, 349, 1436–42.

Olsen, J. (1993). Some consequences of adopting a conditional deterministic causal model in epidemiology. European Journal of Public Health, 3, 204–9.

Olsen, J., Andersen, P.K., Sørensen, T.I.A. et al. (1999). The future of epidemiology. International Journal of Epidemiology, 28, S996.

Ozanne, S.E. and Hales, C.N. (2004). Lifespan: catch-up growth and obesity in male mice. Nature, 427, 411–2.

Ramlau-Hansen, C.H., Thulstrup, A.M., Storgaard, L. et al. (2007). Is prenatal exposure to tobacco smoking a cause of poor semen quality? A follow-up study. American Journal of Epidemiology, 165, 1372–9.

Rose, G. (1992). The strategy of preventive medicine. Oxford University Press, Oxford.

Rothman, K.J. and Greenland, S. (1998) Modern epidemiology. 2nd edn. Philadelphia: Lippincott-Raven.

St. Clair, D., Xu, M., Wang, P. et al. (2005). Rates of adult schizophrenia following prenatal exposure to the Chinese famine of 1959-1961. JAMA, 294, 557–62.

Sharpe, R.M. and Skakkebæk, N.E. (1993). Are oestrogens involved in falling sperm counts and disorders of the male reproductive tract? Lancet, 341, 1392–5.

Tang, K.C., Beaglehole, R., Pettersson, B. (2006). Implementation of the Bangkok Charter on Health Promotion in a Globalized World: experience and challenges of selected high income countries in Europe. Sozial- und Präventivmedizin, 51, 1–3.

The International Early Lung Cancer Action Program Investigators (2006). Survival of Patients with Stage I Lung Cancer Detected on CT Screening. New Engl Journal of Medicine, 355, 1763–71.

UK Childhood Cancer Study Investigators (1999). Exposure to powerfrequency magnetic fields and the risk of childhood cancer. Lancet, 354, 1925–31.

Wang, L., Kong, L., Wu, F. et al. (2005). Preventing chronic diseases in China. Lancet, 366, 1821–4.

Weitz, J., Koch, M., Debus, J. et al. (2005). Colorectal cancer. Lancet, 365, 153–65.

WHO (2001). Macroeconomics and health: investing in health for economic development. Geneva, Switzerland.

WHO (2002). The world health report 2002. Reducing Risks, Promoting Healthy Life. WHO, Geneva.

WHO (2003). STEPS: A framework for surveillance. WHO, Geneva.

WHO (2005). Preventing chronic diseases: A vital investment. WHO, Geneva.

WHO (2006). Comprehensive cervical cancer control. A guide to essential practice. WHO, Geneva.

12.6

Principles of infectious disease control

Robert J. Kim-Farley

Abstract

This chapter provides a global and comprehensive view of the principles of infectious disease control through examination of the magnitude of disease burden, the chain of infection (agent, transmission, and host) of infectious diseases, the varied approaches to their prevention and control (measures applied to the host, vectors, infected humans, animals, environment, and agents), and the factors conducive to their eradication as well as emergence and re-emergence.

Introduction and overview

Ingenuity, knowledge, and organization alter but cannot cancel humanity's vulnerability to invasion by parasitic forms of life. Infectious disease which antedated the emergence of humankind will last as long as humanity itself, and will surely remain, as it has been hitherto, one of the fundamental parameters and determinants of human history. (William H. McNeill 1976)

Infectious diseases remain a leading cause of morbidity, disability, and mortality worldwide. Their control is a constant challenge that faces health workers and public health officials in both industrialized and developing countries. Only one infectious disease, smallpox, was eradicated and stands as a landmark in the history of the control of infectious diseases. The international community is now well down the path towards eradication of poliomyelitis and dracunculiasis (guinea-worm infection). Other infectious diseases, like malaria and tuberculosis, foiled eradication attempts or control efforts and are re-emerging as increasing threats in many countries. Some infectious diseases, such as tetanus, will always be a threat if control measures are not maintained. Newer infectious diseases, like AIDS, demonstrate the truth of McNeill's statement that infectious disease will remain 'one of the fundamental parameters and determinants of human history'. The history of infectious diseases is an exciting story in itself, and readers interested in the subject are referred to McNeill (1976) or the comprehensive work on the history of human diseases (Kiple 1993).

This chapter provides many examples of infectious diseases that illustrate modes of transmission and approaches to infectious disease control; however, it does not attempt to be comprehensive in listing all infectious diseases. Detailed recommendations on control measures for any specific disease are outlined periodically in the updated reports of the American Public Health Association, *Control of Communicable Diseases Manual* (Heymann 2004), the comprehensive two-volume work *Mandell, Douglas and Bennett's Principles and Practice of Infectious Diseases* (Mandell *et al.* 2005), and the textbook *Infectious Diseases* (Gorbach *et al.* 2004). For readers specifically interested in paediatric infectious diseases, there is the comprehensive two-volume *Textbook of Pediatric Infectious Diseases* (Feigin *et al.* 2004); for infectious diseases in emergency medicine settings, there is the textbook on *Infectious Disease in Emergency Medicine* (Brillman & Quenzer 1998); and for tropical infectious diseases, there is *Tropical Infectious Diseases: Principles, Pathogens, and Practice* (Guerrant *et al.* 2006). A comprehensive treatment of the worldwide distribution and diagnosis of infectious diseases is provided in *A World Guide to Infections: Diseases, Distribution, Diagnosis* (Wilson 1991). The Centers for Disease Control and Prevention (CDC) publishes up-to-date disease surveillance information for the United States and recommendations for control measures in the *Morbidity and Mortality Weekly Reports* and provides annual summaries of notifiable infectious diseases in the *Summary of Notifiable Diseases, United States* (CDC 2008). Many other countries have similar types of publications. The World Health Organization (WHO) publishes worldwide surveillance information and recommendations for control measures in the *Weekly Epidemiological Record*. A more detailed background on infectious agents as determinants of health and disease is provided in Volume 1, Chapters 2.7, and Volume 3, Chapters 9.11–9.15, and 9.17.

Definitions of infectious diseases and their control

Infection occurs when an infectious agent enters a body and develops or multiplies. *Infectious agents* are organisms capable of producing inapparent infection or clinically manifest disease and include bacteria, rickettsia, chlamydiae, fungi, parasites, viruses, and prions. An *infectious disease*, or communicable disease, is an infection that results in a clinically manifest disease. Infectious disease may also be due to the toxic product of an infectious agent, such as the toxin produced by *Clostridium botulinum* causing classical botulism. As this is a textbook of public health, the infectious diseases considered are those that manifest in human hosts and are a result of the interaction of people, animals, and their environment. Infectious diseases may be due to infectious agents exclusively found in human hosts such as rubella virus, in the environment such as *Legionella pneumophila*, or primarily in animals such as *Brucella abortus*.

Control of infectious diseases refers to the actions and programmes directed toward reducing disease incidence (new infections), reducing disease prevalence (infections in the community at any given point in time), or completely eradicating the disease. Control aimed at reducing the incidence of infectious disease can be considered as *primary prevention* of infectious disease. Primary prevention protects health through individual and community-wide measures, including such actions as maintaining good nutritional status, keeping physically fit, immunizing against infectious diseases, providing safe water, and ensuring the proper disposal of faeces.

Control aimed at reducing the prevalence by shortening the duration of infectious disease can be considered as *secondary prevention* of infectious disease. Secondary prevention corrects departures from good health through individual and community-wide measures, including such actions as early detection of disease, prompt antibiotic treatment and ensuring adequate nutrition. It should be noted that such control efforts in secondary prevention in a group of infected individuals may also result in primary prevention in uninfected persons. For example, prompt and specific drug therapy for tuberculosis patients resulting in sputum conversion to culture negative status renders them no longer a source of infection to others.

Control aimed at reducing or even eliminating long-term impairments of infectious disease can be considered as *tertiary prevention* of infectious disease. Tertiary prevention reduces or eliminates disabilities, minimizes suffering, and promotes adjustment to permanent disabilities through such actions as providing orthopedic appliances, counselling and vocational training, and prevention of opportunistic infections. For example, the prevention of opportunistic infections in HIV infection can be considered as tertiary prevention (Osterholm *et al.* 2005).

Global burden of infectious diseases

A World Health Organization (WHO) analysis of the global burden of disease estimates that infectious diseases caused 14.9 million deaths, accounting for 26 per cent of total global mortality of 57.0 million deaths in 2002 (WHO 2004a). Five diseases, respiratory infections, AIDS, diarrhoeal diseases, tuberculosis and, malaria, account for some 77 per cent of the total infectious disease burden. Most infectious disease (some 95 per cent, or 14.1 million) deaths occur in the economically developing group of countries where approximately one in three deaths (14.1 out of 43.6 million) are due to an infectious cause. However, infectious diseases are also of importance in more developed countries. In the United States, for example, AIDS rose to become the leading cause of death in persons aged 25–44 years in the late 1980s and early 1990s, and still ranks as an important cause of death in this age group.

The current magnitude of morbidity and mortality due to infectious diseases worldwide is highlighted by the WHO as follows (WHO 2004a):

- *Acute respiratory infections*, including pneumonia and influenza, cause some 451 million episodes of illness each year and result in 4 million deaths annually. These infections are the highest cause of infant and child mortality in developing countries.

- *HIV* newly infects about 2 million people each year and causes an estimated 2.7 million AIDS-related deaths annually. There are now about 33 million people living with HIV as of the end of 2007 (UNAIDS 2007).

- *Diarrhoeal diseases* are also a major cause of morbidity and mortality in infants and children in developing countries. Each year there are some 4.5 billion episodes with 1.8 million deaths due to diarrhoeal disease, of which the vast majority are among children under five years of age.

- *Tuberculosis*, caused by *Mycobacterium tuberculosis*, infects about one-third of the world's population. It is estimated that there are approximately 7.6 million people who develop clinical disease and 1.6 million who die of tuberculosis each year.

- *Malaria* is estimated to cause some 408 million cases of acute illness. An estimated 1.3 million deaths per year worldwide are attributable to malaria, mainly in children under the age of five years.

- *Influenza* epidemics, caused by influenza A and B viruses, are estimated to kill from 500 000 to 1 million people worldwide each year. Influenza pandemics, of which there were three in the last century, have killed as many as 40–50 million people (as occurred during the 1918–1919 'Spanish flu' pandemic) and, as with the current concerns regarding avian influenza (H5N1), continue to threaten to re-emerge as a major public health emergency.

Chain of infection: Agent, transmission, and host

The chain of infection is the relationship between an infectious agent, its routes of transmission, and a susceptible host. The prevention and control of infectious diseases depend on the interaction of these three factors that may result in the human host clinically manifesting disease.

Agent

The infectious agent is the first link in the chain of infection and is any micro-organism whose presence or excessive presence is essential for the occurrence of an infectious disease. Examples of infectious agents include the following:

- *Bacteria:* For example, spirochetes such as *Treponema pallidum* causing syphilis, curved bacteria such as *Borrelia burgdorferi* causing lyme disease, Gram-negative rods such as *Yersinia pestis* causing plague, Gram-positive cocci such as *Streptococcus pyogenes*, group A causing erysipelas, and Gram-positive rods such as *Mycobacterium tuberculosis* causing tuberculosis

- *Rickettsiae:* For example, *Rickettsia rickettsii* causing Rocky Mountain spotted fever, and *Rickettsia prowazekii* causing epidemic louse-borne typhus fever

- *Chlamydiae:* For example, *Chlamydia psittaci* causing psittacosis, and *Chlamydia trachomatis* causing trachoma and genital infections

- *Fungi*: For example, *Trichophyton schoenleinii* and *Microsporum canis* causing tinea capitis, and *Trichophyton rubrum*, *Trichophyton mentagrophytes* and *Epidermophyton floccosum* causing tinea pedis

- *Parasites:* For example, helminths such as *Trichinella spiralis* causing trichinosis, filaria such as *Brugia malayi* causing filariasis, nematodes such as *Enterobius vermicularis* causing enterobiasis (pinworm disease), trematodes such as *Clonorchis sinensis* causing clonorchiasis (oriental liver fluke disease), cestodes such as

Taenia solium causing taeniasis (beef tapeworm disease), and protozoa such as *Trypanosoma cruzi* causing American trypanosomiasis (Chagas' disease)

◆ *Viruses:* For example, Paramyxoviridae such as measles virus which causes measles, Togaviridae such as rubella virus which causes rubella, and arthropod-borne viruses (arboviruses) such as dengue viruses which cause dengue fever

◆ *Prions:* Small proteinaceous infectious particles which cause such diseases as kuru, Creutzfeldt–Jakob disease (and its variant associated with exposure of humans to the bovine spongiform encephalopathy, or 'mad cow', agent), and the Gerstmann–Straussler–Scheinker syndrome (see Volume 3, Chapter 9.11)

There is increasing evidence that some infectious agents, often with cofactors, are associated with human tumours. Examples include *Shistosoma haematobium* with bladder cancer, *Shistosoma japonicum* with colorectal cancer, *Clonorchis sinensis* with cholangiocarcinoma, hepatitis B and C viruses with hepatocellular carcinoma, *Helicobacter pylori* with gastric cancer, and human papillomaviruses with cervical cancer. Cancers attributed by the International Agency for Research on Cancer (IARC) to infectious agents are considered to account for some 26 per cent and 8 per cent of the total number of cancers in the developing world and industrialized world, respectively (WHO 2003).

Agents can be described by their ability to cause disease (pathogenicity) as well as their ability to cause serious disease (virulence). The *pathogenicity* of an infectious agent is the extent to which clinically manifest disease is produced in an infected population and is measured by the ratio of the number of persons developing clinical illness to the total number infected. Examples of highly pathogenic infectious agents are the measles virus and the human (α) herpesvirus 3 (varicella-zoster), causing measles and chickenpox, respectively, in which most infected susceptible persons will manifest disease.

The *virulence* of an infectious agent is the extent to which severe disease is produced in a population with clinically manifest disease. It is the ratio of the number of persons with severe and fatal disease to the total number of persons with disease. An example of a highly virulent infectious agent is HIV whereby nearly all untreated persons with AIDS will die.

Characteristics of infectious agents that effect pathogenicity include their ability to invade tissues (invasiveness), produce toxins (intoxication), cause damaging hypersensitivity (allergic) reactions, undergo antigenic variation, and develop antibiotic resistance. An example of an infectious agent with high *invasiveness* is the *Shigella* organism which can invade the submucosal tissue of the intestine and cause clinically manifest shigellosis (bacillary dysentery). An example of an infectious agent that has a high degree of ability to *produce toxins* is the *Clostridium botulinum* organism which can elaborate toxins in inadequately prepared food and cause classical botulism. An example of an infectious agent that is highly *allergenic* is the *Mycobacterium tuberculosis* organism which can cause tuberculosis. An example of an infectious agent that has a high degree of *antigenic variation* is the type A influenza virus which frequently experiences minor antigenic changes—antigenic 'drift'. Influenza A viruses, on an irregular basis, may also undergo a major antigenic change creating an entirely new subtype—antigenic 'shift'. Antigenic shifts that have the characteristic of high transmissibility between persons may result in an influenza pandemic when large numbers of individuals are exposed to the new subtype for which they have no prior immunity. An example of an infectious agent that can develop *antibiotic resistance* that challenges control efforts is *Neisseria gonorrhoeae* that has both chromosomally mediated and resistance transfer plasmid mediated genetic factors for antibiotic resistance.

The *infective dose* of an infectious agent is the number of organisms needed to cause an infection. The infective dose may vary depending on the route of transmission and host susceptibility. An example of an infectious agent that need only a very low infective dose (as few as 10 organisms) is *Escherichia coli* O157:H7 which causes enterohaemorrhagic diarrhoea.

Control measures for infectious diseases directed at inactivating the agent are designed according to the type of agent and its reservoirs and sources. For example, an agent like *Vibrio cholerae* can be inactivated through adequate chlorination of the water supply. This is a chemical method for provision of safe water to control cholera. An agent like hepatitis B virus can be inactivated through adequate autoclaving of injection and surgical equipment. This is a sterilization method to control hepatitis B. Details of these and other methods of control directed at the agent are provided in the sections in this chapter on control measures applied to the agent and the environment.

Routes of transmission

Control efforts are often designed to break the routes of transmission, the mechanisms by which infectious agents are spread from reservoirs or sources to human hosts. A *reservoir* of an infectious agent is any person, other living organism, or inanimate material in which the infectious agent normally lives and grows. The *source* of infection for a host is the person, other living organism or inanimate material from which the infectious agent came. *Horizontal transmission* refers to transmission between individuals whereas *vertical transmission* refers to the specific situation of transmission between parent to offspring (for example, transplacentally *in utero*, during passage through the birth canal, or through breast milk). The routes of transmission have been summarized in the *Control of Communicable Diseases Manual* (Heymann 2004) as follows:

Direct transmission

Direct and essentially immediate transfer of infectious agents to a receptive portal of entry through which human or animal infection may take place. This may be by direct contact as touching, biting, kissing, or sexual intercourse, or by the direct projection (droplet spread) of droplet spray onto the conjunctiva or onto the mucous membranes of the eye, nose or mouth during sneezing, coughing, spitting, singing or talking (usually limited to a distance of about 1 m or less). It may also occur through direct exposure of susceptible tissue to an agent in soil or through the bite of an animal, or transplacentally.

Indirect transmission
Vehicle-borne

Contaminated inanimate materials or objects (fomites) such as (a) toys, handkerchiefs, soiled clothes, bedding, cooking or eating utensils, surgical instruments or dressings; (b) water, food, milk, and biological products including blood, serum, plasma, tissues, or organs; or (c) any substance serving as an intermediate means by which an infectious agent is transported and introduced into a susceptible host though a suitable portal of entry. The agent may or may not have multiplied or developed in or on the vehicle before being transmitted.

Vector-borne

Mechanical: Includes simple mechanical carriage by a crawling or flying insect through soiling of its feet or proboscis, or by passage of organisms through its gastrointestinal tract. This does not require multiplication or development of the organism.

Biological: Propagation (multiplication), cyclic development, or a combination of these (cyclopropagative) is required before the arthropod can transmit the infective form of the agent to humans. An incubation period (extrinsic) is required following infection before the arthropod becomes infective. Maintenance of infectious agents may occur within vectors through transovarian or transstadial transmission. In transovarian transmission, the infectious agent is passed vertically to succeeding generations (for example, an important mechanism for maintaining *Rickettsia rickettsii* in nature is the through infected eggs passed by an infected adult female tick which will hatch into infected larvae). In transstadial transmission the infectious agent is maintained in the vector as the vector passages from one stage of its lifecycle to another (for example, ticks infected with *Rickettsia rickettsii* can remain infected with this agent as they passage from nymph to adult stages). Transmission may be by injection of salivary gland fluid during biting, or by regurgitation or deposition on the skin of faeces or other material capable of penetrating through the bite wound or through an area of trauma from scratching or rubbing. This transmission is by an infected non-vertebrate host and not simple mechanical carriage by a vector as a vehicle. However, an arthropod in either role is termed a vector.

Airborne transmission

It is the dissemination of microbial aerosols to a suitable portal of entry, usually the respiratory tract. Microbial aerosols are suspensions of particles in the air consisting partially or wholly of microorganisms. They may remain suspended in the air for long periods of time, some retaining and others losing infectivity or virulence. Particles in the 1–5 μm range are easily drawn into the alveoli of the lungs and may be retained there. Microbial transmission through droplets and other large particles that promptly settle out of the air is considered as direct, not airborne, transmission.

Droplet nuclei: Usually the small residues which result from evaporation of fluid from droplets emitted by an infected host. They also may be created purposely by a variety of atomizing devices, or accidentally as in microbiology laboratories or in abattoirs, rendering plants or autopsy rooms. They usually remain suspended in the air for long periods.

Dust: The small particles of widely varying size which may arise from soil (for example, fungus spores), clothes, bedding, or contaminated floors.

Control measures for infectious diseases directed at interrupting transmission are designed according to the type of transmission for the agent. Direct transmission of an agent like *Neisseria gonorrhoeae*, for example, can be reduced by using condoms as a barrier method of control of gonorrhoea. Vector-borne transmission of an agent like *Plasmodium falciparum* can be reduced by using a residual insecticide against *Anopheles* mosquitoes as a chemical vector control method for malaria. Airborne transmission of an agent like

Mycobacterium tuberculosis from sputum-positive pulmonary tuberculosis patients in hospital can be reduced by the use of special ventilation in the patient's room as an environmental method of control of tuberculosis. It should be recognized that some infectious agents may have more than one route of transmission. Poliovirus, for example, can be spread via direct transmission through the faecal–oral route and pharyngeal spread, or indirect transmission through contaminated food or other materials. Details of these and other methods of control directed at interrupting transmission are provided in the sections on control measures in this chapter.

Host

The human host is the final link in the chain of infection. The infectious agent may enter the host through the following portals of entry.

- *Respiratory tract:* Infectious agents can be inhaled into the respiratory tract and will be deposited at different levels of the pulmonary tree according to the size of the aerosol, droplet nuclei or dust particles. For example, *Mycobacterium tuberculosis* in airborne droplet nuclei, 1–5 μm in diameter, may be inhaled into the alveoli of the lungs of a vulnerable host and result in tuberculosis.

- *Intact skin:* Some infectious agents, such as *Necator americanus* which causes hookworm disease, can penetrate the intact skin.

- *Gastrointestinal tract:* An infectious agent, such as *Vibrio cholerae* which causes cholera, may enter via the gastrointestinal tract. Persons who have a compromised gastric function, such as gastric achlorhydria, may be at increased risk of disease.

- *Mucous membranes:* Infectious agents, such as measles viruses, may be deposited on mucous membranes, including the conjunctiva of the eye, by droplet spread or by direct contact with infected persons or contaminated objects.

- *Urinary tract:* Some infectious agents, such as *Escherichia coli* which causes urinary tract infections, can enter the urinary tract via an ascending route from the urethra colonized with the organism. Structural abnormalities of the urinary tract and procedures such as urinary catheterization may predispose the host to disease.

- *Placenta:* Certain infectious agents, such as rubella virus which causes congenital rubella syndrome, can cross the placenta resulting in transplacental transmission, a direct route of transmission from the mother to the fetus that is a form of vertical transmission.

Infectious agents also enter the host though mechanisms that get past the body's natural barriers, including wounds that break the integrity of the skin or mucous membranes; invasive procedures, parenteral injections, parenteral infusions, blood transfusions, or organ transplants that may introduce an agent into the body; or insect vectors that may inject agents through the skin.

The most important host factors regarding developing clinically manifest disease and the severity of disease are immune status and age. Infants, young children, and the elderly are at generally higher risk from more severe disease due to immaturity or deterioration of their immune systems, respectively.

Many host defence mechanisms help prevent infection or disease. *Non-specific* host defence mechanisms include the intact skin, nasal cilia, tears, saliva, mucus, and gastric acid. *Specific* host defence mechanisms include naturally acquired immunity from previous infection, tranplacentally acquired passive immunity in the newborn from the mother, artificially acquired active immunity from immunization, and artificially acquired passive immunity from immunoglobulins and antitoxins.

Host responses to infection that prevent or reduce the severity of infectious disease include (a) polymorphonuclear leukocytosis stimulated by some bacterial infections that increases the number of phagocytic white blood cells, (b) fever that may slow the multiplication of some infectious agents, (c) antibody production that may neutralize some infectious agents or their toxins, (d) interferon production that may block intracellular replication of viruses, and (e) cytotoxic immune cell responses that kill cells infected with viruses.

The *manifestation of infection* in the host may vary from inapparent (subclinical) infection to severe disease that may even result in death. The interaction between an infectious agent, routes of transmission, and host factors determines the spectrum of signs and symptoms. Sometimes the host may become an asymptomatic carrier of the infectious agent and be a source of infection for others.

Control measures for infectious diseases directed at the host are designed according to the immune status of the host and the likelihood of host exposure to certain infectious agents. For example, measles disease can be prevented by active immunization with measles vaccine to develop host immunity. Pneumonic plague can be prevented in those in close contact with patients with plague pneumonia by chemoprophylaxis using tetracycline or sulphonamide. Details of these and other methods of control directed at the host are provided in the section on control measures applied to the host in this chapter.

Tools for control of infectious diseases

The primary concern of infectious disease control in public health, whether in developing or industrialized countries, is the reduction, elimination or even eradication of infectious disease. This is accomplished by directing control measures to the agent, the routes of transmission, or the host. Such control measures include: (a) identifying and then reducing or eliminating infectious agents at their sources and reservoirs, (b) breaking or interfering with the routes of transmission of infectious agents, and (c) identifying susceptible populations and then reducing or eliminating their susceptibility.

The tools for control of infectious diseases are related to recognition and evaluation of the patterns of diseases and the results of interventions to control them. In infectious disease control, the most important tool for recognition and evaluation is *surveillance* of disease defined as:

> the process of systematic collection, orderly consolidation, analysis, and evaluation of pertinent data with prompt dissemination of the results to those who need to know, particularly those who are in a position to take action. It includes the systematic collection and evaluation of: (a) morbidity and mortality reports; (b) special reports of field investigations of epidemics and of individual cases; (c) isolation and identification of infectious agents by laboratories; (d) data concerning the availability, use, and untoward effects of vaccines and toxoids, immune globulins, insecticides, and other substances used in control; (e) information

> regarding immunity levels in segments of the population; and (f) other relevant epidemiologic data. A report summarizing the above data should be prepared and distributed to all cooperating persons and others with a need to know the results of the surveillance activities. The procedure applies to all jurisdictional levels of public health from local to international (Heymann 2004).

Surveillance, therefore, is 'information for action'. More detailed information on surveillance or on field investigations is given in Volume 2, Chapters 6.4, 6.17, and 8.3.

Tools for control related to *interventions* include:

◆ *Control measures applied to the host:* Active immunization, passive immunization, chemoprophylaxis, behavioural change, reverse isolation, barriers, and improving host resistance.

◆ *Control measures applied to vectors:* Chemical, environmental, and biological.

◆ *Control measures applied to infected humans:* Chemotherapy, isolation, quarantine, restriction of activities, and behavioural change.

◆ *Control measures applied to animals:* Active immunization, isolation, quarantine, restriction or reduction, chemoprophylaxis, and chemotherapy.

◆ *Control measures applied to the environment:* Provision of safe water, proper disposal of faeces, food and milk sanitation, and design of facilities and equipment.

◆ *Control measures applied to infectious agents:* Cleaning, cooling, pasteurization, disinfection, and sterilization.

Achieving maximum impact on control of a specific infectious disease may involve more than one of these interventions. For example, the control of hepatitis A infection can be achieved through interventions that may include: Active immunization, passive immunization, food preparation and handwashing behaviours, provision of safe water, food sanitation, and proper disposal of faeces.

The tools for control can also be considered according to the level at which they are applied: Individual, institutional, or community-based. At the *individual level*, control measures, usually initiated by a clinician, are directed toward the specific infectious disease threats to the particular individual. Examples include chemoprophylaxis to prevent wound infection, pre-exposure prophylactic immunization against rabies for a veterinarian, and use of diphtheria antitoxin in a patient with diphtheria.

At the *institutional level*, control measures, usually initiated by the officials of the institution, are directed to a group of people who are in close contact with each other, such as persons in daycare centres, schools, military barracks, hospital wards, nursing homes, and correctional facilities. Examples include (a) administering amantadine hydrochloride or rimantadine for chemoprophylaxis or chemotherapy of influenza A in a high-risk institutional population; (b) quarantining institutionalized young children during a measles outbreak; and (c) hepatitis B immunization of staff and clients of institutions for the developmentally disabled.

At the *community level*, control measures, usually initiated by local, state or national public health agencies, are directed to the community at large. Examples include childhood immunization programmes, provision of safe water, regulation of food supplies, and recall of contaminated food products.

It should be noted that some control measures, such as immunization, may take place at all levels while others, such as the provision of safe water to a community, are more specifically applied at a particular level.

The tools for the control of infectious diseases and their relationship to the chain of infection are the main focus of the remainder of this chapter.

Control measures applied to the host

Control measures applied to the host range from relatively easily administered immunization to behavioural changes that may be extremely difficult for an individual to accept and practice. This section details the types of control measures applied to susceptible hosts and gives examples of their application in the control of selected infectious diseases.

Active immunization

One of the most efficient control measures applied to a host is one that renders the host immune from infectious disease by an infectious agent. Active immunization is a cornerstone of public health measures for the control of many infectious diseases and is considered one of the most cost-effective methods of individual, institutional and community protection for vaccine-preventable infectious diseases. The most powerful example of the potential impact of active immunization against an infectious disease is that of smallpox vaccination. Mobilization of political will on a worldwide basis, coupled with full application of the strategies of active surveillance and containment immunization against smallpox, ultimately resulted in the complete global eradication of the disease and cessation of transmission of the infectious agent, variola virus.

Active immunization is usually considered synonymous with the term vaccination, and is the process of administration of an antigen that can induce a specific immune response that protects a susceptible host from an infectious disease. Some draw a distinction between the two terms. Narrowly defined, *vaccination* is the process of administration of an antigen and *immunization* is the development of a specific immune response. Administering an antigen without evoking an immune response is possible, since no vaccine is 100 per cent effective. Conversely, someone can become immunized even if they were not administered an antigen. For example, the live, attenuated oral polio vaccine viruses can be transmitted from the recipient to other close contacts.

Active immunization can be accomplished through different types of antigens, including the following:

- *Inactivated toxins:* Diphtheria toxoid is an example of a formaldehyde-inactivated preparation of diphtheria toxin that protects against clinically manifest disease, although the immunized person may still become infected with toxin-producing strains of *Corynebacterium diphtheria*. Tetanus toxoid and *Clostridium perfringens* toxoid (pig bel vaccine) are other examples of inactivated toxin preparations.

- *Inactivated complex antigens:* Whole-cell pertussis vaccine is an example of a heat or chemically treated preparation of killed whole pertussis bacteria that protects against clinically manifest disease, although the immunized person may still become infected with *Bordetella pertussis*. Inactivated polio vaccine and inactivated influenza vaccine are other examples of inactivated vaccines.

- *Purified antigens:* Acellular pertussis vaccine is an example of a vaccine composed of isolated and purified immunogenic pertussis antigens. Other vaccines with purified components include polyvalent capsular polysaccharide pneumococcal, polysaccharide meningococcal, protein–polysaccharide conjugate *Haemophilus influenzae* type b, and plasma-derived hepatitis B vaccines.

- *Recombinant antigens:* Hepatitis B recombinant vaccine is an example of a vaccine composed of hepatitis B surface antigen sub-units made through recombinant DNA technology. Human Papilloma Virus vaccine is another example of a DNA recombinant vaccine.

- *Live, attenuated vaccines:* Measles vaccine is an example of a vaccine containing live infectious agents that are of reduced virulence, but induce protective antibodies against measles viruses. Other live, attenuated vaccines include oral polio, mumps, rubella, yellow fever, and bacille Calmette–Guérin (BCG) vaccines.

Protective *antibody responses* usually take 7–21 days to develop. Although most vaccines must be given before exposure to be effective, some vaccines may protect even if administered after exposure to an infectious agent. For example, measles vaccine may provide protection against measles disease if given within 72 h of exposure. This occurs since the percutaneous route of administration of the antigen evokes an immune response faster than the measles virus results in disease through the respiratory route of natural exposure.

Duration of protection varies from only months, such as with killed whole-cell cholera vaccine, to years or even life with some live attenuated vaccines, such as measles vaccine. Some inactivated toxoids and vaccines, such as tetanus toxoid, may require a priming series of doses to be optimally effective and additional booster doses to maintain protective antibodies. Many new technologies are being explored that may increase the number and efficacy of vaccines available against infectious disease, including immune stimulating complexes, live viral or bacterial vector vaccines, and timed-release vaccines.

It should be recognized that vaccines vary in their efficacy and that no vaccine is 100 per cent effective. *Vaccine efficacies* vary with type of vaccine, manufacturing techniques, storage and handling conditions, skill of administration, age of vaccination, and other host factors. Vaccines for routine use are safe. However, no vaccine is 100 per cent safe. Potential vaccinees, or their parents or guardians, should be screened for contraindications and be informed of potential side-effects.

Immunization schedules for the routine control of infectious diseases preventable by immunization vary between countries and are usually based on expert advice to governments and physicians. For example, recommended policies for immunization in the United States are provided by the Advisory Committee on Immunization Practices (ACIP) and are published in the *Morbidity and Mortality Weekly Report* (ACIP 2006). In addition, the American Academy of Pediatrics periodically publishes comprehensive immunization recommendations in its *Report of the Committee on Infectious Diseases* (Committee on Infectious Diseases 2006). At the global level, the WHO publishes recommended immunization schedules and control strategies for vaccine-preventable diseases that are periodically updated by expert advisory groups in the WHO *Weekly Epidemiological Record*.

In *outbreak settings*, immunization schedules may be modified. For example, the age of immunization for measles may be lowered to

6 months of age during an outbreak. In such situations, persons receiving vaccine before the routinely recommended age of immunization should be immunized again at the recommended age since immunization at the earlier age may not have been optimally effective.

Immunization programmes include vaccines for routine child, routine adult, travel, selected high risk populations, and occupational settings. For example, tetanus toxoid is universally recommended; yellow fever vaccine is only recommended in geographic areas of epidemiologic risk; typhoid fever vaccine is only recommended for individuals subject to unusual exposure to typhoid, including persons living in the same household as known carriers; and anthrax vaccine is only recommended for veterinarians and persons occupationally exposed to possibly contaminated industrial raw materials.

Beyond protection of the individual, vaccination may also provide a degree of community protection. This phenomenon is known as herd immunity. *Herd immunity* is the relative protection of a population group achieved by reducing or breaking the chains of transmission of an infectious agent because most of the population is resistant to infection through immunization or prior natural infection. Herd immunity is a complex phenomenon and varies according to the infectious agent, its routes of transmission, the degree to which immunization protects against infection versus only clinically manifest disease, and the distribution of immunization in the population (for example, groups of persons with low vaccination coverage vulnerable to disease introduction may exist within populations with high average levels of vaccination coverage). The mechanisms of herd immunity are several, including 'direct protection of vaccinees against disease or transmissible infection and indirect protection of nonrecipients by virtue of surreptitious vaccination, passive antibody, or just reduced sources of transmission and, hence, risks of infection in the community' (Fine 1993).

A particularly difficult problem for vaccine-preventable infectious disease control programmes is complacency by the population that can result from the very successes of the programmes. Low rates of vaccine-preventable infectious disease may mistakenly lead parents to consider that vaccination is no longer important for maintaining their children's health and may result in political leaders reducing funding for immunization programmes. Low disease rates may also focus undo attention on the relatively rare serious side-effects of vaccination in relation to current rates of disease. Such side-effects should only be compared in relation to rates of disease and its complications that would occur without immunization programmes.

A comprehensive treatment of active immunization is given by Plotkin and Orenstein (2004).

Passive immunization

Passive immunization is a temporary immunity in a host due to the protection afforded by antibody produced in another host. Passive immunity may be acquired either naturally or artificially.

Naturally acquired passive immunity is achieved through transfer of maternal antibodies via the placenta. It is the way that newborn infants are provided with a temporary immunity against many infectious diseases for which the mother is immune. This immunity wanes over time and eventually leaves the infant susceptible to these diseases.

An important use of transplacental immunity as a control measure is in the prevention of tetanus neonatorum (neonatal tetanus) by immunization of women before or during pregnancy with tetanus toxoid. The disease typically occurs when the umbilical cord is cut with an unclean instrument contaminated with tetanus spores or when substances contaminated with tetanus spores are placed on the umbilical stump after delivery. Control by active immunization of the infant cannot be achieved in sufficient time since the average incubation period is only 6 days (with a range from 3 to 28 days). An adequately immunized mother, however, will usually effectively transfer maternal antibodies against tetanus across the placenta to her newborn and prevent tetanus neonatorum.

Another example of naturally acquired passive immunity is the relative protection against measles disease in a young infant born to a mother who previously had the disease. Typically, such infants are immune for approximately 6–9 months or more after birth, depending upon how much residual maternal antibodies are present at the time of pregnancy. Other diseases for which there is usually an effective transplacental immunity in infants, for variable amounts of time, include diphtheria, mumps, poliomyelitis, rubella, and varicella (chickenpox). It should be noted that if the mother is not immune, or if residual maternal antibodies have significantly waned, then the infant may be susceptible to disease.

Research is ongoing as to other infectious diseases that may be preventable in the neonate or infant though immunization of the mother before or during pregnancy. Examples include *Haemophilus influenzae* type b, group B streptococcal and meningococcal diseases (Insel *et al.* 1994). Many diseases, however, are not prevented by transplacental immunity.

Breastfeeding is a form of naturally acquired passive antibody transfer to neonates and infants. Breast milk and colostrum contain secretory immunoglobin A (IgA) antibodies that may play a protective role in the prevention of infections with such agents as respiratory syncytial virus, rotavirus and *Haemophilus influenzae* type b.

Artificially acquired passive immunity is acquired through administration of an antibody-containing preparation, antiserum, or immune globulin. It has a place in the control of certain infectious diseases in special situations. This immunity also wanes over a relatively short period of time.

Examples of the use of artificially acquired passive immunity to control infectious disease include the following:

◆ *Rabies:* Natural immunity to rabies in humans does not exist. Susceptible individuals bitten by an animal known or suspected to be rabid should receive rabies immune globulin to neutralize the rabies virus in the wound. It should be noted that, besides passive immunization with rabies immune globulin, such individuals should also receive active immunization with rabies vaccine.

◆ *Hepatitis A:* In areas where sanitation is poor, hepatitis A infection commonly occurs at an early age and therefore most adults in developing countries are already immune. However, epidemics may occur in industrialized countries. Passive immunization with immune globulin may be given to: (a) all household and sexual contacts of patients with hepatitis A; (b) other food handlers in an establishment where hepatitis A has occurred in a food handler; (c) all individuals in an institution where a focal outbreak of hepatitis A has occurred; and (d) persons from industrialized countries travelling to highly endemic areas. It should be noted that vaccines for active immunization for hepatitis A are available.

- *Diphtheria:* Treatment of this disease is an example of the use of an antibody containing product (diphtheria antitoxin) produced in an animal (only diphtheria antitoxin from horses is available) administered as part of the treatment regimen for secondary prevention of disease. In suspected cases of diphtheria, the antitoxin must be given as soon as possible because it is only effective in neutralizing diphtheria toxins not yet bound to cells.

- *Other important infectious diseases, including hepatitis B, measles, tetanus, varicella:* Depending upon the circumstances of exposure, susceptibility of the host, and status of the host's general immune system there are circumstances under which hepatitis B immune globulin, tetanus immune globulin, varicella-zoster immune globulin, or immune globulin may be warranted.

Chemoprophylaxis

Chemoprophylaxis is the prevention of infection or its progression to clinically manifest disease through the administration of chemical substances, including antibiotics. Chemoprophylaxis can also consist of the treatment of a disease to prevent complications of that disease (Solomon *et al.* 2004). Chemoprophylaxis may be specifically directed against a particular infectious agent or it may be non-specifically directed against many infectious agents. The use of antibiotics before surgical procedures is an example of non-specific chemoprophylaxis to prevent wound infections in the postoperative period. Examples of specific chemoprophylaxis are given below.

The use of chemoprophylaxis to *prevent development of infection* is illustrated by using chloroquine to prevent malarial parasitemia caused by *Plasmodium vivax, Plasmodium ovale, Plasmodium malariae* and chloroquine-sensitive strains of *Plasmodium falciparum.* For some chloroquine resistant strains of *Plasmodium falciparum,* alternative regimens include mefloquine alone, doxycycline alone, primaquine alone, or an atovaquone/proguanil combination. Primaquine may be given to reduce the risk of a relapse from intrahepatic forms of *Plasmodium vivax* and *Plasmodium ovale* after discontinuation of chemoprophylaxis with any chemosuppresive drugs other than primaquine. Determination of a specific malaria chemoprophylactic regimen is complex. It must take into account the geographic area, the possibility of pregnancy, the weight of an individual (dose size for children is determined by body weight), and the risks of adverse reactions to the chemoprophylactic regimen.

Other examples of prevention of development of infection include the following:

- The use of silver nitrate, erythromycin or tetracycline instilled into the eyes of a newborn to prevent gonococcal ophthalmia by transmission of *Neisseria gonorrhoeae* from an infected mother during birth

- The use of tetracycline, sulphonamides (including sulphadiazine and trimethoprim-sulphamethoxazole), chloramphenicol or streptomycin in close contacts of confirmed or suspected cases of plague pneumonia to prevent plague pneumonia by transmission of *Yersinia pestis*

- The use of benzathine penicillin in those in sexual contact with confirmed cases of early syphilis to prevent syphilis by transmission of *Treponema pallidum*

An example of the use of chemoprophylaxis to 'prevent the progression of an infection to active manifest disease' is the use of isoniazid (INH) to prevent the progression of latent infection with *Mycobacterium tuberculosis* to clinical tuberculosis. Persons less than 35 years of age who are tuberculosis test positive should receive isoniazid to prevent clinical tuberculosis. The decision to use isoniazid, especially in individuals more than 35 years of age, must be determined based on such information as length of infection, closeness of association with a current case, status of the immune system, presence of acute liver disease, possibilities of pregnancy and risks of adverse reactions.

Other examples of prevention of progression of an infection to active manifest disease through the use of chemoprophylaxis include the following:

- Co-trimoxazole or pentamidine to prevent subclinical latent infection with *Pneumocystis carinii* from progressing to clinically manifest pneumocystis pneumonia in immunosuppressed persons such as HIV-infected individuals

- Mebendazole, albendazole, or pyrantel pamoate to prevent infection with *Necator americanus, Ancylostoma duodenale,* and *Ancylostoma Ceylanicum* from progressing to the clinically manifest anaemia of hookworm disease

- Pyrimethamine combined with sulphadiazine and folinic acid (to avoid possible bone marrow depression) to prevent asymptomatic infants congenitally infected with *Toxoplasma gondii* from progressing to clinically manifest chorioretinitis and other sequelae of congenital toxoplasmosis

In some situations, establishing *screening* programmes to detect and treat asymptomatic or unrecognized infections in defined populations is useful. An example is the screening for *Chlamydia trachomatis* in sexual partners of persons infected with *Chlamydia Trachomatis,* women with mucopurulent cervicitis, sexually active women 25 years of age or younger, and women older than 25 years of age with risk factors for chlamydia. A more detailed background on screening as a public health function is given in Volume 3, Chapter 12.7.

An example of the use of chemoprophylaxis to 'treat an infectious disease to prevent complications of the disease' is the use of penicillin (or erythromycin in penicillin-sensitive patients) to treat streptococcal sore throats caused by *Streptococcus pyogenes* group A to prevent acute rheumatic fever.

Other examples of prevention of complications of an infectious disease through the use of chemoprophylaxis include the following:

- Tetracycline for adults, or penicillin for children, for treatment of lyme disease caused by *Borrelia burgdorferi* in the erythema chronicum migrans stage to prevent or reduce the severity of late cardiac, arthritic or neurologic complications

- Benzathine penicillin for treatment of syphilis in its primary, secondary, or early latency period to prevent late manifestations of the disease such as cardiovascular syphilis

- Ketoconazole for treatment of blastomycosis caused by *Blastomyces dermatitidis* in its early stages to prevent progression of chronic pulmonary or disseminated blastomycosis that may lead to death

Potential problems with the use of chemoprophylaxis may include compromise of the host's own non-specific defence mechanisms, other replacement infectious agents causing disease by growing in the place of the infectious agent affected by the specific chemoprophylactic regimen, and emergence of resistant strains of the infectious agent. The development of antibiotic resistance can be reduced by using antibiotics only when needed, selecting the proper antibiotic (or, in some situations, the appropriate multidrug therapy) for the infectious agent, and ensuring compliance with the appropriate regimen for the duration of treatment.

Behavioural change

Perhaps the most challenging tool for the control of infectious diseases, and sometimes one of the most powerful and cost-effective, is behaviour change in the host that reduces or eliminates risk of exposure to an agent. Everyone has developed habits of living (lifestyles) that are not easily changed. Some of these behaviours are protective against infectious diseases. Others render the individual at higher risk of infection.

Examples of higher risk of exposure to infectious agents through behaviour, and behaviour changes that can have an impact on the chain of transmission, include the following.

Sexual behaviour

Many infectious agents are transmitted by the direct transmission route through sexual contact, including *Chlamydia trachomatis* causing chlamydial genital infections, *Neisseria gonorrhoeae* causing gonorrhoea, *Treponema pallidum* causing venereal syphilis, *Calymmatobacterium granulomatis* causing granuloma inguinale, *Heamophilus ducreyi* causing chancroid, herpes simplex virus causing herpes simplex, *Trichomonas vaginalis* causing trichomoniasis, human papillomaviruses causing condyloma acuminate, and HIV causing AIDS.

Abstinence behaviour, i.e. refraining from sexual activity with other persons, eliminates the risk of transmission of these agents through sexual contact. The delaying of age of first sexual activity avoids the risk of transmission of these agents at an early age. Restricting sexual contact to only between two uninfected persons who do not have sexual activity with any other persons virtually eliminates the risk of transmission of these agents through sexual behaviours. The exceptions are due to other routes of transmission of some of these agents (for example, HIV acquired through intravenous drug use in one partner being transmitted through sexual contact to the other partner). Limiting the number of sexual partners, and limiting those sexual partners to persons who also have few sexual partners, reduces the risk of exposure. However, at the individual level, if one of these sexual partners has an infectious agent transmissible by sexual contact, the risk of transmission may still be high. Finally, condom use during sexual activity in high risk situations will markedly reduce, but not eliminate, transmission. A more detailed background on sexually transmitted diseases is provided in Volume 3, Chapters 9.12 and 9.13.

Intravenous drug use behaviour

Injection of drugs using non-sterile needles or syringes previously used by other intravenous drug users may transmit infectious agents in blood through the vehicle-borne route of indirect transmission, including HIV causing AIDS; hepatitis B virus causing viral hepatitis B; and *Plasmodium vivax, Plasmodium malariae,* and *Plasmodium ovale* causing malaria.

Abstinence behaviour, i.e. refraining from intravenous drug use, eliminates the risk of transmission of such agents through contaminated needles and syringes. Using a sterile needle and sterile syringe for intravenous drug use will break the chain of transmission of these infectious agents through this route. Some community public health programmes, in addition to promoting drug abstinence and drug rehabilitation, conduct needle and syringe exchanges and education regarding methods of decontamination to help promote the use of sterile injection equipment among intravenous drug users (see Volume 3, Chapter 10.2).

Eating behaviour

Eating certain foods may result in exposure to infectious agents through the vehicle-borne route of indirect transmission. These behaviours include consuming raw molluscs by which an infectious agent like the hepatitis A virus can cause viral hepatitis A, eating raw eggs by which an infectious agent like a *Salmonella* serotype can cause salmonellosis, and consuming raw beef by which an infectious agent like *Taenia saginata* can cause beef tapeworm infection.

Although food and diet are strongly ingrained behaviours, modification of dietary patterns is possible. Cooking foods like beef, pork, and eggs can markedly reduce risk of transmission of infectious agents. In addition, reducing risks by elimination of infectious agents from the food may be possible (see the section on control methods applied to the environment). Handwashing before eating also reduces risk of transmission of many infectious agents that are spread through direct or indirect routes of faecal–oral transmission, such as *Shigella dysenteriae, Shigella flexneri, Shigella boydii,* and *Shigella sonnei* which may cause shigellosis (bacillary dysentery).

Working behaviour

In certain occupations, many behaviours may result in exposure to infectious agents and should be targets for control programmes in occupational safety and health settings. Specific examples include the following:

◆ Dental workers performing procedures with bare hands may result in exposure to hepatitis B viruses from infected patients.

◆ Health workers improperly handling used needles may result in needle-stick injuries leading to exposure to HIV from infected patients.

◆ Hospital laboratory workers improperly processing specimens containing infectious agents without appropriate glove or eyewear protection may result in exposure to these agents.

◆ Veterinarians who do not properly handle animals may result in brucellosis (undulant fever) due to exposure to *Brucella abortus, Brucella melitensis, Brucella suis,* or *Brucella canis.*

Occupational hazards related to non-infectious materials may predispose an individual to increased risk of infectious diseases. For example, working conditions and behaviours in industrial plants and mines that lead to silicosis due to long-term inhalation of free crystalline silica dust will greatly increase the risk of developing tuberculosis.

Working behaviours appropriate for the particular occupational setting may include wearing protective clothing, eyewear and gloves; handwashing and changing clothes after work; meticulous adherence to needle disposal and equipment sterilization procedures; and using hooded laboratory benches when handling highly infectious specimens.

Other behaviours

Other behaviours that may reduce the transmission of infectious agents include the following:

◆ Scheduling outdoor activities at periods of low vector activity, applying insect repellents and sleeping under bednets reduce the indirect transmission of vector-borne agents of infectious diseases like malaria

♦ Searching oneself for attached ticks every 3–4 h when playing or working in tick-infested areas reduces the indirect transmission of vector-borne agents of infectious diseases like Rocky Mountain spotted fever

♦ Avoiding sharing of utensils, cups, toothbrushes, or towels reduces the indirect transmission of vehicle-borne agents of infectious diseases like mononucleosis

♦ Wearing of shoes reduces the direct transmission of infectious agents like those causing hookworm disease

♦ Frequently bathing and regular washing of clothes in hot soapy water controls body lice

♦ Breastfeeding reduces diarrhoeal diseases in the infant, although it may transmit HIV from HIV-infected mothers

♦ Handwashing after defecation or touching potentially contaminated surfaces, persons, or animals prior to preparing food or touching ones own eyes, mucus membranes, or mouth reduces the risk of direct or indirect transmission of a wide variety of infectious agents

♦ Large family sizes and crowding may facilitate airborne transmission of infectious agents in droplet nuclei for infectious diseases like tuberculosis

Some of these other behaviours, like crowding, are conditioned by circumstances such as poverty that are not easily or directly amenable to programmes promoting behavioural change.

Reverse isolation

Certain rare circumstances exist where a means of avoiding transmission of an infectious disease to a highly susceptible host is to provide reverse, or protective, isolation. Such isolation attempts to protect infection-prone patients from potentially harmful infectious agents. Reverse isolation procedures range from provision of a private room with the use of masks, gloves and gowns by all persons entering the room, to elaborate facilities with laminar airflow rooms and sterilization of all food. Protective isolation is usually conducted for a limited time until the normal immune system recovers, a regimen of passive immunization is begun, or a bone marrow transplant is successful.

Examples of persons who may need periods of reverse isolation include those who have such diseases as X-linked agammaglobulinemia, DiGeorge's syndrome, and severe combined immunodeficiency; or those who have received therapies, such as some forms of cancer chemotherapy, that have severely compromised the person's immune system.

Barriers

One tool of control that can be applied to the host is the use of barriers between the host and the infectious agent. The effectiveness of such barriers, however, may be dependent on the behaviour of the host to use them consistently. Examples of barriers include the following:

♦ Screens, bednets (including bednets impregnated with pyrethroid insecticides such as permethrin), long-sleeved shirts and trousers (with the cuffs tucked into boots as a mechanical barrier), and repellents (such as *N,N*-diethyl-meta-toluamide known as

DEET) to prevent transmission of malaria through the bite of infected female *Anopheles* mosquitoes or West Nile virus through *Culix* mosquitoes

♦ Condoms to prevent transmission of HIV and other sexually transmitted infectious agents through sexual intercourse

♦ Masks (air-purifying respirators) to prevent transmission of tuberculosis through airborne droplet nuclei from patients with sputum-positive pulmonary tuberculosis

General improvement in host resistance

Improving host resistance though general improvement of the immune system is a non-specific approach, but may be important in certain settings. Kwashiorkor, marasmus, and other forms of malnutrition debilitate the host's immune system and may make an individual more susceptible to infectious diseases. Moreover, persons who are malnourished and succumb to an infectious disease are at higher risk of the disease being of greater severity and leading to other complications.

Malnutrition also encompasses micronutrient deficiencies. Vitamin A deficiency, for example, has been linked to higher rates of mortality associated with measles disease. Correcting vitamin A deficiency, through programmes of supplementation, fortification, and dietary modification in high-risk populations, can reduce mortality rates due to measles.

A complex interaction exists between infectious diseases, such as diarrhoeal diseases and malnutrition. A downward spiral of infection may lead to malnutrition that, in turn, leads to more infections, and so on. If unchecked, especially in developing countries, this downward spiral can ultimately result in death.

International travel

The special situation of international travel combines many control measures applied to the host already mentioned. The increase in the numbers of travellers, the speed of travel, and the ability to reach areas previously infrequently visited have reduced the effectiveness of surveillance for infectious diseases at ports of arrival and increased infectious disease risks. Advice for prevention against infectious diseases must be both general and specific.

General advice includes such issues as avoidance of eating and drinking potentially contaminated food or drink (including ice) and swimming or bathing in polluted water. Specific advice must be provided based on information about the area to be visited and may include such measures as active immunization against yellow fever, active or passive immunization against hepatitis A, chemoprophylaxis against malaria, repellents against potentially infected mosquitoes, and not walking barefoot in areas of risk for infection with hookworms *Strongyloides stercoralis* and *Strongyloides fuelleborni*. A more detailed background on international travel and health is provided in the annually updated WHO publication on *International Travel and Health* (WHO 2008).

Control measures applied to vectors

Vector-borne transmission is the only or main route of transmission for many infectious diseases. There exist more than 100 arthropod-borne viruses that may produce clinically manifest diseases in humans. Control of vector-borne diseases includes measures to: (a) Change behaviour and create barriers to the susceptible host; (b) reduce or break the chain of transmission of the infectious agent from an infected host to the vector; and (c) directly control the vector population itself. Chemical, environmental, and biological controls are the primary means of directly controlling the vector population.

Chemical control

Chemicals used in the control of vectors include minerals, natural plant products (botannicals), chlorinated hydrocarbons, organophosphates, carbamates, and fumigants. Chemical control measures include the following public health interventions:

◆ Spraying chemical insecticides such as organochlorine insecticides (for example, dichlorodiphenyltrichlorothane, or DDT, and dieldrin), organophosphorus insecticides (for example, malathion and fenitrothion), and carbonate insecticides (for example, propoxur and carbaryl) to prevent malaria through control of mosquitoes

◆ Spraying chemical biodegradable insecticides such as temephos (Abate®) to prevent onchocerciasis through control of *Simulium* fly vectors

◆ Using traps impregnated with decamethrin to prevent African trypanosomiasis (sleeping sickness) through reduction of the population of infective species of *Glossina* (tsetse fly) vectors

◆ Treating snail breeding places with chemical molluscicides to prevent schistosomiasis due to the free-swimming cercariae (larval forms) of *Schistosoma mansoni, Schistosoma haematobium, and Schistosoma japonicum* that develop in snails

◆ Treating step-wells and ponds with chemical insecticides such as temephos (Abate®) to prevent dracunculiasis due to infected cyclops (a crustacean copepod)

◆ Suppressing rat populations by poisoning, preceded or accompanied by measures to control fleas, as an additional measure to supplement environmental sanitation to control rodent populations to prevent human plague

The use of spraying for control of mosquitoes is complicated due to concerns of environmental contamination by chemicals such as DDT and dieldrin which have lead to their being banned in many countries. In addition, the emergence of mosquito vectors resistant to the insecticides diminishes their effectiveness in many areas. New methods of application, such as ultra low-volume spraying of malathion, reduce the amounts of insecticide used.

Environmental control

Environmental control of vectors includes the following public health interventions:

◆ Eliminating breeding sites of mosquito larvae by filling and draining areas of stagnant water and removing objects around houses that may collect water

◆ Destroying the habitats of the tsetse fly vector

◆ Properly implementing landfill procedures, placing lids on rubbish bins, covering food for human consumption, screening privies, cleaning up spilled food, and appropriately storing food

◆ Placing roach and fly traps

◆ Constructing rat-proof houses

◆ Eliminating rodent habitats

It is also important to note that certain development projects may have an impact on the environment that facilitates the growth of vector or intermediate host populations and results in increased infectious diseases. Construction of artificial waterways may serve as breeding sites for *Simulium* fly vectors that can transmit *Onchocerca volvulus* resulting in onchocerciasis. Irrigation schemes can foster the growth of snail intermediate hosts required for the transmission of species of *Schistosoma* resulting in schistosomiasis. Carefully conducted environmental and health impact studies that consider the impact of a construction project on the vector and intermediate host populations, and ways to modify the project to reduce such populations, are important environmental control measures.

Biological control

Biological control of vectors includes the following public health interventions.

◆ *Introduction of predators and parasites:* The introductions of *Gambusia affinis*, a small fish that feeds on mosquito larvae, and of *Coelomomyces*, a fungal parasite, are examples of control measures that are effective against *Aëdes* mosquitoes.

◆ *Insect growth regulators*: The use of such regulators may result in death or sterility of vectors by interfering with normal insect development. An example is the use of methoprene (Altosid®) to control flood water mosquitoes.

◆ *Genetic modification*: Although still at an experimental phase, researchers have developed transgenic, or genetically modified, mosquitoes that are malaria resistant with higher survival rates that could eventually replace mosquitoes that carry malaria parasites.

Control measures applied to infected humans

Control measures may be applied to infected persons at the individual level, in the institutional or hospital setting, and at the community level.

Hospital infection control

The hospital setting is a unique situation that requires special efforts to prevent and control nosocomial infections, or healthcare-associated infections (HAIs), which are infections that originate or occur in a hospital or other healthcare setting. HAIs are a major problem world-wide. In the United States alone, some 2 million HAIs occur annually resulting in an estimated 90 000 deaths and US$4.5 billion in excess healthcare costs (McKibben 2005).

Infection control programmes for hospitals should ideally include the following elements:

◆ An infection control committee responsible for overall co-ordination of infection control activities

◆ One or more infection control practitioners responsible for nosocomial disease surveillance, analysis of data, consultation and training of hospital staff

◆ A hospital epidemiologist to supervise the infection control practitioners, oversee data collection and analysis, and implement any needed emergency infection control measures

◆ An engineer to direct engineering and preventive maintenance operations, especially ventilation equipment

- A sanitarian to develop procedures for proper disposal of liquid and solid wastes; and sanitation of water, ice, and food
- Effective guidelines for patient care practices
- Surveillance of patient care practices, patient infections, and environmental contamination by infectious agents
- Co-ordination with other departments (microbiology laboratory, central services, housekeeping, food service, and laundry)
- Vector control
- Thorough investigation of problems

Examples of specific control measures that may be applied to infected humans at the individual, institutional, and community levels are detailed in the next section.

Chemotherapy

Treatment of persons with infectious diseases or subclinical infections may be a control tool for some infectious diseases. Such treatment may or may not have an impact on disease progression in the patient. It should be noted that rapid case detection and prompt application of appropriate chemotherapeutic agents are needed to limit infectivity.

Some important examples of control by chemotherapy include the following:

- Treatment of patients with sputum-positive pulmonary *tuberculosis* with appropriate multi-drug therapy will usually result in sputum conversion rendering them non-infectious to others within a few weeks. Recommended treatment regimens include isoniazid (INH) combined with one or more of the following antibiotics: Rifampin, streptomycin, ethambutol, and pyrazinamide. The WHO has recommended that adherence to a complete course of multi-drug therapy be directly observed by another responsible person as part of the DOTS (directly observed treatment, short-course) global strategy for the control of tuberculosis.

- Patients with *leprosy* treated with appropriate multi-drug therapy are considered no longer infectious within 3 months of regular and continued treatment. Recommended treatment regimens for multibacillary leprosy include the following antibiotics: Rifampicin, dapsone and clofazimine.

- Treatment of patients with *streptococcal sore throats* with penicillin (or erythromycin for penicillin-sensitive patients) will usually render them no longer be infectious after 24 to 48 hours.

- Patients with *pertussis* treated with antibiotics such as erythromycin or trimethoprim-sulphamethoxazole, although they may not affect the patient's symptoms, will usually result in the patient no longer being infectious after 5–7 days.

Of special note is the situation of treatment of persons who are carriers. A *carrier* is

a person or animal that harbors a specific infectious agent without discernible clinical disease and serves as a potential source of infection. The carrier state may exist in an individual with an infection that is inapparent throughout its course (commonly known as healthy *or* asymptomatic carrier*), or during the incubation period, convalescence, and post-convalescence of an individual with a clinically recognizable disease (commonly known as* incubatory carrier *or* convalescent carrier*). Under either*

circumstance the carrier state may be of short or long duration (temporary *or* transient carrier, *or* chronic carrier*)* (Heymann 2004).

A chronic carrier of diphtheria, for example, may shed the infectious agent *Corynebacterium diphtheriae* for 6 months or more, but appropriate antibiotic therapy will usually promptly stop the carrier state. Another example is that of untreated patients with typhoid fever due to *Salmonella typhi*. Between 2 and 5 per cent of such patients will become permanent carriers. Treatment with appropriate antibiotics may be effective in ending the carrier state.

Antibiotic treatment may not always eliminate a carrier state for some infectious agents. For example, the treatment of persons with salmonellosis with an antibiotic may not terminate the period of communicability and can even result in emergence of antibiotic-resistant strains. However, antibiotic therapy may be still warranted under certain circumstances.

In some situations, establishing screening programmes in defined target populations for identification of asymptomatic or unrecognized infections that could be transmitted to others may be appropriate. Such screening should include the necessary follow-up with appropriate chemotherapy and counselling. An example would be screening close contacts of diphtheria patients with nose and throat cultures for the presence of *Corynebacterium diphtheriae*. Identified carriers with positive cultures should be treated with appropriate antibiotic therapy.

Isolation

Isolation is the 'separation, for the period of at least equal to the period of communicability, of infected persons or animals from others in such places and under such conditions as to prevent or limit the direct or indirect transmission of the infectious agent from those infected to those who are susceptible to infection or who may spread the agent to others' (Heymann 2004).

The Centers for Disease Control and Prevention (CDC), USA, and the Hospital Infection Control Practices Advisory Committee (HICPAC) have provided guidelines for isolation precautions in hospital settings (HICPAC 1996). There are two levels of isolation precautions, namely, (a) a standard precautions level designed for the care of all hospitalized patients, and (b) a transmission-based precautions level designed for the care of hospitalized patients that are suspected or confirmed to be infected by agents spread by contact, droplet, or airborne routes of transmission. These are summarized from HICPAC (1996) as follows.

Standard precautions are universally applied precautions designed to reduce the risk of transmission by infectious agents from blood; body fluids, secretions, and excretions; non-intact skin; and mucous membranes. The essential elements of standard precautions include handwashing; use of gloves; appropriate application of mask and eye protection or a face shield; utilization of gowns; proper handling of patient-care equipment; adequate environmental control measures for routine care, cleaning and disinfection of frequently touched surfaces; appropriate handling, transporting, and processing of used linen; proper handling and disposal of needles, scalpels, and other sharp instruments; and placement of patients who contaminate the environment in private rooms.

Airborne precautions are used, in addition to standard precautions, in settings where patients are suspected or confirmed to be infected by agents transmitted by airborne droplet nuclei.

The essential elements of airborne precautions include placement of patients in a private room that has monitored negative air pressure (if necessary, it is possible to use cohorting of patients with the same active infections); use of mask respirators (N-95 air-purifying respirators); and limiting patient movement and transport from the room (placing a surgical mask on the patient if they are being moved for an essential purpose). An example of an infectious disease for which patients are recommended to be placed under airborne precautions is a patient in hospital with measles through the fourth day of rash. Although isolation of patients with measles not in hospital is not practical in the general population, schoolchildren should remain out of school through at least the fourth day of rash.

Droplet precautions are used, in addition to standard precautions, in settings where patients are suspected or confirmed to be infected by agents transmitted by droplets. The essential elements of droplet precautions include placement of patients in a private room (if necessary, it is possible to use cohorting of patients with the same active infections or maintaining a spatial separation of at least 3 feet between the infected patient and other patients and visitors); use of a mask when working within 3 feet of the patient; and limiting patient movement and transport from the room (placing a surgical mask on the patient if they are being moved for an essential purpose). Examples of infectious diseases for which patients are recommended to be placed under droplet precautions include pharyngeal diphtheria caused by *Corynebacterium diphtheriae* and pneumonic plague caused by *Yersinia pestis*.

Contact precautions are used, in addition to standard precautions, in settings where patients are suspected or confirmed to be infected or colonized by agents transmitted by direct or indirect contact. The essential elements of contact precautions include placement of the patient in a private room (if necessary, it is possible to use cohorting of patients with the same active infections); use of gloves when entering the patient's room and removing them before leaving the room; wearing a gown when entering the patient's room and removing the gown before leaving the room; limiting patient movement and transport to essential purposes only; and, when possible, dedicate the use of patient-care equipment to a single patient (if necessary, it is possible to use such equipment on a cohort of patients with the same active or colonized infections). Examples of infectious diseases for which patients are recommended to be placed under contact isolation precautions include cutaneous diphtheria caused by *Corynebacterium diphtheriae*, rubella, and disseminated herpes simplex caused by herpes simplex virus.

Quarantine of potentially infected persons

Quarantine is the 'restriction of the activities of well persons or animals who have been exposed (or are considered to be at high risk of exposure) to a case of communicable disease during its period of communicability (i.e. contacts) to prevent disease transmission during the incubation period if infection should occur'. Two categories of quarantine are as follows (Heymann 2004):

- *Absolute* or *complete quarantine*. The limitation of freedom of movement of those exposed to a communicable disease for a period of time not longer than the longest usual incubation period of that disease, in such manner as to prevent effective contact with those not so exposed.

- *Modified quarantine*. A selective, partial limitation of freedom of movement of contacts, commonly on the basis of known or presumed differences in susceptibility and related to the assessed risk of disease transmission. It may be designed to accommodate particular situations. Examples are exclusion of children from school, exemption of immune persons from provisions applicable to susceptible persons, or restriction of military populations to the post or to quarters. Modified quarantine includes: *Personal surveillance*, the practice of close medical or other supervision of contacts to permit prompt recognition of infection or illness but without restricting their movements; and *segregation*, the separation of some part of a group of persons or domestic animals from the others for special consideration, control or observation; removal of susceptible children to homes of immune persons; or establishment of a sanitary boundary to protect uninfected from infected portions of a population (known as a *cordon sanitaire*).

Examples of diseases where quarantine may be considered include the following:

- *Pneumonic plague:* Persons who have been in the same household or in face-to-face contact with patients with pneumonic plague and who do not accept chemoprophylaxis should be placed under *absolute quarantine* with strict isolation, including careful surveillance, for 7 days.

- *Measles:* Although absolute quarantine is impractical, a *modified quarantine* is recommended in settings where young children are living in dormitories, wards or institutions. When measles occurs in such institutional settings, strict *segregation* of infants is recommended.

- *Lassa fever:* Close *personal surveillance* of all close contacts is recommended. Such persons include those who live or are in close contact with lassa fever patients as well as laboratory personnel testing specimens from such patients.

Restriction of activities

Controlling infectious disease transmission by restriction of the activities of persons in the community who are potentially infectious to others may be appropriate in certain circumstances. Examples include the following:

- Individuals with a diarrhoeal disease should be excluded from handling food and caring for patients in hospital, children, and elderly persons.

- Known carriers of *Salmonella typhi* should be excluded from foodhandling and care of patients.

- Persons with staphylococcal disease should avoid contact with debilitated persons and infants.

- Persons with rubella should be excluded from school or work for seven days after the onset of rash and from contact with pregnant women.

Behavioural change

Behaviour change in an infected person to protect others may be difficult to accomplish. However, this should be considered in preventing the transmission of infectious agents in the following situations.

Sexual behaviour. Examples of infectious agents transmitted through sexual activities are discussed in the section above on control measures applied to the host and in more detail in Volume 3, Chapter 9.12. Individuals who suspect that they may have a sexually transmitted disease should be encouraged to have health-seeking behaviours. Persons with a sexually transmissible infectious agent should be treated and asked to co-operate with health officials to trace their sexual contacts. Patients with diseases such as lymphogranuloma venereum and syphilis, for example, should refrain from sexual contact until all lesions are healed. HIV-infected individuals should be counselled to treat genital ulcer disease promptly since such disease may increase transmissibility of HIV. Also, HIV-infected persons should avoid sexual intercourse with HIV-negative individuals. For a more detailed overview of HIV and AIDS see Volume 3, Chapter 9.13.

Intravenous drug use behaviour. In addition to counselling to abstain from intravenous drug use and establishing drug rehabilitation programmes to help individuals who wish to abstain, promoting behaviour change in the use of injection equipment is important. Discouraging the sharing of injection equipment and education on methods for the decontamination of needles and syringes for intravenous drug use reduce risks of transmission of infectious agents through contaminated injection equipment.

Food preparation behaviour. Individuals who should be restricted from handling food (for example, carriers of *Salmonella typhi*) should be counselled regarding their condition and potential to infect others if they handle food. Foodhandlers who have an infectious disease that is potentially transmissible through the vehicle-borne means of food should be discouraged from handling food for others. The importance of hand washing, especially after defecation and before handling food, should be stressed.

Other behaviours that may reduce risk of transmission of infectious agents to other persons include the following:

* *Cough and sneeze behaviour:* Patients with infectious diseases directly transmitted by droplet spread or airborne transmitted by droplet nuclei (for example, patients with sputum-positive tuberculosis) should cover their mouth and nose when coughing or sneezing;

* *Avoidance of contaminated drinking water:* Persons suffering from dracunculiasis should avoid entering a source of drinking water if they have an active ulcer or blister;

* *Avoidance of vector bites:* Patients with the vector-borne disease of African trypanosomiasis (sleeping sickness) with trypanosomes in their blood should prevent tsetse flies from biting; and

* *Avoidance of donating organs or bodily fluid by certain persons:* Individuals who are infected with HIV or who have sexual and other behaviours that have placed them at increased risk for HIV infection should not donate blood, plasma, tissues, cells, semen for artificial insemination, or organs for transplantation.

Control measures applied to animals

A zoonosis is any infectious agent or infectious disease that may be transmitted under natural conditions from vertebrate animals, both wild and domestic, to humans. A detailed approach to zoonoses is given in the comprehensive work *CRC handbook series in zoonoses*

(Beran & Steele 1994). In the control of zoonoses many approaches are used that are applied to animals, including the following:

Active immunization

Active immunization, or vaccination, of selected animals may protect susceptible animal hosts from certain infectious diseases. This protection of animals, in turn, prevents susceptible humans from exposure to the infectious agent of those diseases from animals. An example of an infectious disease in animals in which some control can be achieved through immunization in selected animal populations is rabies. The reservoir of the rabies virus is varied and includes dogs, foxes, wolves, skunks, raccoons and bats. Preventive measures include efforts to vaccinate all dogs.

Other examples of immunization of animals under certain conditions include: (a) immunization of young goats and sheep using a live attenuated strain of *Brucella melitensis* and calves using a strain of *Brucella abortus* in areas of high endemicity for brucellosis; and (b) immunization of animals at risk for acquiring infection with *Bacillus anthracis* that could be transmitted to man causing anthrax.

Restriction or reduction

Restriction is the limiting of the movement of animals and includes isolation and quarantine. Reduction is the killing, known as culling, of selected animals. Selective use of restriction of animals or reduction of animal populations that are infected, or potentially infected, with a zoonotic infectious agent are methods used to decrease or eliminate the opportunity of exposure of susceptible humans, or other animals, to such animals.

The example of rabies can also be used to illustrate the use of restriction or reduction of an animal population to help control an infectious disease. Heymann (2004) recommends that a comprehensive rabies control programme include:

> register, license, and immunize all dogs in enzootic countries; collect and sacrifice ownerless animals and strays; educate pet owners and the public on the importance of restrictions for dogs and cats (for example, pets must be leashed in congested areas when not confined on owner's premises; strange-acting or sick animals of any species, domestic or wild, should not be picked up/handled; reporting of such animals and animals that have bitten a person or another animal to the police/local health department; confinement and observation of such animals as a preventive measure; and wild animals should not be kept as pets). Immediately sacrifice unimmunized dogs or cats bitten by known rabid animals; if detention is elected, hold the animal in an approved secure pound or kennel for at least 6 months under veterinary supervision, and immunize against rabies 30 days before release. If previously immunized, reimmunize and detain (leashing and confinement) for at least 45 days. Cooperative programmes with wildlife conservation authorities to reduce fox, skunk, raccoon and other terrestrial wildlife hosts of sylvatic rabies may be used in circumscribed enzootic areas near campsites and areas of human habitation. If such focal depopulation is undertaken, it must be maintained to prevent repopulation from the periphery.

In epizootic situations, 'in urban areas of industrialized countries, strict enforcement of regulations requiring collection, detention and killing of ownerless and stray dogs, and of non-immunized dogs found off owners' premises, and control of the dog population by castration, spaying or drugs have been effective in breaking transmission cycles' (Heymann 2004).

Other examples of restricting or reducing of animal populations include the following:

- Rat-proofing dwellings and reduction of the rat population to prevent rat bites that may transmit the infectious agents *Streptobacillus moniliformis* and *Spirillum minus* causing the rat-bite fevers of streptobacillosis and spirillosis, respectively

- Rat suppression by poisoning (after achieving flea control) in rodent populations with a high potential for epizootic plague

- Culling of domestic poultry flocks that are infected with highly pathogenic avian influenza, such as H5N1

- Elimination of animals infected with *Brucella abortus*, *Brucella melitensis*, *Brucella suis*, and *Brucella canis* by segregation or slaughter to prevent brucellosis

- Slaughtering dairy cattle that test positive for infection with *Mycobacterium bovis*, the infectious agent of bovine tuberculosis

Chemoprophylaxis and chemotherapy

Chemoprophylaxis of an animal is using chemical substances (e.g. antibiotics) that prevent infection or its progression to clinically manifest infectious disease in the animal. Chemotherapy of an animal is using these chemical substances to treat an infectious disease in an animal. Both chemoprophylaxis and chemotherapy are control measures that may be used to reduce or prevent the opportunity of an infectious agent from being transmitted from an animal to susceptible humans.

Psittacosis is an example of a zoonosis controlled by chemoprophylaxis or chemotherapy in selected animal populations. The infectious agent, *Chlamydia psittaci*, may be directly transmitted to humans from infected birds when the dried droppings, secretions, or dust from the feathers of such infected birds are inhaled. Imported psittacine species of birds should be placed under quarantine and receive an appropriate antibiotic chemotherapeutic regimen such as chlortetracycline administered in their feed for 30 days.

Another example is chemoprophylaxis in selected dogs at high risk of infection with *Echinococcus granulosus*. This infectious agent can be transmitted to humans through hand to mouth transmission of the tapeworm eggs from dog faeces causing echinococcosis due to *Echinococcus granulosus*, or cystic hydatid disease. Such high-risk dogs (for example, sled dogs) should periodically receive antihelminth treatment with a chemotherapeutic agent such as praziquantel (Biltricide®). Routine use of chemoprophylaxis in cattle, feed lots, and poultry farms, however, can promote serious drug-resistance problems.

Control measures applied to the environment

Control measures applied to the environment are designed to interrupt the routes of transmission by which an infectious agent may be spread through the environment. Just as the routes of transmission are varied, so, too, are the control methods that can be applied. Control measures that affect transmission that can be applied to the host, agents, vectors, infected humans and other animals are reviewed elsewhere in this chapter. Environmental factors may also have a direct impact on the host, agent, or vector. For example, low humidity may predispose to certain infections due to a greater permeability of mucus membranes in the host; cold, dry climates inhibit development of the infective larvae agent of hookworm disease; and higher altitudes and colder climates limit the mosquito vector.

The recognition of the relationship between disease and filth led to a sanitary revolution in industrialized countries that markedly reduced infectious diseases even before the arrival of the antibiotic era. Improved methods for storing and preserving food, better housing, and smaller families with a resultant decrease in the risk of infections at an early age all contributed to reductions in infant and child mortality rates.

This section focuses on general environmental control measures not mentioned elsewhere. Some of these methods, such as provision of safe water, have the potential to prevent several different infectious diseases and significantly reduce rates of disease in the community.

Provision of safe water

It has been estimated that about 1.3 billion people in the developing world lack access to clean and plentiful water (World Bank 1993). Contaminated drinking water, sometimes the result of poorly designed or maintained systems of sewerage, may lead to the water-borne indirect transmission of such infectious agents as *Giardia lamblia* causing giardiasis, pathogenic serotypes of *Salmonella* causing salmonellosis, and *Cryptosporidium* species causing cryptosporidosis.

Purification of water can occur though natural methods or human intervention. Examples of natural methods that contribute to water purification include the processes of evaporation and condensation, filtration through the earth, plant growth, aeration, and reduction and oxidation of organic material by bacteria. Purification of water for public consumption is conventionally done through such processes as coagulation of colloids by aluminium salts or with other techniques; filtration through such materials as coal, sand, or diatomaceous earth; and disinfection with such chemicals as chlorine derivatives. In special situations, boiling and distillation can be used for purification (Solomon *et al.* 2004).

Proper disposal of faeces

It has been estimated that nearly 2 billion people in the developing world do not have an adequate system for proper disposal of faeces (World Bank 1993). Infectious agents in faeces that may result in infectious diseases include poliovirus causing poliomyelitis; *Shigella dysenteriae*, *Shigella flexneri*, *Shigella boydii*, and *Shigella sonnei* causing shigellosis; and *Entamoeba histolytica* causing amebiasis.

Infectious agents in faeces may be transmitted by the direct transmission route (including the faecal–oral mode), the vehicle-borne route (including water as noted in the previous section) and the vector-borne route (including the simple mechanism of flies carrying infected faeces on their feet). Public health environmental control measures to interrupt these routes of transmission by ensuring the proper disposal of faeces include the following:

- Appropriate on-site disposal through such means as properly constructed sanitary privies in rural areas with no sewerage systems.

- On-site disposal of domestic wastewater (such as use of septic tanks or cesspools).

- Sewerage systems with treatment of wastewater. Such treatment may include preliminary treatment, sedimentation, chemical coagulation and flocculation, biological treatment (such as activated sludge units and trickling filters), stabilization ponds, sludge management, and disinfection (usually with chlorine) of effluents discharged into drinking, bathing, or shellfish-growing waters.

The importance of personal-health-promoting behaviours of using toilets, keeping toilets clean, and handwashing after defecation are a part of control efforts aimed at the proper disposal of faeces.

Food sanitation

Food-borne infectious diseases remain a problem in both industrialized and developing countries. In the United States alone, an estimated 76 million persons are affected each year, resulting in some 5000 deaths annually. Significant food-borne outbreaks and sporadic cases continue to occur due to such factors as the following:

- Contamination of meat, poultry and eggs with infectious agents, including pathogenic serotypes of *Salmonella*, *Yersinia pseudotuberculosis* and *Yersinia entercolitica*, and *Listeria monocytogenes*.

- Contamination of vegetables, especially lettuce and leafy green vegetables, with the infectious enterohaemorrhagic strain of *Escherichia coli* O157:H7. Other outbreaks in fruits, juices, and vegetables have been due to contamination with hepatitis A and pathogenic serotypes of salmonella.

- Problems in food storage, handling, and preparation in commercial eating places and in homes.

- Larger and more centralized production and processing facilities, coupled with increasingly extensive distribution networks, which may result in transmission of infectious agents to many persons if a commercial product becomes contaminated.

Industrialized countries have significantly reduced the transmission of some infectious agents through major public health programmes in food sanitation, including: (a) inspecting eating and drinking establishments; (b) inspecting meat and poultry; (c) improving shellfish sanitation; and (d) promoting adequate cooking, canning and refrigeration methods. Some cities and counties have instituted restaurant grading systems based on inspection reports, including required public display of the restaurant's grade as a guide for consumers.

Examples of vehicle-borne indirect transmission of infectious agents through food that can be controlled though a comprehensive public health food sanitation programme include the following:

- Pathogenic serotypes of *Salmonella* transmitted by ingesting food made from infected animals or contaminated by the infectious agent in faeces that may cause salmonellosis. Control is achieved through '(a) handwashing before, during and after food preparation; (b) refrigerating prepared foods in small containers; (c) thoroughly cooking all foodstuffs derived from animal sources, particularly poultry, pork, egg products and meat dishes; (d) avoiding recontamination within the kitchen after cooking is completed; and (e) maintaining a sanitary kitchen, protecting prepared foods against rodent and insect contamination. Inspect for sanitation and adequately supervise abattoirs, food-processing plants, feed-blending mills, egg-grading stations and butcher shops' (Heymann 2004).

- *Staphylococcus aureus* causing staphylococcal food intoxication by ingesting food containing the staphylococcal enterotoxin. Control is achieved through means to '(a) educate food handlers about strict food hygiene, sanitation and cleanliness of kitchens, proper temperature control, handwashing, cleaning of fingernails; (b) the danger of working with exposed skin, nose and eye infections and the need to cover wounds; (c) reduce food handling time (from initial preparation to service) to a minimum, with no more than 4 h at ambient temperature. If they are to be stored more than 2 h, keep perishable foods hot (above 60°C/140°F) or cold (below 7°C/45°F; best is below 4°C/39°F) in shallow containers and covered; and (d) temporarily exclude people with boils, abscesses and other purulent lesions of hands, face or nose from food handling' (Heymann 2004).

- *Trichinella spiralis* transmitted by ingesting raw or improperly cooked meat or meat products, mainly pork, containing infectious encysted larvae that may cause trichinosis. Control is achieved through means to '(a) educate the public on the need to cook all fresh pork and pork products and meat from wild animals at a temperature and for a time sufficient to allow all parts to reach at least 71°C/160°F, or until meat changes from pink to grey, which allows a sufficient margin of safety. This should be done unless it has been established that these meat products have been processed either by heating, curing, freezing or irradiation adequate to kill trichinae; (b) grind pork in a separate grinder or clean the grinder thoroughly before and after processing other meats; (c) adopt regulations to encourage commercial irradiation processing of pork products. Testing carcasses for infection with a digestion technique and immunodiagnosis of pigs with an approved ELISA test are both useful; (d) adopt and enforce regulations that allow only certified trichinea-free pork to be used in raw pork products that have a cooked appearance or in products that traditionally are not heated sufficiently to kill trichinea during final preparation; and (e) adopt laws and regulations to require and enforce the cooking of garbage and offal before feeding to swine' (Heymann 2004).

Milk sanitation

Milk may be a vehicle for indirect transmission of infectious agents like: *Mycobacterium bovis* causing tuberculosis, *Corynebacterium diphtheriae* causing diphtheria, *Listeria monocytogenes* causing listeriosis, and *Campylobacter jejuni* and *Campylobacter coli* causing campylobacter enteritis.

Public health control measures to break the chain of transmission of infectious agents through milk include:

- Mechanization and sanitization of milking processes

- Refrigeration of milk

- Pasteurization of milk through high-temperature short-time, batch, ultra-pasteurization, or ultra-high-temperature methods

- Monitoring milk quality by testing for bacteria using a standard bacterial plate count, by testing for density of coliform organisms, and by use of the phosphatase test to assay for pasteurization

- Periodic testing of cows for tuberculosis and brucellosis

The use of raw milk for human consumption as well as post-pasteurization contamination of milk may result in outbreaks of milk-borne diseases.

Design of facilities and equipment

The design and proper maintenance of buildings, rooms, and equipment can help break the chain of transmission of infectious agents. Laminar airflow hoods in laboratory workbenches, ventilation systems in hospitals, and disposable intravenous equipment are examples of systems designed to reduce risk of transmission. Routine maintenance needed to retain the original design standards for control of transmission of infectious agents include: (a) replacement of air filters; (b) cleaning of cooling towers; (c) monitoring of positive pressure rooms and airlocks; and (d) replacement of in-dwelling peripheral venous catheters.

Examples of infectious agents whose transmission can be reduced through proper design and maintenance include the following:

- *Legionella* species, the infectious agents responsible for legionellosis, are usually transmitted through airborne transmission via aerosol-production. Transmission of the agent from cooling towers can be reduced by periodically cleaning off any scale or sediment, routinely using biocides to kill slime-forming organisms, and draining such towers when not in use.

- *Staphylococcus aureus*, the infectious agent responsible for staphylococcal disease in medical and surgical wards of hospitals, can be controlled by enforcing strict aseptic techniques, including procedures to change intravenous infusion sites at least every 48 h and replace indwelling peripheral venous catheters every 72 h.

- *Bacillus anthracis*, the infectious agent responsible for anthrax, can be transmitted, among other ways, through inhalation of anthrax spores. Proper design of industrial plants that handle raw animal fibres include providing facilities for adequate ventilation and control of dust, washing and changing clothes after work, and eating away from the places of work.

Other methods

In addition to the environmental methods of control of transmission of infectious agents already mentioned, the following are other methods, some specific and some general, that should also be noted.

- Improvement of housing conditions to *reduce crowding* (as measured by the number of persons per room and not total population density). Reduction in crowding is a general measure that can reduce the transmission of infectious agents, especially direct transmission from direct contact or direct projection (droplet spread).

- *Improvement in working conditions* can affect the risk of infectious disease. For example, control of particulate matter by proper ventilation in occupations such as textile mill workers, metal grinders, and pottery factory workers can reduce inflammation of the lungs and thus decrease the risk of developing tuberculosis. Excessive physical exertion and the stress of exhausting work can also increase the risk of tuberculosis.

- Improved *irrigation* and agricultural practices and *removing vegetation* or *draining* and *filling* of snail-breeding sites can reduce or eliminate the freshwater snail hosts of such infectious agents as *Schistosoma mansoni*, *Schistosoma haematobium*, and *Schistosoma japonicum* that cause schistosomiasis in humans.

- *Adequate screening* of blood, serum, plasma, tissues or organs can break the chain of vehicle-borne transmission from such biological products. Examples include screening for hepatitis B surface antigen and HIV antibodies in donated blood to prevent transmission of hepatitis B and HIV, respectively.

- Installation of *screened living* and *sleeping quarters* and the use of *bednets*, including bednets impregnated with a synthetic pyrethroid such as permethrin, can reduce exposure to mosquitoes infected with the infectious agents of malaria.

Control measures applied to the agent

Control of some infectious diseases can be achieved through means that remove the infectious agents from the environment or inactivate the agents. Physical measures (such as heat, cold, ultraviolet light, and ionizing radiation) and chemical measures (such as liquid disinfectants and antiseptics, gases, and chlorination) can be used. Examples of control measures applied to infectious agents include the following:

- *Cleaning* is the removing of infectious agents from surfaces through such physical actions as vacuum cleaning or washing and scrubbing using soap or detergent and hot water. Cleaning also helps remove organic materials that might support the growth or survival of infectious agents.

- *Cooling* may inhibit bacterial multiplication and some infectious agents, such as *Trichinella* cysts and *Taenia solium* larvae (cysticerci), which can be killed by freezing temperatures.

- *Pasteurization* is heating to a temperature of 75°C/167°F for 30 min to kill pathogenic vegetative bacteria. It does not inactivate bacterial spores. Pasteurization is a commonly used process to help ensure safety of milk and to prolong its storage quality.

- *Disinfection* is the reduction or killing of vegetative harmful bacterial infectious agents outside the body or on objects. Disinfection may not inactivate all bacterial spores and viruses. *Disinfectants* are used to eliminate pathogenic bacteria from the skin surface and from contaminated inanimate surfaces and include: (a) alcohols; (b) halogens such as iodine and chlorine; (c) surface active compounds such as the quaternary ammonium compound benzalkonium chloride; (d) phenolics; and (e) alkylating agents such as glutaraldehyde and formaldehyde. *Antiseptics* are a class of disinfectant that can be applied on body surfaces; they have a lower toxicity than environmental disinfectants and are usually less effective in killing micro-organisms.

- *Sterilization* is the complete removal or killing of all infectious agents in, or on, an object. Sterilization of equipment for surgery and wound dressings; parenteral administration of drugs, vaccines, or nutrients; catheterization; and dental work are all important means of controlling infectious diseases by killing infectious agents. Sterilization can be accomplished through use of fire, steam (such as in an autoclave), heated air, certain gases (such as ethylene oxide), ultraviolet light, ionizing radiation, liquid chemicals, and filtration. The method of sterilization chosen depends on the type of equipment to be sterilized.

The use of sterilized *disposable equipment*, such as disposable needles, syringes, and catheters, has the potential to reduce the risk of transmission of infectious agents. However, it must be assured that such equipment is disposed of properly and is not reused. For example, disposable syringes cannot be properly resterilized because the plastic from which they are made cannot withstand the heat necessary for sterilization. Technologies, such as the single-use disposable needle and syringe developed for immunization programmes, help assure such disposable equipment is not reused.

Control and prevention programmes

The preceding sections have considered the issues and given examples of control measures for infectious diseases at individual, institutional and community levels and the tools for control directed at the host, routes of transmission, and the agent. Control and prevention programmes using these tools must be developed according to a number of factors including: (a) the risk of disease; (b) the magnitude of disease burden (as measured by mortality, degree of disability, morbidity, and economic costs); (c) the feasibility of control strategies; (d) the cost of control measures; (e) the effectiveness of such measures (on current levels of disease and impact on future cases or outbreaks); (f) the adverse effects or complications of the control measures; and (g) the availability of resources. Public heath planning for the control of infectious diseases must consider these issues to design optimal, evidence-based control and prevention programmes.

The tools of disease surveillance for recognition and evaluation of the patterns of disease can provide the information on the risk and magnitude of disease burden to individuals, persons in institutions, subgroups of populations, and the community at large. Establishment and maintenance of the infrastructure for surveillance, including a system for the reporting of notifiable infectious diseases and unusual events, must be a high priority.

Feasibility of possible control and prevention strategies must be assessed through operational research, pilot projects, or from field experience. The fact that a particular measure can help control a disease does not mean it can be applied on a sufficient scale to have the desired impact. The cost of control activities (in both human and material resources) can be assessed through costing studies that can also provide the data needed to conduct more rigorous cost-benefit and cost-effectiveness analyses. A costly measure, even if it provides a high degree of control for an infectious disease, may not be affordable to the society or reasonable to apply in the light of other less expensive alternative strategies. Effectiveness of control measures may be assessed through epidemiologic studies to find out their impact on reduction in the incidence or prevalence of disease.

The availability of resources for prevention and control programmes forces public health planners to set priorities by taking into account all these factors and then designing programmes that have maximum impact within available resources. Planners have a responsibility to mobilize additional necessary resources by raising public awareness and generating political will. Effective communication of disease burden and the results achievable through well-managed and effective control programmes can be a powerful tool for advocacy. Ideally, communities or their representatives should actively participate in the planning, execution, and evaluation of public health programmes.

Prevention effectiveness is 'the measure of the impact on health (including effectiveness, safety and cost) of prevention policies, programmes, and practices. The assessment of prevention effectiveness is the ongoing process of applying evaluation tools to prevention practices' (CDC 1995). Recognizing that systems for assessing the effectiveness of prevention strategies (including prevention strategies for infectious diseases) are weak or non-existent in both developing and industrialized countries alike, the CDC has suggested the following objectives for prevention effectiveness activities: 'evaluate the impact of prevention, use results of evaluation research to establish programme priorities, and establish or apply standardized methods to compare the benefits and effectiveness of alternative prevention strategies' (CDC 1995).

The current situation of *international migration* of many people worldwide presents an additional complexity to the design of programmes for the control of infectious diseases. Pertinent issues include refugee camps, legal status of migrants in recipient countries, and temporary return migration. Public health officials must consider the most effective mix of combined control measures applied to the host, agent, and routes of transmission when designing suitable control and prevention programmes (Gellert 1993).

International commerce and transportation are important areas of concern for public health infectious disease control programmes, especially as the speed of travel has increased. The tools of control include such measures as:

◆ Spraying insecticides effective against mosquito vectors of malaria in aircraft before departure, in transit, or on arrival

◆ Rat-proofing or periodic fumigation to control rats on ships, docks, and warehouses to prevent plague

Specific international control measures relating to aircraft, ships, and land transportation for infectious diseases are detailed in the *International Health Regulations (2005)* (WHO 2005).

The challenge facing infectious disease control programmes is to design an optimal set of interventions at local, institutional, community, national, and international levels supported and accepted by the political leadership and the persons to whom these measures are applied.

Eradication

A unique endpoint in the control of infectious diseases is that of eradication. Eradication is the cessation of all transmission of an infectious agent by extermination of that agent. To date, only one infectious disease, *smallpox*, has been eradicated. The WHO World Health Assembly in May 1980 confirmed its global eradication some three years after the last naturally acquired case of smallpox in October 1977 (Fenner *et al.* 1988). The magnitude of this accomplishment is appreciated when one realizes that, in the early 1950s, it was estimated 50 million cases of smallpox still occurred each year in the world, some 150 years after Edward Jenner had performed the first vaccination and wrote: 'it now becomes too manifest to admit of controversy, that the annihilation of the Small Pox, the most dreadful scourge of the human species, must be the final result of this practice' (Fenner *et al.* 1988).

The goal of global eradication has been set by the World Health Assembly for two other infectious diseases, poliomyelitis caused by wild poliovirus and dracunculiasis (guinea-worm infection), the latter caused by the infectious agent *Dracunculus medinensis*. A high level of sustained political will, aggressively applied disease surveillance, and effective control measures are the required elements to achieve eradication of the infectious agents for these diseases.

Impressive progress has been made toward the global *eradication of poliomyelitis* since the 1988 World Health Assembly set the goal for its eradication. The entire region of the Americas succeeded in interrupting transmission of indigenous wild poliovirus since August 1991. The Western Pacific region succeeded in interrupting transmission since 1997. In other regions of the world, countries endemic for poliomyelitis are carrying out the necessary strategies to eradicate the poliovirus. Poliomyelitis control measures that will lead to eradication include the following:

◆ Achieving and maintaining high levels of routine coverage of infants with at least three doses of oral polio vaccine.

◆ Mass application of oral polio vaccine in countries where poliomyelitis is endemic through national immunization days, usually by providing oral polio vaccine to every child less than 5 years of age twice each year, separated by 4–6 weeks, and conducted during the low season of poliovirus transmission.

◆ 'Mopping-up' operations after the use of national immunization days has reduced transmission of disease to defined focal geographic areas, usually by providing oral polio vaccine house-to-house to all children less than 5 years of age on two occasions separated by 4–6 weeks.

◆ Aggressive action-oriented surveillance for acute flaccid paralysis. Such surveillance includes: (a) case investigation; (b) a laboratory network for isolation and characterization of polioviruses in suspect cases of poliomyelitis and people in close contact with them; and (c) limited outbreak response immunization providing one house-to-house round of oral polio vaccine to children less than 5 years of age living in the same village or neighborhood of the patient.

Significant strides in the *eradication of dracunculiasis* have also been made. Over the last decade the total number of dracunculiasis cases have declined by more than 95 per cent. The disease is now limited to only certain parts of some African countries in a band between the Sahara desert and the equator. India was certified as dracunculiasis free in the year 2000. Dracunculiasis control measures that are leading to its ultimate eradication include the following:

◆ Establishing a national programme office, conducting baseline surveys and preparing and refining a national plan of action.

◆ Educating the population in endemic areas that the source of guinea-worm comes from their drinking water.

◆ Ensuring that persons with blisters or emerging worms do not enter sources of drinking water through behaviour changes and by converting step-wells into draw-wells.

◆ Promoting the boiling or filtering of water through a fine mesh cloth to remove copepods. Treating drinking water with chlorine or iodine will also kill the copepods and infective larvae.

◆ Providing non-infected water through construction of wells or rainwater catchments.

◆ In selected endemic villages, controlling copepod populations with temephos (Abate®) insecticide placed in reservoirs, tanks, ponds, and step-wells.

◆ Implementing an intensified surveillance and aggressive case-containment strategy as programmes get close to achieving eradication.

The eradication of a disease requires a unique set of conditions, including the following: (a) a defined, accessible reservoir of the infectious agent; (b) affordable and effective control measures that can interrupt the chain of infection directed at the host, agent or route of transmission; and (c) a surveillance mechanism adequate to monitor and ultimately certify the disappearance of the infectious agent.

It is likely that measles may be targeted for global eradication in the future. Some countries and geographic regions have already targeted measles for elimination—a term sometimes used to describe the eradication of a disease from a large geographic area. Other diseases that may potentially be targeted for eradication in the future include: Mumps, rubella, hepatitis B, leprosy and diphtheria.

Emerging infectious diseases

New, emerging, and re-emerging infectious diseases have become a focus for the attention of public health prevention and control programmes in both industrialized and developing countries. Such infectious diseases have thwarted any expectation that infectious diseases will soon be eliminated as public health problems and resulted in a widening spectrum of diseases, many of which were once thought to be almost conquered. Krause has reflected on this as follows:

> *Microbes and vectors swim in the evolutionary stream, and they swim faster than we do. Bacteria reproduce every 30 min. For them, a millennium is compressed into a fortnight. They are fleet afoot, and the pace of our research must keep up with them, or they will overtake us. Microbes were here on earth 2 billion years before humans arrived, learning every trick for survival, and it is likely that they will be here 2 billion years after we depart.* (Krause 1998)

Many factors contribute to the emergence of new or re-emergence of those previously known (Lederberg *et al.* 1992; CDC 1994; Murphy 1994), including: Human demographic change; breakdowns of sanitary and other public health measures; economic development and changes in the use of land; climate change; other human behaviours (such as increased use of child-care facilities, sexual and drug use behaviours, and patterns of outdoor recreation); international travel and commerce; changes in food processing and handling; evolution of pathogenic infectious agents; development of resistance of infectious agents; resistance of the vectors of vector-borne infectious diseases to pesticides; imunosuppression of persons; and deterioration in surveillance systems for infectious diseases, including laboratory support, to detect new or emerging disease problems at an early stage.

An aggressive public health response to these new, emerging and re-emerging infectious disease threats must be made to characterize them better and to mount an effective response for their control. For example, the 1999 outbreak of West Nile fever in New York City and surrounding areas that, within a 4-year period, spread throughout the United States demonstrates how a viral encephalitis, initially classified as St. Louis encephalitis and later confirmed to be due to West Nile virus, can reach far beyond its normal setting.

The WHO has outlined the following high priority areas (WHO 1995):

◆ Strengthen global surveillance of infectious diseases

◆ Establish national and international infrastructures to recognize, report, and respond to new disease threats

◆ Further develop applied research on diagnosis, epidemiology, and control of emerging infectious diseases

◆ Strengthen the international capacity for infectious disease prevention and control

Emerging infectious diseases are addressed in detail in Volume 3, Chapter 9.17.

Bioterrorism: The deliberate use of biological agents to cause harm

Another unfortunate source of an infectious disease threat is the spectre of biological warfare or bioterrorism, especially in an age where terrorist acts are frequent events (Christopher *et al.* 1997). The 2002 World Health Assembly resolution urges member states 'to treat any deliberate use, including local, of biological and chemical agents and radionuclear attack to cause harm also as a global public health threat, and to respond to such a threat in other countries by sharing expertise, supplies and resources in order rapidly to contain the event and mitigate its effects' (WHO 2002).

The WHO recommends the following (WHO 2004b):

◆ Public health authorities, in close cooperation with other government bodies, should draw up contingency plans for dealing with a deliberate release of biological or chemical agents intended to harm civilian populations. These plans should be consistent or integral with existing plans for outbreaks of disease, natural disasters, large-scale industrial or transportation accidents, and terrorist incidents.

◆ Preparedness for deliberate releases of biological or chemical agents should be based on standard risk-analysis principles, starting with risk and threat assessment in order to determine the relative priority that should be accorded to such releases in comparison with other dangers to public health in the country concerned. Considerations for deliberate releases should be incorporated into existing public health infrastructures, rather than developing separate infrastructures.

◆ Preparedness for deliberate releases of biological or chemical agents can be markedly increased in most countries by strengthening the public health infrastructure, and particularly public health surveillance and response, and measures should be taken to this end.

◆ Managing the consequences of a deliberate release of biological or chemical agents may demand more resources than are available, and international assistance would then be essential.

Many countries are developing rapid response capability to deal with such contingencies, especially in the light of the 2001 bioterrorist attack using anthrax in the United States.

Conclusion

In summary, the aggressive application of the principles of infectious disease control outlined in this chapter (including the measures applied to the host, vectors, infected humans, animals, environment, and agents), is needed to control, eliminate, or even eradicate infectious diseases. The public's health is continually at risk for infectious disease and we must ensure that our guard against these diseases is not let down and, in fact, is continually

raised as the factors that favour emerging infectious diseases result in new challenges for their control.

It is only through worldwide concerted action will the effort to control infectious disease be effective. We have now in an era where, as Nobel Laureate Dr. Joshua Lederberg has stated, 'The microbe that felled one child in a distant continent yesterday can reach yours today and seed a global pandemic tomorrow' (quoted in CDC 1994). As Hans Zinsser stated over 60 years ago:

Infectious disease is one of the few genuine adventures left in the world. The dragons are all dead and the lance grows rusty in the chimney corner . . . About the only sporting proposition that remains unimpaired by the relentless domestication of a once free-living human species is the war against those ferocious little fellow creatures, which lurk in the dark corners and stalk us in the bodies of rats, mice and all kinds of domestic animals; which fly and crawl with the insects, and waylay us in our food and drink and even in our love. (Hans Zinsser 1934 quoted in Murphy 1994)

References

ACIP (Immunization Practices Advisory Committee) (2006). General recommendations on immunization. *Morbidity and Mortality Weekly Report*, **55**, RR 15.

Beran, G.W. and Steele, J.H. (ed) (1994). *Handbook series of zoonoses*. CRC Press, Boca Raton, FL.

Brillman, J.C. and Quenzer, R.W. (ed.) (1998). *Infectious disease in emergency medicine* (2nd ed). Lippincott-Raven, Philadelphia, PA.

CDC (Centers for Disease Control and Prevention) (1994). *Addressing emerging infectious disease threats: a prevention strategy for the United States*. CDC, Atlanta, GA.

CDC (Centers for Disease Control and Prevention) (1995). *Prevention effectiveness: making prevention a practical reality*. CDC, Atlanta, GA.

CDC (Centers for Disease Control and Prevention) (2008). Summary of notifiable diseases, United States, 2006. *Morbidity and mortality weekly report*, **55**(53), 2–94.

Cristopher, G.W., Cieslak, T.J., Pavlin, J.A. *et al.* (1997). Biological warfare: A historical perspective. *Journal of the American Medical Association*, **278**, 412–7.

Committee on Infectious Diseases (2006), *American Academy of Pediatrics: report of the committee on infectious diseases*, (25th ed). American Academy of Pediatrics, Elk Grove Village, IL.

Evans, A.S. and Kaslow, R.A. (ed.) (1997). *Viral infections of humans: Epidemiology and control*, (4th ed). Plenum Press, New York.

Evans, A.S. and Brachman, P.S. (ed.) (1998). *Bacterial infections of humans: epidemiology and control* (3rd ed). Plenum Press, New York.

Fenner, F., Henderson, D.A., Arita, I. *et al.* (1988). *Smallpox and its eradication*. World Health Organization, Geneva.

Feigin, R.D. *et al* (ed.) (2004). *Textbook of pediatric infectious diseases* (5th ed). W.B. Saunders, Philadelphia, PA.

Fine, P.E. (1993). Herd immunity: history, theory, practice. *Epidemiologic reviews*, **15**, 265–302.

Gellert, G.A. (1993). International migration and control of communicable diseases. *Social Science and Medicine*, **37**, 1489–99.

Gorbach, S.L., Bartlett, J.G., and Blacklow, N.R. (ed.) (2004). *Infectious diseases* (3rd ed). Lippincott Williams and Wilkins, Philadelphia, PA.

Guerrant, R.L., Walker, D.H., and Weller, P.F. (ed.) (2006). *Tropical infectious diseases: Principles, pathogens, and practice* (2nd ed). W.B. Saunders, Philadelphia, PA.

Heymann, D.L. (ed.) (2004). *Control of communicable diseases manual*, (18th ed). American Public Health Association, Washington.

HICPAC (Hospital Infection Control Practices Advisory Committee) (1996). Guideline for isolation precautions in hospitals part II. Recommendations for isolation precautions in hospitals. *Am J Infect Control*, **24**:32–52.

Insel, R.A., Amstey, M., Woodin, K. *et al.* (1994). Maternal immunization to prevent infectious diseases in the neonate or infant. *International Journal of Technology Assessment in Health Care*, **10**, 143–53.

Jamison, D.T. *et al.* (ed.) (2006). *Disease control priorities in developing countries* (2nd ed). Oxford University Press, New York.

Kiple, K.F. (ed.) (1993). *The Cambridge world history of human disease*. Cambridge University Press.

Krause, R.M. (ed.) (1998). *Emerging infections*. Biomedical Research Reports, Academic Press, New York.

Last, J.M. *et al.* (ed.) (2001). *A dictionary of epidemiology* (4th ed). International Epidemiological Association. Oxford University Press, New York.

Lederberg, J., Shope, R.E., and Oaks, S.C. Jr. (ed) (1992). *Emerging infections: microbial threats to health in the United States*. National Academy Press, Washington, D.C.

McKibben, L. *et al.* (2005). Guidance on public reporting of healthcare-associated infections: recommendations of the Hospital Infection Control Practices Advisory Committee). *Am J Infect Control*, **33**, 217–26.

McNeill, W.H. (1976). *Plagues and peoples*. Anchor Press/Doubleday, Garden City, New York.

Mandell, G.L., Bennett J.E., and Dolin, R. (ed.) (2005). *Mandell, Douglas and Bennett's principles and practice of infectious diseases* (6th ed). Elsevier Churchill Livingstone, New York.

Murphy, F.A. (1994). New, emerging, and reemerging infectious diseases. *Advances in Virus Research*, **43**, 1–52.

Osterholm, M.T. and Hedberg C.W. (2005). Epidemiolologic principles. In *Mandell, Douglas and Bennett's principles and practice of infectious diseases* (6th edn) (ed. G.L. Mandell, J.E. Bennett and R. Dolin), pp. 158–68. Elsevier Churchill Livingstone, New York.

Plotkin, S.A. and Orenstein, W.A. (ed) (2004). *Vaccines*. (4th ed.). W.B Saunders, Philadelphia.

Ryan, K.J. and Ray, C.G. (ed.) (2004). *Sherris Medical microbiology: an introduction to infectious diseases* (4th ed). McGraw-Hill, New York.

Solomon, S.L., Fraser, D.W., and Kaplan, S.L. (2004). Public health considerations. In *Textbook of pediatric infectious diseases*, (ed. R.D. Feigin *et al*) (5th edn), pp. 3221–44. W.B. Saunders, Philadelphia, PA.

UNAIDS (Joint United Nations Programme on HIV/AIDS) (2007). *UNAIDS/ WHO AIDS epidemic update: December 2007*. UNAIDS, Geneva.

Wilson, M.E. (1991). *A world guide to infections: diseases, distribution, diagnosis*. Oxford University Press, New York.

World Bank (1993). *World Bank development report: investing in health*. World Bank, Washington.

WHO (World Health Organization) (1995). *Communicable disease prevention and control: new, emerging, and re-emerging infectious diseases*, No. A48/15. WHO, Geneva.

WHO (World Health Organization) (2002). Global public health response to natural occurrence, accidental release or deliberate use of biological and chemical agents or radionuclear material that affect health. World Health Assembly Resolution, WHA55.16, WHO, Geneva.

WHO (World Health Organization) (2003). *Communicable disease 2002: global defence against the infectious disease threat*. WHO/CDS/2003.15, WHO, Geneva.

WHO (World Health Organization) (2004a). *World health report 2004*. WHO, Geneva.

WHO (World Health Organization) (2004b). Public health response to biological and chemical weapons. WHO, Geneva.

WHO (World Health Organization) (2005). *International health regulations (2005)*. WHO, Geneva.

WHO (World Health Organization) (2008). *International travel and health*. WHO, Geneva.

Population screening and public health

Allison Streetly and Walter W. Holland

Abstract

Screening is concerned with actively identifying disease or pre-disease conditions in individuals who presume themselves to be healthy but may benefit from early treatment. Population screening should be distinguished from the testing of individuals to facilitate case finding in clinical settings. The chapter begins by outlining the historical development of screening as a health intervention. It then discusses the properties of screening tests and the criteria that must be fulfilled before a screening programme is introduced. The initiation of a screening programme raises a number of ethical questions that must be addressed at the level of the health system and the screening programme, as well as at the level of the individual subject who may be offered a screening test. The meaning and limitations of informed choice are discussed. The practical problems that must be negotiated when organizing the delivery of a screening programme are outlined. Processes of quality assurance are described. The final section of the chapter summarizes recommendations for screening at different stages of life.

Introduction

The concept of screening, that is actively identifying a disease or pre-disease condition in individuals who presume themselves to be healthy but may benefit from early treatment, sounds easy and attractive. The presumption is that if this is done the clinical course of the disease will be altered and the prognosis will be improved for the person who has been screened. Unfortunately, the reality of screening is more difficult and screening programmes, like other healthcare interventions, may do harm (Raffle & Gray 2007). Unlike most other healthcare interventions, screening programmes are offered to individuals who consider themselves to be healthy and the harms caused by screening programmes are therefore particularly difficult to accept. Consequently, it is important to appreciate what screening can and cannot achieve, and the conditions required for a cost-effective programme. Public health scientists and practitioners contribute by providing and appraising evidence concerning the benefits and harms of screening, managing screening programmes, and informing the expectations of the public and other stakeholders. This chapter outlines the principles that underpin the development and implementation of screening programmes.

It also provides a brief summary of screening applications at different stages of life.

History of screening

The benefits of screening were first demonstrated by the use of mass miniature radiography (MMR) for the identification of individuals with tuberculosis (TB). The use of MMR became common in many countries after the introduction of effective treatment for TB after 1946. With the reduction in the burden of tuberculosis, the application of screening to other chronic conditions began to be considered. This was particularly so in the United States, where a law on the control of chronic diseases and the availability of screening was passed in the late 1950s. Lester Breslow, head of the Division of Chronic Diseases in the California State Health Department (later its Commissioner for Health), was a particularly enthusiastic advocate. A Commission on Chronic Illness was founded in 1957 and a major review published in the Journal of Chronic Disease (Breslow & Roberts 1955). Raffle and Gray (2007) identified Horace Debell, a London physician, who promoted comprehensive periodical examinations in the nineteenth century and exhorted people to prevent disease. He suggested that physicians should give advice on living conditions and other necessary measures and thus prevent the progression of disease. While the concept of routine comprehensive periodic medical examinations was adopted most avidly in the United States, the use of routine medical examinations was also developed by industry, in order to identify those who already had a disease and should not be employed, and by insurance companies, in order to identify those with excess risk (Raffle & Gray 2007).

One of the first comprehensive reviews of screening was published by Thorner and Remein (1961) of the United States Public Health Service; much of this is still relevant. Morris Collen (1988), Medical Director of the Kaiser Permanente Health Maintenance Organization in Oakland, California, was also a great advocate of regular screening and comprehensive medical examinations of adults for chronic disease. Collen believed that regular screening could reduce healthcare costs and utilization of medical care. Screening was introduced as a component of subscribing to the Kaiser Permanente HMO. Unfortunately, no clear benefits to subscribers could be demonstrated.

In the United Kingdom, there was initially much less enthusiasm for the concept of screening. Nonetheless, the concept and belief in the benefits of screening was soon apparent, largely because of the growth of cervical cytology screening for the early identification of the precursors of cancer of the cervix. This was greatly promoted by the women's movement in the early 1960s. The ease of performing these smears meant that these were very popular; only Ahluwahlia and Doll (1968) and Knox (1982) raised critical comments concerning questions of effectiveness. As a result, pathology services were required to devote increasing resources to cervical cytology and rapidly became overwhelmed and other pathology services suffered.

The Ministry of Health in England recognized the importance of the growth of demand for screening as a component of preventive medical services. Dr J.M.G. Wilson was despatched to the United States to review the situation, and he and Jungner, a Swedish biochemist, developed their view and published under the auspices of the WHO, a landmark publication (Wilson & Jungner 1968) that outlined some of the criteria under which a screening programme might be adopted.

In the past 40 years, professional attitudes towards screening have changed. At the start of the period, health professionals were enthusiastic of the promise that early diagnosis could provide in the improvement of prevention and reduction of morbidity from chronic diseases. This enthusiasm has become much more tempered with the appreciation that screening also has disadvantages and should only be applied for certain defined conditions and in carefully controlled circumstances (Holland & Stewart 1990, 2005b).

By contrast, and in spite of widely quoted mishaps, screening has become much more popular with the general public. In recent years, the population has become much more health conscious and, with the growth of the Internet, knowledgeable about health matters. This has increased the demand for health interventions. A firm belief has developed that the earlier a diagnosis is made, the better will be the outcome. The parallel of the annual test for roadworthiness of motor vehicles (MOT) is often quoted. This belief in the efficacy of screening is fuelled through the advocacy of charities concerned with individual diseases, such as prostate cancer; by private clinics and private providers who may have good intentions but can see a way to make money; and by some doctors and politicians, who are anxious to publicize their belief in the importance and value of prevention. Screening has become a commercial enterprise, not only in terms of the promotion of procedures but also in terms of the supply of reagents and equipment. It has become a process driven by financial incentives of services, the promotion of unproven tests and the presence of booths or mobile screening units in supermarkets. Governments are often willing to 'invest' in screening services, even at relatively high cost and with relatively small benefits, as for example in screening for breast cancer, in order to show that they care. Critics who advocate caution in particular instances have been undermined or attacked (Holland & Stewart 1990, 2005b).

The concept of screening

Definitions of screening

McKeown (1968) defined screening as 'medical investigation which does not arise from a patient's request for advice for a specific complaint'. This definition of screening may encompass: (i) research for the validation of a procedure; or (ii) tests done for the promotion of the public health, for example, to identify a source of infection in a food outbreak; or (iii) as a direct contribution to the health of the individual. It is this last, prescriptive screening, which is now the most common objective.

There have been a number of modifications of this definition since 1968. The UK National Screening Committee (2000) defined screening as 'a public health service in which members of a defined population, who do not necessarily perceive that they are at risk of, or already affected by, a disease or its complications are asked a question or offered a test to identify those individuals who are more likely to be helped than harmed by further tests or treatment to reduce the risk of disease or its complications'.

Clinical practitioners commonly use the term 'screening' when they systematically apply tests to their patients in order to detect evidence of elevated risks or early-stage complications as, for example, when diabetic patients are examined annually for signs of retinal disease or peripheral nerve damage. The term 'screening' is also used inappropriately when individuals are offered tests nonsystematically, as when they are tested for infectious diseases. However, these approaches are more correctly termed 'testing' (Gostin 2000) or 'opportunistic screening' or 'case finding'. The term 'screening' should only be used when populations, or groups of people who are thought to be at risk, are systematically offered screening tests as in national programmes for cancer of the breast and cervix.

Criteria for introducing a screening programme

The basic criteria to be fulfilled before the introduction of screening for a condition are fundamental to the screening process. The criteria proposed by Wilson and Jungner (1968) were widely accepted and quoted for many years and these provide the basis for a more elaborate set of the necessary criteria listed in the UK National Screening Committee's Second Report (2000) (Box 12.7.1). The condition sought should be an important health problem whose whole natural history should be understood. The condition must have a recognizable early or latent stage. The diagnosis should be made by a suitable acceptable test and there should be agreement as to whom to regard as a patient. There must be acceptable, effective treatment or intervention for individuals found to have the disease or pre-disease condition and facilities for this must be available. The cost of case finding (including diagnosis and treatment) should be economically balanced in relation to possible expenditure on medical care as a whole. As well as meeting the above criteria and principles there must be adequate, on-going evaluation and quality control.

Properties of screening tests

Screening tests must be applied to large numbers of healthy individuals most of whom will be identified as screen negative. This means that screening tests must be evaluated and judged in lowprevalence settings and not just in the high-prevalence settings, as in hospitals, where they are often developed. Cochrane and Holland (1971) listed some desirable characteristics of screening tests including the requirement that they should be acceptable to screened subjects, safe, rapidly and easily applied and not too costly.

A screening test is not a diagnostic test. Instead, screening tests separate individuals into groups who have either a low probability or a high probability of disease being present. This is commonly misunderstood by members of the public who assume that a positive

Box 12.7.1 UK National Screening Committee criteria for adopting a screening programme

Ideally, all the following criteria should be met before screening for a condition is initiated:

1. The condition should be an important health problem.

2. The epidemiology and natural history of the condition, including development from latent to declared disease, should be adequately understood, and there should be a detectable risk factor, disease marker, latent period, or early symptomatic stage.

3. All the cost-effective primary prevention interventions should have been implemented as far as practicable.

4. If the carriers of a mutation are identified as a result of screening, the natural history of people with this status should be understood, including the psychological implications.

5. There should be a simple, safe, precise, and validated screening test.

6. The distribution of test values in the target population should be known, and a suitable cut-off level defined and agreed.

7. The test should be acceptable to the population.

8. There should be an agreed policy on the further diagnostic investigation of individuals with a positive test result and on the choices available to those individuals.

9. If the test is for mutations, the criteria used to select the subset of mutations to be covered by screening, if all possible mutations are not being tested, should be clearly set out.

The treatment

10. There should be an effective treatment or intervention for patients identified through early detection, with evidence of early treatment leading to better outcomes than late treatment.

11. There should be agreed evidence based policies covering which individuals should be offered treatment and the appropriate treatment to be offered.

12. Clinical management of the condition and patient outcomes should be optimized in all healthcare providers prior to participation in a screening programme.

The screening programme

13. There should be evidence from high-quality randomized controlled trials that the screening programme is effective in reducing mortality or morbidity. Where screening is aimed solely at providing information to allow the person being screened to make an 'informed choice' (e.g. Down's syndrome, cystic fibrosis carrier screening), there must be evidence from high-quality trials that the test accurately measures risk. The information that is provided about the test and its outcome must be of value and readily understood by the individual being screened.

14. There should be evidence that the complete screening programme (test, diagnostic procedures, treatment/intervention) is clinically, socially, and ethically acceptable to health professionals and the public.

15. The benefit from the screening programme should outweigh the physical and psychological harm (caused by the test, diagnostic procedures, and treatment).

16. The opportunity cost of the screening programme (including testing, diagnosis and treatment, administration, training, and quality assurance) should be economically balanced in relation to expenditure on medical care as a whole (i.e. value for money).

17. There should be a plan for managing and monitoring the screening programme and an agreed set of quality assurance standards.

18. Adequate staffing and facilities for testing, diagnosis, treatment and programme management should be available prior to the commencement of the screening programme.

19. All other options for managing the condition should have been considered (e.g. improving treatment, providing other services), to ensure that no more cost effective intervention could be introduced or current interventions increased within the resources available.

20. Evidence-based information, explaining the consequences of testing, investigation, and treatment, should be made available to potential participants to assist them in making an informed choice.

21. Public pressure for widening the eligibility criteria for reducing the screening interval, and for increasing the sensitivity of the testing process, should be anticipated. Decisions about these parameters should be scientifically justifiable to the public.

22. If screening is for a mutation, the programme should be acceptable to people identified as carriers and to other family members.

Source: National Screening Committee (2000).

result is 'bad news' and a negative result is the 'all clear'. This can result in considerable anxiety for the individuals concerned if these perceptions are not addressed appropriately. A positive screening test result must usually be followed up by appropriate confirmatory tests to establish whether the screening result was a true positive, confirming the diagnosis and need for treatment, or more commonly that the result was a 'false positive' and the individual can be reassured.

The classification of individuals which results from a screening test result may be compared with true disease status obtained using a reference method or 'gold standard' (Fig. 12.7.1). Important characteristics to be assessed before any screening test can be considered for use in a screening programme include specificity and sensitivity. Specificity is defined as the proportion of disease-free subjects who are classified as true negatives by the test. Sensitivity is defined as the proportion of subjects with the condition of interest who are classified as true positives by the test. Ideally, both measures should be high. A common misperception among clinicians is that high sensitivity is more important than specificity, in other words, a case must not be 'missed'. In reality, all screening programmes will 'miss' some true positive cases and specificity is as, if not more, important for an effective and acceptable programme because a high rate of false positives can outweigh the benefits to the few true positives identified, with negative consequences for individuals who test false-positive. This is an important issue for programmes such as breast screening. It is generally more important if the prevalence of condition to be identified is low.

The positive predictive value of a test is the proportion of subjects with a positive test result who have the condition of interest. The positive predictive value is determined by the relative proportions of true positives and false positives and, with sensitivity and specificity remaining constant, the positive predictive value depends on the prevalence of the condition of interest. When the condition is common, true positives will be frequent but if the condition is rare, true positives will be infrequent. Conditions that are sought by screening programmes commonly have a prevalence lower than 1 per cent, consequently the positive predictive value of a screening test will be low unless both sensitivity and specificity are extremely high (Table 12.7.1). In practical terms, this means that false positive results may outnumber true positive results, and the impact of screening on those who do not have the condition of interest is an important concern.

As an example, a cut-point for mean cell haemoglobin (MCH) of 27 pg is used in the detection of beta thalassaemia. This has been shown to have a sensitivity of 100 per cent in a sample of 6314 results with 104 carriers from two London hospitals that serve a high-prevalence population (Wald and Leck 2000, p. 255). At this prevalence, the positive predictive value in this sample is approximately 77.4 per cent. In lower-prevalence areas, the predictive value of the same cut-point was estimated to range from 1.3 to 30 per cent (NHS Sickle Cell and Thalassaemia Screening Programme 2008). Using HbA2 estimation, in combination with the MCH result, to increase the specificity of the testing procedure, resulted in important reductions in the workload associated with follow-up of screen positives without compromising detection rate. In the detection of maternal alpha zero carriers, use of a MCH cut-point of 25 pg gives a predictive value, in a research setting with results validated against DNA analysis, of 1:424 with 100 per cent sensitivity. Use of the MCH cut-point in combination with a question about family origins to increase specificity gives an estimated predictive value of 1:3 [12/36] (Sorour et al. 2007). Applying this approach in practice reduces partner recall from 1:61 requiring follow up to 1:1497 requiring partner follow-up (a 96 per cent reduction in partner recall). These examples show how important the predictive value is as a measure of the impact of screening test on programme workload. These examples also demonstrate that when conditions are of low prevalence attending to the specificity of a test is extremely important if staff and public commitment to a programme are to be maintained.

When a screening test generates a quantitative measure, rather than a binary classification, the cut-point used to separate 'normal' from 'abnormal' may be varied. This is illustrated in Fig. 12.7.2 which presents data for prostate-specific antigen (PSA) in relation to later development of prostate cancer (Thompson et al. 2005). Sensitivity and specificity have been estimated and plotted for different PSA cut-points. A low cut-point will give a high sensitivity but low specificity, as the cut-point is increased the sensitivity decreases and the specificity increases. Thus, there is a reciprocal relationship between sensitivity and specificity. The area under the ROC curve is used as a summary measure of test performance. Note that, in this example, PSA test performance is better for detecting tumours that are Gleason grade 8 or higher, these are poorly differentiated tumours that are more likely to spread rapidly and be clinically and prognostically important. The authors of the study observed that lowering the PSA cut-point sufficiently to ensure detection of high-grade tumours would not only have the effect of increasing false positive diagnoses, but would also increase detection of tumours that might be of less clinical importance (Thompson et al. 2005).

In general, the performance of a screening procedure may be improved by modifications that increase both sensitivity and specificity. This can sometimes be achieved by combining several tests

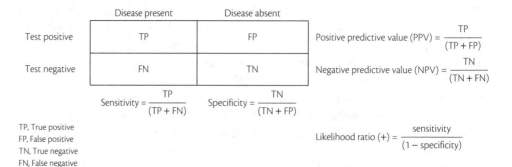

Fig. 12.7.1 Properties of a screening test.

Table 12.7.1 Positive predictive values (PPV) at different values for sensitivity and specificity and disease prevalence

Prevalence	PPV (%) if sensitivity = 75% and specificity = 75%	PPV (%) if sensitivity = 95% and specificity = 95%
10%	25.0	67.9
1%	2.94	16.1
0.1%	0.30	1.9
0.01%	0.03	0.2

together, as in the 'quadruple test' used in antenatal screening for Down syndrome. Wald *et al.* (2003) compared combinations of two, three, or four biochemical measures in the detection of Down's syndrome pregnancies. They reported that the 'double', 'triple', or 'quadruple' tests gave detection rates of 57, 62, and 70 per cent, respectively, while the odds of being affected given a positive result were 1:56, 1:52, and 1:45, respectively.

The likelihood ratio of a positive test provides another measure for analysing measure of test performance. The post-test odds of disease are given by the product of the likelihood ratio of a positive test and the pre-test odds of disease. The likelihood ratio provides a measure of the relative increase in frequency of the disease in subjects who test positive compared with the untested population. The likelihood ratio of a positive test is given by sensitivity divided by (1 − specificity) (Fig. 12.7.1).

Benefits and disadvantages

As noted earlier, screening may cause harm to individuals and populations (Raffle & Gray 2007). It is therefore essential to be aware

Table 12.7.2 Potential benefits and disadvantages of screening programmes

Benefits	Disadvantages
Improved prognosis for some cases detected	Longer morbidity for cases whose prognosis is not altered
Less radical treatment which cures some early treated cases	Over-treatment of questionable abnormalities
Resource savings	Resource costs
Reassurance for those with negative test results	False reassurance for those with false negative results
	Anxiety and sometimes morbidity for those with false positive results
	Hazards of screening test itself

Source: Chamberlain (1984).

of both the benefits and possible harms of screening (Table 12.7.2) (Chamberlain 1984). Some of the problems of screening are not easy to communicate to the public. If thousands of tests are done, 'errors' are bound to occur. All programmes must be subject to continuing quality control to minimize such 'errors'. Yet, even under optimal conditions, some individuals will be labelled as positive and yet not have the condition sought and others labelled as negative and yet have the condition sought. Thus, individuals will be wrongly labelled, stigmatized, and may become anxious, while others are falsely reassured. There is thus a great need to appreciate the ethics of screening. Cochrane and Holland (1971) emphasized that screening differs from other forms of healthcare in that it is the healthcare provider who offers a test with the implicit promise that undergoing this test may provide benefit, in contrast to the normal situation, where the individual seeks the help of the provider. It is thus essential that screening services are only introduced if the necessary principles and criteria are met. In countries other than the United Kingdom, including the United States and Canada, national and professional bodies have published the tests and conditions for which screening must be justified, often with appropriate reviews. There is a national body in the United Kingdom, the National Screening Committee, responsible for the review and ongoing assessment of those screening tests that meet the necessary criteria and the responsibility for their introduction and use in the NHS that provides a model approach to these issues.

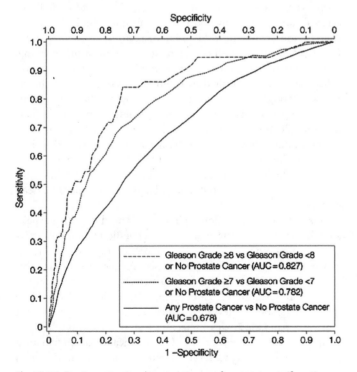

Fig. 12.7.2 Receiver-operating characteristic curve for prostate-specific antigen (PSA) and different grades of prostate cancer. AUC, area under curve.

Legend in figure:
- Gleason Grade ≥8 vs Gleason Grade <8 or No Prostate Cancer (AUC = 0.827)
- Gleason Grade ≥7 vs Gleason Grade <7 or No Prostate Cancer (AUC = 0.782)
- Any Prostate Cancer vs No Prostate Cancer (AUC = 0.678)

Ethics and screening

Lawrence Gostin (2000) observed that 'screening is far from a neutral scientific pursuit. Rather, screening is political . . . fraught with complex choices and weighing values—cost, efficiency, autonomy, and justice' (p. 201). This challenging perception shows that screening must be viewed within its social and ethical context. However, the ethical framework for screening can be considered at more than one level. The traditional biomedical ethical approach, which primarily considers the individual level, is arguably not the most relevant level at which to consider the ethics of screening. All relevant levels, including the level of the screening programme and the health system or society, must be considered to ensure that introduction of a screening programme is as consistent as possible, with a given society's values. This section of the chapter outlines some key ethical questions that must be negotiated if a screening programme is to be introduced.

At the *health system* or *societal* level, the implementation of screening raises questions concerning resource allocation and prioritization. Any screening programme is associated with an opportunity cost that represents the healthcare foregone through allocating resources to screening. The criteria used to justify screening programme implementation are generally oriented towards increasing efficiency, a utilitarian value of ensuring the greatest good for the greatest number given available resources. However, the valuation of different outcomes may present difficult problems. For example, in Down's syndrome screening, it may be feasible to estimate the cost per affected birth prevented but it is difficult, and in some societies unacceptable, to weigh this cost against the cost of treatment and care of affected individuals. This issue is discussed in more detail in a later section.

Allocation of resources to screening programmes also raises questions of equity because the proposed health benefits of screening may be differentially distributed to certain groups in the population. Some men's groups argue that since screening programmes are implemented to detect women's cancers, including breast and cervical cancer screening, fairness requires that screening programmes should also be implemented to detect cancers that affect men, including cancer of the prostate, even if considerations of efficiency do not support this. More generally, screening programmes may be differentially utilized by higher socio-economic groups, with lower-income groups and minorities showing lower uptake. Screening, thus, has the potential to increase inequalities in health while improving the overall health of the total population. Screening outcomes, and inequalities in outcomes, should be important measures for quality assurance of screening programmes.

At the level of the *screening programme*, the selection of population groups to be screened, the choice of screening procedures, the value attached to different screening outcomes and the nature of available treatment services might appear to be purely technical issues, but these processes also raise ethical questions. A screening programme may be either universal or targeted. If a targeted strategy is chosen, then there is a risk of stigmatizing the target population as being particularly associated with an undesirable health outcome, such as a sexually transmitted disease. If the target population is defined on grounds of age, as is done for breast cancer screening, then this raises questions concerning the 'right to health' of women who are either younger or older than the proposed age cut-points. While efficiency arguments may favour a more focused strategy, considerations of equity favour a more universal approach (Sassi *et al.* 2001).

As discussed earlier, screening tests often have low-positive predictive values and this means that there may be large numbers of subjects with false positive results and a smaller number of subjects with true positive results. Subjects with false positive results may be exposed to significant harm through the communication of anxiety producing information and through follow-up tests that may be risky and uncomfortable. Major benefits from screening are shared by a few true positives and these benefits must be balanced against potential harm to many false positives. As a minimum, this indicates an ethical requirement for adequate quality assurance to ensure the reliability and validity of testing procedures, the safety of diagnostic

services, and the adequacy of information communication to screened subjects.

The selection of screening outcomes also requires careful consideration. This is especially true for screening processes that may impact on reproductive outcomes. The possibility of making diagnoses before birth and giving parents informed choice over reproductive outcomes appear to be positive developments. However, these processes may be related to the concept of 'eugenics'. The term 'eugenics' literally means 'well-born'. It is a social philosophy which advocates the improvement of human hereditary traits through various forms of intervention (Osborn 1937; Wikipedia 2008). Although, the notion of eugenics was introduced with good intentions, the concept of eugenics now has negative connotations that mainly date from the Nazi period from 1933 to 1945. Contemporary developments in genetics have increased the potential for genetic screening, but there is now a 'guarded attitude towards eugenics, which had become a watchword to be feared rather than embraced' (Wikipedia 2008).

Finally, it is ethically unjustified to initiate screening unless adequate treatment services are available to provide treatment and care for subjects identified through the screening programme. The resources required for treatment services may seldom be provided through a screening programme, and those advocating the programme must also advocate for investment in appropriate treatment services.

At the level of the *individual subject*, ethical issues are raised concerning the autonomy of the individual. Most screening programmes are voluntary and should be offered to individuals, enabling them to make an informed choice whether to participate in screening or not. In reality, as Gostin (2000) describes, voluntary population screening programmes are offered as routine interventions with limited opportunities for individuals to opt-out of participation. Family practices in the United Kingdom are performance managed against a nationally agreed target for uptake of cervical cancer screening and this target implies limited recognition of the scope for individual discretion in participation. Consequently, there has been increasing interest in the meaning, measurement and value of 'informed choice'. Marteau and colleagues (2001) identified two components of informed choice, relevant good quality information and a choice reflecting the values of the person making the decision. These are present in their proposed definition of informed choice as one 'that is based on relevant knowledge, consistent with the decision-maker's values and behaviourally implemented' (p. 100). According to this definition, choices are uninformed if subjects either lack information or their attitudes are not reflected in their behaviour (Marteau *et al.* 2001).

What kind of information do individuals need in order to make an informed choice? The answer to this question varies for different screening programmes. In antenatal screening programmes in which screening may have consequences for reproductive choices and reproductive outcomes, it is particularly important that the potential implications of undergoing a screening test should be fully understood. In newborn-screening programmes, there is a move to expand the range of screening tests offered so as to include a range of different conditions. The significance of information provided by screening varies for different conditions, leading to a situation in which the concept of informed choice becomes difficult and impractical (Nijsingh 2007).

In the context of cancer screening, potential benefit of screening may be communicated in terms of the 'number needed to screen', which is the inverse of the absolute risk reduction (Welch 2001). Rembold (1998) estimated that the 'number needed to screen' to prevent one death from colon cancer was 1374 over 5 years and for mammography, to prevent one death from breast cancer was 2451 over 5 years for women aged 50–59 years. From the individual's perspective, these statistics are not encouraging, however, understanding the limitations of screening and the potential for harm from screening are equally, if not more, important (Welch 2001). More aggressive cancers are most likely to be missed by screening programmes; these cancers are often diagnosed by clinical services as 'interval' cancers between screening rounds. Screening tests are not diagnostic tests and typically have a low-positive predictive value. This means that a positive screening test may lead on to more invasive procedures that may be associated with negative consequences. Screening may identify abnormalities that might never have caused clinical disease, leading to unnecessary treatment. This is exemplified by prostate cancer screening because sub-clinical prostate cancer is a frequent finding in older men. Histopathological definitions of cancer are unreliable contributing to incorrect diagnoses and unnecessary treatment in some cases or under-treatment in others (Welch 2001).

The information required to inform an individual's choice to participate in screening is technically complex and wide-ranging. Consequently, there may be limited opportunities for truly informed choice in routine screening programmes. In democratic societies, it may be legitimate for the state to make decisions on the implementation of screening programmes through what the Nuffield Council on Bioethics (2007) terms the state's 'stewardship' role. It is through the stewardship role that states discharge their obligation to protect and fulfil their citizens' right to health. However, this should also include promoting citizens' capacity to make informed choices through better public education about screening. Helping individuals, who may have little understanding of the issues, to make decisions at difficult times in their lives should not be the sole or even main approach (Nijsingh 2007). It may be more helpful to increase people's awareness of relevant issues from before they plan families or are offered screening tests. More needs to be done to develop an educated public which can benefit from screening programmes, whose focus should not be limited to technical issues while broader social perspectives are neglected.

Organizing and delivering screening programmes

Challenges in implementing screening programmes

Introducing and sustaining screening programmes

The first step in implementing a screening programme should be a formal review of the evidence to evaluate whether this supports the introduction of screening or not (Box 12.7.1). This step is sometimes omitted and screening may be initiated by enthusiasts with testing diffusing into routine practice without formal evaluation. This is particularly likely to occur with tests that are not costly and have broad public support. As noted earlier, this was exemplified by the introduction of the 'pap smear' for cervical screening. Even when there is good evidence to support such a programme, converting existing variable local practices into a standard programme

across a region or country may be more difficult than introducing a new planned programme *de novo*.

The decision to introduce a programme must be viewed in the context of a particular time and place. This is illustrated by international differences in approach. For example, screening for toxoplasmosis in pregnancy is recommended in France but not in the United Kingdom. This difference may be attributed to the different prevalence and epidemiology of the condition in these two countries associated with different meat eating habits. A screening programme that is considered cost-effective in a high-income country may often be unaffordable in a middle- or low-income country.

Temporal variations in the need for screening are illustrated by the example of antenatal syphilis screening in the United Kingdom. Syphilis declined dramatically after World War II, following the introduction of antibiotics to treat the disease. By the 1990s, there were calls for the antenatal screening programme for syphilis to be stopped. However, a 1999 review argued against this because of recent outbreaks of the disease. On the basis of this review, the decision was made to continue screening and rates of syphilis have increased since that time, albeit mostly in men (Connor *et al.* 2000).

Clarifying aims and objectives of the programme

Clarifying the aims and objectives of the screening programme represents another important step. This is not merely a technical exercise but one that should involve professionals, users and the voluntary sector. A classic example of a well-meaning approach to introducing screening that miscarried was the US Sickle Cell Act of 1970. This was intended to help identify those with sickle cell disease and provide care for them. However, the programme was introduced without adequate public education or planning. As a result, carriers identified by the programme were stigmatized, sometimes being refused jobs or losing employment due to misunderstanding of the differences between the disease and carrier states. Ultimately, the public refused to be tested because of the negative impacts of testing (Anionwu 2001). An important lesson from this experience is that the public need to be well informed, educated and continuously engaged, if the implementation of screening programmes is to achieve the potential benefit and be well-accepted with sustained support.

Defining the scope of the programme

Defining the scope of a screening programme should be considered prior to more detailed planning because if this is not considered carefully and comprehensively, some aspects of required service development may be omitted, causing difficulties later. In the United Kingdom, the term 'screening programme' is defined as 'the whole system of activities needed to deliver high-quality screening. This encompasses identifying and informing those to be offered screening through to the treatment and follow-up of those found to have an abnormality, as well as support for those who develop disease despite screening' (National Screening Committee 2000). A key criterion for the introduction of a screening programme is that 'clinical management of the conditions and patient outcomes should be optimized by all healthcare providers prior to participation in a screening programme' (National Screening Committee 2000). For example, the introduction of a newborn hearing programme requires planning and development of a service of adequate capacity and quality in tertiary specialist centres if the programme is to be effective and achieve its goal of timely appropriate treatment of screen positive children. These aspirations have seldom been achieved by the time screening is introduced.

Planning implementation

Planning and implementing the programme should cover a range of aspects such as education and training and standardization of testing procedures. These processes require project planning skills and the overall co-ordination and sequencing of programme implementation is important. Clinical services may be overwhelmed if a screening programme were to suddenly start, placing significantly increased demands on their services. On the other hand, if services are set up and referrals do not occur relatively quickly, then there may be disillusionment and disinvestment. It may be optimal if services do experience some increase in demand early on to ensure that there is a recognition of the increased service need that will be forthcoming but without overwhelming them. Another area that requires sequencing and will take some time to implement is professional and public education. Professional education and training should be implemented before a screening programme undertakes public awareness campaigns in order to avoid difficulties for front-line professionals. The UK experience and approach to planning and implementation are discussed in detail by Raffle and Gray (2007).

Information systems

The importance of adequate information and information systems should not be neglected in the planning and budgeting for a screening programme. Information systems are needed to manage the process of screening. Information systems are also required to provide fail-safe systems and to monitor the outcomes of screening.

Information systems are an important part of ensuring that adequate fail-safe processes are in place to guarantee the benefits of the programme, follow-up those with positive screening tests and assure the safety and quality of the programme. A characteristic of an effectively delivered screening programme is that fail-safe systems operate independently of the individual practitioners who are responsible for patient care. These systems should ensure that all those eligible are offered screening, that those with inconclusive, missing or screen positive results are followed up and managed appropriately. Problems with these processes should be rapidly identified and addressed. In the cervical screening programme in the United Kingdom, a series of fail-safe actions are identified at the level of the call–recall system, the general practice, the cytology laboratory and the colposcopy clinic that follows up cases requiring further management (NHS Cancer Screening Programmes 2004). These fail-safe actions are intended to ensure that errors are minimized in calling women for screening, monitoring test uptake, repeating smears, referring women for colposcopy with the required degree of urgency and ensuring that necessary treatment is received. Screening programmes that do not operate such systems are unsafe and risk high-level failures of process with consequent disengagement of population support.

Data derived from information systems are also important in the quality assurance (QA) of programmes and in monitoring programmes' success against specified objectives and criteria in terms of population outcomes. Failures of process may be less visible in the early stages of the programme but may cause problems later on. In addition, without adequate information, it may be difficult to demonstrate the benefits of the programme and hence to maintain investment.

Quality assurance in screening programmes

Importance of quality assurance

Quality assurance and performance management should be an integral part of any organized screening programme. Screening offers the promise of benefiting individuals and populations by identifying health problems about which they are unaware, unlike the usual situation in which an individual presents for healthcare. Screening is also offered to, and taken up by, many individuals from large populations. Consequently, failures of systems or processes can cause harm to many individuals, and the promise of screening may not be fulfilled. The overall aim of quality assurance should be to ensure that a screening programme achieves the potential health benefits while minimizing associated risks and harms. The processes of quality assurance should include assessment of all relevant risks, particularly those that are most likely to have adverse effects on subjects who are screened.

The process of quality assurance

The term 'quality assurance' is used to refer to the process by which the quality of a screening programme, in all its key dimensions, can be evaluated and improved. Variations in quality should be identified and addressed, so as to correct problems or implement improvements. Quality assurance is not a passive process; therefore, it requires the potential to intervene so as to address any problem that may be identified. According to Donabedian (2003), a narrow definition of quality assurance requires the collection and interpretation of information, followed by making adjustments to the system. A wider definition includes processes of system design or redesign, linked to resource allocation so as to address problems, as well as including educational and motivational activities to modify the behaviour of health professionals. Quality assurance should be cyclical; moving from assessment of performance, to action, followed by review. Quality assurance has little meaning if it operates only as a monitoring and reporting cycle, in isolation from those able to make real changes and allocate resources to address problems. A well-developed quality management system should specify when and how any task is to be undertaken and by whom (Balmer et al. 2000). A named individual should be identified as responsible for the quality of each component of the screening process, with involvement of the whole organization to plan, deliver, and evaluate quality of services (Moullin 2002). Strong user involvement in the process is recommended. Service quality is dynamic and standards should be continually reviewed and tightened so that quality is maintained and progressively increased, particularly in response to rising expectations from patients. Communication is a key aspect of maintaining quality and good partnerships between service providers are required (Moullin 2002).

Dimensions of quality

The processes of quality assurance should address several dimensions of quality (Donabedian 2003). *Effectiveness* should be enhanced so as to optimize the benefits or health gains from screening. *Efficiency* is required to ensure that the maximal benefits are obtained from available resources. The *equity* of screening uptake and screening outcomes should be evaluated to ensure that screening is accessible to all eligible groups and benefits are fairly distributed. The *safety* of screening programmes is important to ensure that errors are avoided and harms are minimized. The *acceptability* of the screening programme to the public and service users should be ensured. Standards for any programme should encompass each relevant dimension of quality.

Measuring and monitoring quality: Developing criteria and standards

A first step for successfully measuring and monitoring the quality of a programme is determining what to monitor. Clarifying and agreeing the aims and objectives for a programme should be the first step, using the evidence that supports the introduction of the programme as a starting point. Following from this, key priorities for monitoring should be identified including structures, processes, and outcomes (National Screening Committee 2003).

Raffle and Gray (2007) recommend defining the objectives of a programme to encapsulate what a 'good' programme should look like. Box 12.7.2 gives an example from the sickle cell and thalassaemia screening programme in England. A similar approach has been used in the United Kingdom for other programmes including the breast screening and diabetic retinopathy programmes. Once objectives are defined, ways of measuring the achievements of these

---

Box 12.7.2 Example of screening programme aims and objectives. (NHS Sickle Cell and Thalassaemia Screening Programme, 2006)

NHS newborn sickle cell screening programme

Programme aims

◆ To achieve the lowest possible childhood death rate and to minimize childhood morbidity from sickle cell disorders

Overall outcome to be achieved at national level

◆ Mortality rate in children with sickle cell disorders under 5 years of less than 4 per 1000 person years of life (2 deaths per 100 affected infants) by 2010

◆ To accurately diagnose infants born with specific conditions where early intervention is likely to be beneficial

Programme objectives

◆ To offer screening for sickle cell disorders to all infants

◆ To process tests in a timely manner

◆ To identify and arrange timely follow-up of infants identified as needing further investigation

◆ To ensure effective and acceptable follow-up, care and support for affected infants and their carers

◆ To offer treatment and start parental education in a timely manner

◆ To minimize the adverse effects of screening—including failure to follow-up screen positive infants, inaccurate or inadequate information, unnecessary investigation and follow-up, inappropriate disclosure of information and failure to communicate results to parents (normal and carrier)

◆ To ensure that responsibility, accountability, and performance management for all aspects of the programme are clear and that these link together from local to national level and between the newborn and antenatal programme

---

objectives need to be identified. This requires the development of criteria and standards to measure achievement of each objective; criteria and standards are the tools by which quality of care is measured. A criterion is defined 'as an attribute of structure, process, or outcome that is used to draw an inference about quality' (Donabedian 2003, p. 60). A standard is defined as 'a specified quantitative measure of magnitude or frequency that specified what is good or less so' (Donabedian 2003, p. 60). Criteria, therefore, should cover the key dimensions of quality to be assured. Standards then specify exactly what is to be expected for each dimension.

Setting standards for a screening programme should follow from a baseline assessment of performance where possible. Standards are then set using informed judgement of the level of performance that should be achieved. Standards may include both minimum standards, to be achieved by all, and achievable standards that might be reached by the top quartile of programmes. Minimum standards indicate an acceptable level of service below which services should not fall. Achievable or developmental standards target attainment in an environment of increasing expectations. The process of setting standards is iterative and continuous, requiring regular review, particularly in the early years following the development and implementation of a programme. Once standards have been set, it is necessary to identify the interventions required to meet the standards, to monitor service delivery against standards and aim for continuous improvement of services. Standards should also be based on an understanding of patients' requirements and expectations. Moullin (2002) recommends that standards should be realistic and achievable within available resources; service users should contribute to the development process with user involvement, an indicator of quality; and standards must be measurable and capable of being monitored.

The measurement of outcomes for screening programmes can be a particular challenge but is important in evaluating the extent to which a programme has achieved its aims. Measurement of outcomes of a programme may be treated as an overall national- or state-wide evaluation of the programme and not part of the quality assurance process which mostly deals with structural and process measures which are more useful for assessing the operation of a programme at a local or unit level. Table 12.7.3 gives an example of the outcome standards set for the newborn screening programme for sickle cell disease in England (NHS Sickle Cell and Thalassaemia Screening Programme 2006).

Different types of programmes present different challenges

The challenges of screening are typically presented in relation to screening for cancer, but this is not the only type of screening programme. Four different types of programme are considered, including infections, genetic conditions, vascular screening, and cancers.

Infections

Examples of screening for infection include pre-conception syphilis screening as recommended in the United States; Hepatitis B, rubella susceptibility and HIV screening in pregnancy in the United Kingdom; or toxoplasmosis screening in pregnancy in France. The purpose of screening should be clarified as, depending on the purpose, different actions may be required. Screening for infection may identify susceptibility, as in the case of rubella screening that may indicate a need for immunization to prevent infection in a future pregnancy. Screening may identify past infection and

Table 12.7.3 Outcome measures for a newborn sickle cell screening programme in England

Outcome	Criteria	Minimum standard	Achievable standard
Best possible survival for affected infants detected by the programme	Mortality rates expressed in person years	Mortality rate in children under 5 of less than four per 1000 person-years of life (two deaths per 100 affected children)	Mortality rate in children under 5 of less than two per 1000 person years of life (one death per 100 affected children)
Accurate detection of all infants born with major clinically significant abnormalities	Sensitivity of the screening programme	99% for HbSS 98% for HbSC 95% for other variants	99.5% for HbSS 99% for HbSC 97% for other variants

Source: NHS Sickle Cell and Thalassaemia Screening Programme (2006).

sero-conversion, as in the case of hepatitis B and HIV, with potential benefits of intervention for the infant (Hepatitis B) or both mother and infant (HIV) (Department of Health 1998). In pregnancy, there may be benefits either for the mother and/or the baby. Without clarity as to the purpose of screening, the potential benefits of the programme may not be realized. For example, while surveillance of infections is important, screening for this reason can be offered at any stage in pregnancy. Most of the benefits to the infant will be gained if infections, such as syphilis, are identified before pregnancy, as is the policy in the United States, rather than later in pregnancy, when the infection may already have affected the infant. If test information is only to be used for surveillance purposes, this point may be lost and result in a programme that does not deliver optimal benefit.

Another challenge for such programmes is ensuring that information identified as relating to the mother can be transferred to the infant's record to ensure that it receives appropriate care. For example, infants of HIV-infected mothers should receive anti-viral drugs and the mother should be counselled not to breast-feed. In the United Kingdom, well-intentioned data protection legislation has made the transfer of such information very difficult, on occasion effectively preventing the benefits of the screening programme being achieved.

A specific problem for screening programmes for infections, such as HIV in pregnancy, is that the screen performed only relates to a specific point in time and any non-immune individual can subsequently become infected at any point after this screen. This also relates, for example, to screening of migrants for tuberculosis when subsequent poor living conditions may provide an environment for acquiring and developing an active infection. Screening may also fail to detect very recently infected individuals if the screening test is for sero-conversion rather than acute infection. Screening may, if inappropriately applied as in the case of a meningitis outbreak, identify asymptomatic carriers of a particular organism.

Genetic testing and screening

Developments in genetics have opened up many new possibilities for the diagnosis of a variety of diseases, but it is important to note that the same principles apply as in other forms of screening. If genetic tests are offered to any individual, either there must be an effective intervention available for individuals found to be affected, or the information provided by the result must help the individual or other family members to make better decisions than if the information was not available. There are a number of instances where

genetic testing and screening may be helpful. For example, a child known to have multiple endocrine neoplasia type 2 can be spared medullary carcinoma by undergoing prophylactic thyroidectomy or an adult with hereditary haemochromatosis can avoid cirrhosis by the early initiation of phlebotomy treatment. This section includes the application of genetic tests to individuals and populations, that is, testing and screening.

Uses of genetic tests

Genetic tests may be used in a variety of settings for a number of purposes, including diagnostic testing, to confirm or exclude a genetic disorder in an asymptomatic individual; and predictive testing in asymptomatic individuals who have a family history. This may be presymptomatic, when the gene mutation is present (e.g. Huntingdon's disease), or predispositional, when eventual development of symptoms is possible but not certain (e.g. cancer of the breast). It is important that adequate counselling services be available if predictive testing is used. Testing may be useful at different stages of the life course.

(a) Offering carrier testing or screening to allow identification of couples at risk. Tests can be offered at any time up to early pregnancy and in high-risk groups to enable individuals to make informed choices. Examples include testing for thalassaemia, Tay–Sachs, and sickle cell disease. For autosomal recessive conditions, if both partners are carriers, then there is a one-in-four risk in each pregnancy of an affected infant.

(b) Foetal testing in cases where there is thought to be an increased risk of an affected foetus. This is usually done by amniocentesis or chorionic villus sampling. These tests carry risks and may result in foetal loss. Non-invasive genetic tests of maternal blood are under development but not in routine practice at present (Free Foetal DNA testing).

(c) Pre-implantation genetic diagnosis in early embryos after *in vitro* fertilization to minimize the risk of genetic condition in couples at particular risk. This is the option of choice for some parents who have been identified pre-conception as being a couple at risk of a particular condition. This can be extended to the selection of 'saviour siblings' to allow for earlier bone marrow transplantation.

(d) Newborn screening to identify individuals as early a stage as possible in order to start treatment, where there is evidence of benefit or treatment available, e.g. cystic fibrosis, sickle cell disease.

Some of the tests employed are not strictly *genetic tests* but are biochemical tests used to identify genetic diseases.

(e) In a number of common conditions, preventive genetic testing may contribute to the identification of individuals at high risk; for example, BRCA1 and BRCA2 mutations, which can identify women at particular risk for developing breast cancer. However, positive findings are rare. For example, out of 10 000 women, 1000 will have a mother or a sister who has had breast cancer but only 15 will have a mutation that confers a high risk. Furthermore, it must be noted that it has been estimated that lifetime risk of breast cancer associated with a mutation ranges from 26 to 85 per cent. Testing for BRCA1 and BRCA2 do not meet the criteria for a screening programme.

Problems of genetic screening

Public expectations of genetic screening have been greatly magnified by the human genome project, but it is essential to appreciate the problems and difficulties of genetic screening. The Human Genome has several million single nucleotide polymorphisms, and thus, the 'number of possible genetic associations is limited only by the rate at which laboratories are able to type these polymorphisms' (Colhoun *et al.* 2003). These difficulties are often neglected and it must be realized that associations of a gene with a condition should be treated with the same degree of rigorous assessment as the findings of an environmental risk factor associated with a disease.

As with all screening tests, genetic screening may have psychological consequences, thus adequate counselling services must be provided. For common conditions, genetic screening is unlikely to be of great use in view of the complex interaction between environmental, behavioural, biological, and genetic factors. Its use is likely to be greatest in screening certain high-risk groups and populations for a few clearly defined conditions, e.g. to prevent thalassaemia in a high-risk population in Iran, where the costs of treatment for those affected are considered unaffordable to the society and in general, individuals wish to have the option of prenatal diagnosis and termination because of the economic consequences of having an affected child (Samavat & Modell 2004).

Particular problems arising with newborn screening programmes for both cystic fibrosis (to a lesser degree) and sickle cell disease (to a greater degree) are that the methods used by the programme which aims to detect those with disease but unavoidably also detects the carrier state. In the United Kingdom and the United States, this has resulted in a considerable debate as to the merits of revealing carrier status to parents of infants at a stage in life before a child can make such a decision. In both the United States and United Kingdom, the view that has prevailed is that 'carriers should be reported to parents and follow-up counselling is offered to ensure understanding of the difference between carrier state and disease and also the genetic significance of the carrier state' (Human Genetics Commission 2006; Lin & Barton 2007). The UK Human Genetics Commission (2006) emphasizes that such decisions must at their core reflect societal views and not the views of technical experts.

A second common problem, particularly relevant to newborn screening and carrier testing to identify couples at risk, relates to the potential of such programmes to identify non-paternity if counselling and information sharing is not handled sensitively. This emphasizes the importance of public education and awareness about such programmes.

Vascular screening programmes

Vascular programmes include risk assessments for cardiovascular disease, diabetic retinopathy screening and aortic aneurysm screening. Questions have been raised concerning whether some of these procedures should be identified as screening programmes. Cardiovascular risk assessment, it has been argued, is not a screening programme as all people in a given population are at risk of cardiovascular disease and screening cannot sort individuals into two groups. Diabetic retinopathy screening is not always considered to be a true screening programme as it calls a clinically identified population with diabetes. In other respects, this programme does operate as a population screening programme. Aortic aneurysm screening, followed by surgery for those at risk can result in mortality of screen identified cases through operative mortality. This raises ethical questions about the suitability of a programme that may lead directly to mortality. Overall, however, the life years saved by successful intervention outweigh the risks and, on this basis, the UK National Screening Committee has recommended a national programme which is currently being introduced.

Cancer screening

Cancer screening programmes represent the model in which much screening theory has been developed and which are most familiar to the public. Cancer screening is particularly relevant in high-income countries where cancer contributes most to total mortality. Mature breast and cervical programmes are in place in many European countries and North America. A particular problem with cancer programmes has been the difficulty in demonstrating the impact of screening because of the multiple influences on outcomes. In the case of breast cancer screening, there are changes in disease incidence associated with utilization of hormone replacement therapy as well as changes in case management that may be associated with improving prognosis.

Specific problems for cancer screening are 'length time' and 'lead time' biases. Length time bias refers to the fact that screening is most effective at detecting slow developing cancers which are less likely to be the cause of an individual's death but by detection can cause considerable anxiety. More aggressive tumours are likely to develop rapidly in the intervals between screening rounds. Lead time bias refers to the problem for evaluation of programmes that screening programmes detect cancers earlier than would have been the case with symptomatic screening and may thus appear to lengthen the time from diagnosis to survival when there is no true change in natural course or treatment may even shorten life expectancy.

Screening at different stages of life

This section provides a brief summary of debates concerning screening at different stages of life. Current recommendations from the United Kingdom are used for illustration.

Antenatal and newborn screening

One of the most comprehensive reviews on appropriate procedures in the antenatal and neonatal period is published by Wald

Table 12.7.4 Recommendations for antenatal screening tests to be offered routinely

Recommended	NOT recommended
Maternal anaemia	Bacterial vaginosis
Bacteriuria in pregnancy	Chlamydia
Blood group and RhD status	Cytomegalovirus
Down syndrome	Cystic fibrosis
Foetal anomalies (ultrasound)	Diabetes in pregnancy
Thalassaemia and sickle cell disease	Domestic violence
Haemolytic disease of newborn	Foetomaternal alloimmune thrombocytopaenia
Hepatitis B	Fragile X syndrome
HIV	Hepatitis C
Neural tube defects	Genital herpes
Pre-eclampsia	HTLV1
Placenta praevia	Streptococcus B
Psychiatric illness	Thrombophilia
Rubella immunity	Toxoplasmosis
Syphilis	Postnatal depression
Tay–Sachs disease	

Source: Holland and Stewart (2005).

and Leck (2000). It is at this period of life that screening has been shown to be of particular importance and has been used longest. Even so, there are still questions about certain tests and much still needs to be developed. The accepted recommendations in the United Kingdom are shown in Table 12.7.4. If one examines the recommendations of Wald and Leck (2000), differences of opinion can be seen.

It is important to realize that termination of pregnancy is the only effective intervention for some of the conditions listed in Table 12.7.4. This has implications on the need to provide a clear ethical framework for service availability and delivery and informed decision-making before any tests are done. It also means that timing of offer of tests is important and relevant to informed decision-making. Advice on these issues is often omitted or is of poor quality, and testing may be too late to allow informed decision making (Dormandy 2008).

Foetal ultrasound scanning has greatly increased in popularity and utilization. This test is not as uncomplicated as some obstetricians and mothers might imagine. It requires careful application at defined periods of gestation and skilled interpretation. The arguments about its utility are analysed by Holland and Stewart (2005).

The need to continuously review and appraise antenatal screening procedures is well illustrated by the case of Down syndrome. The diagnosis of this condition has been greatly improved by the use of combined serum tests and ultrasound so that the likelihood of detection is now of the order of 80 per cent (Wald & Leck 2000). Nonetheless, the only treatment is termination of the pregnancy and the necessary diagnostic amniocentesis or chorionic villus sampling carries a risk of foetal damage. Thus, the requirement of informed parental consent is paramount. The timing of testing is important. The quadruple test is offered in the second trimester, but first trimester screening with ultrasound and biochemical markers provides relevant information at an earlier stage of pregnancy, is therefore more acceptable to women, and is now recommended in the United Kingdom.

A further ethical concern has also arisen over time. Whereas 20–30 years ago the prognosis for Down syndrome children was very poor—few lived beyond puberty and almost all were not educable—now many such children live to early middle age, are able to participate in education and are able to pursue a simple occupation and become self-sufficient—hence the need for very careful balanced advice in every case before tests are done.

Newborn screening

Screening of newborn infants consists of routine biochemical tests on an infant's blood spot and physical examination including testing for hearing impairment (Table 12.7.5). Bloodspot screening should be done in the first week of life. In the United Kingdom, current recommendations are for testing for phenylketonuria, congenital hypothyroidism, cystic fibrosis, sickle cell disease and, Medium Chain Acyl-CoA Dehydrogenase deficiency (UK Newborn Screening Programme Centre 2005). Physical examination and testing for hearing loss are performed in the first year of life. It is important that methods of routine physical examination are properly standardized, that individuals performing them are trained in these methods and that the programme is kept under continuous review.

Table 12.7.5 Recommendations for newborn screening tests to be offered routinely in the United Kingdom

Condition	Comment
Blood spot for	
Phenylketonuria	
Congenital hypothyroidism	
Cystic fibrosis	
Sickle-cell disease	
Medium chain acyl-CoA dehydrogenase deficiency (MCADD)	In process of introduction for all newborns
Physical examination	
Congenital heart disease	Training programme in physical examination being developed
Congenital cataract	
Cryptorchidism	
Congenital dislocation/dysplasia of the hip	
Other tests	
Hearing impairment	Automated otoacoustic emission (AOAE) test used as first-line screening method in England
Under review	
Additional biochemical screening on the newborn blood spot for fatty acid disorder and amino acid metabolism defects introduced in the United States but currently not recommended in the United Kingdom	

Source: Adapted from Holland and Stewart (2005).

Examination is for signs of congenital heart disease, congenital cataract, cryptorchidism, congenital dislocation or developmental dysplasia of the hip, as well as other congenital malformations. Screening for congenital dislocation of the hip has been the subject of much controversy, but evidence of the effectiveness of ultrasound as a screening method is now accumulating. A national screening programme for hearing impairment has been implemented in the United Kingdom.

Screening in childhood

Screening in childhood is important, both to follow up findings from the neonatal period and to identify remediable defects or problems. A large number of bodies recommend a variety of procedures at different stages. Screening for hearing and visual impairment and congenital displacement of the hip is straightforward, but there is also a need to identify children from deprived and disadvantaged households in order to identify those children who are at particular risk to develop both physical and behavioural impairments—a matter often neglected.

Screening in adolescence

The major need at this stage of life is to build on the findings of the schoolchild examinations and to provide confidential accessible health services to aid the adolescent to confront and deal with such problems as fertility and sex, drugs and alcohol use. All opportunities should be taken to educate the adolescent in methods of healthy living, personal safety, nutrition, exercise, etc. The only opportunistic screening procedure that may be recommended is for chlamydia, a common, curable sexually transmitted disease which is often asymptomatic but can lead to life threatening ectopic pregnancy, pelvic inflammatory disease and infertility. However, evidence about the effectiveness of screening or the best way to deliver this service is limited.

Screening in adults

As we have already stated, screening in adults is big business. Media interest in health is insatiable and politicians have capitalized on public expectations and attitudes in the belief that 'prevention is better than cure'. This has been the mantra of many advocates, who carefully abstain from reminding people that death cannot be avoided. It is therefore essential to consider what screening procedures actually can do in all cases and to appreciate that there are also disadvantages in all the cases. In the United Kingdom, there is a National Screening Committee charged with the task of continuously reappraising the evidence and research to identify those procedures that meet the criteria we have enunciated and to monitor the application of these approved tests. In this chapter, most attention is given to those tests that meet the criteria and principles enunciated. It is essential to realize that these are not 'set in stone' but are subject to continuous research and evaluation. Recommendations are also context-dependent. It is also emphasized that all procedures must be subject to quality control, audit, and evaluation.

Cancer

As the second largest cause of mortality in the high-income countries, it is obviously a candidate for screening. Screening for cervical cancer was one of the main driving forces for the introduction of screening in healthcare. It is thus not surprising that cancer screening has been the subject of a great deal of attention.

Breast cancer

The major trials of breast cancer screening have been done in the United States (Shapiro et al. 1982) and Sweden (Taban et al. 1985, 1989). Other trials have been done in the United Kingdom, which before introducing a national scheme of breast cancer screening, had a major public enquiry (Forrest 1987). Screening for breast cancer is a highly emotive subject which has been the subject of very critical analysis (Gøtzsche & Olsen 2000). Under experimental conditions, as in the two original studies (Shapiro et al. 1982; Taban et al. 1985), there is a reduction in breast cancer mortality following mammographic screening. The reduction of total mortality in the test group is not so marked. The benefits in practice are smaller than in the experimental studies. There are arguments about which age range of women should be included in the scheme, the methods of mammography, the interval between repeat screening and the interpretation of mammograms. There is no doubt that for the scheme to be effective, there needs to be a good organization, careful quality control of both mammography and the subsequent breast biopsy as well as good expert-specialized treatment services including surgery, radiotherapy, and chemotherapy. The scheme, if properly executed, is costly, and critics suggest that the resources could be better used on clinical breast cancer treatment services. The major problems with the services are poor information to participants, increased anxiety in those screened, particularly the false positives, side effects from the biopsy and the risks of radiation exposure. Details of the pros and cons are summarized by Holland and Stewart (2005), who follow the UK National Screening Committee guidelines and accept screening 50–70-year-old women every 3 years as worthwhile. In view of the popularity of breast cancer screening, it would be a daring policy-maker who would suggest that the scheme should cease.

Cervical cancer

A programme of screening was first proposed in the mid-1960s. The original scheme was wasteful, including any woman attending any gynaecological service or family planning. In the United Kingdom, since 1998, the service has been re-launched on the basis of a call–recall system based on the GP patient register. Women are first invited at the age of 25 years and then recalled every 3 years until age 50 when the interval is increased to 5 years. About 80 per cent of the eligible women are screened, comparable to breast cancer screening coverage. Although mortality from cervical cancer has fallen considerably, it is worthwhile appreciating that an enormous effort is required. Raffle (2004), in an analysis of screening records of 348 419 women in Bristol, calculated that 1000 women need to be screened for 35 years to prevent one death, over 80 per cent of women with high-grade cervical intra-epithelial neoplasia will not develop invasive cancer, but all will need to be treated, and for each death that is prevented, over 150 women have an abnormal result, over 80 women are referred for investigation, and over 50 women receive treatment.

The method of cytological examination used is also subject to development. Straightforward cytological examination has been superseded by liquid-based cytological examination and now by human papilloma virus (HPV) culture. This is, of course, in order to automate the procedure. Cervical cancer prevention through screening may be superseded by the use of an HPV vaccine which is now being introduced for girls aged 13 years.

Colorectal cancer

A number of studies have shown that early detection by screening can reduce mortality (Hardcastle *et al.* 1996; Kronborg *et al.* 1996). As a result, screening for individuals aged more than 50 years is gradually being introduced in the United Kingdom (UK Colorectal Cancer Screening Pilot Group 2004). Individuals are mailed a filter paper which tests for faecal occult blood (FOBT). These filter papers are then returned to the centre. If the screening test is positive, then a colonoscopy and/or double contrast barium enema are done. The alternative advocated by some is flexible sigmoidoscopy. Followed if necessary by colonoscopy and/or double contrast barium enema. It is suggested that the screening tests are done at a five yearly intervals. Some authorities advocate screening by colonoscopy, however, it is important to note that this is found to be a very unpleasant procedure by many and carries a risk of bowel perforation of 0.5–5 per cent. It is important that the necessary surgical facilities and pathological and radiological facilities are available for those positives identified.

Prostate cancer

Although a biochemical screening test—prostate specific antigen (PSA) and digital rectal examination and transrectal ultrasound are available, confirmation by biopsy is essential.

Prostate cancer is one of the commonest cancers in men, particularly, the elderly. It has therefore become a 'cause celebre' in screening arguments. Many groups, particularly prostate charities, male advocacy groups and commerce are strong advocates. It has been the subject of intense argument and review. Although it is a very common cancer, many more men die with the cancer than of it (Martin 2007). Many studies have not shown any evidence that mortality is reduced or postponed if screening is undertaken in asymptomatic individuals. In our view, with present knowledge, there is no case for screening well individuals but those with prostate symptoms of frequency nocturia, inadequate voiding, etc. should be investigated.

Other cancers

Lung cancer is the commonest cancer in the United Kingdom. Unfortunately symptoms develop late. Trials of sputum cytology and chest x-ray have not shown any benefit with mortality of those screened compared with controls not improved. Diagnosis is too late. Major trials of spiral-computed tomography are ongoing and offer possible hope of an effective screening tool but the results are not yet available. Far more effective is to persuade smokers to give up smoking.

Ovarian cancer screening is the subject of at least three large randomized trials. Results are awaited before any recommendations can be given. Skin cancer and melanoma are a significant cause of morbidity. Theoretically, they seem a suitable condition for screening. However, no empirical evidence has yet been provided to suggest that benefits outweigh disadvantages. Protection from the sun and by suitable health education is preferable.

Coronary heart disease, stroke, and abdominal aortic aneurysm

Cardiovascular and related diseases are now the commonest causes of death in most developed Western countries and are rapidly catching up with infectious diseases as the main cause of death in developing countries. Since diabetes and cardiovascular diseases are closely related, it is worthwhile to consider them together.

The most effective preventive strategy for these conditions is not to smoke, improve the diet by reducing and maintaining cholesterol level of less than 4 mmol/l, increase the amount of physical exercise and reduce levels of blood pressure to 76-mm Hg diastolic or below. To achieve these goals, the most important changes that need to be made are to behaviour and attitude. As the important risk factor, exposures are so common in the general population, whole population screening programmes are unlikely to be an effective use of resources. Since, in all countries, most of the population has contact with the health services at least annually, it is essential that this contact should be used to reduce these risk factors. Populations with organized primary care systems can develop patient registers on which risk factor details should be noted. Any individual consulting should be advised and helped to stop smoking, have blood pressure measured and if necessary antihypertensive treatment instituted, have cholesterol and weight measured and if necessary given advice re-diet and anti-cholesterol drug treatment (statin) instituted. In addition, of course, appropriate public health measures should be taken to aid people in their decision to stop smoking; for example, by reducing cigarette advertising; banning smoking in public places; improving the provision and reducing the cost of healthy food particularly in deprived areas; providing and encouraging the use of public open spaces, cycling and running tracks, etc.; and labelling food so that people can make better informed choices.

Recent controlled trials and a systematic review have demonstrated the effectiveness of ultrasound screening of men aged 65–74 years for abdominal aortic aneurysm, linked with appropriate vascular surgical services (Cosford & Leng 2007). It is, however, important to note that the risk from surgery is high, and renal disease can result in a minority of cases.

Type 2 diabetes and diabetic retinopathy

Type 2 diabetes is not uncommon. There are divided views about the usefulness of screening for this condition. Wareham and Griffin (2001) do not advocate universal screening. This has also been the view of the National Screening Committee in the United Kingdom. We do not consider that population screening is worthwhile, but as stated above, those considered to be at risk should be tested, and treated if necessary. Spijkeman and colleagues (2002) used a simple validated questionnaire—the Cambridge risk score shows that these individuals are at high risk of mortality and suggests that direct public health interventions may be helpful.

Diabetic eye disease is the most common cause of preventable visual loss in the UK working population. Different methods of screening for diabetic retinopathy are available and have been evaluated by Squirrel and Talbot (2003). These use retinal photography and screening by optometrists. They are certainly worthwhile, but must be subject to stringent quality control and audit. They are quite difficult to establish satisfactorily although a successful programme has been implemented in the United Kingdom.

Mental illness

Depression is the third commonest reason for consultation in UK general practice. A variety of questionnaires have been proposed for screening for this condition. Unfortunately, none of them have met the criteria for an effective instrument. Arrol *et al.* (2003) in New Zealand found two questions: 'During the past month, have you often been bothered by feeling down depressed or hopeless?' and 'During the past month, have you often been bothered by little interest or pleasure in doing things?' detected most cases of depression.

There is a case for opportunistic screening for depression using such a simple questionnaire in general practice. There do not appear to be appropriate indications for screening for other mental conditions or personality disorders or alcohol misuse or domestic violence.

Occupational health

In view of the changes in the distribution of manufacturing and industry, there is now much less concern with the hazards of coal mining and steel production in high-income countries. Thus, in Western countries, most work-site screening is concerned with emphasis on lifestyles, etc., rather than pneumoconiosis or 'bent knees'. This continues to be of importance in areas where heavy industry is common. Thus, in work-site screening, the main concerns are to:

◆ Assess fitness for the task pre-employment or pre-placement for a specific task, e.g. food handler crane operators.

◆ Assess fitness during routine exposure to hazards, e.g. specific chemical, noise, radiation, vibration, etc.

◆ Assess general health risks from history or lifestyle, e.g. smoking, entry to a pension plan.

◆ Assess capability, e.g. taking drugs.

◆ Genetic screening—this is still in development and raises major ethical concerns but may be useful to 'screen out' individuals at particular risk for a specific hazard, e.g. chemical exposure.

Screening in the elderly

This is an important issue in view of the increasing proportion of elderly in many societies. There is little scientific evidence of the benefits of screening in this age group largely because of a lack of clear objectives.

In a randomized controlled trial over a period of 3 years in Denmark, Hendricksen et al. (1984 and 1989) showed reduced mortality resulting from a programme of home visits and three monthly intervals that led to an improvement in the provision of home helps, equipment, and modifications to the home. Although this incurred costs, they reckoned to have saved about twice as much because of the reduction in hospital nursing home care.

Since most elderly persons have most contact with primary care services than any other age group, these contacts should be used for opportunistic case finding. Obviously, search should be made for potentially treatable condition including hypertension, hearing loss, and visual impairment. It is also worthwhile considering symptomatic conditions such as bacteriuria and incontinence. In addition, a common condition which causes distress are foot problems. Behavioural concerns such as inappropriate medication, lack of physical exercise, depression, dementia, alcohol problems, and social isolation should be considered. Home visits to those aged over 75 years may make one aware not only of inappropriate housing, hazards in the home which may cause falls, but also social isolation under-nutrition and elder abuse. Thus, screening in this age group is concerned with case finding and improvement in quality of life.

Conclusion

The concept of screening for disease offers the possibility of bringing the benefits of health interventions to apparently healthy subjects, free from known disease. This chapter has discussed some of the difficulties associated with this approach. These problems must be analysed from several different disciplinary perspectives. The epidemiological approach is required to analyse problems of screening test performance, as well as questions of the effectiveness of intervention through screening. Applying screening techniques raises important ethical questions concerning the relationships between individuals, screening programmes, and the wider society. These reflect uncertainty and disagreement as to how the benefits and harms from intervening through screening should be valued and distributed. Developing a screening programme represents a complex technical challenge and sound planning and project management strategies should be employed for implementation. Ongoing screening programmes should be continuously improved through application of quality assurance and the implementation of systems to minimize errors and harm. Application of these principles to different screening programmes in the main areas of infections, genetic conditions, vascular disease, and cancer, and at different stages of life, requires detailed knowledge, and the reader is referred to specialist texts for further information.

Further reading

Holland, W.W. and Stewart, S. (1990). *Screening in healthcare*. The Nuffield Provincial Hospitals Trust, London.

Holland, W.W. and Stewart, S. (2005a). *Screening in Europe*. Copenhagen, European Observatory on Health Systems and Policy. World Health Organization.

Holland, W.W. and Stewart, S. (2005b). *Screening in disease prevention. What works?* Radcliffe Publishing, Oxford.

Raffle, A.E. and Muir Gray, J.A. (2007). *Screening: evidence and practice*. Oxford University Press, Oxford.

Wald, N. and Leck, I. (eds.) (2000). *Antenatal and neonatal screening (2e)*. Oxford University Press, Oxford.

References

Ahluwahlia, H.S. and Doll, R. (1968). Mortality from cancer of the cervix uteri in British Columbia and other parts of Canada. *British Journal of Preventive and Social Medicine*, **22**, 161–4.

Anionwu, E. (2001). *The politics of sickle cell and thalassaemia*. Open University Press, Milton Keynes.

Arrol, B., Khin, N., and Kerse, N. (2003). Screening for depression in primary care with two verbally asked questions. Cross sectional study. *British Medical Journal*, **327**, 1144–6.

Balmer, S., Bowens, A., Bruce, E., Farrar, H., Jenkins, C., and Williams, R. (2000). *Quality management for screening*. University of Leeds, Leeds. Available at http://www.leeds.ac.uk/hsphr/ nuffield_publications/ documents/screening.pdf. Accessed at http://www.nsc.nhs.uk/uk_nsc/ uk_nsc_ind.htm.

Breslow, L. and Roberts, D.W. (eds.) (1955). Screening for asymptomatic disease. *Journal of Chronic Disease*, **2**, 363–490.

Chamberlain, J.M. (1984). Which prescriptive screening programmes are worthwhile? *Journal of Epidemiology and Community Health*, **38**, 270–7.

Cochrane, A.L. and Holland, W.W. (1971). Validation of screening procedures. *British Medical Bulletin*, **27**, 3–8.

Colhoun, H.M., McKeigue, P.M., and Davey Smith, G. (2003). Problems of reporting genetic associations with complex outcomes. *The Lancet*, **361**, 865–72.

Collen, M.F. (1988). *History of the Kaiser Permanente Medical Care Programme*. An interview conducted with Sally Smith Hughes. Regional Oral History Office. Bancroft Library. University of California, Berkeley.

Connor, N., Roberts, J., and Nicoll, A. (2000). Strategic options for antenatal screening for syphilis in the United Kingdom: a cost effectiveness analysis. *Journal of Medical Screening*, **7**, 7–13.

Cosford, P.A. and Leng, G.C. (2007). Screening for abdominal aortic aneurysm. *Cochrane Database of Systematic Reviews* (2):CD002945.

Department of Health (1998). *Screening of pregnant women for hepatitis B and immunisation of babies at risk (Health Service Circular: HSC 1998/127)*. Department of Health, London.

Donabedian, A. (2003). *An introduction to quality assurance in healthcare*. Oxford University Press, Oxford.

Dormandy, E., Gulliford, M.C., Reid, E.P. *et al.* (2008) Delay between pregnancy confirmation and sickle cell and thalassaemia screening: a population-based cohort study, *British Journal of General Practice*, **58**, 154–9.

Forrest Report. (1987). *Breast cancer screening. Report to the Health Ministries of England Wales Scotland and Northern Ireland by a working group chaired by Sir Patrick Forrest*. HMSO, London.

Gostin, L.O. (2000). *Public health law. Power, duty, restraint*. University of California Press, Berkeley and Los Angeles.

Gøtzsche, P.C. and Olsen, O. (2000). Is screening for breast cancer with mammography justifiable? *The Lancet*, **355**, 129–34.

Hardcastle, J.D., Chamberlain, J.O., Robinson, M.H., Moss, S.M., Amar, S.S., Balfour, T.W., James, P.D., and Mangham, C.M. (1996). Randomised controlled trial of faecal-occult-blood screening for colorectal cancer. *The Lancet*, **348**, 1472–7.

Hendriksen, C., Lund, E., and Tromgaard, E. (1984). Consequences of assessment and intervention among elderly people a three year randomised controlled trial. *British Medical Journal*, **289**, 1522–4.

Hendricksen, C., Lund, E., and Stromgaard, E. (1989). Hospitalisation of elderly people a three year controlled trial. *Journal American Geriatric Society*, **37**, 119–22.

Human Genetics Commission (2006). *Making babies: reproductive decisions and genetic technologies*. Human Genetics Commission, London. Available at http://www.hgc.gov.uk/UploadDocs/DocPub/Document/Making%20Babies%20Report%20-%20final%20pdf.pdf accessed 13 April 2008.

Knox, E.G. (1982). *Cancer of the uterine cervix*. In Trends in cancer incidence (ed. J. Magnus). Hemisphere, Washington.

Kronborg, O., Fenger, C., Olsen, J., Jørgensen, O.D., and Søndergaard, O. (1996). Randomised study of screening for colorectal cancer with faecal-occult-blood-test. *The Lancet*, **348**, 1467–71.

Lin, K. and Barton, M. (2007). Screening for haemoglobinopathies in newborns. Reaffirmation update for the US Preventive Services Taskforce. Evidence synthesis No. 52. Agency for Health Care Quality, Rockville. AHRQ Publication Number 07-05104-EF-1. Available at http://www.ahrq.gov/cliic/serfiles.htm#sicklecell accessed 13 April 2008.

Marteau, T.M., Dormandy, E., and Michie, S. (2001). A measure of informed choice. *Health Expectations*, **4**, 99–108.

Martin, R.M. (2007). Commentary: prostate cancer is omnipresent, but should we screen for it? *International Journal of Epidemiology*, **36**, 278–81.

McKeown, T. (ed.) (1968). *Screening in medical care: reviewing the evidence*. Oxford University Press for Nuffield Provincials Hospital Trust, Oxford.

Moullin, M. (2002). *Delivering excellence in health and social care*. Open University Press, Buckingham.

National Health Service Cancer Screening Programme (2004). *Guidelines on failsafe actions for the follow-up of cervical cytology reports*. NHS Cancer Screening Programmes, Sheffield.

National Health Service Sickle Cell and Thalassaemia Screening Programme (2006). *Standards for the linked antenatal and newborn screening programmes*. NHS Sickle Cell and Thalassaemia Screening Programme, London. Available at http://www.sickleandthal.org.uk/Documents/ProgrammeSTAN.pdf accessed 13 April 2008.

National Screening Committee (2000). Second Report of the National Screening Committee. Department of Health, London. Available at http://www.nsc.nhs.uk/pdfs/secondreport.pdf accessed 13 April 2008.

National Screening Committee (2003). *New world symphony – screening and quality management in the reorganised NHS in England*. Available at www.nsc.nhs.uk accessed 13 April 2008.

Nijsingh, N. (2007). Informed consent and the expansion of newborn screening. In *Ethics, prevention and public health* (eds. A. Dawson and M. Verweij). Oxford University Press, Oxford.

Nuffield Council on Bioethics (2007). *Public health: ethical issues*. Nuffield Council on Bioethics, London.

Osborn, F. (1937). Development of a Eugenic Philosophy. *American Sociological Review*, **2**, 389–97.

Raffle, A. (2004). Cervical screening. *British Medical Journal*, **328**, 1272–3.

Rembold, C.M. (1998). Number needed to screen: development of a statistic for disease screening. *BMJ*, **317**, 307–12.

Samavat, A. and Modell, B. (2004). Iranian national thalassaemia screening program. *British Medical Journal*, **329**, 1134–7.

Sassi, F., Le Grand, J., and Archard, L. (2001). Equity versus efficiency: a dilemma for the NHS. *British Medical Journal*, **323**, 762–3.

Shapiro, S., Venet, W., Strox, P. *et al.* (1982). Ten to fourteen year effect of screening on breast cancer mortality. *Journal of the National Cancer Institute*, **69**, 349–55.

Sorour, Y., Heppinstall, S., Porter, N., Wilson, G.A., Goodeve, A.C., Rees, D. and Wright, J. (2007). Is routine molecular screening for common a-thalassaemia deletions necessary as part of antenatal screening programme? *Journal of Medical Screening*, **14**, 60–1.

Spijkeman, A., Griffin, S., Dibben, J., Nijpels, G., and Wareham, N.J. (2002). What is the risk of mortality for people who are screen positive in a diabetes screening programme but who do not have diabetes on biochemical testing? Diabetes screening programmes from a public health perspective. *Journal of Medical Screening*, **9**, 187–90.

Squirrel, D.M. and Talbot, J.F. (2003). Screening for diabetic retinopathy. *Journal of the Royal Society of Medicine*, **96**, 273–6.

Streetly, A., Clarke, M., Downing, M. *et al.* (2008). Implementation of the newborn screening programme for sickle cell disease in England: results for 2003–2005. *Journal of Medical Screening*, **15**, 9–13.

Taban, L., Gad, A., Holmberg, L.H. *et al.* (1985). Reduction in mortality for breast cancer after mass screening with mammography. *The Lancet*, **ii**, 829–32.

Taban, L., Fagerberg, G., Gunman, D. *et al.* (1989). The Swedish two county Trial of mammographic screening for breast cancer: recent results and calculation of benefit. *Journal of Epidemiology and Community Health*, **43**, 107–14.

Thompson, I.M., Ankerst, D.P., Chi, C., Lucia, M.S., Goodman, P.J., Crowley, J.J., Parnes, H.L., and Coltman, C.A., Jr. (2005). Operating characteristics of prostate-specific antigen in men with an initial PSA level of 3.0 ng/mL or lower. *Journal of the American Medical Association*, **294**, 66–70.

Thorner, R.M. and Remein, Q.R. (1961). *Principles and procedures in the Evaluation of screening for disease*. PHS Publication No. 846. Public Health Monograph No. 67. Public Health Service, Washington DC.

UK Colorectal Cancer Screening Pilot Group (2004). Results of the first round of a demonstration pilot of screening for colorectal cancer in the United Kingdom. *British Medical Journal*, **329**, 133.

UK Newborn Screening Programme Centre (2005). Newborn blood spot screening in the UK Policies and Standards. Available at www.newbornscreening-bloodspot.org.uk. Accessed 13 April 2008

Wald, N.J., Huttly, W.J., and Hackshaw, A.K. (2003). Antenatal screening for Down's syndrome with the quadruple test. *The Lancet*, **361**, 835–6.

Wareham, N.J. and Griffin, S.J. (2001). Should we screen for type 2 diabetes? Evaluation against national screening committee criteria. *British Medical Journal*, **322**, 986–8.

Welch, H.G. (2001). Informed choice in cancer screening. *Journal of the American Medical Association*, **285**, 2776–8.

Wikipedia (2008). *Eugenics*. Available at http://en.wikipedia.org/wiki/Eugenics#_note-Osborn1937 accessed 13 April 2008.

Wilson, J.M.G. and Jungner, G. (1968). *Principles and practice of screening for disease*. Paper Number 34. World Health Organization, Geneva.

Environmental health practice

Lynn R. Goldman and Elma B. Torres

Abstract

Environmental health practice occurs within the context of physical, chemical, biological, social, and psychosocial processes in the environment that impact health, and actions to modify these factors to promote health for present and future generations. There are many professional disciplines and players in the environmental health practice arena, all of whom have important roles in the process. Environmental health practice is a three-phase process involving health impact assessment, policy development, and assurance that action is taken. Developing countries have a greater focus on prevention of infectious diseases and on efforts to reduce poverty, but their priorities are shifting along with economic transitions. Prevention of global environmental impacts is of increasing priority.

Several international policy goals have been adopted in principle, including sustainable development, the precautionary principle, and the concept of 'polluter pays'. Policy approaches include: Use of best available technology to control pollution, requirements for environmental impact reviews, consideration of economic impacts and equity (environmental justice), and ability to address issues across entire ecosystems. Assuring that policies are carried out largely depends on the strength of the rule of law in a country. Approaches include command and control, pollution prevention, and environmental monitoring. More recently, countries have increased the use of 'right-to-know' approaches. Environmental education plays an important role in strengthening the awareness and role of individuals. Increasingly, international agreements are being used to curb harmful environmental practices, for example, the Montreal Protocol to phase out ozone-depleting chemicals. Such global capacity building is occurring on a number of fronts, for example, control of greenhouse gases and management of chemical in commerce.

The rapid pace of global change, including, population growth, economic globalization, natural resource depletion, and climate change, is creating challenges for environmental health practice, even as economic transitions are creating new opportunities in developing countries.

Introduction

Environmental health practice can be best understood within an overall context of health. In 1993, the World Health Organization (WHO) stated that 'environmental health comprises those aspects of human health, including quality of life, that are determined by physical, chemical, biological, social, and psychosocial processes in the environment. It also refers to the theory and practice of assessing, correcting, controlling, and preventing those factors in the environment that can potentially affect adversely the health of present and future generations' (World Health Organization 1994). Thus, as defined, environmental health encompasses a wide array of determinants that can impact the health of the individual. Elsewhere in this textbook (Volume I, Chapter 2.5 'Water and sanitation', Chapter 2.6 'Food and nutrition', and Chapter 2.8 'The global environment'), chapters provide overviews of the environmental determinants of health. Also, Volume II, Chapter 8.1 ('Environmental health issues in public health') provides a general overview of environmental health issues.

This chapter will focus on the practice of environmental health with respect to non-occupational environmental exposures. It will also focus on those aspects of the environment that are largely not under the control of individuals, such as contaminants in food, drinking water, and indoor and outdoor air. It will not cover voluntary exposures like smoking nor will it cover injury prevention and control of radiation hazards, which are covered in other chapters. This chapter will not cover occupational health, which is discussed in Volume II, Chapter 8.5 ('Occupational health').

Many factors modify the relationship between environment and health. The practice of environmental health should take into account the variability in individual responses to the environment. Differences in age, gender, and individual genetic make-up influence both exposure and susceptibility to environmental agents. Gene–environment interactions are presented in Volume III, Chapter 9.1. A challenge in environmental health is the consideration of all age groups, as well as the very ill and the very healthy, in evaluation of hazards. Behaviour is also important and can have a major impact on exposure. In addition, social differences can affect exposure. For example, diets vary greatly across different cultural groups. People who live in poverty may experience multiple environmental threats, dietary inadequacies, and other factors that contribute to increased risk from environmental exposures.

The practice of environmental health is inextricably involved with the prevention of chronic diseases such as, cancers, asthma, and birth defects as well as acute illnesses such as viral gastroenteritis. The general state of knowledge about causation of many chronic diseases is less advanced than for communicable diseases so that while outbreaks or statistical excesses (so-called 'clusters') of chronic disease are often attributed by the public to environmental exposures, in many cases, the cause is unknown. Thus, practitioners of environmental health are often called upon to address not only known exposures and links to disease but also diseases of unknown aetiology and public concern about the potential for environmental links. How to investigate such issues is outlined in Volume II, Chapter 6.4 ('Principles of outbreak investigation'). In the United States, the Centers for Disease Control (CDC) National Center for Environmental Health and the Agency for Toxic Substances and Disease Registries (ATSDR), as well as state and local public health agencies, are often called upon to address such community outbreaks.

From the outset, it is important to emphasize that certain environmental health problems are much more serious in developing countries; for example, drinking water contamination with microorganisms and toxic substances is much more prevalent and consequent morbidity and mortality more serious. Indoor and outdoor air pollution are much more impacted by the burning of coal, wood, and other biomass fuel sources for cooking and heating homes. Air is much more polluted because many of the controls and technological changes that have been required in developed countries have not yet been applied. Chemical spills and plant accidents are more common and there are fewer means to protect nearby communities and passers-by. Not covered in this chapter, but very important worldwide, is disaster prevention and management. Worldwide there are large numbers of unnecessary deaths and injuries due to earthquakes, storms, and floods, which are completely preventable with appropriate environmental measures like construction standards for homes and buildings.

Environmental health practice in developing countries will follow a unique course according to traditions, culture, and legal structures. Because poverty is at the root of many environmental health problems, elimination of poverty is in itself a major component of environmental health policy-making. Thus, the eradication of extreme poverty and hunger by 2015 globally, a key target of the United Nations Millennium Development Goal, would be expected to result in a number of environmental health improvements (United Nations Millennium Summit 2000).

As developed countries successfully combated most, if not all, communicable diseases and a number of non-communicable diseases, the developing world is still coping with the control of both communicable and non-communicable diseases. This situation is further aggravated by global ecological changes affecting habitats of disease vectors such as those for malaria, Lyme disease, and tick-borne encephalitis (Yassi et al. 2001). Further, the global technological progress and ease of travel have likewise facilitated the occurrence and transmission of emerging diseases such as severe acute respiratory syndrome (SARS) and avian flu.

Control of non-communicable diseases is an even bigger hurdle for developing societies to surmount than communicable diseases. This is largely because non-communicable diseases lack a single aetiology and involve numerous factors including environmental exposures, individual behaviours, and other modifying factors, as described above. In developing countries, there is scarcity of information generated from local environmental epidemiological research, thus, making environmental health practice highly dependent on international standards. Although this approach has

achieved progress in environmental health, it is open to criticism as to the appropriateness and relevance of using data from more developed countries with different cultures, climates and lifestyle, for assessing local exposures and health risks.

In 1965, Rene Dubos noted that indices of environmental health are 'expressions of the success or failure experienced by the (human) organism in its efforts to respond adaptively to environmental challenges' (Dubos 1965). This effort to respond adaptively to environmental challenges becomes ever more complex as the environment is changed by humans at a very rapid pace. Despite the difficulty of adapting to an environment that has been changed dramatically within just a few generations, there is evidence of remarkable success in this century. The sanitation movement of the 1800s resulted in enormous reductions in mortality due to infectious diseases and marked increases in life expectancy. This has resulted in much of the increase in life expectancy in the United States, from 47 years in 1900 to almost 77 in 1997.

In the last 30 years, in the industrialized nations, stronger environmental laws have resulted in cleaner air, safer drinking water, and recovery of some water bodies that in 1970 had unacceptable levels of pollution for fishing and recreation. In developing countries, on the other hand, economic development and the rapid pace of urbanization have resulted in opposite trends with alarming increases in pollution of air and water and in the generation of municipal and hazardous wastes.

The global trends in environmental health are more disturbing and indicative of a failure to adapt to a changing environment (McMichael et al. 2006). (This is further covered in Chapter 2.8 'The global environment'.) On a global basis, the trend for pollution of air and drinking water supplies is upward. Drinking water is under pressure both from pollution and from consumption and in many parts of the world, there are serious shortages of drinkable water today. Even in the United States, there are shortages of potable drinking water in many parts of the country, shortages which may become more chronic with the onset of global warming. Climate extremes associated with global warming are associated with increased risk of epidemics of heat related mortality, increased severity of major weather events and resultant impacts on human health and wellbeing and changes in ranges of vector borne diseases. In addition, over fishing and pollution of water bodies is posing an increasing threat to fish harvests. In most of the world, there is little control of chemicals and pesticides in commerce and chemical waste disposal, even while development is moving forward at a very rapid pace.

Even in developed nations, there are numerous challenges that remain. To a great extent, the easiest problems have been addressed, leaving environmental threats that are much more difficult to control and require more participation from a broader range of society. Often the problems that must be faced today involved multiple small sources of pollutants rather than a few large and visible ones. Many of these small sources are from sectors, like agriculture and small business, which are less familiar with environmental regulations and often resistant to change. Clearly, they will need to be involved; yet, they do not have the resources of large industries to address environmental issues. As automobile emissions become a larger component of air pollution, land use and transportation planning and urban sprawl are becoming greater concerns. Further, problems like non-point source pollution engage everyone in society from the farmer to the weekend car mechanic who needs to know how to properly dispose of used motor oil. All of this means that new tools for assessing and managing environmental hazards will be needed in order to continue to achieve gains in environmental health.

In 1988, the US Institute of Medicine published a report *The Future of Public Health*, which defined three major functions for the practice of public health practice: Assessment, policy development, and assurance (Institute of Medicine 1988). This chapter will take this approach in describing the practice of environmental health. The general principles underlying the practice of environmental health do not differ between developed and developing nations, however, the methods and tools distinctly vary according to the individual country's social, cultural and demographic attributes, economic development, trends in science and technology, management of natural resources, and by the institutional and policy framework that the country supports.

Environmental health assessment

Environmental health assessment is necessary in preventing diseases attributable to environmental exposures. The impact of environment on health is significant. In 2006, WHO estimated that 24 per cent of the global disease burden and 23 per cent of all deaths can be attributed to environmental factors and that developing regions carry a disproportionately heavy burden for communicable diseases and injuries (Pruss-Ustun & Corvalan 2006). Some developing countries have initiated efforts to estimate the burden of communicable diseases attributable to environmental factors using regularly collected national statistics (census, demographic, health, and environmental) and available epidemiological data. Whenever epidemiological and surveillance data are limited, expert opinions from the health and non-health sectors are sought particularly in setting exposure scenarios.

The weight of evidence approach employed in environmental health inevitably involves a multitude of disciplines. Toxicology is the study of how chemicals and pollutants can be hazardous to humans and other organisms. Environmental epidemiologists study and interpret the distributions and relationships among diseases and exposure in the environment. Exposure assessors and industrial hygienists have expertise in measuring and estimating human exposure to contaminants. Analytic chemical laboratories are important for measuring levels of pollutants whether in human blood and tissues or in environmental samples such as air, food, water and soil. Statistics and modelling experts contribute an understanding of how to utilize the often-immense quantity of data in order to inform decision-making. Many science disciplines, ranging from environmental and atmospheric chemistry to hydrogeology, which looks at the dynamics of flow of water in the environment, are needed to understand how pollutants move in the environment and the ultimate fate in terms of exposures to humans and ecosystems. There are many fields of engineering involved: Chemical engineers who can design processes to minimize, eliminate or treat wastes, sanitary engineers who can design treatment systems for wastewater, and so forth. Engineering may play a role not only in the management of environmental hazards but also in the development of standards, as described below.

Thus, environmental health assessment requires specialists from a range of science disciplines and branches of medicine, engineering, and chemistry as well as facilities such as chemical and analytical laboratories. However, many developing countries are constrained in undertaking human health risk assessments, environmental health monitoring and epidemiological studies due to shortage of trained environmental health professionals and practitioners. In addition, support infrastructures and equipment such as chemical analytical laboratories are not widely available and whenever available, are poorly managed and maintained. This problem becomes apparent particularly during reported 'outbreaks' of environmental diseases such as cholera and other gastroenteritis, malaria, paralytic shellfish poisoning, etc. and when community health concerns are raised during industrial 'disasters' such as chemical spills and leaks contaminating air, water and food sources. Developing countries often seek technical assistance from the international community in order to address and manage such situations, but, in the near term, need support to build such capacity.

Generally, the assessment of environmental health threats involves the identification of hazards that may lead to disease states, on the one hand and measurement or monitoring of exposures or doses to the population. *Hazard* is a measure of the intrinsic ability of the stressor to cause harm. *Dose* is the amount of the stressor delivered to the person, organism, or ecosystem. *Effect modifiers* are other factors that influence the relationship between exposure to a hazardous agent and health. These include biologic factors like age and gender, socioeconomic factors such as poverty, and exogenous agents such as exposure to other environmental agents, tobacco, alcohol, drugs, and pollutants.

The principles are those used in the evaluation of epidemiology, the nine Bradford Hill principles: Strength of association, consistency, specificity, temporality, biological gradient, biological plausibility, coherence of evidence, experimental evidence, and reasoning by analogy. A strong association between hazard and dose is one where the risk or odds of disease is relatively large. A consistent association is one that is demonstrated in different studies and perhaps using different methods. Specificity is the extent to which the effect is uniquely associated with a disease. For example, vinyl chloride is the only exposure known to cause a rare cancer, angiosarcoma of the liver. Temporality has to do with the relationship between time of exposure and time of disease. Some diseases like cancer may have long latency periods, as much as 10 or more years. Other diseases are caused by more immediate exposures, for example, pesticide poisoning from carbamates occurs within an hour of exposure. Biological gradient refers to the ability to demonstrate that there is a dose–response between the exposure and the disease. Biological plausibility is the extent to which the association is consistent with what is already known about the response to the exposure and/or the disease. Coherence of evidence has to do with the fit between the studies and what else is known that is relevant to the association and experimental evidence is evidence from controlled experiments that is relevant. Reasoning by analogy is the extent to which the observed pattern is similar to known exposure/disease relationships. For example, knowledge about how benzene causes cancer has been helpful in interpreting data for similar compounds, with similar results from animal studies, but which lack the epidemiologic information available for benzene.

Hazard identification

Hazard identification generally relies on two types of information, data from epidemiologic studies, and data from animal testing and other scientific studies of animals. There are many sources of hazard

Table 12.8.1 Sources of hazard information

Data	Observational studies	Controlled studies
Human	Epidemiology	Dosing studies
	Case reports	Clinical trials
	Surveillance	
	Disease	
	Exposure	
	Case control studies	
	Prospective studies	
Environmental/ animal	Incident reports	In vitro studies
	Emissions inventories	General toxicity
	Field studies	Specialized toxicity
	Environmental monitoring	
	Ecological impacts	

information (Table 12.8.1). *Environmental epidemiology* is defined as 'the study of the effect on human health of physical, biologic, and chemical factors in the external environment, broadly conceived. By examining specific populations or communities exposed to different ambient environments, it seeks to clarify the relationship between physical, biologic or chemical factors and human health' (National Research Council 1991).

Environmental health surveillance is an important tool for community environmental health; it is defined as the ongoing systematic collection, analysis, and interpretation of data on specific health events affecting a population (Thacker & Stroup 1994). Surveillance of hazards and exposures, as well as diseases, is critical to the practice of environmental health (Wegman 1992). By tracking exposures and diseases we can identify and respond to different kinds of public health problems. Surveillance and monitoring are also essential to the assurance function, that is, the follow-up to make sure that the treatment for the community is effective (Thacker *et al.* 1996). Examples of environmental health surveillance include air pollution monitoring, blood lead monitoring, poison centre surveillance for pesticide and chemical ingestions, pesticide illness reports, asthma surveillance and birth defects registries. All of these are tools for monitoring trends, and identifying opportunities to prevent and control environmental disease and exposures. Another form of surveillance is post-market monitoring for adverse effects. In the United States, there are provisions under both the pesticide and chemicals laws for reporting to the Environmental Protection Agency (EPA) of adverse health (as well as environmental) effects of toxic chemicals. This can be an important safety mechanism for chemicals approved as a result of animal testing alone since such limited testing cannot detect effects that are expected to occur in a small percentage of the population, especially idiosyncratic effects that are not completely dose-dependent.

It is important to recognize that environmental health monitoring is not the same as environmental quality monitoring. Although many of these data systems have other important uses for enforcement and administrative purposes as well as for assessment of ecological systems, it is clear that environmental health assessments need to be better informed by information about both exposure and disease rates in populations. There are examples of remarkable successes that have resulted in application of the public health

model for surveillance in environmental health. The Centers for Disease Control and Prevention (CDC) surveillance of lead levels in children in the United States demonstrated the benefits of the US phase-out of lead in gasoline at a time when this was in doubt and there were efforts to overturn the decision. Despite this and other successes, the capacity for environmental surveillance at the federal, state, and local level is quite limited.

Environmental epidemiology suffers from some limitations. For one, it cannot detect risks of concern when there is little variation in exposure across the population. For example, dioxin exposures are difficult to evaluate in the general population because most people have dioxin body burdens within a narrow range. Second, epidemiology cannot be applied before approving the introduction into commerce of a chemical, product, or technology. Third, studies of environmental exposures often rely on measurements for the ambient environment as a whole rather than measurements of individual exposures. Such studies are known as *ecologic studies* and they are often the only feasible way to study exposures; air pollution is often studied this way. Generally, the larger the area over which exposures are averaged, the greater are the methodological limitations with these studies. The major limitation of ecologic studies is the *ecological fallacy*, which in some circumstances can result from making causal inferences based on ecological data (Morgenstern 1982). Issues related to use of ecological data in epidemiology are discussed in Section II, Chapter 6.2 ('Ecologic variables, ecologic studies, and multilevel studies in public health research').

Animal *toxicity testing* allows examination of a wide range of exposures, use of experimental controls to limit the possibility of confounding and pre-market prediction of hazards. In the practice of environmental health, governments have established regulatory standards or guidelines to ensure that any testing required by the law meets strict standards for quality of the data generated. The international standard that is available, and employed by most industrialized nations, is the set of internationally harmonized guidelines developed by the Organization for Economic Cooperation and Development (OECD). Test guidelines attempt to assay toxic properties of chemicals in a manner that is valid, reproducible, standardized between different laboratories, and is as humane to laboratory animals as possible. In countries, specific requirements for testing vary with the type of substance and the statute under which the substance is covered. In the United States, the most highly tested substances are food-use pesticides, for which numerous health tests are required including: Tests of acute and chronic toxicity, neurotoxicity tests, cancer bioassays, and multiple generation studies to assess reproductive and developmental toxicity. In addition, there are new requirements for tests of immunotoxicity, developmental neurotoxicity, and endocrine toxicity that are being implemented by the EPA. The OECD is currently developing new and enhanced assays for endocrine disruption for oestrogen, androgen, and thyroid effects. Because most chemicals and pesticides are marketed in many countries, the OECD has also established an agreement for Mutual Acceptance of Data to avoid unnecessary duplication of tests.

Toxicity testing is done under *good laboratory practices* (GLP), standards established by governments to eliminate extraneous factors, such as poor nutrition of animals, sloppy laboratory practices, or unclean environments, which would tend to bias or distort the results of laboratory tests. These practices also include record-keeping requirements that allow intensive peer review of studies to ensure their quality. There is an internationally agreed upon set of GLP for chemicals adopted by the OECD.

Despite efforts to carry out accurate toxicity tests, these tests have limitations. To be cost-effective and humane, they are designed with as few animals as statistically possible, while dosing animals at high levels. Outcome measures have been refined over the years but may be cruder than the measurements that can be taken in humans; for example, a mouse cannot report a headache. There can be phenomena that occur in the high-dose groups that are not relevant to human risk assessment. Thus, expert judgement is needed to interpret such data and it is important that scientists review all of the evidence before making a judgement. Unfortunately, there is a perception that animal testing is irrelevant. When we have both epidemiological and animal testing data, there is a striking concordance between the two with respect to relevance to risk assessment. Further, most chemicals that have been subjected to high-dose testing do not cause cancer, refuting the often-made assertion that 'everything causes cancer if you give a high enough dose'.

Despite the availability of accepted tests and practices to assess hazards, the truth is that we know very little about the chemicals in commerce worldwide. The industrialized nations belonging to the OECD have for years been collaborating on an effort to obtain at least screening information about such chemicals (Organization for Economic Co-operation and Development and Environment Directorate 1991).

Exposure assessment

Assessment of exposure involves numerous factors. Usually, in risk assessment, one does not have access to precise measurements of all of these exposure attributes, and yet they are all important in being able to calculate an average daily lifetime exposure. We would like to know the rate and duration of exposure and the amount absorbed, as well as the body weight. Issues related to assessment of human exposures are examined in Chapter 8.4 ('The science of human exposures to contaminants in the environment').

Almost never available to decision-makers are direct measurements of exposure to the human population. It is recognized that such direct measurements, in combination with better information about environmental sources and levels, would be a vast improvement over the current methods for modelling and estimating exposure. In the United States, the National Health Assessment and Nutrition Examination Survey (NHANES) has conducted some population monitoring of exposures and the CDC is beginning to publish data about trends (Centers for Disease Control and Prevention 2005).

As a practical matter, actual exposure measurements are often replaced by defaults. At the US EPA, the policy is to assess a *reasonable high-end exposure*—that is, an exposure at the upper 90th or 95th percentile. Summation of numerous high-end exposures can greatly overestimate exposure, however. Exposure to pesticides in food is a good example of this. Adding up the upper 90th percentile bound for all foods would result in a theoretical individual who eats 5000 calories/day—not exactly a reasonable high-end estimate of exposure. If there are data on distributions of food consumption and on pesticide levels in the food, it is possible to use *probabilistic modelling*, which incorporates those distributions for all foods to compute the distribution of exposure to pesticide residues in the food. Most frequently, this is done using Monte Carlo modelling

techniques, not only for pesticide residues on food but also for other aggregate exposure situations. Monte Carlo and other probabilistic modelling techniques simulate the distributions of individual combinations of multiple exposures, to produce a theoretical distribution of an aggregate exposure to the population.

There is not currently a process underway for international harmonization of exposure assessment. This is probably because of the large differences—cultural, dietary, climatic, and others—which can lead to differences in exposures for different countries. For example, in a hot equatorial climate, there is more consumption of drinking water; in the Arctic among traditional societies there is more consumption of marine mammals.

Effect modification

Assessment of effect modification involves a number of considerations. Are there age or life stage 'windows of vulnerability' that need to be taken into consideration (as described below)? It is important to consider whether there are higher (or lower) exposures during these vulnerable times. Another factor is whether there are concurrent exposures or other situations in the population. For example, children exposed to lead may be more vulnerable if they also have iron or calcium deficiency. For another example, risk of cancer from exposure to asbestos is magnified by concurrent exposure to tobacco smoke. Such considerations are especially important in developing countries. Poverty, which by itself is a consequence of the country's economy and social structures, exerts tremendous consequences on health status of individuals. Malnutrition, poor access to water supply, sanitation and garbage disposal, exposures to pollution of air, water, soil and food are the major health concerns brought about by poverty. These factors often occur in combination.

Risk assessment

There are a number of tools used for integrating and summarizing information about environmental health hazards. Environmental health relies extensively on the use of *risk assessment* to evaluate environmental stressors. Use of risk assessment allows us to extrapolate either between human populations or from laboratory animals to humans. It involves weighing all of the evidence in order to develop estimates of the risks to populations who may be exposed. The current practice of risk assessment in environmental health is largely based on a set of principles developed by the National Research Council (1983). Risk is a function of hazard and dose. Four steps in risk assessment have been delineated: Hazard identification, dose–response evaluation, exposure assessment, and risk characterization (National Research Council 1983). These are laid out in detail in Volume II, Chapter 8.7 ('Toxicology and risk assessment in the analysis and management of environmental risk'). Some aspects of hazard and exposure assessment have been addressed above. The section below discusses some aspects of dose–response evaluation and risk characterization that are important to the practice of environmental health.

The practice of *dose–response assessment* differs significantly between a carcinogen and a non-carcinogen. *Cancer assessment* is one of the most established areas of risk assessment. There are several authoritative bodies, all of which conduct cancer risk assessment in a similar fashion. On the international level, there is the International Agency for Research in Cancer (IARC), which publishes monographs on assessments of individual carcinogens.

There are many bodies in the United States, but the most important is the National Toxicology Program, which in its *Biennial Report on Carcinogens* reviews the evidence and lists substances likely to be carcinogenic (US Department of Health and Human Services and National Toxicology Program 2005).

At the present time, hazard assessments for cancer are done in a roughly similar fashion worldwide. At the hazard assessment phase, all studies relevant to the assessment of cancer are reviewed. If there is definitive human evidence of cancer causation, all of these bodies rate the chemical as a human carcinogen. A substance can also be rated as a human carcinogen when the human evidence alone does not prove a causal relationship, but the weight of the evidence is convincing. (This is a change from the past, when only human data could be used to make this judgement.) When there is strong evidence, but not probative, of carcinogenicity to humans, the substance is considered to be a 'probable' human carcinogen. Most systems then have a category for 'possible' carcinogens, those with weaker evidence and non-carcinogens, chemicals that despite testing show no evidence for carcinogenicity.

At the dose–response assessment phase, the default assumption is that the dose–response curve is linear at low doses and starts at zero. This means that we assume that for every additional exposure there is additional cancer risk. In other words, we generally assume that if 20 out of 100 people exposed at 1 part per 1000 in air will get cancer, the risk for an exposure to a much lower level of 1 part per million would be 200 cancers for every 1 million people exposed. This relationship is assumed unless there is compelling evidence for a different dose–response relationship at low doses.

There are many mechanisms for carcinogenicity and it is believed that not all of these mechanisms have linear dose–response relationships at low doses. However, there are rigorous criteria for accepting arguments to depart from the low-dose linear model, and most carcinogens are still considered to have linearity at low doses. Whether from human or from animal data, the dose–response curve is modelled using statistical techniques that extrapolate the curve from the higher doses in the occupational or laboratory setting to the lower doses that are often of concern in environmental settings. Because of the uncertainties in extrapolating from high to low doses, and to account for the variability in the general human population, the dose–response curve is plotted with 95 percentile confidence limits and the upper 95th percentile bound is generally used for risk assessment. This estimate is combined with the exposure assessment to give a probabilistic estimate of risk, e.g. 10^{-3}, 10^{-5}, 10^{-6}.

Non-cancer risk assessment generally involves use of the *reference dose* (RfD) or *acceptable daily intake* (ADI) approach. It is important for decision-makers to understand that a reference dose is a dose considered safe with a margin of uncertainty rather than a bright line for toxicity. A chronic RfD is an estimate of a daily exposure to a population, which, over a 70-year life span, is likely to have no significant deleterious effects (Barnes & Dourson 1988). An acute RfD considers a 1-day exposure only. Generally, the RfD for an acute exposure may be much higher than the RfD for a chronic exposure, but this is very much dependent on the nature of the chemical and effects under study.

Susceptible populations

Children and other susceptible populations pose a special challenge for assessment of environmental hazards. Children are not just small adults. Children develop very rapidly in the first few years of life, their diets vary from those of adults, and they require more caloric intake, oxygen, and water for their body weights than adults. Children's metabolism changes over the first few years of life, affecting how their systems handle pharmaceuticals and toxic substances. Normal childhood behaviour includes intense exploration of the environment and hand-to-mouth activities that can lead to increased exposures to contaminants in soil and around the home. Children lack judgement and thus cannot avoid exposures unless adults ensure that their environments are safe (Rogan 1995).

These differences between children and adults influence toxicity and exposure assessments for children, as well as options for risk management. A National Research Council (NRC) committee in its 1993 report *Pesticides in the Diets of Infants and Children* concluded that the toxicity of, and exposures to, pesticides are frequently different for children and adults. It found that, despite a wealth of scientific information to warrant addressing risks to children, the EPA rarely did so in making regulatory decisions about pesticides. The committee advised EPA to incorporate information about dietary exposures to children in risk assessments, and augment pesticide testing with new assessments of neurotoxicity, developmental toxicity, endocrine effects, immunotoxicity, and developmental neurotoxicity. It recommended that the EPA include cumulative risks from pesticides that act via a common mechanism of action and aggregate risks from non-food exposures when developing a tolerance for a pesticide. Since that time, there has been a major undertaking by government to incorporate these recommendations into federal management of the use of pesticides (National Research Council 1993).

While this is good in theory, children in developing countries may have much more emergent environmental health risks that need to be addressed. A recent review identified unsafe drinking water, lack of sanitation, and household burning of fossil fuels as being responsible for huge number of completely preventable childhood deaths every year: 49 700 in Latin America and the Caribbean, 0.8 million in South Asia, and 1.47 million in sub-Saharan Africa (Gakidou *et al.* 2007).

There are other vulnerable populations as well, many of whom are not in the workplace. Those who live in poverty are very vulnerable because of the potential to multiple exposures, poorer diets, and lack of access to medical care (Institute of Medicine and Committee on Environmental Justice 1999). For example, children who are relatively deficient in iron or calcium absorb more lead per gram of intake than children who have adequate nutrition. The elderly population may be particularly susceptible to some environmental exposures and may have slower elimination of many toxicants. Those who have chronic illnesses are often more susceptible as well. For example, people who have human immunodeficiency virus (HIV) infections or are immunosuppressed as a result of cancer therapy are much more at risk for serious infections from pathogens in drinking water or food. Pregnant women are at risk not only from the perspective of exposure to the developing child but also because of altered physiology and metabolism of many toxic agents. For women, menopause may be another time of vulnerability. For example, there is evidence that at the time of menopause, blood lead levels increase because of liberation of stored lead from bones.

It is easy to conclude that the process of dose–response assessment has become ever more complex, given considerations of the increasing sophistication in understanding of mechanisms of toxicity as well as increased appreciation that there are some in the population that are more vulnerable. This is creating challenges for practitioners in environmental health in developing a language that can be used and understood by stakeholders as well as decision-makers to achieve the public involvement and transparency that are so important in environmental health practice.

Risk characterization

The *risk characterization* is the final step of the risk assessment process. No additional scientific information is added during this phase, which involves estimating the magnitude of the public health or environmental problem. Much judgement is needed in appropriate selection of populations and exposure levels for analysis. In addition, it is important that relevant statistical and biological uncertainties are made clear at this stage. This part of the risk assessment process is the largest nexus between risk assessment and risk managers, and it is important that risk managers receive a complete set of information to guide decisions. This is where the very complex interactions between scientists, decision-makers and the public occur and yet where some of the most difficult communication issues occur as well. Issues related to risk communication are described in Section II, Chapter 8.8 ('Risk perception and communication').

The International Program for Chemical Safety, which is a collaborative effort between the World Health Organization (WHO), the United Nations Environment Program (UNEP), the International Labor Organization (ILO), and the Food and Agriculture Organization (FAO), publishes Environmental Health Criteria documents which are intended to serve as international characterizations of risk for substances. In addition, there is information available in the ILO Chemical Safety Cards, in the WHO/FAO pesticide assessments and in summary form on the UNEP Global Information Network. Many nations make risk assessments widely available via the Internet and other means but it is important to emphasize that the exposure assessment may differ between countries, as mentioned above. While all of this information is helpful, it is also true that the best efforts to accurately characterize risk are hobbled by the great variability in risk among different populations, the uncertainties in our models for assessing risk, and the enormous knowledge gaps that remain even after the most thorough assessment.

Environmental health policy-making

For the most part, environmentally induced diseases and injuries are completely preventable, using pollution prevention, product design, engineering controls, personal protection, housing policies, consumer product safety, and education—all within the context of supportive policy environments including engagement of various industry sectors, government at all levels, as well as the general public, in active efforts to protect the environment. So much of environmental health practice falls outside the realm of traditional medicine because the focus is generally on primary prevention, preventing exposures before the development of disease. At the same time, other interventions flow directly from a physician encounter that diagnoses the health problem and forms a connection between that problem and an environmental exposure (for example, childhood lead poisoning, pesticide poisoning, and

asthma exacerbation by air pollution). As with occupational disease, single or small numbers of diagnosed cases can be sentinels for more widespread population exposures and disease. However, environmental health requires a broad range of disciplinary approaches and the application of engineering, sanitation, public health nursing, education and communication, epidemiology, toxicology, statistics, laboratory, administration, enforcement and legal expertise as well as the expertise of public health generalists and physicians. This is therefore a complex web of scientific expertise and information and much of the science of environmental policymaking involves the job of weaving together information from multiple disciplines in order to define problems and develop alternative approaches to solving them.

Who makes environmental health policy? The players

Who makes environmental health policy? Nearly everyone at some level is involved with decisions related to the environment and health. At all the levels, decisions about planning of towns and cities, road building, and economic development all have an impact on environmental health. Much of the time, the policy-makers may not be aware of the environmental health implications of these decisions. Yet, there is a need for more input of public health assessment data into such decision-making processes at all levels. For example, health experts are rarely engaged in discussions about transportation planning in the United States. Involvement of 'stakeholders', literally those with a stake in the outcome of decision-making, is important in environmental health policy-making. In a sense, since everyone wants to be able to breathe clean air, drink safe drinking water and eat healthful food, all are stakeholders in environmental policy-making. Much of the art of environmental health practice is in not only informing but also involving stakeholders in all stages of the decision-making process, from problem definition through selection of alternative solutions to the problem at hand (The Presidential/Congressional Commission on Risk Assessment and Risk Management 1997). It also involves no small amount of political will to see solutions through since by its very nature environmental health protection inevitably involves either costs to taxpayers, costs to industry or both. At the same time, environmental health practice usually creates winners as well as losers and planning for transition from more to less polluting activities is at the heart of environmental health policy-making at its best.

The role of various players in environmental health policymaking is recognized by many nations. It has been promoted internationally as exemplified by the UNCED (United Nations Conference on Environment and Development) Principles of Sustainable Development in 1992 (United Nations Conference on Environment and Development 1992) the Health and Environment Linkages Initiative launched by the WHO and UNEP during the World Summit on Sustainable Development in Johannesburg, South Africa in 2002, and the UN Millennium Development Goals of 2000 (United Nations Millennium Summit 2000). These initiatives are global efforts to promote and facilitate inter-sectoral partnerships and networking in reducing environmental threats to human health in concert with support of sustainable development objectives.

For example, as a commitment to the UNCED principles, the Philippine government enacted a 1992 Executive Order that created the National Interagency Committee on Environmental Health to develop environmental health policies addressing those threats confronting the country (Office of the President and Republic of the Philippines 1992). The Committee is chaired by the Department of Health and vice-chaired by the Department of Environment and Natural Resources. Other sectors represented in the committee are agriculture, public works and highways, science and technology, trade and industry, transportation and communication, labour, economic development, and public information. A successful policy developed by the Committee and put into action is the reduction of paralytic shellfish poisoning morbidity and mortality. Participation of other sectors in the Committee such as non-governmental organizations, the industry sector, and the private sector are sought by the Committee whenever issues concern these sectors. To manage environmental health concerns of various administrative regions of the country, the Committee created the Regional Interagency Committee on Environmental Health; these address local environmental issues and thus support the national policy- and decision-making processes.

Environmental health policy principles adopted by governments

In 1992, more than 100 nations signed the United Nations Commission on Environment and Development (UNCED) treaty that formally adopted the goal of *sustainable development* and 27 principles of sustainable development (Table 12.8.2). Chief among these is principle 1, which states: 'Human beings are at the centre of concerns for sustainable development. They are entitled to a healthy and productive life in harmony with nature'. The second principle is also very fundamental; it describes a 'sovereign right' of states 'to exploit their own resources pursuant to their own environmental and developmental policies, and the responsibility to ensure that activities within their jurisdiction or control do not cause damage to the environment of other States or of areas beyond the limits of national jurisdiction' (United Nations Conference on Environment and Development 1992). The outcomes of UNCED were reviewed in the 2002 World Summit on Sustainable Development (WSSD) held in Johannesburg. The WSSD identified six major environmental treaties that flowed directly from UNCED: The Framework Convention on Climate Change with the Kyoto Protocol; the Convention on Biological Diversity with the Cartagena Protocol; the Convention to Combat Desertification; the Convention on Persistent Organic Pollutants; the Convention on Straddling and Highly Migratory Fish Stocks; and the Convention on the Prior Informed Consent (PIC) Procedure for Certain Hazardous Chemicals and Pesticides in International Trade. All of these directly or indirectly involve environmental health and some are discussed further. At the same time, fighting poverty was a major theme of the WSSD meeting and particularly the urgent need to strengthen the UN institutions working on sustainable development. The WSSD called for a focus on provision of safe drinking water and sanitation, more sustainable sources of energy, and addressing economic and social imbalances in world trade rules and the ecological impacts of the globalized economy in order to contribute to sustainable development (World Summit on Sustainable Development 2002). Thus, while in theory development leads to economic improvements that enhance health, there are enormous problems related to overconsumption, pollution, poverty and inequities that will continue to create challenges for generations to come.

The *precautionary principle* is another UNCED principle for environmental policy-making. As governments agreed in 1992: 'In order to protect the environment, the precautionary approach shall be widely applied by States according to their capabilities. Where there are threats of serious or irreversible damage, lack of full scientific certainty shall not be used as a reason for postponing cost-effective measures to prevent environmental degradation' (United Nations Conference on Environment and Development 1992). For example, the pesticide dichlorodiphenyltrichloroethane (DDT) was banned in the United States long before its precise mechanisms of action had been described by scientists. Despite the agreement to this principle at UNCED, there has been a great deal of disagreement on its applicability within other global contexts, none more evident than in the context of the disputes by the United States and Canada versus the European Union over Europe's ban of hormones fed to farm animals (Carlarne 2007).

Another important principle, adopted in many nations, is the principle of *polluter pays* (United Nations Conference on Environment and Development 1992). Put very simply, this means that those who profit from pollution should pay the price for cleaning it up. More recently, this has evolved to the concept of *economic instruments* such as pollutant trading systems that seek to shift the societal cost of pollution to the polluter, in order to ratchet down the overall levels of pollution. While these principles are important, it is obvious, from the trends that have been mentioned above, that they have not been put in place consistently and that, too often, it is possible to profit at the expense of the health of others as well as the degradation of resources that are needed for human well-being. Worldwide, the practice of environmental health involves not only the application of science but also policy approaches to shift the costs of pollution onto the shoulders of the polluter, because this is one of the most effective ways to prevent pollution.

Environmental health policy tools

There are a number of tools that are used in environmental policy-making. In some cases, an *economic analysis* of costs or feasibility in developing standards is an important driver in decision-making. Economic analyses can play a number of roles including attempting to weight costs and benefits of an action (so called cost-benefit analysis) weighing the relative *cost effectiveness* of alternative solutions to a problem and identification of economic inequities in impact that can inform decision-making.

Pollution and its consequences are not distributed equally in society, and thus it is important to consider *environmental justice* issues in assessment of hazard (Institute of Medicine and Committee on Environmental Justice 1999). Unfortunately, in the past there was a failure to do so, accounting for concentrations of polluting industries, sources of air pollution, and waste disposal operations in certain low income and minority communities. In addition, there are higher rates of many diseases in poor and minority communities globally, lending support to the notion of differential exposure and risk (Goldman & Tran 2002).

Another important tool at a community level is an *ecosystem-based* approach or a *community-based* approach to environmental protection. For air pollution control, it has long been recognized that, for many communities, it would not be possible to meet standards unless management is undertaken for an entire air shed. This approach is now being adopted for protection of large

Table 12.8.2 UNCED principles of sustainable development most relevant to environmental health

Principle 1	Human beings are at the centre of concerns for sustainable development. They are entitled to a healthy and productive life in harmony with nature.
Principle 2	States have, in accordance with the Charter of the United Nations and the principles of international law, the sovereign right to exploit their own resources pursuant to their own environmental and developmental policies, and the responsibility to ensure that activities within their jurisdiction or control do not cause damage to the environment of other States or of areas beyond the limits of national jurisdiction.
Principle 3	The right to development must be fulfilled so as to equitably meet developmental and environmental needs of present and future generations.
Principle 4	In order to achieve sustainable development, environmental protection shall constitute an integral part of the development process and cannot be considered in isolation from it.
Principle 5	All States and all people shall cooperate in the essential task of eradicating poverty as an indispensable requirement for sustainable development, in order to decrease the disparities in standards of living and better meet the needs of the majority of the people of the world.
Principle 10	Environmental issues are best handled with the participation of all concerned citizens, at the relevant level. At the national level, each individual shall have appropriate access to information concerning the environment that is held by public authorities, including information on hazardous materials and activities in their communities, and the opportunity to participate in decision-making processes. States shall facilitate and encourage public awareness and participation by making information widely available. Effective access to judicial and administrative proceedings, including redress and remedy, shall be provided.
Principle 11	States shall enact effective environmental legislation. Environmental standards, management objectives and priorities should reflect the environmental and developmental context to which they apply. Standards applied by some countries may be inappropriate and of unwarranted economic and social cost to other countries, in particular developing countries.
Principle 13	States shall develop national law regarding liability and compensation for the victims of pollution and other environmental damage. States shall also cooperate in an expeditious and more determined manner to develop further international law regarding liability and compensation for adverse effects of environmental damage caused by activities within their jurisdiction or control to areas beyond their jurisdiction.
Principle 14	States should effectively cooperate to discourage or prevent the relocation and transfer to other States of any activities and substances that cause severe environmental degradation or are found to be harmful to human health.
Principle 15	In order to protect the environment, the precautionary approach shall be widely applied by States according to their capabilities. Where there are threats of serious or irreversible damage, lack of full scientific certainty shall not be used as a reason for postponing cost-effective measures to prevent environmental degradation.
Principle 18	States shall immediately notify other States of any natural disasters or other emergencies that are likely to produce sudden harmful effects on the environment of those States. Every effort shall be made by the international community to help States so afflicted.
Principle 19	States shall provide prior and timely notification and relevant information to potentially affected States on activities that may have a significant adverse transboundary environmental effect and shall consult with those States at an early stage and in good faith.
Principle 22	Indigenous people and their communities and other local communities have a vital role in environmental management and development because of their knowledge and traditional practices. States should recognize and duly support their identity, culture and interests and enable their effective participation in the achievement of sustainable development.
Principle 24	Warfare is inherently destructive of sustainable development. States shall therefore respect international law providing protection for the environment in times of armed conflict and cooperate in its further development, as necessary.
Principle 25	Peace, development and environmental protection are interdependent and indivisible.

and complex watersheds both within countries and internationally. Increasingly, it is recognized that *non-point sources* of pollution to air and water—that is, sources that are diffuse rather than from large industrial incinerator stacks and water disposal outfalls—are important. Ecosystem-based approaches are more effective than individual permitting activities in controlling such sources. Across the world today of increasing concern is agricultural runoff from confined animal feeding operations, which can release harmful pathogens and nutrients to aquatic environments. Aquaculture, if not done properly, may directly pollute aquatic ecosystems with animal waste as well as antibiotics and nutrient loadings from feeds. The nutrients in turn have been associated with blooms of harmful organisms like toxic algal blooms and with the production of 'dead zones', areas of hypoxia which damages health by diminishing the productivity of fish and other seafood. Only watershed based management schemes can address this kind of pollution.

Global environmental health policy issues

The threats of large-scale changes to the *global environment*, such as destruction of the tropospheric ozone layer and global climate change, are encouraging nations to cooperate on environmental policy issues. For example, air pollutants can persist and travel long distances, creating environmental damage. Hazardous wastes can be transported across borders and into nations with little or no capacity to handle them. Pollution to large water bodies like the Great Lakes or the Baltic Ocean can affect the quantity and quality of food available to neighbouring nations. Clearly, when pollutants cross boundaries environmental decision-making must occur on an international basis.

Another international issue in environmental policy is the emergence of a global economy, and along with it, a global trading system that is more open than in the past. Although trading agreements have recognized past environmental agreements, there is always the possibility of trade taking precedence over future environmental actions. Environmental policy-making today must take into account not only national economic interests but international ones as well, while upholding the sovereign right of nations to establish their own health and environmental standards as agreed in UNCED.

Environmental health assurance

Environmental health assurance is a complex process that involves a multitude of players. In most nations, there are a number of governmental entities that carry out the process of providing environmental health protection. Generally, there is a national environmental ministry that carries out most national environmental regulatory responsibilities. In the United States, this function is divided between the Department of the Interior and the Environmental Protection Agency (EPA), but this is the exception rather than the rule. Generally, there are separate regulatory authorities for food safety that are either located in the health or agriculture ministry or, in the case of the United States, both. In addition, in many nations, the health or labour ministry also has some responsibility in the area of management of chemicals. There may be separate radiation safety and consumer products agencies as well. There may also be a justice agency (in the United States, the Department of Justice), with additional enforcement responsibilities.

In addition to agencies with direct responsibility for environmental health, there are many others who may become involved because of how regulations affect economic interests in society. Thus, in the United States, the Departments of Energy, Commerce, and Defense, the Office of Management and Budget, the Small Business Administration, and others all become involved where their interests may be affected by regulations. Therefore, at a national level, assurance of environmental health involves a complex web and much of the practice of environmental health involves learning how to coordinate and work effectively within this kind of complex environment.

In most nations, environmental regulation is delegated to state and local government levels. For example, municipal waste disposal is primarily a state and local function in the United States. At a local level in the United States, environmental assurance primarily is in the hands of environmental health divisions within local health agencies. However, there are many other players, including those as diverse as environmental agencies, fire departments, and agriculture departments. Whereas activities at a national level may focus on assuring that there is a minimum standard for clean air, drinking water and food, on a local level there are different responsibilities, such as, inspection of food preparation establishments, rat control, sanitation services, spill cleanups, lead poisoning prevention, and the like.

Command and control approaches to environmental health management

In most of the world, much environmental health assurance is via a *command and control* approach that involves the development and enforcement of *laws*, *regulations* and *standards*. For example, there may be rules against leaking septic tanks or creating cross connections between water and sewer lines in cities. In addition, for chemicals and pesticides there are licensing functions like new

chemicals approvals and pesticide registrations. *Environmental impact assessments* allow the review of proposed projects to ensure compliance with environmental standards prior to the commitment of resources for new development and construction. *Permitting* of facilities for air emissions, water discharges, and waste disposal are essential to controlling point sources of pollution as is a strong environmental *enforcement* presence. Generally, enforcement is targeted to specific goals; hopefully goals that are informed by priorities for protection of health and ecosystems. Generally, the first line of responsibility for enforcement is with local and state health and environmental agencies. Command and control approaches require a strong infrastructure including adherence to rule of law, standards setting ability and authorities, and strong monitoring and enforcement capacities.

The *environmental impact assessment* is one of the best ways of achieving goals related to sustainable development. While the ultimate goal of economic development is the attainment of the highest possible level of well-being of its citizens, and while economic development has brought improvements to general health status, it has likewise brought an array of new and complex health problems. Thus, many countries, including developing countries, have enacted environmental laws related to economic development, environmental degradation and impact on human health. Such laws required environmental impact assessments (EIAs) before development projects are implemented. Impact on health is generally based on secondary health data sets which cover communicable diseases and only limited information on environmentally-induced chronic diseases. Often, a major focus of EIA in the developing world is the social acceptability to communities primarily impacted by the development project. As an example of EIAs in developing countries, in the Philippines, the Health Department developed a National Framework and Guidelines for Environmental Health Impact Assessment (EHIA) (DOH 1997) to strengthen EIAs. The EHIA is integrated into the EIA system and helps assure that human health is considered in economic development in the case of environmentally critical projects (resource extractive industries, power generation, heavy industries and infrastructure projects) and for projects in critical locations (national parks and watersheds, areas where indigenous cultural communities reside, and areas frequently hit by natural calamities such as earthquakes, volcanic activities and floods). The WHO Regional Office for Western Pacific (WPRO) has also commissioned a similar study to develop a regional EHIA framework and guidelines for reference of its member states where about 80 per cent are developing countries (WHO/WPR1997). It is too soon to evaluate these nascent efforts, however. They should provide significant benchmarks for later assessment of impacts of such projects as well as informing decisions about future projects.

Much of command and control regulation is premised on the establishment of environmental standards. Environmental standards may be *risk-based*, that is, wholly or in part based upon assessments of environmental or public health risks. Many environmental standards are *technology-based*. There are many examples of regulatory programs based on *best available technology*, such as the air toxics Maximum Achievable Control Technology (MACT) standards under the US Clean Air Act and similar Best Available Technology (BAT) standards in many European countries. Technology standards can be combined with risk based standards. For example, for hazardous air pollutants, the US EPA was directed by Congress to regulate using MACT standards and then to assess the 'residual risks' and tighten the regulations if necessary. While technology standards can speed the development of regulations they do not help with controlling substances in other media. For example, a MACT standard reducing air emissions of a chemical from a toy manufacturer will not reduce the amount of the chemical in the toys.

Environmental health management tools

There are a number of tools that are used in risk management. *Environmental engineering* has played a very important role in identifying alternative methods for pollution prevention and control.

Pollution prevention is an important tool for environmental management as well as for policy. Increasingly, it is understood that trying to address environmental problems one medium at a time can result in just moving pollutants from water to air to land to water, without a net reduction in risk. The rungs of the pollution prevention ladder go from the most preferable strategy, reduction of pollution at the source (source reduction), to waste minimization, reuse, recycling, emissions controls, and, least preferably, clean-up. It is generally less expensive to reduce pollution at the source and thus avoid costs of emissions controls and environmental cleanup. So called multimedia approaches look at all of the impacts of decisions. Pollution prevention can also be an important driver for decision-making. Often changes that involve source reduction occur over a longer production life cycle than more incremental changes. In the United States, pollution prevention is used in both regulatory and also voluntary approaches to environmental assurance. As an example of the latter in the United States, there is a Presidential Award called the Green Chemistry Challenge, a contest in which companies and universities compete to be recognized for innovative new chemistries that reduce waste and are safer for health and the environment.

Environmental monitoring is also an important tool for evaluating the success of efforts and for targeting future regulatory and enforcement actions. Monitoring can involve reporting by regulated entities or actual sampling and analysis of pollutants in the air, water, food, etc. Such monitoring can be enforcement driven or at random to reflect population exposure. While important for environmental health assurance, environmental monitoring that is directly relevant to human health can feed back into the assessment process and inform future environmental health practice.

Right to know and the power of information

Community right to know is a powerful driver for reducing pollution. It was first introduced at a national level in the United States with passage of the 1986 Emergency Preparedness and Community Right to know Act (EPCRA) and establishment of the Toxic Release Inventory (TRI), which initially required the manufacturing industry to report releases of some 300 chemicals to the public. In the rest of the world, such reporting systems are called *Pollutant Release and Transfer Registries (PRTRs)*. Like the material safety data sheets (MSDSs) in workplaces, community right to know is designed to empower citizens to make informed decisions either as individuals or as a community. Community right to know is a powerful tool not only to inform citizens but also workers within plants as well as plant and corporate managers. In the United States, the TRI helped industry recognize that it often was more cost-effective to prevent the pollution by better managing the flows of materials into, in,

and through facilities. In the United States, the TRI was also the basis for a voluntary pollution reduction programme in which industry reduced TRI emissions of several toxic air contaminants by 33 per cent by 1992 and 50 per cent by 1995 from the TRI baseline year of 1988. Canada and Mexico have developed PRTRs that are similar to TRI and work is underway for a North American PRTR that would combine the data for the three countries. Other nations that have developed PRTRs include Australia and the United Kingdom (Kyesku 2003).

Today, with the increasing availability of information online, we will probably continue to see expanded availability of information. A challenge for environmental health professionals will be keeping up with the available information, and helping communities and individuals sift through it to understand what is important and relevant for their communities and how to place it into perspective. Keeping up with and understanding this information is a critical part of environmental health practice. Industry has long been concerned that provision of information is damaging to competitiveness. There are other concerns that information can be easily taken out of context and misunderstood by communities. Clearly, while there is an appropriate balance between providing information and other concerns, right to know has proven to be a useful tool for environmental health protection. Since it is here to stay, an important role of environmental health practitioners is to promote the right to understand as well as the right to know, that is, to provide the context for information so that communities can understand it as well as acquiring it.

Another powerful force in assuring environmental health is the private right of action. This varies with the legal system in countries but in the United States, the tort liability system sometimes has been a powerful driver toward prevention of exposures to environmental pollutants. In some instances, US environmental statutes give the public the right to sue the US EPA to enforce standards (called 'citizen suits' provisions). Completely unique in the United States is California's Proposition 65, which combined the right to know and the citizen suit approach. In a nutshell, companies must label products: (1) if they may cause more than a 1 in 100 000-lifetime cancer risk; or (2) if they may cause reproductive toxicity and have exposures at levels greater than 1000 times the level where no effects are seen (the 'no observed effect level'). Citizens can sue the companies if they fail to provide such warning. Proposition 65 has prompted numerous product reformulations inspired by a desire to avoid having to use the label.

Environmental education also plays an important role in the management of environmental hazards. In the United States, hazards like radon gas in homes and environmental tobacco smoke have largely been managed, on a federal level, by providing education to the public. Environmental educators can also play an important role in helping to translate complex hazard and prevention information so that it is better understood by the public.

International agreements and the emergence of international standards for chemicals

A number of international organizations are responsible for aspects of environmental health practice (Table 12.8.3). As is true for nations, this too is a complex web of activity. Already mentioned are the roles of international organizations in the assessment and policy-making functions of environmental health practice. There are global and regional agreements to prevent climate change,

Table 12.8.3 International organizations involved in environmental protection

Acronym	Organization	Environmental health scope
UNEP	United Nations (UN) Environment Program	Environmental agreements, chemical information systems, technical assistance, right to know
WHO	World Health Organization	Toxicology and epidemiology, IARC, technical assistance
UNCED	UN Commission for Environment and Development	Implementation of Agenda 21 treaty signed in 1992
UNDP	UN Development Program	Sustainable development, growth and population issues
FAO	Food and Agriculture Organization	Pesticides and other agricultural health issues. Food safety (Codex Alimentarius)
IMO	International Maritime Organization	Seafood safety and protection of the seas
OECD	Organization for Economic Cooperation and Development	Harmonization of chemicals testing and classification, good laboratory practices for chemicals, cooperation on waste disposal, climate and other issues
IPCC	International Program on Climate Change	Scientific assessment of climate change
IFCS	Intergovernmental Forum on Chemical Safety	Cooperation on global chemical safety issues
ILO	International Labor Organization	Workplace health and safety; chemicals labelling in the workplace (MSDSs)
SAICM	Strategic Approach to International Chemicals Management	Carries out Global Plan of Action for international management of chemicals
UNCTDG	UN Commission on Transport of Dangerous Goods	Harmonization of classification and labels for chemicals in transport

control emission of ozone-depleting chemicals and decrease acid rain. These include: The Montreal Protocol on Substances that Deplete the Ozone Layer (United Nations Environment Programme, Secretariat for The Vienna Convention for the Protection of the Ozone Layer, and The Montreal Protocol on Substances that Deplete the Ozone Layer 2000), the Rotterdam Convention on Prior Informed Consent, for import of certain toxic chemicals (United Nations Environment Programme 1998) and the Stockholm Convention on Persistent Organic Pollutants (United Nations Environment Programme 2001).

Given the reality of the extensive global trade in chemicals, an internationally-harmonized approach to classification and labelling, which was called 'Globally Harmonized System of Classification and Labeling of Chemicals (GHS)', has recently been adopted. The 2007 edition of the GHS is published at http://www.unece.org/trans/danger/publi/ghs/ghs_welcome_e.html. It is a voluntary system for hazard classification of chemicals. Implementation by nations will require several years but will be important for public health protection and right to know internationally.

Only in recent years have pollutant release and transfer registers begun to be established globally. Under the Aarhus Convention on Access to Information, Public Participation in Decision-making and Access to Justice in Environmental Matters of the UN Economic Commission for Europe (UNECE), there is a protocol for pollutant release and transfer registries that was adopted in 2003. It is not yet in force but is open for participation by all countries globally.

These developments are evidence of a gradual emergence of *international standards*. However, it is important to emphasize that all environmental agreements in existence today recognize the sovereign right and responsibility of nations to set their own standards and tend to get involved only with transboundary issues such as movement of pollutants, trade in hazardous goods and trade in hazardous wastes. For example, the Basel Convention on the Control of Transboundary Movements of Hazardous Wastes and their Disposal contains no provisions relevant to the proper handling and disposal of such wastes generated within a country. As another example, under the Rotterdam Convention on Prior Informed Consent, the covered chemicals may be manufactured and distributed within a country without any prior consent.

In the chemicals arena, the SAICM (Strategic Approach to International Chemicals Management) has developed an *overarching policy strategy* that established objectives for international chemicals risk reduction, knowledge and information, governance, capacity-building and technical cooperation and illegal international traffic, as well as underlying principles and financial and institutional arrangements. Coordinated by UNEP the SAICM Global Plan of Action, which sets out proposed 'work areas and activities' for implementation of the Strategic Approach (http://www.chem.unep.ch/saicm/). Additionally, the Intergovernmental Forum on Chemical Safety contributes to the implementation of the Strategic Approach to International Chemicals Management (SAICM) and the work of other chemicals-related international organizations and institutions by providing an open and inclusive forum where governments and nongovernmental organizations can bring forth new issues with regards to chemicals management (http://www.who.int/ifcs/en/).

Environmental management in developing countries

Environmental health policies and laws are the major driving forces in the prevention of environment-related diseases. Many developing countries are signatories to international treaties and agreements as to environmental protection, sustainable development and health protection and promotion. However, achieving the goals of these agreements is, in many instances, very difficult for these countries.

As primary prevention of disease, some developing countries have enacted and enforced environmental laws covering areas such as water resources, clean air, toxic chemicals, pesticides, hazardous waste management, and solid waste management. However, specific policy-making and environmental standard setting efforts are limited by the lack of relevant epidemiological data and control measures to underpin strategies for preventing the health effects of environmental pollution. For example, indoor air pollution has taken its toll on children's health in many developing countries. Indoor smoke from biomass cooking fuel and second-hand cigarette smoke are significant triggers for asthma attacks (Etzel 2003; Desai *et al.* 2004). The lack of local epidemiological and exposure data deters the development of environmental standards for indoor air pollutants, so that pollution abatement strategies are difficult if not impossible to implement.

Another example for developing countries is the lack of remediation goals for sites contaminated by chemicals. There are insufficient local epidemiological, exposure and environmental data to support development of environmental clean-up standards to reduce the contamination to practically reasonable levels by which health risks are minimized. Moreover, many contaminated sites—such as vacant lot or open spaces or rivers, where wastes have been dumped or buried—have no known legal 'owners' and there are no funds for the government to clean these sites.

Conclusions

In conclusion, the practice of environmental health has come a long way in the last several decades. Although there is still much to be learned about environmental health risks, today, we do possess not only a tremendous fund of knowledge but also a number of tools, and areas of expertise, that can be brought to bear to address the most hazardous environmental conditions. We can point to many achievements that have been gained over the years such as, improvements in sanitation, alleviation of some of the worst sorts of air pollution, prevention of lead poisoning and removal of some of the most hazardous substances from consumer and household products. At the same time, the job is not done and there is a tremendous need for strengthening the practice of environmental health on a global basis. Particularly, those living in poverty continue to be deprived of safe drinking water, food, air, housing and consumer products. The rapid pace of several factors involved with global change, including, population growth, economic globalization, natural resource depletion, and climate change, are likely to create even more challenges to assuring safe environments globally. At the same time, these same conditions are opening up new opportunities. As economies transition, there can be more opportunities to engage in efforts to improve environmental health, as well as to expand the opportunities for training environmental health professionals in developing countries. Likewise, the global nature of many of the challenges we face today are likely to promote further action to develop global governance systems for assuring environmental health (Carpenter 2003).

Key points

- Environmental health practice is best understood within a broader context of efforts to improve health of communities, but it involves a much broader range of interests and stakeholders than other areas of public health practice.

- A critical component of environmental health practice is assuring a healthy environment through environmental management efforts, which involve a broad range of disciplines (medical, engineering, public health) as well as approaches (based on engineering controls, risk-based standards setting, information-based efforts and pollution prevention).

- Environmental health impact assessment is an important tool for review of development projects in order to determine the likely environmental and health consequences before decisions are taken.

- Environmental health policy development occurs at all levels of government and, internationally; it is informed by scientific evidence, economic analyses, considerations of justice, and principles of sustainable development, such as, the precautionary principle and the polluter pays principle.

- Environmental health assessment and monitoring provide important feedback to practitioners in developing priorities for action and assessing the efficacy of past efforts; numerous data are relevant, including risk assessments, environmental health surveillance, and monitoring levels of pollutants in air, water, food, and products.

References

Barnes, D. and Dourson, M. (1988). Reference dose (RfD): description and use in health risk assessments. *Regulatory Toxicology and Pharmacology*, **8**, 471–86.

Carlarne, C. (2007). From the USA with love: sharing home-grown hormones, GMOs, and clones with a reluctant Europe. *Environmental Law*, **37**(Spring), 301–36.

Carpenter, D.O. (2003). The need for global environmental health policy. *New Solutions*, **13**(1), 53–9.

Centers for Disease Control and Prevention (2005). *Third National Report on human exposure to environmental chemicals*. CDC, Atlanta.

Desai, M., Mehta, S., and Smith, K. (2004). Indoor smoke from solid fuels: assessing the environmental burden of disease at national and local levels. *Environmental Burden of Disease Series*, (4). World Health Organization, Protection of the Human Environment, Geneva.

Dubos, R. (1965). *Man adapting*. Yale University Press, New Haven.

Etzel, R.A. (2003). How environmental exposures influence the development and exacerbation of asthma. *Pediatrics*, **112**(1 Pt 2), 233–9.

Gakidou, E., Oza, S., Vidal Fuertes, C. et al. (2007). Improving child survival through environmental and nutritional interventions: the importance of targeting interventions toward the poor. *JAMA*, **298**(16), 1876–87.

Goldman, L.R. and Tran, N. (2002). *Preventable tragedies: the impact of toxic substances on the poor in developing countries: a report to the World Bank*. The World Bank, Washington, DC.

Institute of Medicine (1988). *The future of public health*. National Academy Press, Washington, DC.

Institute of Medicine and Committee on Environmental Justice (1999). *Toward environmental justice: research, education and health policy issues*. National Academy Press, Washington, DC.

Kyesku, P. (2003). The evolution of the pollution inventory. *Environmental Information Bulletin*, **128**, 12–5.

McMichael, A.J., Woodruff, R.E., and Hales, S. (2006). Climate change and human health: present and future risks. *Lancet*, **367**(9513), 859–69.

Morgenstern, H. (1982). Uses of ecologic analysis in epidemiologic research. *American Journal of Public Health*, **72**(12), 1336–44.

National Research Council (1983). *Risk assessment in the federal government: managing the process*. National Academy Press, Washington, DC.

National Research Council (1991). *Environmental epidemiology: public health and hazardous wastes*. National Academy Press, Washington, DC.

National Research Council (1993). *Pesticides in the diets of infants and children*. National Academy Press, Washington, DC.

Office of the President and Republic of the Philippines (1992). *Executive Order No. 489. Institutionalizing the Inter-agency Committee on Environmental Health.*

Organisation for Economic Co-operation and Development and Environment Directorate (1991). *Decision-recommendation of the council on the co-operative investigation and risk reduction of existing chemicals C(90)163/final.* Organisation for Economic Co-operation and Development, Paris.

Pruss-Ustun, A. and Corvalan, C. (2006). *Preventing disease through healthy environments.* World Health Organization, Geneva.

Rogan, W.J. (1995). Environmental poisoning of children – lessons from the past. *Environmental Health Perspectives*, **103** (Suppl. 6), 19–23.

Thacker, S.B. and Stroup, D.F. (1994). Future directions for comprehensive public health surveillance and health information systems in the United States. *American Journal of Epidemiology*, **140**(5), 383–97.

Thacker, S.B., Stroup, D.F., Parrish, R.G., and Anderson, H.A. (1996). Surveillance in environmental public health: issues, systems, and sources [see comments] [published erratum appears in Am J Public Health 1996 Nov;86(11):1526]. *American Journal of Public Health*, **86**(5), 633–8.

The Presidential/Congressional Commission on Risk Assessment and Risk Management (1997). *Framework for Environmental Health Risk Management*, Washington, DC.

U.S. Department of Health and Human Services and National Toxicology Program (2005). *Report on carcinogens, Eleventh Edition.* U.S. Department of Health and Human Services, Public Health Service, Research Triangle Park.

United Nations Conference on Environment and Development (1992). *Rio declaration on environment and development.* United Nations, Rio de Janeiro.

United Nations Environment Programme (1998). *Convention on the prior informed consent procedure for certain hazardous chemicals and pesticides in international trade.* UNEP, Rotterdam.

United Nations Environment Programme (2001). *Convention on persistent organic pollutants.* UNEP, Stockholm.

United Nations Environment Programme, Secretariat for The Vienna Convention for the Protection of the Ozone Layer, and The Montreal Protocol on Substances that Deplete the Ozone Layer (2000). *The Montreal protocol on substances that deplete the ozone layer.* United Nations Environment Programme, Nairobi.

United Nations Millennium Summit (2000). *United Nations millennium declaration. Millennium development goals.* UN, New York.

Wegman, D. (1992). Hazard surveillance. In *Public health surveillance* (eds. W. Halperin and E.J. Baker), pp. 62–75. Van Nostrand Reinhold Co, New York.

World Health Organization (1994). Action plan for environmental health services in Eastern and Central Europe and the Newly Independent States: Report on a WHO Consultation, Sofia, Bulgaria, 19–22 October 1993. WHO Regional Office for Europe, Copenhagen.

World Health Organization.(1997). *EHIA Framework for the Western Pacific Region.*

World Summit on Sustainable Development (2002). *World summit declares 'fault line' between rich and poor threatens prosperity, adopts broad measures to alleviate poverty, protect environment (17th Plenary Meeting (PM) and Round-up) ENV/DEV/J/35.* UN Department of Public Information, Johannesburg; News and Media Services Division, New York.

Yassi, A., Kjellstrom, T., de Kok, T., and Guidotti, T. (2001). *Basic environmental health.* Oxford University Press, New York.

Structures and strategies for public health intervention

Don Nutbeam and Marilyn Wise

Abstract

The earlier chapters of this book confirm that the scientific basis for public health is well developed and evolving in response to emerging public health challenges. However, to achieve the goal of improving the health of populations and improving equity in health, this science must be applied both within the health sector and more broadly in society in ways that have an impact on the social determinants of health.

The application of the science of public health is dependent upon the existence of an infrastructure for public health action that provides strategic and technical public health leadership, and contributes directly to the development and implementation of policies and programmes that are necessary to deliver improvements in the health of populations. Such infrastructure must also include the capacity to form partnerships with communities and with organizations across different sectors that support the delivery of public health services and programmes, as well as the capacity to evaluate and report routinely on progress.

This chapter analyses and describes key elements of an infrastructure for public health that have been found to be effective in guiding national action, and the components of an infrastructure and delivery system required to design, deliver, and evaluate public health interventions. Public health intervention requires a complex mix of science, art (of practice), and politics. Four key challenges for the future emerge from this analysis: The need to address all determinants of health, the importance of gaining greater public visibility for public health, the need to increase our capacity to work across sectors to develop policy and plans to improve health, and the importance of working with all the people and organizations that have a role in improving or protecting the health of populations.

Introduction

Current and emerging public health problems require the application of existing knowledge and strategies within the health sector and more broadly in society in ways that have an impact on the key determinants of health such as environment, education and employment. The greatest contemporary public health challenge is to ensure that there is action to achieve equity—to eliminate the unjust gaps in life expectancy and health across the life span that have proven to be persistent within wealthy and poor nations and, of course, between nations.

The most explicit sign of a nation's commitment can be found in the extent to which public policy and investment are linked explicitly to achieving improved population health and reducing inequity. Examples of this type of commitment can be observed in countries such as Sweden, Canada, and the United Kingdom (Agren 2003; Public Health Agency of Canada 2007; Wanless 2004). But in addition to policy, action is needed. The translation of policy (and resources) into effective action is dependent upon the existence of an infrastructure for public health action that provides both strategic and technical public health leadership, and that contributes directly to the development and implementation of policies and programmes that are necessary to deliver improvements in the health of populations. Such infrastructure must also include the capacity to form partnerships with communities, and with organizations across different sectors that support the delivery of public health services and programmes, as well as the capacity to evaluate and report routinely on progress.

Figure 12.9.1 provides an overview of the essential elements of such a system, and provides the structure for this chapter. Based on analysis of experiences in several countries, the Figure traces the steps which link identification of the determinants of health, through definition of priorities and development of policy, to the infrastructure and delivery systems required by countries and regions to guide and implement effective public health action (International Union for Health Promotion and Education 1999; National Health and Medical Research Council 1997; Mittelmark et al. 2007).

Figure 12.9.1 describes an infrastructure and delivery system that enables countries or regions to apply public health science both to the identification and analysis of the determinants of public health problems, and to the design, delivery and evaluation of public health interventions. The infrastructure includes the capacity to link evidence of the effectiveness of these public health actions with regular review and re-definition of problems and priorities for public health and for related policy, and to a system of public accountability for progress (Australian Institute of Health and Welfare 2006a; NSW Health 2007).

Following the structure in Fig. 12.9.1, the chapter explores the need for an initial analysis of the determinants of public health problems—economic and social, alongside behavioural and environmental—and of their distribution across populations and communities. These analyses then provide the raw material for political, professional and community debate on the issues/problems to be given greatest priority, and to identify the most effective interventions to address their causes and health consequences. This will often include action with sectors other than the health sector in the development of public policy interventions.

Expanding the vision of national health policies beyond the provision of health care services has proved to be consistently challenging around the world. This is especially the case in attempting to develop 'health policies' that address the underlying determinants of health that are often outside of the scope and immediate influence of Health Ministries or Health Ministers. The chapter begins with examples of different initiatives taken to date by governments. It goes on to identify the explicit components of infrastructure and capacity needed by the health sector in particular (and government in general) to direct and guide action to achieve improved population health and reductions in inequity.

Policies and interventions to address the determinants of health in populations

Earlier chapters in this book describe the range of personal, social, economic and environmental factors that are related to increased risk of disease, and of adverse outcomes from disease. Analysis of the determinants of the health of populations is essential to clarify the relative importance of each, and to identify those that are modifiable through public health intervention.

These determinants include individual characteristics and behaviours, such as smoking, physical activity, hypertension or diet, which have been the focus for the majority of public health interventions in high-income countries to reduce the burden of non-communicable disease in the population over recent decades. Epidemiological analysis also reveals major differences in the disease experiences of different groups in populations with different social, economic and environmental circumstances. Although some of these differences can be explained by differences in individuals' health-related behaviours (such as tobacco use and food choices), more of the difference is explained by the different social, economic and environmental circumstances in which people live and work (Raphael 2007; Marmot & Wilkinson 1999).

For example, in the case of coronary heart disease Marmot's work in the United Kingdom has indicated that a high proportion of the variance in premature deaths between different social groups cannot be adequately explained by known behavioural and other personal risk factors. Other factors, related to differences in the social status and economic conditions of different groups within a population, clearly play a major role in determining the health status of populations. The distribution of these conditions is socially determined and is beyond the control of individuals, and is not amenable to change through health sector related activities alone.

However, it is increasingly clear that policies and interventions to modify these social, economic, and environmental conditions have

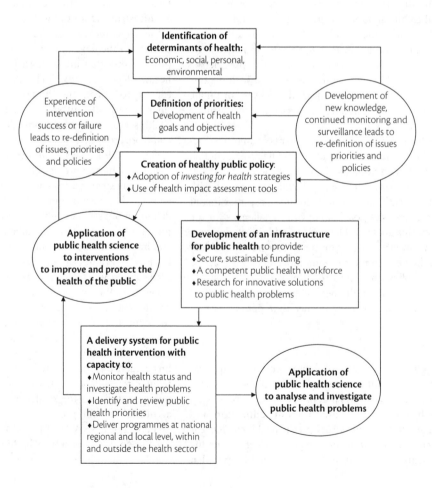

Fig. 12.9.1 Overview of an infrastructure for public health intervention.

the potential to produce even greater gains in health status than those attributed to changes in lifestyles and improved health care in many high-income countries in the past two decades.

This is not a new discovery. Creating supportive environments for health has been a major goal of public health policy and action for the past 150 years. Environmental interventions to provide clean water and waste disposal, safe food, and safe living and working conditions led to major improvements in public health in industrialized countries. Programmes to improve maternal and child health, and effective mass immunization programmes have been effective in reducing morbidity and mortality among children in most countries throughout the twentieth century.

However, over the course of the twentieth century the very success of public health policy, research and practice meant that it became 'invisible' in many countries. In industrialized countries, the public health policies, strategies and structures that had been so effective in reducing mortality and morbidity across their populations were in decline by the middle of the twentieth century. In most countries the great proportion of health sector investment has been (and remains) in biomedical intervention. In high-income countries, in particular, public health interventions have tended to become marginalized within the health sector, and rather narrowly focused on the identification of biological and behavioural risk factors for non-communicable diseases—followed by interventions that aimed to change individuals' lifestyles.

This has meant that progress toward improving the health of populations has been limited and that the benefits have been distributed unequally and unfairly. Limited public health interventions to address behavioural risks have had an impact on the lifestyles of those who are wealthier and better educated—those best placed to make personal changes in their lifestyles. But there is evidence that these interventions may also have had an unintended effect of exaggerating existing differences in health status between social groups.

The need to expand health policy to include explicit commitment to improving the health of populations (and not, simply, to responding to disease and injury), and to eliminating unjust inequalities in the distribution of health was identified more than 30 years ago by the World Health Organization (WHO). The concept of *Health for All* was adopted as the main social target of governments and the WHO at that time (World Health Organization 1980). This resolution represented a commitment to explore new avenues to solve public health problems and gave prominent attention to the need to reduce growing health inequalities between and within countries. *Health for All* provided a major focal point for a renaissance in public health action, and impetus for a long overdue examination of health policy, infrastructure, capacity and evidence.

However, even with the evidence and WHO leadership it has proven difficult for health sectors (and governments) in most countries to use this knowledge to design and implement the interventions necessary to achieve the goal of *Health for All*, and to build the infrastructure and capacity to deliver these effectively and efficiently.

Designing effective interventions

All health problems in any population have multiple causes or determinants. Finding ways of taking action that effectively address these represents a major challenge for governments and public health systems in all countries. In the 1980s, WHO led a series of processes designed to reinvigorate public health practice by bringing a wider range of disciplinary perspectives to public health interventions. These reforms were in response to changes in the disease profile in most high-income countries resulting from the emergence of health problems that have their origins in individual behaviours and social conditions. This 'new public health' methodology was referred to as *health promotion*. For many, a significant turning point in the conversion of this renewed interest and understanding into public health action came through the *Ottawa Charter for Health Promotion* (World Health Organization 1986). The Charter advocated a 'new' approach to public health, where public health intervention had come to be understood as action which is directed towards improving people's control over all modifiable determinants of health.

The late twentieth century saw the growth of evidence confirming that it is possible to act purposefully to improve the health of populations—to reduce the incidence of acute and chronic conditions, to reduce the prevalence of some conditions, and to reduce deaths associated with these (International Union for Health Promotion and Education 1999; Centers for Disease Control and Prevention 1999; Wanless 2004). Although progress has been achieved through interventions that are highly targeted to the needs of specific population groups, on its own, this is neither optimally effective nor efficient in achieving the shift in population risk first described by Geoffrey Rose (1992). Taking smoking as an example, although there are some good targeted interventions (e.g. for pregnant women) the greatest progress in reducing the prevalence of smoking in a population has been achieved by combining efforts to communicate to people the benefits of not smoking with a wider set of measures to reinforce and sustain this healthy lifestyle choice. This has meant taking action to reduce demand through restrictions on promotion and increases in price, to reduce supply by restrictions on access (especially to minors), and to reflect social unacceptability through environmental bans (Bonnie *et al.* 2007). Such a comprehensive approach addresses the underlying social and economic determinants of individuals' behavioural choices, and was recognized formally in the world's first international public health treaty—the Framework Convention on Tobacco Control (2003) that was adopted at the World Health Assembly in 2003.

This same comprehensive approach to implementing a complex array of actions to address public health problems is being highlighted in contemporary efforts to reduce or at least slow the advance of obesity in populations across the globe (Popkin 2007).

However, such actions, although successful in reducing the prevalence of some major diseases and behavioural risk factors across populations (on average), have not, as yet, proven to be effective in reducing the pre-existing inequities in the distribution of the social determinants of health within populations. The need to expand action to more overtly address these social determinants is now being recognized (Norwegian Ministry of Health and Care Services 2007). Evidence-based actions to address the impact of social determinants of health are gradually emerging (Raphael 2007; Whitehead 2007; World Bank Povertynet 2007; Cutler & Lleras-Muney 2007; Kawachi *et al.* 1999). More needs to be done to convert our understanding of the causes of inequalities into practical, politically manageable policies and actions. In 2003, the World Health Organization established a Commission on the Social Determinants of Health to focus more precisely on identifying actions to address the social determinants of health effectively, and to stimulate governments, the private sector and civil society to take these actions (World Health Organization 2006). The WHO Bangkok Charter (2005) affirmed that policies and partnerships to empower communities and to improve health and health equality should be at the centre of global and national development.

Determining directions and priorities for public health intervention

The 1980s saw the development of national health policy in several countries that incorporated, for the first time, national health goals and objectives—expressed as quantifiable, population-wide health outcomes. The US national health objectives (US Department of Health and Human Services 1980) and the World Health Organization European Region promoted health targets as a mechanism for defining the outcomes expected of nations' investment in 'health', as a mechanism for defining differences in health status between populations and as a mechanism for targeting reductions in these differences—the central tenet of *Health for All* (World Health Organization, Regional Office for Europe 1985, 1999). Several other nations followed these leads in the 1980s and 1990s (Nutbeam & Wise 1996).

The initial rationale for setting national health goals and targets was to link national health investment with improved population health outcomes. In specifying this link, it was intended that the role of public health interventions (in addition to the provision of health care services) would become more prominent—highlighting the need for interventions to prevent the onset of disease and occurrence of injury, in addition to the interventions to diagnose, treat, and rehabilitate people with symptoms or established illness. For the first time, nations were establishing *a priori* benchmarks against which to measure the effectiveness and efficiency of their investments in the health of populations. In itself, this shift in focus was a significant conceptual step for governments, for health professionals and populations—from a focus on the provision of health care services to a focus on the achievement of population health outcomes.

Although there are similarities in the rationale for setting national health goals and targets across nations, there has been considerable strategic and technical variation in their development, in their scope, and in their intended impact. It is useful to analyse some of these variations in order to identify the strengths and weaknesses of the different approaches, and to assess their implications for the future.

Developing national health goals and targets is a significant technical undertaking, and the process in most countries has revealed the need for expanded national health information systems to gather, analyse and report on the health of their populations over time. This has required clarity in understanding of the links between health outcomes and their determinants. It has also required the definition of indicators that measure health outcomes (mortality and morbidity, life expectancy and quality of life), as well as indicators of the social and behavioural determinants of the health of populations, and of the distribution of health in populations. These challenges in turn have highlighted strengths and weaknesses in national health data and in the data available from other sectors that impact on health determinants.

Setting health objectives and targets also requires some form of explicit prioritization—inevitably it involves identification of objectives and targets in relation to a relatively defined range of health issues, population groups or settings that would receive greatest attention and investment.

Australia's experience in setting national health goals and targets provides an example of these processes. Work on national targets began in 1987, resulting in a narrowly defined group of priority health issues and behavioural risk factors in 1988 (Health Targets and Implementation Committee 1988). But in 1993 a major revision expanded the scope of the targets beyond the limited range of the initial report (Nutbeam *et al.* 1993). This work saw the inclusion of two new categories of health targets concerned with *personal health literacy* and *healthy environments*, and a section focusing explicitly on the role of health services in achieving the overall goals and targets.

Figure 12.9.2 is derived from the report and provides an illustration of the framework for the targets, showing how each of three key determinants of health—health literacy, health behaviours, and healthy environments—is inextricably linked to the other. The report made a strong case for coordinated public health action to address all of the determinants, particularly by adding to existing efforts to promote health literacy and healthy lifestyles with matching attention to the creation of healthy environments.

The Australian experience provides an example of the ways in which health targets can be used to highlight and address the social, economic and environmental determinants of health status. The report was also structured partly to reflect the way in which government was organized into Ministries (e.g. housing, employment, environment), and partly to build upon existing working relations between the health sector and other sectors (e.g. health promoting schools). Such an approach was seen as important both in defining the respective roles of the different sectors, in establishing a workable model for monitoring progress, and determining accountability for the achievement of targets (Nutbeam *et al.* 1993).

More recently, other governments have been strong advocates of the use of targets in all sectors to set priorities, and to make explicit expectations for change over time. In England two 'headline' targets were set to reduce health inequalities over a 10-year period. These medium-term targets are backed by a set of 12 short-term indicators that were adopted as a way of assessing progress within 10 years through several ministries in addressing the underlying determinants of health across a range of sectors (Department of Health 2003). Table 12.9.1 lists the two headline targets and 12 national indicators.

A further distinction among the goals and targets set by different nations exists in the extent to which the process was used to identify the strategies (policies and programmes) that would be necessary to achieve them, and to allocate responsibility for action. In the United States for example, the implementation of policies and programmes to achieve the objectives was substantially a responsibility of each individual state (and not of the Federal government), and of organizations/agencies of civil society as well as the private sector that had contributed to setting the goals and targets, and to establishing priorities.

By contrast, the targets and indicators established in England have been developed following a Treasury review of spending by different ministries to assess the extent to which their respective policies and programmes contributed to the action necessary to reduce health inequalities. This review led to a cross-government strategy that specifies the actions and responsibilities of different

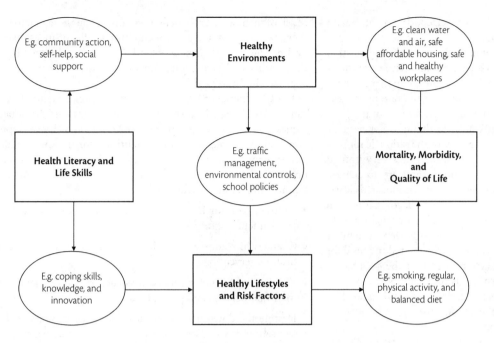

Fig. 12.9.2 The relationship between the four groups of health targets. Examples of targets are shown in oval boxes.
Source: Nutbeam *et al.* (1993).

Table 12.9.1 English health inequalities targets, and headline indicators

Health inequalities targets

1. Infant mortality
   A 10% reduction in the relative gap (i.e. percentage difference) in infant mortality rates between the 'routine and manual' socioeconomic group and England as a whole from the baseline year of 1998 (the average of 1997–1999) to the target year 2010 (the average of 2009–2011).

2. Life expectancy
   A 10% reduction in the relative gap (i.e. percentage difference) in life expectancy at birth between the fifth of areas with the worst health and deprivation indicators and England as a whole.

Headline indicators

1. Preventable deaths
   Age-standardized death rates per 100 000 population for the major killer diseases (cancer, circulatory disease), ages under 75 (for the 20% of areas with the highest rates compared with the national average.

2. Teenage pregnancies
   Rate of under-18 conceptions comparing differences by area of deprivation.

3. Road accident casualties
   Road accident casualties comparing differences by area of deprivation.

4. Access to primary care
   Number of primary care professionals per 100 000 population comparing differences by area of deprivation.

5. Uptake of flu vaccinations
   Percentage uptake of flu vaccinations by older people (aged 65+) comparing differences by area of deprivation.

6a. Prevalence of smoking
   Prevalence of smoking among people in manual social groups.

6b. Prevalence of smoking among pregnant woman
   Prevalence of smoking among pregnant woman comparing differences by area of deprivation.

7. Educational attainment
   Proportion of those aged 16 who get qualifications equivalent to five GCSEs at grades A to C comparing national average with schools in the most disadvantaged communities

8. Fruit consumption
   Proportion of people consuming five or more portions of fruit and vegetables per day in the lowest quintile of household income distribution.

9. Housing quality
   Proportion of households living in non-decent housing comparing private and social housing status.

10. Physical activity
   Percentage of schoolchildren who spend a minimum of two hours each week on high-quality PE and school sport and beyond the curriculum comparing national average with schools in the most disadvantaged communities

11. Poverty
   Proportion of children living in low-income households.

12. Homelessness
   Number of homeless families with children in temporary accommodation

Source: Department of Health (2006). *Tackling health inequalities: Status report on the program for action 2006, Update on headline indicators.* London, DOH.

ministries and agencies of government (Department of Health 2002; Department of Health 2003).

Despite the significant conceptual and technical progress that has been achieved, the twenty-first century has seen less enthusiasm for the use of goals and objectives as a core component of their national health policy. It is important, however, to examine the reasons for this shift and to reflect on its meaning for the future.

The Australian experience was similar to that of other nations. Although there was widespread acceptance of the rationale for preparing national health goals and targets, there was very limited investment in the infrastructure or actions necessary to achieve them. Responsibility for their achievement was not allocated clearly in the ensuing health policy environment. Instead, governments in Australia invested in a relatively small public health programme to address some priority issues (Commonwealth Department of Human Services and Health 1994) but largely ignored the need for their own commitment to lead action to address the social, economic and environmental determinants of health. Nor was there any investment in reorienting health services to align their work to ensure that they accounted for their contributions to the achievement of population health outcomes.

Other nations' experiences mirrored these. Busse and Wismar (2002) highlighted the fact that in no country or region did the health goals and targets policy outline the scale and redistribution of health sector resources that would be necessary to achieve the health goals and targets. Nor did the policies identify the health service and public health infrastructure and capacity necessary to lead and deliver interventions, or to report on progress.

Reviewing experience in eight countries, Allin *et al.* (2004) concluded that, to date, health goals and targets remain political constructs that have been a source of inspiration rather than explicit benchmarks against which to account for progress in improving a nation's health. As with all political processes to set priorities for spending, changes in government, or even changes in Ministers, have led to reinterpretation of the nature and purposes of the targets, and substantial dislocation of any actions that had been previously committed to (Nutbeam & Wise 1996; Beaglehole & Davis 1992; Wismar 2002).

The processes of establishing goals and targets have contributed significantly to the technical development of public health. The conceptual frameworks, the indicator development, the evolution of national and local health information systems to report on social and economic determinants of health in addition to the biological and behavioural determinants, and the development of a much stronger body of research identifying and tracking inequalities in the health status of populations are all positive outcomes of the initiatives to establish national health goals and targets. So, too, is the growing body of evidence of effective interventions, and the routine public reporting on the health of populations that provides governments, organizations and communities with the information necessary to guide future investment. This applies not only at the national level but also at the state/province/regional level (NSW Health 2007). In the United States, the objectives offered a benchmark against which changes in population health status could be observed over time, and acted as a catalyst for response (US Department of Health and Human Services 1995, 2006).

Conceptually, health goals and targets are the proposed outcomes of a nation's entire investment in the health of its population.

Much of their potential benefit, therefore, lies in the extent to which they are used to guide and measure the results of investments in health. The example from England that involved leadership from the Treasury, and a cross-government response offers a much clearer approach in this regard.

The US experience has suggested that national health objectives can survive changes in government provided they are developed by a quasi-independent agency, are based on good technical support, and are supported by strong coalitions for action outside of government. Overall, in those countries that have adopted health objectives or targets, the objectives appear to have played an important role in focusing on the need for:

♦ A broad base for health policy across the different sectors of government

♦ Changes in resource allocation to develop capacity for public health intervention

♦ The development of methods and structures which enable action to promote health and prevent disease

Despite the downturn in enthusiasm in recent years goal and target setting is still used as a tool for determining priorities, and achieving accountability for health outcomes. One example of great public health significance has been the commitment of countries and international organizations to the Millennium Development Goals (MDGs). The MDGs are intended to provide a mechanism through which to join public health initiatives to engage with the global organizations, industries and social movements that make global economic, social, environmental, and trade decisions, in particular (United Nations. 2000).

Developing public policy for health: Health in all policies

Whilst setting goals for improvement in the underlying determinants of health that are outside the health sector have provided a useful stimulus in some situations, other mechanisms need to be utilized as an alternative, or to complement and extend this approach. Actions to improve and protect the health of the public have to be grounded in a policy structure which is sensitive to the impact on health policy decisions across all government sectors, and which maximises opportunities for matching economic and social development goals with health development goals and objectives.

This logic is the basis for WHO's *Investment for Health* strategy which offers a model for achieving a 'whole of government' approach to improving public health. This strategy is described as:

> *a practical approach based on the rationale that resources are best applied in a way that not only addresses the main causes of ill-health in a credible, effective and ethical manner, but also furthers the achievement of goals for social and economic development.*

The key elements of the *Investment for Health* concept concern achieving a strong commitment to health in policy making across all government ministries, a commitment to intersectoral working, and a continued focus on equity (World Health Organization 2002). Health improvement will not always be the primary policy goal, but the strategy represents a commitment to assess the *population health impact* (both positive and negative) of public policy decisions, development strategies and investment decisions, particularly those with social and economic implications. Economic development becomes a means of improving both the social infrastructure and people's health. Tools for *health impact assessment* are essential to support this element of the strategy and there is a growing body of evidence on the use of formal health impact assessment and its impact on policy-making (Kemm 2006).

Though the rationale for the health sector to work with other sectors is strong, the experience with working in partnership with other sectors has highlighted the need for the health sector to avoid imposing its own priorities on the core business of other sectors and to ensure that all partners are able to identify the benefits that will flow from working in collaboration. Building on existing common ground between sectors, combined with transparency in purpose, and investment in building inter-organizational and interpersonal relationships appear to offer a basis for developing effective partnerships that are required to advance health and achieve greater equity in health by addressing its underlying determinants (Padgett *et al.* 2004). Where progress has been achieved it has, most often, been through bilateral partnerships between the health services and other sectors. In the latter case such action is most achievable where there is obvious mutual benefit, and where the roles and responsibilities of each sector and are clearly defined (Harris *et al.* 1996).

The WHO has revived its focus on equity through the work of the Commission on the Social Determinants of Health. The work of the commission is directed toward improving understanding of the social determinants of health and their unequal impact on health between and within populations, and between countries. Equity in this case implies that all people will have equal opportunity to develop and maintain their health through a fair distribution of the resources and opportunities that support health. A mix of programmes to address fundamental differences in opportunity and access to resources, as well as targeted programmes for disadvantaged individuals and communities, is required to support this element of the strategy.

Achieving such a substantial commitment to health is by no means an easy political task. The European Office of the WHO carried out national *Investment for Health* Appraisals in several countries including Slovenia, Hungary, Romania, and Malta (Ziglio *et al.* 2000). This involved external appraisal and reporting back to the Health Ministry and/or Parliament on:

- The strategy needed to improve the health status of the population

- The potential for investment for health in the country

- The infrastructure needed to build, support, and sustain *Investment for Health*

Each part of the appraisal identified the opportunities to promote health more effectively through key economic and social development policies. This strategy represented a sophisticated attempt to put into public health practice the logical consequences of contemporary analyses of what determines health in populations. Although the approach has been implemented for less than a decade, it illustrates the important challenge facing public health advocates and practitioners. This challenge is to engage government, civil society, and the private sector in dialogue about the health impact of policies and practices, and to consider the scope for a synergistic relationship between health, economic, and social development strategies.

Like health goals and targets, the *Investing in Health* strategy is not a substitute for investment in a public health infrastructure in countries. Rather, it is a mechanism that facilitates the dialogue needed to link investment for health with economic and social development, and support action across sectors to improve the health of the public. One recent example of this mechanism at work is that of the European Commission, which has taken action to ensure that there is a high level of human health protection in all Community activities, and has codified this as a central part of the Community's responsibilities (WHO European Office for Investment in Health and Development 2007; Stahl *et al.* 2006).

Developing infrastructure and delivery systems for public health interventions

To be effective, the science of public health must be 'applied'. The science, strategies, and tools used in public health are too often used only to describe and analyse public health problems, and to develop policy. To enjoy the fruits of this analysis, and of health-oriented public policy, it is essential that attention is also given to the development of the organizational capacity for effective public health intervention. This capacity is most often concentrated in the health sector but can be found in other sectors of government and in the non-government sector. The public health interventions include the health education and health promotion strategies described in previous chapters, as well as other forms of public health intervention required to assist people and communities *improve their control over the determinants of health*.

The limited shifts in government investment and action to support the achievement of their national health goals and priorities are both a cause and consequence of the frailty of the infrastructure for public health intervention in many countries. Although the last two decades have seen a rejuvenation of interest and investment in public health in many countries, it is still the case that much of that investment has been and continues to be *ad hoc*—in targeted programmes and services rather than in a well-resourced, sustained public health infrastructure that is capable of programme development and implementation and for routinely reporting on progress (Baker *et al.* 2005).

Creating a sustainable, specialized infrastructure for public health has proven to be a complex undertaking. Although there is strong evidence that the greatest improvements in the health of populations have arisen from social and economic developments that have an impact on health, modern health sectors have evolved to diagnose and treat diseases, their symptoms, and injuries. As a result, the 'health' debate and investment in most countries continues to centre on the accessibility and quality of health care services. The need for an effective public health service tends to be invisible both to governments and to the public except in times of crisis, and is often oriented towards the control of infectious diseases (such as the SARS epidemic). There is relatively limited public demand for a strong public health service (compared with demand for health care services) in all but exceptional circumstances (Grossman & Scala 1993). However, the evolution of health policy to include recognition of the social determinants of health and to commit governments to tackle non-communicable diseases has stimulated action by a number of countries to review and strengthen their infrastructure for public health.

Although there remain significant unanswered questions about the most effective systems or structures through which to design and deliver public health interventions, there are emerging models for defining priorities for action, for working across government to address determinants of health, and for establishing elements of an effective public health infrastructure.

The range of activities and sectors in which practitioners need to act, and the broad range of disciplines that can be said to make up the field of public health have made it challenging to define the 'core business' of public health. Several recent initiatives have sought to identify these 'core functions' (Population Health and Wellness 2005; Institute of Medicine 2003). Within these lists of core functions, essential services, and public health practices there is still a considerable lack of conceptual consistency. A mix of intended outcomes, interventions (or strategies), and principles for good practice is represented in all the lists. To help untangle these conceptual inconsistencies the distinction is made in Fig. 12.9.1 between the essential **infrastructure** required to lead the development of policy and interventions to achieve priority health goals and targets, and the **delivery system** required to develop and execute public health interventions.

Key elements of infrastructure for public health

The components of public health infrastructure are similar to those needed by all organizations to conduct their core business. In addition to the strategic direction and priority setting outlined in previous sections in this chapter, the infrastructure for public health is made up of material resources, a skilled workforce, and information from research and evaluation, that are then combined by organizations to develop and implement policies and to deliver services or interventions that promote, protect, and maintain the health of populations, and to account for progress (Baker & Koplan 2002).

Figure 12.9.1 highlights three essential components of an **infrastructure** for public health including secure and sustainable funding, a well-trained workforce, and supportive research.

Secure and sustainable funding

Aside from the *investing for health* strategy discussed earlier, secure, recurrent financial resources are required to support a public health infrastructure within the health sector. Without such investment in a dedicated infrastructure there is little chance to build a sustainable infrastructure, and even where one exists, experience has shown that the public health system can quickly lose capacity if investment declines (National Health and Medical Research Council 1997; US Department of Health and Human Services 1999).

Public health cannot work if left to market forces. Most countries have recognized the need to invest in a public health infrastructure as a 'public good'. These investments have provided capacity to analyse public health status, guide decision-making on priorities for action, and respond to public health threats, especially infectious disease outbreaks. This latter capacity has been tested considerably in past years with outbreaks of SARS and avian flu, and more general concern with preparedness for bio-terrorism. Despite these dramatic reminders, secure, sustainable funding for the design, delivery and evaluation of public health interventions directed to addressing non-communicable diseases, and to tackling the social determinants of health has proved more elusive.

This secure 'programme funding' necessary to tackle non-communicable diseases is especially vulnerable when interventions run counter to prevailing government policy or ideology, and especially when they contradict economic policy—such as in relation to the sale of alcohol or tobacco, or nutritional programmes which conflict with agricultural practices or with the food supplied by significant food industries. Providing a strong rationale for investing in public health interventions continues to be a major part of the role of public health professionals—requiring the use of science (to demonstrate effectiveness), political argument (to demonstrate professional and community concern) and practical demonstration in the form of case studies (Nutbeam 2003). Achieving sustainable funding may require more active communication and political advocacy. Baker and Koplan (2002) argue for the development of a new language to increase the public's understanding of public health, and the use of case reports and studies to sustain interest in and support for public health infrastructure.

Data on the proportion of national recurrent health sector expenditure that is accounted for by public health infrastructure and programmes in different countries indicate that it is very small, relative to expenditure on acute and chronic health care services. Furthermore, there has been little tangible progress in the last three decades in the proportion of health budgets invested in public health or health promotion. For example, in Australia, recently published data by the Australian Institute for Health and Welfare (2006b) indicates that expenditure on public health activities by Australian health departments in 2004–2005 was approximately 1.7 per cent of total recurrent health expenditure, or A$71 per person. The greatest proportion of public health expenditure (23.6%, or A$338.3 million) was on organized immunization, followed by selected health promotion (A$232.8 million) and communicable disease control (A$232.0 million). While this does not include all the funding invested in public health it provides some indication of the minimal level of public investment through the health sector that might be expected to support public health infrastructure and intervention programmes.

In many countries low levels of funding have meant that it has been necessary to find alternative sources of funding for public health interventions. A growing number of countries have established Health Promotion Foundations based, most commonly, on funding generated by taxation levied by government on the sale of tobacco products. This type of Foundation was first established in Australia as part of a strategy to replace lost income from tobacco company sponsorship of sports, arts, and cultural events. The model has been copied in several countries, both high- and middle-income countries, with general success. Foundations now engage in a diversified range of programmes and have been able to make a significant contribution to funding public health research as well as to actions to address social and environmental determinants of health (International Network of Health Promotion Foundations 2007).

The non-government and community sectors play significant roles in funding research and delivering interventions on issues such as cardiovascular disease prevention, tobacco control, or childhood injury prevention. Organizations such as Heart Foundations and Cancer Councils perform important roles in many countries, not only in raising money for research, but in conducting direct community interventions to promote health and prevent disease. There are limitations imposed by their focus on single issues and by the level of funding that they are able to raise directly from their constituencies (in addition to government support). But their high levels of credibility among health professionals and community members mean that they can also be attractive to partners in developing and implementing public health interventions.

The private sector, too, has begun to take an increasing interest in contributing to public health and social development. In many cases the benefits of partnership are obvious and mutual. For example, in several countries, the insurance industry has contributed significant levels of funding to specific programmes to reduce motor vehicle crashes, and the food industry has committed to a programme to improve consumers' recognition of healthier food options.

It is important to recognise that private sector contributions, in particular, are linked to the needs of business for community support and to assist marketing of specific goods and products. These needs do not automatically clash with public health goals, but the mutual benefit in partnerships with the private sector is not always as apparent as it could be. The WHO Jakarta Declaration provides some useful general guidance on this issue concerning the need for transparency in relationships and clearly defined mutual benefit (World Health Organization 1998). In negotiating partnership agreements with the private sector it is important to ensure that there is no potential conflict between the outcomes required by the company and the intended public health outcomes.

A well-trained, competent workforce, including capacity for leadership to guide and direct action within and outside the health sector

The delivery of essential public health services requires a skilled, competent workforce, often working in partnership with other organizations and the community (Gebbie *et al.* 2000; Gebbie and Turnock 2006; Joint Task Group on Public Health Human Resources 2005). In addition to a specifically trained public health workforce, professionals from many different sectors can be considered as part of the broad public health workforce. There is equal need to support education and professional development for both groups.

Most specialist public health training is provided at the postgraduate level through universities—usually through schools or departments of public health. In some countries medical qualifications have been a prerequisite for entry into public health training; in others a wide range of undergraduate qualifications is accepted. Many disciplines contribute to the body of knowledge that underpins the field, but there is growing agreement about the core competencies required of all members of the specialist public health workforce (Council on Linkages between Academia and Public Health Practice 2006; Joint Task Group on Public Health Human Resources 2005; Commonwealth Department of Health and Aged Care 2000). Within the field there are also several specialities that have developed advanced training programmes—epidemiology and biostatistics, health economics and health promotion being three of the more common speciality groupings. Specific competencies are also being developed in these disciplines within public health (Howat *et al.* 2000; McCracken-Rance 2000).

In some countries, governments have recognized the need to invest in training programmes to ensure that there are adequate numbers of trained public health professionals. In Australia, for example, the Public Health Education and Research Program (PHERP) was established by the Federal Department of Health and Aged Care in 1986 to fund universities to develop Master of Public Health programmes. Later, the PHERP was expanded to include funding to develop the quality and quantity of teaching and research in specific areas of special need, including environmental health, health promotion, mental health, health economics, and public health nutrition. More recently, the Program has funded innovation in developing the public health workforce necessary to meet emerging needs (such as bioterrorism, or SARS, as well as issues such as obesity), and it has expanded its focus on mechanisms to ensure that the public health workforce is 'judgement safe'. These initiatives have led to the expansion of the quality and effectiveness of the public health workforce in Australia—and to recognition of the need for regular review to ensure that the workforce is adequately prepared to meet current and emerging public health challenges (Durham & Plant 2005).

Professional associations, too, make a significant contribution to workforce development. Some of the global professional bodies with members in most countries include: Public Health Associations (linked through the World Federation of Public Health Associations [http://www.wfpha.org]), Epidemiological Associations (linked through the International Epidemiological Association [http://www.dundee.ac.uk/iea]), Health Promotion and Health Education Associations (linked through the International Union of Health Promotion and Education [http://www.iuhpe.org]). The conferences and journals produced by these organizations are essential components of workforce development infrastructure. Such associations are also important in the development of and advocacy for healthy public policy.

The opportunities for collaboration among institutions that are offered by the Internet have resulted in new possibilities to establish national and international programmes and standards of quality in public health workforce training. The Internet also offers students the opportunity to access a wider range of public health training—some of it across national borders (Davies *et al.* 2000).

Public health intervention requires special skills that are different to those required to analyse health problems in a population. Influencing health behaviour in populations, and influencing the structural and environmental determinants of health requires public health specialists to have substantial knowledge and skills in the behavioural, social and political sciences. This will require educational institutions to extend the range of current training in many cases (Institute of Medicine 2003).

This emphasis on intervention also highlights the need for a different style of leadership from senior public health practitioners. Earlier sections in this chapter have pointed to some of the difficulties inherent in collaboration across sectors. Leadership for public health intervention requires practitioners to work more closely with other sectors, to advocate effectively for the development and adoption of healthy public policy, and to create, with communities, a shared vision for the public's health. There are few programmes that explicitly address the need for advanced training for public health leadership. One example is a National Public Health Leadership Institute supported by the Centers for Disease Control and Prevention (CDC) in the United States, and based at the University of North Carolina at Chapel Hill (http://www.phli.org/aboutPHLI/index.htm).

The training of other health professionals is gradually being adapted to provide them with basic knowledge of public health. Professionals in the health sector (doctors, nurses, allied health professionals), and professionals in other sectors (such as teachers, social workers, architects and urban planners) are increasingly being involved in developing policies and programmes that contribute to improvements in the health of the population. This is a major challenge and significant area for development in public health education in the next decade.

The education systems responsible for providing workforce development lie, largely, outside the ambit of the health sector. It is necessary that there be strong links between academic institutions and agencies responsible for public health. Examples of efforts to achieve this can be seen in the United States, by the formation of the Council on Linkages between Academia and Public Health Practice, and in Australia by the Public Health Education and Research Programme.

Supportive research policy, funding, and training

Public health research and development is central to continuous improvement in the relevance, quality and impact of public health intervention. An effective system for public health research is dependent upon a national/organizational research policy that highlights the need for specific public health research—as distinct from biomedical research. It then depends upon the availability of funds specifically for public health research, and upon a strong system of peer review by qualified public health researchers. Furthermore, the strength of the research system depends on there being high-quality research training available to young researchers, and upon a career development path for public health researchers.

Research funding for public health can come from many sources. However, competition for health research funding is fierce, and public health research often competes poorly through institutions which are dominated by biomedical and health services research. Within public health research, there is also a strong bias towards descriptive/investigative epidemiological research at the cost of adequate investment in intervention research (Millward *et al.* 2003). It is important to ensure that research addresses priority health/structural issues, population groups and settings and that it also addresses the need for methodological development specific to public health intervention.

Although no single model has been identified to ensure the funding and conduct of policy-driven research that is necessary to supplement the investigator-driven research in public health, there has been growing recognition of the need for research funding bodies to ensure the balance between biomedical and public health research funding (Wanless 2004). Experience has shown that there is a continuous need for review of research funding criteria so that nations are able to develop the information they need to make effective, efficient decisions on health and medical policies and practices. But within this generic concern to find balance, strong advocacy for public health research, in particular, is required. The need for research on the systems needed to design and deliver optimal public health interventions and services to defined populations at different levels of jurisdiction has been identified (Institute of Medicine 2003). This is in addition to research on strengthening health systems more generically (Travis *et al.* 2004).

Even within the discipline of public health there has been tension between the twin intellectual approaches to public health practice—with many public health researchers focusing on the development of knowledge rather than on the actions required to solve public health problems (Hunter & Berman 1997). The most obvious manifestation of this can be seen in the overwhelming investments made in monitoring and surveillance, and in research focused on improving knowledge about public health problems and their causes, rather than on research that improves knowledge of effective

action to resolve the problems (Millward *et al.* 2003). In reviewing the available information on research funding and publication in the public health literature, it is hard to escape the conclusion that the policies of research funding agencies need to give greater weight to 'intervention' and evaluation research, and ensuring that the peer review process includes reviewers with appropriate knowledge and skills in such research.

Because effective public health interventions include a complex set of actions to bring about widespread social change there is a need for the development of research and evaluation methods that better 'fit' the context of the intervention (Nutbeam & Bauman 2006; Rootman *et al.* 2001). Several efforts are being made to identify frameworks and criteria to ensure that the quality of evidence to guide public health interventions meets the highest possible standards of scientific rigour within this more complex environment (Weightman *et al.* 2005).

The infrastructure for public health is not, on its own, sufficient to ensure that effective public health interventions are developed, delivered and evaluated. The infrastructure must then work to develop organizational capacity within and beyond the health sector to create a *delivery system* for public health intervention referred to in Fig. 12.9.1. The components of the delivery system include population health surveillance, mechanisms for priority setting, programme delivery systems, and mechanisms for quality control, as discussed in the succeeding sections.

A system for population-wide health monitoring and surveillance

Understanding the complex and changing health status of the population is a cornerstone of public health. A national, comprehensive system for population-wide health monitoring and surveillance is an essential component of public health infrastructure. Such a system should facilitate on-going, systematic collection, analysis and interpretation of national or local population data relevant to the national public health effort. Such data need to be collected at national or more local levels repeatedly over time. This 'health intelligence' is needed to identify problems, to set priorities for action, and to monitor progress (National Health and Medical Research Council 1997). The US Centers for Disease Control and Prevention are a widely recognized example of an organization with this important function.

Health information in many countries is largely restricted to data on mortality, morbidity and health system use. This information is vitally important for epidemiological investigation, and to provide broad guidance on public health priorities and policy, but has limitations in its usefulness for planning and monitoring public health interventions (Nutbeam & Bauman 2006). For this a much wider range of information is needed, including information that is either national in coverage or has relevance nationally such as:

◆ Measures of health status in the population (including mortality and morbidity data)

◆ Measures of the determinants of the population's health, including those in the external environment (physical, biological, social, cultural and economic) and those internal to individuals (such as knowledge, behaviour, disease risk factors)

◆ Measures of the distribution of health in the population, and measures of the distribution of the determinants of a population's health

◆ Health interventions or health services, including interventions provided directly to individuals and those provided to communities, covering information on the nature of interventions, management, resourcing, accessibility, use, and effectiveness

◆ The relationships among these elements (National Health and Medical Research Council 1997)

Any type of health information system should enable analysis of the needs and progress of specific population sub-groups, with particular emphasis on disadvantaged groups. It must be capable of identifying inequities in health status and their determinants.

The system for monitoring and surveillance should also be responsible for reporting on the 'state of the health of the population'—on progress toward achieving health goals and targets, and on emerging issues or gaps. There are some useful examples of such reports being used effectively to highlight progress and the need for specific investment in action to address the needs of socially and economically marginalized populations. In the United Kingdom, the regular reports of the Chief Medical Officer (e.g. Department of Health 2005), and in the United States, Reports of the Surgeon General (http://www.surgeongeneral.gov/reportspublications. html) are practical examples of well-researched public health reports that are produced largely independent of the political administration

Examples of efforts to improve the relevance and range of health status indicators are beginning to emerge. To measure the influence of social, economic and environmental factors on the health of populations an expanded range of information is needed in national systems of monitoring and surveillance. The importance of developing a broader set of health indicators is strongly supported by the work of the WHO Commission on the Social Determinants of Health (2007), particularly through its Knowledge Networks.

A system for identifying national, regional, local priorities for action, and for regular review and redefinition of priorities

The identification of priorities for investment in public health interventions remains one of the most contentious issues in contemporary public health. The use of different criteria for establishing priorities leads to very different priorities for action (Nutbeam & Bauman 2006). Nationally determined priorities do not always resonate with local needs and perceptions of what actions are important to improve health.

Among the different approaches to priority development are those determined by epidemiological, economic, and community perspectives. Although not mutually exclusive, each of these perspectives places 'value' on different outcomes and processes.

To date, epidemiological analysis has dominated priority setting at national levels. The national health goals and targets identified by many nations and regions discussed earlier have given priority to leading causes of preventable deaths and morbidity. Criteria that have been used to identify priorities include: Analysis of the incidence, prevalence, costs to the health care system and to society associated with the disease/injury, and an assessment of the feasibility of acting to prevent or reduce the incidence or prevalence of the condition. Actions that are linked through epidemiological analysis to a reduction in disease are valued in such an analysis (Lopez 2003).

Increasingly, economic principles of efficiency are being proposed as a means of identifying priorities for public health intervention (Woodley 2001). Efficiency is used here to mean obtaining optimal gain from investment. However to use the concept of 'efficiency' as a criterion for identifying public health priorities, it is important to distinguish between two components of 'efficiency'. The first component has to do with ensuring that the services to address a particular issue or problem (e.g. cardiovascular disease) are organized and resourced. This means placing investment across the range of interventions (preventive, curative, palliative, or all three) for a particular condition to maximise individual and community health gain. It is called 'technical efficiency'. It means giving the greatest proportion of investment to the 'part' of the service that produces the greatest health gains—sometimes this will be prevention; sometimes it will be treatment. The evidence is also continually changing, and needs to be applied to readjust the balance of investment.

However, even if investment within a programme area (e.g. cardiovascular disease) is efficient, it is possible that investment across the range of health issues and population groups is not well-balanced. The second component of efficiency is 'allocative' efficiency. The analysis of the balance of investment based on assessment of allocative efficiency helps to identify priority issues or problems across the whole range of potential programme or service areas. At its most basic it is a tool for ensuring that a significant issue (such as mental illness) does receive adequate resources compared with other equally prevalent, severe issues. More sophisticated analyses will link investment in programme areas to predetermined population health outcomes, making decisions about the relative level of investment across different service/programme areas.

The third approach to priority setting reflects the growing evidence that the most effective and sustainable public health interventions have been characterized by high levels of community, organizational and political support. This is particularly true at the local level, which is also where national priorities are often seen to be remote from local concerns. Criteria for establishing priorities at local levels include: Extent of community concern about an issue, the capacity of the community to act to address the issue, and the capacity of local institutions, organizations, and people to contribute to action (Hancock & Minkler 1998). The process of participation in decision-making, and perceived responsiveness to local priorities are valued through such an analysis (Perrons & Skyler 2003).

These three perspectives on setting priorities are not mutually exclusive, and are best combined to achieve a sound basis for effective action that is nationally relevant, locally sensitive and financially sound.

Further, the development of priorities for public health intervention should not be considered a one-off event. The 'health intelligence' system established for defining priorities should also be capable of use in the review and redefinition of priorities. This is to ensure that there is capacity to redirect resources (as well as to increase the pool of resources) to address new priorities.

Programme delivery systems at national, regional, local levels of jurisdiction—within and outside the health sector

As indicated earlier, epidemiological analysis of priorities for intervention has generally led public health intervention towards reducing risk factors and behaviours in individuals. This in turn has led frequently to highly differentiated, vertical programmes within health sectors to tackle specific risks, such as tobacco use, or diseases such as coronary heart disease. Such programmes tend to have their own goals, resources, workforces, and research programmes (National Health and Medical Research Council 1997). As a consequence there is limited scope for integrated programmes to address the social, economic and physical environmental determinants of health. In contrast to disease/risk factor-specific programmes, such integrated programmes are more likely to focus on policy and institutional changes, in addition to public information, education and mobilization programmes.

Recently in Europe and in Australia there are examples of processes being implemented that, amongst other things, are intended to encourage the redefinition of priorities to include greater emphasis on the underlying factors and environments that are 'shared' across different causes of disease and injury. The significant burden of chronic disease being experienced by so many nations has led to the development of 'integrated' chronic disease-prevention programmes. The WHO has organized its work into chronic diseases and health promotion, together with a series of 'issue-specific' programmes. And, encouragingly, there is evidence of countries exploring initiatives to shift the focus of their public health programmes and funding away from vertical programmes to address the underlying determinants of health (Department of Health 2003). Again, WHO has established a structure on equity, poverty and social determinants of health to lead work on these 'cross-cutting' issues. Although vertical programmes continue to be the dominant organizational structure guiding public health investment and intervention, these new initiatives are interesting attempts to link funding with the more contemporary analysis of determinants of health and the need for explicit efforts to achieve equity.

The comprehensive programmes that are needed to bring about the wide-scale changes in the health of populations require public health infrastructure and action at national, regional and local levels of jurisdiction. Experience has demonstrated the need for clear role delineation and mechanisms for coordinating activity—particularly where the focus of the activity is change in legislation, policy, or programmes in sectors other than health. The exact nature of infrastructure needed at each level of jurisdiction has not been defined.

In most countries the greater part of the systems for programme delivery are devolved to state, regional, or local levels. A significant factor in improving the infrastructure for programme delivery in some countries, including the United Kingdom and Australia, has been the establishment of sub-regional administrative structures within the health sector that are responsible for protecting, promoting and maintaining the health of defined geographic populations. Within these structures, there have been initiatives to draw together the parts of the health care system that have the greatest 'affinity' with public health. This has been an effective means of ensuring an ongoing public health service at local and regional levels. However, it has been less effective in refocusing public health action to address inequalities in health and the determinants of health, and it has not been an effective mechanism through which to increase the proportion of health sector spending on public health action.

In addition to its specialist public health services, the health sector has many other opportunities to make significant contributions to improving the health of the population—through its hospitals, general practitioners, nursing homes, and early childhood services, for example. The sector also has a more direct role in public health—as a major employer, as a consumer of non-renewable resources, and as a physical and social setting that can influence the health of patients, staff, visitors and the community (Coote 2002; Swedish National Institute of Public Health 2006). Mobilizing this significantly untapped resource remains a major challenge for specialist public health practitioners.

As noted above, non-government, community and professional organizations also play significant roles in the design and delivery of public health interventions. Many of these are linked to specific health issues, e.g. sudden infant death syndrome, HIV/AIDS, or schizophrenia. Others focus on the needs of specific population groups, e.g. older people, immigrants, or indigenous people. Such organizations have specific knowledge, experience, and access to individuals and communities that is often difficult for government agencies to obtain.

Local government, too, has a key role in public health. The *Healthy Cities* movement is based, largely, on this level of government. Municipal public health planning has been found to be an effective mechanism to bring together local government, communities and key government agencies (including health) to define steps that each can take separately and together to improve the health of the population (Bagley *et al.* 2007; Lenihan 2005.) In the United Kingdom, a derivation of the healthy cities concept in the form of Health Action Zones represents a deliberate attempt to bring together the different agencies for public health at a local level (Barnes *et al.* 2005). It is through this type of organizational structure that other sectors can be more successfully engaged in public health action. The health sector's role in such relationships varies, depending on the context and the issue being addressed (Harris *et al.* 1996). However, a nation's public health infrastructure must include people with the knowledge, skills and resources (including power) to work effectively with other sectors. This is particularly important as the emphasis of public health action shifts from programmes developed and delivered by and within the health sector, to influencing public policy and organizations and programmes delivered by other sectors.

Systems for quality control, evaluation, promotion of best practice

Public health interventions need to be evaluated. The frameworks for assessing the quality of evidence to guide public health interventions referred to above are a component of an effective public health infrastructure. However, such frameworks have tended to focus on the quality of research design, and methods, rather than on the quality of the interventions (relevance, use of evidence and theory, practicality of implementation, etc.). There is a growing body of evidence that defines the characteristics of effective public health interventions (International Union for Health Promotion and Education 1999; McQueen & Jones 2007; Jackson & Waters 2005). It is a base from which to develop standards of quality for the design and implementation of public health interventions in relation to specific issues or population groups. The National Institute for Clinical Excellence (NICE) in the United Kingdom and the Centers for Disease Control and Prevention in the United States have developed standards for application to national and regional intervention programmes (Zaza *et al.* 2005). Use of such standards and guidelines in the development and implementation of public health interventions will be vitally important in improving the quality and impact of public health intervention in the future.

Concluding remarks: Key tasks to improve structures and strategies for public health intervention into the twenty-first century

This chapter has described key elements of health policy and strategy that have been found to be effective in guiding national public health action, and the components of an infrastructure and delivery system required to design, deliver and evaluate public health interventions. Public health intervention requires a complex mix of science, art (of practice), and politics. The emergence of high rates of non-communicable diseases in most high-income countries has required a radical re-appraisal of what determines health, and what public health responses are most appropriate and effective. In addition, many low- and middle-income countries are now experiencing both high rates of communicable and of non-communicable diseases. Four key challenges emerge from this chapter:

- **Addressing all determinants of health:** It is increasingly apparent that, in many cases, public health practitioners need to expand the range of research methods used to identify public health problems and their causes. As well as using the traditional public health tools of epidemiology and demography, it is necessary to use the social, behavioural and environmental sciences to obtain a more complete picture. More complex analysis of patterns of disease in populations, and of the determinants of disease will lead to better informed and potentially more effective interventions as a response.

In addition, knowledge of current infrastructure and existing strengths in communities is a powerful platform from which to build effective public health interventions (Labonte 1999). Identifying this capacity within communities also requires the use of a wider range of research and consultation methods (McKnight & Kretzmann 1998). It also emphasises the key role of communities in defining and prioritizing problems and in developing solutions, and is particularly important when working with communities that are disadvantaged or socially excluded.

- **Gaining visibility for public health:** It is also clear from the analyses in this chapter that public health action often involves political processes. Public health practitioners need to better use health data to influence these political processes. Reporting on ever more sophisticated analyses of public health problems and their determinants will not, on its own, result in any action. However, this data is of great use in raising public and political awareness of health problems, and in highlighting the obligation of governments to develop policy that enables action to improve the health of the population. This includes engaging politicians in dialogue to identify priorities for efficient health sector investment, and when appropriate, advocating for action to support investment in public health interventions in the face of pressure for increased investment in health care services.

- **Influencing policy and plans for improving public health:** The range of determinants of health means that public health practitioners will be required increasingly to provide technical advice on the impact on health of policies and practices in sectors other than the health sector. *Health impact analysis* is a relatively new

and underdeveloped tool to assist this process. Such technical advice will inevitably lead to conflict in some cases that will require the public health practitioner to act as an advocate for health in the face of competing pressures.

More positively, as evidence grows of the effectiveness of public health interventions it will be necessary for public health practitioners to operate across different sectors of government at national, regional and local levels. Public health practitioners need skills in identifying the policy relevance of the evidence and in identifying the most effective ways to ensure the use of evidence in the development and implementation of public policy.

- **Working with people and organizations to improve health:** Public health practitioners need to be able to engage people and organizations in practical action to address the determinants of health. Such action will often occur at a local level. The capacity to develop and deliver interventions within local communities and through different settings (such as schools and worksites) is an essential public health skill. The chapter by Kickbusch and McQueen (and other chapters) provides practical guidance on the type of skills and strategies required of public health practitioners to achieve change for public health at this level.

The development of effective organizational structures through which to bring together the components of an effective public health infrastructure within the health sector (in particular) to provide the capacity to 'orchestrate' public health action is a major challenge for the twenty-first century. It is important, however, to reflect on the fact that having the technical capacity to develop and deliver effective interventions is not sufficient, on its own. Without political commitment, action to promote health is, at best, difficult—at worst, impossible. The national infrastructure for promoting health must include people and strategies aimed at building and maintaining political support both for public health in general as a key area of government activity, as well as for the specific actions that must be taken, if we are to succeed in improving the health of the population.

References

Agren G. (2003). *Sweden's new public health policy: national public health objectives for Sweden*. Stockholm: Swedish National Institute of Public Health.

Allin S., Mossialos E., McKee M., and Holland W. (2004). *Making decisions on public health: a review of 8 countries*. European Observatory on Health Systems and Policies. Copenhagen, Denmark: World Health Organization (on behalf of the European Observatory on Health Systems and Policies.

Australian Institute of Health and Welfare(2006a). *Australia's Health 2006. The tenth biennial health report of the Australian Institute of Health and Welfare*. Canberra: Australian Institute of Health and Welfare.

Australian Institute of Health and Welfare (2006b). *National public health expenditure report 2000–2001 to 2003 – 4*. Health and welfare expenditure series no. 26. Canberra: Australian Institute of Health and Welfare.

Bagley P., Lin V., Sainsbury P., Wise M., Keating T., and Roger K. (2007). In what ways does the mandatory nature of Victoria's municipal public health planning framework impact on the planning process and outcomes? *Australia and New Zealand Health Policy* **4**. Available at: www.anzhealthpolicy.com/content/4/1/4 (accessed on 1 July 2007).

Baker E., Potter M., Jones D., Mercer S., Cioffi J., Green L. *et al.* (2005). The public health infrastructure and our nation's health. *Annual Review of Public Health* **26**, 303–18.

Baker E. and Koplan J. (2002). Strengthening the nation's public health infrastructure: historic challenge, unprecedented opportunity. *Health Affairs* **21**, 15–27.

Barnes M., Baule L., Benzeval M., Judge K., MacKenzie M., and Sullivan H. (2005). *Building capacity for health equity*. London, Routledge.

Beaglehole R. and Davis P. (1992). Setting national health goals and targets in the context of a fiscal crisis: the politics of social choice in New Zealand. *International Journal of Health Services*, **22**, 417–28.

Bonnie R., Stratton K., Wallace R. (eds.) (2007). *Ending the tobacco problem: a blueprint for the nation*. Washington DC, The National Academies Press.

Busse R. and Wismar M. (2002). Health target programmes and health care services – any link? A conceptual and comparative study (Part 1). *Health Policy* **59**, 209–221.

Centers for Disease Control and Prevention (1999). *An ounce of prevention . . . what are the returns?* 2nd ed. revised. Atlanta, Centers for Disease Control and Prevention, US Department of Health and Human Services.

Commonwealth Department of Human Services and Health (1994). *Better health outcomes for Australians: national goals, targets and strategies for better health outcomes into the next century*. Canberra, Australian Government Publishing Service.

Commonwealth Department of Health and Aged Care (1999). *Independent review of the public health education and research program*. Report to the Commonwealth Department of Health and Aged Care. Canberra, Department of Health and Aged Care.

Commonwealth Department of Health and Aged Care (2000). *National Public Health Education Framework*. Public Health Education and Research Program. Canberra, Department of Health and Aged Care.

Coote A., ed. (2002). *Claiming the health dividend: unlocking the benefits of NHS spending*. London, King's Fund.

Cutler D., Lleras-Muney A. (2007). *Education and health: evaluating theories and evidence*. National Poverty Centre. Policy Brief 9. Gerald R. Ford School of Public Policy, University of Michigan. Available at: www. npc.umich.edu/publications/policy_briefs/brief9/policy_brief9/pdf (accessed 1 July 2007).

Davies J., Colomer C., Lindstrom B., Hospers H., Tountas Y., Modolo M., and Kannas L. (2000). The EUMAHP Project – the development of a European Masters programme in health promotion. *Promotion and Education*, **VII**, 15–18.

Department of Health (2002). *Tackling health inequalities – 2002 cross-cutting review 2002*. London, Department of Health.

Department of Health (2003). *Tackling health inequalities: a programme for action*. London, Department of Health.

Department of Health (2005). *The Chief Medical Officer on the state of public health. Annual Report 2006*. London, Department of Health.

Department of Health (2006). *Tackling health inequalities: Status report on the program for action 2006, Update on headline indicators*. London, DOH.

Health Inequalities Unit, Department of Health (2006). *Tackling health inequalities: status report on the programme for action – 2006 update of headline indicators*. London, Department of Health.

Durham G. and Plant A. (2005). *The Public Health Education and Research Program Review 2005: strengthening workforce capacity for public health*. Canberra, Commonwealth of Australia.

Gebbie K., Rosenstock L., and Hernandez L. (eds.) (2000). *Who will keep the public healthy? Educating public health professionals for the 21st century*. Washington D.C, The National Academies Press.

Gebbie K. and Turnock B. (2006). The public health workforce 2006: new challenges. *Health Affairs*, **25**, 923–933.

Grossman R. and Scala K. with the assistance of Untermarzoner D. (1993). *Health promotion and organizational development: developing settings for health*. European Health Promotion Series No. 2. Vienna, World Health Organization, Regional Office for Europe and IFF Health and Organizational Development.

Hancock T. and Minkler M. (1998). Community health assessment or healthy community assessment: whose community? whose health? whose assessment? In Minkler M. *Community organizing and community building for health*, pp. 139–156. New Jersey, Rutgers University Press.

Harris E., Wise M., Hawe P. *et al.* (1996). *Working together: intersectoral action for health*. Canberra/Sydney, National Centre for Health Promotion and Commonwealth Department of Human Services and Health.

Health Targets and Implementation Committee (1998). *Health for all Australians*. Report to the Australian Health Ministers' Advisory Council and the Australian Health Ministers' Conference. Canberra, Australian Government Publishing Service.

Howat P., Maycock B., Jackson L. *et al.* (2000). Development of competency-based university health promotion courses. *Promotion and Education*, **VII**, 33–38.

Hunter D., and Berman P. (1997). Public health management. Time for a new start? *European Journal of Public Health*, **7**, 345–349.

Institute of Medicine (2003). The governmental public health infrastructure. In: *The future of the public's health in the 21st century*. Washington DC, Institute of Medicine of the National Academies.

International Network for Health Promotion Foundations (2007). Available at: www.hp-foundations.net (accessed on 5 June 2007).

International Union for Health Promotion and Education (1999) *The evidence of health promotion effectiveness. Shaping public health in a new Europe. A report for the European Commission* (2nd edition). Brussels/Luxembourg, The European Commission.

Jackson N. and Waters E. (2005). Criteria for the systematic review of health promotion and public health interventions. *Health Promotion International*, **20**, 367–374.

Joint Task Group on Public Health Human Resources (2005). *Building the public health workforce for the 21st century*. A Pan-Canadian framework for public health human resources planning. Ottawa, Advisory Committee on Health Delivery and Human Resources, Advisory Committee on Population Health and Health Security.

Kawachi I., Kennedy B. and Wilkinson R. (eds.) (1999). *Income inequality and health: a reader*. New York, New Press.

Kemm J. (2006) Health impact assessment and health in all policies. In Stahl T., Wismar M., Ollila E., Lahtinen E., Leppo K. (eds.) (2006). *Health in all policies: prospects and potentials*. Helsinki, Finnish Ministry of Social Affairs and Health.

Labonte R. (1999). Health promotion in the near future: remembrances of activism past. *Health Education Journal* **58**, 365–377.

Lenihan P. (2005). MAPP and the Evolution of Planning in Public Health Practice. *Journal of Public Health Management and Practice*, **11**, 381–386.

Lopez A. (2003). Evidence and information for health policy: a decade of change. *Medical Journal of Australia*, **179**, 396–7.

McCracken-Rance H. (2000). Developing competencies for health promotion training in Aotearoa-New Zealand. *Promotion and Education*, **VII**, 40–3.

McKnight J. and Kretzmann J. (1988). Mapping community capacity. In Minkler M. *Community organizing and community building for health*, pp. 157–174. Rutgers University Press, New Jersey.

McQueen D. (2000). Perspectives on health promotion: theory, evidence, practice and the emergence of complexity. *Health Promotion International*, **15**, 95–97.

McQueen D. and Jones C. (2007). *Global Perspectives on Health Promotion Effectiveness*. New York, Springer Science & Business Media.

Marmot M. and Wilkinson R. (eds.) (1999). *Social determinants of health*. Oxford, Oxford University Press.

Millward L., Kelly M. and Nutbeam D. (2003). *Public health intervention research – the evidence*. London, Health Development Agency.

Mittelmark M., Wise M., Nam E.W. *et al.* (2007). Mapping national capacity to engage in health promotion: overview of issues and approaches. *Health Promotion International*, **21** (S1).

National Health and Medical Research Council (1997). *Promoting the health of Australians: a review of infrastructure support for national health advancement.* Canberra, National Health and Medical Research Council.

NSW Department of Health (2007*). The health of the people of New South Wales*: Report of the Chief Health Officer 2006. Sydney, NSW Department of Health.

Norwegian Ministry of Health and Care Services (2007). *National strategy to reduce social inequalities in health.* Report No. 20 (2007–7) to the Storting. Oslo: Norwegian Ministry of Health and Care Services.

Nutbeam D., Wise M., Bauman A. *et al.* (1993). *Goals and targets for Australia's health in the year 2000 and beyond.* Canberra, Australian Government Publishing Service.

Nutbeam D. and Wise M. (1996). Planning for Health for All: international experience in setting health goals and targets. *Health Promotion International*, **11**, 219–226.

Nutbeam D. (1996). Achieving 'best practice' in health promotion: improving the fit between research and practice. *Health Education Research*, **11**, 317–325.

Nutbeam D. (1998). Evaluating health promotion – progress, problems and solutions. *Health Promotion International*, **13**, 27–44.

Nutbeam D. (2003). How does evidence influence public policy? Tackling health inequalities in England. *Health Promotion Journal of Australia*, **14**: 154–8.

Nutbeam D. and Bauman A. (2006). *Evaluation in a nutshell.* Sydney, McGraw Hill.

Padgett S., Bekemeier B. and Berkowitz B. (2004). Collaborative partnerships at the state level: promoting systems changes in public health infrastructure. *Journal of Public Health Management Practice*, **10**, 251–257.

Perrons D. and Skyers S. (2003). Empowerment through participation? Conceptual explorations and a case study. *International Journal of Urban and Regional Research*, **27**, 265–285.

Popkin B. (2007). Understanding global nutrition dynamics as a step towards controlling cancer incidence. *Nature*, **7**: 61–67.

Population Health and Wellness (2005). *A framework for core functions in public health. Resource Document.* Province of British Columbia, Canada, Population Health and Wellness, Ministry of Health Services.

Public Health Agency of Canada (2007). *About the Agency.* Available at: http://www.phac-aspc.gc.ca/about_apropos/index.html (accessed 3 July 2007).

Raphael D. (2007). *Poverty and policy in Canada: Implications for health and quality of life.* Toronto, Canadian Scholars' Press.

Rootman I., Goodstadt M., Hyndman B. *et al.* (2001). *Evaluation in health promotion: principles and perspectives.* Who Regional Publications, European Series No. 92. Denmark, World Health Organization.

Rose G. (1992). *The strategy of preventive medicine.* Oxford, New York, Tokyo, Oxford University Press.

Stahl T., Wismar M., Ollila E. *et al.* (eds.) (2006). *Health in all policies: prospects and potentials.* Helsinki, Finnish Ministry of Social Affairs and Health.

Swedish National Institute of Public Health (2006). *Towards a more health-promoting health service.* Stockholm, Swedish National Institute of Public Health.

Travis P., Bennett S., Haines A., Pang T., Bhutta Z., Hyder A. *et al.* (2004). Overcoming health-systems constraints to achieve the Millennium Development Goals. *The Lancet*, **364**, 900–906.

United Nations (2000) Millennium Development Goals. New York. Available at: http://www.un.org/millenniumgoals (accessed 7 August 2008).

US Council on Linkages (1999). *Competencies.* Available at: www.TrainingFinder.org/competencies (accessed 8 August 2007).

US Department of Health and Human Services (1980). *Promoting health/ preventing disease: objectives for the nation.* Washington D.C, Department of Health and Human Services, Public Health Service.

US Department of Health and Human Services (1995). *Healthy people 2000. Midcourse review with 1995 revisions.* US Department of Health and Human Services, Public Health Service. Washington DC, US Government Printing Office.

US Department of Health and Human Services (1999). *The Public Health Functions Project.* Available at: http://www.healthypeople.gov/document/HTML/Volume2/23PHI.htm (accessed 9 August 2007).

US Department of Health and Human Services (2006). *Midcourse Review: Healthy people 2010.* Washington, DC: US Government Printing Office.

Wanless D. (2004). *Securing good health for the whole population. Final report.* HM Treasury. London: HMSO.

Weightman A., Ellis S., Cullum A. *et al.* (2005). *Grading evidence and recommendations for public health interventions: developing and piloting a framework.* Support Unit for Research Evidence, Information Services (Cardiff University) and Health Development Agency. London, Health Development Agency.

Whitehead M. (2007). A typology of actions to tackle social inequalities in health. *Journal of Epidemiology and Community Health*, **61**, 473–478.

Wismar M. and Busse R. (2002). Outcome-related health targets – political strategies for better health outcomes. A conceptual and comparative study (Part 2). *Health Policy*, **59**, 223–241.

Woodley P. (2004). *Health financing and population health.* Occasional papers. Health Financing Series Vol. 7. Canberra, Population Health Division, Commonwealth Department of Health and Aged Care.

World Bank Povertynet (2007). *Poverty and health.* Available at: http://web.worldbank.org/WBSITE/EXTERNAL/TOPICS/EXTPOVERTY (accessed 3 July 2007).

World Health Organization (1980). *Global strategy for Health for All.* Geneva, World Health Organization.

World Health Organization.(1985). *Targets for Health for All.* Copenhagen, World Health Organization, Regional Office for Europe,.

World Health Organization, Health and Welfare Canada, Canadian Public Health Association (1986). *Ottawa Charter for Health Promotion.* (Available through) Copenhagen, World Health Organization, Regional Office for Europe.

World Health Organization (2002). *Investment for health: a discussion of the role of economic and social determinants.* WHO Regional Office for Europe. Copenhagen, World Health Organization.

World Health Organization (1998). *Jakarta Declaration on leading health promotion into the 21st century.* Geneva,World Health Organization.

World Health Organization (1999). *Health 21 – health for all in the 21st century.* Copenhagen, World Health Organization.

World Health Organization (2003). *WHO Framework Convention on Tobacco Control.* Geneva, World Health Organization.

World Health Organization (2006). *Commission on the Social Determinants of Health.* Geneva, World Health Organization.

World Health Organization (2005). The Bangkok Charter for Health Promotion in a globalized world. *Health Promotion Journal of Australia*, **16**, 168–171.

WHO European Office for Investment in Health and Development (2007). http://www.euro.who.int/ihd (accessed 3 July 2007.)

World Health Organization (2007). *Knowledge Networks. How the knowledge networks work?* Commission on the Social Determinants of Health. Available at: www.who.int/social_determinants/knowledge_networks/how_kn_operate/en/index.html (accessed 3 July 2007).

Zasa S., Briss P. and Harris K. (2005). *The guide to community preventive services: what works to promote health?* Oxford, New York, Oxford University Press.

Ziglio E., Hagard S., McMahon L. *et al.* (2000). Principles, methodology and practices of investment for health. *Promotion and Education*, **VII**, 4–15.

Strategies for health services

Martin McKee, Ellen Nolte, and Josep Figueras

Abstract

This chapter starts from the premise that a health system should, fundamentally, seek to improve population health. It first reviews the evidence that modern healthcare can impact positively on population health. Employing the concept of avoidable mortality, which identifies deaths that should not occur in the presence of timely and effective care, it shows that modern healthcare does make an important contribution to health but it also notes that some care provided is either ineffective or even harmful. It continues by examining the many factors that are acting on health systems and to which they must respond. One factor is the changing economic situation, with increasing evidence that investment in health promotes economic growth. Another is the evolving burden of disease, characterized in particular by the growing number of people with multiple complex disorders. Others include changing beliefs about the relationship between the individual and the state, and greater knowledge and expectations among actual and potential users. It then examines what public health professionals can do to maximize the amount of effective care provided to those in need while minimizing what is ineffective or harmful. It identifies a series of strategies. One is priority setting, which should be based on evidence and underpinned by explicit values, including the pursuit of equity in healthcare funding and delivery. Another is optimal allocation of resources, based on the quest to maximize health gain, which includes assessment of need and intelligence-led purchasing of appropriate care. Another is defining models of service delivery, ensuring that care is provided in the most appropriate setting and in ways that achieve optimal outcomes. Finally, the chapter examines some of the ways in which health systems can provide a setting for prevention and health promotion. It concludes by arguing that public health professionals must engage in the debate about how healthcare is funded and delivered if they are to maximize population health.

Introduction

The inclusion of this chapter in a textbook of public health begs a question. Why should public health professionals be interested in health services? This seemingly naïve question brings to the fore a more fundamental question; what are health services for? The answer one gets will vary according to whom the question is addressed. A financial analyst on Wall Street, viewing with pleasure the return on capital of an American for-profit hospital chain will see the provision of healthcare as an economic activity like any other service industry, no different, fundamentally, from running chains of hotels, theme parks or even casinos. A regional development agency may view a healthcare facility as something that enhances the attraction of a run down post-industrial area, an essential element of infrastructure similar to a road network, an airport, and high-speed Internet links, a view endorsed by those responsible for the European Union's structural funds, which actively support investment in health infrastructure. A trade union representing healthcare workers may see it as a source of employment for its members.

From a public health perspective, however, this chapter draws on a framework set out initially in the seminal 2000 World Health Report (World Health Organization 2000) and used subsequently by other writers. In it, the key functions of a health system are to improve population health, to collect the necessary money in a way that is fair, thus protecting people from catastrophic expenditure when they fall ill, and to respond to their legitimate expectations about how a health service should be provided. Public health professionals have a crucial role in ensuring that health systems achieve these objectives, but especially the first of these. To do so, they must promote the equitable use of interventions that are effective and appropriate for the population in question, reduce interventions that are ineffective or harmful, and thus maximize the health gain obtained with the available resources.

Yet, they must do so within a changing environment. This brings both opportunities and threats for public health professionals. On the one hand, change offers the possibility to challenge existing arrangements and maximize the contribution of health services to population health. On the other hand, it brings threats as those responsible for health policy may seek to meet other objectives, such as the narrow pursuit of profit or the exclusion of those in need. Consequently, this chapter explores the changing nature of health services, the roles that public health professionals can play in these processes, and the strategies that they can pursue to enhance health gain and promote equity. It begins by assessing the contribution that health services make to population health.

Do health services affect population health?

There is little argument that some interventions, most obviously immunization against diseases such as smallpox, poliomyelitis and measles, but also some low-technology strategies such as integrated management of childhood illness, have been remarkably successful in reducing mortality in many parts of the world. However, there is much less agreement about many other elements of health services.

At the risk of simplification, the debate has become somewhat polarized. Thus, some have argued that healthcare contributes little to population health, a view that is associated most closely with the work of McKeown (1979). He argued that three-quarters of the decline in mortality in England and Wales between 1841 and 1971 had been due to a reduction in deaths from infectious disease, yet three-quarters of this reduction had preceded the widespread introduction of immunization or antibiotics. This, he contended, demonstrated that the main drivers of improvements in health had been nutrition, environment, and behaviour. A different, but related, perspective is offered by those who argue that it is unrealistic to expect healthcare to contribute significantly to population health because so little of it has been adequately evaluated and found to be effective (Chappell 1993).

To others, however, it is not just that healthcare has little impact on health. Instead, it may actually damage it. This view receives some support from studies that have related healthcare inputs to outputs. If anything, these have suggested that there is an inverse association, with greater healthcare resources leading to worse overall health (Cochrane et al. 1978). One explanation advanced for this observation is that scarce resources are being channelled into healthcare rather than sectors such as education where they might have a greater, albeit less immediately obvious, impact on health. Another is that healthcare has a direct and adverse effect on health, a view advanced by Illich (1976), who coined the term iatrogenesis to describe the adverse consequences of prescribed drugs, hospital-acquired infections, poorly performed surgery, and the harm done by following up spurious abnormalities found among the vastly increased number of laboratory investigations being undertaken.

These views have elicited a range of responses. Some physicians have simply dismissed them, arguing that they are completely at odds with the everyday experience of clinicians who see the results of the care that they provide. In contrast, others have argued that the existing level of healthcare provision in some countries is excessive (Lavis & Stoddart 1994) and that politicians should shift expenditure from healthcare to sectors such as education, housing, and employment.

This debate has considerable implications for the role of public health professionals. Thus, if the major determinants of health lie outside the healthcare sector, is the involvement of public health professionals in the delivery of healthcare at best an irrelevance and, at worst, a diversion from the more important roles of advocacy and mobilizing inter-sectoral action (Whitty & Jones 1992)? Or have public health professionals a role in ensuring that healthcare is provided effectively and efficiently, on the basis that this will maximize population health?

However, the debate has to be interpreted in the light of the context within which it was held. Thus, while Illich and McKeown may have been correct in the 1960s and 1970s when they were developing their arguments, the intervening period has seen major changes, with many formerly fatal conditions now amenable to treatment. Furthermore, many of the criticisms made by Illich concerning unnecessary and inappropriate investigations and treatment have now been addressed by the greater acceptance of evidence-based healthcare. In this scenario, healthcare is seen as an important determinant of health of a population. It is thus worthy of the attention of public health professionals, who have a role in enhancing access to effective care and reducing exposure to ineffective and dangerous care.

Quantifying the contribution of healthcare to population health

It is important to recall that healthcare has changed remarkably in a relatively short time. Many new treatments have been shown, in high-quality evaluative research, to be able to prolong life. Examples include effective treatment for hypertension and heart failure, secondary prevention following myocardial infarction and chemotherapy for many childhood cancers. There has also been, in many countries, a revolution in the approach to evidence in making treatment decisions. These changes are part of a long-term trend. Beeson (1980) showed how many treatments advocated in a 1927 edition of a major textbook of medicine were, at the time he was writing, known to be either ineffective or harmful. By the time that the 1975 edition was published there was a major shift to treatments that had been proven to be effective. However, the pace of change has accelerated during the 1980s and 1990s. There has been a much greater willingness to challenge professional judgement where it is not supported by evidence of effectiveness and to question whether clinical performance is optimal. This has led from early pioneers of the medical audit to the enormous expansion of evidence-based healthcare (see below). It encompasses a wide range of activities which together have helped to eliminate many interventions that do not work and have increased the uptake of those that are effective. Thus there is a case that if healthcare had made little contribution to population health during the period that McKeown was looking at, up to the mid-1960s, it may now be doing so. The following section asks whether this has actually happened.

Rutstein et al. (1976) asked an expert panel to identify a list of conditions from which death should not occur in the presence of timely and effective care. These deaths were deemed to be 'preventable' although subsequent writers have also used the terms 'avoidable' and 'amenable to medical care'; and were interpreted as a measure of the quality of the healthcare system. This concept was later applied empirically by other researchers, with publication of regional atlases permitting cross-national comparisons. A seminal study by Mackenbach et al. (1988) related changes in deaths from particular causes to the time that various interventions were introduced. By doing so, they were able to show that the impacts of specific treatments were observable as accelerating falls in mortality from the conditions they were intended to treat. They concluded that the healthcare interventions they examined added 2.9 years to life expectancy at birth for men and 3.9 years for women in the Netherlands between 1950 and 1984.

More recently, Nolte and McKee (2004) undertook a systematic review of the evidence that deaths from specific causes of death could be avoided. This enabled them to update the previous lists of 'avoidable' causes, taking account of advances in medical knowledge and technology, while extending the upper age limit to 75 years of age. Figure 12.10.1 shows the age standardized death rates in 2003 in a range of industrialized countries.

A comparison of trends over time in selected European countries showed that reductions in avoidable mortality contributed substantially to increasing life expectancy in Western European countries

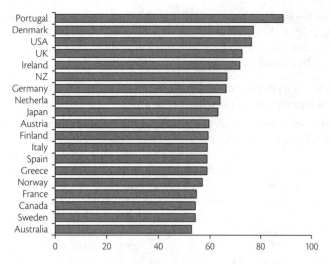

Fig. 12.10.1 Age-standardized death rates (0–74 years per 100000) from conditions amenable to care (2003 or most recent year).
Source: Authors' calculations using data from the WHO mortality database.
Note: Denmark 2001, Italy, Sweden, United States 2002.

during the 1980s. They continued to do so during the 1990s, although by then the contribution was greater in southern European countries such as Italy and Spain, suggesting some catching up with their northern neighbours. In contrast, the then communist countries in central and eastern Europe saw little benefit from healthcare during the 1980s but this changed in the 1990s and has continued, with further substantial reductions in avoidable mortality in the first decade of the twenty-first century (Nolte *et al.* 2004). Finally, a comparison of Russia and the United Kingdom shows how the two countries had very similar rates of avoidable mortality in the mid-1960s, a time when there were relatively few modern pharmaceuticals available in either country. The rate in the United Kingdom then began to fall steadily while they remained steady in Russia, which during the Soviet era never managed to develop a modern pharmaceutical system and where the principles of evidence-based care were essentially unknown (Andreev *et al.* 2003).

Further evidence that healthcare can impact positively on population health comes from studies of particular causes of death. Beaglehole (1986) estimated that 42 per cent of the decline in deaths from cardiovascular disease in New Zealand between 1974 and 1981 could be attributed to advances in medical care. The long-term decline in mortality from coronary heart disease in the Netherlands between 1969 and 1993 accelerated significantly after 1987, coinciding with the wider availability of interventions such as coronary care units and thrombolysis (Bonneux *et al.* 1997).

Thus, while there is increasing evidence for a positive impact of healthcare on population health, it is also important not to dismiss Illich's views entirely. The thalidomide scandal in the 1960s, in which what was thought to be a safe sedative was found later to cause serious limb deformities in the children of mothers who took it while pregnant, confirmed the potential for an effective drug to cause harm to susceptible individuals. Subsequently other apparently safe drugs have been shown to have caused unanticipated long-term side effects. For example, the growing burden of multi-drug resistant tuberculosis is entirely a creation of healthcare, providing a classic example of iatrogenesis. In some countries, the

1990s have seen a marked increase in the rate of resistance among hospital-acquired infections. Rates vary markedly between countries, and there is compelling evidence that they are related to the approach taken to the prescribing of antibiotics. Thus, hospitals and other healthcare facilities in which prescribing is uncontrolled and haphazard represent a threat to the wider population, and not only in the country concerned. Unfortunately, surveillance systems are often weak, even in many industrialized countries. It is easy to forget that, until the early twentieth century, one's probability of dying was increased by coming into hospital because of the risk of infection and the growth of iatrogenic antibiotic resistance is perhaps one of the greatest challenges facing public health professionals today.

It is also important to recognize the accumulating evidence of patient harm resulting from medical errors, with one analysis suggesting this could account for as much as 44000 deaths among Americans each year (Institute of Medicine 2000). Finally, it is salutary to recall that even well-established interventions may be ineffective or even harmful, as in the example of albumin, long given to patients with burns and multiple trauma on the basis, incorrectly, of an intuitive belief that it was likely to be beneficial (Alderson *et al.* 2004). In this context, it is necessary to consider the specific situation in the countries of the former Soviet Union. Its isolation from international developments during the Soviet era led to the widespread adoption of many entirely ineffective treatments based on various forms of electromagnetic and ionizing radiation, many of which remain in widespread use (McKee 2007).

Healthcare and health equity

The health impact of health services raises the important issue of equity. When healthcare had little measurable impact on health, socio-demographic inequalities in access to care may have been of little importance. Indeed, it is arguable that the wealthy, exposed at considerable personal expense to such painful and ineffective treatments as cupping and bleeding were actually disadvantaged compared with the poor who patiently waited for the inevitable death spared such indignities. The present situation is quite different. If healthcare does contribute materially to population health, then lack of access to it will exacerbate health inequalities (Arblaster *et al.* 1996).

There is considerable evidence from many countries that such inequalities exist and that they have an impact on health. This is intuitive in healthcare systems where there is not universal access to care, such as the United States. For example, American research has found that people living in deprived areas with poor access to care have high rates of hospital admission with chronic medical conditions, such as asthma, heart failure, and diabetes that, if detected and treated early should not require admission to hospital (Billings *et al.* 1996). Death rates from many chronic disorders responsive to healthcare are very much higher among African Americans than white Americans (Kunitz & Pesis-Katz 2005), with similar differences in survival from many cancers, reflecting both later presentation (itself a reflection of access to primary care) and lower rates on intervention once a diagnosis has been made (Morris *et al.* 2006).

Inequalities are, however, also seen in countries offering universal coverage. In the United Kingdom, women, people from minority ethnic populations, older people, and those living in deprived areas are all disadvantaged in access to surgical interventions for coronary artery disease.

Differential access is a factor in the observation that social class gradients are substantially greater for causes amenable to medical care than other causes of death (Marshall *et al.* 1993).

Inequitable access to care can disadvantage many groups of people other than those listed above (Healy & McKee 2004). Thus, those living in rural areas may be disadvantaged unless specific measures are taken to ensure their access to care. This will often require innovative delivery models, taking advantage of technological developments such as near-patient testing and telemedicine to compensate for the increasing pressure to centralize facilities. Prisoners in many countries receive poor quality care, while disabled people may face structural obstacles in accessing health facilities and obtaining services. At a global level there are enormous inequalities in access to basic, but essential, treatments such as immunization and life-sustaining drugs such as anti-retrovirals and insulin.

This section has highlighted how, unlike the situation prior to the 1970s, healthcare can make a substantial difference to population health. However, as the World Health Organization noted in the Ottawa Charter (World Health Organization 1986), health services are only one of the determinants of health, others being genetic predisposition, individual behaviour and lifestyle, and environmental circumstances (Lalonde 1974), whose importance are recognized in the creation by the World Health Organization, in March 2005, of a Commission on Social Determinants of Health.

Public health professionals must look at the wider picture and take into account these other determinants but it is important that, in taking a broad perspective, they do not lose sight of the contribution that healthcare can make to population health, ensuring that what care is provided is effective and is provided equitably. The remainder of this chapter explores the changing nature of health services, the impact that various policies have, and the role that public health professionals can play in maximizing the health gain that health services can provide.

Why are health systems changing?

Health systems face a range of pressures, from both within and outside. External factors include the macroeconomic climate and the evolving framework of values of the society within which the system is located. Internal factors include the changing pattern of health in the population being served, upward pressures on expenditures arising from ageing populations and technological change, a search for improvements in the quality of healthcare that is delivered, and the expansion of information technology. These will be considered in turn.

Macroeconomic factors

Health systems are influenced strongly by their economic environments. One is the nature of the market within which resources are procured. In general, the costs of some inputs into health services have tended to reflect local market conditions, such as salaries for healthcare professionals. Others, such as pharmaceuticals and technology, have tended to reflect world market prices although, in practice, the situation is not quite so simple. Thus, the cost of employing health professionals will reflect the market within which they function. Those in countries where few speak one of the major international languages may still be operating in what is essentially a national market, allowing salaries to remain low. Conversely, where most speak a language such as English, French, or Spanish,

health workers operate increasingly in a global market, so that healthcare providers must pay high salaries if they are to retain them. The inability to do so has contributed to the emigration of vast numbers of health professionals from low-income countries. In the case of pharmaceuticals, the price paid in a low-income country may actually be several times higher than in a developed one because of the fragmentation of the purchasing function and multiple mark-ups along the supply chain (Mossialos *et al.* 2004). The different costs of inputs will shape the pattern of care that is provided.

A second consideration relates to the resources available for healthcare. There are two issues to be considered. The first is the overall state of the economy. The second is the share of the economy devoted to health.

Clearly, the healthcare system is likely to come under pressure during an economic crisis. Examples include events in some Latin American countries in the 1980s and 1990s, in the countries of the former Soviet Union in the years following 1991 or, in many low-income countries, in the face of externally imposed structural adjustment policies. The effects may be seen in death rates from treatable conditions. Thus, deaths from diabetes among young people increased many times in the former Soviet Union during the early 1990s (Telishevka *et al.* 2001) while child mortality has increased in countries facing structural adjustment.

These circumstances are, however, unusual and economic swings are typically much less severe. Yet, they still impact on the health system. An economic downturn, especially where it leads to long-term unemployment, will increase demand for many elements of healthcare at a time when financial resources are scarce, although, paradoxically, death rates from cardiovascular disease, traffic injuries, and cirrhosis increase during an economic boom.

The share of the economy devoted to healthcare is, inevitably, the result of the interplay between market forces and political choices. Regardless of the funding system in place, governments in all industrialized and middle-income countries play an important role in determining how much will be spent. This is easiest in countries where healthcare is financed from taxation but governments in countries with social insurance systems are usually partners to negotiations on contribution levels, salaries, or pharmaceutical prices, simply because of the important macroeconomic implications. Even in a country such as the United States, where the role of the government in healthcare is often considered to be minimal, almost 50 per cent of the population have their healthcare paid from government funds.

The way in which healthcare expenditure is viewed has changed over the past decade. During the 1980s and 1990s it was often regarded as a drain on the economy, with high social costs damaging national competitiveness. In particular, the cost of healthcare was sometimes cited as a reason for trans-national corporations to relocate production in a country where the costs were less (Stephens *et al.* 1999). This was exacerbated in some places by specific factors. In the mid-1990s, the countries of Southeast Asia suffered a major economic crisis. However, countries responded in different ways, providing a valuable natural public health experiment. Thailand and Indonesia followed advice from the World Bank to cut back on public expenditure while Malaysia did not (Hopkins 2006). There was a short-lived but detectable increase in mortality in the first two countries but not in Malaysia, highlighting the importance of maintaining social safety nets at times of economic crisis.

More recently, there are signs of a change of direction in the prevalent thinking. Research, initially in low-income countries (World Health Organization and Commission on Macroeconomics and Health 2001), but later confirmed in high-income countries (Suhrcke *et al.* 2006), has highlighted the contribution of good health to economic growth, with better health leading to greater wages, higher labour force participation, higher savings, and greater investment in one's own education.

Historical improvements in health and nutrition have contributed substantially to the favourable economic status of today's advanced industrialized countries (Fogel 1994). People who are healthy are more likely to remain in the workforce, where they are more productive. They are likely to save more, increasing the resources available for capital investment, and to invest in their own skills. Furthermore, there is a growing recognition that investment in timely care can reduce the frequency of complications, which are much more expensive to treat (Billings *et al.* 1996). One example of this new thinking is the Wanless Report (Wanless 2001), commissioned by the United Kingdom Treasury. This report showed how investment in better health now would lead to a substantial reduction in expenditure in the future.

While, in most cases, public health professionals must work within the constraints imposed by the macroeconomic context in which they find themselves, they also have a major role, as advocates for the public's health, in shaping the debate, arguing for sustained investment in health on the basis of its contribution to future economic growth.

Norms and beliefs

A second set of factors driving change in healthcare systems relate to the underlying norms and beliefs of the society within which the system is embedded (Contandriopoulos *et al.* 1998). Healthcare systems act as mirrors reflecting deeply rooted social and cultural expectations of the population that they serve. Although these norms and beliefs are generated outside the formal structure of the healthcare system, they play a major role in defining the system's overall characteristics.

The impact of different norms and beliefs is apparent when comparing the United States, where healthcare is generally seen as a commodity to be bought and sold, and Europe, where healthcare is seen predominantly as a social or collective good, in which citizens benefit when an individual receives effective care (McKee 2002).

Societies thus have dominant belief systems (Benson 1975). This does not imply that a single view is held by all members of that society; rather, the tension and negotiation that exist between various beliefs and values have some stability. A useful approach to understanding belief systems sees these tensions as grouped around four poles (Habermas 1987): Values, understanding of phenomena, definition of jurisdictions and allocation of resources, and logic of regulation. Values include tensions and trade-offs between equity, individual autonomy, and efficiency (Clark 1998). Understanding of phenomena relates to how concepts such as life, death, sickness, health, and pain are interpreted and thus viewed as relating to the objectives of a healthcare (Gillett 1995). Definition of jurisdictions and allocation of resources comprise the perceptions of the role and functions of those responsible for and working in the healthcare sector, as well as the allocation of resources between prevention and cure and between healthcare and broader determinants of health. The logic of regulation relates to how society chooses to regulate

the delivery of healthcare (Contandriopoulos *et al.* 1998). This may be technocratic, with trained experts guiding the system on the basis of their knowledge and position within the hierarchy; professional self-regulatory, which has the physician, as the best agent of the patient, at the centre of the system; the market-based model, in which regulations reflect supply and demand in a competitive market; or the democratic model, in which the population, either directly or, more often, through elected or appointed representatives, is responsible for setting out the framework for delivery of healthcare.

Although dominant belief systems have some stability, they are in a state of constant tension as different classes and groups within society struggle for ascendancy, a phenomenon most clearly seen in the fluctuating electoral success of political parties. In some societies, the process of change will be evolutionary and incremental. In others, as exemplified by the countries in Central and Eastern Europe after the collapse of communism, it will be abrupt. An understanding of the dominant belief system in a society is important for public health professionals as it contributes to knowledge of why systems are as they are, how they have changed, and the objectives that individuals within the healthcare system are pursuing. It will also influence the choice of strategies that should be adopted to bring about change.

Changing burden of disease

Although it would be naive to think that the health needs of the population are the only factor driving the configuration of health services, they do play an important role. For example, the creation of public health services in many industrialized countries was a direct result of the global epidemics of cholera in the mid-nineteenth centuries. Recognition of the infectious nature of tuberculosis led, somewhat controversially, to the creation of sanatoria in rural areas. As the need for surgery for tuberculosis declined, thoracic surgeons turned first to undertaking mitral valvotomies for rheumatic heart disease, and then to more advanced forms of cardiac surgery, explaining why some world-famous cardiac surgical hospitals are currently situated on their own in open countryside. More recently, the discovery of the agent responsible for hepatitis B and, especially, the emergence of the HIV virus, have both had significant implications for the organization of systems designed to reduce cross-infection in healthcare facilities, and in the latter case, the approaches taken to issues of patient consent and confidentiality.

The burden of disease worldwide is dynamic (Mathers & Loncar 2006). One factor is the changing age structure of the population. In many populations, the number of old people, and especially the very old, is increasing. This is something to be celebrated, especially as there is growing evidence that it is associated with compression of morbidity, so that people are living even longer in good health. Yet, when coupled with the ability to maintain people with chronic diseases in good health, this is leading to a situation wherein there are many more people with multiple chronic diseases (McKee & Nolte 2004). This will be perhaps the greatest challenge to health systems in the twenty-first century. Yet traditionally, health services have been based on a model of individual self-limiting illnesses in which a patient is attended to by a single health professional. This model is inappropriate in a situation where a patient must navigate a complex maze of health facilities and health professionals. In such circumstances, the patient (or his or her carer, where the patient has cognitive impairment) may be the only person who has a comprehensive view of the total package of care.

Recognition of these challenges has led to the development of new models of care, especially in the United States where, as already noted, outcomes of chronic disease are poor. One of the best known, the Chronic Care Model, illustrates many of the issues related to these new models of care (Wagner *et al.* 1999). Most other models are variations on the same theme. The Chronic Care Model comprises four interacting system components: Self-management support, delivery system design, decision support and clinical information systems. Evaluations have linked individual components to improvements in some process or outcome measures, such as perceived quality of care, patient outcomes, pathways to care, and reduced cost (Tsai *et al.* 2005). However it is less clear whether this is a consequence of applying the model as a whole, or whether the same benefits can be achieved using only some of the components (Bodenheimer *et al.* 2002). The message to emerge from this body of work is that appropriate care for the growing number of people with multiple chronic disorders requires systems that empower patients and help them to navigate through a complex system, secure in the knowledge that the care available is co-ordinated and based on evidence of effectiveness.

There are, however, many other ways in which the burden of disease is changing that have implications for health services. To a considerable extent this reflects changing risk factors. It is increasingly likely that the epidemic of tobacco-related disease will be seen as a transient phenomenon of the twentieth and early twenty-first century, at least in industrialized countries. Other changes are a result of a general improvement in living conditions, such as the long-standing decline in stomach cancer, reflecting falling rates of infection with *Helicobacter pylori* in childhood. Still others are more complex. Death rates from cardiovascular disease have fallen by about 50 per cent in many industrialized countries over the past three decades, reflecting a combination of lower rates of smoking, improved diet (in part a result of global trade), and improved understanding of risk factors. Yet, not all changes are so encouraging. A combination of energy-rich diets and reduced levels of exercise are leading to a rapid increase in obesity in many countries, with an accompanying rise in the prevalence of type II diabetes. Finally, successes against some infectious diseases, such as measles, contrast with failures with others, exemplified by increasing rates of HIV infection and drug-resistant bacteria in many places.

The key message for public health professionals is that they have a central role in tracking and predicting these emerging trends, in designing mechanisms that address them, and in supporting the changes in service delivery that are required.

Upward pressure on healthcare expenditure

The debate on the future of health systems often seems to be dominated by discussion of the cost of providing care. This is an issue that is surrounded by a great deal of mythology. For example, the observation that healthcare costs increase with age is often used to support the argument that an ageing population will render the provision of universal healthcare unsustainable. However, it is now clear that age per se does not increase costs but rather proximity to death (McGrail *et al.* 2000). In fact, in the United States, Medicare data show that payments associated with an additional year of death fall as age at death increases (Lubitz *et al.* 1995) and that the most costly patients are those who die young, possibly because, for a variety of reasons, they are more intensively treated. An ageing population will, however, incur increased costs for social care,

largely reflecting the effects of cognitive decline (Meerding *et al.* 1998). However, when looking to the future it is necessary to take account of evidence that tomorrow's elderly population is likely to be considerably healthier than today's, as they will have benefited from a lifetime of better nutrition and social conditions. This is known as compression of morbidity (Fries 2003). For these reasons, simplistic extrapolation of cross-sectional cost data to a future population with a longer life expectancy is flawed.

The changing composition of the population does, however, have one important consequence. In many countries ageing populations are coinciding with falling birth rates, leading to an increasing old-age dependency ratio (ratio of people 65 and over to those aged 15–64). These changes vary greatly between countries. Some countries, such as Germany and Japan, face substantial challenges while others, such as the United Kingdom, will be somewhat less affected, at least until the middle of the twenty-first century. This development, taken with the evidence of compression of morbidity noted above, is leading several countries to explore the possibility of raising the retirement age as a means of addressing what would otherwise be a shrinking share of the population in working ages. Projections indicate that a relatively small increase in retirement age, coupled with efforts to increase the participation in the workforce of people over 50, would overcome many of the anticipated problems.

Another area where there appears to be considerable misunderstanding relates to the oft-quoted statement that healthcare costs inevitably rise at a faster rate than the economy, or in economic terms, that healthcare is a luxury good. This is often linked to a view, usually implicit, that it is legitimate to restrict health expenditure because the additional expenditure is not yielding proportionate health gains. However, cost estimates are only as good as the underlying data and models used. Thus, Parkin and colleagues have shown it is possible to derive widely differing figures for the elasticity of health spending on national income in industrialized countries, depending on whether exchange rates or purchasing power parities are used and on how the model is specified (Parkin *et al.* 1987). Furthermore, analyses inside countries consistently indicate that healthcare is not a luxury good.

A third issue is the introduction of new pharmaceuticals and technology. The pace of change in healthcare is steadily accelerating. The growth of healthcare technology is widely held to have contributed substantially to the upward pressure on healthcare expenditure, for several reasons, although its precise contribution is controversial (Mossialos & Le Grand 1999). New technologies can be more expensive than the ones they replaced. Even where the actual technology is less expensive, it may lead to increased costs as other aspects of the service are reorganized to reflect changing patterns of treatment. The introduction of new treatments may lead to an expansion in the number of individuals with indications for treatment, either because a previously untreatable condition becomes treatable or, as side-effects or contraindications are reduced, the threshold for treatment falls. Finally, the diffusion of technology from tertiary centres, in some cases into primary care, can markedly reduce barriers to access and thus increase uptake. In response to the increasing use of expensive new technologies, many countries have established health technology assessment programmes and related systems to control introduction and diffusion. One example is the United Kingdom's National Institute for Health and Clinical Excellence, which looks beyond specific technologies to evaluate a wide range of health interventions. It assesses evidence of cost-effectiveness, typically recommending the adoption of interventions where the cost of an additional quality-adjusted life year gained is under about £30 000 (€44 000). It also identifies gaps in the available research. While some of its decisions not to recommend interventions or products have attracted considerable controversy, it has also been credited with increasing the uptake of innovations of proven effectiveness.

Fourth, consumers have increased their expectations about the services provided by the healthcare system, in some cases encouraged by governments. As noted above, the development of new and more expensive technologies coupled with the increased access to information via the Internet have led people to demand a wider range of services of high quality from healthcare providers, an issue dealt with in more detail below.

Each of these issues has implications for public health professionals. Public health professionals must contribute to the process of anticipating future health needs. This requires an understanding of the relationship over time between a change in exposure and its corresponding outcome. This may be very short, as was seen following the collapse of the USSR where rapid fluctuations in mortality were driven by large-scale changes in alcohol consumption (Shkolnikov et al. 2001). In contrast, there is a delay of many years between an increase in smoking in a population and the development of many tobacco-related diseases. It is, however, important to recognize that relationships may be asymmetrical, with reductions in exposure leading to rapid declines in disease or death.

Public health professionals must also contribute to discussions on how health services can be reconfigured to meet the increasingly complex needs of the elderly population with multiple disease processes, as well as how to invest effectively in prevention so as to extend the years that people live in good health. Discussions about new health technology require inputs from public health professionals, drawing on skills such as epidemiology and economics, to assess appropriateness and cost-effectiveness. However, it is also important to stress that attention to these issues may lead to a conclusion that there is a need for greater expenditure on healthcare, as was the case in the United Kingdom, where the Wanless Report demonstrated how the National Health Service was underperforming because of long-term underinvestment (Wanless 2001).

The quest for enhanced quality of care

Research undertaken in the 1970s and 1980s drew attention to widespread geographical variations in the use of common procedures (McPherson 1989) and led to a questioning of clinical judgements about the appropriateness of healthcare interventions. The International Cochrane Collaboration has played a major part in this process by highlighting the extent to which much care that was provided was ineffective, while effective interventions were not adopted widely (Chalmers & Altman 1995). Similar findings have emerged from the health technology assessment activities discussed above. More recently, there has been growing attention to patient safety, in the light of research showing unacceptably high levels of patient injury and death due to clinical errors (Institute of Medicine 2000).

These developments reflect a change in dominant belief systems, challenging traditional models based on clinical autonomy. They are contributing to a range of changes in healthcare systems that include not only the elimination of ineffective treatments and adoption of effective ones but also new organizational structures to bring about change. Again, public health professionals have key roles to play because of their skills in healthcare evaluation and the management of change. Strategies to ensure quality of care are discussed in more detail below.

The information society

The 1980s and 1990s have seen an unparalleled revolution in the pace and volume of communication. This brings both challenges and opportunities for health systems, discussed in more detail in Chapter 5.3 (Web-based public health information dissemination and evaluation).

Strategies for health services

Given these changing circumstances, coherent strategies are needed to enable health systems to respond appropriately. Four such strategies are considered here. The first includes those that address resource scarcity, which here includes the process of setting priorities for healthcare. The second relates to healthcare funding, focusing on the issue of equity and, specifically, the tension between competition and solidarity. The third includes those designed to achieve a more effective allocation of resources, here including assessment of healthcare need and purchasing healthcare. The final set includes strategies designed to achieve more cost-effective and higher-quality care.

Tackling scarcity of resources

Upward pressures on healthcare costs in the face of limited resources confront governments with two interconnected options. One is to increase the resources for healthcare by shifting funds from other areas of public sector expenditure or by increasing taxation, social insurance contributions, or direct payments. The second is to seek to control healthcare expenditure by pursuing strategies that influence either the demand for or the supply of healthcare. Strategies that act on supply of health services include reducing the number of healthcare professionals or facilities, setting global budgets for providers, giving professionals incentives to reduce the amount of care provided, and reducing access to care (Abel-Smith et al. 1995).

Strategies acting on demand include priority setting to ration access to certain services, the use of cost-sharing, incentives to encourage greater private expenditure, such as tax concessions, and the right to opt out of the statutory system.

Each of these measures seeks to reduce demand by shifting some portion of healthcare costs to the individual. They have all been discussed elsewhere (Mossialos & Le Grand 1999) and here only one approach, that of setting priorities, is considered as it is the one in which public health professionals have played the greatest role.

During the 1990s, many countries addressed the issue of explicit rationing of publicly funded healthcare. The debate has been lengthy and complex, with many different views. Perhaps the only issue where there is a degree of unanimity is that, in all healthcare systems, some form of rationing has always taken place although, in most cases, this was implicit, inextricably linked to clinical judgement. Beyond this, the consensus breaks down as illustrated by the situation in the United Kingdom where there was fundamental disagreement between politicians and others about even the choice of the terms 'rationing' or 'priority setting' as a means of describing the process.

In this debate, some commentators have argued that rationing should not be necessary if either sufficient funding was made available typically by redirecting it from other areas of public expenditure or raising taxes or by ensuring that available resources are used more efficiently. However, others have argued that the continuing upward pressure on healthcare costs has made explicit rationing of effective care necessary. For these commentators, the key issue is transparency.

Concerns about the affordability of healthcare have led, in several countries, to initiatives that examine priority setting on a more systematic and explicit basis. These processes have brought together a wide range of individuals, including public health professionals, managers, politicians, economists and philosophers.

Explicit setting of priorities involves making decisions at different levels within the healthcare system, ranging from the overall funders of healthcare to the treatments available to individual patients. If explicit priority setting is to be undertaken, a co-ordinated, strategic approach is most effective to integrate decision-making at these different levels.

Decisions may lead to blanket exclusions of intervention, or of condition–intervention combinations, as in the approach taken in Oregon in the United States, or production of guidelines, such as those developed by the National Institute of Health and Clinical Excellence in the United Kingdom. The experience of Oregon was especially interesting because of the technical and ethical issues it raised (Oregon Health Services Commission 1991). It was designed to create a list of condition intervention pairs, ranked on the basis of cost-benefit, with a cut-off point based on available resources below which combinations would not be funded. The idea was that this would maximize the return on resources invested in healthcare. However, the process was extremely problematic when it became clear that many of the data required were unavailable and some results were quite counterintuitive—for example, appendectomy was rated lower than cosmetic dentistry.

An alternative approach was used in the Netherlands. There the Dunning Committee (Dunning 1992) proposed four criteria that an intervention to be funded from social health insurance should meet. These were necessity, effectiveness, efficiency, and whether treating the condition should be a matter of individual rather than community responsibility. As a result of this process, it was recommended that services such as dentistry for adults, homeopathic treatment, *in vitro* fertilization and physiotherapy for sports injuries should be excluded.

This debate has created a recognition that the priority-setting process must include government, providers, the public and patients, as well as evidence on health needs and on the cost and effectiveness of available interventions (Ham 1993). Priority setting cannot be reduced to a technical exercise and should be combined with a thorough public debate about the values underpinning the choices to be made. This is seen in the approach taken in Sweden (McKee & Figueras 1996), which focused on the need to reach a shared view of the ethical basis on which priorities should be set. This rejected a narrow economic approach and gave priority to the treatment of life-threatening conditions. It also emphasized the importance of social solidarity.

Ultimately, while public health professionals have an important role in providing the evidence on which any debate on priority setting must be based and on examining the consequences of any decisions for equity, priority setting in a publicly funded system is the responsibility of politicians. Decision-making inevitably involves trade-offs between objectives as a balance is sought among universal coverage, comprehensiveness of services, equity, efficiency, cost-containment, and broader social values. However, it is also important to note that, despite enormous efforts being devoted to the setting of priorities, it has been extremely difficult for any health system ostensibly providing universal coverage to exclude any treatments except for a few on the margin, such as cosmetic surgery.

Equitable funding of health systems

Whitehead (1988) has shown how access to services is a key element of strategies designed to reduce health inequalities. Throughout the twentieth century the steady expansion of coverage in many countries has served to improve access to healthcare for those in greatest need, based on the principle of solidarity, in which individual financial contributions are related to ability to pay and are not dependent on the individual's health status.

At present, however, certain developments threaten to undermine the principle of solidarity. One is the pressure from advocates of market-based policies to establish competition among healthcare insurers. A second is the development of information technology and, increasingly, the use of genetic profiling, enabling individual risks to be predicted more accurately and permitting exclusion or higher premiums for those at greatest risk, although this is raising enormous technical and ethical issues. A third is the failure, by some governments, to collect sufficient taxes or social insurance contributions from the wealthy to fund the system. This has several causes. One is a neo-liberal agenda that argues that, for countries to attract inward investment and employment, they must reduce taxes. A second cause, which is especially problematic in, but not exclusive to, low- and middle-income countries, is widespread tax avoidance by the wealthy.

Each of these issues has important implications for equity and thus for public health professionals. The third is beyond the scope of this chapter, but the first and second, which are linked in that competitive insurers have a strong incentive to identify the risks attached to those they accept, are relevant as public health professionals may have to work with such competitive systems.

Competition between health insurers (whether private or public) tends to erode solidarity in healthcare financing, since health insurers seek to select good risks. In the absence of regulation, older people and those with pre-existing illness or even a strong family history of illness are either excluded from coverage or charged higher premiums. As noted above, advances in information technology and genetics are making this ever easier, although this is raising enormous ethical issues. For example, should an insurer be permitted to know an individual's genotype?

Two responses are open to policy-makers. One is mandatory open enrolment, so that insurers are unable to refuse coverage to an individual. This is typically linked to regulation of the level of contributions, such as community ratings. The second is the use of risk-adjustment schemes that redistribute the health insurance system's revenue among competing health insurers on the basis of the risk profile of those enrolling with each insurer.

While these responses might work in theory, they are much more problematic in practice. Apparently open enrolment can be distorted in many subtle ways by targeting promotional activities or manipulating access so that insurers tend to 'cream skim'. Risk pooling requires development of valid formulas, which have proved elusive, with several systems relying purely on crude measures such as age.

If politicians choose to introduce competitive markets in health-care financing, despite a widespread consensus from health economists and others that such initiatives are fraught with danger, public health professionals have an important role in monitoring and responding to any effects on equity. Maintaining solidarity in healthcare financing while introducing competition among insurers is an ambitious and difficult undertaking. The 'safety-net' for solidarity has to be designed very carefully, and such an undertaking requires experienced supervision of healthcare markets. Moreover, several crucial questions have not yet been answered. Whether competition among insurers really leads to more efficient and more effective healthcare has yet to be demonstrated (Chinitz et al. 1998), not least because of the need for expensive regulatory and risk adjustment systems, as has the question of whether mechanisms seeking to combine solidarity with competition can succeed.

Optimal allocation of resources

Upward pressure on costs and an increasing willingness of politicians, managers and the public to challenge established patterns of care have placed an increased emphasis on the optimal allocation of scarce healthcare resources. Several interconnected strategies are available to health policy-makers. These include ensuring that the health services provided reflect the health needs of the population that they serve, enhance the efficiency with which services are delivered, and control the cost of key inputs such as pharmaceuticals and technology. Public health professionals can play an important role in both the assessment of health needs and, increasingly, in the process of intelligent purchasing of healthcare so as to maximize health gain for a given set of inputs.

Assessing need for healthcare

Assessment of healthcare needs has arisen from recognition that, left to itself, the pattern of health services will frequently reflect only partially the health needs of the population it is serving, and often those whose needs are greatest will receive least, a phenomenon described by Tudor Hart (1971) as the Inverse Care Law. Instead, other factors come into play, such as, the specialist interests of individual physicians, the structure of financial incentives, and the ease of interacting with different groups of patients. Three types of needs assessment have been described: Epidemiological, comparative, and corporate (Stevens & Gabbay 1991). These are examined in detail in Chapter 12.2 (Needs assessment: A practical approach). Public health professionals play a central role in assessment of need, drawing on the skills they possess, especially where there is a major epidemiological perspective.

Intelligent purchasing

In an increasing number of countries intelligent purchasing is seen as an instrument to implement health policy objectives, including ensuring that health services closely reflect the health needs of the population that they serve (Øvretveit 1995). Purchasing acts as a co-ordinating mechanism that offers an alternative to a traditional command-and-control approach. Its essential characteristic is that it separates purchasers from providers but binds each party by means of contracts to explicit commitments, with creation of the economic motivation to fulfil these commitments.

Contracts have always been a feature of those healthcare systems based on social insurance systems, with complex institutional structures developed to represent health insurers and physicians in negotiations over payment schedules. Governments have often played some role in these discussions, typically to ensure cost containment and preservation of solidarity. However, both insurers and governments are increasingly using contracts as a means of reorienting the focus of health services, to ensure that they reflect health needs and provide cost-effective care.

In contrast, in most tax-based systems, relationships between health authorities and providers have traditionally been based on hierarchies. This is also changing as policy-makers seek new ways of influencing provider behaviour, based on a clearer identification of the objectives of the health system.

In systems where private insurance plays an important role, similar changes are taking place. Instead of simply reimbursing costs incurred retrospectively, insurers are introducing what is described as managed care, in which entitlements are defined in advance and treatment patterns are closely scrutinized.

From a public health perspective, interest in purchasing relates to whether or not it can achieve health gain and promote equity. Whether it does so will depend on both the objectives being pursued and on the quality of the contracting process. Contracts bring many potential benefits but also some risks.

For purchasing to promote health gain it must be based on an assessment of health needs coupled with a strong focus on the cost-effectiveness of clinical interventions and the organizational context within which they are delivered. Conversely, if it is based primarily on cost-saving, it will reduce health gain.

Purchasing can support equity if, through needs assessment, they take explicit account of vulnerable and disadvantaged groups as well as under-served communities. From this perspective, purchasers represent the interests of their populations, allocating resources and purchasing services in accordance with their needs. However, purchasing also carries the risk of undermining equity if providers are able to underemphasize or phase out services that are less profitable. Purchasing also offers a means for enhancing participation by the population in the organization of healthcare, thus increasing the accountability of governments and the medical profession and making health policy more relevant to the needs and priorities of society.

In some countries, especially where public health professionals have played a central role in the contracting process, it has been possible to use contracts to develop intersectoral responses to health problems or to reorient healthcare providers so that they integrate prevention with curative care. The opportunities for doing so are discussed in more detail below.

Implementation of an intelligent purchasing system is a complex process requiring a high level of skills and well-developed information systems (Figueras et al. 2005). At a minimum, information is required on patient flow, cost, and utilization information across specialties or diagnostic groups, and demographic and risk groups. It is important that expectations of what can be achieved are realistic. Medical care is extremely complex. Diagnostic labels are often imprecise and clouded by a degree of legitimate uncertainty. Decisions on clinical management incorporate values and beliefs relating to factors such as attitude to risk and the utility placed on different health states. Contracts must incorporate sufficient flexibility and reflect the views of all those concerned if they are to retain any credibility.

Purchasing also involves transaction costs to cover activities such as needs assessment, performance analysis, negotiating, and monitoring. A substantial increase in quality and efficiency is required to justify these additional costs. If transaction costs can be minimized without compromising the pursuit of the objectives of equity and health gain, intelligent purchasing can provide a formidable instrument to promote population health.

Efficient and effective service delivery

The increasing use of intelligent purchasing is focusing the attention of public health professionals on the delivery of healthcare. Evaluative research has highlighted the extent of use of treatments that are unsupported by evidence of effectiveness and the importance of appropriate organizational structures and cultures in the provision of high-quality care. This section examines three areas in which public health professionals can play an important role: The design of systems that ensure that patients are managed at the level of the healthcare system that is most appropriate, the creation of mechanisms that identify and promote high-quality clinical care, and the reorientation of curative services towards prevention.

Shifting interfaces

Health services are typically organized on different levels, reflecting the need to balance two competing objectives. On the one hand, dispersion permits easy access to those facilities in which most people receive care and where they can obtain an initial contact with the system. On the other hand, concentration of specialized resources required by relatively small numbers of patients optimizes scarce resources, with potential gains in effectiveness and efficiency, although the relationships are complex and often counterintuitive (Ferguson *et al.* 1997). Movement between the various levels (primary, secondary, tertiary, and community care) typically involves passage across an interface that is governed by rules of varying degrees of formality. Examples include referral to hospital by a primary care physician or discharge from an acute hospital to a long-stay facility.

The nature of these interfaces is steadily changing in the face of the new circumstances discussed above. Upward pressure on costs is causing policy-makers to ensure that patients are treated in the most cost-effective settings. Changing patterns of disease, coupled with evolving patient beliefs about the nature of healthcare, are challenging established ways of delivering care. New technologies in fields such as imaging, diagnosis, surgery, pharmaceuticals, and information are having a substantial impact on clinical practice. Healthcare professionals are developing new and different sets of skills.

These changes involve a process of substitution, by which there has been a continual regrouping of resources across care settings to exploit the best available solutions. This can take many forms. One typology differentiates three kinds of substitution: Moving the location of care, introducing new technologies, and shifting the mix of staff and skills (Warner 1996).

From a public health perspective, substitution brings the potential of both benefits and risks. Benefits include increased patient satisfaction, improved clinical outcomes, greater efficiency, and more appropriate management of certain diseases. Risks include fragmentation of services, loss of specialized skills, increased costs, and wasteful duplication of expensive technology. Each case must be assessed on its merits as initiatives that have seemed intuitively better than what they replaced have often, on detailed evaluation, failed to live up to the initial expectations.

Effective substitution policies require co-ordination, with clear strategic objectives. A system-wide perspective is necessary to identify unintended consequences for other services. Too often substitution involves simply changing the location, without an appropriate shift in skills and technology or without a reallocation of resources. However, substitution offers a valuable tool to public health professionals to make services more accessible and appropriate to the population and to ensure that care is provided as cost-effectively as possible.

Improving outcomes

As noted above, former deference to medical judgement about how to deliver healthcare is giving way, in the face of wide variations, to how care is delivered (Institute of Medicine 2001). The view expressed by the editor of *The Lancet* in 1951, that central guidance on clinical care should be rejected because of the harm that it would do to the sense of personal responsibility of the physician (Fox 1951), is no longer tenable.

Variations in clinical practice have many causes, the most important being clinical uncertainty about the most appropriate treatment in any given circumstance. Studies of treatment patterns reveal both over-treatment, where patients receive treatments that are ineffective, and under-treatment, where those who would benefit are denied effective treatment. This has led to four related questions. Firstly, which treatments can be expected to produce improved health outcomes? Secondly, does a treatment that has been shown to be efficacious in evaluative research achieve the intended objective in routine clinical practice? Thirdly, why are treatments of known effectiveness not used in circumstances where they would achieve health improvement? Finally, how does one change professional behaviour so as to ensure that the most effective, efficient, and humane treatments are provided? Together, these questions contribute to the quest for what is termed 'evidence-based healthcare'.

Four aspects of quality assurance are relevant. The first is that it should be based on evidence, typically organized as guidelines or protocols. While these should take full account of local circumstances, there are a number of international collaborations seeking to achieve economies of effort. Second, it is a continuous process, involving repeated cycles of setting standards, introducing change to meet those standards, and review of the results of change. The third is that it is necessary to differentiate three types of quality measures (Donabedian 1966). Measures of structure relate to inputs such as facilities and the availability of trained staff. Measures of process include adherence to agreed good practice. Measures of outcome assess the extent to which the objectives of treatment are achieved. A fourth relates to the question of whether quality assurance should be internal or external.

Quality assurance activities often deal with structures and processes of care rather than outcomes. Ideally, the focus would be on outcomes, but outcomes are typically more difficult to measure and may only become apparent long after the intervention took place. Some outcomes may also be rare and the sample size required to detect a deviation from what is expected may be very large. For example, Mant and Hicks (1995) showed, on the basis of knowledge of effective treatment for myocardial infarction, that, in a comparison of two typical hospitals, it would take 73 years of data to detect a significant 3 per cent reduction in mortality. In contrast, a significant difference in process measures, here uptake of treatments, would emerge after only 4 months. Where process or structure measures are used there should be evidence that they correlate with a good outcome. Measures based on structure can be of some value, based on the assumption that high-quality care cannot be provided in the absence of basic prerequisites, such as adequately trained staff, but this is a necessary rather than a sufficient measure and should normally be supplemented by measures of either process or outcome.

Internal and external forms of quality assurance have quite different characteristics. In the former, the activity is conducted by those undertaking the clinical activities concerned, such as the physicians in a hospital. They are responsible for setting standards and implementing change. This has the advantage of fostering a sense of ownership and is less open to opportunistic manipulation of results. However, it does require a culture in which it is accepted that clinical practice should be open to examination by one's peers. Professional bodies have often played a major role in promoting this approach.

External quality assurance involves a body outside the healthcare facility examining measures of quality. This typically focuses on structure, largely because this is so much easier to measure than process or outcome. A typical example is hospital accreditation. Accreditation is especially important for countries seeking to establish a mix of private and public health services, as it offers a means of reassurance that all facilities meet an agreed minimum level of quality. In some countries there is growing pressure to make public assessments of the performance of individual health professionals and facilities yet there is now considerable evidence that comparisons can be highly misleading (Jacobson *et al.* 2003) and that they can create strong incentives for perverse behaviour (Green & Wintfeld 1995). Such behaviour includes imaginative use of disease coding to increase the apparent severity of patients' conditions, refusal to operate on patients at high risk, and even frank distortion of data.

Perhaps the greatest challenge facing those seeking to improve the quality of healthcare is how to change clinical behaviour. An increasing volume of research on this topic is being brought together by the work of the Cochrane Collaboration on Effective Practice and Organization of Care. This has examined behavioural, financial, and organizational approaches to changing practice. It has shown how many traditional approaches, such as conferences and short educational events, are of little value. Educational outreach visits have a small effect, and financial and organizational initiatives, such as the introduction of co-payments, tend to reduce appropriate and inappropriate care to a similar extent. The most successful strategies involve combing a range of behavioural approaches, such as audit and feedback, production of guidelines, and, where appropriate, computer-generated reminders (Grimshaw *et al.* 2006). However, the main conclusion of this research is that change is very difficult and requires carefully targeted sustained action.

Public health professionals have played a key role in the development of evidence-based healthcare, although its elements, from research through dissemination to implementation, are in place in only a few countries and health policy discussion often remains focused on issues of financing and organization.

Health services as a setting for promoting health

Public health professionals have a particularly important role in promoting the reorientation of health services to address the broader determinants of health. Health services are important settings in which it is possible actively to promote health through primary preventive strategies. Health professionals have an important role as opinion formers, both in individual patient encounters and,

among the wider public, as respected advocates for healthy public policies (Chapman & Lupton 1994). Conversely, contradictory images, such as physicians and nurses smoking while they advise their patients to quit, can do much to undermine public health messages.

Relatively simple approaches, such as brief interventions by health professionals, can often be very effective. Yet it is not sufficient to assume that such approaches are always going to be effective, and, as with treatment interventions, each must be assessed individually. For example, while advising patients to take more exercise or eat more nutritious food may seem intuitively beneficial, there is little evidence that it is effective. There is no evidence that attempts to reduce the risk of coronary heart disease through multiple risk factor interventions have an impact on either total or coronary heart disease mortality (Ebrahim & Smith 1997), and fiscal and legislative measures seem more appropriate.

Many people come into contact with healthcare facilities, either as patients or staff. This provides an important opportunity to demonstrate support for health-promoting policies by means of an ethos based on healthy lifestyles. Most obviously, it is no longer acceptable for healthcare facilities to permit smoking on their premises (McKee *et al.* 2003). Ideally, smokers should be seen several weeks before admission and supported with advice and nicotine replacement therapy (Moller *et al.* 2002). In contrast, failure to ban smoking provides an implicit message that health promotion is simply not taken seriously and the obvious conflict between the culture of the organization and the advice given to patients will make behavioural change more difficult.

There is, however, much more that can be done to create a healthy environment. For example, patients and staff should be able to choose healthy diets. The provision of cycle parks, gyms, and showers will encourage staff to cycle to work. Many of these ideas have been brought together in the WHO's Health-Promoting Hospitals project, which seeks to increase participation in health-promoting activities by patients, staff, and others outside the hospital, as well as improving communication and reorienting hospitals towards health promotion.

Finally, the contribution that health services can make to health by employing people should not be ignored. The adverse health effects of unemployment are well recognized (Bartley 1994), in particular the impact of job insecurity and anticipation of unemployment (Ferrie *et al.* 1995). Health services have always been labour intensive. Healthcare reforms in many countries have led to substantial reductions in staff numbers, either through redundancy or, in some countries, transfers to private sector agencies where levels of pay and conditions of service are substantially worse. While reducing the direct costs to the health service, such policies often increase overall government expenditure through increased social costs. However, some governments are recognizing the role of health services as a source of employment, as illustrated by the use of the European Union's structural funds to support investment in healthcare infrastructure.

The contribution of public health to health services

This chapter began by showing how healthcare can no longer be regarded as peripheral to attempts to improve the health of populations. Notwithstanding the importance of tackling the wider determinants of health, modern medical care offers new opportunities to reduce mortality and improve quality of life. Healthcare is also taking on a greater importance as evidence emerges of how differential access can increase health inequalities.

Health services are changing, bringing new opportunities for public health to increase its impact on this process by reorienting health services towards the maximization of health gain. However, if public health professionals are to take full advantage of these new opportunities, they will need to have a thorough understanding of the pressures that are driving the health services change.

This chapter has highlighted the contributions that they can make to the response to the changing demands on healthcare systems. These various strategies can be summarized through a conceptual shorthand suggested by Saltman and Figueras (1998). This approach compresses activities into two traditional economic parameters: Policy interventions instituted on the demand side as against those instituted on the supply side of the healthcare system.

The demand side incorporates all strategies that influence funding of the healthcare system and more specifically the relationships between the consumer and the third-party payers. A number of health system strategies have concentrated on the demand side by introducing measures shifting costs to the patient, such as cost-sharing arrangements or limiting the public package of care, and by introducing market competition incentives among third-party insurers. Many of these have led to inequities. The role of public health here is twofold: First to ensure that solidarity in the health system is not harmed by these measures which tend to reduce access and coverage particularly for the most vulnerable groups in our society, and second to shift the policy-makers' agenda from these individual patient-based demand policies towards strategies dealing with aggregate population-based demand. Indeed, the latter is very much at the core of a public health role.

The introduction of effective health promotion and primary prevention strategies will ultimately reduce the total demand for healthcare services and healthcare costs. However, health promotion has not played a central role in the health reform agenda. Public health professionals need to strive to develop more and better ways to evaluate health promotion that satisfies the needs of policy-makers, managers and clinicians so the full potential of health promotion can be realized.

The supply side includes strategies forming a continuum that moves from the allocation of health resources to the delivery of health services. Some of the key strategies include the introduction of quality-oriented strategies, and the integration and substitution of services across the hospital and primary healthcare sectors. In many instances, these reforms have met with considerable success (Saltman & Figueras 1998), but the extent of their success will depend on the availability of a series of skills traditionally linked to the public health profession. These include assessing the health needs of the population, evaluating and monitoring interventions, assessing health outcomes, and reorienting healthcare delivery so that the focus is on prevention as well as cure.

Health services can make an important contribution to improving the health status of populations. This chapter has identified mechanisms through which public health can have a major role in maximizing the health gain obtained from health services, but much will depend on the ability of the public health profession to adapt and bring its portfolio of tools and skills to bear on rapidly changing health services.

Key points

- Modern healthcare has the potential to make a substantial contribution to population health and has been doing so in high-income countries for at least four decades.

- While much healthcare that is provided is effective in improving health, some is ineffective or even harmful.

- Healthcare systems must continually adapt to changing circumstances, including the economic situation, the burden of disease and scope for intervention, and public expectations.

- Expenditure on improved health should be seen not as a drain on the economy but as an investment in future growth.

- Public health professionals have a critical role to play in maximizing the health gain achieved by healthcare.

References

Abel-Smith, B., Figueras, J., Holland, W. *et al.* (1995). *Choices in health policy: An agenda for the European Union* Aldershot, Dartmouth Press/Office for Official Publications of the European Communities.

Alderson, P., F. Bunn, C. Lefebvre. *et al.* (2004). Human albumin solution for resuscitation and volume expansion in critically ill patients. *Cochrane Database Syst Rev* (4): CD001208.

Andreev, E.M., E. Nolte, V.M. Shkolnikov. *et al.* (2003). The evolving pattern of avoidable mortality in Russia. *Int J Epidemiol* **32**, 437–46.

Arblaster, L., M. Lambert, V. Entwistle. *et al.* (1996). A systematic review of the effectiveness of health service interventions aimed at reducing inequalities in health. *J Health Serv Res Policy* **1**, 93–103.

Bartley, M. (1994). Unemployment and ill health: understanding the relationship. *J Epidemiol Community Health* **48**, 333–7.

Beaglehole, R. (1986). Medical management and the decline in mortality from coronary heart disease. *Br Med J (Clin Res Ed)* **292**, 33–5.

Beeson, P.B. (1980). Changes in medical therapy during the past half century. *Medicine* **59**, 79–99.

Benson, J.K. (1975). The interorganisational network as a political economy. *Administrative Science Quarterly* **20**, 229–49.

Billings, J., G.M. Anderson and L.S. Newman (1996). Recent findings on preventable hospitalizations. *Health Aff* **15**, 239–49.

Bodenheimer, T., E.H. Wagner and K. Grumbach (2002). Improving primary care for patients with chronic illness. *JAMA* **288**, 1775–9.

Bonneux, L., C.W. Looman, J. J. Barendregt. *et al.* (1997). Regression analysis of recent changes in cardiovascular morbidity and mortality in the Netherlands. *BMJ* **314**, 789–92.

Chalmers, I. and D.G. Altman (1995). *Systematic reviews*. London, BM Publications.

Chapman, S. and D. Lupton (1994). *The fight for public Health*. London, BMJ Publications.

Chappell, N.L. (1993). The future of health care in Canada. *Journal of Social Policy* **22**, 495.

Chinitz, D., Preker A., and Wasem J. (1998). Balancing competition and solidarity in health care financing. *Critical challenges for health care reform*. R.B. Saltman, J. Figueras and C. Sakellarides. Buckingham, Open University Press: xvi, p. 424.

Clark, D.G. (1998). Autonomy, personal empowerment and quality of life in long-term care. *Journal of Applied Gerontology* **7**, 279–97.

Cochrane, A.L., A.S. St Leger and F. Moore (1978). Health service 'input' and mortality 'output' in developed countries. *Journal of Epidemiology and Community Health* **32**, 200–5.

Contandriopoulos, A.P., M. Lauristin and E. Leibovich (1998). Values, norms and the reform of health care systems. *Critical challenges for health care reform*. R. B. Saltman, J. Figueras and C. Sakellarides. Buckingham, Open University Press: 339–62.

Donabedian, A. (1966). Evaluating the quality of medical care. *Milbank Mem Fund Q* **44**(3), Suppl,166–206.

Dunning, A. (1992). Choices in health care: a report by the Government Committee on Choices in health care. Rijkswijk, the Netherlands, Ministry of Welfare, Health and Culture.

Ebrahim, S. and G.D. Smith (1997). Systematic review of randomised controlled trials of multiple risk factor interventions for preventing coronary heart disease. *BMJ* **314**(7095), 1666–74.

Ferguson, B., T. Sheldon, and J. Posnett (1997). *Concentration and choice in health care.* Glasgow, Royal Society of Medicine Press.

Ferrie, J.E., M.J. Shipley, M.G. Marmot. *et al.* (1995). Health effects of anticipation of job change and non-employment: longitudinal data from the Whitehall II study. *Bmj* **311**(7015), 1264–9.

Figueras, J., R. Robinson, and E. Jakubowski (2005). *Purchasing to Improve Health Systems Performance.* European Observatory Series. Maidenhead. Open University Press. McGraw Hill Education.

Fogel, R.W. (1994). Economic Growth, Population Theory, and Physiology: the bearing of long-term process on the making of economic policy. *American Economic Review* **84**(3), 369–395.

Fox, T.E. (1951). Professional freedom. *Lancet* **2**(3), 115–9.

Fries, J.F. (2003). Measuring and monitoring success in compressing morbidity. *Ann Intern Med* **139**(5 Pt 2), 455–9.

Gillett, G. (1995). Virtue and truth in clinical science. *J Med Philos* **20**(3), 285–98.

Green, J. and N. Wintfeld (1995). Report cards on cardiac surgeons. Assessing New York State's approach. *New England Journal of Medicine* **332**, 1229–32.

Grimshaw, J., M. Eccles, R. Thomas. *et al.* (2006). Toward evidence-based quality improvement. Evidence (and its limitations) of the effectiveness of guideline dissemination and implementation strategies 1966-1998. *J Gen Intern Med* **21 Suppl 2**, S14–20.

Habermas, J. (1987). *Theorie de l'agir communicationnel.* Paris, Fayard.

Ham, C. (1993). *Priority setting in the NHS: reports from six districts. Rationing the action.* London, BMJ Publications.

Healy, J. and M. McKee (2004). *Accessing healthcare: responding to diversity.* Oxford, Oxford University Press.

Hopkins, S. (2006). Economic stability and health status: evidence from East Asia before and after the 1990s economic crisis. *Health Policy* **75**(3), 347–57.

Illich, I. (1976). *Limits to medicine: medical nemesis, the expropriation of health.* London, Boyars.

Institute of Medicine (2000). *To err is human: building a safer health system.* Washington, D.C., Institute of Medicine.

Institute of Medicine (2001). *Crossing the quality chasm: a new health system for the 21st century.* Washington DC, Institute of Medicine.

Jacobson, B., J. Mindell and M. McKee (2003). Hospital mortality league tables. *British Medical Journal* **326**, 777–8.

Kunitz, S.J. and I. Pesis-Katz (2005). Mortality of white Americans, African Americans, and Canadians: the causes and consequences for health of welfare state institutions and policies. *Milbank Q* **83**(1), 5–39.

Lalonde, M. (1974). *A new perspective on the health of Canadians: a working document.* Ottawa, Department of Health and Welfare.

Lavis, J. and G.L. Stoddart (1994). Can we have too much health care? *Daedalus* **123**, 43–60.

Lubitz, J., J. Beebe, and C. Baker (1995). Longevity and medical care expenditures. *New England Journal of Medicine* **332**, 999–1003.

Mackenbach, J.P, C.W.M. Looman, A.E. Kunst. *et al.* (1988). Post-1950 mortality trends and medical care: gains in life expectancy due to declines in mortality from conditions amenable to medical interventions in the Netherlands. *Soc Sci Med*; **27**, 889–94.

Mant, J. and N. Hicks (1995). Detecting differences in quality of care: the sensitivity of measures of process and outcome in treating acute myocardial infarction. *BMJ* **311**(7008), 793–6.

Marshall, S.W., I. Kawachi, N. Pearce. *et al.* (1993). Social class differences in mortality from diseases amenable to medical intervention in New Zealand. *Int J Epidemiol* **22**(2), 255–61.

Mathers, C.D. and D. Loncar (2006). Projections of global mortality and burden of disease from 2002 to 2030. *PLoS Med* **3**(11), e442.

McGrail, K., B. Green, M.L. Barer. *et al.* (2000). Age, costs of acute and long-term care and proximity to death: evidence for 1987-88 and 1994-95 in British Columbia. *Age Ageing* **29**(3), 249–53.

McKee, M. (2002). Values, beliefs and implications. *Health targets in Europe.* M. Marinker. London, BMJ Books: 181–205.

McKee, M. (2007). Cochrane on Communism: the influence of ideology on the search for evidence. *Int J Epidemiol* **36**(2):269–73.

McKee, M. and J. Figueras (1996). Setting priorities - can Britain learn from Sweden? *BMJ* **312**, 691–4.

McKee, M., A. Gilmore and T. Novotny (2003). Smoke-free hospitals. *BMJ* **326**, 941–2.

McKee, M. and E. Nolte (2004). Responding to the challenge of chronic diseases: ideas from Europe. *Clin Med* **4**(4), 336–42.

McKeown, T. (1979). *The role of medicine: drama, mirage or nemesis?* Oxford, Blackwell.

McPherson, K. (1989). International comparisons in medical care practices. *Health Care Financing Review* **Annual supplement**, 9–20.

Meerding, W. J., L. Bonneux, J. J. Polder. *et al.* (1998). Demographic and epidemiological determinants of healthcare costs in Netherlands: cost of illness study. *Bmj* **317**(7151), 111–5.

Moller, A. M., N. Villebro, T. Pedersen *et al.* (2002). Effect of preoperative smoking intervention on postoperative complications: a randomised clinical trial. *Lancet* **359**(9301), 114–7.

Morris, A. M., Y. Wei, N. J. Birkmeyer and J. D. Birkmeyer (2006). Racial disparities in late survival after rectal cancer surgery. *J Am Coll Surg* **203**(6), 787–94.

Mossialos, E. and J. Le Grand (1999). Cost containment in the EU: An overview. *Health care and cost containment in the European Union.* E. Mossialos and J. Le Grand. Aldershot, Ashgate: 1–154.

Mossialos, E., M.F. Mrazek, and T. Walley (2004). *Regulating pharmaceuticals in Europe: striving for efficiency, equity and quality.* Maidenhead, Open University Press.

Nolte, E. and M. McKee (2004). *Does healthcare save lives? Avoidable mortality revisited.* London, The Nuffield Trust.

Nolte, E., V. Shkolnikov, R. Scholz. *et al.* (2004). Progress in health care, progress in health? Patterns of amenable mortality in central and eastern Europe before and after political transition. *Demographic Research* **Special Collection 2**, 139–162.

Oregon Health Services Commission (1991). Prioritization of health services. Salem, Or, Oregon Health Commission.

Øvretveit, J. (1995). *Purchasing for health: a multidisciplinary introduction to the theory and practice of health purchasing.* Buckingham, Open University Press.

Parkin, D., A. McGuire, and B. Yule (1987). Aggregate health care expenditures and national income. Is health care a luxury good? *J Health Econ* **6**(2), 109–27.

Rutstein, D. D., W. Berenberg, and T. C. Chalmers (1976). Measuring the quality of medical care: a clinical method. *New England Journal of Medicine* **294**, 582–8.

Saltman, R. B. and J. Figueras (1998). Analyzing the evidence on European health care reforms. *Health Aff (Millwood)* **17**(2), 85–108.

Shkolnikov, V., M. McKee, and D. A. Leon (2001). Changes in life expectancy in Russia in the 1990s. *Lancet* **357**, 917–21.

Stephens, C., G. Leonardi, S. Lewin. *et al.* (1999). The multilateral agreement on investment. Public health threat for the twenty-first century? *European Journal of Public Health* **9**(3–5).

Stevens, A. and J. Gabbay (1991). Needs assessment needs assessment. *Health Trends* **23**(1), 20–3.

Suhrcke, M., M. McKee, R. S. Arce. *et al.* (2006). Investment in health could be good for Europe's economies. *BMJ* **333**(7576), 1017–9.

Telishevka, M., L. Chenett and M. McKee (2001). Towards an understanding of the high death rate among young people with diabetes in Ukraine. *Diabet Med* **18**(1), 3–9.

Tsai, A. C., S. C. Morton, C. M. Mangione. *et al.* (2005). A meta-analysis of interventions to improve care for chronic illnesses. *Am J Manag Care* **11**(8), 478–88.

Tudor Hart, J. (1971). The inverse care law. *Lancet* **1**(7696), 405–12.

Wagner, E. H., C. Davis, J. Schaefer. *et al.* (1999). A survey of leading chronic disease management programs: are they consistent with the literature? *Manag Care* Q **7**(3), 56–66.

Wanless, D. (2001). Securing our future: taking a long-term view. An interim report, London, HM Treasury.

Warner, M. (1996). *Implementing health care reforms through substitution.* Cardiff, Welsh Institute for Health and Social Care.

Whitehead, M. (1988). *The health divide.* Harmondsworth, Penguin.

Whitty, P. and I. Jones (1992). Public health heresy: a challenge to the purchasing orthodoxy. *BMJ* **304**(6833), 1039–41.

World Health Organization (1986). *Ottawa Charter for Health Promotion: First International Conference on Health Promotion. WHO/HPR/HEP/95.1.* Geneva, World Health Organization.

World Health Organization (2000). *Health systems: improving performance.* Geneva, W.H.O.

World Health Organization and Commission on Macroeconomics and Health (2001). *Macroeconomics and health: investing in health for economic development.* Geneva, World Health Organization.

12.11

Public health workers

Suwit Wibulpolprasert and Piya Hanvoravongchai

Go to the people.
Live among them. Learn from them.
Plan with them. Work with them.
Start with what they know. Build on what they have.
Teach by showing. Learn by doing.
Not a showcase, but a pattern.
Not odds and ends, but a system.
Not piecemeal, but integrated approach.
Not to conform, but to transform.
Not relief, but release.

Dr Y.C. James Yen

The Constitution of the World Health Organization (WHO) defines 'health' as: 'A state of complete physical, mental, social well-being, and not merely the absence of diseases and infirmity'. This broad perspective of health underscores its multi-factorial nature. Health improvement depends much on the educational status (particularly of women), and other socioeconomic development, as well as on the development of healthcare systems (Roemer 1991; World Health Organization 1999) (Fig. 12.11.1).

'Health workers', as defined in the World Health Report (2006), includes 'all people engaged in actions whose primary intent is to enhance health'. According to the Joint Learning Initiative (2004) and the WHO (2006), health workers are a crucial component of the health sector because they manage all other financial and non-financial resources. Workers are also the key to improve performance of the health system in regards to quality, efficiency and accessibility of health services.

Moreover, spending on health workers accounts for a large share of public health spending in most countries (Joint Learning Initiative 2004). On an average, a country spends over 40 per cent of its public health budget on its health workforce (World Health Organization 2006). Many developing countries spend more than half of their public health funding on salaries and remuneration. For example, Ecuador in 1995 and the Dominican Republic in 1996 spent 72 per cent and 67 per cent, respectively, of their Ministries of Health's budget on health workforce salaries (Berman et al. 1999).

History has proved that health workers, especially public health workers, are essential for effective disease control programmes and increases in child survival (Beaglehole & Dal Poz 2003; Joint Learning Initiative 2004). Therefore, the current weakness of health workforce systems in many countries are major obstacles to the provision of necessary health services in order to achieve national health targets and internationally agreed upon health-related development goals (Chen et al. 2004; Haines & Cassels 2004; Kober & Van Damme 2004; Travis et al. 2004; World Health Organization 2006). In addition, many global health initiatives, such as the Global Fund to fight AIDS, tuberculosis, and malaria, and the Global Alliance on Vaccine and Immunization, are vertical programmes that have put tremendous pressure on the already weak health workforce and diverted limited resources from other important public health problems.

This chapter focuses on an important group of health workers, the public health workforce. They are at the core of the health system in delivering public health interventions to achieve health goals. This chapter is divided into four sections: (1) background on public health workers, including the definition, their roles and functions, and their importance to public health; (2) key management principles necessary for an effective, efficient, and equitable public health workforce system; (3) a specific case of frontline public health workers, namely, community health workers (CHWs); and (4) definition, history, and functions of CHWs, as well as the keys to successful and efficient management of this group. It concludes by addressing key challenges to public health workforce development.

Who are the public health workers and what are their roles?

Defining public health workers

The term 'public health worker' has been used in at least three different ways: (1) the *sector* in which a person works (public sector); (2) their *functions*, referring to all workers whose goal is to improve public health, but does not distinguish whether the workers are employed by public, private, or non-government agencies; and (3) the work *setting* where the workers are employed. In this case, all workers in the agencies that work primarily for public health would be defined as public health workers.

Sometimes 'public health workers' is limited to a group of workers based on their *credentials*. This would include all workers with a degree in public health. However, the term 'public health professional' is more frequently used. For example, the US Institute of

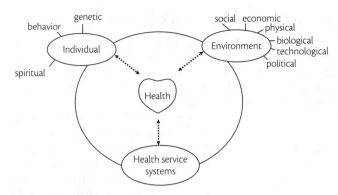

Fig. 12.11.1 Multifactorial relationship of health and its determinants. *Source*: Wibulpolprasert (2006).

Medicine defines a public health professional as 'one educated in public health or related discipline who is employed to improve health through a population focus' (Gebbie *et al*. 2003).

The most commonly used operational definition of various agencies and among scholars is the one based on their functions; i.e. those whose work is primarily for public health (Box 12.11.1).

Public health workers' functions

Through broad definition, the public health workforce is a diverse and complex group of workers. Their education can range from primary level to graduate degrees. They could be from the professional sector, the popular sector, or the folk sector. Their occupational backgrounds could be as wide-ranging as farmers, teachers, social scientists and health professionals such as physicians, nurses, and laboratory technicians. What characterizes them as public health workers are their primary functions in public health (Box 12.11.2).

Another way to understand the scope of public health workers' functions is to look at the classification of public health workers. Based on the types and areas of work, public health workers can be classified into various categories (US Bureau of Labor Statistics 2007). A sample list includes the following:

- Health educators
- Community health workers, public health and community social workers

---

Box 12.11.2 US public health workers' functions

- Monitor health status to identify community health problems
- Diagnose and investigate health problems and health hazards in the community
- Inform, educate, and empower people about public health issues
- Mobilize community partnerships to identify and solve health issues
- Develop policies and plans that support individual and community health efforts
- Enforce laws and regulations that protect health and ensure safety
- Link people to needed personal health services and ensure the provision of health care when otherwise unavailable
- Ensure a competent public health and personal health care workforce
- Evaluate effectiveness, accessibility and quality of personal and population-based health services
- Conduct research for new insights and innovative solutions to health problems

Source: US Department of Health and Human Services (1994).

- Occupational safety technicians/technologists
- Environmental engineers/technicians/technologists/scientists/specialists
- Health services managers/administrators
- Public health policy analysts, health planners
- Public health administrative or clerical staff
- Health information systems specialists
- Biostatisticians/health economists/public health researchers
- Epidemiologists
- Public health physicians/nurses/dentists/dental workers/veterinarians/nutritionists
- Mental health and substance abuse social workers/counsellors

Roles of public health workers

Public health workers contribute to the improvement of population health worldwide. Smallpox eradication is an example that would not have been successful without active contributions by public health workers (Joint Learning Initiative 2004). When properly trained and provided with appropriate incentives and resources, non-professional public health workers and community health workers are capable of effectively delivering health interventions to reduce child mortality in developing countries (Bryce *et al*. 2003; Haines *et al*. 2007). For ongoing health efforts such as the eradication of polio or prevention and control of the burden of non-communicable diseases, public health workers have a major contributory role in their success.

Box 12.11.1 Defining public health workers based on their functions

'A public health worker is one for whom a significant portion of work content advances or contributes to accomplishing one or more of the ten essential public health services identified by the Public Health System Performance Standards' (Tilson and Gebbie 2004).

'Public health workers are defined as all those responsible for providing the essential services of public health regardless of the organization in which they work' (US Department of Health and the US Department of Health and Human Services 1994; cited in Gebbie *et al*. 2002).

The effectiveness of improving the population's health in Shasta Shabikas by community workers in Bangladesh, the Lady Health Workers in Pakistan, and the Brazilian Community Health Agents, is well documented (Joint Learning Initiative 2004). In Africa, community health workers from Gambia, South Africa, Tanzania, Zambia, Madagascar, and Ghana cost-effectively improved health programme performance at the community level (Gericke *et al.* 2003; Lehmann *et al.* 2004).

In addition, frontline workers such as community health workers and village health staff improved coverage and increased health equity. They are generally better distributed geographically (Berman *et al.* 1987; Chapman *et al.* 2005). They are also more accessible and acceptable to communities, resulting in an increase in health service utilization, especially among poorer households (Berman 1984). Extending services through community health workers is seen as a way to reduce inequity in child health (Victora *et al.* 2003; Masanja *et al.* 2005).

Public health workers can also contribute to strategic policy development, planning and regulation, and organization, delivery and evaluation of health.

Enumerating public health workers

Despite the importance of public health workers, information about numbers and dynamics of public health workers is very limited. The problem of limited data availability occurs in both poor and rich countries (Cioffi *et al.* 2004; World Health Organization 2006). Additionally, quantification of public health workers is not an easy task, given the diversity in occupational backgrounds, education and experience, as well as functions.

The World Health Report of 2006 provides the latest counts of the health workforce in member countries estimated from available surveys, censuses and other national statistics (World Health Organization 2006). The actual numbers of public health workers are estimated to be much higher than those reported, because they do not include public health workers from countries with no data and they are limited only to some cadres. In addition, some public health workers may have reported their occupations in different categories that were not captured as public health workers in the surveys or censuses. The information provided is mostly for key health professionals such as nurses, physicians, pharmacists and dentists. Data on the numbers of environmental and public health professionals are available for 70 countries, totalling 655 415 professionals. Similarly, data on numbers of community health workers are available in only 40 countries, totalling 563 348 community workers worldwide. This figure is definitely an underestimate, as village health volunteers in a country such as Thailand totalled more than 800 000 in 2007.

Even in a wealthy country such as the United States, information is limited, and mostly restricted to public health professionals. The latest information on US public health professionals employed to deliver public health services in the country, estimated from employer and employee surveys, is approximately 500 000 persons (US Health Resources and Services Administration 2000). It has been found that nurses are the largest professional group in public health (Gebbie *et al.* 2002). However, this figure does not include approximately 2.8 million volunteers who are engaged in unspecific public health activities (Gebbie & Merrill 2001). The total number of public health workers in the United States could therefore be over three million, or more than one per 100 population.

Towards effective public health workers

To function properly, the health worker system needs to fulfil its three objectives: Coverage, motivation, and competence (Joint Learning Initiative 2004). As presented in (Fig. 12.11.2) strategic management of health workers is required to lead to better health system performance and health outcomes.

Coverage is not limited to the physical, but also includes social accessibility. There should be numeric adequacy and appropriate skill mixes of the health workforce. They should be located within accessible geographical distances, with no social barriers to access. *Motivation* is influenced by various elements, including personal beliefs, financial and non-financial incentives, support provided by the system, and work environment. *Competency* is the result of education, training, and experience that can be fostered prior to their recruitment, as well as while they are in service in the field (Kennedy & Moore 2001; Joint Learning Initiative 2004; World Health Organization 2006). To achieve these three workforce objectives, the system requires active strategic management and health workforce development and concerted action.

Public health worker education and training

Health worker education and training is aimed at ensuring numeric adequacy of a well-qualified and appropriate mix of staff. A set of knowledge and skills that are recommended for public health workers is proposed, and transformed into the appropriate mode of recruitment, education and training. Appropriate policy interventions to empower and guide public health education and training are needed.

Public health worker competency

Competency of public health workers includes adequate *knowledge* and *skills* that are necessary for their functions.

Knowledge: Afifi and Breslow (1994) proposed that public health knowledge essential to public health functions is comprised of five major disciplines: Epidemiology, biostatistics, behavioural and social sciences, environmental health, and health services management. Recent advancement in science and technology means that additional knowledge in areas such as informatics and genomics would be beneficial to their work (Tilson & Gebbie 2004).

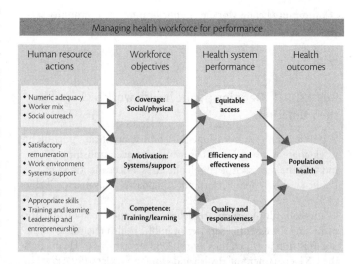

Fig.12.11.2 Health workforce actions and objectives.
Source: Joint Learning Initiative (2004).

Similarly, the increasing importance of social determinants of health requires that public health workers be knowledgeable in the areas of law and public policy. Global health is also an emerging area, with threats from emerging diseases.

Skills: A core set of public health workers' skills should encompass eight domains: (1) critical analysis and assessment; (2) policy development and programme planning; (3) communication; (4) cultural competency; (5) community dimensions of practice; (6) basic public health science; (7) financial planning and management; and (8) leadership and systems (Tilson & Gebbie 2004). For each of these eight domains, the level of proficiency required for frontline staff, senior level staff, and supervisory and management staff could vary from being aware, being knowledgeable and being proficient in that skill.

In addition to the core skill set, additional skills are required for each public health worker that differ by his/her function and responsibility. Moreover, each public health worker should have general work skills such as computer literacy, presentation skills and writing skills. These skill sets can be grouped or classified in several ways. An example is the competencies framework for public health workers as proposed by the US Center for Disease Control (Box 12.11.3).

Education for public health workers

Public health education can be carried out through various mechanisms and at different phases. The training could occur before recruitment (pre-service training) or after workers are already working (in-service training). It could be through formal public health degree programmes or through specific training courses for specific tasks.

Schools of public health

Schools of public health are a product of the twentieth century. Before having public health schools, most professional public health training occurred in medical schools through a department of preventive or community medicine. The emergence of schools of public health in many countries is the result of the demand for workforce training to support public health campaigns (World Health Organization 2006). In the United States, establishment of

---

Box 12.11.3 US CDC key competency sets for public health workers

- Core: Basic public health skills (skills needed to perform the essential functions of public health)

- Function-specific: For example, leadership, management, supervisory, and support staff

- Discipline-specific: For example, community dentistry for public health dentists, other professionals or technical specialists

- Subject-specific (within a discipline): Maternal and child health, sexually transmitted diseases, vaccine preventable diseases, cancer, other chronic diseases

- Workplace basics: Required of all personnel, including literacy, writing, and presentation skills, and computer literacy

Source: Appendix E: Competencies for Public Health Workers: A Collection of Competency Sets for Public Health-Related Occupations and Professions (Institute of Medicine 2002).

---

schools of public health was a result of a conference in 1914 that designed the educational system for the public health profession and was presented in the Welch-Rose Report on Schools of Public Health by the Rockefeller Foundation in 1915 (Fineberg *et al.* 1994). The number of public health schools then increased significantly thereafter. It is claimed that in the United States, 'the emergence of schools of public health was a major factor in the development of public health' (Gordon & McFarlane 1996).

The WHO estimated that there are 375 schools of public health globally (World Health Organization 2006). However, more than half of them are located in the Americas and Europe. In South Asia, with a major share of the global population and the burden of disease, there are less than 10 schools of public health. More than half of the countries in Africa also have no graduate training programme in public health (Joint Learning Initiative 2004).

Schools of public health are not the only source of training for professional public health practitioners. There are many public health programmes outside schools of public health (Gordon & McFarlane 1996; Tulchinsky & Bickford 2006). These programmes are offered in other health professional schools, such as medical and nursing schools, as well as by users, such as the health ministries.

Other modes of public health training

Since most schools of public health are usually under the control of education ministries or independent universities, their isolation from ministries of health and health providers is a major concern as a weakness of the system. Public health education through an institution-based model may be far from actual field experience, and the knowledge learned may be irrelevant to real-world practices and health problems in the community (Beaglehole & Dal Poz 2003). Additionally, the students or trainees may lack public health skills that could have been gained from public health programme implementation and practices.

One innovative project to address the weakness described above is by the Rockefeller Foundation, which initiated the Public Health Schools Without Walls Initiative in many developing countries (Beaglehole & Dal Poz 2003). It uses a broad-based, integrative and adaptive model, with focus on community-based services and practical health problems. The curricula incorporate a large proportion of field training, with close collaboration with the ministry of health. Students gain competence in key areas through actual work in the field, such as health problem investigation, health programme management and workplace communications.

Distance education in public health

Another mode of public health education that is increasingly popular is the use of distance education. Distance education occurs when teachers and the students are distant from each other (Keegan 1996; Knebel 2001). Distance could refer to geographical distance or time difference or both. The instructors use various form of media, such as printed materials, electronic devices, and audio and video to deliver pedagogical messages to the students.

The advantages of distance education for public health training are numerous. First, it expands the access of health education programmes to the prospective students who are unable to physically attend classes at schools or colleges. Second, most distance learning programmes allow for flexibility of times so it is more convenient for many, especially those who have full-time jobs. Third, good distance learning programmes for health workers can benefit from a closer link between training and actual field experiences for the students.

Fourth, distance education programmes are generally less expensive for students, with savings on travel expenses and infrastructure (such as buildings). The cost to the educators also decreases with the number of students, as instructional media development costs are fixed. Availability of distance education is also compatible with the concept of life-long learning that is recommended for all public health workers.

The distance education approach also has its limitations. It is based on limited personal contact, with no active face-to-face interactions, so communication errors can occur. These could be complicated by cultural differences between the instructors and students in the case of cross-regional or cross-country programmes. The lack of personal interaction also means that the style of teaching will be more formal, which could be less stimulating to some students. Also, for distance education, teachers need to play additional roles as facilitators, coaches, and mentors. Their workload is generally greater than in traditional modes of education. More importantly, this method generally has lower graduation rates, as the programme relies heavily on the responsibility and motivation of the students.

Nevertheless, distance education is continually gaining in popularity in the public health sector. Since the first distance education programme in health in the 1960s, many public health training programmes have been offered through distance learning (Knebel 2001). In both developed and developing countries, distance education has been used for pre- and in-service education, for degree programmes, and for short courses. Several public health schools are now offering masters of public health programmes through distance education.

Numerous studies have shown that distance education programmes in health are equally effective as traditional training programmes, with lower costs and greater satisfaction of the students (Knebel 2001). However, pre-service training by distance education may be less attractive to some because of the lack of peer interaction and the lower prestige compared to traditional university education.

Policies on education of public health workers

There are several health workforce education policies that can be used to influence the performance of the health workforce system:

◆ First, there should be an adequate link between the public health education system and the healthcare system.

◆ Second, the policy on public health education, especially the number of trainees and their required mix of skills, should consider the current and future demand for the health workforce in the country.

◆ Third, public health education policy could contribute to improving equity in health service provision in several ways. The geographical location of training institutions could affect the practice location of the workforce once they are trained. Additionally, the recruitment policy based on the socioeconomic and geographical backgrounds of the students may also influence the population they will serve.

◆ Fourth, financing policy for public health education as well as its social ties after graduation may be effective tools to ensure better distribution and fairness of financial burden.

◆ Fifth, public health education should be expanded to other health and public policy professions. Professors and medical specialists, as well as other non-public-health persons, can serve as very strong advocates for public health if they are sensitized to it. Thus, building a 'public health mind' for non-public health individuals may be as important as training public health workers.

System for effective management of public health workers

A study in the United States shows that competency comprises about 2–20 per cent of service performance (Mayer 2003), which suggests that larger roles may be played by other factors, including individual, organizational and social influences. This section describes key factors of health workforce and health system management that can influence the effectiveness and performance of the health workforce. They are remuneration and financial incentives, non-financial incentives and system support, policy and regulation, and monitoring and evaluation.

Remuneration and financial incentives

Satisfactory remuneration is considered an important factor to promote workplace motivation. However, in some developing countries, the level of payment for public health workers is based on the civil service system, and is very low and may not be enough for living expenses. Inadequate or late payments may lead public health workers to pursue informal or unwanted economic activities that contribute to inefficiency and lower health service accessibility.

There are several forms of dubious coping strategies that public health workers have been known to use in such cases (McPake *et al.* 1999; Van Lerberghe *et al.* 2002; Muula & Maseko 2006). These include requesting informal payments or under-the-counter fees for services that are meant to be free, misusing or stealing drugs, overtime work at public facilities for private income, and treating private patients during official and non-official work hours. Ensuring a timely and adequate level of remuneration is therefore important.

Payment mechanisms to remunerate public health workers is another area for policy decision. Salaries provide a secure source of income, but may not create incentive for active service provision. Case-based payments could increase motivation and reflect workloads for which the workers are responsible but may lead to excessive provision of unnecessary services. The use of a mixed payment system, such as providing basic salary with top-up payments based on performance, could combine the benefit of both payment mechanisms.

Financial incentives could also be formulated to influence decisions on practice locations of the health workforce. There is a tendency for health workers, especially health professionals, to be concentrated in highly populated and affluent areas. Providing extra monetary incentives specifically for service in deprived areas or to those specialists in shortage has been used to recruit and maintain health workers in under-served areas or unpopular specialties (Wibulpolprasert & Pengpaibon 2003).

Non-financial incentives, work environment and system support

Social recognition, fairness of management and the opportunity to fulfil self-determination, as well as work environment and system support, play significant roles in the performance of the health workforce (World Health Organization 2006). Dieleman and colleagues indicated that the main motivating factors for health workers, in addition to stable jobs and income, are appreciation by managers, colleagues and the community, and availability of continued training (Dieleman *et al.* 2003).

Work environments can be improved in many ways. Good management and leadership in the health system are seen as a simple step to improve individual and organization performance. Since public health functions require teamwork, good team management is necessary. Having clear job descriptions and responsibilities can reduce tension and increase job satisfaction and compliance. In addition, the public health workforce should also be provided with an opportunity for continuous learning and training to be ready for changing public health demands.

The public health workforce's motivation and performance can also improve with better system support, such as an effective information and communication system. The availability of a functioning infrastructure, necessary supplies, and a safe workplace can promote the workforce's functions. In many cases, provision of support to the families of the workforce, such as safe housing for the family and good schooling for their children, is a very effective incentive for health workers to work and remain in underserved areas.

Roles of certification and credentials

One emerging issue in public health workforce management is certification and credentials of public health professionals. Certain members of the health sector, such as clinical scientists, doctors, nurses and technicians, are required to have certain certification or credentials before they can practice. However, in public health, this issue has only been recently raised in some countries. In the United States, only the state of New Jersey requires licensure of public health administrators employed to run a local health department, while the state of Illinois is moving to certify directors of local health departments.

Proponents of certification argue that it has several benefits (Akhter 2001; Tilson & Gebbie 2004). Certification can help identify professionals with adequate training experience and appropriate competency to deliver public health functions successfully. The establishment of national competency standards and certification could influence health workers to participate in lifelong learning activities to be qualified. It could also facilitate recognition and respect of the profession by the public, and could be used for job promotions or as one of the criteria for remuneration increases.

On the other hand, requiring credentials could mean rising costs of health professional employment. It may also limit the number of people willing to work in public health from a previously open arena. The majority of those practising public health do not have specific training or public health competency, but may have speciality training in other fields such as medicine or nursing.

There is also a practical difficulty in the public health certification process, as the scope of public health is very broad and entails several disciplines. The effort could also face political resistance from other professions perceiving certification as a threat to their scope of practice. In Thailand, there is an effort to legislate for the requirement of credentials of public health officers, but it faces strong resistance from eight professional groups, including medical and nursing councils. The bill introduced in 2007 was finally voted down in the parliament.

Health workforce system monitoring and evaluation

Health workforce system monitoring and evaluation is very important for public health workforce management. The current system is suffering from a lack of data and information for strategic decision-making. With increasing interest in outputs and outcomes of health investment, it is essential that there be more monitoring and evaluation of the health workforce system, especially performance measurement.

To measure performance, it is important to monitor inputs, processes, outputs and/or outcomes in a sound and effective way. The World Health Report of 2006 proposes four dimensions to monitor health workforce performance: Availability, competence, responsiveness, and productivity.

- *Availability* of the health workforce should be monitored in terms of space and time, covering both the distribution and attendance of existing workers.

- *Competence* includes the combination of technical knowledge, skills, and behaviours.

- *Responsiveness* measures how people are treated, regardless of who they are or how ill they are.

- *Productivity* refers to how effective health services and health outcomes are produced, given the existing stock of health workers.

Several methods of data collection are available for public health workforce system monitoring and evaluation. They include routine reporting systems, such as personnel records and health service reports; rapid appraisal methods, such as key informant interviews, focus group discussions, and direct observation; or formal surveys. In the case of performance measurement, it is recommended that all key stakeholders are involved in the planning process, so that the results of the monitoring and evaluation processes are accepted by all.

Planning for an effective public health workforce

Strategic planning for a public health workforce system should be done within the context of overall health workforce and health system planning, as the public health workforce is a part of the overall health system, which is complex and influenced by interactions between multiple players and stakeholders. Health workers are also employed in competitive labour market environments. Public health problems are influenced by demographic and epidemiological changes, changing patterns of public behaviours, and expectations. Innovative strategies and implementation plans are necessary to prepare the public health workforce with an evolving capacity in response to the changing needs of a modern health system. One common mistake in health workforce planning is that it usually focuses on the number and responses to adequate numbers of workers, which does not take into consideration the important issues of motivation, distribution and productivity.

The WHO and its partnerships propose that six interlinking thematic areas should be considered when dealing with public health workforce development and planning (Dal Poz *et al.* 2006). They are human resource management systems, policy, finance, education, partnership, and leadership (Fig. 12.11.3). These six areas should be considered concurrently in health workforce planning, as well as in situation analysis, implementation and monitoring and evaluation.

Specifically regarding public health personnel, Cioffi *et al.* (2004) proposed six strategic elements for public health workforce development, which include: (1) monitoring the workforce composition; (2) identifying competencies/developing curriculum; (3) designing integrated learning systems; (4) using incentives to

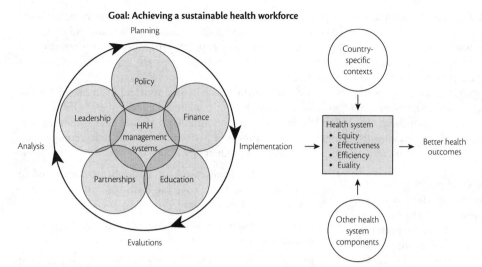

Fig. 12.11.3 Health Workforce Action Framework.
Source: Dal Poz *et al.* (2006).

assure competency; (5) conducting evaluation and research; and (6) assuring financial support.

In addition to the components of the public health workforce system and the strategic elements required, public health workforce planning should also take into account external factors that could affect its functions and roles over time. Since the health workforce is a component of health systems, it is almost always affected by changes in health systems. In many countries, the public health workforce is mostly in the public sector, which is therefore sensitive to any public sector or civil service reform, such as downsizing, decentralization or privatization.

The notion of public sector reform often receives lukewarm and sceptical responses by public health workers. They are generally seen as weakening workers' positions as professionals and undermining job security, which can lower workers' motivation (Kyaddondo & Whyte 2003). In Uganda and Bangladesh, decentralization of health services creates a change in the power structure, with a power struggle between various stakeholders (Ssengooba *et al.* 2004). It is perceived as jeopardizing job security, especially career structure and the opportunity for promotion. In the United States, privatization of public health agencies and the use of temporary workers (Keane *et al.* 2002) are seen by some managers as a cost-control measure, but it could mean a contract-based staff who may not closely adhere to public health principles and are less dedicated to the work and public health goals.

Community health workers (CHWs)

Community health workers comprise a major workforce for public health in many developing countries. Expansion of the roles of CHWs is seen as a model to alleviate the ongoing crisis due to a severe shortage of health workers in many sub-Saharan African countries. This sector uses CHWs as a case to demonstrate the development and effective management of one cadre of public health workers as part of the health system to achieve public health goals.

What is a CHW?

Accessibility to modern healthcare services depends not only on availability, but also on affordability, cultural acceptability, and effectiveness (Fig. 12.11.4) (World Health Organization 1984). Countries usually respond to the problem of inadequate physical access to professional services first by providing a lower level of health personnel. For example, auxiliary midwives and junior sanitarians have been produced in Thailand since 1953. In the United States and Canada, physician assistants and nurse practitioners have been produced since the mid-1960s (Jonas 1998). Nevertheless, even with the expanded services by these auxiliaries, basic health services are still not accessible by large numbers of rural villagers and poor people in urban slums.

The WHO (1978, p. 62; 1987, p. 10) defined CHWs as people with limited education trained in a short time to carry out either a wide range or restricted aspects of healthcare services. They include:

men and women chosen by the community, and trained to deal with the health problems of individuals and the community, and to work in close relationship with the health services.

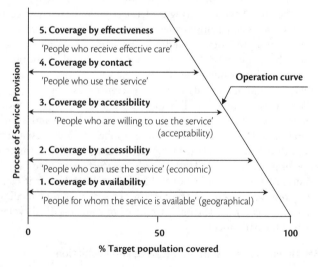

Fig. 12.11.4 Coverage of health services.
Source: Adapted from World Health Organization (1984).

Most CHWs are volunteers and receive short but systematic training. However, some CHWs receive longer-term training and even civil servant status; e.g. auxiliary midwives in Myanmar and community health aides in Jamaica. The WHO (1989) proposed that CHWs should be:

- Members of the communities where they work
- Selected by the communities
- Answerable to the communities for their activities
- Supported by the health system but not necessarily a part of its organization
- Have shorter training than professional workers

CHWs may go by different names in different countries and in different situations, and have different responsibilities. They may be called, for example, community health workers, village health volunteers (VHVs), village health communicators (VHCs), health guides (HGs), sanitation monitors, barefoot doctors, feldschers, health guides, lady health workers, etc. In addition, there may be more than one category of CHWs adopted by a country. Table 12.11.1 shows the various categories of CHWs and community financing schemes for nine elements of PHC in Thailand in 1988.

The origin of community health workers

Inadequate access to basic health services by a large portion of the population prompted many countries to start piloting the creation of systematically trained local CHWs. For example, in Thailand, the first pilot project to involve communities and to appoint CHWs for sanitation activities was started in 1960 (Vacharotai 1978). In DPR Korea, female sanitation monitors were recruited and trained in 1955. However, reliance on pilot or small-scale top-down projects not adapted to local conditions and lacking community participation, local support and resources resulted in disappointments and failures.

In the early 1970s, the health of the Chinese people improved dramatically, partly as a result of what is now called the nationwide primary healthcare approach. One of its guiding principles was the use of CHWs to extend health services to the places where the people live and work, support communities in identifying their own health needs, and helping people solve their own health problems. This new concept that communities should assume substantial responsibility for their own health brought a new dimension to the management of healthcare services. It opened up an opportunity to redraft and expand basic health services in many countries.

The Alma Ata International Conference on Primary Health Care (PHC) in 1978, organized jointly by the WHO and UNICEF, proposed the development of national CHW programmes as an important strategy for improving access to primary healthcare (World Health Organization 1978). Since then, CHW programmes have expanded to many developing countries,

Table 12.11.2 provides a summary of CHWs in nine countries of the WHO's South-East Asia Region.

After several decades of development, ample evidence has been published on the CHW role as a key agent in improving health. In Africa, the use of community health workers has evidently been found to improve health development (World Bank 1994; Gericke *et al.* 2003; Uta Lehmann 2004). Walt (1990) concluded that CHWs not only provide basic health services, but also promote the key principles of primary healthcare; i.e. equity, intersectoral collaboration, community involvement and use of appropriate technology. CHWs have shown that they can reduce mortality and improve other indices of health status. In certain communities, they can satisfy basic healthcare needs that cannot realistically be met by other means (World Health Organization 1989). They are also more accessible and acceptable to communities, resulting in an increase in health service utilization, especially among poorer households (Berman 1984; Berman *et al.* 1987). Extending services through

Table 12.11.1 Categories of CHWs and community financing schemes for nine elements of PHC, Thailand, 1988

Elements	CHWs[a]	Role	Financing schemes[b]
Health education	VHVs/VHCs	Village broadcasts/ education/motivation	–
Control of locally endemic diseases	Some VHVs/VHCs and malaria volunteers	Malaria surveillance, bleeding site control, provision of antimalarials	Mosquito Net Fund
Immunization (EPI)	VHVs/VHCs	Communication for immunization	Health Card Fund
Maternal and child health, family planning	VHVs/VHCs and trained traditional birth attendants	Advocate breast-feeding, supplementary diet, family planning, and maternal and child health; distribute oral pills and condoms	Health Card Fund
Nutrition	Model mother VHVs/VHCs	Nutritional surveillance, demonstration of supplementary diets	Nutrition Fund
Essential drugs and treatment of basic medical problems	VHVs/VHCs	Provision of essential drugs, first aid, and basic medical care	Village Drug Fund
Sanitation	Village sanitary craftsmen	Building latrines and water jars	Sanitation Fund
Dental health	VHVs/VHCs	Education and demonstration of regular and correct tooth brushing	Toothbrush and Toothpaste Fund

Note: VHV, village health volunteer; VHC, village health communicators.
[a] Only VHVs and malaria volunteers still existed in 1999.
[b] Most community financing schemes have diminished and been integrated into multipurpose village development funds.
Source: Adapted and updated from Wibulpolprasert (1991).

Table 12.11.2 Main categories of community health workers/volunteers in nine countries of the WHO's Southeast Asia Region, by country

Country	Category	Date initiated	CHW per number of population (pop) or households (hh)	Duration of training	Percentage of females	Numbers trained
Bangladesh	Village health volunteer	1988	1: 30 hh	4 days	80	38 262
Bhutan	Village health volunteer/worker	1978–1979	1:20–30 hh	12 days	10	1400
Democratic People's Republic of Korea	Sanitation monitor	1955	1:20–30 hh	5 days	100	NA
India	Village health guides	1977	1:1000 pop	3 months	25	416 724 (1985)
	Anganwadi worker	1975	1:1000 pop	3 months	100	NA
Indonesia	Health cadre	1978	1:10 hh	3 days	100	1.8 million (1991)
Myanmar	Community health worker	1977	1:1000 pop	4 weeks	5	36 358
	Auxiliary midwife	1977	1:2266 pop	6 months	100	17 856 (1994)
	Ten-household health worker	1987	1:10 hh	7 days	90	41 643 (1994)
Nepal	Female village health volunteer	1988–1989	1:400 (normal terrain) 1:250 (hill area) 1:150 (mountains)	12 days + 3 days refresher yearly	100	32 000
Sri Lanka	Volunteer health worker	1975–1977	Cluster of hh	6 hours (spread out)	66	40 000 (1996)
Thailand	Village health communicator	1979	1:10–15 hh	5 days	NA	598 908 (abolished in 1994)
	Village health volunteer	1979	1:80–150 hh	15 days	NA	642 532 (1998)
	Village sanitary craftsmen	1982	1:5–10 villages	15 days	NA	4132 (1990)
	Family health leaders	1996	1:1 hh	1 day	NA	1 177 464 (1998)

Notes:
[1] Many countries train traditional birth attendants as volunteer health workers; e.g. Thailand.
[2] Numbers of community health volunteers enlisted are mainly those selected and trained in the government health care system; figures from NGOs are not included.
[3] NA, not available.
Source: Adapted and updated from World Health Organization (1996).

CHWs is seen as a way to reduce inequity in child health (Victora *et al.* 2003; Masanja *et al.* 2005; Haines *et al.* 2007).

Responsibilities of CHWs

CHWs usually serve in roles as educators, communicators, problem detectors, problem-solvers, community organizers, and leaders for health. They serve as the link between the community and the healthcare system. They play an important role in galvanizing communities for action. They provide information that promotes individual and family self-care and responsibility as integral components of everyday life.

Some CHWs support delivery of general basic health services; e.g. village health volunteers in Bangladesh, Bhutan, and Thailand.

Others play more specific roles; e.g. trained traditional birth attendants and village sanitary craftsmen in Thailand, and sanitation monitors in DPR Korea. The specific roles of CHWs are adapted to local situations and health demands. Nevertheless, their roles must be specifically defined. In Pakistan, the lady health workers are female workers recruited from the same community for which they serve, to provide reproductive health services and to promote positive health behaviours.

As a member (and leader) of the community, CHWs can integrate health issues into other community development activities, a role that is difficult for health professionals. In many countries, CHWs combine service and developmental functions that are not confined to the field of health. The relative importance of these two functions varies according to the socioeconomic situation and the availability and accessibility of local health services. The service function is less important where there is ready access to healthcare facilities. The developmental function is useful in all circumstances, and is crucial in less developed communities.

Table 12.11.3 shows the duties of CHWs in 11 different countries (World Health Organization 1987). Most CHWs play education and motivation roles, as well as delivering first aid treatment and dispensing basic medications. More specific or sophisticated service is provided only by CHWs in some countries. For example, CHWs in Columbia and Papua New Guinea also give injections, particularly for immunization. CHWs in Botswana, Sudan, and Yemen provide regular school health activities. CHWs in Botswana, Jamaica, China and Papua New Guinea assist in health centre clinic activities.

Community health workers: Conditions for success

Early evaluation of CHW programmes points to four necessary (but difficult) conditions for success; i.e. CHWs must be well trained, well supervised, provided with logistic support, and linked to functioning district health systems for referral when needed (World Bank 1993). These four conditions are relevant technical and managerial conditions, which require clear policy and leadership support. Experiences with many developing countries point to three necessary conditions for success of CHW programmes; namely, strong political support, intersectoral approaches and active community participation.

Strong political support

Initiating a CHW programme means accepting the health for all policy based on primary healthcare. It also means that the limitations of health professionals and the potential of the community are well accepted. This inevitably means a decision to put more resources into primary healthcare, which includes resources to support activities to establish and strengthen CHWs. It may also mean shifting resources from secondary and tertiary care in urban areas to support basic health services and primary healthcare in rural settings. Shifting of resources is a painful process that requires strong political leadership. Strong political support is also needed for CHW programmes to overcome resistance and win acceptance from health professionals.

The Alma-Ata declaration on health for all policy based on primary healthcare in 1978 provided very strong political support for CHW programmes in many developing countries. The Kenyan community-based healthcare project initiated in 1979 was a good example (Kaseje 1990). Political commitment for further and real decentralization of health services also allows more active participation by the community. At the local level, political leadership support from village leaders, religious leaders, teachers and other informal leaders are crucial to the success of CHW programmes.

Intersectoral approach

The priorities of most rural communities mainly focus on roads, water for agriculture, electricity, schools and employment, rather than on health. To attract higher priority and more community involvement, CHW programmes should be integrated into overall community development programmes. This approach complements the holistic, multifactorial nature and 'All for Health' concept of health.

This intersectoral concept, although not difficult to accept, is not easy to implement. In most developing countries, ministries usually have their own interests in maintaining a vertical bureaucracy. Vertical non-integrated activities are normal phenomena in different ministries or in different departments or divisions within one ministry. Thus, it is not uncommon to see health, education, rural development and agriculture ministries compete for the recruitment of volunteers in villages.

Active community participation

Sustainability of CHW programmes depends heavily upon acceptance by the communities, its relevance to their demands, and their participation. Active community participation should be included in all activities of CHW programmes, including community preparation, selection of CHWs, decisions on types and strategies of health development activities, and management of the programmes.

Active community participation is not easy to achieve in prevailing patron-client relationships between government officials and villagers of most rural communities. Reorientation of health personnel perspectives and the release of community potential are essential for its achievement. This requires not only community preparation, but also active preparation of health personnel. Socioeconomic and political reform of the country toward more decentralization and more participatory democracy is also conducive to its success.

One possibility to increase active community participation is to increase the flexibility of CHW programmes. Most developing countries implement CHW programmes based on a single rigid top-down primary healthcare model. This approach usually leaves little room for lower-level health personnel and the community to make adjustments to fit the local context. A single rigid top-down primary healthcare model implemented on a nationwide scale may yield rapid impressive results, but is usually short-lived.

Leaders in villages, formal or informal, are important resource persons who can actively participate in CHW programmes. Religious leaders, schoolteachers, youth leaders, and leaders of housewife groups are examples of local leaders conducive to CHW programmes. Local health personnel should contact these leaders and seek their opinions and support for the success and sustainability of CHW programmes.

Efficient management of CHW programmes

Even when the rationale for a CHW programme receives high political support and active community participation, managing the programme is not an easy task. Several factors in the programme management need to be addressed.

Preparation of health personnel

Preparation is one of the most crucial components of CHW programmes. Health personnel, particularly at the district level, are the prime (and closest) trainers and supporters of CHWs. Their attitudes and skills for working together with CHWs need to be developed and monitored.

In general, health personnel at the district level health infrastructures (e.g. district hospitals and health centres) are responsible for community preparation, selection and training, providing supervision and support, and direct communication with CHWs. They must be trained as trainers, primary healthcare supporters, and social advocates. Most important is their positive attitude towards CHWs, their respect for the community capacity, and their community skills. They should be able to build friendly relations with community leaders, CHWs and active members of the community.

Table 12.11.3 Duties of community health workers in different countries

Task summary	Benin	Botswana	Colombia	India	Jamaica	Liberia	Papua New Guinea	Philippines	Sudan	Thailand	Yemen
1. First aid, treat accidents and simple illness	/	/	/	/	/	/	/	/	/	/	/
2. Dispense drugs	/	/	/ (including injections)	/	/	/	/ (including injections)	/	/	/	/
3. Pre- and post-natal advice, motivation	/	/	/	/	/	/	/	/	/	/	/
4. Deliver babies	/	X	/	X	X	X	X	X	X	/ (trained TBA)	X
5. Child care advice, motivation	/	/	/	/	/	/	/	/	/	/	/
6. Nutrition motivation, demonstration	/	/	/	/	/	/	/	/	/	/	/
7. Nutrition action (W=weigh children, maintain chart; F=distribute food supplements)	F	W	W	X	W, F	X	W	W, F	F	W, F	X
8. Immunization motivation, assistance during clinics	/	/	/	/	/	/	/	/	/	/	/
9. Immunization—give injections	X	X	/	X	X	X	/	X	/	X	X
10. Family planning motivation	/	/	/	/	/	/	X	/	/	/	/
11. Family planning—distribute supplies	X	/	/	/	X	X	X	/	/	/	X
12. Environmental sanitation, personal hygiene, general health habit motivation	/	/	/	/	/	/	/	/	/	/	/
13. Communicable disease screening, referral, prevention, motivation	/	/	/	/	/	X	/	/	/	/	/
14. Communicable disease follow-up, motivation of confirmed cases	/	/	/	/	X	Sometimes	/	/	/	/	Sometimes
15. Communicable disease action (D=provide drug resupply; M=take malaria slides)	X	D	D, M	M	X	X	D, M	TB sputum smear	D	D, M (Malaria volunteers)	D
16. Assist health centre clinic activities (i.e. not in village)	Occasionally	/	Occasionally	X	/	X	/	X	Occasionally	Occasionally	X
17. Refer difficult cases to health centre or hospital	/	/	/	/	/	/	/	/	/	/	/
18. Perform school health activities regularly	X	/	X	X	X	X	X	X	/	X	/
19. Collect vital statistics	X	/	/	/	X	/	X	/	/	/	/
20. Maintain records, reports	/	/	/	/	/	/	/	/	/	/ (VHV only)	
21. Visit homes on a regular basis	/	/	/	/	/	Sometimes	/	/	/	/	X
22. Perform tasks outside the health sector (e.g. agriculture)	/	/	X	/	X	/	X	/	/	/	/
23. Participate in community meetings	/	/	/	/	/	/	/	/	/	/	/

Note: /, task performed by CHWs; X, task not performed; VHV, village health volunteer; TBA, traditional birth attendant.

Source: Adapted from World Health Organization (1987).

These skills will enable them to be effective supporters of CHWs. Their preparation can be achieved through short courses, on-the-job-training of primary healthcare, CHW programmes, and training methodology.

Training materials and working guides for health personnel should be locally prepared. They may be adapted from the one provided by WHO (McMahon 1980). In addition, reorientation of basic medical education curricula to build understanding, positive attitudes and community skills for health professionals is also very important.

Financial incentives

Schemes based on financial incentives (e.g. Jamaica CHW programme) often collapse when the incentives are discontinued. In the case of needs for financial incentives, the community should be consulted and asked to decide on suitable recompense. For sustainability and acceptance, financial incentives should come more from the community than from the government.

The WHO Study Group (Rohde 1983) warned against a 'fee-for-service' arrangement, because of its tendency to concentrate on curative services for which CHWs can charge fees. However, fee-for-service for preventive and health promotion tasks may be allowed; e.g. fees for distribution of oral pills and condoms. Other additional incentives such as free medical care for CHWs and their family members, and nominal profit from sales of essential drugs may be given. If the time required to carry out the functions assigned is not a significant proportion of their time, direct financial remuneration could be counterproductive, and is therefore not recommended.

Continuing education

Some CHWs with an adequate level of education may be good candidates for recruitment into health personnel training colleges. They usually have better attitudes toward the community, as well as better community skills, than other students in these colleges. Nevertheless, providing this incentive may also have some detrimental effects, and must be carried out with great care and be highly selective. China's barefoot doctors are a good example.

China's barefoot doctors contributed greatly to the success of preventive health that had a proven effect on mortality and morbidity. In the late 1970s and 1980s, as a result of changes in economic policy and in the demand for medical care, they were offered the opportunity to become village doctors through training and qualifying exams. They then provided more sophisticated services and, in many provinces, moved to a fee-for-service financing system. Thus, a national CHW programme evolved to become a private practice model free from any governmental guidance resulting in a decline in preventive and promotion services (Zhu 1989; De Geyndt 1992; Ministry of Public Health 1999).

Resources and support

CHW programmes require initial investment, plus additional reinvestment in training, management, logistics, and supervision. Although the resource need is sizable, it is nevertheless usually a small fraction of the total national health budget.

In addition to public resources, other resources can be recruited from the community. Community financing schemes can be established to support various elements of primary healthcare, or to support integrated community health development activities. These additional resources may be used to provide incentives to CHWs.

For example, in Thailand, the multipurpose village development fund pays the village sanitary craftsmen to build latrines and water jars. The dividend from these community-financing schemes, if sufficient, may also encourage active community participation.

Evaluation of CHW programmes

Evaluating any health programme is a complex and difficult exercise, beginning with the problem of methodology. Although there is some general agreement on the measurements in terms of reduction in morbidity and mortality, the methodology for evaluating social impact is more complex. Qualitative phenomena such as community participation, behaviour, and perceptions are difficult to measure. Some subjectivity and criticism are thus inevitable.

No matter how complex and difficult it is, a built-in system of monitoring and evaluating CHW programmes is needed, from formulation through to implementation. Evaluation is intended not only to measure progress and success, but also to yield necessary proposals for further development. Necessary relevant, valid, and reliable indicators need to be developed to measure the input, processes, and outcomes of the programme. In addition to the built-in system, some periodic external evaluations are helpful to guide further development of the CHW programme.

Information from the built-in monitoring and evaluation system of the Thai primary healthcare programme in 1986 revealed several constraints in the CHW programme; e.g. high drop-out rates, low levels of activity and low morale. This led to a systematic external evaluation in 1988, which resulted in abolishment of village health communicators, an increase in social and financial incentives, and more involvement of village headmen and village committees, as well as further strengthening of health service system support (Wibulpolprasert 1991).

Community management structures

CHWs should not be left alone in the community. Linkages to community infrastructures can gain more acceptability, and also allow CHWs to gain access to community resources conducive to health development. CHWs should be included as members in the community development committee. In Thailand, CHWs are now supported mainly by local administrative authorities rather than by the central government; they are therefore part of the local community.

Sometimes separate village health development committees have been set up. Top-down establishment of village health committees may be unsuccessful or even counterproductive. In the Saradidi project in Kenya, it was learned that reorganizing the community or setting up a new leadership system of the village health committee was not appropriate.

Certain community financing schemes may provide a good basis for the activities of the CHWs in the community development committee. They can also empower their community management skills. The resources generated can be used for further development of CHWs and the community. Figure 12.11.5 shows three important components for community health development; i.e. CHWs, management committees, and community financing schemes.

Conclusions

This chapter has provided an overview of the public health workforce and its roles, functions, and related factors that contribute to its effectiveness. An example of one public health workforce cadre,

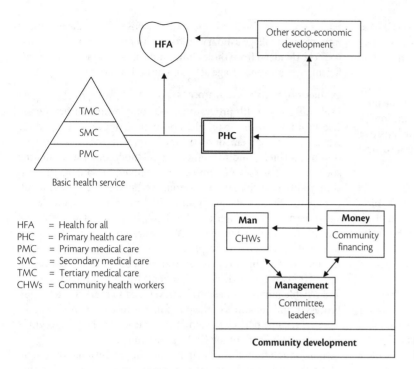

HFA = Health for all
PHC = Primary health care
PMC = Primary medical care
SMC = Secondary medical care
TMC = Tertiary medical care
CHWs = Community health workers

Fig. 12.11.5 Conceptual framework for community development in support of primary health and health for all.

community health workers, is discussed in detail to demonstrate the complexity of workforce development and management, as well as the support required by all factors.

One major challenge to the success of the public health workforce system is the lack of policy and political attention. In most developing countries, there has been a general neglect of both the public health workforce and its related infrastructure, as well as its long-term development. High-profile health professionals working in clinical care, such as doctors and nurses, are generally better organized, and their problems often get media attention more easily.

The Joint Learning Initiative, a global network of public health experts, called for increased attention to current failures in the health workforce system and the necessity to overcome the crisis (Joint Learning Initiative 2004). They indicated five main challenges, including shortages, skill-mix imbalance, geographical maldistribution, poor work environment, and a weak knowledge base. These problems are similarly shared by the public health workforce system, a major component of the overall health workforce, with a stronger intensity of problems in developing countries.

The Fifty-Seventh World Health Assembly in 2004 requested the WHO Director General to include human resources for health development as a top-priority programme area in the organization's General Programme of Work for 2006–2015 (World Health Organization 2004). Development of the public health workforce should be at the core of health workforce development for WHO, as well as all countries. Successful action requires active involvement of the public, communities and all stakeholders inside and outside health system. More importantly, there is a huge shortfall of rigorous research to provide the needed evidence base for policy decision-making regarding the public health workforce, similar to the problems in the public health field in general (Tilson & Gebbie 2004).

Only a strong public-health workforce will be able to respond to the global and national health challenges (Beaglehole et al. 2004).

Acknowledgements

The authors are thankful for research supported by Paichit Pengpaiboon and Sirianong Peyasuntiwong. The chapter also benefits from helpful comments and suggestions by the reviewers.

References

Afifi, A.A. and Breslow, L. (1994) The maturing paradigm of public health. *Annual Review of Public Health*, **15**, 223–35.

Akhter, M.N. (2001) Professionalizing the public health workforce: the case for certification. *Journal of Public Health Management Practice*, **7**, 46–9.

Beaglehole, R. and Dal poz, M. (2003) Public health workforce: challenges and policy issues. *Human Resources Health*, **1**, 4.

Berman, P.A. (1984) Village health workers in Java, Indonesia: coverage and equity. *Soc Sci Med*, **19**, 411–22.

Berman, P.A., Gwatkin, D.R., and Burger, S.E. (1987) Community-based health workers: head start or false start towards health for all? *Soc Sci Med*, **25**, 443–59.

Berman, P., Arellanes, L., Henderson, P., and Magnoli, A. (1999) Health care financing in Eight Latin American and the Caribbean Nations: the first regional national health accounts network. *Latin America and Caribbean Health Sector Reform Initiative*. Bethesda, MD, Partnerships for Health Reform Project, Abt Associates.

Bryce, J., EL Arifeen, S., Pariyo, G. et al. (2003) Reducing child mortality: can public health deliver? *Lancet*, **362**, 159–64.

Chapman, J., Congdon, P., Shaw, S. et al. (2005) The geographical distribution of specialists in public health in the United Kingdom: is capacity related to need? *Public Health*, **119**, 639–46.

Chen, L., Evans, T., Anand, S. et al. (2004) Human resources for health: overcoming the crisis. *Lancet*, **364**, 1984–1990.

Cioffi, J.P., Lichtveld, M.Y., and Tilson, H. (2004) A research agenda for public health workforce development. *J Public Health Management Practice*, **10**, 186–192.

Dal poz, M.R., Quain, E.E., O'neil, M. et al. (2006) Addressing the health workforce crisis: towards a common approach. *Human Resources Health*, **4**, 21.

De geyndt, W., Zhoa, X., Liu, S. (1992) From barefoot doctor to village doctor in rural China. World Bank Technical Paper, No.187. *World Bank Technical Paper*. Washington DC, World Bank.

Dieleman, M., Cuong, P., Anh, L. *et al.* (2003) Identifying factors for job motivation of rural health workers in North Viet Nam. *Human Resources Health*, **1**, 10.

Fineberg, H.V., Green, G.M., Ware, J.H. *et al.* (1994) Changing public health training needs: professional education and the paradigm of public health. *Annual Rev Public Health*, **15**, 237–257.

Gebbie, K.M., Merrill, J., and Tilson, H.H. (2002) The public health workforce. *Health Affairs (Project Hope)*, **21**, 57–67.

Gebbie, K.M. and Merrill, J. (2001) Enumeration of the public health workforce: developing a system. *J Public Health Management Practice*, **7**, 8–16.

Gebbie, K.M., Rosenstock, L., and Hernandez, L.M. (2003) *Who Will Keep the Public Healthy? Educating Public Health Professionals for the 21st Century*, Washington DC, National Academies Press.

Gericke, C., Kurowski, C., Ranson, M.K. *et al.* (2003) Feasibility of Scaling-up Interventions: The Role of Intervention Design. *Disease Control Priority Project Working Paper*.

Gordon, L.J. and Mcfarlane, D.R. (1996) Public health practitioner incubation plight: following the money trail. *J Public Health Policy*, **17**, 59–70.

Haines, A. and Cassels, A. (2004) Can the millennium development goals be attained? *Br Med Assoc*, **329**(7462), 394–397.

Haines, A., Sanders, D., Lehmann, U. *et al.* (2007) Achieving child survival goals: potential contribution of community health workers. *Lancet*, **369**(9579), 2121–2131.

Hongwiwatana, T., Sri-Ngernyuang, L. and Chuengsatiensap, K. (1988) *Alternatives to primary health care volunteers in Thailand*, Bangkok, Sangdad Publishing Co., Ltd.

Institute of Medicine (2002) *The Future of Public Health in the 21st Century*, Washington DC, National Academy Press.

Joint Learning Initiative (2004) *Human resources for health: Overcoming the crisis*, Cambridge, MA, Harvard University Press.

Jonas, S. (1998) *An introduction to the U.S. health care system*. New York, Springer Publishing Company.

Kaseje, D.C.O. (1990) Community-based health care: The Saradidi, Kenya experience. In Walsh, S.H.A.J. (Ed.) *Why Things Work*. Boston, Adams Publishing Group.

Keane, C., Marx, J., and Ricci, E. (2002) Public health privatization: proponents, resisters, and decision-makers. *J Public Health Policy*, **23**, 133–152.

Keegan, D. (1996) *Foundations of Distance Education*, Routledge.

Kennedy, V.C. and Moore, F.I. (2001) A systems approach to public health workforce development. *J Public Health Management Practice*, 7, 17–22.

Knebel, E. (2001) The use and effect of distance education in healthcare: What do we know? *Operations Research Issue Paper*, 2.

Kober, K. and Van damme, W. (2004) Scaling up access to antiretroviral treatment in southern Africa: who will do the job? *Lancet*, **364**, 103–107.

Kyaddondo, D. and Whyte, S.R. (2003) Working in a decentralized system: a threat to health workers' respect and survival in Uganda. *Int J Health Plan Management*, **18**, 329–42.

Lehman, U., Friedman, I., Sanders, D. (2004) Review of the Utilisation and Effectiveness of Community-Based Health Workers in Africa. *Joint Learning Initiative Working Paper*.

Masanja, H., Schellenberg, J.A., De savigny, D. *et al.* (2005) Impact of integrated management of childhood illness on inequalities in child health in rural Tanzania. *Health Policy Plan*, **20** Suppl 1, i77–i84.

Mayer, J.P. (2003) Are the public health workforce competencies predictive of essential service performance? A test at a large metropolitan local health department. *J Public Health Manag Pract*, **9**, 208–213.

Mcpake, B., Asiimwe, D., Mwesigye, F. *et al.* (1999) Informal economic activities of public health workers in Uganda: implications for quality and accessibility of care. *Soc Sci Med*, **49**, 849–65.

Ministry of Public Health (1999) *Health in Thailand 1997-1998*, Bangkok, The Veteran Press.

Muula, A.S. and Maseko, F.C. (2006) How are health professionals earning their living in Malawi? *BMC Health Services Res*, **6**, 97.

Roemer, M.I. (1991) *National Health System of the World*, New York, Oxford University Press.

Rohde, J. (1983) Health for All in China: principles and relevance for other countries. In D. Morley, J.R., G. Wiliams (Ed.) *Practising Health for All*. Oxford, Oxford University Press.

Ssengooba, F., Rahman, A., Hongoro, C. *et al.* (2004) The Impact of Health Sector Reforms on Human Resources in Health in Uganda and Bangladesh.

Tilson, H. and Gebbie, K.M. (2004) The public health workforce. *Annual Rev Public Hlth*, **25**, 341–356.

Travis, P., Bennett, S., Haines, A. *et al.* (2004) Overcoming health-systems constraints to achieve the Millennium Development Goals. *Lancet*, **364**, 900–906.

Tulchinsky, T.H. and Bickford, M.J. (2006) Are schools of public health needed to address public health workforce development in Canada for the 21st century? *Can J Public Health. Revue Canadienne De Sante Publique*, **97**, 248–250.

U.S. Bureau of Labor Statistics (2007) 2000 Standard Occupational Classification. Washington, DC, U.S. Bureau of Labor Statistics.

U.S. Department of Health and Human Services (1994) *The public health workforce: an agenda for the 21 century*, Washington DC, Government Printing Office.

U.S. Department of Health and Human Services, P. H. S., Public Health Functions Steering Committee (1994) *Public Health in America*, Washington, DC, Government Printing Office.

U.S. Health Resources and Services Administration (2000) *The public health workforce:enumeration 2000.*, Washington DC, Bureau of Health Professions, National Center for Health Workforce Analysis.

Vacharotai, S. (1978) *Lampang health development project: a Thai primary health care approach.*, Bangkok, Amarin Press.

Van lerberghe, W., Conceio, C., Van damme, W. *et al.* (2002) When staff is underpaid: dealing with the individual coping strategies of health personnel. *Bull WHO*, **80**, 581–584.

Victora, C.G., Wagstaff, A., Schellenberg, J.A. *et al.* (2003) Applying an equity lens to child health and mortality: more of the same is not enough. *Lancet*, **362**, 233–241.

Walt, G. (1990) *Community Health Workers in National Health Programmes. Just Another Pair of Hands?* Oxford University Press, Oxford.

Wibulpolprasert, S. (1991) Community financing: Thailand's experiences. *Health Policy Planning*, **4**, 354–360.

Wibulpolprasert, S. (2006) *Thailand Health Profile 2001-2004*, Nonthaburi, Bureau of Policy and Strategy, MOPH.

Wibulpolprasert, S. and Pengpaibon, P. (2003) Integrated strategies to tackle the inequitable distribution of doctors in Thailand: four decades of experience. *Human Resources Health*, **1**, 12.

World Bank (1993) *World Development Report 1993. Investing in Health*, Oxford University Press, Oxford.

World Bank (1994) *Better Health in Africa. Experiences and Lessons Learned*. Washington DC, World Bank.

World Health Organization (1978) *Primary Health Care*. Geneva, World Health Organization.

World Health Organization (1984) Evaluating primary health care in South East Asia. *WHO/SEARO technical publication*. World Health Organization, South-East Asia Regional Office, New Delhi.

World Health Organization (1987) *The Community Health Worker*. Geneva, World Health Organization.

World Health Organization (1989) *Strengthening the Performance of Community Health Workers in Primary Health Care*. Report of a WHO study group. *WHO Technical Report Series*. Geneva, World Health Organization.

World Health Organization (1996) *Role of Health Volunteers in Strengthening Action for Health*. Report of an intercountry consultation, Yangon, 20–24 February 1995. New Delhi, World Health Organization.

World Health Organization (1999) *The World Health Report 1999. Making a Difference*. Geneva, World Health Organization.

World Health Organization (2004) International migration of health personnel: a challenge for health systems in developing countries. In the *Proceedings of the 57th World Health Assembly*.

World Health Organization (2006) *The World Health Report 2006: Working Together for Health*, Geneva, World Health Organization.

Zhu, N. (1989) Factors associated with the decline of the Cooperative Medical System and barefoot doctors in rural China. *Bull WHO*, 431–441.

Planning for and responding to public health needs in emergencies and disasters

Khanchit Limpakarnjanarat and Roderico H. Ofrin

Abstract

Natural and man-made disasters have cause significant harm throughout history. However, the frequency and level of devastation caused by disasters appears to be increasing. Disasters not only cause loss of life and property, but also cause tremendous psychological damage, affecting the society and culture of the area as well. Poverty increases the impact of disasters, and developing countries tend to suffer more. The impact of disasters can be mitigated by disaster preparedness planning. To be effective, disaster planning must involve the entire community and must anticipate the range of disasters to which the community is vulnerable. In the modern world, disasters in one region often affect other regions. Thus, there is a need not only for local and national disaster preparedness, but also for international preparedness. The World Health Organization (WHO) has developed the International Health Regulations (IHR-2005), which has been approved by all Member States, and has established the Benchmarks for Emergency Preparedness and Response. The Benchmark provides a framework for systematic monitoring of health systems that comprise preparedness for natural and man-made disasters.

Synopsis

The importance of disasters as a major public health problem is widely recognized (Godschalk *et al.* 1999; Goel 2006). The sudden impact of natural disasters may cause many deaths, injuries, and illness. For example, the earthquake and tsunami in December 2004 resulted in approximately 280 000 deaths in Indonesia, Thailand, Sri Lanka, Southern India, Maldives, and Myanmar, and left 1 723 543 homeless (Kohl *et al.* 2005; World Health Organization 2005). The impact on the health system can also be drastic: Disaster can destroy health infrastructures, health staff may perish in the event, and funds must be re-allocated to support relief efforts. Surveillance systems need to be scaled up and public health interventions have to be re-prioritized quickly. Consequently, national healthcare goals may be set back for years (Noji 1997).

At the global level, the natural disasters continue to cause substantial loss of lives and property, despite scientific and material progress in disaster management. In 1989, the United Nations General Assembly declared the decade 1990–2000 as the International Decade for Natural Disaster Reduction with the objective to reduce loss of lives and property through international actions especially in developing countries (United Nations Department of Economic and Social Affairs 1996).

Human culture is also vulnerable to destruction. As a result of disasters, ancient structures and sometimes traditional customs can disappear due to the impact of an event or its related effects such as relocation and displacement (Cuny 1993).

The damage from natural and man-made disasters tends to be more severe if there is no proper preparedness in place (Lechat 1990). The goal of preparedness is to strengthen a public health system to be more efficient and effective at a time when special and immediate needs have to be addressed such as those in an emergency. This can be achieved if the approach is based on well-organized scientific principles of vulnerability and risk analyses. The approach can make prevention more effective, relief more relevant, and management more efficient at the local, national, and international levels. Overall, this will help save more lives and prevent avoidable morbidity (Armenian 1986).

The aim of public health disaster preparedness is prevention and control of unnecessary morbidity and mortality (Pan American Health Organization 1983). Therefore, application of effective prevention strategies can minimize the effects of disasters on public health. Preparedness can make a difference to minimize the destruction caused by natural disasters. As with all public health interventions, emergency preparedness and response requires involvement of many sectors. The involvement of sectors such as infrastructure, water and sanitation, finance, disease control, media and legal sectors can ensure that lives are saved.

In many instances, when city planning ignored building codes, communities were located in dangerous areas, warnings were not issued or followed, or a plan was not tested prior to the events, disasters caused more harm than necessary. Understanding the risks of people who died or were injured in disaster is a prerequisite for preventing and reducing deaths and injuries from future disasters (Guha-Sapir & Lechat 1986a). This chapter will review the basic concepts of disasters, provide a global review of the epidemiology of disasters, identify key public health problems in specific scenarios, and present the WHO strategic recommendations for emergency planning and response.

Classification of disasters

We can divide disasters into two broad categories: Natural and human generated (Rutherford *et al.* 1983).

◆ Natural events arise from hazards whose origin is from nature, such as earthquakes, volcanic eruptions, hurricanes, floods, fires, tornadoes, and extremes of temperature (Goel 2006).

◆ Man-made disasters fall into two categories (Pan American Health Organization 1982). The first are results from accidental destructive activity. Such events may be acute, as with aeroplane crashes, explosions, fires, and intoxications, or they may be chronic processes like deforestation and the contamination of the environment. Accidental man-made disasters, which usually pose little, if any, additional risk of communicable disease to the community, are beyond the scope of this chapter. The second category consists of man-made disasters caused by warfare, economic or social disruption and civil disturbances. Warfare is frequently subdivided into the conventional type, including siege and blockade, and the non-conventional type, including biological, chemical (toxic gas) and nuclear warfare. Experience with the effect of non-conventional warfare on communicable disease is limited. Public health handles biological agents capable of producing epidemics that incapacitate military or civilian populations (e.g. anthrax and plague) through taking the same measures as those used for naturally occurring outbreaks.

Other authors (Goel 2006) further specify these broad classifications as: (a) Complex emergencies usually involving situations in which civilian populations suffer casualties and loss of property, loss of basic services, and a means of livelihood as a result of war, civil unrest, or other political conflict. In many instances, people are forced to leave their homes temporarily or permanently, others become refugees in other countries; (b) technological disasters are those in which large numbers of people, property, infrastructure, or economic activity affected by major industrial accidents, severe pollution, unplanned nuclear release, major fires, or explosions from hazardous substances, e.g. fuel, chemicals, explosive, or nuclear materials; and (c) other disasters such as transportation (vehicular), material shortages resulting from energy embargoes, and dam breaks that are not caused by natural hazards but that occur in human settlements.

The distinction between natural and man-made disasters may not be clear-cut. A natural disaster may trigger secondary disasters—such as fires after an earthquake, hazardous air pollution may result from temperature inversion, or release of toxic chemicals into the environment in the aftermath of floods.

Natural disasters and those generated by people can be divided into acute- or sudden-impact events, such as earthquake and tropical cyclones, and those of chronic- or slow genesis, such as droughts leading to famine or chronic exposure to harmful chemicals from local industry or radiation from toxic disposal sites by community (Noji 1997).

Global overview of epidemiology of disasters

Trends show that events leading to emergencies and disasters are increasing as shown from data from the Center for Research on the Epidemiology of Disasters. Figure 12.12.1 shows the number of natural disasters at the country level during the past two decades has increased four- to fivefold worldwide.

The numbers of affected populations are also increasing. Natural disasters such as earthquakes, tropical cyclones, floods, and volcanic eruptions have claimed approximately 3 million lives worldwide during the past 20 years. They have adversely affected the lives of at least 800 million more displaced people. They have also caused more than US$50 billion in property damage.

The number of people killed in natural disasters in the past decade by continents is reflected in data from World Disaster Report 2006 (International Federation of the Red Cross and Crescent Societies 2006), which shows that disasters in the Asia Pacific region were responsible for 78 per cent of the total deaths globally (Fig. 12.12.2).

Many parts of the world experience major natural disasters which resulted in very high mortality (Table 12.12.1) (Advisory Committee on the International Decade for Natural Hazard Reduction 1987). Worldwide, a major disaster occurs almost daily, and natural disasters that require international assistance for affected populations occur weekly (Binder & Sanderson 1987).

From 1960 to 1990, floods were the most frequent type of natural disaster, accounting for more than one-third of all disasters. Windstorms (e.g. cyclones, hurricanes, and tornadoes) were the next most frequent disaster, contributing one-quarter of the total number. Earthquakes and cyclones caused the greatest devastation in terms of numbers of deaths and economic loss (Berz 1984) (Table 12.12.2). From 1965 to 1992, more than 90 per cent of all natural-disaster-affected persons lived in Asia and Africa. The following is the distribution for major natural disaster occurrences per year: Asia, 15; Latin America and Africa, 10; North America, Europe, and Australia, 1. Whether disasters in a region are measured by economic loss or by numbers of deaths and injuries, data show that Asia is the most natural-disaster-prone area of the world, Latin America and Africa are the second-most prone, and North America, Europe, and Australia are the least prone (IDNDR Promotion Office 1994).

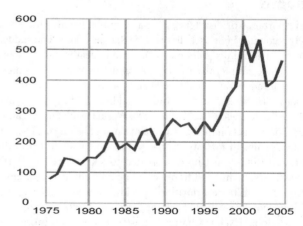

Fig. 12.12.1 Number of disasters from 1975 to 2005.
Source: Center for Research on the Epidemiology of Disasters (2007).

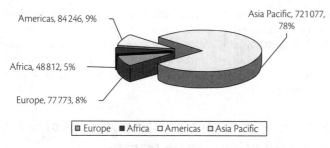

Fig. 12.12.2 Total number of people killed in natural disasters (1996–2005) Numbers.
Source: World Disaster Report (2006).

During the period 1947–1980, cumulative data gathered worldwide showed the top 10 major types of disasters ranked by the number of lives lost to be caused by heavy storms such as cyclones, hurricanes, or typhoons, with an almost equal number caused by earthquakes, followed by floods, thunderstorms and tornadoes, snowstorms, volcanoes, heat waves, avalanches, and landslides, respectively (Table 12.12.3).

Factors that may contribute to a disaster and the severity of its impact, particularly in developing countries, are human vulnerability resulting from poverty and social inequality, environmental degradation resulting from poor land use, lack of sophisticated health structures and disaster preparedness plans, and rapid population growth, especially among the poor. It has been estimated that 95 per cent of the deaths that are the result of natural disasters occur among 66 per cent of the world's population that lives in the poorest countries (Anderson 1991). For example, more than 3000 deaths per disaster occur in low-income countries compared with the average of 500 deaths per disaster that occur in high-income countries. The poor are most at risk because they are least able to afford housing that can withstand earthquake activity, often live

Table 12.12.1 The 10 worst natural disasters worldwide, 1945–2005.

Year	Location	Type of disaster	Number of deaths
1948	USSR	Earthquake	100 000
1949	China	Flood	57 000
1954	China	Flood	40 000
1965	Bangladesh	Cyclone	30 000
1968	Iran	Earthquake	30 000
1970	Peru	Earthquake	70 000
1970	Bangladesh	Cyclone	500 000
1971	India	Cyclone	30 000
1976	China	Earthquake	250 000
1990	Iran	Earthquake	40 000
2004	Indonesia, Sri Lanka, Maldives, India, Thailand, Myanmar, Somalia	Tsunami	280 000

Source: Office of US Foreign Disaster Assistance. (1995). *Disaster history: significant data on major disasters worldwide, 1900–present*; Agency for International Development, Washington DC.

Table 12.12.2 Crude disaster mortality by type of disaster, 1960–1969, 1970–1979, and 1980–1989 (Office of US Foreign Disaster Assistance 1995).

Disaster type	Deaths		
	1960–1969	1970–1979	1980–1989
Floods	28 700	46 800	38 598
Cyclones	107 500	343 600	14 482
Earthquakes	52 500	389 700	53 740
Hurricane			1263
Other disasters			1 011 777
Total			1 119 800

along coasts where storms or tidal waves strike, or live in floodplains subject to flooding. Their economic circumstances force them to live in substandard housing susceptible to landslides or are located near industrial sites. Furthermore, they are not educated about lifesaving behaviours. Risks and vulnerabilities are higher in poor countries and poorer subsets of the population because there is less investment in preparedness. Preparing for emergencies decreases mortality and morbidity from the impact of events. It prevents events from turning into emergencies, and emergencies into disasters (Guha-Sapir & Lechat 1986b).

Hazards, risks, and vulnerabilities

The basis of any preparedness planning is risk and vulnerability analysis. Understanding the dynamics of risks, hazards, vulnerability, and capacities provides essential information for proper prioritization of resources and actions. A definition of these three terminologies is essential (International Strategy for Disaster Reduction 2003).

Hazard A hazard is a potentially damaging physical event, phenomenon or human activity that may cause the loss of life or injury, property damage, social and economic disruption, or environmental degradation.

Table 12.12.3 Ten major types of disasters ranked by the number of lives lost worldwide during the period 1947–1980 (Shah 1983).

Type of disaster	Number of deaths
Tropical cyclones, hurricanes, typhoons	499 000
Earthquakes	450 000
Floods (other than those associated with hurricanes)	194 000
Thunderstorms and tornadoes	29 000
Snowstorms	10 000
Volcanoes	9000
Heat waves	7000
Avalanches	5000
Landslides	5000

Hazards can include latent conditions that may represent future threats and can have different origins: Natural (geological, hydro meteorological and biological) or induced by human processes (environmental degradation and technological hazards). Hazards can be single, sequential or combined in their origin and effects. Each hazard is characterized by its location, intensity, frequency and probability.

Vulnerability comprises the conditions determined by physical, social, economic, and environmental factors or processes that increase the susceptibility of a community to the impact of hazards.

The opposite of vulnerability is *capacity*. It is defined as a combination of all the strengths and resources available within a community, society or organization that can reduce the level of risk or the effects of a disaster. Capacity may include physical, institutional, social, or economic resources, as well as skilled personal or collective attributes such as leadership and management. Capacity may also be equivalent to capability.

Risk is defined as the probability of harmful consequences or expected losses (deaths, injuries, property, livelihoods, economic activity disrupted or environment damaged) resulting from interactions between natural or human-induced hazards and vulnerable conditions. Conventionally, risk is expressed by the notation: Risk = Hazards × Vulnerability.

Some disciplines also include the concept of exposure to refer particularly to the physical aspects of vulnerability.

Beyond expressing a possibility of physical harm, it is crucial to recognize that risks are inherent or can be created or exist within social systems. It is important to consider the social context in which risks occur, and that people do not necessarily share the same perceptions of risk and their underlying causes.

Taking these concepts together—hazards, risks, vulnerabilities, and capacities—will comprise the key information for planning. Knowing risks and vulnerabilities, one will be able to identify what to plan for and what to prioritize. Identifying existing capacities will also inform us of which gaps to fill and what to strengthen.

There are differences in health effects, depending on the hazards that cause an event (Goel 2006) (Table 12.12.4). Planning for disasters and emergencies should be based on analysis of risks, and vulnerabilities, *vis-à-vis* capacities that are in place in the areas where the planning is being conducted (e.g. national, subnational). It would be important to plan to examine all hazards, also known as the all-hazard approach, and developing scenarios around each possible event.

Specific examples

Islands are prone to extremely damaging natural disasters, such as hurricanes and tropical storms, volcanic eruptions, storm surges, landslides, extended droughts, and extensive floods. A recent study of the UN/DHA shows that at least 13 of the 25 most disaster-prone countries worldwide are small island developing country states. The impact of natural disasters is especially severe for islands because of their small size, dependence on agriculture and tourism, narrow resource base, and the pervasive impact of such events on their people, environment and economies, including loss of insurance coverage. For those affected by these natural disasters, these particular characteristics mean that the economic, social, and environmental consequences are long-lasting and the costs of rehabilitation are high. Island nations which are prepared and aware of the consequences they may face suffer less from such events. In Cuba

(Mas Bermejo 2006), every village boards up their homes and stocks up on essential supplies before a storm. In Japan (Shaw *et al.* 2004), another island nation, there are regular drills for earthquakes. Community-performed exercises based on community plans linked to higher levels of authority and administration reduce the impact of disasters.

Factors that determine the potential of communicable disease transmission

One of the most common myths associated with disasters is that epidemics of communicable diseases are inevitable. This myth is often perpetuated by the media and by local politicians who demand mass vaccination campaigns immediately following natural disasters such as hurricanes, earthquakes, and floods. The public perception that disease outbreaks are imminent often derives from its exaggerated sense of the risk posed by dead bodies that remain exposed after an acute natural disaster. The truth is that communicable disease epidemics are relatively rare after rapid onset natural disasters unless large numbers of people are displaced from their homes and placed in crowded and unsanitary camps (Seaman *et al.* 1984; World Health Organization 1986). Six types of adverse changes influence the potential risk of communicable diseases after disasters (Noji 1997). These are changes in pre-existent levels of disease, changes in ecology that are the result of the disaster, changes due to population displacement, changes in population density, changes due to disruption of public utilities, and changes due to interruption of basic public health services.

Changes in pre-existent levels of disease

Usually the risk of a communicable disease in a community affected by a disaster is proportional to the endemic level. There is generally no risk of a given disease when the organism that causes it is not present beforehand. Developing countries frequently have poor systems for reporting communicable diseases; thus, their national authorities lack adequate information about levels of specific organisms. Political pressure nonetheless is sometimes exerted demanding public health measures against diseases such as smallpox, cholera, yellow fever, or other vector-borne diseases in geographic areas considered free of them by communicable disease specialists.

Relief workers can conceivably introduce communicable diseases into areas affected by disasters. Diseases potentially introduced include new strains of influenza, foot-and-mouth disease, and those borne by insect vectors, particularly by *Aedes aegypti*. In addition, non-immune relief workers may be susceptible to endemic diseases to which the local population is tolerant or immune, and may become ill.

Changes in ecology caused by disasters

Natural disasters, particularly droughts, floods, and hurricanes, frequently produce ecological changes in the environment that increase or reduce the risk of communicable diseases. Vector-borne and water-borne diseases are the most significantly affected. A hurricane with heavy rains that strikes the Caribbean coastal area of Central America may, for example, reduce the number of *Anopheles aquasalis* hatched, since the vectors prefer brackish tidal swamps, and increase *A. albimanus* and *A. darlingi*, which breed easily in

Table 12.12.4 Short-term effects of major disasters.

Effect	Earthquakes	High winds (without flooding)	Tidal waves/flash floods	Slow onset floods	Landslides	Volcanoes
Deaths*	Many	Few	Many	Few	Many	Many
Severe injuries requiring extensive treatment	Many	Moderate	Few	Few	Few	Few
Increased risk of communicable diseases	Potential risk following all major disasters (probability rising with overcrowding and deteriorating sanitation)					
Damage to health facilities	Severe (structure and equipment)	Severe	Severe but localized	Severe (equipment only)	Severe but localized	Severe (structure and equipment)
Damage to water systems	Severe	Light	Severe	Light	Severe but localized	Severe
Food shortage	Rare (may occur due to economic and logistic factors)	Rare (may occur due to economic and logistic factors)	Common	Common	Rare	Rare
Major population movement	Rare (may occur in heavily damaged areas)	Rare (may occur in heavily damaged areas)	Common (generally limited)	Common (generally limited)	Common (generally limited)	Common (generally limited)

*Potential lethal impact in absence of preventive measures.

Source: Goel (2006) *Encyclopedia of Disaster Management* (vol. 1—Disaster Management Policy and Administration)—page 6.

fresh, clear water and overflows. The net effect of the hurricane on human malaria, of which both mosquitoes are vectors, would be difficult to predict. Rain from such a hurricane would also cause flooding of streams and canals in rural areas that are often the source of drinking water. Under some circumstances, a water-borne zoonotic disease such as leptospirosis may become more widely disseminated via water-contact or drinking from contaminated sources. There is evidence that the short-term effect of diluting supplies of already contaminated drinking water with rain may reduce the level of disease (Rutherford *et al.* 1983). The population may avoid drinking water contaminated by flooding for a cultural/psychological reason such as the presence of animal carcasses.

Changes due to population displacement

Movement of populations away from the areas affected by a disaster can affect the relative risk for communicable diseases in three ways. If the population moves nearby, the existing facilities and services in the receiving community will be strained. When resettlement occurs at some distance, the chances increase that the displaced population will encounter diseases not prevalent in their own community, to which they are susceptible. For example, non-immunized, rural Andean populations brought together in camps after an earthquake may then be exposed to measles. Alternatively, displaced populations may bring the agents or vectors of communicable diseases with them. The latter concern frequently occurs when populations from low-lying coastal areas with malaria move further inland before a hurricane.

Changes in population density

Population density is a critical factor in the transmission of diseases spread by the respiratory route and through person-to-person contact.

Because of the destruction of houses, natural disasters almost invariably contribute to increased population density. Survivors of severe disasters seek shelter, food, and water in less affected areas. When the damage is less severe, crowding may occur when people move in with other families and congregate in such public facilities as schools and churches. The resulting problems most commonly mentioned are acute respiratory illness, and include influenza and non-specific diarrhoeas.

Changes due to disruption of public utilities

Disasters may interrupt electricity, water, sewage disposal, and other public utilities. In situations with disruption of public utilities, there are promiscuous defecation habits and contaminated sources of water that promote communicable diseases. However, in economically more developed areas, the extended disruption of basic services increases the risks of food- and water-borne disease. Insufficient water for washing hands and bathing promotes the spread of diseases transmitted by contact.

Changes due to interruption of basic public health services

The interruption of basic public health services such as vaccination, ambulatory treatment of tuberculosis, and programmes for the control of malaria and vectors are frequent, but often overlooked factors increase the probability of disease transmission after disaster in a developing country. The risk of transmission increases proportionally to the extent and the duration of the disruption. An outbreak of communicable disease may occur months or years after a drought, famine, or civil disturbance. The interruption causing such an occurrence is usually the result of the diversion of staff and financial resources to the relief effort, beyond the critical period.

In addition or in conjunction with this, the failure to reestablish resources at sufficient levels contributes to the interruption.

Phases of a disaster and its link to sustainable development

The UN International Strategy for Disaster Reduction identifies the phase of a disaster as follows:

Preparedness	Activities and measures taken in advance to ensure effective response to the impact of hazards, including the issuance of timely and effective early warnings and the temporary evacuation of people and property from threatened locations.
Prevention	Activities to provide outright avoidance of the adverse impact of hazards and means to minimize related environmental, technological, and biological disasters.
	Depending on social and technical feasibility and cost/benefit considerations, investing in preventive measures is justified in areas frequently affected by disasters. In the context of public awareness and education, related to disaster risk reduction changing attitudes and behaviour contribute to promoting a 'culture of prevention'.
Recovery	Decisions and actions taken after a disaster with a view to restoring or improving the pre-disaster living conditions of the stricken community, while encouraging and facilitating necessary adjustments to reduce disaster risk.
	Recovery (rehabilitation and reconstruction) affords an opportunity to develop and apply disaster risk reduction measures.
Relief/ response	The provision of assistance or intervention during or immediately after a disaster to meet the life preservation and basic subsistence needs of those people affected. It can be of an immediate, short-term, or protracted duration.
Mitigation	Structural and non-structural measures undertaken to limit the adverse impact of natural hazards, environmental degradation, and technological hazards.

These phases can be better understood as a cycle:

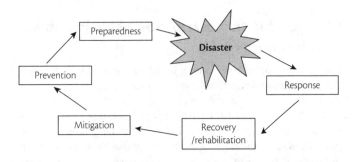

It is important to note that the cycle and its phases should be viewed in terms of managing risks. This cycle illustrates the process by which various stakeholders (e.g. governments, civil society, private sector) plan for, respond to, and conduct activities to reduce the impact of disasters even before they happen. With appropriate legislation, policies, regulations and activities in place at every point in the cycle, then the net effect is contribution to:

◆ Greater reduction of vulnerability of communities

◆ Increased capacities in preparedness

◆ Increased response capacity

◆ Increased resilience in recovery of communities

As the cycle recurs with every event, there is also the opportunity to improve the legislation, policies, regulations, and investments in mitigation, prevention, and preparedness. Events and emergencies will continue to help improve public policies that modify the causes of, or reduce the impacts of disasters on communities. All of which then ensure continuous development.

Indeed, the link between disasters and development becomes crucial as we view the cycle. Managing disasters is all about understanding and managing risks at all points of this cycle and the health sector has much to contribute in this. This being so, it is clear why the health sector plays a key role in disaster and emergency preparedness and response, and development of nations in general.

Sustainable development requires various approaches and among them is risk management of which a safer community is the main end goal. Managing risks goes hand in hand with developing capacity to adequately manage emergencies and disasters when they occur. There is a synergistic and cyclical relationship between disasters and development: The goal of disaster and emergency management is to reduce risks to create safer communities and to safeguard the existing as well as the potential gains of development. Conversely, development that is risk approach-oriented prevents and mitigates the deleterious effects of catastrophic events. A good example would be establishing good hospital systems and training health professionals to attend to affected populations of an earthquake. But then, in many cases, hospitals themselves cannot withstand tremors and earthquakes due to poor construction. It then becomes a case of development creating more risks and vulnerabilities; this should be prevented. This is an example from within the health sector. However, there are development issues impinging on wider areas, such as the environment, urban planning, and migration in which development may generate further risks and disasters if not addressed properly. The health sector does not only act to prepare and respond to disasters but needs to involve itself in other sustainable development issues. After all, a risk to health is a risk to achieving development, with the reverse being true as well. A holistic view of the various phases, how they link, and what are the appropriate interventions that can be done per phase can help in ensuring that health and environment are protected.

Health sector functions in emergencies: Components for planning

The WHO categorizes its functions for emergencies described below. This framework can also apply to the health sector in its preparedness and responses for emergencies. The following are the four major areas:

1. *Capacity building for health responses in disasters*: The concept of capacity building covers a wide range of operational and

disciplinary factors. These can range from the capacity of the government military, civil society groups, and the community response to the capacity of laboratories for providing testing at the approved quality level. It also covers a wide range of activities from building systems and policies to training community members or health staff for specific skills. The goals of building capacity in the health sector are not different from those in other sectors; i.e. autonomy and self-reliance, local capacities, and sustainability:

◆ *Autonomy and self-reliance* is the primary goal for all communities at risk. In this context, building the capacity of local communities is the main strategy to accomplish this objective.

◆ *Local capacities* in the areas of relief and responses are most effective when people in local communities are well trained and the community is well prepared for disasters. Persons at the community level will reach the affected areas the quickest, and are most familiar with local conditions. Thus, the efficiency and effectiveness of the responses are enhanced greatly by improving the capacity of local health professionals. Experienced and skilled international relief workers are useful in disaster management, but require adjustment to the conditions and the customs and characteristics of the area in which the disaster occurs.

◆ Skilled, well-trained local personnel in place can ensure *sustainability*. When the relief efforts stop, these personnel will continue to provide the affected community with long-term recovery.

2. *Assessments*: Needs assessment is one of the most important aspects of disaster responses and relief planning. The main reason to conduct needs assessment is to inform decision-makers about what to do in relation to a given situation. The assessment will help answer five decision-making questions: (1) Should there be an intervention?; (2) What is the nature and scale of intervention needed?; (3) What are the priorities for the allocation of resources?; (4) What are the gaps that need to be filled?; and (5) What is the program design and what planning is required? Several problems can result from poor needs assessment, including unnecessary repetition, lack of coordination, inadequate determination of effectiveness, changes over time, inadequate dissemination, and need for standards.

Assessments are keys in the event of various disasters. The accident at Chernobyl (Ukraine 1986) (World Health Organization 2007), the explosions in fireworks storage (The Netherlands, 2000) (Ruijten 2007), the AZF factory (France, 2001) (Verger *et al.* 2007), fuel explosion (The United Kingdom, 2005) (Russell & Saunders 2007), terrorist attacks on the Twin Towers (United States, 2001) (Herbert *et al.* 2006), the summer 2003 heat wave in Europe (Sardon 2007), the tsunami in Southeast Asia (2004) (World Health Organization 2005) and, most recently, hurricanes Katrina and Rita (United States, 2005) (Blendon *et al.* 2007) and the earthquake in Pakistan (2005) (Laverick *et al.* 2007) all had serious human health, social, and economic effects on human societies. However, no comprehensive strategy for investigating and learning more about health, social, and societal consequences of disasters has been defined at the international level. Health assessment involves exposure and health risk assessment, as well as epidemiologic surveillance and in-depth studies.

Standardization and coordination of assessment activities require consensus at the international, national, and subnational levels.

There is a role for health assessment after an event, as well as using epidemiology to anticipate catastrophes. These evaluations face many difficulties, including lack of pre-disaster health indicator information such as post-traumatic stress disorders (PTSD), availability of soil contamination data, lack of pre-exposure data, relevant demographic databases, loss of follow-up of subjects, etc. Post-disaster assessments and health information systems that are set up shortly after an emergency can provide decision-making support to manage health hazards, screening for specific health problems, and organization of medical follow-up and health surveillance. Public information about health risks must be transparent and available to the media, the public, affected populations, healthcare professionals, and various other stakeholders. Scientific knowledge resulting from research will increase knowledge and improve responses to any future event.

3. *Coordination*: The elements in emergencies that require coordination in the health sector include efforts by affected communities, national and local governments in the affected areas, donor governments (bilateral), multi-lateral agencies (UN and international financial institutions), national and international non-government organization (NGOs), academic institutions, the military, and the media. The national government, especially the Ministry of Health, should coordinate all health responses in emergencies in their respective countries. However, in areas that the national government has failed during the conflict, organizations such as World Health Organization may take a leadership role in health sector coordination to guarantee minimum standard healthcare for the affected populations. Roles of coordinating bodies responsible for medical care and public health functions are:

◆ Working with all players to establish and agree to norms and standards

◆ Leading in emergency preparedness and drills

◆ Actively engaging other players within the sector, sharing information as it becomes available

◆ Integrating health expertise and activities for maximum effectiveness and efficiency

◆ Acknowledging the roles of all of actors

4. *Filling gaps in available services*: To identify gaps in available services, health authorities should consider these general points; i.e. uniqueness of the types of disasters, such as floods, tsunamis, earthquakes. Decision-makers require adequate and accurate needs assessment to generate information, and population data to determine the impact of the event. Gaps in the early phase of relief common to all sudden onset disasters are interventions relating to provision of food, supply of adequate safe water and sanitation facilities, construction of temporary shelters, and rapid restoration of preventive and curative healthcare services. The healthcare services that should be considered as high priority are field hospitals, mental health, and women's health.

New tools to address new challenges for health emergencies

◆ International Health Regulations (2005)

◆ Benchmarks for Emergency Preparedness and Response

Disaster response relies upon the concept of International Health Security. There is a need to reduce the vulnerability of people to the escalation of existing, new, acute, or rapidly spreading risks to health, particularly those that threaten to cross international borders. Health issues present new challenges that go far beyond national borders, and have an impact on the collective security of people around the world.

Globalization with its easy, frequent travel, as well as large-scale trade, offers ample opportunity for disease to spread across borders quickly and easily. Epidemic-prone diseases, both new and re-emerging, humanitarian emergencies, bioterrorism, climate change, and environmental degradation have the potential to become international public health emergencies.

No single institution or country has all the capacities needed to respond to international public health emergencies caused by epidemics, natural hazards, conflicts, or by epidemics of existing diseases, or new and emerging infectious diseases.

The earth's climate is changing. Temperatures are rising, tropical storms are increasing in frequency and intensity, and polar ice caps and permafrost regions are melting. The acute impact of climate change-related events may be local, but the cause is global. When floods contaminate international waters, when people migrate across borders to find food and shelter, when disease patterns change due to an altered climate, the impact is felt internationally. As a result, trends and predictions for changes in morbidity and mortality patterns all point to an increase.

Humanitarian emergencies arise from the effects of crises such as natural hazards, food and water shortages, and armed conflict. Just as these situations affect individuals, they also affect the already stressed health systems that people rely on for maintaining health security. The World Disasters Report 2006 (International Federation of the Red Cross and Crescent Societies 2006) indicates that approximately 58 per cent of the total number of people killed in natural disasters occurred in the Southeast Asia region during the decade of 1996–2005. In this decade, the Asian region had the highest number of natural disasters (1273 reported events) and technological disasters (1387 reported events). Disaster preparedness strategies and humanitarian response operations together can create a balanced approach to alleviating the negative impact of natural disasters. Both rely on planning, collaboration, and coordination of roles of the various sectors involved.

Considering all these elements of International Health Security, *vis-à-vis* risks and hazards in the region, it would be practical to focus on two key aspects: (1) international health regulations; and (2) systematic emergency preparedness and response.

The International Health Regulations (2005) (WHO 2006)

The revised International Health Regulations (IHR) (2005) unanimously adopted by the World Health Assembly of WHO came into force in June 2007. Their implementation will help build and strengthen effective mechanisms for alert and response for events of public health concern at national and international levels.

Member states will work towards the implementation of the IHR (2005) and towards greater collaboration across borders and between sectors to counter the negative influences on health posed by globalization, disasters, climate change, and existing and emerging diseases.

Key elements of the IHR (2005) are as follows:

◆ This legal framework seeks to protect against, control, and provide a mechanism to initiate a public health response to the threat of international spread of diseases of biological, chemical, or radionuclear origin.

◆ IHR (2005) is a major paradigm shift from IHR (1969), and focuses now on:

  ◆ Containment at the source of a possible Public Health Emergency of International Concern (PHEIC) as opposed to only control at borders

  ◆ All public health threats as opposed to a few diseases

  ◆ Adapted responses as opposed to pre-set measures

  ◆ Facilitates development of proactive systems as opposed to reactive ones

As a binding global legal framework, the adoption of the IHR (2005) requires certain requirements for Member States, including:

◆ Designation of a national IHR focal point

◆ Strengthening core capacity to detect, report, and respond rapidly to events that pose a threat to public health

◆ Assessing events occurring in their territory and notifying WHO within 24 h of all events that may constitute a PHEIC

◆ Providing routine inspection and control activities at international airports, ports and some ground crossings

◆ Building a legal and administrative framework in line with IHR (2005) requirements

In accordance with these needs, WHO will support the development of core capacities in health systems for IHR to be fully functional. This includes its own institutional readiness to support Member States with appropriate staffing, conducting global surveillance and health intelligence gathering, providing technical assistance and guidance to Member States, developing guidelines and measures for PHEIC, and updating the IHR (2005) as appropriate to maintain its scientific and regulatory validity.

WHO South-East Asia Region (SEAR) benchmarking framework for emergency preparedness and response (EPR)

The Benchmarks Framework is a response to the collective experiences of five Asian countries affected by the tsunami of 26 December 2004, the recurring emergencies in all SEAR member countries, and the global call for improved emergency preparedness.

Member States formulated the benchmarks to set standards for emergency preparedness through a participatory approach applicable to the specific situations in the countries of the region and other countries in the world. This gap in standards and benchmarks was a clearly identified need after many lessons learned from the tsunami experience.

The benchmarks are the product of a regional consultation in Bangkok in November 2005 (World Health Organization, Regional Office of South-East Asia 2006) involving all 11 SEAR member countries. In addition to Ministries of Health (MOH), a number of other stakeholders were present, notably from Ministries of Home Affairs, Foreign Affairs and Education, as well as UN agencies, the International Federation of Red Cross, International Non-Governmental Organizations (INGO), donors, and universities.

The consultation's main objective was to identify gaps in addressing response, preparedness, and recovery for health needs of affected and vulnerable populations. The 12 benchmarks address the key issues necessary to establish a disaster preparedness mechanism as identified by the participants at the consultation.

Following a regional consultation in Bali in June 2006 (World Health Organization, Regional Office for South-East Asia 2007a), the Benchmarks Framework was further refined to include standards and indicators to make planning, monitoring, and evaluation more accurate.

The following are the 12 benchmarks (World Health Organization, Regional Office for South-East Asia 2007b)

1. A legal framework and functioning coordination mechanisms and an organizational structure in place for health EPR at all levels involving all stakeholders.

2. Regularly updated disaster preparedness and emergency management planning for the health sector and standard operating procedures (SOP) (emergency directory, national coordination focal point) in place.

3. Emergency financial (including national budget), physical and regular human resource allocation and accountability procedures established.

4. Rules of engagement (including conduct) for external humanitarian agencies, based on needs established.

5. Community planning for mitigation, preparedness and response developed, based on risk identification and participatory vulnerability assessment, backed by a higher level of capacity.

6. Community-based response and preparedness capacity developed, and supported with training and regular simulation/mock drills.

7. A local capacity for emergency provision of essential services and supplies (shelters, safe drinking water, food, communication).

8. Advocacy and awareness developed through education, information management and communication, including media relations (pre-, during, and post-event).

9. The capacity to identify risks and assess vulnerability at all levels.

10. Human resource capabilities continuously updated and maintained.

11. Health facilities built/modified to withstand expected risks.

12. Early warning and surveillance systems for identifying health concerns.

Corresponding to each benchmark are standards, indicators and a question/checklist. All these complete the framework for identifying gaps and monitoring progress towards improved emergency preparedness and response.

Each benchmark has two or three standards, and each standard has one to four health sector indicators for which monitoring can take place. The standards denote the technical reference level of quality or attainment of the benchmark. The standards are qualitative, universal in nature, and applicable in any operating environment, as they specify the minimum level to be attained.

Each standard is equipped with tools to measure the progress towards achieving the standards; i.e. a set of indicators. The indicators provide a way to measure and determine progress in achieving the standards. As the indicators are formulated to be very specific to the standards, they can also be used to guide strategic thinking and planning.

The health sector indicators all refer to health-related issues that various partners have a mandate to ensure, including the Ministry of Health, district health authorities, hospitals, UN agencies, NGOs, and community partners,.

For each standard, a set of non-health sector or 'other sectors indicators' has been included. The other sectors indicators refer to essential preparedness issues that are not within the means of the health sector to achieve, but that nonetheless have a crucial impact on the overall preparedness levels of the country.

Although their implementation might not be the mandate of the health sector, they are important to consider when planning and evaluating the health sector emergency preparedness activities. Some of these indicators point to key areas of intersectoral coordination and collaboration, and highlight the importance of including public health concerns in areas such as national emergency planning, capacity building, and community disaster mitigation.

The last tool in the benchmarks framework is a checklist that consists of pertinent questions for each standard that can help guide analysis of the existing situation.

The questions predominantly relate to health sector issues, but also refer to important factors outside the health sector when the absence or presence of these is a potentially determining factor for the overall vulnerabilities and capacities of the national and local systems.

Use of the benchmarks

Other partners are increasingly looking to the SEAR benchmarks. In May 2007, Yale New Haven Center for Emergency Preparedness and Disaster Response (YNH-CEPDR), the Joint Commission, the Pan American Health Organization (PAHO), and the University of Wisconsin, Department of Surgery/World Association for Disaster and Emergency Medicine (WADEM) used six of the benchmarks as the basis for discussion during a workshop on 'The Safe and Resilient Hospitals: Preparing for the Next Disaster'.

The emergency preparedness and response programme in the WHO Regional Office for Europe is planning to introduce the benchmarks as part of the framework of upcoming country assessments of health security capacities. In the initial phase, assessments are planned for three countries (Armenia, Azerbaijan, and either Ukraine or Georgia).

The IHR and the SEAR benchmark frameworks are new tools to measure the progress in improving emergency preparedness and response in more complex contexts that we live in and in which emergencies occur.

References

Advisory Committee on the International Decade for Natural Hazard Reduction (1987). *Confronting natural disasters: an international decade for natural hazard reduction*. Washington DC: National Academy Press.

Anderson, M.B. (1991). Which costs more: prevention or recovery? In *Managing natural disasters and the environment* (eds. A. Kreimer and M. Munasinghe). World Bank, Washington DC.

Armenian, H.K. (1986). Wartime: options for epidemiology. *American Journal of Epidemiology*, July, **124**(1), 28–32.

Berz, G. (1984). Research and statistics on natural disasters in insurance and reinsurance companies. *The Geneva Papers on Risk and Insurance*, **9**, 135–57.

Binder, S. and Sanderson, L.M. (1987). The role of epidemiologist in natural disasters. *Annals of Emergency Medicine*, September, **16**(9), 1081–4.

Blendon, R.J., Benson J.M., DesRoches C.M., Lyon-Daniel K., Mitchell E.W., Pollard W.E. *et al.* (2007). The public's preparedness for hurricanes in four affected regions. *Public Health Reports*, March–April, **122**(2), 167–76.

Center for Research on the Epidemiology of Disasters (2007). *Report of CRED 2007*. Brussels.

Cuny, F.C. (1993). Introduction to disaster management. Lesson 5: technologies of disaster management. *Journal of Prehospital and Disaster Medicine*, **6**, 372–4.

Cuny, F.C., Abrams, S., and America, O. (1983). *Disasters and development*. Oxford University Press, New York.

Godschalk, D.R. *et al.* (1999). *Natural hazard mitigation: recasting disaster policy and planning*. Island Press, Washington DC.

Goel, S.L. (2006). *Encyclopedia of disaster management*. Vol. 1 – Disaster management policy and administration). Deep and Deep Publications, New Delhi.

Guha-Sapir, D. and Lechat, M.F. (1986a). Information systems and needs assessment in natural disasters: an approach for better disaster relief management. *Disasters*, **10**(3), 232–7.

Guha-Sapir, D. and Lechat, M.F. (1986b). Reducing the impact of natural disasters: why aren't we better prepared? *Health Policy and Planning*, **1**(2), 118–26.

Herbert, R. *et al.* (2006). The World Trade Center disaster and the health of workers: five-year assessment of a unique medical screening program. *Environmental Health Perspectives*, December, **114**(12), 1853–8.

IDNDR Promotion Office (1994). *Natural disasters in the world: statistical trends on natural disasters*. National Land Agency, Tokyo.

International Federation of the Red Cross and Crescent Societies (2006). *World disasters report – focus on neglected crises*. International Federation of Red Cross and Red Crescent Societies. Geneva.

International Strategy for Disaster Reduction (2003). Glossary. Geneva. Availabale at http://www.unisdr.org/eng/public_aware/world_camp/2003/english/5_Glossary_eng.pdf, accessed 13 September 2007).

Kohl, P.A. *et al.* (2005). The Sumatra–Andaman Earthquake and Tsunami of 2004: the hazards, events, and damage. *Prehospital and Disaster Medicine*, November–December, **20**(6), 355–63.

Laverick, S. *et al.* (2007). Asian earthquake: report from the first volunteer British hospital team in Pakistan. *Emergency Medical Journal*, August, **24**(8), 543–6.

Lechat, M.F. (1990). Updates: the epidemiology of health effects of disasters. *Epidemiologic Reviews*, **12**(1), 192–7.

Mas Bermejo, P. (2006). Preparation and response in case of natural disasters: Cuban programs and experience. *Journal of Public Health Policy*, **27**(1), 13–21.

Noji, E.K. (1997). *The public health consequences of disasters*. Oxford University Press, New York.

Office of US Foreign Disaster Assistance (1995). *Disaster history: significant data on major disaster worldwide, 1900-present*. Agency for International Development, Washington DC.

Pan American Health Organization (1982). *Epidemiologic surveillance after natural disaster*. PAHO, Washington DC.

Pan American Health Organization (1983). *Health services organization in the event of disaster*. PAHO, Washington DC.

Ruijten, M. (2007). The Dutch experience with health impact assessment of disasters. *European Journal of Public Health*, February, **17**(1), 5–6.

Russell, D. and Saunders, P. (2007). The UK experience with Health Impact Assessment of disasters. *European Journal of Public Health*, February, **17**(1), 4–5.

Rutherford, W.H. *et al.* (1983). The definition and classification of disasters. *Injury*, July, **15**(1), 10–2.

Sardon, J.P. (2007). The 2003 heat wave. *Euro Surveillance*, March 1, **12**(3), 226.

Seaman, J. *et al.* (1984). *Epidemiology of natural disasters*. Karger, New York.

Shah, B.V. (1983). Is the environment becoming more hazardous? A Global survey 1947–1980. *Disasters*, **7**, 202–9.

Shaw, R. *et al.* (2004). From disaster to sustainable civil society: the Kobe experience. *Disasters*, March, **28**(1), 16–40.

United Nations Department of Economic and Social Affairs (1996). *International Decade for Natural Disaster Reduction*. Resolution 196/45 at 52nd plenary meeting, 26 July 1996. Available at http://www.un.org/documents/ecosoc/res/1996/eres1996-45.htm accessed 1 September 2007).

Verger, P. *et al.* (2007). French experiences with Health Impact Assessment of disasters. *European Journal of Public Health*, **17**(1), 3–4.

World Health Organization (1986). Communicable diseases after natural disasters. *Weekly Epidemiological Record*, **11**(14), 79–81.

World Health Organization (2005). *Communicable disease toolkit for tsunami affected areas: surveillance system for emergency phase*. Geneva.

World Health Organization (2006). *International health regulations (2005)*. Geneva.

World Health Organization (2007). *The world health report 2007: a safer future: global public health security in the 21st century*. Geneva.

World Health Organization, Regional Office for South-East Asia (2006). *Health Aspects of Emergency Preparedness and Response: Report of the Regional Meeting Bangkok, 21–23 November 2005*, New Delhi. Document SEA/EHA/13.

World Health Organization, Regional Office for South-East Asia (2007a). *Emergency preparedness and response: from lessons to action: report of the regional consultation, Bali, Indonesia, 27–29 June 2006*, New Delhi. Document SEA/Dis. Prep/3.

World Health Organization, Regional Office for South-East Asia (2007b). *Benchmarking emergency preparedness: Emergency & humanitarian action*, New Delhi: p. 8. Available at http://www.searo.who.int/LinkFiles/EHA_BenchmarkingEPP_Aug07.pdf accessed 1 September 2007).

Private support of public health

Roger Detels and Sheena G. Sullivan

Abstract

Although private funding of health initiatives has existed for some time, in recent years, private investment in health, particularly in developing countries, has increased considerably and has often resulted in improvements in health and alleviation of suffering. However, the donation of large sums of money to address one or a handful of health problems can have, and has occasionally had, unintended repercussions in developing nations. Left unchecked, cause-specific funding may undermine the public health systems of these countries, rather than improving them. The purpose of this chapter is to present the positive and negative aspects of private funding of public health and to make suggestions to minimize the harmful unintended negative impacts and to maximize positive outcomes of donor investments in public health.

History

The late twentieth and early twenty-first centuries have witnessed a huge influx of private support for public health as exemplified by generous gifts from the Bill and Melinda Gates Foundations, Warren Buffett, the William Clinton Foundation, the Carter Center, the Wellcome Trust, industry, professional and non-governmental organizations, and others. However, such generous giving, especially by Americans, actually dates back to the formation of the original foundations in the earliest years of the twentieth century. The earliest foundation in the United States was the Russell Sage Foundation founded in 1906, which had a limited focus on working women and social ills. The establishment of the large, broadly focused foundations began with the founding of the Carnegie Foundation by Andrew Carnegie in 1911 'to do real and permanent good in this world' (Carnegie Foundation 2007) followed by the founding of the Rockefeller Foundation in 1913 (Rockefeller Foundation 2007).

These early gifts had a significant impact on public health. The Rockefeller Foundation, for example, founded the International Health Commission in its first year. This was the first appropriation of funds by private sources for international public health activities and has helped 52 countries on 6 continents and 29 islands to improve their public health systems. In the same year, the Foundation began 20 years of support for the *Bureau of Social Hygiene* which focused on research and education on birth control, maternal health and sex education. Moreover, they played a key role in founding the world's first schools of public health, first at Johns Hopkins, then at Harvard and later in other parts of the United States, as well as in 21 foreign countries. Overseas, they helped to establish the London School of Tropical Medicine and Hygiene with a large gift in 1921, as well as the China Medical Board (1914) and the Peking Union Medical College (1921), both of the latter having played a significant role in the development of public health in China.

Since the establishment of these early foundations, the culture of donation to support public health has increased, particularly in recent years. Now, there are over 40 major foundations based in both the United States and abroad (see Table 12.13.1), as well as countless smaller ones. This increase can be attributed in part to at least two phenomena: The AIDS epidemic and the rise in public pressure for corporate social responsibility.

AIDS and the new culture of donation

With the discovery of therapy that could control the progression of HIV disease came the recognition, strongly expressed at the International AIDS Meeting in 1996, that millions of people, especially in developing countries, were being denied access to treatment because of the cost of the drugs. This realization spurred a tripling of funding for international projects to provide treatment for HIV/AIDS and to address the problems of malaria and tuberculosis, two of the major diseases responsible for loss of life and disability internationally. The increased funding was led by the Global Fund to Fight AIDS, Tuberculosis and Malaria (GFATM 2007) and the Bill and Melinda Gates Foundation (Bill and Melinda Gates Foundation 2007) which by 2006 had total assets of US$33.7 billion, more than the total budget of many developing countries. Every year, the Gates Foundation gives away approximately US$800 million approaching the total budget of the World Health Organization and equivalent to the budget for fighting infectious diseases given by the US Agency for International Development. The commitment of the Gates Foundation stimulated additional large donations by Warren Buffett and the William Clinton Foundation.

Corporate social responsibility (CSR) and public–private partnerships

Concurrent with these increases in funding for health has been the rise of CSR. Although corporations are required to abide by certain laws and regulations to reduce any adverse consequences of their

Table 12.13.1 Wealthiest foundations globally

	US$ (billion)		US$ (billion)
Canada		Whitgift Foundation	0.51
The MasterCard Foundation of Toronto, Ontario	2.2	Nuffield Foundation	0.5
Denmark		Joseph Rowntree Foundation	0.48
Realdania of Copenhagen	5.6	*United States* (according to Foundation Center)	
A.P. Møller og Hustru Chastine Mc-Kinney Møllers Fond til almene Formaal of Copenhagen ca	1.5	Bill & Melinda Gates Foundation (WA)	33.12
		The Ford Foundation (NY)	13.66
Carlsberg Foundation of Copenhagen	1.4	J. Paul Getty Trust (CA)	10.13
Germany		The Robert Wood Johnson Foundation (NJ)	10.09
Robert Bosch Foundation	6	The William and Flora Hewlett Foundation (CA)	8.52
Landesstiftung Baden-Württemberg	3.3	W.K. Kellogg Foundation (MI)	8.40
Volkswagen Foundation	2.7	Lilly Endowment Inc. (IN)	7.60
Deutsche Bundesstiftung Umwelt	2.1	The David and Lucile Packard Foundation (CA)	6.35
Liechtenstein		John D. and Catherine T. MacArthur Foundation (IL)	6.18
Onassis Foundation of Vaduz, Liechtenstein	2.1	The Andrew W. Mellon Foundation (NY)	6.13
The Netherlands		Gordon and Betty Moore Foundation (CA)	5.84
Stichting INGKA Foundation	>36	The California Endowment (CA)	4.41
Norway		The Rockefeller Foundation (NY)	3.81
Sparebankstiftelsen DnB NOR of Oslo	1.8	The Kresge Foundation (MI)	3.33
Institusjonen Fritt Ord of Oslo	0.4	The Starr Foundation (NY)	3.30
Cultiva—Kristiansand Kommunes Energiverksstiftelse of Kristiansand	0.3	The Annie E. Casey Foundation (MD)	3.27
		The Duke Endowment (NC)	2.98
UNIFOR—Foundation of the University of Oslo of Oslo	0.2	The Annenberg Foundation (PA)	2.68
Spain		Charles Stewart Mott Foundation (MI)	2.63
La Caixa	0.32	Carnegie Corporation of New York (NY)	2.53
Sweden		Casey Family Programs (WA)	2.49
Knut and Alice Wallenberg Foundation of Stockholm	3.9	John S. and James L. Knight Foundation (FL)	2.34
Nobel Foundation of Stockholm	0.4	The Harry and Jeanette Weinberg Foundation, Inc. (MD)	2.27
United Kingdom (according to Charities Direct)		Tulsa Community Foundation (OK)	2.26
Wellcome Trust of London	26.57	Robert W. Woodruff Foundation, Inc. (GA)	2.25
The Church Commissioners for England	8.32	The McKnight Foundation (MN)	2.21
Garfield Weston Foundation	6.94	Richard King Mellon Foundation (PA)	2.08
The Leverhulme Trust	2.12	Ewing Marion Kauffman Foundation (MO)	2.07
Esmée Fairbairn Foundation	1.82	The New York Community Trust (NY)	2.04
The National Trust	1.66	Doris Duke Charitable Foundation (NY)	1.95
Bridge House Trust	1.46	*India*	
The Henry Smith Charity	1.4	Tata Trusts	
Wolfson Foundation of London	1.32		

businesses, CSR takes this concept further to encourage corporations to take actions to improve the quality of life of their employees and their families, customers, stakeholders, and the community in general (WBCSD 2000). As part of the Millennium Development Goals (UN 2008), corporations, especially large multinationals, are encouraged to increase their awareness of their impact on the societies in which they operate. Many corporations have since established a CSR division to run social programmes. For example, the Standard Chartered Bank, recognizing the need to maintain a stable and healthy workforce, has an extensive HIV/AIDS programme to provide healthcare and support for staff and their families affected by HIV/AIDS in Africa (Standard Chartered 2006).

General CSR programmes may include production of healthful foods, design and manufacturing of low-emission vehicles with higher standards of safety, improvement of the work environment of workers, control of industrial waste, etc.

In addition, corporations, particularly pharmaceutical companies, have been increasingly signing public–private partnerships. These are generally joint ventures between private industry, government, or international agencies such as the WHO or UN agencies, and civil society including universities or NGOs to achieve a shared health objective (Widdus 2005). There were more than 90 international partnerships in health in 2004 (Nishtar 2004). The majority address infectious diseases, notably AIDS, TB, and malaria. Some involve individual governments or NGOs or both forming an alliance with the for-profit sector. For example, Sanofi-Aventis has an extensive international programme of humanitarian sponsorship, including a partnership with the Nelson Mandela Foundation and the South African Department of Health to provide free tuberculosis treatment in areas badly affected within South Africa (Sanofi-Aventis 2008). Other partnerships may involve many players. The most notable are the global health alliances, such as the Global Alliance for Vaccines and Immunizations, Roll Back Malaria, the Stop TB partnership, the Global Polio Eradication Program, and the International AIDS Vaccine Alliance. They may be principally driven by a company, be legally independent, or hosted by a civil society organization (Nishtar 2004). Stop TB, for example, comprises a network of more than 500 partners, including governments of both developed and developing countries, research and technical health institutes, multilateral organizations, civil society, pharmaceutical companies and other industry partners and is housed within the WHO (Stop TB 2007).

Examples of private support

Private support of public health, given by foundations, industry, pharmaceutical companies, and professional organizations has been directed towards disease control and treatment, poverty alleviation, education, training of health workers, infrastructure development, research, improved agricultural practices, health information dissemination, and sponsorship of the many global health alliances.

Specific examples include the provision of drugs and the reduction of drug prices for developing countries, the earliest example being the Metzican Donation Program by Merck & Co. Inc. for treatment for onchocerciasis (river blindness) in West Africa in 1988 (Mectizan 2008). In 1998, GlaxoSmithKline provided albendazole for treatment of lymphatic filiarisis as part of the Mectizan programme. To date, this ongoing programme has reached more than 40 million people (Mectizan 2008).

Another major contribution has been the establishment of special training programmes and scholarships/fellowships for training health personnel. Many foundations are set up for this purpose alone or as part of a broader portfolio. For example, the Robert Wood Johnson Foundation has a clinical scholars programme for US students (Robert Wood Johnson Foundation 2008). Additionally, foundations may provide gifts to schools, such as equipment or teaching resources.

Another important contribution of private agencies has been to research. The Hughes Medical Institute, for example, was established by Hughes Aviation to conduct research into human illness (HHMI 2008) (although the motivation for doing so has been attributed to tax evasion rather than philanthropy; Wikipedia 2008). The Gates Foundation currently supports a large number of research projects related to HIV prevention strategies including vaccine and microbicide development. There are also the very significant contributions made by pharmaceutical companies to the research and development of vaccines and treatments, both independently and in public–private partnerships. Increasingly, these efforts are focusing on the so-called 'neglected diseases' that disproportionately affect the world's poorest nations.

Industry is realizing that improving the health of the public is in their best interest in the long run. These generous gifts and actions have unquestionably had a very significant impact on the growth of public health in the twentieth century and played a significant role in shaping the character and missions of public health. For these significant contributions to 'promote the well-being of mankind throughout the world', they are to be commended (Rockefeller Foundation Charter 1913).

Unforeseen problems

Many of these very generous gifts have benefited the recipient countries enormously and have achieved goals which otherwise would have been impossible to achieve. There is no question that the recent surge in international giving, which shows no signs of slowing, is a positive step towards reducing the disparities between the rich and poor countries and benefiting all mankind. Why, then, have there been critics of this surge in generosity?

From the beginning, the foundations have determined their goals for giving based on the personal perspectives of their founders and subsequent leaders. Often, they did not consult public health leaders in determining these goals. This strategy has the risk of distorting the public health agenda with the influx of large sums of money, which often dwarfs the national budgets of the recipient countries and cannot be matched by the local government. This presents a myriad of problems for these countries.

First, their public health agenda is being determined by outside agencies. This agenda may not coincide with the country's needs, and may deplete existing resources, especially trained personnel. When a huge donor driven programme is established, it must rapidly acquire an infrastructure for its management. Programmes will often attract qualified personnel by providing higher salaries than can realistically be provided by local government agencies. Thus, much of the staff is drawn from the existing public health infrastructure, leaving fewer staff within government to work on other health priorities. The result—the goals of the donors are met, but at the expense of the country's health system resulting in deterioration of other important public health programmes and exacerbating the existing public health human resource crisis extant in most developing countries. For example, in Haiti, the dramatically improved HIV/AIDS situation has paralleled a decline in other measures of the population's health, including infant mortality (Farmer & Garrett 2006).

Second, the governments, in many developing countries, have invested little of their funds, often less than 5 per cent, in health. Large infusions of donor funds allow these countries to continue to underfund health. Kwame Ampomah, a Ghanaian with the UNAIDS programme in Gaborone, Botswana, asserts that 'you need a clear health system with equity that is not donor-driven' (Garrett 2007).

The influx of huge sum of money can also contribute to corruption, inflation, and destabilization of the economy. In countries with entrenched bureaucracies and rampant corruption, the donor funds may not all be used for implementation of public health programmes. In the absence of any evaluation to measure the benefits of a programme or any auditing to account for spending, donations may simply serve to exacerbate corruption and bureaucracy. In addition, increasing the salaries of some, especially government officials, can widen the rich–poor gap and generate inflation (Garrett 2007).

Further, programmes that appear acceptable to the Western intellect may not be culturally acceptable to people of other countries. For example, family-planning programmes, in order to be successful, had to demonstrate that smaller families meant increased survival for the children and an increased probability that parents would have a viable male to support them in their old age.

Sustainability

The donation of large sums of money to tackle specific health problems does not lend itself to a sustainable solution. For example, the Gates Foundation now provides 17 per cent of the global budget (US$86 million) to eradicate poliomyelitis and also supports vaccine programmes for HIV/AIDS, Japanese encephalitis, and other diseases, as well as research in HIV/AIDS, particularly towards development of female-controlled interventions. In an effort to assist women to become more independent, the foundation has given money to the Grameen Foundation, whose founder recently received the Nobel Peace Prize. With the Rockefeller Foundation, the Gates Foundation has also provided funds to support improved agricultural practices in developing countries. But, when Gates' and other donor monies are discontinued, are these programmes going to be sustained by the local governments which do not have the resources of these large donors?

Currently, massive funding is being injected to provide treatment for HIV/AIDS to those in need, but it is likely that other major health problems will occur in the future which will divert donors' attention away from HIV/AIDS. The countries now receiving these massive infusions of money for treatment programmes for HIV/AIDS patients will not be able to sustain them. Thus, it is unclear what the long-term impact of the huge influx of funds will be on HIV/AIDS. A larger investment in prevention may have a more long-lasting benefit, but currently the majority of donors have concentrated their funds on treatment with little allocated to prevention, in part because it is difficult to show immediate outcomes with prevention.

The implementation of demonstration/pilot projects needs to consider whether the projects can be sustained by the local government if they are demonstrated to be effective, and whether it will be feasible to upscale the project to the point where it will have a significant impact on the health of the country. Often, outside support to maintain a programme is provided without seeking in-country solutions to supply issues, and there is a focus on treatment rather than prevention. In the case of pharmaceuticals, for example, the solution is usually to help countries find cheap avenues for importing drugs, rather than helping them to establish their own pharmaceutical plants to manufacture generic medicines. By supporting development of local industries, donor money can have an impact that reaches far beyond health.

Reliance on imported pharmaceuticals has very real risks for disease control. Cessation of an externally funded programme, including the drug supply, can lead to the resurgence of disease, as was the case in Uganda when sleeping sickness quickly resurfaced once control had apparently been achieved and the project staff withdrew (Widdus 2005). Irregular supply or inadequate storage facilities, both common in developing countries, can lead to treatment failure and subsequent resistance to medications. Simple mismanagement of programmes has also had serious adverse consequences—such as the reckless provision of TB therapy without adequate medical supervision in KwaZulu Natal, which has led to the evolution of the most drug-resistant strains of the mycobacteria (Garrett 2007). Ironically, by providing quick fixes to a problem, some foundations are doing what medicine has long known as unsustainable—treating symptoms without preventing the cause!

Coordination

In some countries, there are so many donors, each targeting their own agendas, that the country's public health professionals are not aware of all the programmes being conducted in their country. Without this information for coordination, national programmes may be duplicating donor programmes while other urgent needs may be unmet. This lack of coordination is exacerbated in countries where the donors feel that the government is corrupt and therefore bypass it. In developed countries, governments that have played a central role in funding health have had better control over growth and may lead to a more efficient health service (Navarro 1985). Thus, external investment in a country's health should prioritize partnering with, improving and supporting existing public infrastructures, and should recognize that a country's elected government may be able to judge its health priorities better than an external organization based in a rich country (Widdus 2003). Donors may also bypass established health authorities who work closely with governments to determine priorities, such as the WHO, which undermines their role in international health and fractures the system further.

For HIV/AIDS, at least, UN agencies have overseen the development of the 'Three Ones' agreement: *One* agreed-upon HIV/AIDS action framework that provides the basis for coordinating the work of all partners; *one* national AIDS coordinating authority, with a broad based multi-sector mandate; and *one* consensus for country-level monitoring and evaluation system (WHO 2004). Similar agreements are needed for donor-supported health projects in general. China provides a unique example of how government authoritarianism has helped achieve this kind of coordination. Although it was motivated by a different purpose, China insists that large donor agencies have government approval before being allowed to work in-country, and thus, the relevant officials have been able to have a direct role in deciding where and how donor money should be channelled.

Dubious motives

Because of charitable tax deductions by the US government, the foundations are able to reduce their tax burden by as much as 25 per cent. The *New York Times* has estimated that charitable deductions cost the US government US$40 billion in lost tax revenue in 2006 (Strom 2007). Thus, to some extent, the foundations, not the US government, are determining where public health funds are spent. Recognizing this fact, Eli Broad, one of the major donors, has said that, 'What smart entrepreneurial philanthropists and their foundations do is get greater value for how they invest their money than if the government were doing it' (*The New York Times*, September 6, 2007). Not everyone would agree with him. Foundations often determine their targets and objectives on emotional grounds rather than an objective assessment of international and national need.

It is well to remember that the founders of many of these large foundations or organizations obtained their massive wealth though questionable business and labour practices—exploitation of the very public that these foundations strive to serve! Thus, it is not surprising that the motives of these organizations are viewed with suspicion (Reich 2000). Several of the large foundations have been criticized because they obtained their funds through questionable business practices and currently derive some of their income from investments that negatively impact the public and the environment (*Los Angeles Times*, January 7, 2007, January 8, 2007). Thus, they help the public with one hand while harming it with the other.

Recommendations

Clearly, the generous giving of the foundations, industry, and private donors has benefited public health greatly. Nonetheless, they have sometimes also had unintended negative consequences. How can the behaviour of the foundations and other donors be modified to maximize the positive impact and minimize the negative? Several changes, suggested below, may contribute to this goal:

- Careful objective assessment of the goals of the foundation *vis-a-vis* the needs of the proposed recipient countries

- Consultation with health leaders of the recipient countries and the World Health Organization on the health priorities/needs of the recipient countries

- Consideration of the impact that the infusion of money and the programme will have on the existing public health structure and economy of the country

- Strengthening the existing national and local public health infrastructures by incorporating foundation programmes into the existing public health system

- Periodic evaluation of the impact of the donor's programmes by an objective group not affiliated with the donors, but including local expertise

- Establishment of advisory committees that include both international and local public health experts from developing countries and targeted areas

- Introducing ethical evaluations, as many universities currently do, in determining in which companies, institutions and commodities to invest, so that investment practices are not counter to the charitable goals of the donor/foundation. Investments in companies, etc. that negatively impact the health and quality of life of the public to make money to do good do not make sense

- Implementation of projects that can be sustained by the local governments when funding is discontinued

- Partnering with countries to contribute to the programmes in an effort to encourage countries to increase their investment in health

- Investment in local businesses to reduce reliance on external sources of health consumables

- Development of clear governance mechanisms, as well as transparent policies and procedural frameworks that facilitate monitoring and evaluation

Many of these recommendations have already been incorporated by the Global Fund to Fight AIDS, Tuberculosis and Malaria and other private donors. Private funding of public health has contributed greatly to the goals of public health. Let us hope that foundations, industry, and other private donors/agencies will continue to generously support public health in ways that will strengthen the public health structures, stability, and well-being of the recipient countries.

References

Bill and Melinda Gates Foundation. (2007). Available at www.gatesfoundation.org/aboutus/, www.gatesfoundation.org/GlobalHealth/, accessed October 2007.

Carnegie Corporation of New York. (2007). Available at http://www.carnegie.org/, accessed October 2007.

Farmer, P., and Garrett, L. (2007). From "marvellous momentum" to health care for all: success is possible with the right programs. *Foreign Affairs*, March/April. Available at http://fullaccess.foreignaffairs.org/20070301faresponse86213/paul-farmer-laurie-garrett/from-marvelous-momentum-to-health-care-for-all-success-is-possible-with-the-right-programs.html, accessed October 2008.

Garrett, L. (2007). The challenge of global health. *Foreign Affairs*, January/February. Available at http://fullaccess.foreignaffairs.org/arp/to_fullaccess?u=%2F20070101faessay86103%2Flaurie-garrett%2Fthe-challenge-of-global-health.html, accessed October 2008.

Global Fund to Fight AIDS, Tuberculosis and Malaria. (2007). Available at www.theglobalfund.org/en/about/record, accessed October 2007.

HHMI: Howard Hughes Medical Institute. (2008). Available at http://www.hhmi.org/, accessed January 2008.

Mectizan Donation Program. (2008). Available at http://www.mectizan.org/, accessed January 2008.

Navarro, V. (1985). The public/private mix in the funding and delivery of health services: an international survey. *American Journal of Public Health*, **75**, 1318–20.

Nishtar, S. (2004). Public–private partnerships in health – a global call to action. *Health Research Policy and Systems*, **2**, 5.

Pillar, C. (2007). Money clashes with mission. *Los Angeles Times*, January 8; Business.

Pillar, C., Sanders, E., and Dixon, R. (2007). Dark clouds over good works of Gates Foundation. *Los Angeles Times*, January 7; National.

Reich, M.R. (2000). Public–private partnerships for public health. *Nature Medicine*, **6**, 617–20.

Robert Wood Johnson Foundation. (2008). Available at http://www.rwjf.org/applications/m accessed January 2008.

Rockefeller Foundation Charter. (1913). Available at http://www.rockfound.org/about_us/Rockefeller_Foundation_Charter.pdf, accessed March 2008.

Rockefeller Foundation. (2007). Available at http://www.rockfound.org/aboutus/aboutus.shtml, accessed October 2007.

Sanofi-Aventis. (2008). *Sanofi-Aventis joins the fight against tuberculosis in South Africa*. http://en.sanofi-aventis.com/ethics_responsibilities/humanitarian_sponsorship/humanitarian_sponsorship.asp, accessed October 2008.

Sanofi-Aventis. (2006). *Humanitarian sponsorship*. http://en.sanofi-aventis. com/group/sponsorship/sponsorship_developpementproject.asp, accessed December 2007.

Standard Chartered. (2006). *Sustainability review 2006 leading the way in Asia, Africa and the Middle East*. Available at http://www. standardchartered.com/_documents/2006-sustainability-review/sc_ 2006_sustainabilityReview.pdf, accessed December 2007.

Stop TB. (2007). *Partnership*. Available at http://www.stoptb.org/stop_tb_ initiative/, accessed December 2007.

Strom, S. (2007). Big gifts, tax breaks and a debate on charity. *New York Times*, September 6; Business.

UN. (2008). *The millennium development goals*. Available at http://www. un.org/millenniumgoals/, accessed January 2008.

WBCSD. (2000). *Corporate social responsibility: making good business sense*. World Business Council for Sustainable Development. Available at

http://www.wbcsd.org/web/publications/csr2000.pdf, accessed October 2008.

WHO. (2004). *"Three Ones" agreed by donors and developing countries*. Available at http://www.who.int/3by5/newsitem9/en/, accessed December 2007.

Widdus, R. (2003). Public–private partnerships for health require thoughtful evaluation. *Bulletin of the World Health Organization*, **81**, 235–6.

Widdus, R. (2005). Public–private partnerships: an overview. *Transactions of the Royal Society of Tropical Medicine and Hygiene*, **995**, S1–8.

Wikipedia. (2008). *Howard Hughes*. http://en.wikipedia.org/wiki/Howard_ Hughes, accessed January 2008.

Global health agenda for the twenty-first century

Adrian Ong, Mary Kindhauser, Ian Smith, and Margaret Chan

Introduction

... the preservation of health is ... without doubt the first good and the foundation of all the other goods of this life.
(*René Descartes*, Discours de la méthode, *1637*)

The right to the highest attainable level of health is enshrined in the charter of the World Health Organization (WHO) (2002a) and many international treaties. It is this aspiration that spurs the work of the Organization and frames the broader global public health agenda for the twenty-first century. It is a tall order. But the right to health is more important today than ever before given the dramatic evolution in the architecture of global public health and the growing prominence of health within the human security, rights, and development agendas.

The past century had witnessed remarkable gains in health, rapid economic growth, and unprecedented scientific advances. These advances have led to major improvements in health care in which millions more lives are protected than ever before. Life expectancy at birth has continued to rise, by almost 8 years between 1950 and 1978, and 7 more years since (WHO 2007c). These transformations are unmatched in history.

Yet, in spite of this optimistic outlook, the international community faces a demanding health agenda. Many public health problems, both new and old, remain to be solved. Despite progress, nearly 2.6 billion people, especially in fragile states, remain in extreme poverty and live on less than US$2 a day. Nearly 10 million children die before their fifth birthday, with approximately four million of these deaths occurring during the neonatal period (UNICEF 2007). Nutrition is a major problem with one-third of all children in developing countries underweight or stunted; half the people in developing countries lack access to improved sanitation (World Bank 2007a). Health inequalities are growing wider between and within countries, between rich and poor, between men and women, and between different ethnic groups.

These stark numbers reinforce the urgent need for collective global action. The United Nations Millennium Declaration in 2000 committed states to a global partnership to reduce poverty, improve health and education, and promote peace, human rights, gender equality, and environmental sustainability by 2015 (UN 2000).

These Millennium Development Goals (MDGs) establish health as a key driver of socioeconomic progress. In so doing, they elevate the status of health within the development agenda and recognize the two-way, though uneven, link between poverty and health. Poverty contributes to poor health, and poor health anchors large numbers of people in poverty. In all countries, poverty is associated with high childhood and maternal mortality, malnutrition, and increased exposure to infectious diseases as well as chronic diseases such as cardiovascular diseases, diabetes, and cancer.

Investments in health must thus work to reduce poverty, ensure the poor have access to health care, and prevent economic ruin as a result of high health expenditures. As the world around us is becoming progressively interconnected and complex, human health is contingent on the integrated outcome of ecological, sociocultural, economic, and institutional determinants. It is increasingly recognized, also in the Millennium Declaration, that broad intersectoral action in tackling these determinants of health is needed to achieve significant and more durable health gains, especially for the poor.

This chapter lays out, in three sections, a strategy and agenda for global public health by assessing the current context, challenges and opportunities in the global health landscape. Many of the issues highlighted are not new. The first section examines current global health problems and the challenges they present. It reviews the revolution in health spurred, in part, by demographic transitions in societies and by globalization and its related nutritional and behavioural transitions. The second section analyses the impediments to scaling up health service delivery and improving access to care. Building upon these lessons and issues, the final section outlines the fundamental principles and means by which health systems can meet the challenges of the twenty-first century.

The evolving global health landscape

The issues and actors in global health today are myriad and complex. Shaped by the potent forces of globalization, demographic changes and emergent diseases, the agenda for health has never been more challenging nor more pressing. This section surveys current trends and phenomena in international health that meaningfully impact the public health agenda for the new century.

Health within the larger human context

Health in its own right is of fundamental importance and, like education, is among the basic capabilities that give value to human life (Sen & Sen 1999). It is an intrinsic right as well as a central input to poverty reduction and socioeconomic development. Health-related human rights are core values within the United Nations and WHO, and are endorsed in numerous international and regional human rights instruments. They are intimately related to and dependent on the provision and realization of other social and economic human rights such as those of food, housing, work, and education. Appreciation of this defining value underscores all efforts to provide equitable health care for all.

Health is also a central element of human security. The WHO Constitution defines health as a state of complete physical, mental and social well-being and not merely the absence of disease or infirmity (2002a). Humanitarian emergencies, including natural and human-made disasters, outbreaks of epidemic-prone diseases, conflicts and complex emergencies, constitute what has traditionally been considered the main threat to health security worldwide. However, wider considerations of human security, with the individual as a focus, also encompass issues of safe food and water, adequate shelter, clean air, poverty-related threats, violence, and the adverse effects of climate change on health (Ogata & Sen 2003). Strengthening the capacity of health and related sectors and improving international coordination can effectively contribute to reducing avoidable morbidity and mortality resulting from these threats to health security.

The pace of global economic integration has accelerated over the past decade, dramatically transforming the world's economic and political landscape. Globalization, with its remarkable acceleration of trade, knowledge, and resource flows, offers unprecedented promise for improving human health. Many experts assumed that as economic conditions within a country improved, health would improve accordingly through income growth, poverty alleviation and the broader availability of health and other social services.

Yet, to date, globalization has had a complex influence on health and results have been uneven. Opinions differ with regard to the economic benefits of globalization and its impact on poverty and health. Some have argued that income inequality has not widened and that the higher growth rates that follow market integration in developing countries have benefited the poor (Ben-David 2000; Dollar 2001; Dollar & Kraay 2002). Others hold that the economic benefits of recent globalization have been largely asymmetrical, creating among countries and within populations, beneficiaries, losers, and growing inequalities between the two with consequent effects on health (Mazur 2000; Wade 2004; Globalization Knowledge Network 2007).

Globalization may thus create wealth but has no rules that guarantee its fair distribution. Economic growth per se does not ensure equitable health improvement for all. Rather, action within and between countries to mitigate and remove structural inequality is the necessary counterpart to worldwide growth itself and the policies that aim to support it (Marmot 2007). New governance policies structured around equity, distributive fairness, and social

justice should be strengthened to minimize the negative externalities of global integration.

A changing world

Populations of the world are experiencing unprecedented demographic change. There are three billion more people today than there were in 1960. Another 2.5 billion will likely be added by 2050 based on mid-range population estimates (UN 2008).

Behind these numbers lie other important demographic trends common to many countries. Women are bearing fewer children, people are living longer and healthier lives, populations are aging, and increasing numbers of migrants are moving from villages to cities and from one country to another in search of better opportunities (UN 2008). A sharp contrast exists between the poorest nations with their rapidly growing and young populations, and the more demographically advanced and richer nations with near zero population growth and aging populations.

In populations with increasing life expectancy, the number and proportion of people reaching old age has risen throughout the world. Every month, one million people worldwide reach the age of 60 years. Of these, 80 per cent live in the developing world (WHO 2006c). Also with improved public health, more children are now surviving into adolescence and adulthood. One in every five people in the world is an adolescent. Out of 1.2 billion adolescents worldwide, about 85 per cent live in developing countries and the remainder live in the industrialized world (UN 2008).

This growth in human numbers is already leading to greater demand for food, water, energy and other natural resources. Importantly, the demographic heterogeneity and transition strongly impacts priorities and resources required to meet the shifting health needs of populations.

Each age category of persons faces a differing burden and nature of diseases. Many adolescents suffer premature deaths arising through accidents (including road crashes), suicide, violence, pregnancy-related complications, and other illnesses. They are exposed to tobacco-related diseases, harmful use of alcohol, substance abuse, sexually transmitted infections, unwanted pregnancy, and other health problems related to behaviour. Every year, an estimated 1.7 million young men and women between the ages of 10 and 19 lose their lives to preventable or treatable causes (WHO 2002b).

In many developing countries, the speed of modernization has outpaced the ability of governments to provide the necessary supporting infrastructures. Road traffic injuries are a growing public health issue, disproportionately affecting the poor and persons in the most economically productive age group. Such events kill an estimated 1.2 million people annually and injure as many as 5.2 million. Over 70 per cent of road traffic fatalities are under 45 years of age (Peden et al. 2004).

Maternal mortality has remained virtually unchanged for the past 20 years. Each year, more than half a million women die from complications of pregnancy and child-birth (Hill et al. 2008). Developing countries account for almost all of maternal deaths. The greatest burden is felt in sub-Saharan Africa, where more than half of all maternal deaths occur; in these countries, a woman is 100 times more likely to die from complications of pregnancy than a woman in the industrialized world. Underlying many of these deaths is the poor availability of health services. Seven in ten of all maternal deaths are estimated to arise from complications requiring emergency obstetric services. Yet, access to these services in many developing countries is limited, making improving health systems and access to assistance from trained attendants during birth imperative for reducing maternal mortality.

Addressing chronic diseases are another major challenge that now has global dimensions. Current demographic trends, together with deteriorating environmental conditions, unhealthy lifestyles and improper nutrition, has led to a rise in non-communicable or chronic diseases, including mental and substance abuse disorders, and a subsequent demand for long-term medical care in many societies (WHO 2006c). In developing countries, this has created a second burden of disease alongside the continuing struggle to control infectious diseases and the HIV/AIDS epidemic.

While the proportion of burden from chronic diseases, including mental disorders, in adults in developed countries remains stable at over 80 per cent, the proportion in middle-income countries has already exceeded 70 per cent. Almost 50 per cent of the adult disease burden in the high-mortality regions of the world is now attributable to chronic diseases (WHO 2003b). The health impact of this 'risk' transition affects all countries, though the effects may be more severe in the developing world, where health services and social support systems are often inadequate to meet the rising needs.

A few common risk factors are responsible for a considerable proportion of the burden of chronic diseases. Attributable causes include improper diet, inadequate exercise, smoking, and excessive alcohol consumption. An intervention that addresses one of these risk factors can possibly reduce the risk for several diseases, thus giving special impetus for health promotion and disease prevention efforts in controlling chronic diseases. The long time lag between the development of high population levels of risk and the emergence of non-communicable disease epidemics, testifies to the importance of intervening now to control the major risk factors, especially in poorer countries where they tend to be neglected in the face of competing priorities.

Tobacco addiction is a global epidemic and remains the second major cause of death in the world, being currently responsible for about one in ten adult deaths—nearly five million deaths each year. By 2030, unless urgent action is taken, tobacco's annual death toll will rise to more than eight million (Mathers & Loncar 2006). Today, almost one in three adults of the global population smoke. Of these, almost 80 per cent live in low- and middle-income countries (WHO 2008c). Due to the increase in the global adult population, coupled with expanded marketing by the tobacco industry, the total number of smokers is expected to reach about 1.6 billion by 2025, making the negative economic and health implications of tobacco use simply staggering. This growth is being driven largely by the rise in tobacco use in low-income countries and, more ominously, among young persons, especially females, in highly-populous countries (WHO 2008c).

Similar disturbing trends are occurring in the area of nutrition. Changes in global dietary patterns involve the increasing consumption of fats, energy-dense and highly processed foods. The world faces in many ways a double burden of nutrition—the co-existence, often in the same country, of under-nutrition and over-nutrition, with both as leading determinants of morbidity and mortality.

The next few decades will also see an unprecedented escalation of urban growth. About half of the world's population now lives in urban areas (UN 2008). In developing countries, 43 per cent of the urban population lives in slums, and in the least developed countries, 78 per cent of urban residents are slum-dwellers, with 30 per cent of families headed by women.

The flow of migrants from villages to cities is so rapid that the population growth in the rural areas of the developing world has virtually stopped. As a result, most of the 3 billion people expected to be added to the world population in the future are going to be added to urban centres and shantytowns in developing countries, further aggravating already overburdened infrastructure and public services (UNFPA 2007). More disturbingly, this urban population growth will be composed to a large extent, of poor people (Garau et al. 2005), the needs of whom are often overlooked in urban planning.

The contribution of human activities to changes in the climate system is irrefutable. Increases in global average air and ocean temperatures, widespread melting of snow and ice, and rising global average sea levels are phenomena associated with the ongoing and accelerating warming of the climate system (Climate Change 2007). Climate change—possibly the defining issue of the new millennium—poses a significant addition to the spectrum of environmental health hazards faced by humankind. The impacts of climate on human health will not be evenly distributed around the world, with the impoverished populations of the developing world being the first and hardest hit (Confalonieri et al. 2007). It will affect, in profoundly adverse ways, the most basic determinants of health—air, water, food, shelter, and freedom from disease—and could vastly increase the current huge imbalance in health outcomes. The implications of climate variability for human health and security are far-reaching, effecting death and disease through heat waves, floods, droughts, and other extreme weather events. Yet, the greatest health impact may not come from such acute shocks, but from the indirect pressure on the natural, economic, and social systems that sustain health, many of which are already under stress in much of the developing world (Parry et al. 2007).

In recent years, there has been a notable rise in the supply and trade of counterfeit and substandard medicines, including useless and, in some cases, even toxic products (WHO 2006b). This is a vast and under-reported problem that particularly affects countries where regulatory and legal oversight is weakest; it is an important cause of unnecessary morbidity, mortality, and negatively impacts public confidence in medicines and the effectiveness of health programmes (Dondorp et al. 2004). The drugs most commonly counterfeited include antibiotics, anti-malarials, hormones, and steroids. Yet, increasingly, more sophisticated and deceptive practices have seen even anticancer and antiviral drugs, including those used to treat HIV/AIDS, being faked. It has been estimated that some 10–30 per cent of medicines on sale in developing countries, especially those in sub-Saharan Africa, are counterfeit (Cockburn et al. 2005). The impact of this exploitive and poorly regulated trade on health outcomes has been enormous.

Similarly, widespread and inappropriate use of antimicrobials has created high levels of drug resistance and a growing crisis in health care management. Mainstay antimicrobials are now failing at a rate that outpaces the development of replacement drugs (Heymann et al. 2001). Hospital-acquired infections with drug resistant organisms are a serious and mounting complication of hospitalization, contributing significantly to morbidity, mortality and health care costs. Formerly curable diseases such as gonorrhoea and typhoid are rapidly becoming difficult to treat, while old killers such as tuberculosis and malaria are now growing increasingly resistant to mainstay therapy (Smith & Coast 2002). Ominously, the emergence of multi-drug resistant tuberculosis, which is 100 times more expensive to treat than susceptible tuberculosis, and extensively drug-resistant tuberculosis, which is virtually impossible to treat, is jeopardizing current control and elimination efforts (Raviglione & Smith 2007). Drug resistance is a deepening and complex problem accelerated by the overuse of antibiotics in developed nations and the paradoxical underuse of quality antimicrobials in developing nations owing to poverty, trade in counterfeit medicines and a dearth of effective health care.

Communicable diseases, crises, and epidemics

Armed conflicts, epidemics, famine, natural disasters, and other major emergencies have a significant impact on populations and their health. Each year, one in five countries experiences a crisis, often overwhelming national capacities to mitigate and manage such emergencies. These complex humanitarian crises often arise unpredictably and cause untold suffering, population displacement and death. The dislocation of large populations creates immense public health challenges with regard to food, water, sanitation, shelter the risk of epidemics in already vulnerable groups of persons, and the provision of routine immunizations, care, and essential medicines.

New infectious diseases have been emerging at the unprecedented rate of about one a year for the past three decades, a trend that is expected to continue (Smolinski *et al.* 2003). The shrinking of the world by technology and economic interdependence has allowed diseases to spread with great speed. The dissemination of HIV/AIDS and SARS are just two contemporary examples.

Constant evolution is the survival mechanism of the microbial world, and these organisms are well equipped to exploit opportunities to adapt and spread. The opportunities are numerous: Through increased population movements via tourism, migration or disasters; growth in international trade in food and biological products; social and environmental changes linked with urbanization, deforestation and alterations in climate; advancement in medical procedures; and changes in animal husbandry and food production methods (Ong & Heymann 2007).

The free movement of goods, capital, and labour in an increasingly interconnected world facilitates the transnational spread of diseases and places all countries at common risk. However, the same globalizing forces that create such rampant opportunities for pathogens can also provide mechanisms for innovative, global efforts to control infectious diseases. Recognition of shared vulnerability to these diseases, and their often considerable economic consequences, has brought a strong global commitment to make their detection, reporting, control, and prevention a collaborative effort (WHO 2007b).

Health actors and partners

Globalization is eroding traditional distinctions between domestic and foreign affairs. The health of populations largely depends on health and welfare policies of national governments. Yet, growing internationalization, migration, and macroeconomic considerations are, to greater extents, influencing the policy space of national governments and their ability to sustain health and welfare policies for their constituencies. Increasingly, health determinants have become more multifaceted, complex and shaped by factors outside the control of the health sector.

Indeed, the framework of international health is no longer dominated by a few organizations, and now involves numerous players. Health activities are now being pursued by more than 40 bilateral donors, 26 UN agencies, 20 global and regional funds, and 90 global health initiatives (Alexander 2007). An increasing number of non-governmental, faith-based and private sector organizations are delivering care and complement the efforts of national health systems. New philanthropists have emerged, and fast-growing economies have become aid givers and international investors. Governments acting alone, or in international partnerships, have initiated programmes and made available new funding. The number of innovative funding mechanisms continues to grow, as does the size of resources they provide. In quantity, aid for health has almost tripled over 10 years and nearly doubled in the last 5 years (OECD 2007).

Public–private partnerships in the area of research are increasingly important, as they often focus on health needs otherwise neglected by market-driven forces. Academic, industrial, government and non-governmental research continue to shape the directions and use of knowledge acquisition. Industry, trade and finance are powerful drivers of research and development and a massive force in producing and distributing goods. They can also influence decisions on health policy.

In just the past 7 years, more than 100 partnerships, focused on individual diseases, have formed. In addition, the formation of public–private partnerships, often involving large donations of medicines, has marked a watershed, by bringing new actors, resources, business models and a sense of urgency to bear on neglected diseases. Partnerships focused on product access have proven remarkably effective in supplying communities with free or reduced cost, quality-assured medicines and vaccines. The Mectizan Donation Program, The Stop TB Global Drug Facility, and the Global Alliance for Vaccines and Immunization (GAVI) provide three examples.

Globally, there has been a down-sizing of government and a marked trend towards privatization of many functions formerly within the public domain. To varying degrees, many countries have experienced a shift from centrally planned and regulated to market-dominated economies.

Health care policy in most developing countries has generally emphasized the development of government-owned health services, largely financed by government tax revenues. However present, evidence indicates that private health care supply is significant and growing rapidly in many countries (Preker *et al.* 2007). Despite public policies promoting universal access to subsidized public services, the majority of health care contacts in developing countries are with private providers on a fee-for-service basis. Private health care is typically dominant for ambulatory treatment of illness, which in developing countries accounts for the largest share of total health care spending. It is usually less dominant for inpatient treatments and limited for preventive and public health services.

The extensive private sector activity in the health sector has seen growing public–private linkages, such as the contracting-out of selected services or facilities, development of new purchasing arrangements, franchising and the introduction of vouchers. Selective contracting out of services to the private sector is often a component of national health policy, leveraging on these private resources in the service of the public sector and to improve the efficiency of publicly funded services (Mills *et al.* 2002). Contracts for primary care with private providers serve as a quick and simple solution to gaps in coverage, especially in areas where government provision is inadequate and there are private providers already practising. The private sector represents a resource that is available and used even in the poorest countries and among lower income groups (Berman 2000). For example, the majority of malaria episodes in sub-Saharan Africa are initially treated by private providers, mainly through the purchase of drugs from shops and peddlers (Goodman *et al.* 2007). For some diseases of high priority, e.g. malaria, tuberculosis and sexually-transmitted infections and where public infrastructure is limited, scaling up of prevention and treatment efforts in the many countries hinges on enhancing utilization of private sector services (WHO 2008a).

Challenges and gaps

Addressing discrimination, equity, and social justice

Inspection of health outcomes through an equity lens reveals that the impressive gains in health experienced in recent decades are unevenly distributed. Aggregate indicators, whether at the global, regional or national level, do not offer sufficient granularity and often hide striking variations in health outcomes between men and women, rich and poor, both across and within countries.

However, health inequities involve more than inequality—in health determinants or outcomes, or in access to the resources needed to improve and maintain health. They also represent a systematic failure to avoid or overcome social differences in health and opportunities for health and their causes (Whitehead 1992; WHO 2006a). Indigenous people, ethnic minorities, people in poor communities, people living with HIV/AIDS, people with disabilities, and migrants suffer most especially from avoidable discriminatory social, economic, and welfare policies and practices. Beyond this, many marginalized groups are also disenfranchised and voiceless in the economic and social policy-making process.

For example, the richest one-tenth of the population of Latin America and the Caribbean earn 48 per cent of total income, while the poorest tenth earn only 1.6 per cent (ECLAC 2005). This inequality in income distribution extends to unequal access to education, health, water and electricity, as well as huge disparities in voice, assets and opportunities (World Bank 2007b). In some countries of Latin America, greater that 97 per cent of the people in the highest income quintile have access to health care services as compared to less than 10 per cent in the lowest quintile. Not surprisingly, 40 per cent of child deaths in the region occur among those living in the poorest quintile whereas the highest quintile accounts for only 8 per cent (*Lancet* 2007). Further, the poorest quintile of the population showed 3–10 times the prevalence of stunted children than the richest quintile in nine countries (Belizan *et al.* 2007).

In the case of health, the disadvantaged position of women in many societies undermines their ability to protect and promote their own physical, mental and emotional health. Women's status and empowerment—as measured by education, employment, household decision-making, intimate partner violence, and reproductive health—strongly influences their effective use of health information and services (Gill *et al.* 2007). Independent of related factors, educated women are more likely than are uneducated women to use antenatal care, to use trained providers and to have safe deliveries (Grown *et al.* 2005). Similarly, education not only results in substantial improvements in a woman's own health as a mother, but also has positive intergenerational effects on the health and nutrition of her children and their households (Bloom *et al.* 2001). For a variety of reasons, health policies and programmes all too often fail to adequately address these issues around women's autonomy but instead perpetuate gender stereotypes.

The dimensions of inequities in health are also evident in the health status and access to health services of populations. The poor availability of drugs that can significantly reduce AIDS-related mortality in regions of the world most affected by AIDS is a case in point.

It is estimated that, globally, over 33 million people are living with HIV, with more than two out of three adults and nearly 90 per cent of children infected with HIV living in sub-Saharan Africa (UNAIDS 2007). Yet, this region still accounts for over 70 per cent of the global unmet antiretroviral treatment need. Worldwide, over 2 million people living with HIV were receiving treatment in resource-poor countries, representing less than a third of the estimated 7.1 million people in need (UNAIDS 2006).

Such stark disparities in health outcomes are not unique to any one country or region. They exist, to a greater or lesser extent, within all societies of all nations. In many societies, overconsumption and obesity coexist with hunger and malnutrition. Great differences in life expectancy can be seen between the social classes, different occupations, ethnic groups and between the sexes in many countries, including those of highly developed economies (Marmot 2005).

Addressing governance and coordination

In recent years, there has been a unprecedented profusion of new actors, partners and sectors involved in the work and delivery of health care. In the past, few global actors possessed the political or financial authority to influence global health agendas. Today, a rich diversity of new institutions is actively reshaping global health priorities for policy and investment. These new partnerships and initiatives have added significant resources for tackling diseases of the poor and benefiting the health of large populations.

At the same time, this crowed health landscape has created a new set of challenges. The multiplicity of actors has led to an increasingly fragmented, reactive, and disparate agenda for international health (Ruger & Yach 2005). Despite efforts towards better global health partnerships, global health governance has been criticized as being too fragmented, uncoordinated, and largely donor driven. Results on the ground have been mixed; lower-income countries are growing increasingly reliant on external assistance; aid frequently does not support health systems or countries' health priorities; and financing is unpredictable and unsynchronized among donors.

Partnerships are by their very nature, issue-specific and results focused; their interventions are not always congruous with recipient countries' national priorities nor do they efficiently leverage national system resources. Non-aligned international aid skews national priorities of recipient countries by imposing those of donor partners. To achieve their narrow issue-specific goals, there is often insufficient consideration of the impact of their activities on the wider health system, including distortion of local wage structures and health worker resources. The lack of harmonization across agencies has led to inefficiency and overlap in implementation; duplication in planning, project-specific monitoring and evaluation, missions and financial management, and parallel systems for health service delivery (e.g. drug procurement and distribution). This increases significantly the transaction costs of these ventures and jeopardizes sustainable health gains.

Historically, the locus of health governance has been at the national and subnational level as governments of individual countries have undertaken primary responsibility for the health of their domestic populations. However, a range of health determinants are increasingly affected by factors outside the remit of the health sector—trade and investment flows, conflict, illicit and criminal activity, environmental change, and communication technologies (Dodgson *et al.* 2002).

Similarly, the health of individuals suffers or benefits not just from the impact of their domestic environment or personal choices, but also from decisions made at national levels and outside their own countries. Yet, ministries of health and even nation states themselves may lack the power to effect change for health due to a range of developments: Decentralization to regional and local health authorities, decisions set by donors or by lending institutions, rules set by international agreements and regimes, and of course the wider forces of globalization.

Globalization has in many ways eroded the boundary between the determinants of public and individual health, and made health a global public good. Many public health goods can no longer be achieved through domestic policy action alone and depend on international cooperation. This has arisen from the international transfer of risk, intensification of cross-border flows of people, goods, services, and ideas and the increasing threat to common resources. Yet, policy-making is still largely organized on a country-by-country basis and there is no international equivalent of the state. As a result, global public goods are increasingly underprovided for and global public bads are increasingly overprovided.

This blurring of health and jurisdictional frontiers is most obvious in the case of communicable disease transmission and the spread of non-communicable disease risk factors.

For example, susceptibility to tobacco-related diseases, once strongly linked to, and blamed on the lifestyle choices of individuals, is also increasingly being attributable to a variety of complex factors with cross-border effects, including trade liberalization, direct foreign investment, global marketing, transnational tobacco advertising, and the international movement of contraband and counterfeit cigarettes (Chen *et al.* 1999; Bettcher *et al.* 2000). In response to this globalization of the tobacco epidemic, the WHO Framework Convention on Tobacco Control (FCTC) (WHO 2003a) was developed to provide both demand- and supply-side strategies for curbing global tobacco consumption. This includes restrictions on tobacco advertising, sponsorship and promotion; raising prices through tax increases; as well as strengthening legislation to clamp down on tobacco smuggling.

The issue of antimicrobial resistance is also illustrative. It is a global problem that must be addressed in all countries as no single nation, however effective it is at containing resistance within its borders, can protect itself from the importation of resistant pathogens through travel and trade. Poor prescribing practices in any country now threaten to undermine the potency of vital antimicrobials everywhere.

Gaps in health services

Health is the final common pathway, contingent on the good functioning of many other processes and sectors. In many cases, the power of global health interventions is not matched by the power of health systems to deliver them to those in greatest need, on an adequate scale or in time. Many low-income countries are facing a double crisis of devastating disease and failing health systems. There is growing awareness in international health groups that weak national health systems limit the gains and opportunities that can be made in many areas of health, including the health MDGs. Chronic under-investments have led to fragile and fragmented health systems that are especially lacking capabilities in key areas such as health financing, information systems, health workforce, and drug supply.

There has been an implicit assumption that through the implementation of narrow disease-specific interventions, broader health systems will be strengthened more generally. Yet, the evidence of benefit for these selective initiatives on national health system capacities has been mixed. Already weak systems may be further compromised by the over-concentration of resources in specific 'vertical' programmes, leaving many other areas further under-resourced. The establishment of many selective and disease-specific initiatives within countries have resulted in competing and overlapping subsystems within the broader health care system. This can lead to duplication of work processes, distortions of local salary and work norms, service disruptions in existing programmes, and distraction from core work activities (Travis *et al.* 2004).

Further, many groups and communities still do not have access to essential public health interventions even when these are known to be cost effective. This is largely due to inadequate allocation of resources to health and disproportionate allocation to curative and high technology services in urban settings. Also, the funds that are committed often do not benefit those who need them most, and remain underutilized. Equitable health systems need financing mechanisms which remove the barriers to health care, specially those confronting disadvantaged groups. Gaps in implementation include, in some cases, too much emphasis on pilot projects and islands of excellence, with inadequate plans and health system capacity to scale up (WHO 2006c).

The role of the private sector

New challenges have emerged with the commoditization of health care and the often unregulated delivery of health care in the non-government health sector. Private health care is expanding rapidly and is acknowledged as an important and often well-resourced provider of health care services in many countries. Yet, this important component of the health care system has received little policy attention. Increasingly, experience with the private sector has indicated a number of problems with the quality, price and distribution of private health services. This has led to a growing focus on the critical role of government in regulation and the orientation of the private sector with public health goals.

The effectiveness of private services is often very low. Poor treatment practices have been reported for diseases such as tuberculosis (Uplekar *et al.* 2001) and sexually transmitted infections (Chalker *et al.* 2000), with implications not only for the individuals treated but also for disease transmission and the development of drug resistance. For example, to improve affordability, partial doses of drugs may be sold as private services are priced to the purchasing power of the client. In Sierra Leone, for example, the price of purchased drugs was almost a third of the cost of treatment at a public health centre (Fabricant et al. 1999). The rise of chronic diseases in the developing world, often bringing with it a life-long need for medication, is expected to compound this problem considerably.

The use of the more expensive private services, or treatment for chronic conditions, can result in households being unable to afford other vital requirements or being driven into poverty through greater out of pocket expenditure. Moreover, rapidly growing private services compete with the public sector for trained human resources, further weakening public services (Mills et al. 2002).

A crisis in human resources for health

Human resources have been described as 'the heart of the health system in any country' (WHO 2006d). Yet, many national health systems are in crisis, with the shortage of workers severely compromising the delivery of essential health services and interventions. Abundant evidence demonstrates that progress in health in the poorest countries will not be possible without strong national health systems for which the work force is essential. The work force determines health outputs and outcomes and drives health systems performance.

Uneven distribution deprives many groups of access to life-saving services, a problem compounded by accelerating migration in open labour markets that draw skilled workers away from the poorest communities and countries. Health workers are leaving poorer areas for wealthier ones, and often leaving the countries that invested in their training to take up jobs abroad. Strikingly, for every Liberian physician working in Liberia, about two live abroad in developed countries; similarly for every Gambian professional nurse working in the Gambia, likewise about two live in a developed country overseas (Clemens & Pettersson 2008).

Many health services are consequently jeopardized by this trend, including childhood immunization, care during pregnancy and childbirth, and access to treatment for HIV/AIDS, tuberculosis, and malaria. The inadequacy of human resources for health significantly correlates with poorer maternal mortality, infant mortality, under five mortality rates (Anand & Barnighausen 2004), and childhood vaccination coverage (Anand & Barnighausen 2007). As the number of health workers declines, survival declines proportionately. Unless the workforce crisis is addressed, neither priority disease initiatives, including those aimed at achieving the health-related MDGS, nor health systems strengthening can succeed.

Sub-Saharan Africa faces the greatest crisis: This part of the world accounts for 11 per cent of the global population and 24 per cent of the global burden of disease, but has only 3 per cent of the world's health workforce (WHO 2006d). Shortages are widespread, with a gap of more than 1 million health workers estimated for Africa alone. Globally, WHO estimates that more than 4 million more health workers are required to achieve the health-related MDGs and has identified 57 countries with critical shortages of health workers—36 of these countries are in Africa.

The causes of these shortages are manifold. There is a limited production capacity in many developing countries as a result of years of underinvestment in health education institutions.

Decades of economic and sectoral reform capped expenditures, froze recruitment and salaries, and restricted public budgets, depleting working environments of basic supplies, drugs, and facilities (Narasimhan et al. 2004). Moreover, the training output is poorly aligned with the health needs of the population. There are also 'push' and 'pull' factors that encourage health workers to leave their workplaces, mainly related to unsatisfactory working conditions, low salaries, political instability and poor career opportunities. Surveys among health workers intending to migrate or already migrated consistently cite issues of remuneration and living conditions as primary reasons for their departure (Vujicic et al. 2004). Other factors contributing to the shortage of health workers include growth of the global population as training of health workers stagnates, the rise in chronic diseases, and the ageing of populations, which increases the need for long-term care. The devastation of HIV/AIDS is also a major force assailing health workers in the hardest hit societies of sub-Saharan Africa, Asia, the Americas, and eastern Europe; it is a triple threat that is increasing workloads on health workers, exposing them to infection, and stressing their morale (Joint Learning Initiative 2004).

Undoubtedly, health workers have a clear human right to emigrate in search of a better life. Yet, people in source countries hard hit by an exodus of health workers also have the right to health in their own countries, and to see a return on their considerable investments in education and training (Robinson & Clark 2008). The space between these two fundamental rights is the area where a clear global framework for response and cooperation is needed. It will require working in partnership and across sectors in both source and recipient countries, to implement and monitor effective strategies to develop a well-performing health workforce (Global Health Workforce Alliance 2008).

Gaps in knowledge

There is growing recognition that research is critical in the fight against disease. Knowledge contributes to the policies, activities, and performance of health systems, and to the improvement of individuals' and populations' health.

However, gaps in research and the dissemination of knowledge and health information are growing ever more acute. International research efforts are poorly coordinated and fragmented. Spending on health research, when viewed from a global perspective, is grossly skewed and under-funded. The landmark findings of the Commission on Health Research for Development (1990) almost two decades ago, highlighted the discrepancy in research funding and priorities—that only 5 per cent of the total global research funds were spent on research addressing the problems of developing countries whose citizens bore greater than 90 per cent of the global burden of preventable conditions affecting health. The magnitude of this discrepancy is an issue of continuing concern (Global Forum for Health Research 2007).

Despite impressive advances in science, technology, and medicine, society has failed to allocate sufficient resources to fight the diseases that particularly affect the poor. There is a dearth of research and development into neglected diseases such as African trypanosomiasis, lymphatic filariasis, schistosomiasis, and Chagas disease, which account for a high burden of disease in disability-adjusted life years. Sex-disaggregated data is important for developing effective and gender-sensitive health services and policies, yet these data are seldom collected. Lack of access to information through modern communications technology in poor parts of the world is hampering the wider dissemination of best practices in diverse fields such as hygiene, injury prevention, tobacco and substance abuse.

The limited resources available can fund only a fraction of the promising research opportunities. Hence, prioritization is essential for health research in order to focus on areas of greatest need. Yet, the degree to which research funding should reflect the burden of disease has been the subject of extensive debate. Even where there is agreement on existing or new research priorities, the best way of financing the discovery, production and delivery of these pubic goods for health, and making them affordable by poor countries, is seldom clear.

Prescription for the new millennium

An agenda for health

As can be appreciated from the above discussion, the world is falling short in winning sustainable and equitable improvements for health. Aggregate global health indicators have improved substantially since the middle of the past century, but gross health inequalities persist. Indeed, the gaps are widening between the world's poorest people and those better placed to benefit from economic development and public health progress. This trend takes place within an evolving global health landscape characterized by a complex and challenging mixture of old and new health problems and greater pluralism in health actors, funding resources and opportunities.

An analysis of the past provides a starting point for defining an agenda for the future. From the gaps thus examined and our understanding of current key challenges and shortfalls in response, it is evident that greater global commitment and solidarity are needed to forge greater health gains. Lasting health progress, including attainment of the health-related MDGs, depends on strong political will, supported by sound, integrated and evidence-based policies and broad participation from actors both within and outside the health sector.

Global efforts to improve health are inseparable from medical science, but social, economic, environmental and political factors also determine health opportunities and outcomes. Although trends in some major determinants of health, such as demographic changes, are relatively predictable, many are not (WHO 2006c). Progress in public health is rarely linear. Health emergencies—whether climatic, seismic, or infectious in nature—illustrate how quickly situations can change and how precarious health can be. The fragility of health gains has repeatedly been shown in response, for example, to economic and social changes and civil disruption. As such, any global public health agenda has to plan for inherent unpredictability and volatility in the health of populations and societies.

The following outline of a global health agenda identifies seven priority areas. The broad agenda borrows from the eleventh general programme of work of the WHO, which was endorsed and adopted by its 193 Member States at the World Health Assembly in May 2006. It serves as a strategic framework and direction for the future work of the Organization and all it Member States in the new millennium. Of the seven areas, the first three frame the fundamental principles and concepts underlying health advancement: Investing in health to reduce poverty; building

individual and global health security; and promoting universal coverage, gender equality and health-related human rights. The remaining four items focus on more strategic and explicit areas of endeavour: Tackling the determinants of health; strengthening health systems and equitable access; harnessing knowledge, science and technology; and strengthening governance, leadership, and accountability.

Establishing the role of health in development and poverty reduction

Elimination of poverty and extreme hunger is foremost among the MDGs. For the poor with few possessions, health is their main, if not their only, asset—if they do not have even that, they have nothing. For many of these people, being healthy means the possibility to work, earn a living and support their families. When the health of the main earner in poor families is compromised, the implications for economically dependent family members, particularly children, are particularly severe. By definition, poor people have few reserves and may be forced to sell what assets they have, including land and livestock, or borrow at high interest rates, to deal with the immediate crisis precipitated by illness. Each option leaves them more vulnerable, less able to recover, and in greater danger of moving down the poverty spiral (Braveman & Gruskin 2003). Poor people are thus caught in a vicious circle: Poverty breeds ill-health, ill-health maintains poverty.

Yet, the escape from poverty rests on more than just one pillar. Having a population that is healthy and educated enough to participate in the global economy is as important as enlightened economic reform. At the international level, priorities for improving public health are clear: Focus on health problems and diseases that affect the poor disproportionately. Health gains require directing programme benefits towards the poor and increasing the quality and availability of health services, especially where they are most scarce (World Bank 2007b).

Good health enables individuals to be active agents of change in the development process, both within and outside the health sector. The provision of health services is no longer viewed merely as a consumer of resources and an onerous obligation of governments. Health is also a producer of economic gains and integral to development in a broader sense. Beyond raising living standards through economic growth, health and development improve human capital through empowerment and enhancement of individual agency (Sen & Sen 1999). As such, health and poverty alleviation hold a prominent place in debates on priorities for development. Countries, at all levels of development, are realizing the need for sustained, equitable increases in health investment as a contribution to prosperity and social stability.

Our understanding of poverty has broadened from a narrow focus on income and consumption. Poverty is now known to encompass many other dimensions—lack of education, inadequate housing, social exclusion, unemployment, and environmental degradation. Each of these elements diminishes opportunity, limits choices and threatens health. Thus, poverty encompasses not just low income, but also lack of access to services, resources and skills; vulnerability; insecurity and powerlessness.

Poor countries, and poor people within countries, suffer from a multiplicity of deprivations that translate into high levels of ill-health. These wide differences in health status are considered unfair, or inequitable, because they correspond to differing societal, cultural, and system-wide constraints and opportunities. Further, these differences lie largely beyond the choice of the individual (Wagstaff 2002). Poverty-oriented health strategies require complementary policies in other sectors (WHO 2003b). These include improving access to education, enhancing the position of women and other marginalized groups, shaping development policies in agriculture and rural development, and promoting open and participatory governance.

Multidimensional poverty is a potent determinant of health risks, health seeking behaviour, health care access and health outcomes. Economic indicators focusing primarily on income alone offer a limited assessment of poverty, and a limited platform for attacking poverty. In contrast, health indicators provide a greater measure of the multi-faceted nature of poverty. For this reason health should be a key measure of the success or failure of development and of poverty reduction policies during this century (Haines et al. 2000).

Government expenditures on health are often designed to give everyone equal access to health care. Yet, in practice, equal access is usually elusive. Health improvements have not been shared equally and health inequalities among and within countries remain entrenched. Publicly financed health care fails to reach the poor in almost all developing countries. Most research conducted in developing countries in the last 20 years has confirmed that publicly financed health care benefits the well-off more than the poor (Devarajan 2003). If access to health services were distributed according to need, the poor would come first. However, in many cases, the 'inverse care law' unduly prevails and, as a result, the availability of good medical care tends to vary inversely with the need for it in the population served (Tudor Hart 1971).

Health services can fail poor people in many ways—in access, in quantity, in quality, and in costs. The striking differences in health status among different economic groups reflect inequalities in access to information, to facilities that provide decent standards of care, and to the means to pay for good care. In most instances, the poor are less educated than the rich and lack knowledge in areas of hygiene, nutrition and good health practices. Regressive patterns of health financing force greater out-of-pocket expenditure, and exacerbate poverty and ill health. For example, poor people often delay health care until a problem is advanced, more difficult or impossible to treat, and much more costly. This well-documented tendency becomes more of a problem with the rise of chronic diseases in low- and middle-income countries, as it jeopardizes early preventive and protective care.

If policy-makers want health to reduce poverty, they cannot allow the costs of health care to drive impoverished households even deeper into poverty. As noted above, the provision of effective and accessible health services helps protect the poor from spiralling into worsening economic problems. To achieve this, propagation of more equitable socioeconomic policies is paramount. Programmes can address barriers to health for the poor in many ways: Through better education and health promotion, better targeting of services to specific groups, improvements in quality of care, incentives for health providers, and financing mechanisms that make care affordable to those most in need (Mundial 2005). Fair health financing schemes promote the alignment of contribution with the ability to pay, and the use of services with the degree of need. An emphasis on prepayment for health care through taxes or insurance, with contribution tied to an individual's disbursement capacity, goes far

in supporting the poor. The emphasis in conditional cash transfer programmes, such as those in Brazil and Mexico, on channelling resources through female household members, shows the importance policy places on supporting their role in protecting children's development and promoting family health (Marmot 2007).

Since demand for health care by poor people is price sensitive, any reduction in the price charged to the user will induce an increase in demand. Yet, access to ostensibly free health care is, for most users, far from free (Gwatkin et al. 2004). Indeed, use of this entitlement has associated participation costs, such as transportation, food expenditure, and loss of time. Ensuring that the poor access and participate in health services may therefore necessitate the employment of various schemes to reduce participation costs. Examples include the use of vouchers, fee waivers, social health insurance and reimbursement for transport and food.

In addition to supply-driven pro-poor schemes, several complementary approaches are being explored. These focus on creating an effective demand and pressure for relevant health services on the part of the poor, to offset the influence of better-off groups that traditionally shape priorities and programmes. Individuals should have the opportunity to participate in political and social decisions about public policies that affect them (Ruger 2003). This strengthens agency, a process that is central to the sustainability of effective health systems and the achievement of broader development goals; it also provides a foundation for cohesive societies. Participation and enablement allow people to hold service providers accountable, both directly and indirectly, through influence and feedback to policy-makers. Community-level programmes that involve beneficiaries in aspects of programme design, implementation and evaluation can achieve better health outcomes through empowerment and creating a greater sense of ownership. The recently introduced approach of community-led total sanitation, which offers no subsidies but relies on communities to make sanitation a priority and devise local solutions, provides a good example of the potential for rapid, community-wide, and sustainable results (Kar & Bongartz 2006).

In addition, models of social protection have been put forward to lessen the vulnerability of the poor to adverse health crises and catastrophic expenses. An array of social safety nets, social assistance programmes such as cash transfers, food-subsidy programmes, public works, and microfinancing schemes can be used to ameliorate adverse shocks and alleviate poverty. Such schemes, which can enhance social security, need to be targeted to reach poor and vulnerable populations.

Good policies and investments in health are not, in themselves, sufficient to ensure growth and poverty reduction. Institutions and governance are additional key determinants. Efforts to improve governance may aim to increase political accountability, strengthen civil society participation, create a competitive private sector, impose institutional restraints on power or improve public sector management. The role of government in all these processes is critical. Poverty reduction strategies, where they exist, also place national governments in a central role, making them responsible for the cross-sectoral implementation of policies specifically designed to tackle the causes and consequences of poverty in their country.

Promoting universal coverage, gender equity, and health-related human rights

Effective public health action needs an ethical position as well as technical competence. To shape a healthier future, public health must be clear about its values, as well as its scientific principles. As enshrined in the WHO constitution and many international instruments of law, the enjoyment of the highest attainable standard of health is one of the fundamental rights of every human being. Appreciation of this defining value underscores all efforts to provide good health for all. The foundation for realizing physical, mental and social well-being is inextricably linked to the protection and fulfilment of human rights. For example, the violation or neglect of human rights, as expressed by torture or violence against women, can lead to ill-health. Conversely, the fulfilment of human rights can reduce a person's vulnerability to ill-health (Mann *et al.* 1999).

The progressive realization of rights to health requires action and policies that make appropriate and affordable health care accessible to those in greatest need in the shortest possible time. The underlying determinants of health also need to be addressed: Access to safe and potable water, adequate sanitation, safe and nutritious food, and housing; healthy occupational and environment conditions; and access to health education and information, also in the area of sexual and reproductive health.

Health and development outcomes are greatly enhanced by employing human rights as an integral dimension in the design, implementation, monitoring and evaluation of health-related policies and programmes. Through this approach, substantive rights-based elements such as attention to vulnerable groups, safeguarding dignity, equality and freedom from discrimination, employing a gender perspective and ensuring accessible health systems, can be considered and addressed.

A pressing problem in many countries is the deficiency in access by poor and marginalized groups to essential health services. A commitment to universal coverage embraces the principle of fair distribution of opportunities for well-being based on people's needs, rather than their social privileges. It implies equitable health systems characterized by accessibility, affordability, quality and acceptability, and prioritized towards the needs of the marginalized and vulnerable population groups—children, women, indigenous and tribal populations; ethnic, religious and national minorities; immigrants, persons with disabilities and people living with HIV/ AIDS. Indeed, some low-income countries with policies that emphasize equitable access to essential care have achieved greater life expectancies than wealthy countries with no such policy objective. These better health outcomes are achieved when equitable access to care is, at the outset, a categorical and unambiguous objective of policy-makers.

Inequities in health occur along several axes of social stratification, including sex, race, ethnic group, language, educational level, occupation, and residence. Whole classes of people whose health is compromised by economic or social disadvantages are beset by many other problems that make their lives miserable; yet their health plight is often invisible to policy-makers and poorly captured in statistics. To better unmask these variations in health, the employment of disaggregated health data that go beyond gross health statistics and national averages allows for a more profound appreciation of inter-group disparities. Such data go far in informing the redistribution of social and economic resources to those in greatest need and in bringing evidence to bear on political choices in health. Further, mitigation of these health inequities serves the dual goals of equity and efficiency for health services.

A rights-based approach to health also recognizes the need for empowerment and participation. All groups, including the vulnerable and marginalized, have the right to participate in the design, implementation and monitoring of health policies, programmes and legislation that can affect their health. However, a characteristic common to marginalized groups is their lack of power to influence their political, social and economic conditions. Thus, to be effective and sustainable, interventions that aim to redress inequities must typically go beyond remedying a particular health inequity. The broader aim is to help empower the target group through systemic changes, such as legislative reform or changes in economic or social relationships, and the reduction of stigma and discrimination.

In recent decades, great strides have been made in the health of women. Yet, in most societies, disadvantages for women persist. Women's health is compromised by the disproportionate prevalence among them of poverty, few prospects of employment beyond the home, the indignities of violence and rape, limited influence on their sexual and reproductive lives and limited power to influence decisions. Goal 3 of the MDGs—to achieve gender equality and empower women—seeks specifically to rectify those disadvantages through policies and programmes that build women's capabilities, improve their access to economic and political opportunities, and guarantee their safety. Complementary health interventions, such as expanding access to sexual and reproductive health care, health information and education, are also needed to ensure sustainable improvements in women's health. Moreover, policies and programmes designed with a gender perspective must explicitly aim to rectify inequalities and disadvantages faced by women. Ample evidence demonstrates that when women are given opportunities to develop their potential, health indicators for families and communities rapidly improve. As noted in the Millennium Declaration, the empowerment of women is an effective way to combat poverty, hunger and disease and to stimulate development that is truly sustainable.

Many countries are working to expand coverage of essential health services by renewing their systems of primary health care, an approach that is again being strongly supported by WHO. A commitment to the values, principles and approaches of primary health care encourages a focus on vulnerable and marginalized populations, promotes population-based and personal care services, emphasizes prevention as well as cure, and strengthens the referral system It also encourages intersectoral action to address the root causes of ill health and helps orient the private sector to public health goals (WHO 2006c).

Building individual and global health security

In recent years, health has been conceptualized as a security issue, both in terms of individual and community health security, expressed as access to the fundamental prerequisites for health, and global health security. Global health security seeks protection from risks and dangers to health that arise from the ways in which nations and their populations interact at the international level.

At the international level, the relationship between health and security faces many new challenges (and opportunities) in an increasingly globalized world characterized by the unprecedented speed and volume of international travel, the interdependence of businesses and financial markets, and the interconnectedness brought on by the revolution in information technology.

Acute threats to human health posed by conflicts, disease outbreaks, natural disasters and zoonoses have become a larger menace in a globalized society. The 2003 outbreak of severe acute respiratory syndrome (SARS)—the first severe new disease of the twenty-first century—demonstrated how much the world has changed in terms of its vulnerability to emerging diseases. SARS spread rapidly along the routes of international air travel and caused enormous economic losses and social disruption well beyond the outbreak zones. As the emergence of diseases is tied to fundamental changes in the way humanity inhabits the planet, more new diseases can be anticipated as this century progresses. In particular, the behaviour of emerging and epidemic-prone diseases has made all nations acutely aware of their shared vulnerability and their shared responsibility for mutual self-protection. Global public health security is thus both a collective aspiration and a mutual responsibility (WHO 2007d).

Public health emergencies throw into sharp relief the strengths and weaknesses of infrastructures designed to protect the public on a daily basis. To ensure global health security, two interrelated strategies are required: A significant strengthening of public health within both developed and developing countries and the establishment of mechanisms that facilitate the collaborative action of countries. The Global Outbreak Alert and Response Network (GOARN), which proved instrumental in the response to SARS, is one such mechanism. The revised International Health Regulations are another. These regulations, which came into force in 2007, are designed to minimize the international consequences of public health emergencies. For those caused by emerging and epidemic-prone diseases, the regulations follow a proactive approach to risk management that aims to stop an outbreak at source, before it has an opportunity to spread internationally. To do so, the regulations further recognize that all countries must posses a set of core capacities for outbreak surveillance and detection, laboratory diagnosis, and response. Meeting these core requirements, as set out in the regulations, would greatly strengthen collective global health security. Unfortunately, the necessary systems and infrastructures in many countries are lacking, making greater investment in capacity building an urgent priority.

The effectiveness of many collective agreements, including the International Health Regulations, depends on transparency and cooperation between national governments and the larger international community. Accordingly, the open and timely sharing of essential health information and knowledge is a central obligation under the revised Regulations that must be honoured by all countries as a prerequisite for collective security. In addition, given the multidimensional challenges to health security, governments must also foster greater cooperation between different sectors and stakeholders. For example, the engagement of sectors such as health, agriculture, trade and tourism is a key element in preparedness plans for a future influenza pandemic.

While conflicts and natural disasters are localized events, they can also take on international dimensions. During such events, routine health services are frequently disrupted; the health consequences can be compounded by breakdowns in water supply and sanitation or interruptions in the supply of essential medicines and equipment. The risk of epidemics increases dramatically when people are crowded together in temporary shelters. Most natural disasters and long-term conflicts will require assistance and cooperation from the international community. Ensuring the capacity for such swift global response reduces avoidable loss of lives and mitigates suffering.

At the level of the individual and the community, more proximal determinants, such as access to food, water, and shelter, healthy environments, and protection from violence, especially for women, are the focus of security concerns. Broader issues in human security, such as education, gender equality, poverty and globalization have consequential effects on health and require the continued action of governments in framing more equitable development and international policies. Climate change is a further contemporary challenge to collective security (CNA Corporation 2007) and demands urgent attention. Numerous adverse effects on health are projected. While the warming of the planet is expected to be gradual, the effects of extreme weather events—more storms, floods, heat waves, and droughts—will be abrupt and acutely felt. Both trends can have profoundly adverse effects on health. WHO has focused attention on five main health consequences of climate change: (1) Increases in malnutrition and in the severity of childhood infectious diseases; (2) increases in death, disease and injury due to extreme weather events; (3) increases in episodes of diarrhoeal disease; (4) increases in the frequency of cardiorespiratory diseases; and (5) altered distribution of vectors responsible for infectious diseases, most notably malaria and dengue (WHO 2008b). To address these challenges, Member States have called on WHO to promote research and pilot projects aimed at health protection, especially in vulnerable countries. While climate change is a global phenomenon, scientists predict that developing countries, especially in sub-Saharan Africa, will experience the earliest and most severe consequences, also for health.

Health systems strengthening and ensuring equitable access

Appropriately constituted and managed health systems provide a vehicle to improve people's lives, protecting them from the vulnerability of sickness, generating a sense of security, and building social cohesion within society; they can ensure that all groups benefit from socioeconomic development and they can generate the political support needed to sustain them.

Patterns of disease, care and treatment are not static. Health systems have to cope with a spectrum of competing health changes and challenges. Their capacity to respond is similarly impacted by many factors operating at different levels. On a more local level, services and programmes are challenged by the availability of resources, both financial and human, as well as government policies in relation to decentralization and the role of the private sector and civil society. With increasing globalization, issues such as migration, transnational spread of disease, and trade, including obligations under international treaties, are constraining the policy and fiscal space of national governments. In the face of multiple objectives and limited resources, governments have to reconcile the competing demands for access and efficiency against those of ensuring affordability and quality. Strategies for strengthening the health sector also need to be linked to broader processes of national development planning, such as civil service reform, public expenditure reviews and reform, decentralization, and poverty-reduction strategies.

As can be appreciated, strengthening health system performance is a wide-ranging subject, requiring action on many levels and management fronts. Given the contextual complexity, there is no one blueprint or single set of best practices that can be put forward as a model for improved performance. Yet, health systems across countries share commonalities in function, services and objectives; they also share some common experiences and face some similar difficulties. By addressing these challenges through a collaborative, coordinated way, driven by desired health outcomes, sustainable system-wide benefits can be achieved. To be most effective, this process must be country-led and based on priorities set out in comprehensive national health plans. It requires attention to the various functions of the health system to achieve the objectives of: Improved health and health equity through accessible, affordable, quality services to all who need them, greater social and financial risk protection, improved efficiency and responsiveness to health needs, and greater patient safety (WHO 2006c).

Strengthening health systems means addressing key constraints related to health worker staffing, governance, infrastructure, health commodities, logistics, tracking progress, and effective financing. Stronger leadership and governance helps ensure good oversight, accountability, attention to regulation and coalition building both within and outside the national health sector. Stewardship in government seeks innovative engagement with civil society and the private sector and to orient programmes and resources towards public health goals. Communities and individuals must be actively engaged to participate in the decision-making process of policies that affect their health. Policy-making needs to be more collaborative, better coordinated and better informed. A well-functioning health information system contributes to this by the generation, analysis and dissemination of timely and critical information on health determinants, status, and performance. Building up managerial skills at all levels and accommodating reform is critically important, as is the delivery of primary health care.

The contributions of primary health care to improvements in many aspects of population and individual health are well documented (Starfield et al. 2005). Evidence demonstrates that health systems oriented towards primary health care—with its underpinning values of universal access, equity, community participation, and intersectoral action—produce better outcomes, at lower costs, and with higher user satisfaction (Doherty & Govender 2004). Its emphasis on health promotion, continuity of care across levels of care and over the life course, use of appropriate technology and care that is 'close-to-client' is central to health policies in many countries. Equally important, especially as a contribution to efficiency, is the provision of as much care as possible at the first point of contact effectively supported by secondary level facilities through a fully functioning referral processes. Large gains in health outcomes have been seen in countries with a strong political commitment to aligning their health system to the principles of primary health care. Such an approach is relevant to both developing and developed countries alike.

The health workforce is central to managing and delivering health services in all countries. The effectiveness of health systems and the quality of the health services depend on a well-functioning workforce that is responsive, motivated and skilled. Yet, the current crisis of human resources, including shortages and mal-distribution, is jeopardizing the delivery of services in all countries, especially those in sub-Saharan Africa. This shortfall is aggravated by skewed distribution geographically between urban and rural areas and between the private and public sector. To address this crisis, governments must exercise leadership in developing holistic national strategic policies for workforce development, based on sound evidence

and participatory feedback. Increased investments to improve performance and productivity are also essential through compensation adjustments, incentives, education, and the provision of safer working conditions. National and international efforts need to be aligned to address the issues of ethical hiring of health workers trained abroad and the negotiation of policies that shape migration and international labour markets (WHO 2006d).

To achieve sustainable funds for health and social protection, regressive patterns of financing need to be addressed. Reducing reliance on out-of-pocket payments where they are high, and by moving towards prepayment systems based on pooling of financial risk across population groups should be encouraged. Additionally, where needed, social protection schemes should be supported to ensure the poor and other vulnerable groups have access to services based on need, while ensuring that health care costs do not lead to financial catastrophe.

Tackling the determinants of health and promoting intersectoral participation

Modern concepts of health recognize that underlying conditions establish the foundation for realizing physical, mental, and social well-being. Health is a consequence of multiple interacting determinants operating in dynamic biological, behavioural, social, and economic contexts that change as a person develops. Health risks are created and maintained by social systems; the magnitude of those risks is largely a function of socioeconomic disparities and psychosocial gradients. Some social circumstances that affect health relate to social exclusion and other multidimensional disadvantages, such as education, gender, poverty, discrimination, and ethnicity. Beyond these, exposure risks such as working environments, living conditions, unsafe sex and the availability of food and water also contribute to health risks. Wider economic, political and environmental determinants include urbanization, intellectual property rights, trade and subsidies, globalization, air pollution, and climate change.

Accordingly, any effort to reduce health disparities cannot be confined to the provision of better access to care and resources alone but must also go beyond to address the underlying determinants. Such an approach supports the advancement of global health equity. Acting on the structural conditions in society affecting health offers a better hope for sustainable and equitable outcomes in health beyond just medical or social interventions alone. As a framework for this, a strategy of health promotion is needed that enables the fulfilment of health through the creation of supportive environments, healthy public policies, access to information, life skills and opportunities for making healthy choices (Charter 1986). Such policy options are expected to increase after the Commission on Social Determinants of Health publishes its findings (Marmot 2005). The work of the Commission will be instrumental for rendering the problem of health inequity real and actionable by institutional authorities and policy practitioners.

Given their aetiology, many of the attributable causes of chronic disease lend themselves to prevention or control. Physical inactivity, improper diets, tobacco use, and excessive alcohol consumption represent major modifiable risk factors. These factors are now recognized as being amenable to alleviation throughout life, even into old age. Just as the risk occurs at all ages, so all ages are part of the continuum of opportunity for prevention. This can be best applied through a life-course approach that includes maternal health, exclusive breastfeeding for six months, health promotion in schools, and in the work-place, sex education, a healthy diet, and regular physical activity from childhood into old age (WHO 2006c).

However, against a backdrop of globalization and changing health risks, the advocacy for change in individual behaviour alone is insufficient by itself. In many instances, the individual and even the health sector have little or no control over many of the powerful influences on health; many of these issues lie within the ambit of governments and commercial responsibilities. Action on these determinants requires the collaborative engagement of multiple stakeholders across many levels—from communities to governments, local to international and private to non-governmental. Cooperation and advocacy must necessarily push the boundaries of public health action to overcome such structural factors.

Governments, and ministries of health in particular, must play a leading role in intersectoral action to secure better public health policies and achieve some control over the transnational forces that affect the health of their populations. The widespread influence of globalization has increased the need for new frameworks of international collaboration, including conventional international law, to address and formulate policy responses to emerging opportunities for and threats to global health (Taylor 2002). International organizations, such as the WHO, play a pivotal role in contributing to the coherent development of greater global dialogue, building effective partnerships, and stimulating effective governmental and intergovernmental action on public health issues.

Multilateral collective strategies, especially the development of international standards and instruments, are central for protecting and promoting public health. Increasingly, international health legislation is proving an important tool for creating global health covenants in promoting cooperative action against shared health challenges. Agreements such as the revised International Health Regulations (2005) have demonstrated the power of multilateral cooperative arrangements to protect against the transnational spread of disease and pathogens. In the same way, governments must move to strengthen corresponding national regulatory and enforcement frameworks and capacities to support and advance many of these same themes.

Health damaging behaviours in particular, such as the use of tobacco, poor diet and sedentary lifestyles, have proven amenable to such collective action. On an international level, a strong model of cooperation and intersectoral action is provided by the WHO Framework Convention on Tobacco Control, an instrument that embraces a social determinants approach to tobacco control and demands broad intersectoral action on matters as diverse as trade, agriculture, education and the environment (Taylor & Bettcher 2000). Similarly, the WHO global strategy on diet, physical activity and health emphasizes community-based approaches and engagement with industry for action on the structural drivers of food availability, accessibility and acceptability at the global and national levels (Chopra et al. 2002).

Contemporary international cooperation efforts have also seen the linkage of health with other traditionally distinct but substantive issues become increasingly common. For example, the fundamental interdependence of sustainable development and health necessitates intersectoral coordination of economic, social, and environmental policies to promote population well-being. Other growing issue linkages to health have been elaborated in international processes on public health, innovation, and intellectual property, as well as conventions on biological diversity, climate change, and sustainable development. In all these, governments must display strong leadership and give equity and health a central place in their agendas.

Strengthening governance, leadership, and accountability

Good national governance, wise leadership, and strong political will are central societal structures underpinning economic growth and equitable development. The gaps between policies and their implementation are often huge. Governments need to bridge these gaps and address deeper sources of policy failure that can undermine health development. Enlightened policy-making brings coherence to the delivery of health services and outcomes. It is important that the health of populations feature as a principal concern of all governments. Experiences shows that as governance improves, fewer women die in childbirth, more physicians exist per population, there is better access to improved water, and life expectancy is longer. Such is its power and importance.

At the national level, ministries of health must exercise stewardship and advocacy to centre health in development planning and secure increased financial allocation to health in the national budget. This implies the ability to formulate strategic policy direction and clarify the roles and responsibilities of the different actors in health; clear policy priorities must be established while maintaining an overview of societal interests and reorienting policies towards pro-poor public health goals. It also implies ensuring good regulation and the tools for implementing it, and to provide the necessary intelligence on health system performance in order to ensure accountability and transparency.

Through intersectoral engagement, ministries must create a platform for coordination and consensus-building across mutually-reliant sectors—public, civil, and private. Such engagement needs to address cross-cutting issues such as civil service reform, social determinants of health, macroeconomic policy, gender equality, and health-related human rights. Where they exist, health targets must be in integrated into poverty reduction strategies, based on comprehensive and equity-based health sector investment plans.

Recent years have also seen greater expansion and commitment in external resources for health. Concomitantly, there has been an upsurge in the number of external agencies involved in the health sectors of developing countries with growing volumes of resources transferred to these health systems. Notwithstanding the beneficial impact of increased resources, recipients and donors must find greater efficiency in the aid policy process to deliver sustainable health development (Buse & Walt 1997).

In countries where there is significant health sector investment by international partners, there is an imperative to develop capacities and policies to coordinate and manage such cooperation. Substantive challenges regarding development assistance revolve around its possible distortion of country priorities, and the issues of volatile and unpredictable aid that impedes long term macroeconomic and sectoral policy formulation (WHO 2007a). In many developing countries, progress towards rationalizing the new flow and mechanisms of such aid has been limited by the lack of comprehensive national health strategies, and critical deficits in national absorptive and planning capacity.

It is recognized that for aid to become truly effective, stronger and more balanced accountability mechanisms are required at different levels. Aid is more effective when partner countries exercise ownership with strong and effective leadership over their development policies and strategies. This fundamental tenet underpins the

Paris Declaration (OECD 2005) and other multilateral initiatives that aim to increase the effectiveness of aid. To strengthen health systems, expand use and coverage of health services and help achieve the MDGs in developing countries, new initiatives such as the International Health Partnerships (IHP) have been successfully launched; an agreement between donors and developing countries, the IHP aims to put the Paris Declaration into practice in the health sector by setting out a process of mutual responsibility and accountability for the development and implementation of national health plans of developing countries (Alexander 2007). Above all, the IHP recognizes that successful and sustainable health initiatives must be country-led and country-owned.

Globalization and the liberalization of trade and services have materially transformed the capacity of governments to monitor and protect public health. As such, governments must effectively assess and respond to the risks and opportunities for population health presented by negotiated international agreements such as the Agreement on Trade Related Aspects of Intellectual Property Rights (TRIPS) and the General Agreement on Trade in Services (Blouin *et al.* 2006). Governments are challenged to remain informed and engaged in a wide range of issues—covering food, insurance, occupational and environmental health conditions, pharmaceuticals, and affordable access to medicines among others—and their deeper implications for health equity and public health.

Harnessing knowledge, science, and technology

Against a backdrop of unprecedented technological and economic resources for health, the stark reality of large inequities in health status looms ever larger. Across many developing countries, the health status of populations has declined, largely as a result of HIV/AIDS, but also because of enduring poverty, an inadequate tax base in many developing countries, a resurgence in infectious diseases, and a upsurge in non-communicable diseases. Indeed a key imperative for health research must be to bring a sharper focus on mitigating these inequities and the unacceptable gap between unprecedented knowledge about diseases and their control, and the implementation of that knowledge, especially in poor countries.

It is recognized that the creation and diffusion of knowledge is one of the major driving forces for health progress and improving health equity (Jamison *et al.* 2006). Evidence derived from scientific knowledge can help transform health, be it through new and better technologies, promoting better health practices, or the application of evidence in health policy formulation.

Gaps in essential health information prevent effective global and country responses to health challenges. Good health metrics and evaluation is vital. It allows comparative health-system research, building the evidence-base for policy, baseline monitoring and programme performance evaluation. Greater investments are needed to produce actionable learning that national leaders and development partners can use to improve health programmes and assess effectiveness.

Even though the greatest burden of ill health and premature mortality occurs in the developing world, only a small fraction of global research funding is devoted to communicable, maternal, perinatal, and nutritional disorders that constitute the major burden of disease in developing countries (WHO 2002b). As such, developing countries need greater investments to build stronger

scientific and institutional capacity to address problems unique to their circumstances. Greater emphasis should be placed on research on the social, economic, and political determinants of ill health and how the structural barriers to application of existing technologies might be overcome. Advocacy for health systems and implementation research needs to be strengthened to bridge the gap between knowledge and action (Sanders & Haines 2006). This demands stronger capacity for indigenous and multidisciplinary health research, to deliver socially and culturally sensitive evidence to inform practical health systems development.

The opportunities created by advances in biomedical science need to be harnessed more effectively to develop new products. The agenda for research should be guided by national and internationally agreed priorities and biased towards the greatest unmet health needs. There is a strong necessity to continue to develop safe and affordable new products for such communicable diseases as AIDS, malaria and tuberculosis, and for other diseases disproportionately affecting developing countries. Insufficient research has been focused on interventions for the poor, such as treatment for neglected tropical diseases, antibiotic delivery mechanisms for children with pneumonia and access to perinatal care (WHO 2007a).

There has been considerable momentum in recent years by governments, industry, charitable foundations, and non-governmental organizations in funding initiatives to develop new products to fight diseases affecting developing countries, and to increase access to new ones. Strong advocacy must continue to sustain the political will and commitment for such initiatives, and the unprecedented opportunities for health they have created. Multilateral finance mechanisms such as the International Finance Facility for Immunization, the use of Advance Market Commitments to stimulate the development of new vaccines, the Global Fund, UNITAID, and the Global Alliance for Vaccines and Immunization provide long-term, sustainable and predictable funding needed to scale up access and reduce prices of drugs, vaccines, and diagnostics for the treatment of diseases disproportionably affecting developing countries.

The sharing of knowledge and research also serves to promote health through its effect on individual behaviour and better health practices. The dissemination of health information, especially through the use of media, on such issues as tobacco use, and sexual and reproductive health in adolescents and young adults, helps raise awareness, and enhance health promoting behaviour. Advances in the use of information and communication technology to provide health care in remote or hard to reach areas, data collection and research remains an expanding and valuable resource.

Conclusion

At the midpoint to 2015—the target year for the achievement of the MDGs at a global level—we are mindful of the significant gaps and challenges in health that still confront us. We cannot afford to fail. To attain these goals requires action on equity and the underlying social determinants that influence health. It also demands our attention to improving the performance of health systems and for better evidence in policy. The impact of our outputs will be measured by the real and qualitative improvement of the health of women and the people of Africa. Progress on these fronts necessitates unwavering political will and global participation. Only then can we hope to achieve true health for all.

References

Alexander, D. (2007). The international health partnership. *The Lancet*, **370**(9590), 803–4.

Anand, S. and Barnighausen, T. (2004). Human resources and health outcomes: cross-country econometric study. *The Lancet*, **364**(9445), 1603–9.

Anand, S. and Barnighausen, T. (2007). Health workers and vaccination coverage in developing countries: an econometric analysis. *The Lancet*, **369**(9569), 1277–85.

Belizan, J.M., Cafferata, M.L., Belizan, M., and Althabe, F. (2007). Health inequality in Latin America. *The Lancet*, **370**(9599), 1599–600.

Ben-David, D. (2000). *Trade, growth and disparity among nations*. WTO Geneva, WTO Secretariat Geneva.

Berman, P. (2000). Organization of ambulatory care provision: a critical determinant of health system performance in developing countries. *Bulletin of the World Health Organization*, **78**(6), 791–802.

Bettcher, D.W., Yach, D., and Guindon, G.E. (2000). Critical reflection global trade and health: key linkages and future challenges. *Bulletin of the World Health Organization*, **78**(4) 521–534.

Bloom, S.S., Wypij, D., and Das Gupta, M. (2001). Dimensions of women's autonomy and the influence on maternal health care utilization in a north Indian city. *Demography*, **38**(1), 67–78.

Blouin, C., Drager, N., and Smith, R. (2006). *International trade in health services and the gats: current issues and debates*. World Bank Publications, Washington D.C.

Braveman, P. and Gruskin, S. (2003). Poverty, equity, human rights and health. *Bulletin of the World Health Organization*, **81**(7), 539–45.

Buse, K. and Walt, G. (1997). An unruly melange? Coordinating external resources to the health sector: a review. *Social Science & Medicine*, **45**(3), 449–63.

Chalker, J., Chuc, N.T.K., Falkenberg, T., Do, N.T., and Tomson, G. (2000). STD management by private pharmacies in Hanoi: practice and knowledge of drug sellers. *British Medical Journal*, **76**(4), 299.

Charter, O. (1986). *Ottawa charter for health promotion*. Paper presented to First International Conference on Health Promotion, Ottawa, viewed 12 March 2008 <http://www.who.int/hpr/NPH/docs/ottawa_charter_hp.pdf>.

Chen, L.C., Evans, T.G., Cash, R.A., Kaul, I., Grunberg, I., and Stern, M. (1999). *Global public goods: International cooperation in the 21st century*. Oxford University Press, Oxford.

Chopra, M., Galbraith, S., and Darnton-Hill, I. (2002). A global response to a global problem: the epidemic of overnutrition. *Bulletin of the World Health Organization*, **80**(12), 952–8.

Clemens, M. and Pettersson, G. (2008). New data on African health professionals abroad. *Human Resources for Health*, **6**(1), 1.

Climate Change. (2007). *The physical science basis. Summary for policymakers. (Contribution of Working Group I to the Fourth Assessment Report of the Intergovernmental Panel on Climate Change)*, Intergovernmental Panel on Climate Change (IPCC), Geneva.

CNA Corporation. (2007). National security and the threat of climate change, viewed 20 April 2008, <http://securityandclimate.cna.org/>.

Cockburn, R., Newton, P.N., Agyarko, E.K., Akunyili, D., and White, NJ. (2005). The global threat of counterfeit drugs: why industry and governments must communicate the dangers. *PLoS Med*, **2**(4), e100.

Commission on Health Research for Development. (1990). *Health research: essential link to equity in development*. Oxford University Press, Oxford.

Confalonieri, U., Menne, B., Akhtar, R., Ebi, K.L., Hauengue, M., Kovats, R.S., Revich, B., and Woodward, A. (2007). Human health. In *Intergovernmental panel on climate change fourth assessment report: climate change impacts, adaptation, and vulnerability* (eds. M.L. Parry, O.F. Canziani, J.P. Palutikof, P.J. van der Linden and C.E. Hanson), pp. 391–431. Cambridge University Press, Cambridge.

Devarajan, S. (2003). *World Development Report 2004: making services work for poor people*. World Bank Publications, Washington DC.

Dodgson, R., Lee, K., and Drager, N. (2002). *Global health governance*.

Doherty, J. and Govender, R. (2004). The cost-effectiveness of primary care services in developing countries: a review of the international literature. *Background Paper: Disease Control Priorities Project*, World Bank, Washington DC, viewed 12 March 2008, <http://www.dcp2.org/file/49/wp37.pdf>.

Dollar, D. (2001). Is globalization good for your health? *Bulletin of the World Health Organization*, **79**(9), 827–33.

Dollar, D. and Kraay, A. (2002). Growth is Good for the Poor, *Journal of Economic Growth*, **7**(3), 195–225.

Dondorp, A.M., Newton, P.N., Mayxay, M., Van Damme, W., Smithuis, F.M., Yeung, S., Petit, A., Lynam, A.J., Johnson, A., Hien, T.T., McGready, R., Farrar, J.J., Looareesuwan, S., Day, N.P.J., Green, M.D., and White, N.J. (2004). Fake antimalarials in Southeast Asia are a major impediment to malaria control: multinational cross-sectional survey on the prevalence of fake antimalarials. *Tropical Medicine & International Health*, **9**(12), 1241–6.

ECLAC. (2005). *Social panorama of Latin America*. Economic Commission for Latin America and the Caribbean, viewed 12 March 2008, <www.eclac.org/publicaciones/xml/4/24054/PSI2005_Cap2_GastoSocial.pdf>.

Fabricant, S.J., Kamara, C.W., and Mills, A. (1999). Why the poor pay more: household curative expenditures in rural Sierra Leone. *The International Journal of Health Planning and Management*, **14**, 179–99.

Garau, P., Sclar, E., and Carolini, G.Y. (2005). *A home in the city: UN Millenium project. Task force on improving the lives of slum dwellers*. UNDP, James & James (Science Publishers) Ltd, London.

Gill, K., Pande, R., and Malhotra, A. (2007). Women deliver for development. *The Lancet*, **370**(9595), 1347–57.

Global Forum for Health Research. (2007). *Global forum update on research for health volume 4. Equitable access: research challenges for health in developing countries*. Pro-Book Publishing Limited, viewed 12 March 2008, <http://www.globalforumhealth.org/filesupld/global_update4/GlobalUpdate4Full.pdf>.

Global Health Workforce Alliance. (2008). *Health workers for all and all for health workers. The Kampala Declaration and agenda for global action*. Paper presented to First Global Forum on Human Resources for Health, Kampala, Uganda.

Globalization Knowledge Network. (2007). *Towards health-equitable globalisation: rights, regulation and redistribution*, viewed 12 March 2008 <http://www.who.int/social_determinants/resources/globlalization_kn_07_2007.pdf>.

Goodman, C., Brieger, W., Unwin, A., Mills, A., Meek, S., and Greer, G. (2007). Medicine sellers and malaria treatment in Sub-Saharan Africa: what do they do and how can their practice be improved? *The American Journal of Tropical Medicine and Hygiene*, **77**(6) (Suppl.), 203.

Grown, C., Gupta, G.R., and Pande, R. (2005). Taking action to improve women's health through gender equality and women's empowerment. *The Lancet*, **365**(9458), 541–3.

Gwatkin, D.R., Bhuiya, A., and Victora, C.G. (2004). Making health systems more equitable. *The Lancet*, **364**(9441), 1273–80.

Haines, A., Heath, I., and Smith, R. (2000). Joining together to combat poverty. *BMJ*, **320**(7226), 1–2.

Heymann, D. L. and Rodier, G. R. (2001). Hot spots in a wired world: WHO surveillance of emerging and re-emerging infectious diseases. *The Lancet Infectious Diseases*, **1**, 345–353.

Hill, K., Thomas, K., AbouZahr, C., Walker, N., Say, L., Inoue, M., and Suzuki, E. (2008). Estimates of maternal mortality worldwide between 1990 and 2005: an assessment of available data. *The Lancet*, **370**(9595), 1311–9.

Jamison, D.T., Mosley, W.H., Measham, A.R., and Bobadilla, J.L. (2006). *Disease control priorities in developing countries*. World Bank Group, Washington DC.

Joint Learning Initiative. (2004). *Human resources for health: overcoming the crisis*. Harvard University Press, Cambridge, viewed 12 March 2008, <www.who.int/hrh/documents/JLi_hrh_report.pdf>.

Kar, K. and Bongartz, P. (2006). *Update on Some Recent Developments in Community-Led Total Sanitation*, viewed 20 April 2008 <http://www.livelihoods.org/hot_topics/docs/CLTS_update06.pdf>.

Lancet. (2007). Editorial: progress and inequity in Latin America. *The Lancet*, **370**(9599), 1589.

Mann, J.M., Gostin, L., Gruskin, S., Brennan, T., Lazzatin, Z., and Fineberg, H. (1999). *Health and human rights health and human rights: a reader*, Routledge, New York.

Marmot, M. (2005). Social determinants of health inequalities. *The Lancet*, **365**(9464), 1099–104.

Marmot, M. (2007). Achieving health equity: from root causes to fair outcomes. *The Lancet*, **370**(9593), 1153–63.

Mathers, C.D. and Loncar, D. (2006). Projections of global mortality and burden of disease from 2002 to 2030. *PLoS Med*, **3**(11), e442.

Mazur, J. (2000). Labor's new internationalism. *Foreign Affairs*, **79**(1), 79–93.

Mills, A., Brugha, R., Hanson, K., and McPake, B. (2002). What can be done about the private health sector in low-income countries? *Bulletin of the World Health Organization*, **80**(4), 325–30.

Mundial, B. (2005). *World Development Report 2006: equity and development*. World Bank Publications, Washington DC.

Narasimhan, V., Brown, H., Pablos-Mendez, A., Adams, O., Dussault, G., Elzinga, G., Nordstrom, A., Habte, D., Jacobs, M., and Solimano, G. (2004). Responding to the global human resources crisis. *The Lancet*, **363**(9419), 1469–72.

OECD. (2005). *Paris declaration on aid effectiveness: ownership, harmonisation, alignment, results and mutual accountability, organization for economic co-operation and development*. OECD High-Level Forum, Paris.

OECD. (2007). *Reporting directives for the Creditor Reporting System*. Development Assistance Committee, Organisation for Economic Co-operation and Development, Paris.

Ogata, S. and Sen, A. (2003). *Human security now. protecting and empowering people*. United Commission on Human Security, Final Report, New York.

Ong, A.K. and Heymann, D.L. (2007). Microbes and humans: the long dance. *Bulletin of the World Health Organization*, **85**, 422–23.

Parry, M.L., Canziani, O.F., Palutikof, J.P., van der Linden, P.J., and Hanson, C.E. (2007). *Climate change 2007: impacts, adaptation and vulnerability*. Contribution of Working Group II to the Fourth Assessment Report of the Intergovernmental Panel on Climate Change.

Peden, M., Scurfield, R., Sleet, D., Mohan, D., Hyder, A.A., Jarawan, E., and Mathers, C. (2004). *World report on road traffic injury prevention*. World Health Organization, Geneva.

Preker, A.S., Liu, X., and Velenyi, E. (2007). *Public ends, private means: strategic purchasing of health services*. World Bank Publications, Washington DC.

Raviglione, M.C. and Smith, I.M. (2007). XDR tuberculosis – implications for global public health. *The New England Journal of Medicine*, **356**(7), 656–9.

Robinson, M. and Clark, P. (2008). Forging solutions to health worker migration. *The Lancet*, **371**(9613), 691–3.

Ruger, J.P. (2003). Health and development. *The Lancet*, **362**(9385), 678.

Ruger, J.P. and Yach, D. (2005). Global functions at the World Health Organization. *BMJ*, **330**(7500), 1099–100.

Sanders, D. and Haines, A. (2006). Implementation research is needed to achieve international health goals. *PLoS Med*, **3**(6), e186.

Sen, A.K. and Sen, A. (1999). *Development as freedom*. Oxford University Press, Oxford.

Smith, R.D. and Coast, J. (2002). Antimicrobial resistance: a global response. *Bulletin of the World Health Organization*, **80**(2), 126.

Smolinski, M.S., Margaret, A., and Lederberg, J. (2003). *Microbial threats to health emergence, detection, and response*. National Academies Press, Washington DC.

Starfield, B., Shi, L., and Macinko, J. (2005). Contribution of primary care to health systems and health. *The Milbank Quarterly*, **83**(3), 457–502.

Taylor, A.L. (2002). Global governance, international health law and WHO: looking towards the future. *Bulletin of the World Health Organization*, **80**(12), 975–80.

Taylor, A.L. and Bettcher, D.W. (2000). WHO Framework Convention on Tobacco Control: a global "good" for public health. *Bulletin of the World Health Organization*, **78**(7), 920–9.

Travis, P., Bennett, S., Haines, A., Pang, T., Bhutta, Z., Hyder, A.A., Pielemeier, N.R., Mills, A., and Evans, T. (2004). Overcoming health-systems constraints to achieve the Millennium Development Goals. *The Lancet*, **364**(9437), 900–6.

Tudor Hart, J. (1971). The inverse care law. *The Lancet*, **297**(7696), 405–12.

UN. (2000). *United Nations millennium declaration (United Nations General Assembly Resolution 55/2)*. United Nations, New York.

UN. (2008). *Department for economic and social affairs, population division. world urbanization prospects: the 2007 revision*. United Nations, New York.

UNAIDS. (2006). *UNAIDS Annual Report. Making the money work*. Joint United Nations Programme on HIV/AIDS (UNAIDS), Geneva.

UNAIDS. (2007). *AIDS epidemic update: December 2007*. Joint United Nations Programme on HIV/AIDS (UNAIDS) and World Health Organizations (WHO), Geneva.

UNFPA. (2007). *State of world population 2007. Unleashing the potential of urban growth*. United Nations Population Fund, New York.

UNICEF. (2007). *Progress for children. A world fit for children. Statistical Review Number 6*. United Nations Children's Fund, New York.

Uplekar, M., Pathania, V., and Raviglione, M. (2001). Private practitioners and public health: weak links in tuberculosis control. *The Lancet*, **358**(9285), 912–6.

Vujicic, M., Zurn, P., Diallo, K., Adams, O., and Dal Poz, M. (2004). The role of wages in the migration of health care professionals from developing countries. *Human Resources for Health*, **2**(1), 3.

Wade, R.H. (2004). Is globalization reducing poverty and inequality? *World Development*, **32**(4), 567–89.

Wagstaff, A. (2002). Poverty and health sector inequalities. *Bulletin of the World Health Organization*, **80**, 97–105.

Whitehead, M. (1992). The concepts and principles of equity and health. *International Journal of Health Services*, **22**(3), 429–45.

WHO. (2002a). Constitution of the World Health Organization. *Bulletin of the World Health Organization*, **80**, 983–4.

WHO. (2002b). *Global forum for health research: The 10/90 report on health research 2001–2002*. World Health Organization, Geneva.

WHO. (2003a). *WHO framework convention on tobacco control*. World Health Organization, Geneva.

WHO. (2003b). *The World Health Report 2003: shaping the future*. World Health Organization, Geneva.

WHO. (2006a). The commission on social determinants of health: tackling the social roots of health inequities. *PLoS Medicine*, **3**(6), e106.

WHO. (2006b). *Counterfeit medicine*. World Health Organization, viewed 12 March 2008 <http://www.who.int/mediacentre/factsheets/fs275/en/index.html>.

WHO. (2006c). *Engaging for health. Eleventh general programme of work 2006–2015. a global health agenda*. World Health Organization, Geneva.

WHO. (2006d). *World Health Report 2006: working together for health*. World Health Organization, Geneva.

WHO. (2007a). *Tough choices: investing in health for development: experiences from national follow-up to the Commission on Macroeconomics and Health*. World Health Organization, Geneva.

WHO. (2007b). *WHA 58.3 Revision of the International health regulations*. World Health Organization, viewed 12 March 2008 <http://www.who.int/gb/ebwha/pdf_files/WHA58/WHA58_3-en.pdf >.

WHO. (2007c). *WHO mortality database: tables [online database]*. World Health Organization, Geneva.

WHO. (2007d). *World Health Report 2007 – a safer future: global public health security in the 21st century*. World Health Organization, Geneva.

WHO. (2008a). *Global tuberculosis control: surveillance, planning, financing*. WHO Report 2008, Geneva.

WHO. (2008b). *Protecting health from climate change – World Health Day 2008*. World Health Organization, viewed 20 April 2008, <http://www.who.int/world-health-day/en/>.

WHO. (2008c). *WHO report on the global tobacco epidemic, 2008. The MPOWER package*, viewed 12 March 2008 <http://www.who.int/tobacco/mpower/en/index.html>.

World Bank. (2007a). *Global monitoring report 2007: confronting the challenges of gender equality and fragile states*. World Bank, Washington DC.

World Bank. (2007b). *World Development Indicators 2007*. Washington DC.

Index

Page numbers in **bold** refer to major sections of the text.

Since the major subject of this title is public health, entries under this keyword have been kept to a minimum, and readers are advised to seek more specific references.

Indexing style
Alphabetical order. This index is in letter-by-letter order, whereby hyphens, en-rules and spaces within index headings are ignored in the alphabetization. Terms in brackets are excluded from initial alphabetization.

Main abbreviations used
AIDS acquired immunodeficiency syndrome
ANOVA analysis of variance
BMI body mass index
CJD Creutzfeldt-Jakob disease
COPD chronic obstructive pulmonary disease
HIV human immunodeficiency virus
SARS sudden acute respiratory syndrome
STIs sexually transmitted infections

Other abbreviations are defined in the index

Haemophilus
 H. ducreyi 1174, 1610
 H. influenzae 201, 203, 206
  vaccine 208, 1607
Hague Appeal for Peace Civil Society
  Conference 1373
HALE 257, 305, 1423, 1500
hand washing 204
hantavirus 1266, 1371
haplotype 139
HapMap project 138
Harvard Trauma Questionnaire 417
Harvard Youth Violence Prevention
  Center 1362
Hawaii, measles persistence *680*
Hayek, Friedrich von 282
Haynes, Brian 581
hazard 901, *902,* 1641
hazard identification 901, 935, 1641, *1642*
 sources of information *1642*
hazardous air pollutants 937
Hazardous Substances Data Bank 432
headache 1133, *1133*
 clinical overview 1133
 cluster 1133
 costs and public health impact 1136
 familial and genetic risks 1134
 prevalence 1133
 risk factors 1135
 stroke and migraine 1135
 tension-type 1133
health 755
 approaches to 755
 definition of 21, 755, 1714
 determinants of *see* determinants of health
 and health care 1671
 measures of 1488
 socio-ecological approach 756
 socioeconomic determinants 1426
health actors 1716
health-adjusted life expectancies *see* HALEs
Health for All 44, 1655
health behaviour
 and gender 1427
 surveys 708
Health Belief Model 125, 728
health care 827, 1670
 access 16, 247–8, 252
  barriers to 251
  equity in *see* health equity
  gender impact 1430
 concepts and values 239
 costs 417
 criteria, access and utilization 279
 definition 238–9
 delivery, impact of gender on 1430
 and disease prevention 1596
 evolution of 398
 expenditure 1673
  actual vs proposed allocation *246*
  by country *240*
  disparities in 68
 financing 46
  developing countries 307
 funding 1671
 and health 1671
 ideological and philosophical drivers 240
 international trends 279
 measuring effects *244*
 misallocation of resources 242

needs assessment 1676
population health 243
provision 16
reform 794
utilization 417
see also health services
health-care need 239
health-care providers 860
 networks 707
health commissioning 277
health education 120, 759
health emergencies 59
health equity 101, 248, 752, 1583, 1670
 access to health care 248, 252
 achieving 1584
 availability of services 249
 developing countries 309–10
 dimensions of 309
 and health determinants 110
 monitoring and evaluation 311
 policy commitment 310
 relevance and effectiveness 252
 utilization of services 251
health expectancy 257
health facilities 417
Health Field Concept 122
health gain 239
health gap 257
health guides 1689
health impact assessment 757, 1659
health improvement 239
health indicators 346, 422
 in data analysis 404, *404*
health inequality 3, 294, 762, 1671
 country perspective 1585
 definition 784
 developing countries **1581**
 effects of climate change 229
 global perspective 1584
 government subsidies *1587*
 high-income countries **1562**
 local vs. global focus 1583
 measurement of 1582
 reduction in 414
 significant factors in 1582
 socioeconomic *see* socioeconomic health
  inequality
 solutions 1587
  geographic targeting 1589
  health service approach 1588
  individual targeting 1589
  social and economic approaches 1587
  targeting by disease and age 1589
health inequity 1581
health information
 science 396
 sources 406
 systems 395, 420
  see also health information systems
health information systems **413**, 708
 application 400
  challenges in 409
  data access and dissemination 405
  data analysis 403
  data collection 401
  public health programs 400
 data collection 401
 facility-oriented 401
 funding 409
 health behaviour surveys 708

high-income countries **395**
 applications in public health 400
 information science 396
 information technology 396–7
 technology and society 398
insurance records 708
low- to middle-income countries 419
 community key informants 419
 demographic surveillance 419
 geographic 420–1, 431
 health care utilization and costs 417
 health facilities and services 417
 health outcomes 416
 health-related 420
 high-income countries 395
 infrastructure 418
 morbidity data 416
 risk factor surveillance 416
 vital registries and census 415
medical examiner and coroner reports 708
person-oriented 400
privacy and confidentiality 409
syndromic surveillance *see* syndromic
  surveillance
transaction-oriented 401
workers' compensation claims 708
health insurance
 developing countries 308
 resource allocation 1675
Health InterNetwork Access to Research
  Initiative *see* HINARI
Health Metrics Network 420
health needs assessment 1543
health outcomes 239, 416
health partners 1716
health personnel
 detection of outbreaks 486
 training 487
Health Plan Employer Data and Information
  Set 405
health planning 46
health policy 3, 46
 developed countries **20**, 282, *285*
 developing countries 299
 research 47, 817
 as stewardship 300
health of the poor 1581
health promotion 57, 752, 1595
 at work 909
 beliefs and assumptions 754
 concept 753
 definition 753
 education 120, 759
 enabling and empowerment 754
 ethics 384
 global 93
 health services as setting for 1678
 history 759
 older people 1504
 political economy of 763
 politics and philosophy 761
 priority action areas 753
 as process 753
 public health 760
 social movements 761
Health Promotion Glossary 756
health reform 44, 302
health-related behaviours 730, 1570
health-related mobility 111
health security 59, 1722